Women's Vascular Health

Women's Vascular Health

Ian A Greer
Regius Professor of Obstetrics and Gynaecology
University of Glasgow, UK

Jeffrey S Ginsberg
Professor of Medicine
McMaster University
Hamilton, Ontario
Canada

Charles D Forbes
Emeritus Professor of Medicine
Ninewells Hospital and Medical School
University of Dundee, UK

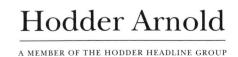

Hodder Arnold

A MEMBER OF THE HODDER HEADLINE GROUP

First published in Great Britain in 2007 by
Hodder Arnold, an imprint of Hodder Education and a member of the
Hodder Headline Group,
338 Euston Road, London NW1 3BH

http://www.hoddereducation.com

Distributed in the United States of America by
Oxford University Press Inc.,
198 Madison Avenue, New York, NY10016
Oxford is a registered trademark of Oxford University Press

Hodder Headline's policy is to use papers that are natural, renewable and
recyclable products and made from wood grown in sustainable forests.
The logging and manufacturing processes are expected to conform to the
environmental regulations of the country of origin.

Whilst the advice and information in this book are believed to be true and
accurate at the date of going to press, neither the author[s] nor the
publisher can accept any legal responsibility or liability for any errors or
omissions that may be made. In particular, (but without limiting the
generality of the preceding disclaimer) every effort has been made to
check drug dosages; however it is still possible that errors have been
missed. Furthermore, dosage schedules are constantly being revised and
new side-effects recognized. For these reasons the reader is strongly
urged to consult the drug companies' printed instructions before
administering any of the drugs recommended in this book.

British Library Cataloguing in Publication Data
A catalogue record for this book is available from the British Library

Library of Congress Cataloging-in-Publication Data
A catalog record for this book is available from the Library of Congress

ISBN-10 0 340 809973
ISBN-13 978 0 340 809976

1 2 3 4 5 6 7 8 9 10

Commissioning Editor: Sarah Burrows
Project Editor: Francesca Naish
Production Controller: Joanna Walker
Cover Design: Nichola Smith

Cover image: © Medioimages/Getty Images

Typeset in 10/12pts Minion by Charon Tec Ltd (A Macmillan Company),
Chennai, India
www.charontec.com
Printed and bound in the UK by CPI Bath

What do you think about this book? Or any other Hodder Arnold
title? Please visit our website: www.hoddereducation.com

In memory of Becky and Andy, who made everything possible.
IG

To my wife, Nancy, and my father-in-law, Archer McEwen.
JG

To my wife, Janette.
CF

Contents

Contributors

Sonia Anand MD, PhD, FRCPC
Associate Professor of Medicine
McMaster University
Hamilton General Hospital
Hamilton, ON
Canada

Philip Baker MBBS, MRCOG, DM
Professor of Maternal and Fetal Health
The Maternal and Fetal Health Research Centre
St Mary's Hospital
Manchester
UK

Kenneth A Bauer MD
Professor of Medicine, Harvard Medical School
Chief, Hematology Section, VA Boston Healthcare System
Director, Thrombosis Clinical Research, Beth Israel Deaconess
Medical Center
Boston, MA
USA

Kitty W M Bloemenkamp MD, PhD
Consultant Obstetrician
Leiden University Medical Centre
Department of Obstetrics
Leiden
the Netherlands

Louise Byrd MBChB, MRCOG
Consultant Obstetrician
The Maternal and Fetal Health Research Centre
St Mary's Hospital
Manchester
UK

Sharon Cameron MD, MRCOG
Consultant Gynaecologist
Simpson Centre for Reproductive Health
Royal Infirmary of Edinburgh
Edinburgh
UK

Hilary A Capell MD, FRCP (Glasgow, Edinb)
Consultant Physician and Rheumatologist
Centre for Rheumatic Diseases
Glasgow Royal Infirmary
Glasgow
UK

Sarah E Capes MD, MSc, FRCPC
Victoria, BC
Canada

Peter Clark BSc, MD, FRCP, FRCPath
Consultant Haematologist and Honorary Senior Lecturer
Department of Transfusion Medicine
Ninewells Hospital and Medical School
Dundee
UK

Jacqueline Conard
Hemostasis-Thrombosis Unit
Hotel-Dieu University Hospital
Paris
France

Krishna Dani BSc (Hons), MBChB
Senior House Officer
Centre for Rheumatic Diseases
Glasgow Royal Infirmary
Glasgow
UK

Bruce L Davidson MD, MPH
Clinical Professor of Medicine
Pulmonary and Critical Care
University of Washington School of Medicine
Swedish Medical Center
Seattle, WA
USA

John R Davies BSc, MBBS, MRCP
Department of Cardiovascular Medicine
Addenbrooke's Hospital
Cambridge
UK

Francesco Dentali MD
Research Fellow
Department of Medicine
McMaster University
St Joseph's Hospital
Hamilton, ON
Canada

James D Douketis MD, FRCPC
Associate Professor
Department of Medicine
McMaster University
St Joseph's Hospital
Hamilton, ON
Canada

Charles D Forbes
Emeritus Professor of Medicine
Ninewells Hospital and Medical School
University of Dundee
UK

Dilys Freeman BSc, PhD
Senior Lecturer
Developmental Medicine
University of Glasgow
Glasgow Royal Infirmary
Glasgow
UK

Sarah Germain MA (CANTAB), MBBS, DPhil (Oxon), MRCP
Medical Specialist Registrar
South East Thames Region
UK

Gregory T Gerotziafas MD, PhD
Assistant Hospitalo-Universitaire
Service d'Hématologie Biologique
Hôpital Hôtel-Dieu de Paris
Paris
France

Hertzel C Gerstein MD, MSc, FRCPC
Associate Professor
Department of Medicine
and
Department of Clinical Epidemiology and Biostatistics
McMaster University
Hamilton, ON
Canada

Jeffrey S Ginsberg MD, FRCPC
Professor of Medicine
McMaster University
Hamilton, ON
Canada

Anne Gompel
Medical Gynecology Unit
Hotel-Dieu University Hospital
Paris
France

Michael Greaves
Professor of Medicine
Department of Haematology and Medicine and Therapeutics
University of Aberdeen
Aberdeen
UK

Ian A Greer MD, FRCP(Glas) FRCPE, FRCP, FRCPI, FRCOG, FMedSci
Regius Professor of Obstetrics and Gynaecology
University of Glasgow
Glasgow
UK

Gareth Griffiths MBChB, MD, FRCS
Consultant Vascular Surgeon
Department of Vascular Surgery
Ninewells Hospital
Dundee
UK

Frans M Helmerhorst MD, PhD
Professor in Reproductive Medicine
Department of Obstetrics, Gynaecology and Reproductive
Medicine
Leiden University Medical Centre
Leiden
The Netherlands

Graham Jackson
Consultant Cardiologist
Guy's and St Thomas' Hospitals NHS Trust
St Thomas' Hospital
London
UK

John G Kelton MD, FRCPC
Canada Research Chair Holder
Department of Medicine
McMaster University
Hamilton, ON
Canada

Louise Kenny MBChB, MRCOG, PhD
Clinical Lecturer
Maternal and Fetal Health Research Center
St Mary's Hospital
Manchester
UK

Homa Keshavarz BSc, MSc, PhD, EIS
Fellow in Women's Health Research
Department of Medicine
McMaster University
Hamilton, ON
Canada

Peter Langhorne PhD, FRCP
Professor
Academic Section of Geriatric Medicine
Glasgow Royal Infirmary
Glasgow
UK

Agnes Y Y Lee MD, MSc, FRCPC
Associate Professor
Division of Hematology
Department of Medicine
McMaster University
Hamilton, ON
Canada

Delphine Levy
Medical Gynecology Unit
Hotel-Dieu University Hospital
Paris
France

Robert S Lindsay MBChB, BSc, PhD, FRCP (Glasg)
Clinical Senior Lecturer in Diabetes and Endocrinology
BHF Glasgow Cardiovascular Research Centre,
University of Glasgow
126 University Place
Glasgow
UK

Gordon D O Lowe
University Department of Medicine
Glasgow Royal Infirmary
Glasgow
UK

Mary Ann Lumsden
Professor of Gynaecology
University of Glasgow
Obstetrics and Gynaecology
Glasgow Royal Infirmary
Glasgow
UK

Rajan Madhok MD, FRCP (Glasgow, Edinb)
Consultant Physician and Rheumatologist
Glasgow Royal Infirmary
Glasgow
UK

Simon J McRae MBBS, FRACP, FRCPA
Clinical Fellow
Thromboembolism Unit
McMaster University Medical Centre
Hamilton, ON
Canada

Scott M Nelson BSc, PhD, MRCOG, DFFP
Clinician Scientist
Reproductive and Maternal Medicine
Division of Developmental Medicine
University of Glasgow
Glasgow
UK

Catherine Nelson-Piercy MA, FRCP
Consultant Obstetric Physician
Guy's and St Thomas' Hospitals Trust
and
Queen Charlotte's Hospital
London
UK

Emmanuel Oger MD, PhD
Department of Internal Medicine and Chest Diseases
Cavale Blanche Hospital
Brest
France

Carlo Patrono MD
Professor of Pharmacology
Department of Pharmacology
University of Rome 'La Sapienza'
Rome
Italy

Jill P Pell MSc, MD
Professor of Epidemiology
BHF Glasgow Cardiovascular Research Centre
University of Glasgow
126 University Place
Glasgow
UK

Geneviève Plu-Bureau MD, PhD
INSERM,
U780
Cardiovascular Epidemiology Section,
Villejuif
France

D Prabhakaran MD, DM
Associate Professor, Department of Cardiology
All India Institute of Medical Sciences
New Delhi
India

Ravendera Ramachandran MB, ChB, MRCP(UK)
Consultant Physician and Rheumatologist
Centre for Rheumatic Diseases
Glasgow Royal Infirmary
Glasgow
UK

Bianca Rocca MD
Adjunct Associate Professor of Pharmacology
Department of Pharmacology
University of Rome 'La Sapienza'
Rome
Italy

Meyer M Samama MD, PharmD
Emeritus Professor of Hematology
Hôtel-Dieu University Hospital
Paris
France

P Sanjay MBBS, MS(Gen Surg), MRCS
Specialist Registrar
Ninewells Hospital and Medical School
Dundee
UK

Naveed Sattar MBChB, PhD, FRCPath, FRCP
Professor of Metabolic Medicine
Section of Vascular Biochemistry
Glasgow Royal Infirmary
Glasgow
UK

Pierre-Yves Scarabin MD
INSERM
U780
Cardiovascular Epidemiology Section
Villejuif
France

Morven M Taylor MBChB, MRCP(UK)
Senior House Officer
Academic Section of Geriatric Medicine
Glasgow Royal Infirmary
Glasgow
UK

Huyen Tran MBBS, FRACP, FRCPA
Clinical Research Fellow
Thromboembolism Unit
McMaster University Medical Centre
Hamilton, ON
Canada

Isobel D Walker MPhil, MD, FRCP (Ed), FRCP (Glasg), FRCPath
Consultant Haematologist
Department of Haematology
North Glasgow University Hospitals NHS Trust
Glasgow Royal Infirmary
Glasgow
UK

Kathryn E Webert, MD, FRCPC
Assistant Professor
Division of Hematology
Department of Medicine
McMaster University
Hamilton, ON
Canada

Peter L Weissberg MD, FRCP
BHF Professor of Cardiovascular Medicine
Division of Cardiovascular Medicine
Addenbrooke's Hospital
Cambridge
UK

Preface

Women's vascular health is an important topic. It has long been recognized that coronary artery disease is a major health issue. In recent years, there has been a dramatic increase in the number of women suffering from this disease and it is no longer unusual to encounter a woman with coronary artery disease in pregnancy. Despite the large number of women affected, the majority of research is focused on the disease in men. It is also being increasingly recognized that the antecedents to the problems of coronary artery disease in women lies in earlier life and impinges on pregnancy and reproductive health. For example, women who suffer from polycystic ovarian syndrome not only suffer from infertility-related problems, but also exhibit metabolic responses that are similar to several of the key risk factors of coronary artery disease. Furthermore, the number of pregnancies a woman has, and a history of preeclampsia, are both associated with an increase in subsequent risk of coronary artery disease. During pregnancy, there are metabolic and haemostatic changes, which are further exaggerated in preeclampsia, that are similar to those seen in established vascular disease. Thus, coronary artery disease in later life may not only be influenced by typical risk factors such as smoking, social deprivation and genetic predisposition, but also by past reproductive experience and problems.

Women's vacular health, of course, encompasses much more than coronary artery disease. Venous disease is also an important problem. It is increasingly recognized that many venous thrombi are associated with congenital or acquired thrombophilic defects. Furthermore, these thrombophilias are not simply associated with venous thrombosis, as there is now increasing evidence linking thrombophilia to pregnancy complications, such as fetal loss, preeclampsia and abruption.

There are also specific problems with vascular disease during pregnancy. Pregnancy is associated with an increase in the risk of venous thromboembolism. Indeed the most common direct cause of maternal death in the UK and other developed countries is pulmonary embolism. Particular vascular complications occur in pregnancy, notably preeclampsia and intrauterine growth restriction. Women with preexisting disease that can impact on the vascular system, also have specific problems in pregnancy. These include women with valvular and congenital heart disease, peripheral or cerebral vascular disease, or underlying connective tissue or renal disease. There are also particular problems with prescribing antithrombotic agents during pregnancy where both the mother and the fetus have the potential to experience side-effects. Furthermore, it is clear that the maternal response to pregnancy may be involved in fetal programming, not simply through established factors such as maternal nutrition and genotype, but also in terms of the maternal response to pregnancy which may be modified by factors such as her body fat distribution, insulin resistance and exercise.

Hormonal therapy in women is also of substantial interest. The use of the combined oral contraceptive pill and hormone replacement therapy (HRT) are associated with increased vascular risk. While the 'pill' is itself a risk factor for thrombosis, many events may be explained by the interaction of the contraceptive pill with an underlying thrombophilia or acquired risk factors for venous thrombosis. Such interaction impacts on contraceptive choice, particularly in women with a personal or family history of venous thrombosis or hereditary thrombopilia. More recently the association between HRT and vascular disease has been established. This has significant implications for the use of HRT and specific guidance is required for patients with a personal or family history of vascular disease.

Hemorrhagic probems are also important to women's vascular health. These range from menorrhagia to congential disorders of coagulation such as von Willebrand's disease, and extend into pregnancy where hemorrhagic problems may ensue through antepartum hemorrhage and disseminated intravascular coagulation or through pre-existing or newly acquired conditions such as idiopathic thrombocytopenic purpura.

Thus, a women's vascular health is relevant throughout her life. Many significant new developments have been made in recent years. All too often, practitioners involved in managing these various problems see only a small aspect of it as it relates directly to their area of expertise. They may not be aware of the wider implications. For example, the obstetrician dealing with the pregnancy-related problems may not appreciate the impact the response to pregnancy may have on the patient's subsequent risk of coronary artery disease and the cardiologist dealing with such a problem may not fully appreciate the antecedents. Thus, we believe there is a need for a book that brings together all aspects of women's vascular health to provide a multidisciplinary resource to give information and advice on the management of these problems with a more holistic view. We believe that this book will go some way to meeting this unmet need, and hope that those who read it not only find it useful, but also enjoy it.

Abbreviations

α_2-M	α_2-macroglobulin	CCP	complement control proteins
ACAT	acid cholesterol-ester hydrolase	CEE	conjugated equine estrogen
ACCP	American College of Chest Physicians	CETP	cholesterol ester transfer protein
ACE	angiotensin-converting enzyme	CHD	coronary heart disease
ACHOIS	Australian Carbohydrate Intolerance Study	CI	confidence interval
aCL	anticardiolipin	CMF	cyclophosphamide, methotrexate, and 5-fluorouracil
ACS	acute coronary syndrome	CLL	chronic lymphotic leukemia
AD	Alzheimer's disease	CLOT	Comparison of Low-molecular-weight heparis versus Oral anticoagulant Therapy (trial)
ADP	adenosine diphosphate		
AFI	amniotic fluid index	CNS	central nervous system
AHA	American Heart Association	COC	combined oral contraceptives
AIDS	acquired immune deficiency syndrome	COMMIT	ClOpidogrel and Metoprolol in Myocardial Infarction Trial
AMI	acute myocardial infarction		
ANA	anti-nuclear antibody	COX	cyclooxygenase
ANCA	antineutrophil cytoplasmic antibody	CR	chemokine receptor
Ang	angiopoietin	CREDO	Clopidogrel for the Reduction of Events During Observation (trial)
Anti-d	anti Rh immunoglobulin		
APC	activated protein C	CRP	C-reactive protein
APCR	activated protein C resistance	CT	computed tomography
APLA	antiphospholipid antibodies	CURE	Clopidogrel in Unstable angina to prevent Recurrent Events (trial)
apo	apolipoprotein		
APS	antiphospholipid syndrome	CUS	compression ultrasonography
aPTT	activated partial thromboplastin time	CVA	cerebrovascular accident
ART	assisted reproductive technology	CVD	cardiovascular disease
ARTEMIS	Arixtra for ThromboEmbolism Prevention in Medical Indications (study)	CVP	central venous pressure
		D&C	dilatation and curettage
ASD	atrial septal defect	DCCT	Diabetes Control and Complications Trial
AST	aspartate aminotransferase	DDAVP	1-deamino-8-D-arginine vasopressin
AT	antithrombin	DIC	disseminated intravascular coagulation
ATP	adenosine triphosphate	DPP	Diabetes Prevention Program
β_2-GP	β_2-glycoprotein	DREAM	Diabetes Reduction Approaches with ramipiril and rosiglitazone Medications Study
BMI	body mass index		
BP	blood pressure		
CABG	coronary artery bypass surgery	DVT	deep vein thrombosis
CAC	coronary artery calcification	EACA	ε-aminocaproic acid
CAD	coronary artery disease	EBCT	electron beam computed tomography
CADASIL	Cerebral Autosomal Dominant, Arteriopathy with Subcortical Infarcts and Leukoencephalopathy	ECAT	European Concerted Action on Thrombosis (study)
		ECG	electrocardiogram
CAMELOT	Comparison of AMlodipine vs. Enalapril to Limit Occurrences of Thrombosis (trial)	ECM	extracellular matrix
		ECST	European Carotid Surgery Trial
		EDTA	ethyl-enediaminetetraacetic acid
CAPRIE	Clopidogrel versus Aspirin in Patients at Risk of Ischaemic Events (trial)	EGIR	European Group for the Study of Insulin Resistance
CASS	Coronary Artery Surgery Study	ELISA	enzyme-linked immunosorbent assay

ENOXACAN	Enoxaparin and Cancer (study)		ICAM	intercellular adhesion molecule
EPT	endogenous thrombin potential		IDF	International Diabetes Foundation
ERA	Estrogen Replacement and Atherosclerosis (study)		IDL	intermediate-density lipoprotein
			IFG	impaired fasting glucose
ERT	estrogen replacement therapy		IFN	interferon
ESPS	European Stroke Prevention Study		IgG	immunoglobulin
ESPRIT	EStrogen in the Prevention of ReInfarction Trial		IGT	impaired glucose tolerance
			IHD	ischemic heart disease
ESR	erythrocyte sedimentation rate		IL	interleukin
ESTHER	Estrogen and ThromboEmbolism Risk (study)		IMT	carotid intima–media wall thickness
			INR	international normalized ratio
EVAR	endovascular repair		IPC	intermittent pneumatic compression
EVTET	Estrogen in Venous Thromboembolism Trial		ISSHP	International Society for the Study of Hypertension in Pregnancy
EXCLAIM	Extended Prophylaxis for Venous ThromboEmbolism (trial)			
			ITP	idiopathic thrombocytopenic purpura
EXPRESS	Expanded Prophylaxis Evaluation Surgery Study		IUCD	intrauterine contraceptive device
			IUGR	intrauterine growth restriction
EXULT	Exanta Used to Lessen Thrombosis (trial)		iv	intravenous
F1+2	prothrombin fragment 1+2		IVC	inferior vena cava
Fc	crystallisable fragment		IVF	*in vitro* fertilization
FEIBA	FVIII inhibitor bypassing agent		IVIG	intravenous immunoglobulin
FIX	coagulation factor IX		IVIg	intravenous immunoglobulin
FpA	fibrinopeptide A		LA	lupus anticoagulant
FSH	follicle-stimulating hormone		LDL	low-density lipoprotein
FVIII	coagulation factor VIII		LETS	Leiden Thrombophilia Study
FVL	Factory V Leiden		LFA	lymphocyte function antigen
GALA	General Anaesthetic versus Local Anaesthetic (trial)		LITE	Longitudinal Investigation of Thromboembolism Etiology (study)
GCS	graduated compression stockings		LMWH	low-molecular-weight heparin
GDM	gestational diabetes mellitus		LNG-IUS	levonorgestrel intrauterine system
GnRH	gonadotrophin-releasing hormone		LP	lipoprotein
GOPEC	Genetics Of Pre-EClampsia (study)		LP(a)	lipoprotein (a)
GP	glycoprotein		LPL	lipoprotein lipase
GRIT	Growth Restriction Intervention Trial		L-TF	low amounts of human tissue factor (transgenic mouse)
GUSTO	Global Utilization Strategies to open Occluded coronary arteries			
			LV	left ventricular
HAPO	Hyperglycaemia and Adverse Pregnancy Outcome (study)		MAP	mean arterial pressure
			MCA	middle cerebral artery
hCG	human chorionic gonadotrophin		MCP	monocyte chemoattractant protein
HDL	high-density lipoprotein		M-CSF	macrophage colony-stimulating factor
HEART	Heart and Estrogen/progestin Replacement Study		MEDENOX	MEDical patients with ENOXaparin (trial)
			METHRO	MElagatran for THRombin inhibition in orthopedic surgery (trial)
HELLP	hemolysis, elevated liver enzyme levels and low platelet count (syndrome)			
			MHC	major histocompatibility complex
HERS	Heart and Estrogen/progestin Replacement Study		MI	myocardial infarction
			MMP	matrix metalloproteinase
HIT	heparin-induced thrombocytopenia		MORE	Multiple Outcomes Raloxifene Evaluation (study)
HIV	human immunodeficiency virus			
HL	hepatic lipase		MPA	medroxyprogesterone acetate
HLA	human leukocyte antigen		MPO	myeloperoxidase
HMG	3-hydroxy-3-methylglutaryl		MRA	magnetic resonance angiography
hMG	human menopausal gonadotrophin		MRI	magnetic resonance imaging
HR	hazard ratio		MTHFR	methylene tetrahydroflate reductase
HRT	hormone replacement therapy		n-APC-sr	normalized APC-sensitivity ratios
HT	hormone therapy		NASCET	North American Symptomatic Carotid Endarterectomy Trial
HUS	hemolytic uremic syndrome			

NCEP-ATP	National Cholesterol Education Programme adult treatment panel
NEFA	nonesterified fatty acid
NEP	neutral endopeptidase
NF	nuclear factor
NHANES	National Health and Nutrition Examination Survey
NIH	National Institutes of Health
NPH	neutral protamine Hagedorn
NSABP	National Surgical Adjuvant Breast and Bowel Project (USA)
NSAID	nonsteroidal anti-inflammatory drug
NYHA	New York Heart Association
OC	oral contraceptive
OGTT	oral glucose tolerance test
OHSS	ovarian hyperstimulation syndrome
OR	odds ratio
PAI	plasminogen activator inhibitor
PAIg	platelet-associated IgG
PARAGON	Platelet IIb/IIIa Antagonism for the Reduction of Acute Coronary Syndrome Events in a Global Organization Network (study)
PC	protein C
PCI	percutaneous coronary intervention
PCOS	polycystic ovarian syndrome
PCR	polymerase chain reaction
PDA	patent ductus arteriosus
PDGF	platelet-derived growth factor
PE	pulmonary embolism
PECAM	platelet endothelial cell adhesion molecule
PEGASUS	PENTasaccharide in Hip-FRActure surgery (trial)
PF	platelet factor
PG	prostaglandin
PGD	preimplantation genetic diagnosis
PGDH	prostaglandin dehydrogenase
PGH	prostaglandin H synthase
PGI_2	prostacyclin
PGM	prothrombin gene mutation
PHASE	Papworth HT Atherosclerosis
PIH	pregnancy-induced hypertension
PMSS	Pregnancy Mortality Surveillance System (USA)
PPAR	peroxisome proliferators-activated receptor
PPCM	peripartum cardiomyopathy
PPS	postphlebitic syndrome
PPT	partial prothrombin time
PREVENT	Prospective Randomized Evaluation of the Vascular Effects of Norvasc Trial
PRIME	Prospective Epidemiological Study of Myocardial Infarction (trial)
PRINCE	PRevention IN Cardiopulmonary Disease with Enoxaparin (trial)
PS	protein S
PT	prothrombin time
PTS	postthrombotic syndrome
PUBS	percutaneous umbilical blood sampling
RA	rheumatoid arthritis
RAS	renal artery stenosis
RATIO	Risk of Arterial Thrombosis in relation to Oral contraceptives (Study)
RCOG	Royal College of Obstetricians and Gynaecologists
RCT	randomized controlled trial
RF	rheumatoid factor
RIND	reversible ischemic neurologic deficit
ROC	receiver operator curve
RR	relative risk
r-tPA	recombinant tissue plasminogen activator
RUTH	Raloxifene Use for the Heart (Trial)
RV	right ventricular
SD	standard deviation
SERM	selective estrogen receptor modulator
SERPINS	serine protease inhibitor superfamily
SFH	symphyseal fundal height
SGA	small for gestation
SHARE	Study of Health Assessment and Risk Evaluation in Ethnic Groups
SHBG	sex-hormone-binding globulin
SMA	superior mesenteric artery
SMR	standardized mortality rate
SNP	single nucleotide polymorphism
SPECT	single photon emission computed tomography
STAR	Study of Tamoxifen And Raloxifene
TAFI	thrombin-activatable fibrinolysis inhibitor
TAT	thrombin–antithrombin complex
TF	tissue factor
TFPI	tissue factor pathway inhibitor
TGF	transforming growth factor
Th2	T helper 2
THS	thyroid-stimulating hormone
TIA	transient ischemic attack
TIMP	tissue inhibitors of matrix metalloproteinase
TNF	tumor necrosis factor
tPA	tissue plasminogen activator
TRIPOD	Troglitazone In the Prevention Of Diabetes (trial)
TTP	thrombotic thrombocytopenic purpura
TTP-HUS	thrombotic thrombocytopenic purpura and hemolytic uremic syndrome
TX	thromboxane
UFH	unfractionated heparin
UKPDS	United Kingdom Prospective Diabetes Trial
uPA	urokinase
V/Q	ventilation/perfusion
VCAM	vascular cell adhesion molecule
VDRL	Venereal Disease Research Laboratory
VEGF	vascular endothelial growth factor
VIP	Vitamins in Pregnancy (trial)
VLA	very late antigen
VLDL	very-low-density lipoprotein
VNTR	variable nucleotide tandem repeat

VSD	ventricular septal defect	vWF	von Willebrand factor
VSMC	vascular smooth muscle cell	WEST	Women's Estrogen for Stroke Trial
VTE	venous thromboembolism	WHI	Women's Health Initiative
vWD	von Willebrand disease	WHO	World Health Organization

Reference annotation

The reference lists are annotated, where appropriate, to guide readers to primary articles, key review papers, and management guidelines, as follows:

- Seminal primary article
- Key review paper
- ★ First formal publication of a management guideline

We hope that this feature will render extensive lists of references more useful to the reader and will help to encourage self-directed learning among both trainees and practicing physicians.

OVERVIEW

Epidemiology of vascular disease in women

JILL P PELL

DISEASE FREQUENCY AND NATURAL HISTORY

In Europe, 41 million life years (47 percent) lost are due to premature death from cardiovascular disease and 11 million (13 percent) are due to premature death from coronary heart disease.[1] Each year there are 213 million admissions to European hospitals due to cardiovascular disease and 69 million due to coronary heart disease. In the United Kingdom, coronary heart disease costs the healthcare system around £1750 million per year and costs the economy a further £5300 million in lost earnings and social care.[2]

Coronary heart disease is commonly perceived as a disease of men by patients and healthcare workers alike,[3,4] because under 55 years of age men are twice as likely as women to die from coronary heart disease. In addition, chest pain is less likely to have a cardiac etiology in women than men. However, the sex difference decreases with increasing age. Coronary heart disease mortality is 50 percent higher in men at 55–65 years of age and 20 percent higher in men at 65–75 years. Beyond 75 years there is no sex difference in mortality from coronary heart disease.[5] In general, the incidence in women lags behind that in men by 10 years for coronary heart disease overall and 20 years for myocardial infarction.[6] Coronary heart disease is far more age dependent in women than in men. In women, both age *per se* and the menopause are risk factors for coronary heart disease. Despite this, young women are by no means free from risk. Nearly 10 percent of coronary heart disease deaths in women occur prior to 65 years of age.[5]

The decline in mortality from coronary heart disease has been slower in women than men. Since 1984, the number of deaths due to cardiovascular disease in American women has exceeded the number in American men.[7] The difference equates to an excess of 67 000 deaths in women each year. In 2001, women represented 54 percent of deaths from cardiovascular disease in the United States and 49 percent of deaths from coronary heart disease.[7] In Europe each year there are 947 420 deaths due to coronary heart disease in women and 943 085 in men.[1] Similarly, there are 2.4 million deaths per annum due to cardiovascular disease in women and 1.9 million in men.[1]

In the United States and Europe, cardiovascular disease accounts for more than half of all deaths in women and coronary heart disease is the overall leading cause of death in women.[1,7,8] In Europe, cardiovascular disease accounts for 54 percent of deaths in all women and 30 percent of deaths in women under 65 years of age.[1] The equivalent figures for men are 43 percent and 30 percent, respectively. In Europe, coronary heart disease accounts for 21 percent of deaths in women of all ages and 12 percent of deaths under 65 years of age. In the United States, 250 000 women died in 2001 from coronary heart disease.[7] The prevalence of angina is higher in women than in men.[7] More than one-fifth of American women have some form of cardiovascular disease.[7] In the United States, between 1970 and 2001, the number of women admitted to hospital for coronary heart disease increased by 49 percent.[7]

Once myocardial infarction occurs, women tend to have a larger infarct size and are more prone to heart failure and cardiogenic shock.[9] Evidence from observational studies and the placebo arms of randomized trials suggests that following myocardial infarction, women are more likely to die than men both immediately and over the subsequent year.[7,9,10–16] The sex difference is only partly explained by the older age at presentation in women. Women under 45 years of age are nearly twice as likely to die in hospital as age-matched men following comparable success at reperfusion.[17] Black women have a particularly poor prognosis following myocardial infarction.[13] Within six years of myocardial infarction, 31 percent of women have a second infarct compared with only 23 percent of men.[18]

The overall incidence of stroke is 19 percent higher in men than women but the sex difference decreases with increasing age,[19] and there are specific instances in which the sex difference is reversed. Women have a higher incidence of subarachnoid hemorrhage than men.[20] Also, among those with a history of transient ischemic attacks, women are at a higher risk of ischemic stroke than men.[21,22] The overall risk of stroke is increased 13–14-fold during the first year following a transient ischemic attack and sevenfold during the first five years. However, the risk in women is twice that in men.[21] Although the lifetime risk of stroke is higher in men, women are more likely to die from stroke, partly due to their older age at presentation. In Europe, 18 percent of all deaths in women are due to stroke compared with 11 percent in men.[1] Five percent of deaths in women under 65 years of age are due to stroke compared with 4 percent in men.[1]

Despite the evidence, few women perceive a significant health risk from cardiovascular disease.[3,4] In general, women perceive breast cancer as a greater threat to their survival. In the United States in 2001, all cardiovascular disease combined claimed the lives of 498 863 women whereas all cancers combined to kill 256 693 women. In young women, chest pain may be dismissed as benign by patients and healthcare workers alike due to perceived low risk and reduced sensitivity of noninvasive investigations among women. These perceptions have been compounded by the fact that women have commonly been excluded from or underrepresented in studies of cardiovascular disease.

RISK FACTORS

In general, the same risk factors predispose to cardiovascular disease in both men and women. However, there are sex differences in the prevalence of many factors. Smoking, excess alcohol consumption and poor diet are more common in men than women.[23,24] In contrast, women undertake less exercise, have higher total cholesterol levels, and are more likely to be overweight and diabetic.[23–25]

The relative risk of coronary heart disease associated with cigarette smoking is similar in men and women. However, because smoking is less prevalent in women, it carries a lower attributable risk.[23] The relative risks associated with body mass index and blood pressure are also similar in men and women.[23] In contrast there are sex differences in the relative risks associated with some risk factors such as diabetes and cholesterol. Overall, premenopausal women have a significantly lower risk of cardiovascular disease than age-matched men. However, the female advantage is attenuated or abolished in women with diabetes mellitus, hyperlipidemia, or multiple risk factors.[6]

Diabetes mellitus

The prevalence of diabetes mellitus is increasing due to a rise in type 2 diabetes associated with obesity. There has been a sixfold increase in the prevalence of diabetes since 1958.[25] Overall, 18 percent of adults over 65 years of age now have diabetes mellitus.[25] However, the prevalence is approximately 10 percent higher in women than men.[25] Diabetes mellitus abolishes the female advantage in respect of the incidence of myocardial infarction, intermittent claudication, and stroke. In the presence of diabetes mellitus, women are at a comparable risk of coronary heart disease to men.[26]

Individual studies have suggested that the presence of diabetes is associated with a twofold to threefold risk of cardiovascular events in men compared with a threefold to sevenfold risk in women.[26–38] Diabetic women have twice the coronary heart disease risk compared with their male nondiabetic counterparts and almost four times the risk of nondiabetic women.[28,29] In men, established coronary heart disease confers a higher risk of coronary heart disease mortality (hazard ratio [HR] 4.2) than diabetes mellitus (HR 2.1). This is reversed in women in whom diabetes mellitus (HR 3.8) is associated with a greater risk of coronary heart disease mortality than established coronary heart disease (HR 1.9).[39] Diabetes mellitus is associated with a threefold risk of stroke in men,[40] and fivefold risk in women.[27] Diabetes mellitus doubles the risk of ischemic stroke.[21] In women, diabetes predicts the occurrence of ischemic rather than hemorrhagic stroke, but not in men.[41] Diabetes increases not only the risk of stroke occurring but also its severity and case fatality.[42]

In diabetic women, endothelial dysfunction may contribute to myocardial ischemia and adverse cardiovascular events. Diabetic premenopausal women are comparable to postmenopausal women and significantly worse than nondiabetic premenopausal women in terms of myocardial blood flow and response to vasodilators and sympathetic stimulation.[43] However, the increased risk associated with diabetes in women is also, in part, due to sex differences in coexisting risk factors such as dyslipidemia and hypertension.[44–46] Dyslipidemia often occurs in association with diabetes. However, the prevalence of dyslipidemia is higher in diabetic women than diabetic men.[26,45,46] Compared with men, women have higher levels of low-density lipoprotein (LDL)-cholesterol and triglycerides, and lower levels of high-density lipoprotein (HDL)-cholesterol.[26,37,45,46] Also, low HDL-cholesterol and high very low-density lipoprotein (VLDL)-cholesterol confer a higher risk of coronary heart disease in women than in men.[44] Women with diabetes mellitus are also more likely to be hypertensive and obese than men with diabetes.[26,45] Women tend to have a higher body mass index than men independent of glucose status. Among those with coronary heart disease, the presence of diabetes mellitus increases the risk of triple vessel disease in men and women alike. However, in women it is also associated with significantly worse stenoses.[26]

Overall, survival is significantly worse in those with coronary heart disease who also have diabetes mellitus.[47,48] However, the effect is greater in women than men. Diabetes doubles the risk of recurrent myocardial infarction in women but has an insignificant effect in men.[49,50] Among nondiabetic patients, the risk of fatal coronary events following acute myocardial infarction is significantly lower in women compared with men.[49] However, in diabetic patients, the risk of recurrent myocardial infarction in women is twice that in men.[49] The temporal decline in coronary heart disease mortality observed in those without diabetes has not been apparent in those with diabetes mellitus.

Hypertension

One in four women over 20 years of age has hypertension.[51] Women differ from men in the incidence and natural history of hypertension. Under 40 years of age, women generally have lower systolic and diastolic blood pressures than men and, therefore, a lower prevalence of hypertension.[51–53] Thereafter, blood pressure prevalence increases more steeply with age in women than men.[54] Therefore, the sex gap narrows. By age 45–65 years more than half of all women are hypertensive.[9,55] The prevalence is even higher in African American women of whom 79 percent are hypertensive beyond 45 years of age.[55] The prevalence of hypertension is comparable in women and men by 70 years of age. Beyond 70 years, the sex difference is reversed with hypertension becoming more common in women.[7,9,52,53,56,57] This is, in part, due to the greater life expectancy in women.[9] Overall, more than 60 percent of those with hypertension are women.[52,56]

Elevated systolic and diastolic blood pressure confer an increased risk of coronary heart disease in both men and women. However, systolic blood pressure is more predictive of future events than diastolic blood pressure. Similarly, there is a 47 percent increase in risk of stroke for every 7 mm Hg rise in diastolic blood pressure.[58] Compared with normotensive individuals, women with hypertension have a fourfold risk of coronary heart disease compared with a threefold risk in hypertensive men.[55,59] Of particular concern are older women who are more prone to develop isolated systolic or wide pulse pressure hypertension, which carries a greater risk of coronary heart disease.[60,61] Isolated systolic hypertension is present in 30 percent of women over 65 years of age.[55] This, combined with the greater prevalence of hypertension in older women, results in a higher population-attributable risk from hypertension in older women than in older men.[13] Hypertension causes stroke more frequently in elderly women than in elderly men of the same age, and it is a more potent risk factor for chronic heart failure even in the absence of coronary heart disease.[62] There is evidence that female sex hormones in premenopausal women protect against genotypic predisposition to hypertension in women. Sibling correlations in hypertension are much stronger in

men and postmenopausal women than premenopausal women.[63] In women, hypertension is associated with a threefold risk of stroke.[64] There is conflicting evidence as to whether the stroke risk reduction from antihypertensive treatment in women is comparable with,[65,66] or less than,[67] that in men.

The overall reduced risk of coronary heart disease in premenopausal women is not apparent in women with multiple risk factors. Hypertension is often associated with other risk factors for cardiovascular disease. In the Framingham Heart Study, less than 20 percent of individuals had isolated hypertension.[68] Approximately 30 percent of the coronary heart disease events in men occurred in individuals with three or more risk factors. The corresponding figure for women was 48 percent. The tendency for risk factors to cluster is higher in individuals who are obese at baseline and those who gain weight subsequently.[68]

Dyslipidemia

Compared with men, cholesterol levels in women tend to be higher,[69] and more age dependent. Following the menopause, there are increases in the levels of total cholesterol, LDL- and VLDL-cholesterol, and triglyceride, and a decrease in the level of HDL-cholesterol.[69–72] There is an increase in small dense LDL particles, which is associated with a particularly high risk of myocardial infarction,[73,74] and a decrease in HDL2-cholesterol subfraction which is more cardioprotective than other subfractions.[70] The increase in LDL-cholesterol is, in part, due to downregulating of hepatic LDL-receptors as a result of the reduction in estrogen level.[70,72,75]

Elevated triglyceride level is associated with an increased risk of coronary heart disease, independent of HDL-cholesterol level and other risk factors.[76–78] The relative risk associated with triglyceride level is higher among women than men.[78–81] A low HDL-cholesterol level is a stronger predictor of coronary heart disease mortality in women than men and has a particularly strong association in women over 65 years of age.[55,82–84] High LDL-cholesterol is associated with increased risk of coronary heart disease in women, especially under 65 years of age.[82] However, the association is weaker than in men. In the Framingham study, the 8-year risk of coronary events increased with total:HDL cholesterol ratio from 7 percent for a ratio under 5 to 12 percent for a ratio of 5–7 to 20 percent for a ratio of over 7.[6] Studies have demonstrated an increased risk of peripheral arterial disease with increased total cholesterol,[85–87] and triglyceride levels.[88] In the Cardiovascular Health Study, total and LDL-cholesterol were inversely associated with ankle–brachial pressure index in women but not in men.[87]

Obesity

Obesity is associated with an increased risk of coronary heart disease.[89] The risk of coronary heart disease is twice as high in women who are moderately overweight (body mass index

$25-29\,kg/m^2$) compared with lean women (body mass index $<21\,kg/m^2$).[89] The association between obesity and coronary heart disease is, in part, due to the confounding effects of blood pressure, dyslipidemia and haemostatic factors. However, in the Nurses Study a body mass index in excess of $25\,kg/m^2$ was associated with an 8 percent increase in coronary heart disease incidence independent of other risk factors.[90] The risk associated with obesity is greater in women than men. A body mass index over $35\,kg/m^2$ increases the risk of coronary heart disease by 42 percent in men compared with 93 percent in women.[89] Similarly, a 20 percent increase in weight increases risk of coronary heart disease by 86 percent in men compared with 360 percent in women.[89]

Central obesity, also known as abdominal or gynecoid obesity, is a greater risk factor for coronary heart disease than android obesity, especially in women.[91–93] In women, waist–hip and waist–height ratios are better predictors of mortality than body mass index.[94] A 0.15 unit increase in waist–hip ratio is associated with a 60 percent increase in relative risk of death independent of other risk factors including body mass index.[94]

Over the past three decades, there has been a dramatic increase in the prevalence of obesity. The increase in obesity has been particularly marked in men, in whom the prevalence has tripled since the mid 1980s.[2] In the United Kingdom, 20 percent of men and 19 percent of women are now obese, and a further 45 percent of men and 34 percent women are overweight.[2] Around 1 in 4 men and 1 in 5 women in the United Kingdom have central obesity.[2] In the United States, 33 percent of all women are now obese and a further 29 percent are overweight.[7] The figures are higher still for black American women with 50 percent obese and a further 28 percent overweight.[7]

Metabolic syndrome

Hypertension, obesity, hyperlipidemia and diabetes mellitus or insulin resistance tend to cluster in individuals and families. The coexistence of these factors, referred to as metabolic syndrome, is more common in women than men. This is particularly so among black Americans in whom the prevalence of metabolic syndrome is 57 percent higher in women than men.[7] In a study of patients with known coronary heart disease, Sprecher and Pearce demonstrated that 8 percent would have been expected to have all four risk factors had they occurred independently of each other.[95] However, clustering occurred in 10 percent of men and 21 percent of women.[95] The risk associated with metabolic syndrome was also greater in women. The hazard ratio for death in the presence of all four risk factors was 2.6 in men compared with 13.4 in women.[95]

Reproductive history

Compared with men, women have a lower overall incidence of coronary heart disease, myocardial infarction, and stroke. These sex differences cannot be fully explained by differences in the prevalence of lifestyle risk factors. The lower risk of cardiovascular disease in women persists even after adjusting for serum cholesterol, diabetes, hypertension, and cigarette smoking.[96] Increasing age is a risk factor for cardiovascular disease in both men and women. However, risk increases with age more steeply in women than men. Prior to the menopause, risk of cardiovascular disease is much lower in women. After the menopause women have a comparable or higher risk to men. Natural menopause confers a threefold risk of coronary heart disease.[6] Premature menopause, resulting from bilateral oophorectomy, is associated with an eightfold risk of coronary heart disease.[97] These findings point to endogenous estrogen being a protective factor for cardiovascular disease in women.

Estrogen acts both directly and indirectly on the endothelium. Estrogen receptors in endothelial and smooth muscle cells mediate potent vasodilatory substances, prostacyclin, and endothelin-derived relaxing factors such as nitric oxide.[98] Estrogen acts as an intrinsic antioxidant, scavenging free radicals, and estrogens may affect vascular cells by modulating gene expression.[98] In addition, estrogen acts indirectly via changes in lipoprotein and glucose metabolism and hemostasis.[99–101]

Menopause is not the only factor influencing estrogen levels. Estrogen levels vary greatly throughout a woman's life. Levels are low before menarche, during breastfeeding, and after menopause. They increase greatly during pregnancy and vary considerably during the menstrual cycle. These patterns are made still more complex by the administration of exogenous estrogens in the form of the combined oral contraceptive pill or hormone replacement therapy. If estrogen levels do play a role in the sex differences observed in cardiovascular disease, there should be associations between the risk of cardiovascular disease and reproductive history, such as age at menarche and menopause, parity, pregnancy losses and menstrual cycle length and regularity. There is strong evidence for an association between age at menopause and both cardiovascular risk factors and cardiovascular disease. Following menopause there are significant increases in the levels of total cholesterol, triglycerides, antithrombin III, factor VII, and fibrinogen as well as an increase in waist–hip ratio.[71,102–114] The risk of dying from coronary heart disease falls by 2 percent for every year by which menopause is delayed.[115,116] The increase in the incidence of cardiovascular disease after menopause is not simply due to the confounding effect of age. In women, age and menopause are independent risk factors for cardiovascular disease. Postmenopausal women have a twofold to threefold higher risk of coronary heart disease than premenopausal women of the same age.[7,97,102,117]

Women who experience menarche at an earlier age are exposed to endogenous estrogen for a longer period. Therefore, one might predict a protective effect of early menarche. However, as yet, there is no clear evidence of a significant inverse association between age at menarche and risk of cardiovascular disease. Women with long or irregular menstrual cycles are likely to have fewer total ovulations and more anovular cycles in which estrogen levels do not reach preovulation levels. Therefore, their mean lifetime estrogen levels will be lower. There is some evidence of an association between irregular and anovulatory cycles and risk of cardiovascular disease.[118,119] There is also some evidence of a possible association between gravidity (total number of pregnancies) and risk of coronary heart disease.[120,121] Studies suggest an association between total number of pregnancy losses and risk of coronary heart disease.[120,122,123] However, the evidence regarding parity (total number of live births) is somewhat conflicting with both positive and negative results having been reported.

Hormone replacement therapy

Although endogenous estrogens are protective against cardiovascular disease, administration of exogenous estrogens may increase risk. Earlier data from cohort studies suggested that postmenopausal hormone replacement therapy was cardioprotective, with metaanalyses reporting relative risks for cardiovascular disease as low as 0.57.[124] These results have subsequently been disputed as a result of three randomized controlled trials that studied the impact of hormone replacement therapy on cardiovascular endpoints. The Heart and Estrogen/progestin Replacement Study (HERS) recruited women with established coronary heart disease.[125] The investigators demonstrated no reduction in coronary heart disease events in treated women despite an 11 percent reduction in LDL-cholesterol and 10 percent increase in HDL-cholesterol. In addition, hormone replacement therapy appeared to predispose to earlier coronary heart disease events. The Women's Estrogen for Stroke Trial (WEST) recruited women with cerebrovascular disease and demonstrated statistically nonsignificant increases in the risk of both coronary heart disease and stroke among treated women.[126]

The Women's Health Initiative (WHI) trial recruited healthy volunteers.[127] It was terminated early due to an excess of breast cancers among treated women. Nonetheless, at 5 years' follow-up, the study demonstrated a small but statistically significant increase in coronary heart disease (relative risk [RR] 1.29, 95 percent confidence interval [CI] 1.02 to 1.63), stroke (RR 1.41, 95 percent CI 1.07 to 1.85), and total cardiovascular events (RR 1.22, 95 percent CI 1.09 to 1.36) among treated women. This equated to 7 excess coronary heart disease deaths and 8 excess stroke deaths per 10 000 person years. Uptake of hormone replacement therapy has fallen following publication of these trials, particularly the WHI trial.[128]

The difference in the results obtained from the observational studies and trials may reflect selection bias whereby the cohort studies recruited atypically healthy women.[124] However, there are also differences in the drug regimens used and the timing of initiation. In general, the gap between menopause and commencement of hormone replacement therapy has been longer in trials than observational studies.

Cigarette smoking

The leading preventable cause of coronary heart disease in women is cigarette smoking.[129] More than 50 percent of myocardial infarctions in middle-aged women can be attributed to cigarette smoking.[55] The risk in heavy smokers (>20/day) is up to five times higher than in nonsmokers but even light smokers (1–4/day) have twice the risk of nonsmokers.[129,130] Following smoking cessation the risk of coronary heart disease falls within months and reaches the level in nonsmokers within 3–5 years.[129] Smoking is also an independent risk factor for stroke. In the Finnmark Study, the risk associated with smoking was higher in women (adjusted RR 2.12) than in men (adjusted RR 1.64).[131] Smoking is the most important risk factor for peripheral arterial disease. The prevalence of peripheral arterial disease is only 6 percent among middle-aged adults who do not smoke, compared with 12 percent in ex-smokers and 18 percent in current smokers.[85]

In Europe and the United States there has been a decline in the overall prevalence of cigarette smoking over the past few decades. However, the decline in smoking prevalence has been less steep in recent years and, in some European countries, prevalence is now starting to rise again.[1] In general, the decline in women has been less marked than that in men and in some countries prevalence among women has not declined. As a result, historical sex differences in smoking prevalence are becoming less apparent. In some countries, the prevalence of smoking in women is now equivalent to that in men.[1] Between the 1970s and 1990s, the prevalence of smoking among adult men in the United Kingdom fell from 51 percent to 28 percent.[1] Over the same period the prevalence in women fell from 41 percent to 26 percent.[1] The most worrying trend is the increase in smoking prevalence among children, particularly young girls. In many European countries girls now smoke more commonly than boys.[1]

Physical activity

Few studies of exercise and coronary heart disease risk have included women. The data that are available suggest that active women have a lower risk of coronary heart disease.[55] Even brisk walking and other moderate intensity activities can substantially reduce coronary heart disease risk.[132] The association with coronary heart disease is, in part, due to the fact that physical activity reduces the risk of obesity. Exercise and dietary modifications resulting in weight loss have beneficial effects on lipid levels even in people with diabetes.[133] Studies in female runners have demonstrated a dose response between level of exercise and HDL-cholesterol level.[133]

Around 25 percent of women report that they have no regular sustained physical activity.[89] Furthermore, level of physical activity declines with age. Only 12 percent of women aged 65–74 undertake regular sustained exercise.[2] It has been calculated that 82 percent of coronary events in women can be attributed to adverse lifestyle.[134] Sixteen percent of the decline in incidence of coronary heart disease between 1980 and 1994 has been attributed to improvements in diet.[90]

Alcohol

High levels of alcohol consumption are associated with increased risk of coronary heart disease, especially if ingested in the form of binge drinking. It is recommended that men consume a maximum of 4 units of alcohol per day and 21 units per week. In the United Kingdom, these limits are exceeded by 39 percent and 29 percent of men, respectively.[2] Twenty-one percent of women exceed the recommended daily limit of 3 units of alcohol and 17 percent exceed the weekly limit of 14 units.[2] Over the past 10 years, the percentage of men consuming excessive amounts of alcohol has remained fairly constant.[2] In contrast, there has been a 50 percent increase in the percentage of women exceeding the recommended limits.[2]

PRESENTATION

There are sex differences in the etiology of chest pain and the presentation of coronary heart disease.

Chest pain

Among patients presenting with chest pain, women are less likely to be diagnosed as having acute myocardial infarction or ischemic heart disease.[133–137] This cannot be explained simply by the less frequent use of diagnostic tests in women or their poorer sensitivity. Among patients undergoing coronary angiography for chest pain, women are less likely to have significant stenoses and more likely to have normal coronary arteries.[138,139] In the Coronary Artery Surgery Study (CASS), half of all women undergoing angiography for suspected coronary heart disease did not have significant obstruction.[138] Even among women who satisfy strict criteria for resting angina and electrocardiographic changes 1 in 4 do not have major obstructive coronary disease.[140] This condition, described variously as syndrome X or variant angina, has been attributed to microvascular endothelial dysfunction not detectable on coronary angiography.[141–143] Around 60 percent of those with no identifiable cause for their chest pain and electrocardiographic anomalies are peri- or postmenopausal women.[144] Women who develop syndrome X while on hormone replacement therapy tend to be on inadequate doses as assessed by plasma estradiol and follicle-stimulating hormone (FSH) levels.[145] Therefore, it has been postulated that estrogen deficiency may play a role in the etiology of syndrome X. Conventional antianginal therapy is less effective in women with syndrome X. However, long-term survival is normal.[44]

Syndrome X is more prevalent in women than men.[146,147] However, there remains an excess of nonischemic chest pain among women. Studies have demonstrated that noncardiac causes of chest pain, such as musculoskeletal and psychosomatic conditions, are over-represented in women.[136,141,142,148] There is also evidence that women generally have a lower threshold for seeking medical attention than men.[149] Some women experiencing chest pain despite normal coronary angiograms may nonetheless have ischemic heart disease.

Coronary heart disease

Among those with coronary heart disease, women are more likely to initially present with angina and less likely to present with acute myocardial infarction compared with men.[150] When women do experience acute myocardial infarction as their first symptom, it is more likely to be silent or unrecognized than in men.[150–152] Sudden cardiac death is a more common first presentation in women than in men.[7] Among women, there is a general shift in presentation after menopause from angina to acute myocardial infarction and sudden cardiac death.[57] As with coronary heart disease, women with peripheral arterial disease are more likely to be asymptomatic compared with men.[153] As a result, they are also less likely to receive hospital treatment.[153]

Compared with men, women with chronic stable angina are more likely to complain of atypical symptoms such as neck pain, nausea, vomiting, fatigue, and dyspnoea.[154] Among those with acute coronary syndromes, women are less likely than men to complain of chest pain and sweating,[155] and more likely to report nonspecific symptoms such as nausea, vomiting, abdominal symptoms, fatigue, palpitations, dizziness, dyspnea, and syncope. Women are more likely than men to feel pain in the arms, neck, back, shoulders, jaw, and epigastrium.[155–157] Chest pain is still the most common presenting symptom among women with coronary heart disease, but it is less frequent than in men.

INVESTIGATIONS

Sex differences have been demonstrated in both access to investigations and the predictive power of the investigations once performed. In general, women are investigated and treated less aggressively than men.[10,158–162] Women are referred less frequently for coronary angiography.[163–165] There is also some evidence that women may have to wait longer than men for examination and investigation, and are more likely to be admitted to a general, rather than specialist, ward.[166]

Many older noninvasive diagnostic tests, such as exercise and pharmacologic stress testing, were developed and tested predominantly on men. Newer noninvasive stress imaging modalities provide greater diagnostic accuracy than traditional exercise stress testing but, in general, the tests are still less accurate for women. The lower accuracy in women reflects a number of factors including a lower prevalence of coronary heart disease, sex differences in pathophysiology and risk factors, different referral patterns and features intrinsic to the test.

Resting and exercise electrocardiography are both less sensitive and less specific in women than men.[167] During exercise testing, false positive electrocardiograph changes, such as ST segment depression in the absence of coronary artery disease, occur more commonly in women than men, particularly among women on hormone replacement therapy.[168–172] The specificity of exercise testing is around 77 percent in men compared with 70 percent in women.[167,173] Exercise testing is also less sensitive in women. In men, the sensitivity is around 68 percent compared with 61 percent in women.[167,173] Women are more likely to experience anginal chest pain during exercise testing.[174] They have poorer exercise capacity than men, and are more likely to fail to achieve the target heart rate and to have repolarization abnormalities.[174,175] Nonetheless, even modified treadmill protocols are less sensitive and less specific in women.[139] When presenting with acute coronary syndromes, women are as likely as men to have some form of electrocardiographic changes. However, women have less marked ST deviation than men and more frequently present with nonspecific electrocardiographic changes.[176]

The combination of imaging techniques and either exercise or pharmacologic testing improves sensitivity and specificity in women. Thallium scanning has a better sensitivity than conventional exercise testing but its specificity is reduced in women because they have smaller heart chambers and the images can be attenuated by breast tissue.[167] Specificity may be better with higher energy isotopes such as technetium where attenuation is less. Radionuclide ventriculography is of limited use in women because of their reduced left ventricular response to exercise compared with men.[177] However, exercise stress echocardiography has greater specificity than exercise electrocardiography and produces comparable results in men and women.[167,178]

TREATMENT

Compared with men, women have lower rates of many coronary heart disease treatments such as thrombolytic therapy and coronary revascularization.[10,179–181] Differences persist after adjustment for demography and disease incidence.[179–181] Some of the residual difference is due to differences in referral and investigation thresholds. Women are less likely than men to undergo coronary angiography.[158,179,182] In one study, 40 percent of men with a positive thallium treadmill test were referred for diagnostic catheterization compared with only 4 percent of women.[158] The higher threshold for investigation in women reflects a number of factors including the perception of lower risk, differences in presentation and the lower sensitivity of noninvasive investigations.

There are conflicting results on whether sex differences persist following a positive coronary angiogram. Some studies suggest that women are less likely to undergo coronary artery bypass grafting after taking account of age and case mix.[183,184] If so, this may reflect the higher risk of perioperative death and neurological complications in women.[184–186] Women are technically more difficult to operate on, due to their smaller coronary arteries.[184,185] Furthermore, some risk factors are associated with a worse prognosis in women than men. The relative risk of inhospital death, periprocedural myocardial infarction, and restenosis attributed to diabetes is higher in women than men.[187] Also, hypertriglyceridemia increases mortality following bypass grafting in diabetic women but not diabetic men.[95] The higher inhospital mortality following surgery in women results in poorer long-term survival after adjustment for age at operation.[188] Periprocedural morbidity and mortality following percutaneous coronary intervention is also three times higher in women than men.[189] Results from the Global Utilization of Streptokinase and Tissue plasminogen activator for Occluded coronary arteries I (GUSTO I) trial demonstrated that thrombolysis for acute myocardial infarction was equally efficacious in women, but women had a higher risk of stroke.[190]

Cardiac rehabilitation produces similar improvements in functional capacity and other outcomes in men and women.[191–193] Despite this, a lower proportion of women attend than men. Following adjustment for age and comorbidity, women are less likely to be invited,[194] are less likely to enroll,[195] and are more likely to drop out early.[195]

FUTURE TRENDS

Both overall life expectancy and survival following cardiovascular events are increasing. Therefore, the population prevalence of cardiovascular disease may increase in the future resulting in an increasing need for investigations, treatment, and hospital admission. In 2001, cardiovascular disease accounted for more than 3 million hospital admissions in the United States. In addition to the growing burden of prevalent disease, the absolute number of deaths due to cardiovascular disease is also increasing.[7]

Over the past 20 years, mortality from coronary heart disease has declined. However, the rate of decline has been slower in women than in men.[7,196] As a result the sex gap operating to women's advantage has reduced. There are a number of trends in cardiovascular risk factors that suggest that the sex gap may reduce still further. Although the prevalence of smoking has fallen overall, the prevalence in young women has increased. In many European countries women now smoke as commonly as men, and a greater percentage of girls smoke than boys.[1] The prevalence of diabetes mellitus is increasing across Europe and the United States and this can be attributed primarily to an increase in type 2 diabetes in women.[1,7] The prevalence of excessive alcohol consumption has remained constant in men but is increasing in women.[2]

Cardiovascular disease is commonly perceived as a less important threat to women than breast cancer.[3,4] In the United States in 2001, cardiovascular disease claimed the lives of 498 863 women compared with 256 693 deaths due to all cancers combined. In the United States, 1 in 5 women now have some form of prevalent cardiovascular disease.[7] Since 1984, the number of cardiovascular disease deaths in women has exceeded those in men. In 2001, women accounted for 54 percent of deaths from cardiovascular disease in the United States. Currently 67 000 more women than men die from cardiovascular disease each year in the United States. In the past cardiovascular disease has been considered a disease of men. This view is becoming increasingly untenable.

KEY LEARNING POINTS

- The overall incidence of cardiovascular disease is lower in women. However, the sex advantage decreases with increasing age, and is diminished in the presence of diabetes mellitus, dyslipidemia, and multiple risk factors.
- Cardiovascular disease is commonly perceived as a disease of men. However, coronary heart disease is the most common cause of death in women. Cardiovascular disease accounts for more than half of all deaths in women and causes a higher absolute number of deaths in women than in men.
- Women are more likely to present with atypical symptoms and are less likely to be investigated. Noninvasive investigations are less sensitive and specific in women.
- Following myocardial infarction and coronary revascularization, women have a worse prognosis than men.
- The decline in mortality from cardiovascular disease has been less dramatic in women than in men. A number of trends in risk factors may reduce the advantage in favor of women still further: in particular increasing type 2 diabetes and excess alcohol consumption in women and increasing smoking prevalence in young women.

REFERENCES

1　Rayner M, Petersen S. *European Cardiovascular Disease Statistics*. Oxford: British Heart Foundation, 2000.

2　British Heart Foundation Statistics Database 2003. Coronary heart statistics. (www.heartstats.org), accessed December 2003.

3　Mosca L, Jones WK, King KB, Ouyang P, *et al.* Awareness, perception, and knowledge of heart disease risk and prevention among women in the United States. American Heart Association Women's Heart Disease and Stroke Campaign Task Force. *Arch Fam Med* 2000; **9**: 506–15.

4　Mosca L, Ferris A, Fabunmi R, Robertson RM; American Heart Association. Tracking women's awareness of heart disease: an American Heart Association national study. *Circulation* 2004; **109**: 573–9.

5　Wenger NK. Coronary heart disease in women: Evolving knowledge is dramatically changing practice. In Julian D, Wenger N, eds. *Women and Heart Disease*. St Louis, MO: Mosby, 1997: 21.

6　Kannel WB, Wilson PWF. Risk factors that attenuate the female coronary disease advantage. *Arch Intern Med* 1995; **155**: 57–61.

7　American Heart Association. *2002 Heart and Stroke Statistical Update*. Dallas, TX: American Heart Association, 2001, www.americanheart.org, 2002.

8　Hoyert DL, Kochanek KD, Murphy SL. Deaths: Final data for 1997. *Natl Vital Statistics Rep* 1999; **47**: 1–107.

9　Anastos K, Charney P, Charon RA, *et al.* Hypertension in women: what is really known? The Women's Caucus, Working Group on Women's Health of the Society of General internal Medicine. *Ann Intern Med* 1991; **115**: 287–93.

10　Hanratty B, Lawlor D, Robinson MB, *et al.* Sex differences in risk factors, treatment and mortality after acute myocardial infarction: An observational study. *J Epidemiol Comm Health* 2000; **54**: 912–16.

11　Gan SC, Beaver SK, Houck PM, *et al.* Treatment of acute myocardial infarction and 30-day mortality among women and men. *N Engl J Med* 2000; **343**: 8–15.

12　MacIntyre K, Stewart S, McMurray JJV, *et al.* Gender and survival: a population-based study of 201,114 men and women following a first acute myocardial infarction. *J Am Coll Cardiol* 2001; **38**: 729–35.

13　Tofler GH, Stone PH, Muller JE, *et al.* Effect of gender and race on prognosis after myocardial infarction: adverse prognosis for women, particularly black women. *J Am Coll Cardiol* 1987; **9**: 473–82.

14　ISIS-1 (First International Study of Infarct Survival) Collaborative Group. Randomized trial of intravenous atenolol among 16,027 cases of suspected acute myocardial infarction: ISIS-1. *Lancet* 1986; **57**: 57–66.

15　The GUSTO Investigators. An international randomized trial comparing four thrombolytic strategies for acute myocardial infarction. *N Engl J Med* 1993; **329**: 673–82.

16　Fibrinolytic Therapy Trialists (FTT) Collaborative Group. Indications for fibrinolytic therapy in suspected acute myocardial infarction: collaborative overview of early mortality and major morbidity results from all randomised trials of more than 1000 patients. *Lancet* 1994; **343**: 311–22.

17　Heer T, Gitt AK, Wienbergen H, *et al.* Do young women with acute myocardial infarction have increased intrahospital mortality? *Circulation* 2000; **102**(Suppl II): 793.

18　American Heart Association. *Heart and Stroke Statistical Update*. Dallas, TX: American Heart Association, 1998.

19 Manolio TA, Kronmal RA, Burke GL, *et al.* Short-term predictors of incident stroke in older adults. The Cardiovascular Health Study. *Stroke* 1996; **27**: 1479–86.

20 Davis P. Stroke in women. *Curr Opin Neurol* 1994; **7**: 36–40.

21 Whisnant JP, Wiebers DO, O'Fallon WM, *et al.* A population-based model of risk factors for ischemic stroke: Rochester, Minnesota. *Neurology* 1996; **47**: 1420–28.

22 Helgason CM, Wolf PA. American Heart Association Prevention Conference IV: prevention and rehabilitation of stroke: executive summary. *Circulation* 1997; **96**: 701–7.

23 Isles CG, Hole DJ, Hawthorne VM, Lever AF. Relation between coronary risk and coronary mortality in women of the Renfrew and Paisley Survey comparison with men. *Lancet* 1992; **338**: 702–6.

24 Fowkes FGR, Pell JP, Donnan PT, *et al.* Sex differences in susceptibility to etiologic factors for peripheral atherosclerosis: the importance of plasma fibrinogen and blood viscosity. *Arteriosoler Thromb* 1994; **14**: 862–8.

25 Centers for Disease Control and Prevention. *National Diabetes Fact Sheet: National Estimates and General Information on Diabetes in the United States. Revised edition.* Atlanta, GA: US Department of Health and Human Services, Centers for Disease Control and Prevention, 1998.

26 Barrett-Connor EL, Cohn BA, Wingard DL, Edelstein S. Why is diabetes mellitus a stronger risk factor for fatal ischemic heart disease in women than in men? *J Am Med Assoc* 1991; **265**: 627–31.

27 Manson JE, Colditz GA, Stampfer MJ, *et al.* A prospective study of maturity-onset diabetes mellitus and risk of coronary heart disease and stroke in women. *Arch Intern Med* 1991; **151**: 1141–7.

28 Kannel WB, McGee DK. Diabetes and cardiovascular risk factors: The Framingham study. *Circulation* 1979; **59**: 8–13.

29 Kannel WB, McGee DL. Diabetes and glucose tolerance as risk factors for cardiovascular disease. *Diabetes Care* 1979; **2**: 120–6.

30 Krolewski AS, Warram JH, Valsania P, *et al.* Evolving natural history of coronary artery disease in diabetes mellitus. *Am J Med* 1991; **90**(Suppl 2A): 56S–61S.

31 Butler WJ, Ostrander LD Jr, Carman WJ, Lamphiear DE. Mortality from coronary heart disease in the Tecumseh study. Long-term effect of diabetes mellitus, glucose tolerance and other risk factors. *Am J Epidemiol* 1985; **121**: 541–7.

32 Pan WH, Cedres LB, Liu K, Dyer A, *et al.* Relationship of clinical diabetes and asymptomatic hyperglycemia to risk of coronary heart disease mortality in men and women. *Am J Epidemiol* 1986; **123**: 504–16.

33 Kleinman JC, Donahue RP, Harris MI, *et al.* Mortality among diabetics in a national sample. *Am J Epidemiol* 1988; **128**: 389–401.

34 Seeman T, Mendes de Leon C, Berkman L, Ostfeld A. Risk factors for coronary heart disease among older men and women: a prospective study of community-dwelling elderly. *Am J Epidemiol* 1993; **138**: 1037–49.

35 Kuusisto J, Mykkanen L, Pyorala K, Laakso M. NIDDM and its metabolic control predict coronary heart disease in elderly subjects. *Diabetes* 1994; **43**: 960–7.

36 Barrett-Connor E, Wingard DL. Sex differential in ischemic heart disease mortality in diabetics: a prospective population-based study. *Am J Epidemiol* 1983; **118**: 489–96.

37 Haffner SM, Lehto S, Ronnemaaa T, *et al.* Mortality from coronary heart disease in subjects with type 2 diabetes and in nondiabetic subjects with and without prior myocardial infarction. *N Engl J Med* 1998; **339**: 229–34.

38 Mosca L, Grundy SM, Judelson D, *et al.* AHA/ACC scientific statement: consensus panel statement. Guide to preventive cardiology for women. American Heart Association/American College of Cardiology. *J Am Coll Cardiol* 1999; **33**: 1751–55.

39 Natarajan S, Liao Y, Cao G, *et al.* Sex differences in risk for coronary heart disease mortality associated with diabetes and established coronary heart disease. *Arch Intern Med* 2003; **163**: 1735–40

40 Stamler J, Vaccaro O, Neaton JD, Wentworth D. Diabetes, other risk factors, and 12 year cardiovascular mortality for men screened in the Multiple Risk Factor Intervention Trial. *Diabetes Care* 1993; **16**: 434–44.

41 Bogousslavsky J, Castillo V, Kumral E, *et al.* Stroke subtypes and hypertension. Primary hemorrhage vs infarction, larger- vs smaller-artery disease. *Arch Neurol* 1996; **53**: 265–69.

42 Biller J, Love BB. Diabetes and stroke. *Med Clin North Am* 1993; **77**: 95–110.

43 DiCarli MF, Bianco-Barlles D, Landon MC, *et al.* Effects of autonomic neuropathy on coronary blood flow in patients with diabetes mellitus. *Circulation* 1999; **100**: 813–19.

44 Goldschmid MG, Barrett-Connor E, Edelstein SL, *et al.* Dyslipidemia and ischemic heart disease mortality among men and women with diabetes. *Circulation* 1994; **89**: 991–7.

45 Cowie CC, Harris ML. Physical and metabolic characteristics of persons with diabetes. In: *Diabetes in America.* Bethesda, MD: National Diabetes Data Group of the National Institute of Diabetes and Digestive and Kidney Disease, National Institutes of Health, 1995: 117–64.

46 Haffner SM, Mykkanen L, Stern MP, *et al.* Greater effect of diabetes on LDL size in women than men. *Diabetes Care* 1994; **17**: 1164–71.

47 Liao Y, Cooper RS, Ghali JK, *et al.* Sex differences in the impact of coexistent diabetes on survival in patients with coronary heart disease. *Diabetes Care* 1993; **16**: 708–13.

48 Zuanetti G, Latini R, Maggioni AP, *et al.* Influence of diabetes on mortality in acute myocardial infarction:

data from the GISSI-2 study. *J Am Coll Cardiol* 1993; **22**: 1788–94.

49   Abbott RD, Donahue RP, Kannel WB, Wilson PW. The impact of diabetes on survival following myocardial infarction in men vs women: The Framingham Study. *JAMA* 1988; **260**: 3456–60.

50   Stone PH, Muller JE, Hartwell T, *et al*. The effect of diabetes mellitus on prognosis and serial left ventricular function after acute myocardial infarction: Contribution of both coronary disease and diastolic left ventricular dysfunction to the adverse prognosis: The MILIS Study Group. *J Am Coll Cardiol* 1989; **14**: 49–57.

51   American Heart Association. *Silent Epidemic: The Truth About Women and Heart Disease*. Dallas, TX: American Heart Association 1995; 9.

52   Burt VL, Whelton P, Roccella EJ, *et al*. Prevalence of hypertension in the US adult population. *Hypertension* 1995; **25**: 305–13.

53   Franklin SS, Guatin WG, Wong ND, *et al*. Hemodynamic patterns of age-related changes in blood pressure: the Framingham Heart Study. *Circulation* 1997; **96**: 306–15.

54   National High Blood Pressure Education Program Working Group. Report on Primary Prevention of Hypertension. *National Institutes of Health Publication* 1993; **93**: 3669.

55   Mosca L, Manson JE, Sutherland SE, *et al*. Cardiovascular disease in women: a statement for healthcare professionals from the American Heart Association. *Circulation* 1997; **96**: 2468–82.

56   Burt VL, Cutler JA, Higgins M, *et al*. Trends in the prevalence, awareness, treatment, and control of hypertension in the adult US population. *Hypertension* 1995; **26**: 60–9.

57   Kannel WB, Gordon T. Evaluation of cardiovascular risk in the elderly: The Framingham Study. *Bull N Y Acad Med* 1978; **54**: 573–91.

58   MacMahon S, Peto R, Cutler J, *et al*. Blood pressure, stroke and coronary heart disease, I. Prolonged differences in blood pressure: prospective observational studies corrected for the regression dilution bias. *Lancet* 1990; **335**: 765–74.

59   Kitler ME. Differences in men and women in coronary artery disease, systemic hypertension and their treatment. *Am J Cardiol* 1992; **70**: 1077–80.

60   Franklin SS, Khan SA, Wong ND, *et al*. Is pulse pressure useful in predicting risk for coronary heart disease? The Framingham Heart Study. *Circulation* 1999; **100**: 354–60.

61   Franklin SS, Jacobs MJ, Wong ND, *et al*. Predominance of isolated systolic hypertension among middle-aged and elderly US hypertensives. *Hypertension* 2001; **37**: 869–74.

62   Levy D, Larson MG, Vasan RS, *et al*. The progression from hypertension to congestive heart failure. *JAMA* 1996; **275**: 1557–62.

63   Giacche J, Vaugnat A, Hunt SC, *et al*. Aldosterone stimulation by angiotensin II: Influence of gender, plasma rennin, and familial resemblance. *Hypertension* 2000; **35**: 710–16.

64   Fiebach NH, Hebert PR, Stampfer MH, *et al*. A prospective study of high blood pressure and cardiovascular disease in women. *Am J Epidemiol* 1989; **130**: 646.

65   Salzberg S, Stroh JA, Frishman WH. Isolated systolic hypertension in the elderly: pathophysiology and treatment. *Med Clin North Am* 1998; **72**: 523–47.

66   Dahlof B, Lindholm LH, Hansson L, *et al*. Morbidity and mortality in the Swedish trial in old patients with hypertension (STOP Hypertension). *Lancet* 1991; **338**: 1281–5.

67   Reynolds E, Baron RB. Hypertension in women and the elderly. *Postgrad Med* 1996; **100**: 58–69.

68   Wilson PWF, Kannel WB, Silbershatz H, D'Agostino RB. Clustering of metabolic factors and coronary heart disease. *Arch Intern Med* 1999; **159**: 1104–09.

69   Johnson CL, Rifkind BM, Sempos CT, *et al*. Declining serum total cholesterol levels among US adults: the National Health and Nutrition Examination Surveys. *JAMA* 1993; **269**: 3002–8.

70   Stevenson JC, Crook D, Godsland IF. Influence of age and menopause on serum lipids and lipoproteins in healthy women. *Atherosclerosis* 1993; **98**: 83–90.

71   Matthews KA, Meilahn E, Kuller LH, *et al*. Menopause and risk factors for coronary heart disease. *N Engl J Med* 1989; **321**: 641–6.

72   Campos H, McNamara JR, Wilson PWF, *et al*. Differences in low density lipoprotein subfractions and apolipoproteins in premenopausal and postmenopausal women. *J Clin Endocrinol Metab* 1988; **67**: 30–35.

73   Austin MA, Breslow C, Hennekens CH, *et al*. Low-density lipoprotein subclass patterns and risk of myocardial infarction. *JAMA* 1998; **260**: 1917–21.

74   Campos H, Blijlevens E, McNamara JR, *et al*. LDL particle size distribution: results from the Framingham offspring study. *Arterioscler Thromb* 1992; **12**: 1410–19.

75   Welty FK. Who should receive hormone replacement therapy? *J Thromb Thrombolysis* 1996; **3**: 13–21.

76   La Rosa JC. Triglycerides and coronary risk in women and the elderly. *Arch Intern Med* 1997; **157**: 961–68.

77   Castelli WP. The triglyceride issue: a view from Framingham. *Am Heart J* 1986; **112**: 432–7.

78   Austin MA, Hokanson JE, Edwards KL. Hypertriglyceridemia as a cardiovascular risk factor. *Am J Cardiol* 1998; **81**: 7B–12B.

79   Bengtsson C, Bjorntorp P, Tibblin E. Ischaemic heart disease in women. *Acta Med Scand* 1973; **549**(Suppl): 1–128.

80   Stensvold I, Tverdal A, Urdal P, Graff-Iversen S. Non-fasting serum triglyceride concentration and mortality from coronary heart disease and any cause of middle-aged Norwegian women. *BMJ* 1993; **307**: 1318–22.

81   Cullen P. Evidence that triglycerides are an independent coronary heart disease risk factor. *Am J Cardiol* 2000; **86**: 943–9.

82   Manolio TA, Pearson TA, Wenger NK, *et al.* Cholesterol and heart disease in older persons and women: review of an NHLBI workshop. *Ann Epidemiol* 1992; **2**: 161–76.

83   Walsh BW, Schiff I, Rosner B, *et al.* Effects of postmenopausal estrogen replacement on the concentrations and metabolism of plasma lipoproteins. *N Engl J Med* 1991; **325**: 1196–204.

84   Corti MC, Guralnik JM, Salive ME, *et al.* HDL cholesterol predicts coronary heart disease mortality in older persons. *JAMA* 1995; **274**: 539–44.

85   Fowkes FG, Dunbar JT, Lee AJ. Risk factor profile of nonsmokers with peripheral arterial disease. *Angiology* 1995; **46**: 657–62.

86   Hiatt WR, Hoag S, Hamman RF. Effect of diagnostic criteria on the prevalence of peripheral arterial disease. The San Luis Valley Diabetes Study. *Circulation* 1995; **91**: 1472–9.

87   Newman AB, Siscovick DS, Manolio TA, *et al.* Ankle-arm index as a marker of atherosclerosis in the cardiovascular heath study. Cardiovascular Health Study (CHS) Collaborative Research Group. *Circulation* 1993; **88**: 937–45.

88   Criqui MH, Langer RD, Fronek A, *et al.* Large vessel and isolated small vessel disease. In: Fowkes FGR, ed. *Epidemiology of Peripheral Vascular Disease.* London: Springer-Verlag; **1991**: 85–96.

89   Manson JE, Colditz GA, Stampfer MJ, *et al.* A prospective study of obesity and risk of coronary heart disease in women. *N Engl J Med* 1990; **322**: 882–9.

90   Hu FB, Stampfer MJ, Manson JE, *et al.* Trends in the incidence of coronary heart disease and changes in diet and lifestyle in women. *N Engl J Med* 2000; **343**: 530–7.

91   Kanaya AM, Vittinghoff E, Shlipak MG, *et al.* Association of total and central obesity with mortality in postmenopausal women with coronary heart disease. *Am J Epidemiol* 2003; **158**: 1161–70.

92   Dalton M, Cameron AJ, Zimmet PZ, *et al.*; AusDiab Steering Group. Waist circumference, waist-hip ratio and body mass index and their correlation with cardiovascular disease risk factors in Australian adults. *J Intern Med* 2003; **245**: 555–63.

93   Ho SY, Lam TH, Janus ED; Hong Kong Cardiovascular Risk Factor Prevalence Study Steering Committee. Waist to stature ratio is more strongly associated with cardio-vascular risk factors than other simple anthropometric indices. *Ann Epidemiol* 2003; **13**: 683–91.

94   Folsom AR, Kaye SA, Sellers TA, *et al.* Body fat distribution and 5-year risk of death in older women. *JAMA* 1993; **269**: 483–7.

95   Sprecher DL, Pearce GL. How deadly is the deadly quartet? *J Am Coll Cardiol* 2000; **36**: 1159–65.

96   Wingard DL, Suarex L, Barrett-Conner E. The sex differential in mortality from all causes and ischemic heart disease. *Am J Epidemiol* 1983; **117**: 165–72.

97   Colditz GA, Willett WC, Stampfer MJ, *et al.* Menopause and the risk of coronary heart disease in women. *N Engl J Med* 1987; **316**: 1105–10.

98   Farhat MY, Lavigne MC, Ramwell PW. The vascular protective effects of estrogen. *FASEB J* 1996; **10**: 615–24.

99   Williams JK, Adams MR, Klopfenstein HS. Estrogen modulates responses of atherosclerotic coronary arteries. *Circulation* 1990; **81**: 1680–7.

100   Herrington DM, Braden GA, Williams JK. Endothelial-dependent coronary vasomotor responsiveness in postmenopausal women with and without estrogen replacement therapy. *Am J Cardiol* 1994; **73**: 951–2.

101   Collins P, Rosano GM, Sarrel PM, *et al.* 17β-Estradiol attenuates acetylcholine-induced coronary arterial constriction in women but not men with coronary artery disease. *Circulation* 1995; **92**: 24–30.

102   Kannel WB, Hjortland MC, McNamara PM, Gordon T. Menopause and risk of cardiovascular disease: the Framingham Study. *Ann Intern Med* 1976; **85**: 447–52.

103   Weiss NS. Relationship of menopause to serum cholesterol and arterial blood pressure: the United States Health Examination Survey of adults. *Am J Epidemiol* 1972; **96**: 237–41.

104   Hjortland MC, McNamara PM, Kannel WB. Some atherogenic concomitants of menopause: the Framingham study. *Am J Epidemiol* 1976; **103**: 304–11.

105   Bush TL, Cowan L, Heiss G, *et al.* Ovarian function and lipid/lipoprotein levels. Results from the Lipid Research Clinics Program. *Am J Epidemiol* 1984; **120**: 489.

106   Witteman JCM, Grobbee DE, Kok FJ, *et al.* Increased risk of atherosclerosis in women after the menopause. *BMJ* 1989; **298**: 642–4.

107   Pansini F, Bonaccorsi G, Calisesi M, *et al.* Influence of spontaneous and surgical menopause on atherogenic metabolic risk. *Maturitas* 1993; **17**: 181–90.

108   Wu Z, Wu X, Zhang Y. Relationship of menopausal status and sex hormones to serum lipids and blood pressure. *Int J Epidemiol* 1990; **19**: 297–302.

109   Jensen J, Nilas L, Christiansen C. Influence of menopause on serum lipids and lipoproteins. *Maturitas* 1990; **12**: 321–31.

110   Beresteijn van ECH, Korevaar JC, Huijbregts PCW, *et al.* Perimenopausal increase in serum cholesterol. A 10-year longitudinal study. *Am J Epidemiol* 1993; **137**: 383–92.

111   Meade TW, Dyer S, Howarth DJ, *et al.* Antithrombin III and procoagulant activity: sex differences and effects of the menopause. *Br J Haematol* 1990; **74**: 77–81.

112   Lindoff C, Petersson F, Lecander I, *et al.* Passage of the menopause is followed by haemostatic changes. *Maturitas* 1993; **17**: 17–22.

113   Edwards DAW. Differences in the distribution of subcutaneous fat with sex and maturity. *Clin Sci* 1951; **10**: 305–15.

114   Ley CL, Lees B, Stevenson JC. Sex- and menopause-associated changes in body-fat distribution. *Am J Clin Nutr* 1992; **55**: 950–4.

115   Rosenberg L, Hennekens CH, Rosner B, *et al.* Early menopause and the risk of myocardial infarction. *Am J Obstet Gynecol* 1981; **139**: 47–51.

116   Schouw van der YT, Graaf van der Y, Steyerberg EW, *et al.* Age at menopause as a risk factor for cardiovascular mortality. *Lancet* 1996; **347**: 714–8.

117   Gordon T, Kannel WB, Hjortland MC, McNamara PM. Menopause and coronary heart disease: the Framingham study. *Ann Intern Med* 1978; **89**: 157–61.

118   La Vecchia C, Decarli A, Franceschi S, *et al.* Menstrual and reproductive factors and the risk of myocardial infarction in women under fifty-five years of age. *Am J Obstet Gynecol* 1987; **157**: 1108–12.

119   Gorgels WJMJ, Graaf van der Y, Blankenstein MA, *et al.* Urinary sex hormone excretion in premenopausal women and coronary heart disease risk. A nested case-referent study in the DOM cohort. *Am J Epidemiol* 1995; **142**: 1157–64.

120   Bengtsson C, Rybo G, Westerberg H. Number of pregnancies, use of oral contraceptives and menopausal age in women with ischaemic heart disease, compared to a population sample of women. *Acta Med Scand* 1973; **89**(Suppl): 75–81.

121   Ness RB, Harris T, Cobb J, *et al.* Number of pregnancies and the subsequent risk of cardiovascular disease. *N Engl J Med* 1993; **328**: 1528–33.

122   Smith GCS, Pell JP, Walsh D. Spontaneous loss of early pregnancy and risk of ischaemic heart disease in later life: retrospective cohort study. *BMJ* 2003; **326**: 423–4.

123   Winkelstein W Jr, Rekate AC. Age trend of mortality from coronary artery disease in women and observations on the reproductive patterns of those affected. *Am Heart J* 1964; **67**: 481–8.

124   Posthuma WF, Westendorp RG, Vandenbroucke JP. Cardioprotective effect of hormone replacement therapy in postmenopausal women: is the evidence biased? *BMJ* 1994; **308**: 1268–9.

125   Hulley S, Grady D, Bush T, *et al.* Randomized trial of estrogen plus progestin for secondary prevention of coronary heart disease in postmenopausal women. Heart and Estrogen/progestin Replacement Study (HERS) Research Group. *JAMA* 1998; **280**: 605–13.

126   Viscoli CM, Brass LM, Kernan WN, *et al.* A clinical trial of oestrogen-replacement therapy after ischemic stroke. *N Engl J Med* 2001; **345**: 1243–9.

127   Roussouw JE, Anderson GL, Prentice RL, *et al.* Risks and benefits of estrogen plus progestin in healthy postmenopausal women: principal results from the Women's Health Initiative randomised controlled trial. *JAMA* 2002; **288**: 321–33.

128   Haas JS, Kaplan CP, Gerstenberger EP, Kerlikowske K. Changes in the use of postmenopausal hormone therapy after the publication of clinical trial results. *Ann Intern Med* 2004; **140**: 184–8.

129   Rich-Edwards JW, Manson JE, Hennekens CH, Buring JE. The primary prevention of coronary heart disease in women. *N Engl J Med* 1995; **332**: 1758–66.

130   Willett WC, Green A, Stampfer MJ, *et al.* Relative and absolute excess risks of coronary heart disease among women who smoke cigarettes *N Engl J Med* 1987; **317**: 1303–9.

131   Njolstad I, Arnesen E, Lund-Larsen PG. Body height, cardiovascular risk factors, and risk of stroke in middle-aged men and women: a 14-year follow-up study of the Finnmark Study. *Circulation* 1996; **94**: 2877–82.

132   Manson JE, Hu FB, Rich-Edwards JW, *et al.* A prospective study of walking as compared with vigorous exercise in the prevention of coronary heart disease in women. *N Engl J Med* 1999; **341**: 650–8.

133   American Diabetes Association. Detection and management of lipid disorders in diabetes. *Diabetes Care* 1996; **19**(Suppl): S96–102.

134   Stampfer MJ, Hu FB, Manson JE, *et al.* Primary prevention of coronary heart disease in women through diet and lifestyle. *N Engl J Med* 2000; **343**: 16–22.

135   Cunningham MA, Lee TH, Cook EF, *et al.* The effect of gender on the probability of myocardial infarction among emergency department patients with acute chest pain. *J Gen Intern Med* 1989; **4**: 392–8.

136   Karlson BW, Herlitz J, Hartford M, Hjalmarson A. Prognosis in men and women coming to the emergency room with chest pain or other symptoms suggestive of acute myocardial infarction. *Coronary Artery Dis* 1993; **4**: 761–7.

137   Zucker DR, Griffith JL, Beshansky JR, Selker HP. Presentations of acute myocardial infarction in men and women. *J Gen Intern Med* 1997; **12**: 79–87.

138   Kennedy JW, Killip T, Fisher LD, *et al.* The clinical spectrum of coronary artery disease and its surgical and medical management. The Coronary Artery surgery Study. *Circulation* 1982; **66**: 16–23.

139   Lewis LF, McGorray SP, Pepine CJ. Assessment of women with suspected myocardial ischemia: review of findings of the women's ischemia syndrome evaluation (WISE) study. *Curr Womens Health Rep* 2002; **2**: 110–14.

140   Hochman JS, McCabe CH, Stone PH, *et al.* Outcome and profile of women and men presenting with acute coronary syndromes: report from TIMI IIIB. *J Am Coll Cardiol* 1997; **275**: 777–82.

141   Kemp HG, Elliot WC, Grolin T. The anginal syndrome with normal coronary arteriography. *Trans Assoc Am Phys* 1967; **80**: 59–70.

142   Kemp HG, Kronmal RA, Vliestra RE, Frye RL. Seven year survival of patients with normal and near normal coronary arteriograms; a CASS registry study. *J Am Coll Cardiol* 1986; **7**: 479–83.

143   Egashira K, Inoue T, Hirooka Y, *et al.* Evidence of impaired endothelium-dependent coronary vasodilatation in patients with angina pectoris and normal coronary angiograms. *N Engl J Med* 1993; **328**: 1659–64.

144   Kaski JC, Rosano GMC, Collins P, *et al.* Cardiac Syndrome X: clinical characteristics and left ventricular function. *J Am Coll Cardiol* 1995; **25**: 807–14.

145   Rosano GMC, Collins P, Kaki JC, *et al.* Syndrome X in women is associated with oestrogen deficiency. *Eur Heart J* 1995; **16**: 610–14.

146 Kaski JC. Overview of gender aspects of cardiac syndrome X. *Cardiovasc Res* 2002; **53**: 620–6.

147 DeSanctis RW, Clinical manifestations of coronary artery disease: chest pain in women. *Cardiovasc Rev Rep* 1994; **15**: 10–16.

148 Karlson BW, Herlitz J, Pettersson P, *et al.* Patients admitted to the emergency room with symptoms indicative of acute myocardial Infarction. *J Intern Med* 1991; **230**: 251–8.

149 Wingard DL. The sex differential in morbidity, mortality and lifestyle. *Ann Rev Pub Health* 1984; **5**: 433–58.

150 Murabito JM. Women and cardiovascular disease: contributions from the Framingham study. *J Am Med Womens Assoc* 1995; **50**: 35–39.

151 Kannel WB, Abbott RD. Incidence and prognosis of myocardial infarction in women: the Framingham Study In: Eaker ED, Pacard B, Wenger NK, eds. *Coronary Heart Disease in Women.* Bethesda, MD: National Heart, Lung and Blood Institute, National Institutes of Health. 1987.

152 Lerner DJ, Kannel WB. Patterns of coronary heart disease morbidity and mortality in the sexes: a 26-year follow-up of the Framingham population. *Am Heart J* 1986; **111**: 383–90.

153 Powell JT, Golledge J. Peripheral arterial disease in women. In Julian D, Wenger N, eds. *Women and Heart Disease.* St Louis, MO: Mosby, 1997: 374.

154 Maynard C, Litwin PE, Martin JS, Weaver WD. Gender differences in the treatment and outcome of acute myocardial infarction: results from the Myocardial Infarction, Triage, and Intervention Registry. *Arch Intern Mcd* 1992; **152**: 972–6.

155 Goldberg RJ, O'Donnell C, Yarzebski J, *et al.* Sex differences in symptom presentation associated with acute myocardial infarction: a population-based perspective. *Am Heart J* 1998; **136**: 189–95.

156 Meishchke H, Larsen MP, Eisenberg MS. Gender differences in reported symptoms for acute myocardial infarction: impact on prehospital delay time interval. *Am J Emerg Med* 1998; **16**: 363–6.

157 Everts B, Karlson BW, Währborg P, *et al.* Localization of pain in suspected acute myocardial infarction in relation to final diagnosis, age and sex, and site and type of infarction. *Heart Lung* 1996; **25**: 430–7.

158 Tobin JN, Wassertheil-Smoller S, Wexler JP, *et al.* Sex bias in considering coronary bypass surgery. *Ann Intern Med* 1987; **107**: 19–25.

159 Wilkinson P, Laji K, Ranjadayalan K, *et al.* Acute myocardial infarction in women: survival analysis in first six months. *BMJ* 1994; **309**: 566–9.

160 Maynard C, Althouse R, Cerquera M, *et al.* Underutilization of thrombolytic therapy in eligible women with acute myocardial infarction. *Am J Cardiol* 1991; **68**: 529–30.

161 Maynard C, Every NR, Martin JS, *et al.* Association of gender and survival in patients with acute myocardial infarction. *Arch Intern Med* 1997; **157**: 1379–84.

162 Clarke KW, Gray D, Keating NA, Hampton JR. Do women with acute myocardial infarction receive the same treatment as men? *BMJ* 1994; **309**: 63–6.

163 Mark DB, Shaw LK, DeLong ER, *et al.* Absence of sex bias in the referral of patients for cardiac catheterization. *N Engl J Med* 1994; **330**: 1101–16.

164 Wenger NK. Gender, coronary artery disease, and coronary bypass surgery. *Ann Intern Med* 1990; **112**: 557–58.

165 Shaw LJ, Miller DD, Romeis JC, *et al.* Gender differences in the noninvasive evaluation and management of patients with suspected coronary artery disease. *Ann Intern Med* 1994; **120**: 559–66.

166 Heston TF, Lewis LM, with the St Louis Emergency Physicians' Association Research Group. Gender bias in the evaluation and management of acute nontraumatic chest pain. *Fam Pract Res J* 1992; **12**: 383–9.

167 Kwok Y, Kim C, Grady D, *et al.* Meta-analysis of exercise testing to detect coronary artery disease in women. *Am J Cardiol* 1999; **83**: 660–6.

168 Lapidus L, Bengtsson C, Lindquist O, *et al.* Prognosis for women with different symptoms and signs suggesting ischaemic heart disease – a 12 year follow-up. *J Chronic Dis* 1986; **38**: 741–8.

169 Hung J, Chaitman BR, Lam J, *et al.* Noninvasive diagnostic test choices for the evaluation of coronary artery disease in women: a multivariate comparison of cardiac fluoroscopy, exercise electrocardiography and exercise thallium myocardial perfusion scintigraphy. *J Am Coll Cardiol* 1984; **4**: 8–16.

170 Swahn E, Areskog M, Berglund U, *et al.* Predictive importance of clinical findings and a predischarge exercise test in suspected unstable coronary artery disease. *Am J Cardiol* 1987; **59**: 208–14.

171 Melin JA, Wijns W, Vanbutsele RJ, *et al.* Alternative diagnostic strategies for coronary artery disease in women: demonstration of usefulness and efficiency of probability analysis. *Circulation* 1985; **71**: 535–42.

172 Cardiovascular stress testing: a description of the various types of stress tests and indications for their use. Mayo Clinic Cardiovascular Working Group on Stress Testing. *Mayo Clin Proc* 1996; **71**: 43–52.

173 Gianrossi R, Detrano R, Mulvihill D, *et al.* Exercise-induced ST depression in the diagnosis of coronary artery disease: a meta-analysis. *Circulation* 1989; 8087–98.

174 Lauer MS, Pashkow FJ, Snader CE, *et al.* Sex and diagnostic evaluation of possible coronary artery disease after exercise treadmill testing at one academic teaching centre. *Am Heart J* 1997; **134**: 807–13.

175 Cerqueira MD. Diagnostic testing strategies for coronary artery disease: special issues related to gender. *Am J Cardiol* 1995; **75**: 52D–60D.

176 Delborg M, Herlitz J, Emanuelsson H, Swedberg K. Electrocardiographic changes during myocardial ischemia: difference between men and women. *J Electro-cardiol* 1994; **29**(Suppl): 42–5.

177   Moriel M, Rozanski A, Klein J, et al. The limited efficacy of exercise radionuclide ventriculography in assessing prognosis of women with coronary artery disease. Am J Cardiol 1995; 76: 1030–5.

178   Marwick TH, Anderson T, Williams MJ, et al. Exercise echo-cardiography is an accurate and cost-efficient technique for detection of coronary artery disease in women. J Am Cardiol 1995; 26: 335–41.

179   MacLeod MCM, Finlayson AR, Pell JP, Findlay IN. Geographical, demographic and socioeconomic variations in the investigation and management of coronary heart disease in Scotland. Heart 1999; 81: 252–6.

180   Kudenchuk P, Maynard C, Martin J, et al. Comparison of presentation, treatment, and outcome of acute myocardial infarction in men versus women (the Myocardial Infarction Triage and Intervention Registry). Am J Cardiol 1996; 78: 9–14.

181   Weitzman S, Cooper L, Chambless L, et al. Gender, racial, and geographic differences in the performance of cardiac diagnostic and therapeutic procedures for hospitalised acute myocardial infarction in four states. Am J Cardiol 1997; 79: 722–6.

182   Steingart RM, Packer M, Hamm P, et al. For the survival and ventricular enlargement investigators. Sex differences in the management of coronary artery disease. N Engl J Med 1991; 325: 226–30.

183   Khan SS, Nessim S, Gray R, et al. Increased mortality of women in coronary artery bypass surgery: evidence of referral bias. Ann Intern Med 1990; 112: 561–7.

184   Fisher LD, Kennedy JW, Davis KB, et al. Association of sex, physical size, and operative mortality after coronary artery bypass in the Coronary Artery Surgery Study (CASS). J Thoracic Cardiovasc Surg 1982; 84: 334–41.

185   O'Connor GT, Morton JR, Diehl MJ, et al. Differences between men and women in hospital mortality associated with coronary artery bypass graft surgery: The Northern New England Cardiovascular disease Study Group. Circulation 1993; 88(5 Pt 1): 2104–10.

186   Hogue C W, Barzilai B, Pieper K, et al. Sex differences in neurological outcomes and mortality after cardiac surgery. Circulation 2001; 103: 2133–7.

187   Kip KE, Faxon DP, Detre KM, et al. Coronary angioplasty in diabetic patients: The National Heart, Lung and Blood Institute Percutaneous Coronary Angioplasty Registry. Circulation 1996; 94: 1818–25.

188   Davis KB, Chaitman B, Ryan T, et al. Comparison of 15-year survival for men and women after initial medical or surgical treatment for coronary artery disease: a CASS registry study. J Am Coll Cardiol 1995; 25: 1000–9.

189   Bell M, Grill D, Garrat K, Berger PB, et al. Long-term outcome of women compared with men after successful coronary angioplasty. Circulation 1995; 91: 2876–81.

190   Weaver WD, White HD, Wilcox RG, et al. Comparisons of characteristics and outcomes among women and men with acute myocardial infarction treated with thrombolytic therapy. JAMA 1996; 275: 777–82.

191   Ades PA, Waldmann ML, Polk DM, Coflesky JT. Referral patterns and exercise response in the rehabilitation of female coronary patients ages ≥62 years. Am J Cardiol 1992; 69: 1422–5.

192   Cannistra LB, Balady GJ, O'Malley CJ, et al. Comparison of the clinical profile and outcome of women and men in cardiac rehabilitation. Am J Cardiol 1992; 69: 1274–9.

193   Lavie CJ, Milani RV. Effects of cardiac rehabilitation and exercise training on exercise capacity, coronary risk factors, behavioural characteristics, and quality of life in women. Am J Cardiol 1995; 75: 340–3.

194   Pell J, Pell A, Morrison C, Blatchford O, Dargie H. Retrospective study of influence of deprivation on uptake of cardiac rehabilitation. BMJ 1996; 313: 267–8.

195   Thomas RJ, Miller NH, Lamendola C, et al. National survey on gender differences in cardiac rehabilitation programs: patient characteristics and enrolment patterns. J Cardiopulm Rehabil 1996; 16: 402–12.

196   Gillum RF. Trends in acute myocardial infarction and coronary heart disease death in the United States. J Am Coll Cardiol 1994; 23: 1273–7.

2

Pathophysiology of atherosclerosis

JOHN R DAVIES, PETER L WEISSBERG

INTRODUCTION

Atherosclerosis is as an abnormal thickening of the vessel wall comprising lipids, inflammatory cells, and fibrous tissue. Pathologic studies have shown that atherosclerotic lesions appear in infancy,[1] but by adulthood the extent to which the vascular tree is afflicted, the rate of lesion progression, and the microscopic composition of the lesions varies tremendously between individuals. Despite its presence in all adult humans, in the majority, atherosclerosis remains asymptomatic throughout life. In others, complications develop, characteristically from late middle age onwards. Complications such as angina and intermittent claudication are caused by transient episodes of ischemia, as a result of atherosclerotic narrowing of the arterial lumen. Typically, symptoms occur when oxygen demand in the tissue supplied by the obstructed artery is high. Angina brought on by exercise is a typical example. Life-threatening complications such as myocardial infarction (MI) and cerebral infarction are usually a result of sudden severe ischemia caused by thrombotic arterial occlusion.

Pathologic and epidemiologic data, together with interventional and molecular studies, have advanced our understanding of the disease process. Consequently new and more effective prevention and treatment strategies have been developed that have drastically reduced the incidence of clinical complications.[2]

This chapter aims to give an overview of the important pathophysiologic mechanisms that dictate the course of the disease. The first section details the histopathologic changes that take place over the natural history of the disease. This is followed by an in-depth discussion of the important cellular and molecular mechanisms responsible for the initiation and progression of atherosclerosis. The chapter concludes with a brief discussion on the influence of the female sex on the pathophysiologic mechanisms that influence disease progression.

HISTOLOGIC APPEARANCE OF THE ATHEROSCLEROTIC ARTERY

The normal arterial wall has three distinct layers, the intima, media, and adventitia (Fig. 2.1). The intima is the innermost layer and thus lies adjacent to the arterial lumen. It consists of a single layer of endothelial cells supported by an extracellular matrix consisting mainly of proteoglycans in between which lies the occasional vascular smooth muscle cell (VSMC) and macrophage. The boundary between the intima and the media is marked by a ring of elastic tissue, named the internal elastic lamina.

The tunica media surrounds the internal elastic lamina and contains a varying number of spindle-shaped VSMCs. In the normal vessel, medial VSMC contraction is controlled by vasoactive substances released by the adjacent endothelium, such that, together, the VSMCs and endothelium control the tone of the artery and can thus control tissue blood flow. In between the VSMCs of the media lies an extracellular matrix that contains a large number of elastin fibers. This enables the artery to stretch and thus withstand the pressure exerted upon it during the cardiac cycle. The larger 'conduit' arteries that deliver blood to the organs have a large amount of elastin

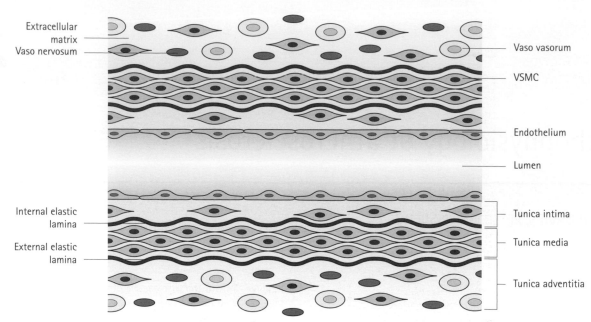

Extracellular matrix
Vaso nervosum
Vaso vasorum
VSMC
Endothelium
Lumen
Internal elastic lamina
External elastic lamina
Tunica intima
Tunica media
Tunica adventitia

Figure 2.1 Schematic representation of the normal artery. VSMC, vascular smooth muscle cell.

and several layers of VSMCs, whereas the smaller 'resistance' arteries which function predominantly to control the volume of blood delivered to the different tissues have little elastin and fewer layers of VSMCs. The outer boundary of the tunica media is marked by another ring of elastic tissue, named the external elastic lamina.

The outermost layer of the artery, the tunica adventitia, comprises connective tissue and fibroblasts which provides support for the vessel. Within this layer run small nutrient vessels, called the vaso vasorum, and nerves, called vaso nervorum.

Atherosclerosis predominantly affects the intimal layer of conduit arteries and is characterized by an increase in both cellular and extracellular material. This invariably leads to an expansion of the intimal layer. However, changes are not necessarily confined to the intima. In some atherosclerotic arteries, the medial and adventitial layers can atrophy leading to a weakening of the arterial wall and aneurysm formation.

Lesion progression is variable both within the same individual and between individuals, highlighting the importance of both systemic and local factors on the natural course of the disease. Thus, at any point in time, atheromatous lesions at differing stages of maturity often coexist in the same individual and even in the same artery. The most commonly used classification of lesion morphology is the American Heart Association (AHA) classification[3,4] which attempts to reflect the cellular, molecular, and mechanical mechanisms that underpin the initiation and progression of atherosclerosis.

American Heart Association classification of atherosclerotic lesions

The AHA classification divides lesions into early (lesion types I and II), intermediate (lesion type III) and advanced (lesion types IV, V, and VI). This reflects the natural history of the disease as early asymptomatic lesions that cause minimal disruption to the arterial wall progress over time to become advanced lesions that cause marked anatomic disarray. However, the AHA classification is of limited use in the clinical arena as disease progression is rarely uniform and predictable, especially in the advanced stages where lesions may progress in different morphogenic sequences, at differing rates, with or without the onset of clinical symptoms.

EARLY LESIONS

Type I lesions, also referred to as 'initial lesions', are the earliest definable lesion in which lipid is found in the intimal layer of the arterial wall. These lesions tend to form in early childhood as eccentric intimal thickenings typically found at arterial bifurcations. Type I lesions can still be found in adults, especially in those who have little atherosclerosis, or in areas of the vasculature that are not particularly prone to the formation of atheromatous lesions. Due to their small size, they are only detectable under the microscope. Histologically, they consist of groups of macrophages, many of which contain lipid droplets and are referred to as foam cells.[1]

The type II lesion (Fig. 2.2) is the first to be visible to the naked eye and is known as the fatty streak. Microscopically, type II lesions consist of layers of macrophage foam cells. In addition, fatty streaks contain intimal VSMCs containing lipid droplets, large numbers of nonlipid-containing macrophages and some T lymphocytes and mast cells. Extracellular lipid is seen for the first time, although not to the extent of that seen within cells. Biochemical analysis has confirmed that the extracellular lipid is made up of cholesterol esters, cholesterol, and phospholipids[5] and derives from apoptotic foam cells and isolated extracellular lipoprotein particles. Type II lesions often do not progress onwards,

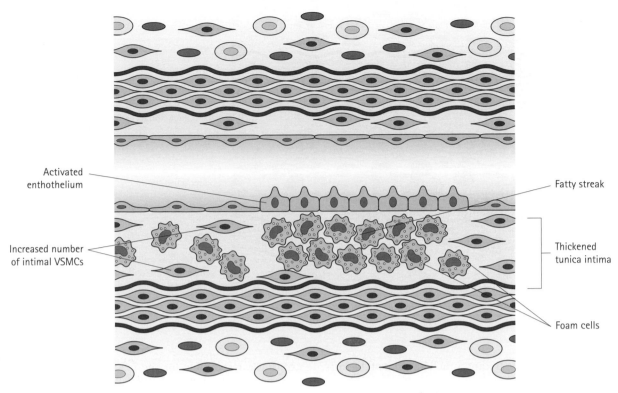

Activated enthothelium

Fatty streak

Increased number of intimal VSMCs

Thickened tunica intima

Foam cells

Figure 2.2   Schematic representation of the 'fatty streak', an early atherosclerotic lesion. VSMC, vascular smooth muscle cell.

especially in people with normal levels of lipoproteins. In the adult, such lesions are often found in areas of the circulation that are not prone to advanced atherosclerosis. Compared with the type II lesions that remain static, those that develop further have a thicker intimal layer consisting of mainly proteoglycan extracellular material and contain numerous VSMCs, foam cells, and nonlipid-containing macrophages. The nonlipid-containing macrophages tend to congregate near the surface, whereas the foam cells are more commonly found at the bottom of the proteoglycan layer, with the extracellular lipid found deeper still.

INTERMEDIATE LESIONS

The type III lesion, also known as the intermediate lesion or preatheroma, bridges the morphologic gap between early asymptomatic lesions and potentially symptomatic advanced lesions. Its characteristic feature is an abundance of extracellular lipid droplets that coalesce to form pools of lipid, which start to replace proteoglycan material and drive the VSMCs of the intimal layer further apart. These lesions contain more free cholesterol, fatty acids, and triglycerides than type II lesions, but do not cause significant structural disruption of the intima, and because of their relatively small volume do not impinge on the vessel lumen.

ADVANCED LESIONS

Atherosclerotic lesions are defined as advanced when accumulation of lipids, cells and extracellular matrix material are associated with structural disorganization, repair, and

thickening of the intima, as well as deformity of the arterial wall. Such lesions may or may not narrow the arterial lumen and may or may not be associated with clinical syndromes.

The type IV lesion is the first of the so-called advanced lesions and is often referred to simply as atheroma. It is characterized histologically by a dense accumulation of extracellular lipid that occupies a large proportion of the intima. This structure is usually referred to as the lipid core, which is formed via the aggregation of lipid pools found in type III lesions.[6] The extracellular matrix overlying the lipid core remains devoid of fibrous tissue and defects in the surface of the lesion are absent. Type IV lesions characteristically first appear in young adults in the atherosclerosis-prone regions. Despite the increasing volume of the lesion, there is rarely a significant effect on the arterial lumen because the artery expands outwards to accommodate the enlarging lesion.[7] The extent to which the artery remodels varies between different individuals and between different segments of artery within a single individual and depends on the rate of plaque growth, endothelial function, and the integrity of the medial and adventitial layers of the artery. In type IV lesions calcification is often seen in association with intimal VSMCs. Calcium particles are also discernable within the lipid core. Between the lipid core and the endothelial surface, reside macrophages and smooth muscle cells with and without lipid inclusions. As with earlier lesions, lymphocytes[8] and mast cells are also present. New vessel formation is a typical feature with fragile capillaries seen particularly at the lateral edges of the lipid core. The extracellular matrix between the lipid core and the surface of the lesion consists

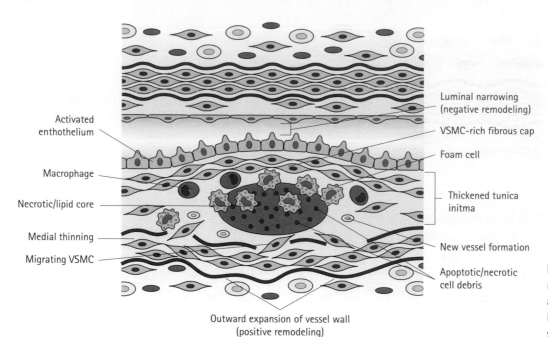

Activated endothelium

Macrophage

Necrotic/lipid core

Medial thinning

Migrating VSMC

Luminal narrowing (negative remodeling)

VSMC-rich fibrous cap

Foam cell

Thickened tunica initma

New vessel formation

Apoptotic/necrotic cell debris

Outward expansion of vessel wall (positive remodeling)

Figure 2.3 Schematic representation of the advanced atherosclerotic lesion. VSMC, vascular smooth muscle cell.

predominantly of proteoglycans, much like that of the intimal layer prior to lesion development.

Despite the fact that type IV lesions rarely impact on the vessel lumen, their clinical significance can be great. This is because the increasing degree of intimal disorganization reduces the tensile strength of the lesion making it less resistant to the sheer stress exerted on it by the flowing blood. If the sheer stress exceeds the tensile strength of the lesion, then surface disruption ensues (the defining characteristic of type VI lesions), drastically increasing the likelihood of thrombotic complications.

Fibrous tissue is often laid down in the extracellular matrix of regions surrounding the lipid core of the type IV lesion. When this happens the plaque is defined as a type V lesion (Fig. 2.3). The region separating the lipid core from the circulating blood in the type V lesion is often referred to as the fibrous cap. Three subdivisions of the type V lesion have been defined:

* The type Va lesion, or the fibroatheroma, describes a lesion which has both lipid core and a surrounding fibrotic extracellular matrix.
* A Type Vb lesion contains significant amounts of calcification in both the lipid core and the surrounding connective tissue, often to the extent that the amount of lipid is decreased.
* A type Vc lesion is one in which the lipid core has been replaced by fibrous tissue to the extent that the remaining core is minimal or completely absent.

The amount of fibrous tissue laid down in type V lesions varies considerably between different lesions both within the same arterial territory and between different arterial territories. The new connective tissue consists mainly of collagen and VSMCs rich with rough endoplasmic reticulum, the

organelle responsible for the manufacture of protein. The newly formed capillaries tend to be larger than in type IV lesions and lymphocytes, monocyte-macrophages and plasma cells are frequently found adjacent to them. Occasionally microhemorrhages are seen surrounding such vessels. Often the medial smooth muscle cells of type V lesions are disarranged and reduced in number leading to a thinning of the medial layer. The media and adventitia may contain lymphocytes, macrophages, and foam cells, which are often seen around the vaso vasorum.[9] Compared with type IV lesions, a higher percentage of type V lesions impinge on the lumen of the vessel causing varying degrees of lumen stenosis. Importantly, as with type IV lesions, surface disruption often occurs in type V lesions, more often in Va lesions which tend to have a weaker fibrous cap than lesion types Vb and Vc. Type Va lesions are often multilayered, with several lipid cores each surrounded by a region of collagen-rich fibrous tissue. These lesions, often referred to as multilayered fibroatheroma, arise either as a result of changing blood flow dynamics as the plaque begins to narrow the arterial lumen[10] or because of repeated episodes of fibrous cap disruption followed by thrombosis, which stimulates a healing process characterized by synthesis of a new fibrous cap.

Type VI lesions (Fig. 2.4) are often referred to as complicated lesions and are defined by the presence of:

* surface disruption (VIa)
* intraplaque hemorrhage (VIb)
* surface thrombus (VIc).

Plaques that exhibit both surface disruption and thrombosis are labeled VIac.

Initially, plaque rupture, where the fibrous cap has been torn away from the underlying vessel wall, was thought to be the only form of surface disruption that predisposed to

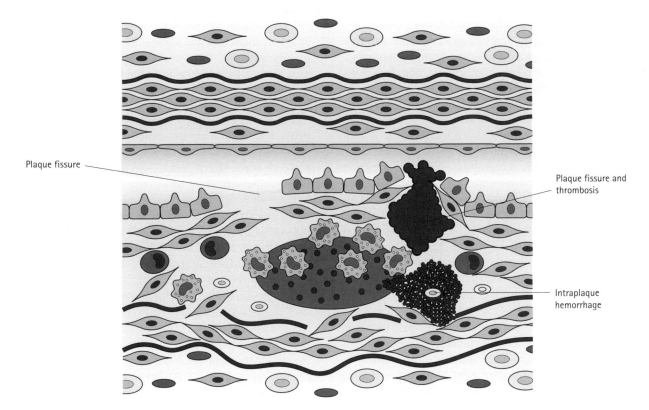

Figure 2.4   Schematic representation of the complicated plaque.

surface thrombosis and its associated clinical manifestations. In early post-mortem studies of sudden coronary death victims plaque rupture was found to be the underlying cause of myocardial infarction and death in the majority of cases. The same studies identified type IV and Va lesions as the commonest precursors to the type VIac plaque.[11–13] Type IV and Va lesions are characterized by a relative excess of extracellular lipid and macrophages, and a paucity of fibrous material and VSMCs. Effectively this translates into lesions with large lipid cores and thin fibrous caps, two features which reduce the tensile strength of the lesion making it vulnerable to rupture.[14]

Surprisingly studies have failed to find a strong correlation between plaque size, degree of luminal stenosis and the occurrence of plaque rupture.[15] In other words, it is the cellular and molecular composition of the plaque that dictates its risk of plaque rupture, rather than its size or impact on the vessel lumen. This notion has since been corroborated by angiographic studies in which it was found that in approximately 70 percent of heart attack victims, a preceding angiographic study had failed to identify a lesion causing >50 percent stenosis.[16,17] The same may also be true in other arterial beds such as the carotid circulation, although the studies have not been done to confirm this. Since these landmark findings further histologic studies have gone on to define two other forms of surface disruption capable of precipitating surface thrombosis, plaque erosion,[18] and calcific nodule exposure.[19] Histologic evaluation of such plaques suggests that the mechanisms that predispose to these two forms of surface disruption are likely to be distinct from those

discussed above that lead to plaque rupture. This is discussed in more detail at the end of the chapter.

The clinical significance of intraplaque hematoma and hemorrhage (type VIb lesions) remains uncertain. It is conceivable that intraplaque hemorrhage could cause sufficient disruption to precipitate an acute clinical event.[20] Plaque hemorrhage is usually due to rupture of fragile newly formed capillaries within the body of advanced lesions. Hematoma can also derive from such an event,[21] but is usually found following surface disruption followed by tracking of blood from the lumen under the surface flap created by plaque rupture.

The immunohistochemical study of atherosclerotic arteries as they change over the course of time highlights the importance of five biologic processes that contribute to atherosclerosis: inflammation, lipid accumulation, fibrosis, calcification, and thrombosis. The next section highlights research carried over the past three decades that has begun to uncover some of the molecular and cellular mechanisms that drive the important biologic processes involved in atherosclerosis.

ENDOTHELIAL DYSFUNCTION AND LESION INITIATION

The endothelium has several functions in the healthy artery.[22] First, it regulates trafficking of cells and molecules from the circulation to the subendothelial layers of the vessel wall. It provides both a physical barrier, by means of adhesive junctions between adjacent endothelial cells, and a functional barrier by upregulating and downregulating various receptors on both its luminal and abluminal surfaces. Second, by synthesizing and releasing antithrombotic factors, the healthy endothelium prevents thrombus formation within the lumen of the artery. Third, the endothelium controls vascular tone by releasing vasoactive mediators such as nitric oxide and prostacyclin which cause vasodilatation, and endothelin, which leads to vasoconstriction.

A variety of both invasive and noninvasive tests have been devised to test the integrity of endothelial function *in vivo*. Such tests have shown that endothelial dysfunction is invariably present in the arteries of humans with established atherosclerosis.[23,24] In addition, endothelial dysfunction has been shown to predict adverse events associated with atherosclerosis.[25–27] Furthermore, there is strong evidence that suggests endothelial dysfunction is a prerequisite for the initiation of atherosclerotic lesions,[28–30] a finding wholly consistent with the modified response to injury hypothesis of atherogenesis proposed by Ross.[31] In its most recent iteration, the hypothesis proposes that mechanical or biochemical injury to the endothelium predisposes the vessel to lipid accumulation which induces an inflammatory response and the development of early atheromatous lesions characterized by lipid and macrophage infiltration. Following the widespread acceptance of this theory, others have gone on to elucidate the molecular mechanisms that facilitate the passage of lipids and monocyte-derived macrophages across the endothelium (Fig. 2.5).[32]

Endothelial function can be perturbed in a wide variety of contexts. There is strong evidence linking atherosclerotic risk factors such as smoking, hypertension, hypercholesterolemia, diabetes, and a family history of premature atherosclerosis, to endothelial dysfunction.[33–35] In addition, more recently recognized risk factors for atherosclerosis such as obesity,[36] systemic inflammation,[37] and infection[38] have also been shown to induce endothelial dysfunction. The mechanisms by which the above insults lead to endothelial injury is not yet clear but increased oxidative stress remains a popular theory.[39]

Endothelial dysfunction in the context of the atherosclerotic lesion has several deleterious effects on vascular homeostasis. First, disruption of normal endothelial function results in abnormal antithrombotic function.[40,41] The production of thromboxane, von Willebrand factor, and tissue factor, and the downregulation of prostacyclin and nitric oxide secretion[42] promote vasoconstriction and the activation of platelets and soluble clotting factors. The result is a luminal surface that increasingly favors thrombosis and vascular occlusion, thus increasing the risk of adverse vascular events such as MI. The propensity to vascular occlusion is further amplified by the increased production of endothelin, a potent vasoconstrictor.[43]

The dysfunctional endothelium also plays an important role in promoting vascular inflammation. Molecules such as oxidized low-density lipoprotein (LDL) activate endothelial cell proinflammatory signaling pathways such as the nuclear factor κB (NF-κB) pathway.[32] Activation of endothelial NF-κB leads to increased transcription and expression of adhesion molecules and chemokines, which attract inflammatory cells to the vessel wall.[44] Adhesion molecules expressed on the endothelium bind to receptors on circulating inflammatory cells such as the monocyte and lymphocyte.[45] The first step in adhesion, the 'rolling' of inflammatory cells along the endothelial surface, is mediated by the interaction between carbohydrate ligands present on the surface of circulating inflammatory cells and selectin molecules (P and E-selectin) expressed on the luminal surface of the endothelium. Firm adhesion to allow the migration of inflammatory cells across the endothelium is then mediated by the interaction of the very late antigen-4 (VLA-4) and lymphocyte function antigen-1 (LFA-1) molecules on circulating cells with vascular cell adhesion molecule-1 (VCAM-1) and intercellular adhesion molecule-1 (ICAM-1), respectively, on the endothelium. *In vitro* and *in vivo* studies have confirmed the importance of adhesion molecules in atherogenesis.[46–48] The accumulation of inflammatory cells is aided by endothelial secretion of chemokines such as monocyte chemoattractant protein-1 (MCP-1) that attract monocytes to sites of atheroma. MCP-1 binds to the transmembrane cc chemokine receptor (CCR)-2 receptor on the surface of circulating monocytes. In MCP-1- and CCR-2-deficient murine models of atherosclerosis, macrophage number and atheroma burden are significantly decreased confirming the important chemotactic role of the MCP-1/CCR-2 interaction.[49,50]

ACCUMULATION OF CHOLESTEROL, AND ITS METABOLISM WITHIN THE ARTERIAL WALL

Cholesterol passively crosses the dysfunctional endothelium predominantly in the form of LDL (see Fig. 2.5). Once LDL particles enter the intima, their retention is dependent on the interaction between the apolipoprotein B (apoB) subcomponent of the LDL complex and matrix proteoglycans.[51] Within the intima, the excess of oxygen-free radicals and relatively low levels of protective antioxidant molecules means that retained LDL particles are prone to progressive oxidation.[52–54] Oxidized LDL particles are able to initiate an inflammatory response within the arterial wall by interacting with endothelial cells and macrophages. Endothelial cell–oxidized LDL interaction increases production of monocyte and macrophage chemokines and growth factors, such as MCP-1 and macrophage colony-stimulating factor (M-CSF) by the dysfunctional endothelium.[55–57] Oxidized LDL also binds to scavenger receptors expressed on the cell surface of plaque macrophages, enabling macrophages to phagocytose and remove oxidized LDL particles from the intima.[54,58,59] Internalization of oxidized LDL particles leads to the formation of lipid peroxides and cholesterol esters resulting in the formation of macrophage foam cells. Enzymes such as acid cholesterol-ester hydrolase (ACAT), 15-lipoxygenase and lipoprotein lipase breakdown oxidize LDL once it has been engulfed by the macrophage.[60] Although the removal of potentially damaging oxidized LDL

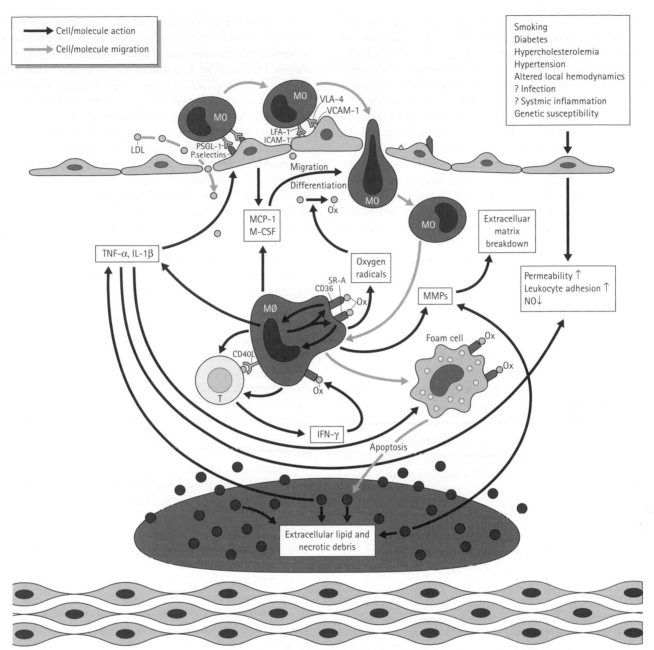

Figure 2.5 A schematic representation of the inflammatory process within the atherosclerotic plaque. CD, cluster differentiation; EC, endothelial cell; ICAM, intracellular adhesion molecule; IFN, interferon; IL, interleukin; LDL, low-density lipoprotein; LFA, lymphocyte function antigen; Mo, monocyte; MØ, macrophage; M-CSF, macrophage colony stimulating factor; MCP, monocyte chemotactic protein; MMP, matrix metalloproteinase; NO, nitric oxide; Ox, oxidized; PPAR, peroxisome proliferator activated receptor; PSGL, P-selectin glycoprotein ligand; SR, scavenger receptor; T, T lymphocyte; TNF, tumor necrosis factor; VCAM, vascular cell adhesion molecule; VLA, very late antigen; VSMC, vascular smooth muscle cell.

particles from the vessel wall is an important protective role of the macrophage, continuing accumulation within the cell can lead to deleterious effects secondary to foam cell activation and secretion of proinflammatory molecules.[61] This is discussed in more detail below.

Therefore, LDL is implicated in both the initiation and maintenance of endothelial dysfunction. In turn this ensures the continual passage of lipid across the endothelium, which further exacerbates endothelial dysfunction, creating a vicious circle. Unless the passage and retention of atherogenic lipid particles within the intima is halted, the vicious circle will continue leading to ongoing inflammatory cell activation and foam cell transformation. The importance of LDL in relation to lesion progression and the onset of atherosclerosis-related complications is highlighted by the beneficial effects of 3-hydroxy-3-methylglutaryl (HMG) co-reductase inhibitors (commonly known as statins) that lower circulating LDL levels.[62–65]

Although LDL is the most important lipid-carrying molecule, there are others that play a role in the atherosclerotic disease process. In direct contrast with LDL, high-density lipoprotein (HDL) protects against atherosclerosis. HDL is responsible for a process known as reverse cholesterol transport, where antioxidant enzymes transported by HDL avert the oxidation of LDL particles preventing its phagocytosis by macrophages, and thus allowing LDL to escape from the intima without causing harm.[66]

Other lipid particles, such as intermediate-density lipoprotein (IDL), and very-low-density lipoprotein (VLDL) are also thought to play a role in atherogenesis. Like LDL, IDL and VLDL undergo oxidative modification and subsequently activate plaque macrophages. Epidemiologic studies have found that a significant proportion of patients who develop atherosclerosis have increased concentrations of triglyceride-rich particles such as VLDL and IDL, and reduced HDL concentrations. This is particularly the case in patients with obesity and late-onset diabetes. This clinical profile is often referred to as the metabolic syndrome.[67] Pharmacologic reversal of the metabolic syndrome has been shown in several clinical studies to improve outcome.[68]

INFLAMMATION – ROLE OF THE MACROPHAGE

Macrophages derive from circulating monocytes and function predominantly as phagocytes and regulators of immune cell activation and the inflammatory process. Their physiologic function is to protect tissues from physical, chemical, and biologic insult by assisting in the detection and removal of pathogens and toxins. The presence of harmful matter activates the macrophage leading to the secretion of proinflammatory chemokines, cytokines, and enzymes designed to remove the offending insult and any damaged tissue. Once the noxious stimulus has been removed, the macrophage downregulates its production of proinflammatory molecules and switches to production of anti-inflammatory cytokines and growth factors which serve to de-activate inflammatory cells in the vicinity and attract cells capable of new tissue production and healing.

MACROPHAGE ACTIVATION AND ITS PROINFLAMMATORY CONSEQUENCES

Macrophages are the most numerous inflammatory cell found in the atherosclerotic lesion.[8,69] Several functions of the macrophage within the plaque have now been elucidated (see Fig. 2.5). The circulating precursor of the macrophage, the monocyte, is encouraged to migrate into the plaque by chemoattractants and adhesion molecules[70,71] expressed by the dysfunctional endothelium. Once the monocytes enter the vessel wall, they transform into macrophages which rapidly become activated by any one of a number of mechanisms including interaction with oxidized LDL,[72] T cell secretion of interferon-γ (IFN-γ),[73] and cell–cell contact regulated by the binding of CD40 ligand with its receptor, CD40.

The interaction between oxidized LDL with scavenger receptors on the cell surface of macrophages has already been touched on in the previous section. Oxidized LDL phagocytosis is facilitated by two scavenger receptors, CD36 and SR-A.[74,75] Oxidized LDL phagocytosis initiates a positive feedback loop that upregulates scavenger receptor expression allowing the further uptake of lipid and the formation of the foam cell. The feedback loop is controlled by the activation of the downstream molecules that make up the peroxisome proliferators-activated receptor-γ (PPARγ) pathway.[76,77] Digestion of oxidized LDL by the macrophage produces breakdown products some of which are transported back to the cell surface where, in conjunction with major histocompatibility complex (MHC) class II molecules, they are presented to naïve CD4 positive T lymphocytes.[78,79] T cells activated in this way undergo clonal proliferation to orchestrate an adapted cell-mediated immune response targeted specifically against the oxidized LDL molecule. Activated T cells produce IFN-γ that has a wide range of effects on the cellular constituents of the plaque such as the upregulation of endothelial adhesion molecules and the activation of nearby macrophages.[80]

Macrophages are also activated by direct cell–cell contact mediated by CD40 receptor binding to its ligand CD40L. Both the receptor and ligand are present on a number of cell types present within the atherosclerotic plaque, suggesting that CD40–CD40L interaction plays an important role in cell activation.[81–84]

Activation of plaque macrophages by any of the above mechanisms leads to the release of cytokines that act in both an autocrine and paracrine fashion to control the inflammatory response. In broad terms these can be divided into those molecules that are proinflammatory and those that are anti-inflammatory. Cytokines that attract other cells to the atherosclerotic plaque are often referred to as chemokines, and those cytokines that stimulate cell proliferation are often termed growth factors.

Tumor necrosis factor-alpha (TNF-α) and interleukin-1β (IL-1β) are the two most extensively investigated proinflammatory cytokines secreted by the activated macrophage.[85,86] They both exert wide-ranging paracrine and autocrine effects designed to amplify the inflammatory response. By increasing the expression of a number of proinflammatory cytokines, their overall effect is to maintain endothelial dysfunction, attract further inflammatory cells to the atherosclerotic plaque, and to encourage proliferation and activation of inflammatory cells in the near vicinity. TNF-α exerts the majority of its effects by binding to two receptors, TNFRSF1A and TNFRSF1B (previously known as TNFR1 and TNFR2, respectively).[87] IL-1β binds to the IL-1 receptor (IL-1R) expressed on the cell surface. Activation of TNFRSF1A, TNFRSF1B and IL-1R all lead to downstream activation of the transcription factor NF-κB, hence the similar actions of TNF-α and IL-1β.[88] The importance of these two molecules has been highlighted by knockout studies in mice, in which absence of the IL-1R and TNFRSF1A receptors led to a reduction in atherosclerotic lesions.[89,90]

Activated macrophages also produce chemokines such as MCP-1, which form a chemical gradient along which other monocytes and macrophages travel to reach sites of plaque inflammation. Indeed, high expression of MCP-1 is found in human atherosclerotic plaques,[91] and studies of MCP-1 overexpression in transgenic mice with a propensity for atherosclerosis showed a threefold rise in oxidized lipid and increased numbers of activated macrophages.[92]

As well as producing molecules that directly affect other cells, macrophages also release enzymes known as matrix metalloproteinases (MMPs) that breakdown the extracellular matrix (ECM) of the plaque. In response to proinflammatory cytokines such as TNF-α,[93] MMP expression is upregulated leading to increased extracellular concentrations capable of overcoming the presence of the constitutively expressed tissue inhibitors of matrix metalloproteinases (TIMPs).[94] Excessive ECM breakdown can lead to weakening of the plaque's structural integrity rendering it more susceptible to the forces exerted on it by the circulating blood.[95] This is discussed in more detail in the section on plaque rupture. Procoagulant molecules such as tissue factor are also released by activated macrophage foam cells. As with MMPs, the release of proinflammatory cytokines and CD40–CD40L interaction have been shown to increase tissue factor elaboration.[82,96] This mechanism is likely to be important in relation to the formation of thrombus on the plaque surface, again a subject that is explained in more detail later.

Cytokines, enzymes, and procoagulant factors are also released as a result of foam cell death. Cell death, either by way of necrosis or apoptosis (programmed cell death) is a common finding in advanced, highly inflamed human plaques.[97] Most evidence points towards toxic intracellular concentrations of free cholesterol as the cause. High concentrations of free cholesterol have been shown to have deleterious effects on membrane function leading to cell death.[98] Whatever the mechanism, cell death releases MMPs, proinflammatory cytokines, and large quantities of cholesterol and necrotic debris, which results in the destruction of the ECM and the formation of a necrotic lipid core.[99–101] Therefore, although beneficial in terms of lipid clearance, persistent macrophage activation leads to gross disruption of the arterial intima and mechanical instability.

DOWNREGULATION OF PROINFLAMMATORY MACROPHAGE ACTIVITY

If endothelial function can be restored to normal by removing or modulating the toxic stimulus (for example, smoking cessation, cholesterol lowering) then lipid and monocyte transport across the endothelium is reduced leading to a reduction in macrophage and foam cell activation. Improved endothelial function also changes the pattern of cytokine release by macrophages and T cells, suppressing expression of proinflammatory molecules and increasing production of anti-inflammatory cytokines (Fig. 2.6).

Two examples of cytokines that downregulate the inflammatory response are IL-1Ra and IL-10.[102] Of these,

IL-1Ra has a strong affinity for the IL-1 receptor but does not induce a cellular response; it is therefore believed to be an endogenous inhibitor of IL-1 signaling.[103] The anti-inflammatory role of IL-1Ra in atherosclerosis has been confirmed by the reduction in foam cell-rich lesions seen in IL-1Ra transgenic mice[104] and apoE knockout mice following IL-1Ra administration. Interleukin-10 has been shown to exert a wide range of anti-inflammatory effects including attenuation of proinflammatory cytokine release by macrophages and T cells,[105–107] suppression of antigen presentation,[108] a decline in release of reactive oxygen species[109] and inhibition of adhesion molecule expression.[110,111] The anti-inflammatory effects of IL-10 in atherosclerosis have been confirmed in an IL-10 knockout and transgenic mouse.[112] Clinical evidence also exists for the protective role of IL-10; patients with unstable angina have been found to have lower levels of circulating IL-10 than patients with chronic stable angina suggesting that IL-10 may have a direct stabilizing effect on atherosclerotic plaques.[113] This theory is supported by the finding that IL-10 suppresses MMP production and increases the expression of TIMPs.[114] Downregulation of the inflammatory process is an important step that must be initiated if the healing process driven predominantly by the VSMC is to ensue.

HEALING – ROLE OF THE VASCULAR SMOOTH MUSCLE CELL

In healthy vessels, VSMCs are more or less exclusively located in the medial layer of the arterial wall. They contain large amounts of contractile proteins and synthesize little extracellular matrix making them well suited to contracting and relaxing to regulate vascular tone. The 'contractile' phenotype is maintained by the influence of medial extracellular proteins on VSMC surface integrins. In the vessel wall of the atherosclerotic artery, VSMCs are also seen in the intimal layer, often surrounded by large amounts of newly formed ECM. Studies suggest that these intimal VSMCs predominantly originate from the medial layer of the arterial wall,[115,116] but there is evidence that some are derived from circulating bone marrow-derived cells.[117] Intimal migration of the VSMC is accompanied by activation of genes responsible for the production of ECM proteins such as collagen and proteoglycans.[118,119] The resulting 'synthetic' phenotype enables the VSMC to adopt a reparative role in which the ECM destroyed by the inflammatory process is replaced by freshly synthesized connective tissue. If the healing process is allowed to continue, then the layers of freshly synthesized ECM proteins become confluent to form a 'fibrous cap' that distances foci of inflammatory cells and extracellular lipid from the luminal surface of the plaque. In a proportion of advanced lesions, continuing repair is even thought to lead to the replacement of extracellular lipid and debris with fibrous tissue. Therefore in response to endothelial dysfunction and intimal disruption, the VSMC plays an important healing role

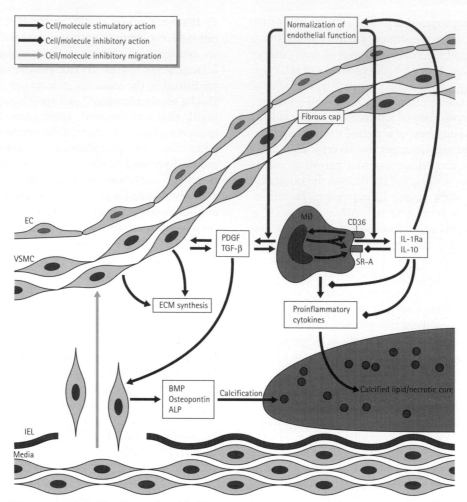

Figure 2.6   Schematic representation of healing and anti-inflammatory mechanisms within the atherosclerotic plaque. ALP, alkaline phosphatase; BMP, bone morphogenic protein; CD, cluster differentiation; EC, endothelial cell; ECM, extracellular matrix; IEL, internal elastic lamina; IL-1Ra, interleukin-1 receptor antagonist; MØ, macrophage; PDGF, platelet-derived growth factor; SR, scavenger receptor; TGF, transforming growth factor; VSMC, vascular smooth muscle cell.

that increases the strength and mechanical stability of the atherosclerotic plaque, although often at the expense of increased lesion size and luminal narrowing.[120]

The healing response is only allowed to proceed if there is sufficient downregulation of the inflammatory process (as described above) and secretion of growth factors to attract VSMCs into the atherosclerotic plaque (see Fig. 2.6). Platelet-derived growth factor (PDGF) and transforming growth factor-beta (TGF-β) are two molecules that appear to be central to the healing process. The PDGF is a potent VSMC chemoattractant produced predominantly by activated macrophages and platelets.[121] Different isoforms of PDGF (A and B) have been shown to induce phenotypic modulation in cultured VSMCs[122] and stimulate proliferation and migration of VSMCs in animal models of atherosclerosis.[123,124] The effects of PDGF on VSMCs are mediated via the PDGFR-α and PDGFR-β receptors on the cell surface, and all isoforms of PDGF and its receptors are expressed in human atherosclerosis.[125,126] The importance of PDGF in atherogenesis has been demonstrated in a

mouse model of atherosclerosis where VSMC recruitment was reduced by 80 percent following injection of an antibody directed against PDGF receptors.[127] Also, atheroma-prone mice deficient in PDGF develop atherosclerotic lesions that are devoid of intimal VSMCs and a mature fibrous cap.

An important cytokine that controls VSMC differentiation, and thus ECM synthesis, is TGF-β.[128] A reduction in TGF-β levels induces de-differentiation from the contractile to synthetic phenotype. De-differentiation is accompanied by a change in receptor expression from the type II to type I TGF-β receptor. Activation of the type I TGF-β receptor results in a massive elevation in ECM production.[129] However, if TGF-β levels do not return to normal or worse still drop further, then ECM matrix production is switched off. In addition, TGF-β also has important anti-inflammatory effects. Gene knockout studies in mice have revealed that a loss of constitutive TGF-β expression leads to widespread leukocyte extravasation into most organs resulting in perinatal death.[130,131] Cell culture studies have identified the anti-inflammatory effects of TGF-β *in vitro* which include suppression of endothelial adhesion molecule expression[132] and reduced uptake of lipid by macrophages.[133] There is also evidence that TGF-β regulates T cell function[134] and by disrupting TGF-β signaling one sees a reduction in T cell number, as well as the number of MHC class II-positive macrophages, in the atherosclerotic plaques of mice.[135] Overall, a reduction in TGF-β provides the atherosclerotic lesion with a 'double hit' by reducing ECM production and increasing inflammatory cell activity. Therefore, TGF-β clearly plays an important protective role in both the normal and atherosclerotic vessels.[136]

In contrast with PDGF and TGF-β, proinflammatory cytokines such as IFN-γ, TNF-α and IL-1β exert a cytostatic effect on the VSMC. The same cytokines can also promote apoptosis possibly by priming the VSMC to macrophage-induced killing via the binding of Fas ligand on the macrophage cell surface to the Fas receptor on the outer membrane of the VSMC.[137,138]

In summary, medial VSMCs de-differentiate and migrate into the plaque under the influence of chemokines and growth factors secreted by inflammatory and endothelial cells. VSMCs play an important role in healing the damage incurred by lipid deposition and the inflammatory response, by synthesizing the ECM that forms the fibrous cap. This provides the plaque with the necessary strength to withstand the sheer forces exerted on it by the circulation.

Plaque calcification

Calcification is an almost universal component of advanced atherosclerotic plaques that has received little attention until recently. Its clinical importance lies in the fact that it can be noninvasively detected by computed tomography (CT). Plaque calcification is now recognized to be a highly organized and regulated process (see Fig. 2.6) and is associated with the presence of various bone-associated molecules such as bone morphogenetic proteins,[139] osteopontin,[140,141] and alkaline phosphatase.[142] It is thought that VSMCs play a central role in the regulation of calcification, having the ability to differentiate down an osteogenic line.[143] The mechanisms involved in the calcification of advanced lesions remain unclear. However, *in vitro* studies have shown that vesicles released into the extracellular matrix following apoptosis act as a nidus for the accumulation of calcium. This would explain the distribution of calcium within advanced lesions, which is found mainly around and within the lipid core where there is a high rate of apoptosis. Proof of concept has been provided by a study showing that by inhibiting apoptosis one can prevent vascular calcification.[144] Heavily calcified plaques rarely contain large numbers of inflammatory cells which is surprising given the link between inflammation and apoptosis. It has therefore been suggested that calcification may represent past inflammation that has 'burnt out'.[145]

PLAQUE DISRUPTION AND THROMBOSIS

Acute vascular events attributable to atherosclerosis occur as a direct consequence of luminal thrombosis caused by plaque rupture, endothelial erosion or calcific nodule eruption. The mechanisms involved are described below.

PLAQUE RUPTURE

Fibrous cap rupture is the most common trigger for acute thrombosis, accounting for approximately 60 percent of coronary thromboses. It occurs when the shear stress exerted upon the cap exceeds its tensile stress. Cap rupture exposes the underlying lipid core to the circulating blood resulting in thrombus formation that is commonly extensive and associated with complete occlusion of the lumen.

Histologic studies have identified three structural features that are commonly present in ruptured plaques, a thin fibrous cap, a reduction in extracellular matrix and a large lipid/necrotic core. This combination of features confers considerable mechanical weakness making the plaque particularly prone to rupture.[13] The terms 'thin cap fibroatheroma', 'unstable', and 'vulnerable' are commonly applied to lesion exhibiting such features, although the latter two can also be applied to other lesion morphologies that also predispose to thrombosis. Immunocytochemical evaluation of the thin cap fibroatheroma, defined as a lesion with a fibrous cap thickness <65 μm, confirmed a significantly lower number of VSMCs and a higher number of macrophages and T lymphocytes compared with that in lesions with a fibrous cap thickness >65 μm.[146] These findings were particularly noticeable at the shoulder regions of the plaque where the fibrous cap lies adjacent to normal arterial wall, the site at which the majority of ruptures are seen. Thus, the likelihood of plaque rupture is directly influenced by the balance between the destructive effects of local inflammation and the healing effect of VSMCs (Fig. 2.7). If the balance tips in favor of inflammation, then the plaque becomes vulnerable to rupture, where as if it tips the other way, then the plaque stabilizes.

ENDOTHELIAL EROSION

In 40 percent of lesions associated with surface thrombus there is no evidence of rupture. In 90 percent of these there is evidence of endothelial erosion, characterized by a focal absence of endothelial cells on the luminal surface of the plaque exposing intimal VSMCs and proteoglycans to the circulation. This form of plaque disruption is more common in the young and in women.[18] The cellular and molecular processes responsible for plaque erosion remain poorly understood, but current theories center on increased propensity to endothelial apoptosis. Durand and colleagues have recently confirmed the importance of endothelial apoptosis in regard to thrombus formation in a rabbit model.[147] Despite the fact that inflammatory cells such as the macrophage and mast cell can induce endothelial cell

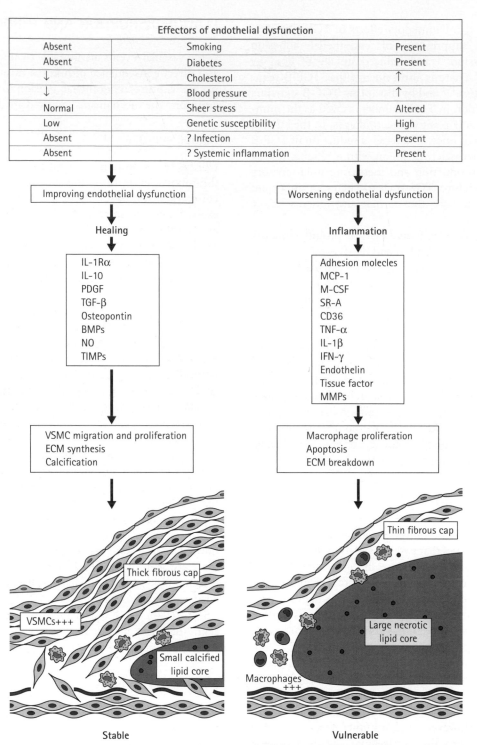

Effectors of endothelial dysfunction		
Absent	Smoking	Present
Absent	Diabetes	Present
↓	Cholesterol	↑
↓	Blood pressure	↑
Normal	Sheer stress	Altered
Low	Genetic susceptibility	High
Absent	? Infection	Present
Absent	? Systemic inflammation	Present

Improving endothelial dysfunction

Worsening endothelial dysfunction

Healing

Inflammation

IL–1Rα
IL–10
PDGF
TGF–β
Osteopontin
BMPs
NO
TIMPs

Adhesion molecles
MCP-1
M-CSF
SR-A
CD36
TNF-α
IL-1β
IFN-γ
Endothelin
Tissue factor
MMPs

VSMC migration and proliferation
ECM synthesis
Calcification

Macrophage proliferation
Apoptosis
ECM breakdown

Thick fibrous cap

VSMCs+++

Small calcified lipid core

Thin fibrous cap

Large necrotic lipid core

Macrophages +++

Stable

Vulnerable

Figure 2.7 The balance between healing and inflammation and its influence on plaque stability. BMP, bone morphogenetic protein; CD, cluster differentiation; ECM, extracellular matrix; IFN, interferon; IL-1Ra, interleukin-1 receptor antagonist; M-CSF, macrophage colony stimulating factor; MCP, monocyte chemotactic protein; MMP, matrix metalloproteinase; NO, nitric oxide; PDGF, platelet-derived growth factor; SR, scavenger receptor; TGF, transforming growth factor; TIMP, tissue inhibitors of matrix metalloproteinases; TNF, tumor necrosis factor; VSMC, vascular smooth muscle cell.

apoptosis, the majority of lesions with evidence of endothelial erosion do not contain significant numbers of inflammatory cells.[148,149] However, differences in ECM composition have been found between eroded and stable plaques. Eroded lesions contain significantly more hyaluronan in the fibrous cap, despite the presence of similar numbers of 'synthetic' VSMCs.[150] This finding has led to speculation that high concentrations of hyaluronan and versican provide a high risk substrate for thrombosis, perhaps by interfering with the integrity of the normal endothelium. For example, apoptosis rates in cultured endothelial cells have been shown to increase in the presence of a hyaluronan substrate.[151] Hyaluronan also appears to increase fibrin polymerization, an important part of the thrombotic process. To date there is no evidence to suggest a difference in VSMC phenotype to explain the differential accumulation of hyaluronan between stable and eroded lesions.

CALCIFIC NODULE EXPOSURE

The calcified nodule is a third, albeit uncommon mechanism by which thrombus forms on the luminal surface of the atherosclerotic plaque. It accounts for approximately 5% of fresh thrombus found in post-mortem studies of sudden coronary death.[19] In such lesions calcium extends from the intima, through the fibrous cap and into the vessel lumen. The majority of eruptive calcific nodules arise from plaques that have evidence of previous thrombotic episodes that have subsequently healed, suggesting that the development of this complication may be dependent on prior inflammation and plaque rupture.

THROMBOTIC MECHANISMS – PLATELETS AND THE COAGULATION CASCADE

For atherosclerosis to cause a clinical event it is necessary for thrombus to form within the lumen of the vessel at the site of plaque disruption. The incidence of atherosclerosis-related thrombosis has been significantly underestimated as a significant proportion of plaque disruption events do not cause overt symptoms.[152–155]

Thrombus that completely occludes the vessel lumen usually causes extensive tissue infarction, and therefore the therapeutic priority is to remove the thrombus and restore blood flow. This is commonly achieved pharmacologically by administering thrombolytic drugs or mechanically by inflating a balloon on the end of an intravascular catheter to dislodge the thrombus, a procedure known as angioplasty. If the thrombus only partially blocks the lumen, then infarction is often averted. However, the force of the blood flow past the freshly formed thrombus can lead to embolization which often causes occlusion in the smaller downstream vessels leading to 'microinfarcts'. This is a particularly common phenomenon in patients with atherosclerotic carotid disease presenting with stroke.[156–158] In this scenario, the aim of initial treatment is to prevent continuing thrombosis that could lead to complete occlusion of the artery and further embolization. This is achieved by using drugs that inhibit thrombosis such as platelet inhibitors and heparin.

The size and stability of freshly formed thrombus play a crucial role in eventual outcome. This is dictated by both local and systemic factors.[159–161] Local factors include blood flow dynamics, endothelial function, and perhaps, most importantly, the potency and persistence of the stimulus provided by plaque contents. For example, tissue factor, a potent activator of the coagulation cascade, is produced in higher quantities by lipid- and macrophage-rich lesions compared with fibrotic plaques.[162] Differences in the size of thrombotic stimulus may explain the higher rates of vascular occlusion, infarction and mortality associated with plaque rupture when compared with endothelial erosion. Systemic factors that affect thrombus formation appear to be of particular importance in those episodes caused by superficial erosion. Systemic triggers include platelet number and function, abnormal production of soluble coagulation factors or endogenous inhibitors, smoking and estrogen/progesterone imbalance. The latter may explain the higher incidence of acute events due to plaque erosion in women than in men.

Importantly, thrombosis also stimulates a healing response, the extent of which dictates future plaque stability and the degree of plaque growth. Fresh thrombus is a rich source of growth factors and cytokines, including PDGF, thrombin and TGF-β, all potent inducers of VSMC migration, proliferation, and matrix synthesis.[31] A vigorous healing response, although beneficial in terms of plaque stability, often leads to a substantial increase in plaque size due to the incorporation of thrombus and newly synthesized extracellular matrix into the body of the plaque. The phenomenon of rupture and repair can explain the propensity of some plaques to grow in a stepwise fashion, and is likely to be responsible for a significant proportion of patients presenting with new onset reversible ischemia both with and without a history of preceding infarction.

ATHEROSCLEROSIS IN WOMEN

Epidemiological studies have consistently shown a lower incidence and prevalence of atherosclerosis-related syndromes in women compared with men.[163] The reasons for this protection are largely unclear, but ovarian hormones have been implicated since at any age, postmenopausal women have a greater cardiovascular risk than premenopausal women.[164] Furthermore, women who undergo bilateral oophorectomy and do not take hormone replacement therapy (HRT) have a five times greater risk of developing atheroma than women with functioning ovaries, even after controlling for age and other cardiovascular risks.[165]

Initial observational studies and small clinical trials of hormone therapy have supported this hypothesis.[166–168] However, in recent years larger studies with improved design have found that HRT increases the incidence of myocardial infarction and stroke, despite clearly having beneficial effects on lipid profiles[169] and endothelial function.[170] In-depth analysis of the latest trial data has revealed that the increase in vascular events seen with HRT predominantly occurred in the first two years after starting therapy. It was also noted that the incidence of other thrombotic events not related to atherosclerosis such as deep vein thrombosis and pulmonary embolus were also increased by

HRT.[171–173] Experts have therefore hypothesized that the potential beneficial effects of improving endothelial function and lipid profile are more than offset by an increased propensity for thrombosis in the first few years of therapy. Studies that clearly show a deleterious effect on several of the circulating coagulation factors and their intrinsic inhibitors following the initiation of hormone therapy provide good evidence to support this hypothesis.[174]

SUMMARY

The molecular and cellular interactions that lead to the initiation and progression of atherosclerosis can be characterized as a chronic inflammatory response to lipids that accumulate in the vessel wall as a consequence of endothelial dysfunction. The aetiology of endothelial dysfunction and therefore the initiation of atherosclerosis are complex and incompletely understood. Factors such as smoking, hypertension, diabetes, hypercholesterolemia, and family history of atherosclerosis-related complications all have a strong association with the development of atherosclerosis and endothelial dysfunction. It is therefore likely that such factors along with as yet undiscovered faults all play a role in initiating the disease process.

The majority of life-threatening events associated with atherosclerosis occur as a result of disruption to the plaque surface, an event that leads to thrombosis and vascular occlusion. Our understanding of the pathophysiologic mechanisms that lead to plaque disruption, especially plaque rupture, has increased dramatically over the two decades but several questions remain unanswered, especially those relating to plaque erosion.

There is little evidence to suggest that the underlying processes are any different in women than in men. However, it is likely that the process of atherogenesis progresses more slowly in women because of the, as yet, uncharacterized protective effects of female hormones. The relation between female hormones and atherosclerosis is likely to be complicated given the increased incidence of atherosclerotic complications seen in recent trials of HRT.

The prevalence of atherosclerosis and its related complications in Western society remains high. Research aimed at addressing the unanswered questions relating to the etiology of endothelial dysfunction, the pathophysiology of plaque disruption and the role of female hormones in atherogenesis and thrombosis holds the key to reducing the morbidity and mortality associated with atherosclerosis in the future.

KEY LEARNING POINTS

- Atherosclerosis is characterized by a pathologic thickening of the arterial wall predominantly affecting the intimal layer of medium- and large-sized arteries.
- Endothelial dysfunction, inflammation, lipid accumulation, plaque disruption, and healing are the five main pathophysiologic processes that contribute to the formation and progression of atherosclerotic plaques.
- Endothelial dysfunction is likely to be responsible for lesion initiation characterized by the passage of lipid and inflammatory cells into the vessel wall.
- The cause of endothelial dysfunction is often multifactorial. Local blood flow dynamics, hypertension, smoking, hypercholesterolemia, diabetes mellitus, and genetic predisposition are known to predispose to endothelial dysfunction
- Inflammation and lipid accumulation is driven predominantly by the plaque macrophage, with the T lymphocyte playing a supporting role.
- Healing is characterized by the synthesis of new extracellular matrix proteins by intimal vascular smooth muscle cells.
- The majority of life-threatening clinical complications, such as myocardial infarction and stroke, are caused by intraluminal thrombosis which arises as a result of disruption to the plaque surface.
- There are three main causes of plaque disruption: plaque rupture, plaque erosion, and eruption of a calcific nodule. Plaque rupture accounts for the majority of plaque disruption.
- The risk of plaque rupture is dictated by the balance between inflammation and healing. Inflammation reduces the mechanical strength of the plaque predisposing to rupture, where as healing increases the tensile strength making the lesion more resistant to rupture.
- Plaque erosion is a poorly understood mechanism of plaque disruption. It is more commonly seen in women and in the relatively young.
- The extent of thrombosis, and therefore the size and severity of tissue infarction is dictated not only by the stimulus provided by the plaque, but also the function of platelets and soluble coagulation factors.
- Premenopausal women have a reduced propensity to form atherosclerotic lesions, thought to be due to the protection afforded by the female sex hormones. However, this is partially offset by an increased thrombotic tendency, which predominantly manifests as clot on the surface of eroded plaques.

ACKNOWLEDGMENT

Funded by the British Heart Foundation.

REFERENCES

1. Stary HC. Macrophages, macrophage foam cells, and eccentric intimal thickening in the coronary arteries of young children. *Atherosclerosis* 1987; **64**: 91–108.

2. Tunstall-Pedoe H, Kuulasmaa K, Mahonen M, *et al.* Contribution of trends in survival and coronary-event rates to changes in coronary heart disease mortality: 10-year results from 37 WHO MONICA project populations. Monitoring trends and determinants in cardiovascular disease. *Lancet* 1999; **353**: 1547–57.

3. Stary HC, Chandler AB, Glagov S, *et al.* A definition of initial, fatty streak, and intermediate lesions of atherosclerosis. A report from the Committee on Vascular Lesions of the Council on Arteriosclerosis, American Heart Association. *Arterioscler Thromb* 1994; **14**: 840–56.

4. Stary HC, Chandler AB, Dinsmore RE, *et al.* A definition of advanced types of atherosclerotic lesions and a histological classification of atherosclerosis. A report from the Committee on Vascular Lesions of the Council on Arteriosclerosis, American Heart Association. *Circulation* 1995; **92**: 1355–74.

5. Insull W, Jr., Bartsch GE. Cholesterol, triglyceride, and phospholipid content of intima, media, and atherosclerotic fatty streak in human thoracic aorta. *J Clin Invest* 1966; **45**: 513–23.

6. Stary HC. Evolution and progression of atherosclerotic lesions in coronary arteries of children and young adults. *Arteriosclerosis* 1989; **9**: I19–I32.

7. Glagov S, Weisenberg E, Zarins CK, *et al.* Compensatory enlargement of human atherosclerotic coronary arteries. *N Engl J Med* 1987; **316**: 1371–5.

8. Jonasson L, Holm J, Skalli O, *et al.* Regional accumulations of T cells, macrophages, and smooth muscle cells in the human atherosclerotic plaque. *Arteriosclerosis* 1986; **6**: 131–8.

9. Mitchell JR, Schwartz CJ. *Arterial Disease.* Philidelphia, PA: FA Davis Co, 1965.

10. Glagov S, Zarins C, Giddens DP, Ku DN. Hemodynamics and atherosclerosis. Insights and perspectives gained from studies of human arteries. *Arch Pathol Lab Med* 1988; **112**: 1018–31.

11. Davies MJ, Thomas AC. Plaque fissuring – the cause of acute myocardial infarction, sudden ischaemic death, and crescendo angina. *Br Heart J* 1985; **53**: 363–73.

12. Falk E. Morphologic features of unstable atherothrombotic plaques underlying acute coronary syndromes. *Am J Cardiol* 1989; **63**: 114E–120E.

13. Falk E. Why do plaques rupture? *Circulation* 1992; **86**: III30–III42.

14. Felton CV, Crook D, Davies MJ, Oliver MF. Relation of plaque lipid composition and morphology to the stability of human aortic plaques. *Arterioscler Thromb Vasc Biol* 1997; **17**: 1337–45.

15. Mann JM, Davies MJ. Vulnerable plaque. Relation of characteristics to degree of stenosis in human coronary arteries. *Circulation* 1996; **94**: 928–31.

16. Ambrose JA, Tannenbaum MA, Alexopoulos D, *et al.* Angiographic progression of coronary artery disease and the development of myocardial infarction. *J Am Coll Cardiol* 1988; **12**: 56–62.

17. Little WC, Constantinescu M, Applegate RJ, *et al.* Can coronary angiography predict the site of a subsequent myocardial infarction in patients with mild-to-moderate coronary artery disease? *Circulation* 1988; **78**: 1157–66.

18. Farb A, Burke AP, Tang AL, *et al.* Coronary plaque erosion without rupture into a lipid core. A frequent cause of coronary thrombosis in sudden coronary death. *Circulation* 1996; **93**: 1354–63.

19. Virmani R, Kolodgie FD, Burke AP, *et al.* Lessons from sudden coronary death: a comprehensive morphological classification scheme for atherosclerotic lesions. *Arterioscler Thromb Vasc Biol* 2000; **20**: 1262–75.

20. Kolodgie FD, Gold HK, Burke AP, *et al.* Intraplaque hemorrhage and progression of coronary atheroma. *N Engl J Med* 2003; **349**: 2316–25.

21. Barger AC, Beeuwkes R, III, Lainey LL, Silverman KJ. Hypothesis: vasa vasorum and neovascularization of human coronary arteries. A possible role in the pathophysiology of atherosclerosis. *N Engl J Med* 1984; **310**: 175–7.

22. Rubanyi GM. The role of endothelium in cardiovascular homeostasis and diseases. *J Cardiovasc Pharmacol* 1993; **22**(Suppl 4): S1–14.

23. Cox DA, Vita JA, Treasure CB, *et al.* Atherosclerosis impairs flow-mediated dilation of coronary arteries in humans. *Circulation* 1989; **80**: 458–65.

24. Ludmer PL, Selwyn AP, Shook TL, *et al.* Paradoxical vasoconstriction induced by acetylcholine in atherosclerotic coronary arteries. *N Engl J Med* 1986; **315**: 1046–51.

25. Schachinger V, Britten MB, Zeiher AM. Prognostic impact of coronary vasodilator dysfunction on adverse long-term outcome of coronary heart disease. *Circulation* 2000; **101**: 1899–906.

26. Suwaidi JA, Hamasaki S, Higano ST, *et al.* Long-term follow-up of patients with mild coronary artery disease and endothelial dysfunction. *Circulation* 2000; **101**: 948–54.

27. Gokce N, Keaney JF, Jr., Hunter LM, *et al.* Risk stratification for postoperative cardiovascular events via noninvasive assessment of endothelial function: a prospective study. *Circulation* 2002; **105**: 1567–72.

28. Sorensen KE, Celermajer DS, Georgakopoulos D, *et al.* Impairment of endothelium-dependent dilation is an early event in children with familial hypercholesterolemia and is related to the lipoprotein(a) level. *J Clin Invest* 1994; **93**: 50–5.

29. Reddy KG, Nair RN, Sheehan HM, Hodgson JM. Evidence that selective endothelial dysfunction may occur in the absence of angiographic or ultrasound atherosclerosis in patients with risk factors for atherosclerosis. *J Am Coll Cardiol* 1994; **23**: 833–43.

30. Jarvisalo MJ, Raitakari M, Toikka JO, *et al.* Endothelial dysfunction and increased arterial intima-media

thickness in children with type 1 diabetes. *Circulation* 2004; **109**: 1750–5.

♦ 31   Ross R. The pathogenesis of atherosclerosis: a perspective for the 1990s. *Nature* 1993; **362**: 801–9.

32   Kinlay S, Libby P, Ganz P. Endothelial function and coronary artery disease. *Curr Opin Lipidol* 2001; **12**: 383–9.

33   Creager MA, Cooke JP, Mendelsohn ME, *et al.* Impaired vasodilation of forearm resistance vessels in hyper-cholesterolemic humans. *J Clin Invest* 1990; **86**: 228–34.

34   Celermajer DS, Sorensen KE, Gooch VM, *et al.* Non-invasive detection of endothelial dysfunction in children and adults at risk of atherosclerosis. *Lancet* 1992; **340**: 1111–15.

35   Celermajer DS, Sorensen KE, Bull C, *et al.* Endothelium-dependent dilation in the systemic arteries of asymptomatic subjects relates to coronary risk factors and their interaction. *J Am Coll Cardiol* 1994; **24**: 1468–74.

36   Steinberg HO, Chaker H, Leaming R, *et al.* Obesity/insulin resistance is associated with endothelial dysfunction. Implications for the syndrome of insulin resistance. *J Clin Invest* 1996; **97**: 2601–10.

37   Fichtlscherer S, Rosenberger G, Walter DH, *et al.* Elevated C-reactive protein levels and impaired endothelial vasoreactivity in patients with coronary artery disease. *Circulation* 2000; **102**: 1000–6.

38   Prasad A, Zhu J, Halcox JP, *et al.* Predisposition to atherosclerosis by infections: role of endothelial dysfunction. *Circulation* 2002; **106**: 184–90.

39   Heitzer T, Schlinzig T, Krohn K, *et al.* Endothelial dysfunction, oxidative stress, and risk of cardiovascular events in patients with coronary artery disease. *Circulation* 2001; **104**: 2673–8.

40   Fuster V, Lewis A. Conner Memorial Lecture. Mechanisms leading to myocardial infarction: insights from studies of vascular biology. *Circulation* 1994; **90**: 2126–46.

41   Libby P, Geng YJ, Sukhova GK, *et al.* Molecular determinants of atherosclerotic plaque vulnerability. *Ann N Y Acad Sci* 1997; **811**: 134–42.

42   Palmer RM, Ferrige AG, Moncada S. Nitric oxide release accounts for the biological activity of endothelium-derived relaxing factor. *Nature* 1987; **327**: 524–6.

43   Lerman A, Holmes DR, Jr., Bell MR, *et al.* Endothelin in coronary endothelial dysfunction and early atherosclerosis in humans. *Circulation* 1995; **92**: 2426–31.

44   Barnes PJ, Karin M. Nuclear factor-kappaB: a pivotal transcription factor in chronic inflammatory diseases. *N Engl J Med* 1997; **336**: 1066–71.

45   Blankenberg S, Barbaux S, Tiret L. Adhesion molecules and atherosclerosis. *Atherosclerosis* 2003; **170**: 191–203.

46   Dong ZM, Chapman SM, Brown AA, *et al.* The combined role of P- and E-selectins in atherosclerosis. *J Clin Invest* 1998; **102**: 145–52.

47   Collins RG, Velji R, Guevara NV, *et al.* P-Selectin or intercellular adhesion molecule (ICAM)-1 deficiency substantially protects against atherosclerosis in apolipoprotein E-deficient mice. *J Exp Med* 2000; **191**: 189–94.

48   Shih PT, Brennan ML, Vora DK, *et al.* Blocking very late antigen-4 integrin decreases leukocyte entry and fatty streak formation in mice fed an atherogenic diet. *Circ Res* 1999; **84**: 345–51.

49   Gosling J, Slaymaker S, Gu L, *et al.* MCP-1 deficiency reduces susceptibility to atherosclerosis in mice that overexpress human apolipoprotein B. *J Clin Invest* 1999; **103**: 773–8.

50   Boring L, Gosling J, Cleary M, Charo IF. Decreased lesion formation in CCR2-/- mice reveals a role for chemokines in the initiation of atherosclerosis. *Nature* 1998; **394**: 894–7.

51   Boren J, Olin K, Lee I, *et al.* Identification of the principal proteoglycan-binding site in LDL. A single-point mutation in apo-B100 severely affects proteoglycan interaction without affecting LDL receptor binding. *J Clin Invest* 1998; **101**: 2658–64.

52   Griendling KK, FitzGerald GA. Oxidative stress and cardio-vascular injury: Part I: basic mechanisms and *in vivo* monitoring of ROS. *Circulation* 2003; **108**: 1912–16.

53   Griendling KK, FitzGerald GA. Oxidative stress and cardiovascular injury: Part II: animal and human studies. *Circulation* 2003; **108**: 2034–40.

♦ 54   Steinberg D, Lewis A. Conner Memorial Lecture. Oxidative modification of LDL and atherogenesis. *Circulation* 1997; **95**: 1062–71.

55   Quinn MT, Parthasarathy S, Fong LG, Steinberg D. Oxidatively modified low density lipoproteins: a potential role in recruitment and retention of monocyte/macrophages during atherogenesis. *Proc Natl Acad Sci U S A* 1987; **84**: 2995–8.

56   Rajavashisth TB, Andalibi A, Territo MC, *et al.* Induction of endothelial cell expression of granulocyte and macrophage colony-stimulating factors by modified low-density lipoproteins. *Nature* 1990; **344**: 254–7.

57   Leonard EJ, Yoshimura T. Human monocyte chemoattractant protein-1 (MCP-1). *Immunol Today* 1990; **11**: 97–101.

58   Khoo JC, Miller E, Pio F, *et al.* Monoclonal antibodies against LDL further enhance macrophage uptake of LDL aggregates. *Arterioscler Thromb* 1992; **12**: 1258–66.

59   Han J, Nicholson AC. Lipoproteins modulate expression of the macrophage scavenger receptor. *Am J Pathol* 1998; **152**: 1647–54.

60   Vainio S, Ikonen E. Macrophage cholesterol transport: a critical player in foam cell formation. *Ann Med* 2003; **35**: 146–55.

61   Berliner JA, Navab M, Fogelman AM, *et al.* Atherosclerosis: basic mechanisms. Oxidation, inflammation, and genetics. *Circulation* 1995; **91**: 2488–96.

● 62   Prevention of cardiovascular events and death with pravastatin in patients with coronary heart disease and a broad range of initial cholesterol levels. The Long-Term

Intervention with Pravastatin in Ischaemic Disease (LIPID) Study Group. *N Engl J Med* 1998; **339**: 1349–57.

63 Randomised trial of cholesterol lowering in 4444 patients with coronary heart disease: the Scandinavian Simvastatin Survival Study (4S). *Lancet* 1994; **344**: 1383–9.

64 MRC/BHF Heart Protection Study of cholesterol lowering with simvastatin in 20,536 high-risk individuals: a randomised placebo-controlled trial. *Lancet* 2002; **360**: 7–22.

65 Nissen SE, Tuzcu EM, Schoenhagen P, *et al.* Effect of intensive compared with moderate lipid-lowering therapy on progression of coronary atherosclerosis: a randomized controlled trial. *JAMA* 2004; **291**: 1071–80.

66 Rader DJ. Regulation of reverse cholesterol transport and clinical implications. *Am J Cardiol* 2003; **92**: 42J-49J.

67 Haffner S, Taegtmeyer H. Epidemic obesity and the metabolic syndrome. *Circulation* 2003; **108**: 1541–5.

68 Grundy SM, Hansen B, Smith SC, Jr., *et al.* Clinical management of metabolic syndrome: report of the American Heart Association/National Heart, Lung, and Blood Institute/American Diabetes Association conference on scientific issues related to management. *Circulation* 2004; **109**: 551–6.

69 Still WJ, Marriot PR. Comparative morphology of the early atherosclerotic lesion in man and cholesterol-atherosclerosis in the rabbit: an electronmicroscopic study. *J Atheroscler Res* 1964; **4**: 373–86.

70 Mach F. The role of chemokines in atherosclerosis. *Curr Atheroscler Rep* 2001; **3**: 243–51.

71 Cybulsky MI, Lichtman AH, Hajra L, Iiyama K. Leukocyte adhesion molecules in atherogenesis. *Clin Chim Acta* 1999; **286**: 207–18.

72 Jovinge S, Ares MP, Kallin B, Nilsson J. Human monocytes/macrophages release TNF-alpha in response to Ox-LDL. *Arterioscler Thromb Vasc Biol* 1996; **16**: 1573–9.

73 Frostegard J, Ulfgren AK, Nyberg P, *et al.* Cytokine expression in advanced human atherosclerotic plaques: dominance of pro-inflammatory (Th1) and macrophage-stimulating cytokines. *Atherosclerosis* 1999; **145**: 33–43.

74 Suzuki H, Kurihara Y, Takeya M, *et al.* A role for macrophage scavenger receptors in atherosclerosis and susceptibility to infection. *Nature* 1997; **386**: 292–6.

75 Podrez EA, Febbraio M, Sheibani N, *et al.* Macrophage scavenger receptor CD36 is the major receptor for LDL modified by monocyte-generated reactive nitrogen species. *J Clin Invest* 2000; **105**: 1095–108.

76 Tontonoz P, Nagy L, Alvarez JG, *et al.* PPARgamma promotes monocyte/macrophage differentiation and uptake of oxidized LDL. *Cell* 1998; **93**: 241–52.

77 Nagy L, Tontonoz P, Alvarez JG, *et al.* Oxidized LDL regulates macrophage gene expression through ligand activation of PPARgamma. *Cell* 1998; **93**: 229–40.

78 Stemme S, Faber B, Holm J, *et al.* T lymphocytes from human atherosclerotic plaques recognize oxidized

low-density lipoprotein. *Proc Natl Acad Sci U S A* 1995; **92**: 3893–7.

79 Nicoletti A, Caligiuri G, Tornberg I, *et al.* The macrophage scavenger receptor type A directs modified proteins to antigen presentation. *Eur J Immunol* 1999; **29**: 512–21.

80 Tau G, Rothman P. Biologic functions of the IFN-gamma receptors. *Allergy* 1999; **54**: 1233–51.

81 Hollenbaugh D, Mischel-Petty N, Edwards CP, *et al.* Expression of functional CD40 by vascular endothelial cells. *J Exp Med* 1995; **182**: 33–40.

82 Mach F, Schonbeck U, Bonnefoy JY, *et al.* Activation of monocyte/macrophage functions related to acute atheroma complication by ligation of CD40: induction of collagenase, stromelysin, and tissue factor. *Circulation* 1997; **96**: 396–9.

83 Schonbeck U, Mach F, Sukhova GK, *et al.* Regulation of matrix metalloproteinase expression in human vascular smooth muscle cells by T lymphocytes: a role for CD40 signaling in plaque rupture? *Circ Res* 1997; **81**: 448–54.

84 Schonbeck U, Mach F, Bonnefoy JY, *et al.* Ligation of CD40 activates interleukin 1beta-converting enzyme (caspase-1) activity in vascular smooth muscle and endothelial cells and promotes elaboration of active interleukin 1beta. *J Biol Chem* 1997; **272**: 19569–74.

85 Aggarwal BB, Natarajan K. Tumor necrosis factors: developments during the last decade. *Eur Cytokine Netw* 1996; **7**: 93–124.

86 Loppnow H, Werdan K, Reuter G, Flad HD. The interleukin-1 and interleukin-1 converting enzyme families in the cardiovascular system. *Eur Cytokine Netw* 1998; **9**: 675–80.

87 Locksley RM, Killeen N, Lenardo MJ. The TNF and TNF receptor superfamilies: integrating mammalian biology. *Cell* 2001; **104**: 487–501.

88 Callaghan MM, Lovis RM, Rammohan C, *et al.* Autocrine regulation of collagenase gene expression by TNF-alpha in U937 cells. *J Leukoc Biol* 1996; **59**: 125–32.

89 Chi H, Messas E, Levine RA, *et al.* Interleukin-1 receptor signaling mediates atherosclerosis associated with bacterial exposure and/or a high-fat diet in a murine apolipoprotein E heterozygote model: pharmacotherapeutic implications. *Circulation* 2004; **110**: 1678–85.

90 Branen L, Hovgaard L, Nitulescu M, *et al.* Inhibition of tumor necrosis factor-alpha reduces atherosclerosis in apolipoprotein E knockout mice. *Arterioscler Thromb Vasc Biol* 2004; **24**: 2137–42.

91 Reape TJ, Groot PH. Chemokines and atherosclerosis. *Atherosclerosis* 1999; **147**: 213–25.

92 Aiello RJ, Bourassa PA, Lindsey S, *et al.* Monocyte chemoattractant protein-1 accelerates atherosclerosis in apolipoprotein E-deficient mice. *Arterioscler Thromb Vasc Biol* 1999; **19**: 1518–25.

93 Rajavashisth TB, Xu XP, Jovinge S, *et al.* Membrane type 1 matrix metalloproteinase expression in human athero-sclerotic plaques: evidence for activation by

proinflammatory mediators. *Circulation* 1999; **99**: 3103–9.

94   George SJ. Tissue inhibitors of metalloproteinases and metalloproteinases in atherosclerosis. *Curr Opin Lipidol* 1998; **9**: 413–23.

95   Galis ZS, Sukhova GK, Lark MW, Libby P. Increased expression of matrix metalloproteinases and matrix degrading activity in vulnerable regions of human atherosclerotic plaques. *J Clin Invest* 1994; **94**: 2493–503.

96   Thompson SG, Kienast J, Pyke SD, *et al*. Hemostatic factors and the risk of myocardial infarction or sudden death in patients with angina pectoris. European Concerted Action on Thrombosis and Disabilities Angina Pectoris Study Group. *N Engl J Med* 1995; **332**: 635–41.

97   Geng YJ, Libby P. Evidence for apoptosis in advanced human atheroma. Colocalization with interleukin-1 beta-converting enzyme. *Am J Pathol* 1995; **147**: 251–66.

98   Kellner-Weibel G, Jerome WG, Small DM, *et al*. Effects of intracellular free cholesterol accumulation on macrophage viability: a model for foam cell death. *Arterioscler Thromb Vasc Biol* 1998; **18**: 423–31.

99   Oliver MF, Davies MJ. The atheromatous lipid core. *Eur Heart J* 1998; **19**: 16–18.

100   Kolodgie FD, Narula J, Burke AP, *et al*. Localization of apoptotic macrophages at the site of plaque rupture in sudden coronary death. *Am J Pathol* 2000; **157**: 1259–68.

101   Kolodgie FD, Narula J, Haider N, Virmani R. Apoptosis in atherosclerosis. Does it contribute to plaque instability? *Cardiol Clin* 2001; **19**: 127–39, ix.

102   Lalani I, Bhol K, Ahmed AR. Interleukin-10: biology, role in inflammation and autoimmunity. *Ann Allergy Asthma Immunol* 1997; **79**: 469–83.

103   Dinarello CA. Interleukin-1. *Cytokine Growth Factor Rev* 1997; **8**: 253–65.

104   Devlin CM, Kuriakose G, Hirsch E, Tabas I. Genetic alterations of IL-1 receptor antagonist in mice affect plasma cholesterol level and foam cell lesion size. *Proc Natl Acad Sci U S A* 2002; **99**: 6280–5.

105   Lang R, Patel D, Morris JJ, *et al*. Shaping gene expression in activated and resting primary macrophages by IL-10. *J Immunol* 2002; **169**: 2253–63.

106   Bogdan C, Vodovotz Y, Nathan C. Macrophage deactivation by interleukin 10. *J Exp Med* 1991; **174**: 1549–55.

107   Fiorentino DF, Bond MW, Mosmann TR. Two types of mouse T helper cell. IV. Th2 clones secrete a factor that inhibits cytokine production by Th1 clones. *J Exp Med* 1989; **170**: 2081–95.

108   de Waal MR, Haanen J, Spits H, *et al*. Interleukin 10 (IL-10) and viral IL-10 strongly reduce antigen-specific human T cell proliferation by diminishing the antigen-presenting capacity of monocytes via downregulation of class II major histocompatibility complex expression. *J Exp Med* 1991; **174**: 915–24.

109   Haddad JJ, Fahlman CS. Redox- and oxidant-mediated regulation of interleukin-10: an anti-inflammatory, antioxidant cytokine? *Biochem Biophys Res Commun* 2002; **297**: 163–76.

110   Mostafa ME, Chollet-Martin S, Oudghiri M, *et al*. Effects of interleukin-10 on monocyte/endothelial cell adhesion and MMP-9/TIMP-1 secretion. *Cardiovasc Res* 2001; **49**: 882–90.

111   Song S, Ling-Hu H, Roebuck KA, *et al*. Interleukin-10 inhibits interferon-gamma-induced intercellular adhesion molecule-1 gene transcription in human monocytes. *Blood* 1997; **89**: 4461–9.

112   Pinderski Oslund LJ, Hedrick CC, Olvera T, *et al*. Interleukin-10 blocks atherosclerotic events *in vitro* and *in vivo*. *Arterioscler Thromb Vasc Biol* 1999; **19**: 2847–53.

113   Smith DA, Irving SD, Sheldon J, *et al*. Serum levels of the antiinflammatory cytokine interleukin-10 are decreased in patients with unstable angina. *Circulation* 2001; **104**: 746–9.

114   Lacraz S, Nicod LP, Chicheportiche R, *et al*. IL-10 inhibits metalloproteinase and stimulates TIMP-1 production in human mononuclear phagocytes. *J Clin Invest* 1995; **96**: 2304–10.

115   Ross R, Glomset JA. The pathogenesis of atherosclerosis (first of two parts). *N Engl J Med* 1976; **295**: 369–77.

116   Ross R, Glomset JA. The pathogenesis of atherosclerosis (second of two parts). *N Engl J Med* 1976; **295**: 420–5.

117   Simper D, Stalboerger PG, Panetta CJ, *et al*. Smooth muscle progenitor cells in human blood. *Circulation* 2002; **106**: 1199–204.

118   Shanahan CM, Weissberg PL. Smooth muscle cell heterogeneity: patterns of gene expression in vascular smooth muscle cells *in vitro* and *in vivo*. *Arterioscler Thromb Vasc Biol* 1998; **18**: 333–8.

119   Owens GK. Regulation of differentiation of vascular smooth muscle cells. *Physiol Rev* 1995; **75**: 487–517.

120   Libby P. Molecular bases of the acute coronary syndromes. *Circulation* 1995; **91**: 2844–50.

121   Heldin CH, Wasteson A, Westermark B. Platelet-derived growth factor. *Mol Cell Endocrinol* 1985; **39**: 169–87.

122   Blank RS, Owens GK. Platelet-derived growth factor regulates actin isoform expression and growth state in cultured rat aortic smooth muscle cells. *J Cell Physiol* 1990; **142**: 635–42.

123   Ferns GA, Raines EW, Sprugel KH, *et al*. Inhibition of neointimal smooth muscle accumulation after angioplasty by an antibody to PDGF. *Science* 1991; **253**: 1129–32.

124   Jawien A, Bowen-Pope DF, Lindner V, *et al*. Platelet-derived growth factor promotes smooth muscle migration and intimal thickening in a rat model of balloon angioplasty. *J Clin Invest* 1992; **89**: 507–11.

125   Tanizawa S, Ueda M, van der Loos CM, *et al*. Expression of platelet derived growth factor B chain and beta receptor in human coronary arteries after percutaneous transluminal coronary angioplasty: an immunohistochemical study. *Heart* 1996; **75**: 549–56.

126 Ueda M, Becker AE, Kasayuki N, et al. In situ detection of platelet-derived growth factor-A and -B chain mRNA in human coronary arteries after percutaneous transluminal coronary angioplasty. Am J Pathol 1996; 149: 831–43.

127 Sano H, Sudo T, Yokode M, et al. Functional blockade of platelet-derived growth factor receptor-beta but not of receptor-alpha prevents vascular smooth muscle cell accumulation in fibrous cap lesions in apolipoprotein E-deficient mice. Circulation 2001; 103: 2955–60.

128 Hautmann MB, Madsen CS, Owens GK. A transforming growth factor beta (TGFbeta) control element drives TGFbeta-induced stimulation of smooth muscle alpha-actin gene expression in concert with two CArG elements. J Biol Chem 1997; 272: 10948–56.

129 McCaffrey TA, Consigli S, Du B, et al. Decreased type II/type I TGF-beta receptor ratio in cells derived from human atherosclerotic lesions. Conversion from an antiproliferative to profibrotic response to TGF-beta1. J Clin Invest 1995; 96: 2667–75.

130 Kulkarni AB, Huh CG, Becker D, et al. Transforming growth factor beta 1 null mutation in mice causes excessive inflammatory response and early death. Proc Natl Acad Sci U S A 1993; 90: 770–4.

131 Shull MM, Ormsby I, Kier AB, et al. Targeted disruption of the mouse transforming growth factor-beta 1 gene results in multifocal inflammatory disease. Nature 1992; 359: 693–9.

132 Gamble JR, Khew-Goodall Y, Vadas MA. Transforming growth factor-beta inhibits E-selectin expression on human endothelial cells. J Immunol 1993; 150: 4494–503.

133 Argmann CA, Van Den Diepstraten CH, Sawyez CG, et al. Transforming growth factor-beta1 inhibits macrophage cholesteryl ester accumulation induced by native and oxidized VLDL remnants. Arterioscler Thromb Vasc Biol 2001; 21: 2011–18.

134 Mallat Z, Tedgui A. The role of transforming growth factor beta in atherosclerosis: novel insights and future perspectives. Curr Opin Lipidol 2002; 13: 523–9.

135 Gojova A, Brun V, Esposito B, et al. Specific abrogation of transforming growth factor-beta signaling in T cells alters atherosclerotic lesion size and composition in mice. Blood 2003; 102: 4052–8.

136 Grainger DJ. Transforming growth factor beta and atherosclerosis: so far, so good for the protective cytokine hypothesis. Arterioscler Thromb Vasc Biol 2004; 24: 399–404.

137 Boyle JJ, Bowyer DE, Weissberg PL, Bennett MR. Human blood-derived macrophages induce apoptosis in human plaque-derived vascular smooth muscle cells by Fas-ligand/Fas interactions. Arterioscler Thromb Vasc Biol 2001; 21: 1402–7.

138 Geng YJ, Wu Q, Muszynski M, et al. Apoptosis of vascular smooth muscle cells induced by in vitro stimulation with interferon-gamma, tumor necrosis factor-alpha, and interleukin-1 beta. Arterioscler Thromb Vasc Biol 1996; 16: 19–27.

139 Bostrom K, Watson KE, Horn S, et al. Bone morphogenetic protein expression in human atherosclerotic lesions. J Clin Invest 1993; 91: 1800–9.

140 Shanahan CM, Cary NR, Metcalfe JC, Weissberg PL. High expression of genes for calcification-regulating proteins in human atherosclerotic plaques. J Clin Invest 1994; 93: 2393–402.

141 Giachelli CM, Bae N, Almeida M, et al. Osteopontin is elevated during neointima formation in rat arteries and is a novel component of human atherosclerotic plaques. J Clin Invest 1993; 92: 1686–96.

142 Shanahan CM, Proudfoot D, Tyson KL, et al. Expression of mineralisation-regulating proteins in association with human vascular calcification. Z Kardiol 2000; 89(Suppl 2): 63–8.

143 Steitz SA, Speer MY, Curinga G, et al. Smooth muscle cell phenotypic transition associated with calcification: upregulation of Cbfa1 and downregulation of smooth muscle lineage markers. Circ Res 2001; 89: 1147–54.

144 Proudfoot D, Skepper JN, Hegyi L, et al. Apoptosis regulates human vascular calcification in vitro: evidence for initiation of vascular calcification by apoptotic bodies. Circ Res 2000; 87: 1055–62.

145 Weissberg PL. Noninvasive imaging of atherosclerosis: the biology behind the pictures. J Nucl Med 2004; 45: 1794–5.

146 Kolodgie FD, Burke AP, Farb A, et al. The thin-cap fibroatheroma: a type of vulnerable plaque: the major precursor lesion to acute coronary syndromes. Curr Opin Cardiol 2001; 16: 285–92.

147 Durand E, Scoazec A, Lafont A, et al. In vivo induction of endothelial apoptosis leads to vessel thrombosis and endothelial denudation: a clue to the understanding of the mechanisms of thrombotic plaque erosion. Circulation 2004; 109: 2503–6.

148 Latti S, Leskinen M, Shiota N, et al. Mast cell-mediated apoptosis of endothelial cells in vitro: a paracrine mechanism involving TNF-alpha-mediated down-regulation of bcl-2 expression. J Cell Physiol 2003; 195: 130–8.

149 Sugiyama S, Kugiyama K, Aikawa M, et al. Hypochlorous acid, a macrophage product, induces endothelial apoptosis and tissue factor expression: involvement of myeloperoxidase-mediated oxidant in plaque erosion and thrombogenesis. Arterioscler Thromb Vasc Biol 2004; 24: 1309–14.

150 Kolodgie FD, Burke AP, Farb A, et al. Differential accumulation of proteoglycans and hyaluronan in culprit lesions: insights into plaque erosion. Arterioscler Thromb Vasc Biol 2002; 22: 1642–8.

151 Relou IA, Damen CA, van der Schaft DW, et al. Effect of culture conditions on endothelial cell growth and responsiveness. Tissue Cell 1998; 30: 525–30.

152 Davies MJ, Thomas A. Thrombosis and acute coronary artery lesions in sudden cardiac ischemic death. N Engl J Med 1984; 310: 1137–40.

153 Davies MJ, Bland JM, Hangartner JR, *et al.* Factors influencing the presence or absence of acute coronary artery thrombi in sudden ischaemic death. *Eur Heart J* 1989; **10**: 203–8.

154 Falk E. Plaque rupture with severe pre-existing stenosis precipitating coronary thrombosis. Characteristics of coronary atherosclerotic plaques underlying fatal occlusive thrombi. *Br Heart J* 1983; **50**: 127–34.

155 Frink RJ. Chronic ulcerated plaques: new insights into the pathogenesis of acute coronary disease. *J Invasive Cardiol* 1994; **6**: 173–85.

156 Sitzer M, Muller W, Siebler M, *et al.* Plaque ulceration and lumen thrombus are the main sources of cerebral microemboli in high-grade internal carotid artery stenosis. *Stroke* 1995; **26**: 1231–3.

157 Carr S, Farb A, Pearce WH, *et al.* Atherosclerotic plaque rupture in symptomatic carotid artery stenosis. *J Vasc Surg* 1996; **23**: 755–65.

158 Golledge J, Greenhalgh RM, Davies AH. The symptomatic carotid plaque. *Stroke* 2000; **31**: 774–81.

159 Zaman AG, Helft G, Worthley SG, Badimon JJ. The role of plaque rupture and thrombosis in coronary artery disease. *Atherosclerosis* 2000; **149**: 251–66.

160 Naghavi M, Libby P, Falk E, *et al.* From vulnerable plaque to vulnerable patient: a call for new definitions and risk assessment strategies: Part II. *Circulation* 2003; **108**: 1772–8.

★ 161 Naghavi M, Libby P, Falk E, *et al.* From vulnerable plaque to vulnerable patient: a call for new definitions and risk assessment strategies: Part I. *Circulation* 2003; **108**: 1664–72.

162 Toschi V, Gallo R, Lettino M, *et al.* Tissue factor modulates the thrombogenicity of human atherosclerotic plaques. *Circulation* 1997; **95**: 594–9.

◆ 163 Rich-Edwards JW, Manson JE, Hennekens CH, Buring JE. The primary prevention of coronary heart disease in women. *N Engl J Med* 1995; **332**: 1758–66.

164 Bush TL, Barrett-Connor E, Cowan LD, *et al.* Cardiovascular mortality and noncontraceptive use of estrogen in women: results from the Lipid Research Clinics Program Follow-up Study. *Circulation* 1987; **75**: 1102–9.

● 165 Witteman JC, Grobbee DE, Kok FJ, *et al.* Increased risk of atherosclerosis in women after the menopause. *BMJ* 1989; **298**: 642–4.

● 166 Stampfer MJ, Colditz GA, Willett WC, *et al.* Postmenopausal estrogen therapy and cardiovascular disease. Ten-year follow-up from the nurses' health study. *N Engl J Med* 1991; **325**: 756–62.

167 Isles CG, Hole DJ, Hawthorne VM, Lever AF. Relation between coronary risk and coronary mortality in women of the Renfrew and Paisley survey: comparison with men. *Lancet* 1992; **339**: 702–6.

◆ 168 Farhat MY, Lavigne MC, Ramwell PW. The vascular protective effects of estrogen. *FASEB J* 1996; **10**: 615–24.

● 169 Beral V, Banks E, Reeves G. Evidence from randomised trials on the long-term effects of hormone replacement therapy. *Lancet* 2002; **360**: 942–4.

170 Herrington DM, Espeland MA, Crouse JR, III, *et al.* Estrogen replacement and brachial artery flow-mediated vasodilation in older women. *Arterioscler Thromb Vasc Biol* 2001; **21**: 1955–61.

171 Writing Group for the Women's Health Initiative Investigators. Risks and benefits of estrogen plus progestin in healthy postmenopausal women: Principal results from the Women's Health Initiative randomized controlled trial. *JAMA* 2002; **288**: 321–33.

172 Hulley S, Grady T, Bush T, *et al.* Randomized trial of estrogen plus progestin for secondary prevention of coronary heart disease in post menopausal women. *JAMA* 1998; **280**: 605–13.

173 Grady O, Herrington D, Bittner V, and Heart and Estrogen/progestin Replacement Study Follow-up (HERS II). Cardiovascular disease outcomes during 6–8 years of hormone therapy. *JAMA* 2002; **288**: 49–57.

◆ 174 Rosendaal FR, Helmerhorst FM, Vandenbroucke JP. Oral contraceptives, hormone replacement therapy and thrombosis. *Thromb Haemost* 2001; **86**: 112–23.

3

Metabolic risk factors for vascular disease in women

HOMA KESHAVARZ, D PRABHAKARAN, SONIA ANAND

INTRODUCTION

Gender differences in health are influenced by social, cultural, and biologic factors. Understanding gender differences in health is important because it increases our understanding of the pathogenesis of disease and informs the creation of prevention strategies. This is especially true for the metabolic syndrome, which affects a substantial proportion of women, and is significantly influenced by lifestyle factors such as high energy intake and physical inactivity.

The metabolic syndrome is characterized by a clustering of cardiovascular disease (CVD) risk factors (that is, abdominal obesity, dyslipidemia, dysglycemia, hypertension, and glucose intolerance) with insulin resistance as the underlying theme. Gender differences in the prevalence of metabolic syndrome have been reported from several populations.[1–3] Although these differences are frequently attributed to the biologic differences between men and women, individual abnormalities comprising the metabolic syndrome occur in different frequencies between men and women, and depending on the definition of the metabolic syndrome used may lead to apparent gender differences in the prevalence of the metabolic syndrome. In this chapter we will review the epidemiology, pathogenesis, and treatment approaches of the metabolic syndrome and highlight the gender differences.

DEFINITION AND FEATURES OF THE METABOLIC SYNDROME

In 1988, Reaven described the insulin resistance syndrome which was characterized by hyperinsulinemia, dyslipidemia

(atherogenic lipid profile), hypertension, abdominal obesity, and glucose intolerance or noninsulin dependent diabetes mellitus.[4–6] In 1999 the World Health Organization (WHO)[7] introduced the name 'metabolic syndrome' to formalize this cluster of factors as a clinical entity. In their definition, diabetes mellitus, *or* glucose intolerance, *or* insulin resistance is an essential feature of the metabolic syndrome, in addition to two or more of the factors listed in Table 3.1.

Additional features of this syndrome, not included in the WHO definition of the metabolic syndrome, include biochemical evidence of inflammation, blood coagulation abnormalities (such as elevated plasminogen activator inhibitor type 1 [PAI-1] and fibrinogen levels), and elevated levels of small dense low-density lipoprotein (LDL)-cholesterol, leptin, and uric acid.[8–11] The WHO

Table 3.1 Formalized metabolic syndrome as a clinical entity in women

Factors	Criteria
a	Arterial hypertension
b	Hypertriglyceridemia (triglycerides $\geqslant$1.7 mmol/L or $\geqslant$152 mg/dL) and or low levels of HDL-cholesterol ($<$1.0 mmol/L or $<$39 mg/dL)
c	Central obesity, waist to hip ratio $>$0.85 and or body mass index $>$30 kg/m^2
d	Microalbuminuria (urinary albumin excretion $>$20 μg/min or urinary albumin/creatinine $\geqslant$20 μg/g)

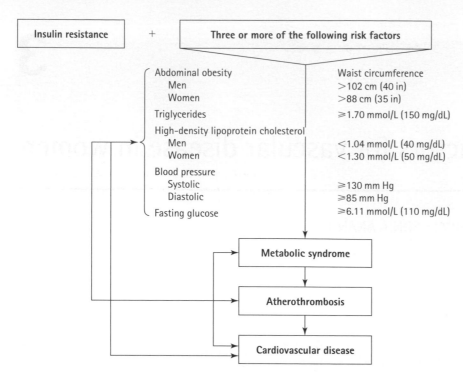

Figure 3.1 Schematic representation of aggregated factors in the metabolic syndrome.

definition was developed as a standardized tool for the purpose of epidemiologic research, and the National Cholesterol Education Programme's adult treatment panel 3 (NCEP-ATP III) describes a set of practical and useful criteria for clinical diagnosis and management of metabolic syndrome.[12] The European Group for the study on Insulin Resistance (EGIR) suggested a set of new criteria to diagnose insulin resistance in nondiabetic individuals. Essentially a modification of the original WHO criteria, this definition excludes microalbuminuria, has a lower threshold for the diagnosis of hypertension, and includes a waist girth of ≥88 cm as evidence of abdominal obesity in women.[13] Despite these variations in the definition of metabolic syndrome, men and women who possess most of these features experience an excess prevalence of CVD compared with individuals without them.[14,15] Although the term 'insulin resistance' is sometimes used interchangeably with the metabolic syndrome, it should be understood that insulin resistance refers to biochemical abnormalities characterized by fasting hyperinsulinemia alone or in combination with hyperglycemia (fasting and postprandial), whereas the metabolic syndrome refers to a clinical entity in which the clustering of both conventional and nonconventional risk factors is associated with a higher likelihood of CVD.

The pathway from insulin resistance to the clinical metabolic syndrome and subsequent development of atherosclerosis is schematically represented in Figure 3.1.

EPIDEMIOLOGY OF METABOLIC SYNDROME

The prevalence of metabolic syndrome in women varies between 20 percent and 50 percent depending on the population studied (Table 3.2). In 8814 men and women aged 20 years or older from the third National Health and Nutrition Examination Survey (NHANES) (between 1988 and 1994), the age-adjusted prevalence of the metabolic syndrome was 24 percent. Worldwide, with the exception of the European population, the prevalence of metabolic syndrome is higher among women than men (Table 3.2). Further a propensity to develop the metabolic syndrome has been observed among populations who are undergoing rapid lifestyle changes characterized by increased energy intake and decreased physical activity, including South Asians, Hispanics, Arabs, and Chinese.[16–19] With increasing urbanization in developing countries, the prevalence of metabolic syndrome is expected to increase severalfold in the coming years. The increasing prevalence of the metabolic syndrome, diabetes, and CVD will have substantial public health implications in these countries, and globally in the following two decades.[17–19]

RISK FACTORS FOR METABOLIC SYNDROME

Environmental factors

OBESITY

Weight gain and overweight are the critical determinants of the metabolic syndrome.[20,21] The primary 'cause' of the weight gain leading to the metabolic syndrome appears to be a change in lifestyle characterized by increased energy intake and decreased energy expenditure. Overweight is predictive of developing metabolic syndrome.[22–24] In the NHANES III survey the group with a body mass index

Table 3.2   Variation in the prevalence of metabolic syndrome by gender and ethnicity

Definition	Country	Age-adjusted prevalence %			Population (study years)
		Women	Men	Both	
NCEP–ATP III guidelines	USA[20]	23.4	24	23.7	US civilians
	White	22.8	24.8	23.8	(1988–94)
	Mexican American	35.6	28.3	31.9	
	African American	25.7	16.4	21.6	
	USA[21]	–	–	55.2	American Indians aged 45–74 years (1989–95)
	Canada[22]			25.8	Random sample of Canadian adults (1996–2000)
	Native Indian	45.4	41.3	41.6	
	South Asian	28.3	23.4	25.9	
	European	14.3	28.8	22.0	
	Chinese	7.1	15.9	11.0	
	India[23]	–	–	–	Urban and rural adult North Indian population, 35–64 years (1991–94)
	Urban	33.4	26.8	30.2	
	Rural	11.6	10.6	11.1	
	Turkey[24]	38.6	27	–	Turkish men and women (1997–2001)
	Finland[25]	–	–	14.2	Middle-aged Finnish men in the Kuopio province (1984–89)
WHO criteria	Finland and Sweden[26]	10.0	15.0	10.0	Finnish and Swedish men and women 35–70 years, with NGT[†](1990)
	Europe[27]	14.2	15.7	15.0	11 prospective European cohort, 30–89 years, (1971–94)
Any three of five risk determinants*	USA[28]	34.0	–	–	Migrant Filipino women in San Diego, USA (1992–99)
IRS[†]	France[29]	12.0	23.0	12.0	French adults 35–64 years (1994–97)
Clustering of hyperglycemia, HT and dyslipidemia[§]	China[30]	–	–	–	Adult Chinese 20–94 years (1998–2000)
N/A	China[31,32]	14.2	12.7	14.2	Adult Chinese 35–64 years (1992)

*Risk determinants: (i) waist circumference >88 cm; (ii) triglycerides ⩾150 mmol/L; (iii) HDL-cholesterol <50 mmol/L; (iv) systolic BP ⩾130 mm Hg or diastolic BP ⩾85 mm Hg or (v) fasting glucose ⩾110 mmol/L.

[†]NGT, Normal glucose tolerance.

[†]IRS, insulin resistance syndrome. Its presence was determined by HOMA ⩾3.8 and presence of antidiabetic drug treatment and/or fasting blood glucose ⩾6.1 mmol/L with at least two of the following: (i) anthropometrical data: BMI ⩾30 kg/m² or a waist-to-hip ratio ⩾0.95 for men or ⩾0.85 for women; (ii) blood pressure (BP) systolic BP >140 or diastolic BP >90 or the presence of antihypertensive treatment; (iii) dyslipidemia: triglyceride level >1.70 mmol/L or HDL level <0.9 mmol/L or triglyceride-lowering drug therapy.

[§]Hyperglycemia: diabetes, impaired fasting glucose or impaired glucose tolerance; HT (hypertension): systolic blood pressure 140 mm Hg or greater and diastolic blood pressure 90 mm Hg or greater; dyslipidemia: triglycerides ⩾1.7 mmol/L or HDL <0.9 mmol/L.

(BMI) greater than 35 kg/m² had a 67.7-fold odds (95 percent confidence interval [CI] 40.5 to 113.3) of having metabolic syndrome as compared with the group with normal BMI.[20] In Canada, the difference in body weight between individuals with and without the metabolic syndrome was reported to be 15 kg (33 lb).[25] Physical inactivity, a common feature among obese individuals, is strongly and inversely associated with obesity and metabolic syndrome.[25,26] The essential role of lifestyle factors in 'causing' the metabolic syndrome is highlighted from studies in

which the prevalence of metabolic syndrome has been reduced with weight loss and regular physical activity.[26,27]

Among nondiabetic adults, waist circumference as a signal detector appears to be the best predictor of metabolic syndrome in both men and women. The optimal cutpoint chosen for waist circumference is similar to NCEP. However, certain components of the metabolic syndrome interact with waist circumference differently in men and women, when predicting the future incidence of metabolic syndrome. Whereas high-density lipoprotein (HDL) levels

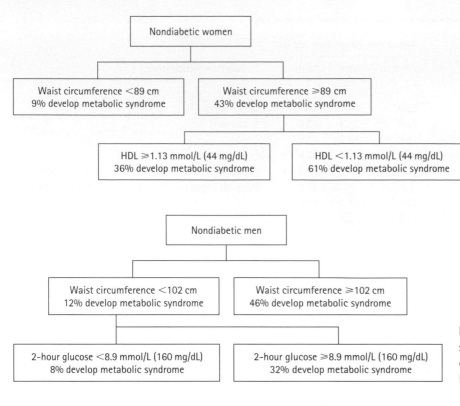

Figure 3.2 Incident of metabolic syndrome in women stratified by waist circumference and high-density lipoprotein (HDL).

Figure 3.3 Prevalence of metabolic syndrome in men stratified by waist circumference and high-density lipoprotein levels.

appear to be a strong predictor of the incidence of metabolic syndrome among nondiabetic women with high waist circumferences, glucose abnormalities contribute to the excess risk for future metabolic syndrome among nondiabetic men with nor-mal waist circumferences. For example, among women 61 percent of the subgroup with waist circumference >89 cm and HDL-cholesterol <1.13 mmol/L (44 mg/dL) developed the metabolic syndrome. Among men the highest risk group is those with waist circumference ≥102 cm (in this group the prevalence of metabolic syndrome is 46 percent)[28–30] (Figs 3.2 and 3.3).

PHYSICAL ACTIVITY AND INACTIVITY

Ecologic data suggest that physical inactivity may be one of the main modifiable risk factors in the etiology of the metabolic syndrome.[31] As physical activity is inherently difficult to measure precisely, epidemiologic studies have primarily demonstrated the association of metabolic risk with self-reported participation in recreational activities.[7,13,32–34] Further, total physical activity (measured as habitual energy expenditure) and fitness (measured as maximal oxygen consumption per kilogram) have independent effects on the components of metabolic syndrome.[35] Body weight and physical fitness modulate insulin action, a core feature of metabolic syndrome. This modulation of metabolic syndrome by physical inactivity may be a plausible biologic pathway through which the risk of coronary heart disease (CHD) is enhanced.[36] The association between physical inactivity and the metabolic syndrome is further supported by the observation that vigorous activity reduces the odds of having metabolic syndrome by approximately 50 percent

compared with those at risk individuals who remain sedentary. Moderate levels of physical activity also reduce the odds of developing the metabolic syndrome by 22 percent.[37,38]

TOBACCO EXPOSURE

Tobacco exposure has been implicated in the pathogenesis of insulin resistance. Smoking impairs insulin action and induces insulin resistance,[39,40] whereas smoking cessation increases insulin sensitivity (measured after 8 weeks of cessation).[41] In a population-based study of 1280 Canadians, those with the metabolic syndrome were significantly more likely to smoke compared to those without the metabolic syndrome.[25] Given the increasing numbers of women who smoke cigarettes worldwide, combined with increased energy intake and decreased physical activity leading to weight gain, an increasing incidence of the metabolic syndrome among women is expected in the next decade (Table 3.3).[42]

Genetic factors

A genetic basis for the metabolic syndrome (insulin resistance) is supported by several lines of reasoning.[43–46] However, genes for the metabolic syndrome have not been clearly identified, except for the rare and heritable forms of insulin resistance, which manifest early in infancy and childhood. Cluster analyses of two large studies, the Kaiser Permanente women twins study[47] and the Framingham offspring study,[48] reveal that only two to three factors

Table 3.3 Risk factors and contributory causes of metabolic syndrome (modified from Grundy[11])

Risk factors	Contributory causes
Atherogenic dyslipidemia	Obesity (especially
Elevated triglycerides (>1.7 mmol/L or 150 mg/dL)	truncal)
Small LDL particles (LDL pattern B)	
Borderline high-risk LDL cholesterol (3.33–4.08 mmol/L or 130–159 mg/dL)	
Low HDL cholesterol (<1.03 mmol/L or 40 mg/dL in men and <1.28 mmoL/L or 50 mg/dL in women)	
• High normal blood pressure (130–139/85–89 mm Hg)	Physical inactivity, obesity, dietary factors
• Insulin resistance ± impaired fasting glucose (6.1–7 mmol/L or 110–126 mg/dL)	Diet, physical inactivity, smoking, aging
• Proinflammatory state*	Unidentified
• Prothrombotic state†	Insulin resistance
• Cigarette smoking	Behavioral and societal factors

*Indicated by elevated high sensitivity C-reactive protein (hs-CRP; >3.0 mmol/L).
†Indicated by elevated plasminogen activator inhibitor-1, elevated fibrinogen, elevated homocysteine (≥1.5 μmol/L), or clotting factor VIIc HDL, high-density lipoprotein; LDL, low-density lipoprotein.

contribute significantly to the variance in the insulin resistance syndrome. These factors include body weight, glucose and insulin, and blood pressure.[49] Hanley and colleagues, who studied 1087 multiethnic nondiabetic men and women (African American, Hispanic and non-Hispanic white) from four clinical centers in the United States, identified two principal factors:

- a 'metabolic factor' comprising BMI, waist circumference, fasting and 2-hour post-load glucose and HDL.
- a 'blood pressure factor' comprising systolic and diastolic blood pressure.

Although this suggests that two independent pathophysiologic processes determine insulin resistance, recent studies suggest that more than two factors may be operative in determining metabolic syndrome.[50–52] Specific gene–environmental interactions may account for the increased prevalence of the metabolic syndrome in certain populations. The etiology of most complex diseases such as obesity, diabetes, and CVD, which affect large numbers of people, is heavily influenced by environmental factors. These may act alone or in combination with specific genetic factors to cause disease states.[53] However, among selected subgroups the susceptibility to a given environment may be modified by their genes.[54] Further a twin pair study has demonstrated a higher genetic influence on glucose intolerance and systolic blood pressure and a lower genetic influence on low HDL-cholesterol and diastolic blood pressure among male twins compared with female twins. This was a small study comprising 303 twin pairs. Therefore the role of genes, and their interactions with environmental factors in influencing gender-specific differences in the pathogenesis of metabolic syndrome, requires further investigation.[54]

Fetal influences

Recently the influence of the maternal–fetal environment has been advocated as an explanatory factor for type 2 diabetes and the metabolic syndrome. The 'Barker hypothesis' suggests that adult-onset cardiovascular risk factors and the insulin resistance syndrome are predicted by birth weight.[55] There is substantial evidence linking low birthweight to the development of adult-onset diabetes and insulin resistance.[56–59] Possible explanations for this include: maternal malnutrition, which results in fetal undernutrition; and compensatory fetal hyperinsulinemia. This produces an efficient utilization of nutrients in fetal life. Although this fetal programming may initially provide a survival advantage, it may also result in an increased propensity in low birthweight babies to develop type 2 diabetes, and CVD, during adulthood. This mechanism is frequently attributed to the burgeoning epidemic of diabetes and CVD (which is determined by many components of the metabolic syndrome) in developing countries.[17] Although this hypothesis is intriguing, it does not sufficiently explain the rural–urban differences in the prevalence of type 2 diabetes in developing countries, the differences in prevalence of type 2 diabetes between native and migrant populations (from developing to developed), or the low prevalence of type 2 diabetes and CVD in Africa where the prevalence of low birthweight is common. Further, recent evidence suggests that it may be rapid catch-up growth rather than low birthweight that is associated with insulin resistance, and this finding is more significant among girls than among boys. Specifically, the EarlyBird study reported that insulin resistance at 5 years was not related to birthweight, but was correlated with current weight and weight catch-up in both sexes, although more strongly so in girls) ($r = 0.33$, $P < 0.001$ vs. $r = 0.18$, $P = 0.03$).[60]

Polycystic ovary syndrome

Polycystic ovarian syndrome (PCOS) is a heterogeneous clinical entity characterized by signs and symptoms of hyperandrogenism and anovulatory disorders, often associated with infertility and obesity. The underlying pathogenesis remains uncertain, although key components of the syndrome may be insulin resistance and hyperinsulinemia.[61,62] Chronic hyperinsulinemia is hypothesized to act synergistically with luteinizing hormone on the ovaries to produce excessive quantities of androgens, resulting in anovulatory disorders. Further, hyperinsulinemia directly reduces serum levels of sex-hormone-binding globulin in obese women with PCOS.[62] Increased androgens may be associated with an increased ratio of visceral to subcutaneous fat, which is significantly correlated with markers of insulin resistance.[63] Recently, data from, two large prospective cohort studies, showed that those women who reported usually irregular or very irregular cycles had a significantly increased risk for CHD and type 2 diabetes.[64,65] They concluded that menstrual cycle irregularity, the most frequent cause of which is PCOS, may be a marker of metabolic abnormalities predisposing to an increased risk for CVD.

PATHOPHYSIOLOGIC FEATURES OF THE METABOLIC SYNDROME

Glucose abnormalities

Insulin resistance, especially among diabetic and obese people, is believed to result from multiple mechanisms including defective insulin signaling, alterations in insulin receptor concentrations, and abnormalities in glucose transport.[66] Elevated blood glucose in the nondiabetic range, referred to as dysglycemia, especially impaired glucose tolerance (IGT), is an important component of the metabolic syndrome.[6] Hyperglycemia is believed to precede overt type 2 diabetes by many years.[67] Therefore it is attractive to speculate that insulin resistance is central to the progression from 'normoglycemia' to 'dysglycemia' (elevated glucose in the nondiabetic range) and from IGT to overt type 2 diabetes. Initial peripheral resistance to insulin action may lead to a state in which there is an increased production of insulin by β cells to maintain normoglycemia. Subsequently the β cells may fail to maintain the required rate of insulin secretion to compensate for the peripheral insulin resistance leading to IGT and diabetes. Dysglycemia in the nondiabetic range has been linked to the progression of atherosclerosis despite the absence of overt diabetes.[68,69] In the Study of Health Assessment and Risk Evaluation in Ethnic Groups (SHARE), the degree of carotid wall atherosclerosis, measured by B-mode carotid ultrasound, was related to the level of HbA_{1c} irrespective of the diabetic status and independent of abdominal obesity and other markers of metabolic syndrome.[70] Similarly in the San Antonio Heart Study, hyperinsulinemia predicted the development of type 2 diabetes, dyslipidemia and hypertension over an 8-year follow-up period.[71]

Although glucose abnormalities are part of the various definitions of metabolic syndrome and are believed to broadly represent insulin resistance, the NCEP criteria may underestimate insulin resistance in metabolic syndrome. This is because the NCEP criteria use impaired fasting glucose (IFG) to represent insulin resistance. Impaired fasting glucose has been postulated to result from a raised hepatic glucose output and a defect in early insulin secretion. Thus

it may not reflect insulin resistance accurately.[72] Impaired glucose tolerance is characterized by peripheral resistance to insulin action and can be used as a surrogate for insulin resistance. Despite these intriguing associations, the exact pathogenesis of insulin resistance leading to impairment in insulin action has not been clearly delineated. However, certain differences between men and women have been noted in the risk of CHD imposed by glucose abnormalities.

Diabetic women have been shown to be at an increased risk of CVD compared with men, with relative risk for CHD varying between 3 and 7 in women and 2 and 3 in men.[73] The reason for this increased risk is unclear. Presence of other established risk factors, such as tobacco smoking may contribute to the increased risk of CHD among women with diabetes.[74]

Lipids

As the metabolism of glucose and fatty acids is associated, it is not surprising that specific lipid abnormalities are widely prevalent among diabetic patients and among nondiabetic people who have insulin resistance.[75–77] These lipid abnormalities primarily include hypertriglyceridemia, and low HDL-cholesterol concentration. Additional lipid abnormalities observed among people with the metabolic syndrome include elevated small dense LDL particles and non-HDL cholesterol fractions: intermediate-density (IDL) and very-low-density lipoproteins (VLDL). Insulin plays a key role in the metabolism of free fatty acids by suppressing their release from adipose tissue, resulting in an increased concentration of plasma free fatty acids.[76,77] Excess plasma free fatty acids lead to an increased flux of free fatty acid to the liver resulting in an increase in hepatic triglyceride VLDL and cholesterol ester synthesis and secretion.[77–79] Also the lipoprotein lipase activity that is already impaired by insulin resistance leads to decreased catabolism of chylomicrons and VLDL. This reduced catabolic activity of lipoprotein lipase leads to a decreased release of lipoprotein particles (which have a surface coat comprising phospholipids, free cholesterol, and apo proteins) that are necessary components in the formation of HDL-cholesterol,[9,80] leading to low HDL-cholesterol levels. Other mechanisms for low HDL-cholesterol in patients with metabolic syndrome include altered or reduced activity of lecithin cholesterol acyltransferase (induced by the altered lipid fractions such as raised VLDL-cholesterol and increased triglycerides)[68,81] and elevated levels of cholesterol ester transfer protein (CETP).[82] In addition to producing these lipid abnormalities, excess plasma free fatty acids are believed to decrease glucose utilization by skeletal muscle, and decrease insulin removal and promote gluconeogenesis in the liver. Sniderman et al. suggest that all these three factors may be critical in the development of insulin resistance and diabetes mellitus.[83] Additional abnormalities include elevated small dense LDL particles, which are highly atherogenic and known to coexist with hypertriglyceridemia and low

HDL levels.[84] The levels of small dense LDL-cholesterol are also directly proportional to the blood glucose levels. The mean LDL size decreases and its subclass distribution is altered when individuals with normal glucose tolerance are compared with people with IGT and diabetes.[85] Lipid abnormalities, diabetes, and insulin resistance have been shown to coexist in many studies[2] and the host of metabolic abnormalities found in the metabolic syndrome may only reflect the interrelationship between the metabolism of lipids and glucose, some of which are understood, others which are not.

Data from NHANES III show that in 1999 over 53 million adult women had total cholesterol levels ≥5.13 mmol/L (200 mg/dL), with an age-adjusted prevalence of 43.3 percent that is roughly equal among ethnic groups. Although women tend to have more favorable lipid profiles than men from the age of 20 to 50 years, after the onset of the menopause cholesterol levels increase in women; as men age, cholesterol levels remain steady. In women under the age of 65 years, high levels of LDL have been shown to be strongly correlated with CHD, and in women over 65 years low levels of HDL appear to be a stronger risk factor. Hypertriglyceridemia also appears to be a significant risk factor in women, especially older women.[86,87]

Elevated blood pressure

Elevated blood pressure (BP) is a key component of the metabolic syndrome and is the most widely studied factor in relation to insulin resistance.[78,88] However, the relation between increased BP and the metabolic syndrome is controversial, as not all people who meet the definition of the metabolic syndrome have elevated BP. Due to the association between blood pressure and body weight, obesity could be a major confounder in the association between elevated BP and insulin resistance. High BP alone is unlikely to be a major cause of insulin resistance as is evident from the lack of association with insulin resistance. It is plausible that insulin resistance could cause an elevation of blood pressure given that hyperinsulinemia increases renal sodium and water reabsorption leading to extracellular volume expansion enhanced sympathetic activity,[89,90] intracellular hypernatremia and vasoconstriction.[91,92] Although the association of insulin resistance and blood pressure in the white Caucasian population is strong, no such relation has been observed in African Americans or Pima Indians, among whom insulin resistance and diabetes are prominent.[93] Factor analysis of a large population from Kinmen in China revealed that hypertension was linked to the metabolic syndrome in women but not in men.[94] The reason for these differences is not known.

Abnormalities in coagulation markers

Several prothrombotic factors (Box 3.1) are abnormal among people with the metabolic syndrome.[77] These

Box 3.1 Coagulation markers increased in metabolic syndrome

- PAI-1
- tPA
- Factor VIIc
- von Willebrand factor
- Factor VIII
- Factor IXc
- Factor Xc
- Fibrinogen
- Homocysteine levels
- Platelet aggregability

abnormalities include: elevated PAI-1, tissue plasminogen activator (tPA), factor VIII, von Willebrand factor, factors VII: C, IX: C, X: C, and fibrinogen.[66] The primary inhibitor of the fibrinolytic system is PAI-1, and it is increased among people with insulin resistance and type 2 diabetes.[10] It has also been associated with CVD in experimental,[95,96] clinical[97,98] and epidemiologic studies.[99] Elevated plasma PAI-1 has been associated with increased cardiovascular events such as angina pectoris, myocardial infarction (MI) and restenosis after coronary angioplasty. In the European Concerted Action on Thrombosis and Disabilities (ECAT) study PAI-1 and tPA antigen did not emerge as predictive factors for CVD after adjustment for other variables contributing to insulin resistance. Elevated levels of tPA predict future MI and stroke both in healthy individuals and in those with type 2 diabetes, IGT, and CHD.[98,99] In the Physician's Health Study, the tPA antigen level increased in a stepwise fashion depending on the number of clinical characteristics associated with insulin resistance.[100]

More recently the clot lysis time, a functional test of fibrinolysis, has been demonstrated to be prolonged among people with the metabolic syndrome compared to those without the metabolic syndrome.[24] In addition, von Willebrand factor and factor VIII levels are positively associated with diabetes, BMI, waist-to-hip ratio, serum insulin, and plasma triglycerides – all components of the metabolic syndrome.[101] Homocysteine, another prothrombotic factor, has been demonstrated to be elevated in patients with the metabolic syndrome,[81,102–104] and is also pathophysiologicaly linked to microalbuminuria, an important component of the metabolic syndrome.[105,106] Some of the procoagulant factors have been demonstrated to be elevated and to predict metabolic syndrome in certain ethnic groups. For example, fibrinogen, tPA, von Willebrand factor, factor XIII and its subunit B have been shown to be increased among insulin-resistant South Asians and to correlate with the components of metabolic syndrome.[107] Insulin also has been shown to influence platelet activity, which plays a key role in the pathogenesis of acute coronary syndromes. The normal platelet inhibitory action of insulin has been demonstrated to be blunted or absent in obese individuals when compared with nonobese individuals.[108] Although the association of prothrombotic factors with insulin resistance is evident, the exact mechanism by which they contribute to CVD appears to be complex, and is currently unclear.

Inflammation

Recently inflammation has emerged as an important predictor of diabetes and CVD.[109] Highly sensitive C-reactive protein (CRP) is a mediator of the acute phase response of inflammation. It is primarily derived from interleukin-6 (IL-6) stimulated hepatic biosynthesis and both IL-6 and CRP are independent predictors of CVD.[110] Elevated levels of IL-6 and CRP are found in patients with insulin resistance and overt type 2 diabetes,[80,110] and elevated CRP, in particular, is an independent predictor of diabetes and future CHD among apparently healthy men and women.[52,111,112] Ridker and colleagues demonstrated that CRP was an independent predictor of future CVD among apparently healthy women in the Women's Health Study who had the metabolic syndrome.[113] Other inflammatory mediators, including tumor necrosis factor-α (TNF-α), and TNF receptor are also elevated in individuals with the metabolic syndrome.[114,115] Thus inflammation may play a role in the pathophysiology of metabolic syndrome through its association with type 2 diabetes or by its association with obesity-mediated cytokine production,[116,117] or both. In this regard adiponectin, a protein secreted by the adipocytes has anti-inflammatory and antiatherogenic properties and has been closely linked to the regulation of CRP and IL-6.[118] Low adiponectin levels have been implicated in the pathogenesis of obesity, linked to the presence of major cardiovascular risk factors such as hypertension and diabetes. Further studies of the role of IL-6, IL-18, and CRP as markers of inflammation in atherosclerosis, endothelial dysfunction, and type 2 diabetes mellitus, as well as their interaction with adiponectin, are required to define the association between inflammatory markers and atherosclerosis, endothelial dysfunction and the metabolic syndrome, and also to define risk stratification criteria and explore the reasons for the differences in risk between genders.

Other factors

Recently leptin, serum uric acid levels, and microalbuminuria have been implicated as risk factors for metabolic syndrome. Some ethnic variability also has been demonstrated with leptin as a risk factor. The operative mechanisms of these factors have not been clearly delineated. Whether uric acid and microalbuminuria are confounders for underlying renal dysfunction or diabetic nephropathy is not clear and requires further investigation.

RISK OF CARDIOVASCULAR DISEASE AND METABOLIC SYNDROME

Individuals with the metabolic syndrome have an increased prevalence of CHD than people without the metabolic syndrome. In the Botnia study,[119] which included people from Sweden and Finland, the relative risk of CHD among those with the metabolic syndrome was 2.96 (95 percent CI 2.36 to 3.72). For MI the relative risk was 2.63 (95 percent CI 1.86 to 3.72) and for death related to cardiovascular causes it was 1.81 (95 percent CI 1.24 to 2.65, $P = 0.002$). Several other studies have demonstrated an increased risk for CHD associated with the metabolic syndrome.[25,120–122] Generally women appear to have higher risk for CHD especially when other risk factors are present. A large, prospective cohort study among women in the United States evaluated the risk of future cardiovascular events among those with the metabolic syndrome. The study found that the risk was increased among those who also had high CRP levels.[115] The age-adjusted relative risk among women with metabolic syndrome who had low and high CRP levels was 2.3 (95 percent CI 1.6 to 3.3) and 4.0 (95 percent CI 3.0 to 5.4), respectively, compared with women without the metabolic syndrome who had low CRP levels at baseline.

The results of a metaanalysis of the risk of CVD mortality associated with the metabolic syndrome defined by different sets of its components are summarized in Table 3.4. In women, with different definitions of the metabolic syndrome, multivariate-adjusted overall hazard ratios (HRs) associated with the presence of the metabolic syndrome ranged from 1.56 to 2.78. In men, the corresponding HRs ranged from 1.74 to 2.26 for CVD mortality.[123]

There continue to be few prospective studies on the relations between the metabolic syndrome and CVD risk. Some of these indicate that the increase in the relative risk associated with the metabolic syndrome is similar in men and women.[124,125]

Table 3.4　Metaanalysis of the Association of the Metabolic Syndrome with the risk of cardiovascular mortality*

Definition of metabolic syndrome	Cardiovascular disease mortality	
	Women	Men
≥2 of the component	1.56 (0.93–2.60)	1.75 (1.28–2.39)
≥3 of the components	2.17 (1.13–4.19)	1.74 (1.19–2.55)
Hyperinsulinemia plus any two or more of the other components	2.78 (1.571–4.94)	2.26 (1.61–3.17)
Hyperinsulinemia plus any three or more of the other components	2.74 (1.21–6.20)	1.98 (1.27–3.10)

*Data are given as hazard ratios (95% confidence interval) adjusted for age, cholesterol levels, and smoking.

MANAGEMENT OF METABOLIC SYNDROME

The goals of treatment and management of the metabolic syndrome are similar between men and women with few exceptions. These include lifestyle modifications, such as caloric restriction and increased physical activity, and drug therapy when indicated. Key issues are the early detection and treatment of the underlying risk factors which make up the syndrome. In particular, there is a need for aggressive management of underlying factors such as hypertension or a mild elevation of blood glucose in patients with metabolic syndrome as compared with their management when they occur in isolation. We do not recommend routine insulin measurements to diagnose metabolic syndrome due to:

- the inability of fasting plasma insulin levels to accurately reflect insulin resistance
- nonavailability of a single standard for assaying plasma insulin levels
- wide variability in the normal range of insulin values
- lack of a universal cut-off point for normal insulin levels
- the complexities involved with HOMA measurements.[126]

Once a clinical diagnosis has been made, decreasing energy intake and increasing physical activity remains the cornerstone of therapy for metabolic syndrome. These factors also play an important role in preventing the development of metabolic syndrome and its components.[127–128] Recent data suggest that long-term consumption of foods with a high glycemic load may increase the risk of CHD by worsening glucose intolerance and dyslipidemia.[133–134] The adverse effects of a high dietary glycemic load are particularly prominent in individuals who are obese and insulin resistant. Various strategies are available, but the most common approach for an overweight person with the metabolic syndrome is a balanced-calorie diet. Several excellent reviews are available detailing the approaches to the dietary modifications of metabolic syndrome.[131] Decreasing dietary glycemic load by reducing the intake of high-glycemic beverages and replacing refined grain products and potatoes with minimally processed plant-based foods such as whole grains, fruits, and vegetables may reduce CHD incidence among people with metabolic syndrome. Other measures include nutritional therapy. Recommendations call for a low intake of saturated fats, *trans*-fats, and cholesterol, reduced consumption of simple sugars, increased intakes of fruits, vegetables, and whole grains, and an avoidance of extremes in carbohydrate or fat intakes. If lifestyle modification is ineffective, drug therapy may be required to achieve treatment goals.[132]

Exercise has the potential to bring about weight loss, increase insulin sensitivity, alter the plasma lipoprotein profile, and improve fibrinolytic activity.[133] These favorable effects likely result from changes in the activity of insulin-sensitive glucose transporters and of skeletal muscle lipoprotein lipase. Aerobic exercise, resistance training and weight loss improves blood pressure and other metabolic factors among obese, sedentary, middle-aged men and women.[132,134] Although the beneficial effects of vigorous physical activity have been documented extensively, recent data suggest that even long-term, moderate, nonvigorous physical activity may be equally effective in reducing the adverse consequences of the metabolic syndrome.[135]

Drug therapy

Appropriate drug therapy should be initiated for the management of clinical hypertension and dyslipidemia, especially among women with PCOS who require control with drugs. The choice of drug should be based on established guidelines for the management of hypertension, dyslipidemia, and diabetes initiated. Modulation of insulin resistance is possible by two classes of drug: the thiazolidinediones and metformin. Apart from their glucose-lowering effects, the thiazolidinediones have multiple nonglucose metabolic effects.[136,137] These novel oral antihyperglycemic agents reduce insulin resistance through binding to and activation of the nuclear receptor, peroxisome proliferator-activated receptor-gamma (PPARγ), with subsequent effects on the glucose and lipid homeostasis. Troglitazone, in the TRoglitazone In the Prevention Of Diabetes (TRIPOD) trial, delayed or prevented the onset of type 2 diabetes during a median follow-up of 30 months, among high-risk Hispanic women with insulin resistance.[138] However, troglitazone was withdrawn in the United Kingdom voluntarily by the manufacturer and in the United States on the directive of the Food and Drug Administration. Two other thiazolidinediones, rosiglitazone and pioglitazone, have been approved for the treatment of type 2 diabetes mellitus and on average lower HbA_{1c} by 1–2 percent. Unlike troglitazone, these drugs have not been associated with liver toxicity.[139] A large clinical trial is underway to determine if these drugs will convert individuals with IGT to normal glucose tolerance, reduce insulin resistance, and prevent diabetes (the Diabetes REduction Approaches with ramipril and rosiglitazone Medications [DREAM] study), thereby becoming the drug of choice among people with the metabolic syndrome.[140]

Metformin, a biguanide, significantly improves glycemic control and lowers insulin resistance and improves plasma lipid levels among those with dysglycemia, polycystic ovarian disease and human immunodeficiency virus infection.[135,141,142] Therefore, metformin could be the drug treatment of choice for people with dysglycemia, especially among those who have failed lifestyle modification. In patients with IGT, lifestyle interventions which bring about weight loss can significantly reduce the incidence of diabetes compared with metformin and control. Recently, the Diabetes Prevention Program randomized trial demonstrated that reducing postprandial hyperglycemic peaks, by a program of weight loss through an improvement of diet (low fat and low calorie), and a moderate increase of physical exercise, lowers the risk for development of type 2 diabetes by 58 percent (95 percent CI 48 to 66; $P < 0.001$) compared with placebo. Treatment with metformin was less effective than lifestyle modification, but was also associated with an average reduction of risk of type 2 diabetes of 31 percent (95 percent CI 17 to 43; $P < 0.001$) compared with placebo.[135,143] These results were also supported by the Finnish diabetes prevention study,[134,144] in which an intensive dietary modification and exercise program was demonstrated to prevent the development of type 2 diabetes among people with IGT. Metformin is used extensively in the management of type 2 diabetes and can reduce peripheral insulin concentrations while improving glucose tolerance and metabolism. A number of studies have shown significant improvements in insulin sensitivity and hyperinsulinemia in obese women with PCOS after metformin administration.[145,146]

Other drugs

Other drugs which have the potential to control glucose abnormalities associated with the metabolic syndrome include the prandial oral antidiabetic agents such as α-glucosidase inhibitors (acarbose, miglitol) and the rapidly acting insulin secretagogues (nateglinide, repaglinide). These drugs improve the control of postprandial hyperglycemia and offer an exciting treatment opportunity.[147,148] The approach of treating patients with IGT with medications to prevent or delay diabetes is rapidly evolving and its benefits need to be confirmed in large, prospective clinical trials.

Patients with diabetes derive substantial benefits from low-dose aspirin as an antiplatelet agent to prevent vascular disease. It also has been shown to be useful in patients with hypertension.[149] However, aspirin when used in a primary prevention strategy for preventing CHD has produced mixed results, especially in women.[150–152] Aside from its use in diabetic people, the role of aspirin in nondiabetic people with the metabolic syndrome is uncertain.

CONCLUSIONS

The metabolic syndrome affects a quarter of women and men in Western countries, and is disproportionately higher among women compared with men of nonwhite ethnicity. The primary determinants of the metabolic syndrome include high energy intake in the face of physical inactivity, which leads to weight gain. Women and men with central adiposity appear to be at particularly high risk of the metabolic syndrome. Weight loss and increased physical activity are effective in reversing many of the metabolic derangements of this syndrome, and drug therapy is reserved for those individuals who are unsuccessful at making these changes.

KEY LEARNING POINTS

- The metabolic syndrome affects a substantial proportion of women, with a worldwide prevalence ranging between 20 percent and 50 percent depending on the population studied and the definition used for the diagnosis.
- The metabolic syndrome appears to be disproportionately high among women from nonwhite ethnic groups.
- The prevalence of metabolic syndrome is enhanced by high energy intake and physical inactivity, which are amenable to preventive strategies.
- The future risk of CVD-related mortality appears to be higher among women as compared with men with the metabolic syndrome.
- Weight loss and increased physical activity are effective in reversing the metabolic derangements in the metabolic syndrome.
- Obese and overweight women should be targeted for prevention and management of the metabolic syndrome.

REFERENCES

1 Srinivasan SR, Wattigney W, Webber LS, Berenson GS. Race and gender differences in serum lipoproteins of children, adolescents, and young adults – emergence of an adverse lipoprotein pattern in white males: the Bogalusa Heart Study. *Prev Med* 1991; **20**: 671–84.

2 Wing RR, Jeffery RW. Effect of modest weight loss on changes in cardiovascular risk factors: are there differences between men and women or between weight loss and maintenance? *Int J Obes Relat Metab Disord* 1995; **19**: 67–73.

3 Beregi E, Regius O, Nemeth J, *et al*. Gender differences in age-related physiological changes and some diseases. *Z Gerontol Geriatr* 1995; **28**: 62–6.

4 Ford ES. The metabolic syndrome and mortality from cardiovascular disease and all-causes: findings from the National Health and Nutrition Examination Survey II Mortality Study. *Atherosclerosis* 2004; **173**: 309–14.

5 Reaven GM. Banting Lecture 1988. Role of insulin resistance in human disease. 1988. *Nutrition* 1997 Jan; **13** (1): 65; discussion 64, 66.

6 Reaven GM, Chen YD. Role of abnormal free fatty acid metabolism in the development of non-insulin-dependent diabetes mellitus. *Am J Med* 1998 Nov 28; **85** (5A): 106–12.

7 Alberti KG, Zimmet PZ. Definition, diagnosis and classification of diabetes mellitus and its complications. Part 1: diagnosis and classification of diabetes mellitus provisional report of a WHO consultation. *Diabet Med* 1998; **15**: 539–53.

★ 8 Yip J, Trevisan R. Microalbuminuria and insulin resistance. In: Reaven MG, ed. *Laws A Insulin Resistance. The Metabolic*

Syndrome X, Contemporary Endocrinology. New Jersey: Totowa, Humana Press, 1999: 309–16.

9 Timar O, Sestier F, Levy E. Metabolic syndrome X: a review. *Can J Cardiol* 2000; **16**: 779–89.

10 Juhan-Vague I, Alessi MC. PAI-1, obesity, insulin resistance and risk of cardiovascular events. *Thromb Haemost* 1997; **78**: 656–60.

11 Grundy SM. Small LDL, atherogenic dyslipidemia, and the metabolic syndrome. *Circulation* 1997; **95**: 1–4.

12 Expert Panel on Detection, Evaluation, and Treatment of High Blood Cholesterol in Adults. Executive Summary of The Third Report of The National Cholesterol Education Program (NCEP) Expert Panel on Detection, Evaluation, And Treatment of High Blood Cholesterol In Adults (Adult Treatment Panel III). *JAMA* 2001; **285**: 2486–97.

13 Balkau B, Charles MA. Comment on the provisional report from the WHO consultation. European Group for the Study of Insulin Resistance (EGIR). *Diabet Med* 1999; **16**: 442–3.

14 Hulthe J, Bokemark L, Wikstrand J, Fagerberg B. The metabolic syndrome, LDL particle size, and atherosclerosis: the Atherosclerosis and Insulin Resistance (AIR) study. *Arterioscler Thromb Vasc Biol* 2000; **20**: 2140–7.

15 Young MH, Jeng CY, Sheu WH, *et al.* Insulin resistance, glucose intolerance, hyperinsulinemia and dyslipidemia in patients with angiographically demonstrated coronary artery disease. *Am J Cardiol* 1993; **72**: 458–60.

16 Grundy SM. Obesity, metabolic syndrome, and coronary atherosclerosis. *Circulation* 2002; **105**: 2696–8.

17 Reddy KS, Yusuf S. Emerging epidemic of cardiovascular disease in developing countries. *Circulation* 1998; **97**: 596–601.

18 Yusuf S, Reddy S, Ounpuu S, Anand S. Global burden of cardiovascular diseases: Part II: variations in cardiovascular disease by specific ethnic groups and geographic regions and prevention strategies. *Circulation* 2001; **104**: 2855–64.

19 Yusuf S, Reddy S, Ounpuu S, Anand S. Global burden of cardiovascular diseases: part I: general considerations, the epidemiologic transition, risk factors, and impact of urbanization. *Circulation* 2001; **104**: 2746–53.

20 Park YW, Zhu S, Palaniappan L, *et al.* The metabolic syndrome: prevalence and associated risk factor findings in the US population from the Third National Health and Nutrition Examination Survey, 1988–1994. *Arch Intern Med* 2003; **163**: 427–36.

21 Reaven G. Metabolic syndrome: pathophysiology and implications for management of cardiovascular disease. *Circulation* 2002; **106**: 286–8.

22 Duncan BB, Chambless LE, Schmidt MI, *et al.* Correlates of body fat distribution. Variation across categories of race, sex, and body mass in the atherosclerosis risk in communities study. The Atherosclerosis Risk in communities (ARIC) Study Investigators. *Ann Epidemiol* 1995; **5**: 192–200.

23 Meigs JB, Wilson PW, Fox CS, *et al.* Body mass index, metabolic syndrome and risk of Type 2 diabetes or

cardiovascular disease. *J Clin Endocrinol Metab* 2006 May 30.

24 Freedman DS, Williamson DF, Croft JB, *et al.* Relation of body fat distribution to ischemic heart disease. The National Health and Nutrition Examination Survey I (NHANES I) Epidemiologic Follow-up Study. *Am J Epidemiol* 1995; **142**: 53–63.

25 Anand SS, Yi Q, Gerstein H, *et al.* Relationship of metabolic syndrome and fibrinolytic dysfunction to cardiovascular disease. *Circulation* 2003; **108**: 420–5.

26 Case CC, Jones PH, Nelson K, *et al.* Impact of weight loss on the metabolic syndrome. *Diabetes Obes Metab* 2002; **4**: 407–14.

27 Irwin ML, Ainsworth BE, Mayer-Davis EJ, *et al.* Physical activity and the metabolic syndrome in a tri-ethnic sample of women. *Obes Res* 2002; **10**: 1030–7.

28 Wei M, Gaskill SP, Haffner SM, Stern MP. Waist circumference as the best predictor of noninsulin dependent diabetes mellitus (NIDDM) compared to body mass index, waist/hip ratio and other anthropometric measurements in Mexican Americans – a 7-year prospective study. *Obes Res* 1997; **5**: 16–23.

29 Palaniappan L, Carnethon MR, Wang Y, *et al.* Predictors of the incident metabolic syndrome in adults: the Insulin Resistance Atherosclerosis Study. *Diabetes Care* 2004; **27**: 788–93.

30 Janssen I, Katzmarzyk PT, Ross R. Body mass index, waist circumference, and health risk: evidence in support of current National Institutes of Health guidelines. *Arch Intern Med* 2002; **162**: 2074–9.

31 Laws A, Reaven GM. Insulin resistance and risk factors for coronary heart disease. *Baillieres Clin Endocrinol Metab* 1993; **7**: 1063–78.

32 Pouliot MC, Despres JP, Lemieux S, *et al.* Waist circumference and abdominal sagittal diameter: best simple anthropometric indexes of abdominal visceral adipose tissue accumulation and related cardiovascular risk in men and women. *Am J Cardiol* 1994; **73**: 460–8.

33 Bloomgarden ZT. American Association of Clinical Endocrinologists (AACE) consensus conference on the insulin resistance syndrome: 25–26 August 2002, Washington, DC. *Diabetes Care* 2003; **26**: 1297–303.

34 Bloomgarden ZT. American Association of Clinical Endocrinologists (AACE) consensus conference on the insulin resistance syndrome: 25–26 August 2002, Washington, DC. *Diabetes Care* 2003; **26**: 933–9.

35 Wareham NJ, Hennings SJ, Byrne CD, *et al.* A quantitative analysis of the relationship between habitual energy expenditure, fitness and the metabolic cardiovascular syndrome [see comment]. *Br J Nutr* 1998; **80**: 235–41.

36 Brunner EJ, Marmot MG, Nanchahal K, *et al.* Social inequality in coronary risk: central obesity and the metabolic syndrome. Evidence from the Whitehall II study. *Diabetologia* 1997; **40**: 1341–9.

37 Rennie KL, McCarthy N, Yazdgerdi S, *et al.* Association of the metabolic syndrome with both vigorous and

moderate physical activity. *Int J Epidemiol* 2003; **32**: 600–6.

38 Cheal KL, Abbasi F, Lamendola C, *et al.* Relationship to insulin resistance of the adult treatment panel III diagnostic criteria for identification of the metabolic syndrome. *Diabetes* 2004; **53**: 1195–200.

39 Attvall S, Fowelin J, Lager I, *et al.* Smoking induces insulin resistance – a potential link with the insulin resistance syndrome. *J Intern Med* 1993; **233**: 327–32.

40 Bennet AM, Brismar K, Hallqvist J, *et al.* The risk of myocardial infarction is enhanced by a synergistic interaction between serum insulin and smoking. *Eur J Endocrinol* 2002; **147**: 641–7.

41 Eliasson B, Attvall S, Taskinen MR, Smith U. Smoking cessation improves insulin sensitivity in healthy middle-aged men. *Eur J Clin Invest* 1997; **27**: 450–6.

42 Carroll S, Cooke CB, Butterly RJ, Gately P. Associations of leisure-time physical activity and obesity with atherogenic lipoprotein-lipid markers among non-smoking middle-aged men. Scandinavian *J Med Sci Sports* 2001; **11**: 38–46.

43 Elbein SC, Maxwell TM, Schumacher MC. Insulin and glucose levels and prevalence of glucose intolerance in pedigrees with multiple diabetic siblings. *Diabetes* 1991; **40**: 1024–32.

44 Haffner SM, Stern MP, Hazuda HP, *et al.* Increased insulin concentrations in nondiabetic offspring of diabetic parents. *N Engl J Med* 1988; **319**: 1297–301.

45 Lillioja S, Mott DM, Zawadzki JK, *et al. In vivo* insulin action is familial characteristic in nondiabetic Pima Indians. *Diabetes* 1987; **36**: 1329–35.

46 Mitchell BD, Kammerer CM, Blangero J, *et al.* Genetic and environmental contributions to cardiovascular risk factors in Mexican Americans. The San Antonio Family Heart Study. *Circulation* 1996; **94**: 2159–70.

47 Edwards KL, Austin MA, Newman B, *et al.* Multivariate analysis of the insulin resistance syndrome in women. *Arterioscler Thromb* 1994; **14**: 1940–5.

48 Meigs JB, D'Agostino RB, Sr, Wilson PW, *et al.* Risk variable clustering in the insulin resistance syndrome. The Framingham Offspring Study. *Diabetes* 1997; **46**: 1594–600.

49 Hanley AJ, Karter AJ, Festa A, *et al.* Factor analysis of metabolic syndrome using directly measured insulin sensitivity: The Insulin Resistance Atherosclerosis Study. *Diabetes* 2002; **51**: 2642–7.

50 Hanley AJ, Connelly PW, Harris SB, Zinman B. Adiponectin in a native Canadian population experiencing rapid epidemiological transition. *Diabetes Care* 2003; **26**: 3219–25.

51 Novak S, Stapleton LM, Litaker JR, Lawson KA. A confirmatory factor analysis evaluation of the coronary heart disease risk factors of metabolic syndrome with emphasis on the insulin resistance factor. *Diabetes Obes Metab* 2003; **5**: 388–96.

52 Shen BJ, Todaro JF, Niaura R, *et al.* Are metabolic risk factors one unified syndrome? Modeling the structure of the metabolic syndrome X. *Am J Epidemiol* 2003; **157**: 701–11.

53 Prentice AM. Obesity and its potential mechanistic basis. *Br Med Bull* 2001; **60**: 51–67.

54 Barsh GS, Farooqi IS, O'Rahilly S. Genetics of body-weight regulation. *Nature* 2000; **404**: 644–51.

55 Barker DJ. Fetal origins of cardiovascular disease. *Ann Med* 1999; **31**(Suppl 1): 3–6.

56 Curhan GC, Willett WC, Rimm EB, *et al.* Birth weight and adult hypertension, diabetes mellitus, and obesity in US men. *Circulation* 1996; **94**: 3246–50.

57 Fall CH, Stein CE, Kumaran K, *et al.* Size at birth, maternal weight, and type 2 diabetes in South India. *Diabet Med* 1998; **15**: 220–7.

58 Valdez R, Athens MA, Thompson GH, *et al.* Birthweight and adult health outcomes in a biethnic population in the USA. *Diabetologia* 1994; **37**: 624–31.

59 Zimmet PZ, Alberti KG. The changing face of macrovascular disease in non-insulin-dependent diabetes mellitus: an epidemic in progress. *Lancet* 1997; **350**(Suppl 1): SI1–SI4.

60 Wilkin TJ, Metcalf BS, Murphy MJ, *et al.* The relative contributions of birth weight, weight change, and current weight to insulin resistance in contemporary 5-year-olds: the EarlyBird Study. *Diabetes* 2002; **51**: 3468–72.

61 Burghen GA, Givens JR, Kitabchi AE. Correlation of hyperandrogenism with hyperinsulinism in polycystic ovarian disease. *J Clin Epidemiol Metab* 1980; **50**: 113–16.

62 Korhonen S, Hippelainen M, Niskanen L, *et al.* Relationship of the metabolic syndrome and obesity to polycystic ovary syndrome: a controlled, population-based study. *Am J Obstet Gynecol* 2001; **184**: 289–96.

63 Bhasin S. Effects of testosterone administration on fat distribution, insulin sensitivity, and atherosclerosis progression. *Clin Infect Dis* 2003; **37** (Suppl 2): S142–9.

64 Tsai EC, Matsumoto AM, Fujimoto WY, Boyko EJ. Association of bioavailability, free, and total testosterone with insulin resistance: influence of sex hormone-binding globulin and body fat. *Diabetes Care* 2004 Apr; **27**(4): 861–8.

65 Solomon CG, Hu FB, Dunaif A, *et al.* Long or highly irregular menstrual cycles as a marker for risk of type 2 diabetes mellitus. *JAMA* 2001 Nov 21: **286**(19): 2421–6.

66 Kohler HP. Insulin resistance syndrome: interaction with coagulation and fibrinolysis. *Swiss Med Wkly* 2002; **132**(19–20): 241–52.

67 Haffner SM. The prediabetic problem: development of non-insulin-dependent diabetes mellitus and related abnormalities. *J Diabetes Complications* 1997; **11**: 69–76.

68 Gerstein HC, Yusuf S. Dysglycaemia and risk of cardiovascular disease. *Lancet* 1996; **347**: 949–50.

69 Gerstein HC, Pais P, Pogue J, Yusuf S. Relationship of glucose and insulin levels to the risk of myocardial infarction: a case-control study. *J Am Coll Cardiol* 1999; **33**: 612–19.

70 Gerstein HC, Anand S, Yi QL, et al. The relationship between dysglycemia and atherosclerosis in South Asian, Chinese, and European individuals in Canada: a randomly sampled cross-sectional study. Diabetes Care 2003; **26**: 144–9.

71 Mitchell BD, Haffner SM, Hazuda HP, et al. The relation between serum insulin levels and 8-year changes in lipid, lipoprotein, and blood pressure levels. Am J Epidemiol 1992; **136**: 12–22.

72 Unwin N, Shaw J, Zimmet P, Alberti KG. Impaired glucose tolerance and impaired fasting glycaemia: the current status on definition and intervention. Diabet Med 2002; **19**: 708–23.

73 Gotto AM. Lipid management in diabetic patients: lessons from prevention trials. Am J Med 2002; **112**: Suppl-26S.

74 Al Delaimy WK, Manson JE, Solomon CG, et al. Smoking and risk of coronary heart disease among women with type 2 diabetes mellitus. Arch Intern Med 2002; **162**: 273–9.

75 Meigs JB. Epidemiology of the metabolic syndrome, 2002. Am J Manag Care 2002; **8**(11 Suppl): S283–S292.

76 McKenney JM. Understanding and treating dyslipidemia associated with noninsulin-dependent diabetes mellitus and hypertension. Pharmacotherapy 1993; **13**: 340–52.

77 Grundy SM. Hypertriglyceridemia, insulin resistance, and the metabolic syndrome. Am J Cardiol 1999; **83**(9B): 25F–29F.

78 Reaven GM. Syndrome X: 6 years later. J Intern Med Suppl 1994; **736**: 13–22.

79 den Boer MA, Voshol PJ, Kuipers F, et al. Hepatic glucose production is more sensitive to insulin-mediated inhibition than hepatic VLDL-triglyceride production. Am J Physiol Endocrinol Metab 2006 Jul 18.

80 Patsch JR, Karlin JB, Scott LW, et al. Inverse relationship between blood levels of high density lipoprotein subfraction 2 and magnitude of postprandial lipemia. Proc Natl Acad Sci U S A 1983; **80**: 1449–53.

81 Dieplinger H, Zechner R, Kostner GM. The in vitro formation of HDL2 during the action of LCAT: the role of triglyceride-rich lipoproteins. J Lipid Res 1985; **26**: 273–82.

82 Bagdade JD, Lane JT, Subbaiah PV, et al. Accelerated cholesteryl ester transfer in noninsulin-dependent diabetes mellitus. Atherosclerosis 1993; **104**(1–2): 69–77.

83 Sniderman AD, Scantlebury T, Cianflone K. Hypertriglyceridemic hyperapob: the unappreciated atherogenic dyslipoproteinemia in type 2 diabetes mellitus. Ann Intern Med 2001; **135**(6): 447–59.

84 Gray RS, Robbins DC, Wang W, et al. Relation of LDL size to the insulin resistance syndrome and coronary heart disease in American Indians. The Strong Heart Study. Arterioscler Thromb Vasc Biol 1997; **17**: 2713–20.

85 Austin MA, Mykkanen L, Kuusisto J, et al. Prospective study of small LDLs as a risk factor for non-insulin-dependent diabetes mellitus in elderly men and women. Circulation 1995; **92**: 1770–8.

86 Mazza A, Tikhonoff V, Schiavon L, Casiglia E. Triglycerides plus high-density lipoprotein-cholesterol dyslipidaemia, a coronary risk factor in elderly women: the CArdiovascular STudy in the ELderly. Intern Med J 2005 Oct; **35**(10): 604–10.

87 Bello N, Mosca L. Epidemiology of coronary heart disease in women. Prog Cardiol Dis 2004; **46**: 287–95.

88 Rowe JW, Young JB, Minaker KL, et al. Effect of insulin and glucose infusions on sympathetic nervous system activity in normal man. Diabetes 1981; **30**: 219–25.

89 Blaustein MP. Sodium ions, calcium ions, blood pressure regulation, and hypertension: a reassessment and a hypothesis. Am J Physiol 1977; **232**: C165–C173.

90 Sowers JR, Epstein M. Diabetes mellitus and associated hypertension, vascular disease, and nephropathy. An update. Hypertension 1995; **26**(6 Pt 1): 869–79.

91 Canessa M, Brugnara C, Escobales N. The Li+-Na+ exchange and Na+-K+-Cl- cotransport systems in essential hypertension. Hypertension 1987; **10**(5 Pt 2): I4–10.

92 Saad MF, Lillioja S, Nyomba BL, et al. Racial differences in the relation between blood pressure and insulin resistance. N Engl J Med 1991; **324**: 733–9.

93 Weyer C, Pratley RE, Snitker S, et al. Ethnic differences in insulinemia and sympathetic tone as links between obesity and blood pressure. Hypertension 2000 Oct; **36**(4): 531–7.

94 Chen CH, Lin KC, Tsai ST, Chou P. Different association of hypertension and insulin-related metabolic syndrome between men and women in 8437 nondiabetic Chinese. Am J Hypertens 2000; **13**(7): 846–53.

95 Carmeliet P, Stassen JM, Schoonjans L, et al. Plasminogen activator inhibitor-1 gene-deficient mice. II. Effects on hemostasis, thrombosis, and thrombolysis. J Clin Invest 1993; **92**: 2756–60.

96 Carmeliet P, Bouche A, De Clercq C, et al. Biological effects of disruption of the tissue-type plasminogen activator, urokinase-type plasminogen activator, and plasminogen activator inhibitor-1 genes in mice. Ann N Y Acad Sci 1995; **748**: 367–81.

97 Salomaa V, Stinson V, Kark JD, et al. Association of fibrinolytic parameters with early atherosclerosis. The ARIC Study. Atherosclerosis Risk in Communities Study. Circulation 1995; **91**: 284–90.

98 Juhan-Vague I, Pyke SD, Alessi MC, et al. Fibrinolytic factors and the risk of myocardial infarction or sudden death in patients with angina pectoris. ECAT Study Group. European Concerted Action on Thrombosis and Disabilities. Circulation 1996; **94**(9): 2057–63.

99 Meade TW, Ruddock V, Stirling Y, et al. Fibrinolytic activity, clotting factors, and long-term incidence of ischaemic heart disease in the Northwick Park Heart Study. Lancet 1993; **342**: 1076–9.

100 Ridker PM, Vaughan DE, Stampfer MJ, et al. Endogenous tissue-type plasminogen activator and risk of myocardial infarction. Lancet 1993; **341**: 1165–8.

● 101   Coca M, Cucuianu M, Hancu N. Effect of abdominal obesity on prothrombotic tendency in type 2 diabetes. Behavior of clotting factors VII and VIII, fibrinogen and von Willebrand Factor. *Rom J Intern Med* 2005; **43**(1–2): 115–26.

● 102   Hoogeveen EK, Kostense PJ, Beks PJ, *et al.* Hyperhomocysteinemia is associated with an increased risk of cardiovascular disease, especially in non-insulin-dependent diabetes mellitus: a population-based study. *Arterioscler Thromb Vasc Biol* 1998; **18**: 133–8.

★ 103   Giltay EJ, Hoogeveen EK, Elbers JM, *et al.* Insulin resistance is associated with elevated plasma total homocysteine levels in healthy, non-obese subjects. *Atherosclerosis* 1998; **139**: 197–8.

● 104   Meigs JB, Jacques PF, Selhub J, *et al.* Fasting plasma homocysteine levels in the insulin resistance syndrome: the Framingham offspring study. *Diabetes Care* 2001; **24**: 1403–10.

● 105   Choi HS, Ryu SH, Lee KB. The Relationship of Microalbuminuria with Metabolic Syndrome. *Nephron Clin Pract* 2006 Jun 19; **104**(2):c85–c93.

● 106   Bonnet F, Marre M, Halimi JM, Stengel B, Lange C, Laville M, Tichet J, Balkau B; DESIR Study Group. Waist circumference and the metabolic syndrome predict the development of elevated albuminuria in non-diabetic subjects: the DESIR Study. *J Hypertens* 2006 June; **24**(6): 1157–63.

● 107   Kain K, Catto AJ, Young J, *et al.* Increased fibrinogen, von Willebrand factor and tissue plasminogen activator levels in insulin resistant South Asian patients with ischaemic stroke. *Atherosclerosis* 2002; **163**: 371–6.

● 108   Westerbacka J, Yki-Jarvinen H, Turpeinen A, *et al.* Inhibition of platelet-collagen interaction: an *in vivo* action of insulin abolished by insulin resistance in obesity. *Arterioscler Thromb Vasc Biol* 2002; **22**: 167–72.

● 109   Ridker PM, Hennekens CH, Buring JE, Rifai N. C-reactive protein and other markers of inflammation in the prediction of cardiovascular disease in women. *N Engl J Med* 2000; **342**: 836–43.

◆ 110   Blake GJ, Ridker PM. Inflammatory bio-markers and cardiovascular risk prediction. *J Intern Med* 2002; **252**: 283–94.

● 111   Bermudez EA, Rifai N, Buring J, *et al.* Interrelationships among circulating interleukin-6, C-reactive protein, and traditional cardiovascular risk factors in women. *Arterioscler Thromb Vasc Biol* 2002; **22**: 1668–73.

◆ 112   Albert MA, Ridker PM. The role of C-reactive protein in cardiovascular disease risk. *Curr Cardiol Rep* 1999; **1**: 99–104.

● 113   Ridker PM, Buring JE, Cook NR, Rifai N. C-reactive protein, the metabolic syndrome, and risk of incident cardiovascular events: an 8-year follow-up of 14 719 initially healthy American women. *Circulation* 2003; **107**: 391–7.

◆ 114   Sethi JK, Hotamisligil GS. The role of TNF alpha in adipocyte metabolism. *Semin Cell Dev Biol* 1999; **10**: 19–29.

● 115   Moon YS, Kim DH, Song DK. Serum tumor necrosis factor-alpha levels and components of the metabolic syndrome in obese adolescents. *Metabolism* 2004 Jul; **53**(7):863–7.

● 116   Gabriely I, Ma XH, Yang XM, *et al.* Removal of visceral fat prevents insulin resistance and glucose intolerance of aging: an adipokine-mediated process? *Diabetes* 2002; **51**: 2951–8.

● 117   Stefan N, Stumvoll M, Vozarova B, *et al.* Plasma adiponectin and endogenous glucose production in humans. *Diabetes Care* 2003; **26**: 3315–19.

● 118   Whitehead JP, Richards AA, Hickman IJ, *et al.* Adiponectin – a key adipokine in the metabolic syndrome. *Diabetes Obes Metab* 2006 May; **8**(3): 264–80.

● 119   Isomaa B, Almgren P, Tuomi T, *et al.* Cardiovascular morbidity and mortality associated with the metabolic syndrome. *Diabetes Care* 2001; **24**: 683–9.

★ 120   Resnick HE, Strong HS. Metabolic syndrome in American Indians. *Diabetes Care* 2002; **25**: 1246–7.

● 121   Araneta MR, Wingard DL, Barrett-Connor E. Type 2 diabetes and metabolic syndrome in Filipina-American women: a high-risk nonobese population. *Diabetes Care* 2002; **25**: 494–9.

● 122   Lakka HM, Laaksonen DE, Lakka TA, *et al.* The metabolic syndrome and total and cardiovascular disease mortality in middle-aged men. *JAMA* 2002; **288**: 2709–16.

● 123   Hu G, Qiao Q, Tuomilehto J, *et al.* Prevalence of the metabolic syndrome and its relation to all-cause and cardiovascular mortality in nondiabetic European men and women. *Arch Intern Med* 2004; **164**: 1066–76.

● 124   Maggi S, Noale M, Gallina P, Bianchi D, Marzari C, Limongi F, Crepaldi G; ILSA Working Group. Metabolic syndrome, diabetes, and cardiovascular disease in an elderly Caucasian cohort: the Italian Longitudinal Study on Aging. *J Gerontol A Biol Sci Med Sci* 2006 May; **61**(5): 505–10.

● 125   Hu G; DECODE Study Group. Gender difference in all-cause and cardiovascular mortality related to hyperglycemia and newly-diagnosed diabetes. *Diabetologia* 2003 May; **46**(5): 608–17.

● 126   Matthews DR, Hosker JP, Rudenski AS *et al.* Homeostasis Model Assessment – Insulin Resistance and Beta-Cell Function from Fasting Plasma-Glucose and Insulin Concentrations in Man. *Diabetologia* 1985: **28**(7): 412–19.

◆ 127   Buemann B, Tremblay A. Effects of exercise training on abdominal obesity and related metabolic complications. *Sports Med* 1996; **21**: 191–212.

● 128   Dengel DR, Pratley RE, Hagberg JM, *et al.* Distinct effects of aerobic exercise training and weight loss on glucose homeostasis in obese sedentary men. *J Appl Physiol* 1996; **81**: 318–25.

◆ 129   Liu S, Willett WC. Dietary glycemic load and athero-thrombotic risk. *Curr Atheroscler Rep* 2002; **4**: 454–61.

● 130   Liu S, Willett WC, Stampfer MJ, *et al.* A prospective study of dietary glycemic load, carbohydrate intake, and risk of coronary heart disease in US women. *Am J Clin Nutr* 2000; **71**: 1455–61.

131   Jenkins DJ, Kendall CW, Augustin LS, *et al.* Glycemic index: overview of implications in health and disease. *Am J Clin Nutr* 2002; **76**: 266S–273S.

132   Dengel DR, Hagberg JM, Pratley RE, *et al.* Improvements in blood pressure, glucose metabolism, and lipoprotein lipids after aerobic exercise plus weight loss in obese, hypertensive middle-aged men. *Metabolism* 1998; **47**: 1075–82.

133   Mayer-Davis EJ, D'Agostino R, Jr, Karter AJ, *et al.* Intensity and amount of physical activity in relation to insulin sensitivity: the Insulin Resistance Atherosclerosis Study. *JAMA* 1998; **279**: 669–74.

134   Tuomilehto J, Lindstrom J, Eriksson JG, *et al.* Prevention of type 2 diabetes mellitus by changes in lifestyle among subjects with impaired glucose tolerance. *N Engl J Med* 2001; **344**: 1343–50.

135   Knowler WC, Barrett-Connor E, Fowler SE, Hamman RF, Lachin JM, Walker EA *et al.* Reduction in the incidence of type 2 diabetes with lifestyle intervention or Metformin. *N Engl J Med* 2002; **346**: 393–403.

136   Schmitz OE, Brock B, Madsbad S, Beck-Nielsen H. [Thiazolidinediones – a new class of oral antidiabetics]. *Ugeskr Laeger* 2001; **163**: 6106–11.

137   Lebovitz HE. Rationale for and role of thiazolidinediones in type 2 diabetes mellitus. *Am J Cardiol* 2002; **90**(5A): 34G–41G.

138   Buchanan TA, Xiang AH, Peters RK, *et al.* Preservation of pancreatic beta-cell function and prevention of type 2 diabetes by pharmacological treatment of insulin resistance in high-risk hispanic women. *Diabetes* 2002; **51**: 2796–803.

139   Fuchtenbusch M, Standl E, Schatz H. Clinical efficacy of new thiazolidinediones and glinides in the treatment of type 2 diabetes mellitus. *Exp Clin Endocrinol Diabetes* 2000; **108**: 151–63.

140   The DREAM trial Investigators. Rationale, design and recruitment characteristics of a large, simple international trial of diabetes prevention: the DREAM trial. *Diabetologia* 2004 Sep; **47**(9): 1519–27. Epub 2004 Aug 21.

141   Leclair C, Patton PE. Advances in polycystic ovary syndrome treatment: Metformin and ovarian diathermy. *Curr Womens Health Rep* 2002; **2**: 333–7.

142   van Wijk JP, de Koning EJ, Cabezas MC, *et al.* Comparison of rosiglitazone and metformin for treating HIV lipodystrophy: a randomized trial. *Ann Intern Med* 2005 Sep 6; **143**(5): 337–46.

143   Haffner SM. Can reducing peaks prevent type 2 diabetes: implication from recent diabetes prevention trials. *Int J Clin Pract Suppl* 2002: 33–9.

144   Uusitupa M, Louheranta A, Lindstrom J, *et al.* The Finnish Diabetes Prevention Study. *Br J Nutr* 2000; **83**(Suppl 1): S137–S142.

145   Acbay O, Gundogdu S. Can metformin reduce insulin resistance in polycystic ovary syndrome? *Fertil Steril* 1996; **65**: 946–9.

146   Ehrmann DA, Cavaghan MK, Imperial J, *et al.* Effects of metformin on insulin secretion, insulin action, and ovarian steroidogenesis in women with polycystic ovary syndrome. *J Clin Epidemiol Metab* 1997; **82**: 524–30.

147   Davies MJ. Insulin secretagogues. *Curr Med Res Opin* 2002; **18**(Suppl 1): s22–s30.

148   Chiasson JL, Josse RG, Gomis R, *et al.* Acarbose for prevention of type 2 diabetes mellitus: the STOP-NIDDM randomised trial. *Lancet* 2002; **359**: 2072–7.

149   Hansson L, Zanchetti A, Carruthers SG, *et al.* Effects of intensive blood-pressure lowering and low-dose aspirin in patients with hypertension: principal results of the Hypertension Optimal Treatment (HOT) randomised trial. HOT Study Group. *Lancet* 1998; **351**: 1755–62.

150   Final report on the aspirin component of the ongoing Physicians' Health Study. Steering Committee of the Physicians' Health Study Research Group. *N Engl J Med* 1989; **321**: 129–35.

151   Peto R, Gray R, Collins R, *et al.* Randomised trial of prophylactic daily aspirin in British male doctors. *Br Med J (Clin Res Ed)* 1988; **296**: 313–16.

152   Cook NR, Lee IM, Gaziano JM, *et al.* Low-dose aspirin in the primary prevedntion of cancer: the Women's Health Study: a randomized controlled trial. *JAMA* 2005 Jul 6; **294**(1): 47–55.

4

Genetic factors in vascular disease

DILYS FREEMAN

INTRODUCTION

The study of genetic factors in vascular disease is complex. Vascular diseases have many clinical manifestations (phenotypes) that vary in severity and with age of onset. This is due to the multiple biologic pathways underlying the pathology. These pathways are influenced by many genes with small, and overlapping, individual contributions to disease risk. Furthermore the pathways are influenced by environment to varying extents. Because of the complex interactions between multiple genetic and environmental factors, it is difficult to identify genes influencing susceptibility to common polygenic disorders such as vascular disease. Nevertheless, genetic studies are of value because they afford the opportunity to identify determinants of disease that are likely to be causative.

The study of genetics also allows identification of novel molecular targets against which therapeutic interventions might be designed. An individual is born with their genotype, and it does not change throughout life. Thus assessment of genotype is not open to confounding by the disease process itself or the form of expression the disease takes in an individual. Recent technological and bioinformatic advances made in sequencing the human genome and cataloging polymorphic markers throughout its length have brought new possibilities to the study of genetics in vascular disease.

This chapter will address the usefulness of genetics as diagnostic tests and the most common types of genetic study. The literature on genetic studies in vascular disease is inundated with small, inconclusive, and underpowered studies. Therefore in attempting to summarize genetic factors in vascular disease in women the discussion will be limited, where possible, to large metaanalyses. The focus will be on cardiovascular disease (CVD), which is of increasing prevalence in women; venous thromboembolism (VTE), which is of particular importance to women as a complication of pregnancy and due to the interaction of the disease with exogenous sex hormones; and preeclampsia, a poorly understood vascular condition of pregnancy associated with both poor maternal and poor fetal outcomes.

GENETICS AS A DIAGNOSTIC TEST

Most commonly, genetic variants have been studied to identify diagnostic tests to add to the repertoire of biochemical screening tests for disease. Genetic factors are inherently useful screening tools as they are not influenced by diet, physiology, or concomitant medications. They are also easy and quick tests to carry out once DNA is available. The hope is to identify genotypes, perhaps composite, which might identify an individual's risk of disease. Developing strategies to identify at-risk individuals to target intervention is an important public health challenge.

Much resource has been directed toward research into identifying genes that are robust and reproducible predictors for complex diseases but the investment has not yet paid off in terms of diagnostic tests. Just because it is now much easier to carry out genomic research does not mean that such an approach is useful in all disorders. Merikangas and Risch[1] discuss the characteristics of complex disorders which are most amenable to study by genomics research and conclude that complex diseases with the strongest evidence for a genetic etiology (familial aggregation), where there is limited ability to modify environmental risk factors, and with the highest public health impact should be targeted. Interventions focused on genes associated with rare diseases will have little impact on public health, whereas even a small reduction in risk for common diseases may have major public health implications. From these considerations vascular diseases are good candidates for study.

The value of genetic tests for assessing risk of disease has recently been discussed comprehensively.[2] It is not yet a given that genetic testing will be more useful clinically over and above the current phenotypic, usually blood biochemistry, tests that are available. In the review by Humphries et al.[2] this point is demonstrated admirably by the example of apoE genotype and prediction of coronary heart disease (CHD) events. Addition of apoE genotype to PROCAM risk score (comprising age, body mass index [BMI], total cholesterol, triglycerides, systolic blood pressure, and family history) in a receiver operator curve (ROC) analysis of CHD event prediction did not add significant improvement to the accuracy of the ROC value of PROCAM score alone despite apoE genotype being significantly associated with CHD risk (see Table 4.1 below). Analogous to current clinical tests, a genetic test must be easily measured, inexpensive and have high reproducibility and reliability. Genotypes can predict levels of an intermediate trait that confers risk for disease but may not provide any additional risk information. Indeed, the intermediate trait can often be influenced by environmental factors and as such may provide better prediction than the genotype alone.

TYPES OF GENETIC STUDY

The study of genetic factors in vascular disease is longstanding and much research was carried out long before the introduction of new genomic technologies. Different approaches have different advantages and disadvantages that relate to the number of genes that contribute to disease risk and the size of effect of each individual gene. If the number of genes contributing to disease are few and have large effects then these should be easier to find than if there are many contributing genes with smaller effects on disease.

Family history

Recording of family history has long been used as a tool to assess risk of disease and is a method of assessing genetic susceptibility, albeit in a rather blunt fashion. A family history reflects genetic susceptibility in addition to other potential environmental factors (or in utero factors) and as such can be a useful tool for assessing risk. As family history

reflects both environmental and genetic risk factors it may be a better indicator than genetic risk factors alone. There are problems associated with using a family history.

- A lack of a standard definition of the disease can lead to misclassification errors.
- Often it is difficult to verify the self-report of disease and recall bias comes into play.
- The level to which family history should be extended, that is, parents only or first, second or third generation family members is not clear.
- It is also difficult to assess the levels of confounding factors.

Nonetheless, the presence of a family history for premature cardiovascular disease death has been listed as a risk factor by the National Cholesterol Education Program.[3]

Linkage studies

Linkage studies examine the coinheritance of common sections of chromosome with disease between family members. If the genetic effects are large, then family linkage studies are effective ways of finding genes associated with a disease trait and this has been the common method of identifying genes involved in single-gene disorders. However, when the disease has relatively low heritability as in vascular disease, large scale linkage studies are less effective. For example it is unlikely that one major gene contributes to the risk of preeclampsia. Genome-wide linkage scans have identified a number of chromosomal regions of interest: 9p13, 10q22,[4–6] and several locations on chromosome 2.[4,7,8] The observations linking chromosome 2 to preeclampsia have been replicated in a number of populations prompting a call for the preeclampsia-linked locus on chromosome 2 to be designated 'PREG1'.[8] The linkage approach has recently identified a new candidate gene for preeclampsia located on 10q22, STOX1, that controls polyploidization of extravillous trophoblasts.[6] However, these chromosomal loci only explain a small proportion of the overall cases of preeclampsia.

Twin studies

Twin studies compare the concordance for disease between pairs of monozygotic and dizygotic twins. If monozygotic twins share a similar risk of disease to a greater extent than dizygotic twins, then this indicates that there is a genetic contribution to the etiology of the disease. The assumption in these studies is that twins have similar environments. However this does not always hold up and consequently, twin studies can overestimate the genetic contribution to a disease. In the case of CHD, a large twin study[9] indicated a significant contribution of genetics to CHD. If male monozygotic twins were compared, the relative risk for the second twin having fatal CHD, if the first had died of CHD before the age of 55, was 8.1 (95 percent confidence interval [CI] 2.7 to 24.5). However, if male dizygotic twins were compared, the relative risk was only 3.8 (95 percent CI 1.4 to 10.5). When female twins were compared the relative risk of fatal CHD in the second twin, when the first twin had died of CHD before the age of 65 was 15.0 (95 percent CI 7.1 to 31.9) for monozygotic twins and 2.6 (95 percent CI 1.0 to 7.1) for dizygotic twins. The difference in relative risk between monozygotic and dizygotic twins became less pronounced as the age at which the fatal event took place increased. This suggests that the risk attributable to genes is larger at younger ages and becomes less pronounced in older individuals.

Genetic association studies

The most frequently used genetic studies in vascular disease research are the genetic association studies. Because of their widespread use, it is worth going into some detail about the caveats of such studies. Genetic association studies attempt to correlate the presence of a specific allele of a gene with disease within a population. When a disease has relatively low heritability as in vascular disease, such large-scale population association studies can be effective because they have greater power to resolve small effects.

The most common approach to genetic association studies has been the candidate gene approach. An hypothesis, usually based on current biologic understanding of the disease process, is generated to select a candidate gene which, should the activity of its product be altered, might be expected to influence the expression of the disease trait. Genetic variants or polymorphisms in, or near, the candidate gene are identified. These variants are often common single nucleotide polymorphisms (SNPs), which occur when one of two different nucleotides is present at corresponding positions on different chromosomes. On average, SNPs are present once every 100 base pairs throughout the genome.[10] Other types of polymorphism such as insertion/deletion polymorphisms and variable length repeat sequences (variable nucleotide tandem repeats [VNTRs]) are also present. Polymorphisms are selected that are known to have, or might potentially have, effects on gene product level or function either by being located in a coding sequence or in the promoter region of a gene. A population under study is then genotyped for the candidate polymorphism and statistical methods are used to determine whether a particular gene allele is associated with the disease phenotype of choice. Candidate gene studies subscribe to the 'common disease – common variant model' where the variants within a candidate gene conferring susceptibility to disease will be common within the population (>5 percent).[11] It is likely that the effect of any given polymorphism on risk of disease will be small. Using the candidate gene approach, outcomes selected can either be the intermediate phenotype or a disease endpoint. There is some advantage to selecting disease endpoints because these are ostensibly easier to measure than complex biomolecules in plasma and indeed many intermediate phenotypes are not yet possible to measure in biologic populations, for example, apoptosis. Also the clinician requires an assessment of the risk for disease event and not a surrogate or intermediate. If genes are associated with disease endpoints then it raises the possibility of intervention in the biologic pathway identified.

Many polymorphisms are studied that do not have direct effects on gene product expression or function, but are in linkage disequilibrium with other polymorphisms that do. The term linkage disequilibrium refers to a nonrandom relation between two alleles that typically arises because those alleles are closely sited on the same chromosome and therefore infrequently separated from one another by recombination at meiosis. Recently it has been shown for the human genome that linkage disequilibrium is structured in blocks of variable lengths (up to tens of kilobases).[12,13] Within these blocks there exists substantial linkage disequilibrium between polymorphic markers. The blocks are interspersed with recombination 'hotspots' where there is marginal disequilibrium.[12,13] Some ethnic populations, for example, African populations, have less extensive blocks of linkage disequilibrium than others.[14,15] It has been suggested that these linkage disequilibrium differences between populations might be exploited by using populations with a greater degree of linkage disequilibrium to coarse map genes and then repeating analyses in a low linkage disequilibrium population for finer mapping.[16] This approach has been used to narrow down the location of a quantitative trait locus near the ACE gene for plasma angiotensin-converting enzyme (ACE) levels.[16]

With technological advances it is increasingly easy to type numerous SNPs. Taking together the large databases containing SNP locations and the existence of blocks of linkage disequilibrium raises the possibility that 'large hypothesis' experiments could be carried out.[11] This would consist of a genome-wide survey of SNPs in vascular disease with no a priori knowledge of the potential role of the genes in the disease. This would allow an unbiased assessment of the contribution of all genes to vascular disease and could identify novel risk pathways. Such an approach is currently limited by cost and throughput, and the lack of appropriate bioinformatic and biostatistical approaches to interpret the huge volume of data that would be generated. Most candidate genes identified so far contribute very little to overall risk of disease. In order to reliably detect such small risk estimates large studies need to be undertaken to achieve reliable risk estimates with small confidence intervals. Basing clinical management decisions on unreliable data is inadvisable and the data generated from the majority of studies in the literature are just not robust enough. Often metaanalyses have been used to try to circumvent this problem and obtain more accurate estimates of risk.

A number of criticisms might be leveled at genetic association studies,[17,18] including lack of reproducibility and generation of false-positive associations using high throughput methods. However, many concerns can be alleviated by good study design. Confirmation of positive associations in independent secondary populations, large study sizes with adequate power and supporting phenotypic information from the same population, that is, plasma levels or activity of the gene product or an appropriate plasma marker are all hallmarks of robust genetic association studies. The large majority of published genetic association studies suffer from small sample size and lack of statistical power. Statistical evidence for associations between polymorphic markers and disease may be due to chance. A good review of factors affecting statistical power in the detection of genetic association was published recently by Gordon and Finch.[19] It has been recommended that a minimum requirement for a genetic marker to be included in a cardiovascular risk assessment would be a metaanalysis based on data from a minimum of three different independent studies with at least a total of 1000 cases.[2] This would be appropriate for a relatively common polymorphism (frequency > 0.3) and would provide 80 percent power to detect a relative risk of 1.25 at $P < 0.05$. However for more infrequent polymorphisms, the total number of cases may need to rise dramatically.[2] The bottom line is that studies should be designed to have the highest possible power.[19]

Another problem with genetic association studies is phenotype error, a common problem in complex diseases. The most frequent form of this is due to locus heterogeneity. Individuals with phenotypically indistinguishable forms of a disease may have mutations in different genes leading to expression of the same phenotype. This might be explained by the fact that a disrupting polymorphism in any gene forming part of a disease pathway can result in the same disease phenotype. A further limitation of risk estimates obtained is that the majority have been determined in Caucasian males and so estimates in women and in other ethnic groups are often not available. This is obviously particularly relevant for women's vascular health as the effect of a genetic polymorphism on a quantitative trait may be influenced by gender. An example of this type of effect is seen with variation at the *APOE* gene where relative to ε3,3 homozygotes, ε3,2 heterozygote women are protected and ε4,3 and ε4,4 men are more susceptible to CHD.[20] In addition, the effects of variation at *APOE* on lipid metabolism are manifest differently in women from men and change throughout the woman's life cycle.[21] Women overall are at lower risk of vascular disease than men, thus it is not apparent that risk estimates for genes derived from a high risk male population will be applicable to the female population.

GENETIC FACTORS IN CARDIOVASCULAR DISEASE, VENOUS THROMBOEMBOLISM, AND PREECLAMPSIA

To form an impression of the consensus of studies assessing the contribution of genetic factors to cardiovascular disease, venous thromboembolism, and preeclampsia, data from some recent metaanalyses which adhere to the criteria recommended by Humphries,[2] that is, a minimum of three different independent studies with at least a total of 1000 cases, have been summarized where available. Metaanalyses attempt to summarize data and compensate for small underpowered studies. There are many more studies in the literature of numerous candidate genes but the power of the data is insufficient to make a good assessment of the contribution of these genes to disease. It should be kept in mind that metaanalyses are open to publication bias where positive associations are most likely to be published thus leading to overestimate of the true effect. Agema *et al.*[22] show evidence for such publication bias in their metaanalysis of the association between the insertion/deletion polymorphism in the *ACE* gene and restenosis (Table 4.1). In order to avoid this in future, Colhoun *et al.*[18] have recommended that an automated form of metaanalysis based on web-based submission of data would be a useful way forward.

Cardiovascular disease

The candidate gene approach has been used widely in the study of cardiovascular disease and there is an abundance of data in the literature incorporating a variety of candidate genes and studies of various sizes. It is beyond the scope of this chapter to cover all these studies in detail. Genetic association studies in the field of cardiovascular research have benefited from the large numbers of biobanks of DNA and associated phenotypic data available from epidemiologic studies and clinical trials. However, most of these studies have been carried out in men. The data from a number of metaanalyses are presented in Table 4.1 to give an overall impression of the strength of some of the genetic associations observed.

Candidate genes studied represent a wide variety of pathologic pathways including coagulation, lipid metabolism, blood pressure, inflammation, homocysteine metabolism, and vascular function (see Table 4.1). The affect on risk afforded by the gene variants is, as has been anticipated, small for each individual gene, for example, in the order of 10–30 percent. However, as can be seen for situations where more than one metaanalysis is available, usually using overlapping datasets, consistent effects can be observed, for example, in the *ACE* and *PON* genes.

Venous thromboembolism

The R506Q mutation in the factor V gene, commonly known as factor V Leiden (*FVL*), is associated with risk of venous thrombosis. This mutation has a high prevalence and penetrance and there are many advocates that genetic screening for this mutation in certain situations is required. This mutation occupies ground between that of a monogenic high penetrance mutation (such as familial hypercholesterolemia) and the common gene polymorphisms with relatively modest contributions to disease. As venous thrombosis can be fatal and there is a high risk of recurrence,

Table 4.1   Metaanalyses of candidate gene polymorphisms and cardiovascular disease

Study	Disease	Metaanalysis size No. studies (n cases/ n controls)	Candidate genes	Odds ratio (95% [*99%] confidence intervals)
Coagulation				
Iacoviello et al., 1998[23]	MI	9 (1521/2120)	PAI-1 promoter −675 (4G/5G)	1.30 (1.07 to 1.58)
Di Castelnuovo et al., 2001[24]	CAD and revascularization	34 (9095/12508)	Glycoprotein IIIa (PLA1/PLA2)	CAD 1.10 (1.03 to 1.18) Revas 1.31 (1.10 to 1.56)
Wu and Tsongalis 2001[25]	CAD	8 (1818/3789)	Factor II (G20210A)	1.15 (0.84 to 1.59)
		9 (2323/3108)	Factor V Leiden	1.24 (0.96 to 1.60)
		6 (1258/1316)	Factor VII (R353Q)	0.78 (0.65 to 0.93)
		9 (3788/4132)	Glycoprotein IIIa receptor (PI$^{A1/A2}$)	1.12 (1.01 to 1.24)
		10 (2419/3225)	MTHFR (C677T)	1.30 (1.11 to 1.52)
Burzotta et al., 2004[26]	CHD	19 (4944/7090)	Prothrombin G20210A	1.21 (0.99 to 1.59)
Lipid metabolism				
Wilson et al., 1996[27]	CVD	9 (2383/3972)	Apo E ε2 (referent ε3)	0.98 (0.85 to 1.14)
			ε4	1.26 (1.13 to 1.41)
Song et al., 2004[28]	CHD	48 (15492/32965)	Apo E ε2 (referent ε3)	0.98 (0.66 to 1.46)
			ε4	1.42 (1.26 to 1.61)
Chiodini et al., 2003[29]	CAD, MI	20 (2731/3346)	Apo B XbaI	1.14 (0.88 to 1.48)
		15 (1816/2054)	Apo B Eco RI	1.32 (1.14 to 1.54)
		22 (6007/5609)	Apo B SpIns/Del	1.15 (1.06 to 1.24)
Boekholdt et al., 2005[30]	CHD	7 (2857/8815)	CETP *TaqIB*	0.78 (0.66 to 0.93)
Mackness et al., 2001[31]	CHD	19 (not quoted)	PON R192	1.16 (1.00 to 1.35)
Lawlor et al., 2004[32]	CHD	39 (10738/17068)	PON R192	1.14 (1.08 to 1.20)
Wheeler et al., 2004[33]	CHD	43 (11212/12786)	PON R192	1.12 (1.07 to 1.16)
Blood pressure				
Samani et al., 1996[34]	MI	15 (3394/5479)	ACE DD	1.26 (1.15 to 1.39)
Agerholm-Larsen et al., 2000[35]	MI	19 (4192/14472)	ACE DD	1.21 (1.11 to 1.32)
Bonnici et al., 2002[36]	Coronary restenosis	16 (1683/2948)	ACE DD	1.23 (1.03 to 1.46)*
Agema et al., 2002[22]	Coronary restenosis	12 (1077/2073)	ACE DD	1.22 (1.04 to 1.44)*
Inflammation				
Allen et al; 2001[37]	CHD	4 (1585/1418)	TNFα -308	0.98 (0.85 to 1.13)
Homocysteine				
Wald et al., 2002[38]	MI	48 (12193/11945)	MTHFR C677T	1.21 (1.06 to 1.39)
Vascular function				
Casas et al., 2003[39]	MI	26 (9867/13161)	eNOS E298D	1.31 (1.13 to 1.51)

CAD, coronary artery disease; CHD, coronary heart disease; CVD, cardiovascular disease; MI, myocardial infarction.

identification of high-risk patients who are genetically susceptible to deep vein thrombosis (DVT) would be clinically useful. *FVL* carriers occur with a frequency of around 5 percent in European populations (2–11 percent).[40] Around 16–30 percent of individuals who have a DVT are *FVL* carriers.[41–43] Another prothrombotic mutation, the prothrombin *F2* G20210A mutation, is more weakly associated with recurrent DVT.[44,45] Carriers of both mutations are at considerably increased risk for DVT compared with noncarriers.[46–48] Screening may potentially be useful and could be of benefit

to a patient with a DVT to suggest earlier or more aggressive treatment. However, although screening for the *FVL* mutation has a good positive predictive value and a low false-positive rate, it has not been proved to be cost effective for men or women with a first DVT.[49–51] Since the *FVL* mutation only accounts for a small proportion of the total DVT events then a negative result for a genetic screen for the mutation is relatively meaningless.

Pregnancy will expose mothers to a number of factors which may interact with her genetic makeup. Thus her risk of disease may be increased, or decreased, in ways that would not have been observed had she remained nulliparous. *FVL* is also associated with vascular complications of pregnancy. Recently, a systematic review of heritable forms of thrombophilia and pregnancy outcome was carried out,[52] in which 80 studies were included. The main heritable forms of thrombophilia reviewed were antithrombin deficiency, protein C deficiency, protein S deficiency, the *FVL* mutation, prothrombin G20210A polymorphism and the methylene tetrahydrofolate reductase (*MTHFR*) C677T polymorphism. Strong associations for VTE in pregnancy for *FVL* (odds ratio [OR] 34.40, 95 percent CI 9.86 to 120.05) and prothrombin G20210A (OR 23.89, 95 percent CI 1.13 to 507.08) were observed. Other vascular pregnancy complications were also associated with the *FVL* and prothrombin G20210A inherited thrombophilias including early pregnancy loss, late pregnancy loss, preeclampsia (additionally associated with *MTHFR* C677T), placental abruption, and intrauterine growth restriction. Thus women with a genetic thrombophilia are more likely to experience an adverse pregnancy outcome. Pregnant women who are *FVL* 506Q carriers could be offered prophylactic anticoagulant therapy. However in a similar manner to the situation described for VTE in the nonpregnant population, it has also not been proved to be cost effective to screen for *FVL* in pregnant women.[53]

An interaction of gender with polymorphisms in the factor VII gene has been described.[54] Polymorphisms in the *FVII* gene affecting plasma factor VII had larger effects on plasma levels in men rather than women and a statistically significant interaction term was found for gender. Gender-specific genetic effects may occur because of the potential of polymorphisms in the estrogen receptor to affect clinical outcome of estrogen administration.[55] Furthermore interaction between prothrombotic mutations such as the *FVL* and prothrombin genes and the exogenous estrogen in oral contraceptive and hormone replacement therapy formulations can occur. The risk for VTE associated with *FVL* is amplified by exposure to oral contraceptives and the risk associated with activated protein C resistance is amplified by hormone replacement therapy use.[56,57] Similarly, hormone replacement therapy is associated with an increased risk of atherothrombotic disease in the presence of the prothrombin G20210A mutation.[58] More dramatically, Psaty *et al.*[59] studied a subgroup of postmenopausal women with hypertension. In this group the prothrombin G20210A mutation was associated with an increased risk for myocardial infarction (OR 4.32, 95 percent CI 1.52 to 12.1). However, when they compared nonusers of hormone replacement therapy with wild-type prothrombin G20210A genotype to current users who carried the rare prothrombin mutation, the latter women were at nearly 11-fold increased risk of a nonfatal myocardial infarction (OR 10.9, 95 percent CI 2.15 to 55.2). However the numbers in these groups were very small (n = 8 events) and so these data should be interpreted with caution. It has been advocated[55] that these interactions may contribute to the increased risk for arterial disease shortly after commencing hormone replacement therapy and the pattern of early harm and late benefit seen in the Heart and Estrogen/progestin Replacement Study (HERS) trial.[60] Large-scale studies looking at different genetic effects in men and women have not been carried out and the observations seen in small studies may be due to chance.

Preeclampsia

Preeclampsia is a complication of pregnancy described elsewhere in this book. The question here is: To what extent is preeclampsia genetic? Like cardiovascular disease, the contribution of genetic factors to preeclampsia is indicated by family history of the disease as a risk factor.[61–63] However, there is a low concordance for preeclampsia in monozygotic twins and there is a recognized increased risk in multiparous gestations with different fathers which suggest that the fetal genotype may also contribute to the genetic risk for preeclampsia.[64] This is supported by the fact that both men and women whose mother had preeclampsia during pregnancy are at increased risk of having a child in whom pregnancy is complicated by preeclampsia.[65] A recent population-based study of 1 118 207 births in Sweden[66] indicated a genetic component in the development of preeclampsia. Full sisters and mother-daughters were more likely to both have preeclampsia (OR 3.3, 95 percent CI 3.0 to 3.6 and OR 2.6, 95 percent CI 1.6 to 4.3, respectively) than maternal half-sisters (OR 1.4, 95 percent CI 0.9 to 2.2) and paternal half-sisters (OR 1.0, 95 percent CI 0.6 to 1.6). The heritability estimate for preeclampsia was 31 percent.

Many candidate genes have been proposed to contribute to genetic risk of preeclampsia: *MTHFR*, *APOE*, *LPL*, *eNOS*, and *FVL* among others. However, the majority of studies have been small and the case selection diverse. Good-sized populations for genetic association studies are difficult to collect for preeclampsia because of its relatively infrequent, sudden presentation and the many clinical forms it may take, which makes standardized clinical diagnosis difficult. Few metaanalyses have been carried out to try to clarify the literature. Studies have indicated a role for *FVL* in the development of preeclampsia[52,67,68] but only one of these,[52] the largest, found an association with the prothrombin mutation. Similarly, such metaanalyses disagree with regard to the role of the *MTHFR* mutation[52,67,69,70] with again just the larger metaanalysis showing an association[52] and other smaller metaanalyses only further confusing the issue.[69,70] Many of these metaanalyses of genetic associations in preeclampsia highlight the heterogeneity between studies.[68,69]

There is clearly a need for large multicenter studies for the genetic analysis of preeclampsia. In preeclampsia there is the additional complication of trying to assess the contribution of fetal genotype. The Genetics of Pre-Eclampsia (GOPEC) study was set up to address the need for large studies.[71] Additionally this collaborative group set out to analyse the contribution of fetal genotype. The group looked at variation in the maternal and fetal genes coding for angiotensinogen, the angiotensin receptors, *FVL*, *MTHFR*, *NOS*, and *TNFA*, and concluded that none conferred a high risk of preeclampsia.

CONCLUSIONS

The study of genetic factors in vascular disease in women to date has been rather unsatisfactory for a number of reasons. First, many genetic studies of vascular disease have been carried out in all-male populations, and it is not clear whether results can be extrapolated to females. Many studies, especially of vascular disease in pregnancy, are just too small and underpowered to provide any conclusive data. Metaanalyses of genetic effects in cardiovascular disease have demonstrated some consistent effects of genes, however, in the case of vascular complications of pregnancy for which data are much more sparse the results of metaanalyses have been rather inconsistent. In vascular complications of pregnancy, case ascertation has presented problems as diagnostic criteria are not universal and often the contribution of fetal genotype is not assessed. Advances in technology allow for the speedier, cheaper analysis of many polymorphisms simultaneously. The challenge facing the researcher is to accumulate large biobanks of material comprising sufficient numbers of samples to allow adequately powered studies. It is likely that researchers will need to collaborate both nationally and internationally to achieve this aim.

KEY LEARNING POINTS

- Genetic studies can provide clues on the etiology of a disease, provide screening tests, identify those most at risk from environmental factors, or those who might most benefit from intervention.
- Most genetic association data in vascular disease have been collected from male populations.
- Metaanalyses show that the contribution of many genes to disease risk is small.
- The majority of published genetic association studies are too small and underpowered to provide meaningful data.
- Gene–environment interactions may be particularly relevant in women when taking exogenous estrogens.
- There is an urgent need for large biobanks of material from women with vascular disease, including in pregnancy, with clearly agreed diagnostic criteria and accompanying phenotypic data.

REFERENCES

1 Merikangas KR, Risch N. Genomic priorities and public health. *Science* 2003; **302**: 599–601.

2 Humphries SE, Ridker PM, Talmud PJ. Genetic testing for cardiovascular disease susceptibility: a useful clinical management tool or possible misinformation? *Arterioscler Thromb Vasc Biol* 2004; **24**: 628–36.

3 Summary of the second report of the National Cholesterol Education Program (NCEP) Expert Panel on Detection, Evaluation, and Treatment of High Blood Cholesterol in Adults (Adult Treatment Panel II). *JAMA* 1993; **269**: 3015–23.

4 Laivuori H, Lahermo P, Ollikainen V, *et al.* Susceptibility loci for preeclampsia on chromosomes 2p25 and 9p13 in Finnish families. *Am J Hum Genet* 2003; **72**: 168–77.

5 Oudejans CB, Mulders J, Lachmeijer AM, *et al.* The parent-of-origin effect of 10q22 in pre-eclamptic females coincides with two regions clustered for genes with down-regulated expression in androgenetic placentas. *Mol Hum Reprod* 2004; **10**: 589–98.

6 van Dijk M, Mulders J, Poutsma A, *et al.* Maternal segregation of the Dutch preeclampsia locus at 10q22 with a new member of the winged helix gene family. *Nat Genet* 2005; **37**: 514–19.

7 Arngrimsson R, Sigurardóttir S, Frigge ML, *et al.* A genome-wide scan reveals a maternal susceptibility locus for pre-eclampsia on chromosome 2p13. *Hum Mol Genet* 1999; **8**: 1799–805.

8 Moses EK, Lade JA, Guo G, *et al.* A genome scan in families from Australia and New Zealand confirms the presence of a maternal susceptibility locus for pre-eclampsia, on chromosome 2. *Am J Hum Genet* 2000; **67**: 1581–5.

9 Marenberg ME, Risch N, Berkman LF, *et al.* Genetic susceptibility to death from coronary heart disease in a study of twins. *N Engl J Med* 1994; **330**: 1041–6.

10 Woodage T, Venter JC, Broder S. Application of the human genome to obstetrics and gynecology. *Clin Obstet Gynecol* 2002; **45**: 711–29.

11 Keavney B. Genetic epidemiological studies of coronary heart disease. *Int J Epidemiol* 2002; **31**: 730–6.

12 Daly MJ, Rioux JD, Schaffner SF, *et al.* High-resolution haplotype structure in the human genome. *Nat Genet* 2001; **29**: 229–32.

13 Jeffreys AJ, Kauppi L, Neumann R. Intensely punctate meiotic recombination in the class II region of the major histocompatibility complex. *Nat Genet* 2001; **29**: 217–22.

14 Johnson GC, Esposito L, Barratt BJ, *et al.* Haplotype tagging for the identification of common disease genes. *Nat Genet* 2001; **29**: 233–7.

15 McKenzie CA, Julier C, Forrester T, *et al.* Segregation and linkage analysis of serum angiotensin I-converting enzyme levels: evidence for two quantitative-trait loci. *Am J Hum Genet* 1995; **57**: 1426–35.

16 McKenzie CA, Abecasis GR, Keavney B, *et al.* Trans-ethnic fine mapping of a quantitative trait locus for circulating angiotensin I-converting enzyme (ACE). *Hum Mol Genet* 2001; **10**: 1077–84.

17 Tabor HK, Risch NJ, Myers RM. Opinion: Candidate-gene approaches for studying complex genetic traits: practical considerations. *Nat Rev Genet* 2002; **3**: 391–7.

18 Colhoun HM, McKeigue PM, Davey SG. Problems of reporting genetic associations with complex outcomes. *Lancet* 2003; **361**: 865–72.

19 Gordon D, Finch SJ. Factors affecting statistical power in the detection of genetic association. *J Clin Invest* 2005; **115**: 1408–18.

20 Frikke-Schmidt R, Tybjaerg-Hansen A, Steffensen R, *et al.* Apolipoprotein E genotype: epsilon32 women are protected while epsilon43 and epsilon44 men are susceptible to ischemic heart disease: the Copenhagen City Heart Study. *J Am Coll Cardiol* 2000; **35**: 1192–9.

21 Frikke-Schmidt R, Sing CF, Nordestgaard BG, Tybjaerg-Hansen A. Gender- and age-specific contributions of additional DNA sequence variation in the 5' regulatory region of the APOE gene to prediction of measures of lipid metabolism. *Hum Genet* 2004; **115**: 331–45.

22 Agema WR, Jukema JW, Zwinderman AH, van der Wall EE. A meta-analysis of the angiotensin-converting enzyme gene polymorphism and restenosis after percutaneous transluminal coronary revascularization: evidence for publication bias. *Am Heart J* 2002; **144**: 760–8.

23 Iacoviello L, Burzotta F, Di Castelnuovo A, *et al.* The 4G/5G polymorphism of PAI-1 promoter gene and the risk of myocardial infarction: a meta-analysis. *Thromb Haemost* 1998; **80**: 1029–30.

24 Di Castelnuovo A, de Gaetano G, Donati MB, Iacoviello L. Platelet glycoprotein receptor IIIa polymorphism PLA1/PLA2 and coronary risk: a meta-analysis. *Thromb Haemost* 2001; **85**: 626–33.

25 Wu AH, Tsongalis GJ. Correlation of polymorphisms to coagulation and biochemical risk factors for cardiovascular diseases. *Am J Cardiol* 2001; **87**: 1361–6.

26 Burzotta F, Paciaroni K, De Stefano V, *et al.* G20210A prothrombin gene polymorphism and coronary ischaemic syndromes: a phenotype-specific meta-analysis of 12 034 subjects. *Heart* 2004; **90**: 82–6.

27 Wilson PW, Schaefer EJ, Larson MG, Ordovas JM. Apolipoprotein E alleles and risk of coronary disease. A meta-analysis. *Arterioscler Thromb Vasc Biol* 1996; **16**: 1250–5.

28 Song Y, Stampfer MJ, Liu S. Meta-analysis: apolipoprotein E genotypes and risk for coronary heart disease. *Ann Intern Med* 2004; **141**: 137–47.

29 Chiodini BD, Barlera S, Franzosi MG, *et al.* APO B gene polymorphisms and coronary artery disease: a meta-analysis. *Atherosclerosis* 2003; **167**: 355–66.

30 Boekholdt SM, Sacks FM, Jukema JW, *et al.* Cholesteryl ester transfer protein TaqIB variant, high-density lipoprotein cholesterol levels, cardiovascular risk, and efficacy of pravastatin treatment: individual patient meta-analysis of 13,677 subjects. *Circulation* 2005; **111**: 278–87.

31 Mackness B, Davies GK, Turkie W, *et al.* Paraoxonase status in coronary heart disease: are activity and concentration more important than genotype? *Arterioscler Thromb Vasc Biol* 2001; **21**: 1451–7.

32 Lawlor DA, Day IN, Gaunt TR, *et al.* The association of the PON1 Q192R polymorphism with coronary heart disease:

findings from the British Women's Heart and Health cohort study and a meta-analysis. *BMC Genet* 2004; **5**: 17.

33 Wheeler JG, Keavney BD, Watkins H, *et al.* Four paraoxonase gene polymorphisms in 11212 cases of coronary heart disease and 12786 controls: meta-analysis of 43 studies. *Lancet* 2004; **363**: 689–95.

34 Samani NJ, Thompson JR, O'Toole L, *et al.* A meta-analysis of the association of the deletion allele of the angiotensin-converting enzyme gene with myocardial infarction. *Circulation* 1996; **94**: 708–12.

35 Agerholm-Larsen B, Nordestgaard BG, Tybjaerg-Hansen A. ACE gene polymorphism in cardiovascular disease: meta-analyses of small and large studies in whites. *Arterioscler Thromb Vasc Biol* 2000; **20**: 484–92.

36 Bonnici F, Keavney B, Collins R, Danesh J. Angiotensin-converting enzyme insertion or deletion polymorphism and coronary restenosis: meta-analysis of 16 studies. *BMJ* 2002; **325**: 517–20.

37 Allen RA, Lee EM, Roberts DH, *et al.* Polymorphisms in the TNF-alpha and TNF-receptor genes in patients with coronary artery disease. *Eur J Clin Invest* 2001; **31**: 843–51.

38 Wald DS, Law M, Morris JK. Homocysteine and cardiovascular disease: evidence on causality from a meta-analysis. *BMJ* 2002; **325**: 1202.

39 Casas JP, Bautista LE, Humphries SE, Hingorani AD. Endothelial nitric oxide synthase genotype and ischemic heart disease: meta-analysis of 26 studies involving 23028 subjects. *Circulation* 2004; **109**: 1359–65.

40 Juul K, Tybjaerg-Hansen A, Steffensen R, *et al.* Factor V Leiden: The Copenhagen City Heart Study and 2 meta-analyses. *Blood* 2002; **100**: 3–10.

41 Ridker PM, Miletich JP, Stampfer MJ, *et al.* Factor V Leiden and risks of recurrent idiopathic venous thromboembolism. *Circulation* 1995; **92**: 2800–2.

42 Simioni P, Prandoni P, Lensing AW, *et al.* The risk of recurrent venous thromboembolism in patients with an Arg506→Gln mutation in the gene for factor V (factor V Leiden). *N Engl J Med* 1997; **336**: 399–403.

43 Eichinger S, Pabinger I, Stumpflen A, *et al.* The risk of recurrent venous thromboembolism in patients with and without factor V Leiden. *Thromb Haemost* 1997; **77**: 624–8.

44 Miles JS, Miletich JP, Goldhaber SZ, *et al.* G20210A mutation in the prothrombin gene and the risk of recurrent venous thromboembolism. *J Am Coll Cardiol* 2001; **37**: 215–18.

45 Ridker PM, Hennekens CH, Miletich JP. G20210A mutation in prothrombin gene and risk of myocardial infarction, stroke, and venous thrombosis in a large cohort of US men. *Circulation* 1999; **99**: 999–1004.

46 Margaglione M, D'Andrea G, Colaizzo D, *et al.* Coexistence of factor V Leiden and Factor II A20210 mutations and recurrent venous thromboembolism. *Thromb Haemost* 1999; **82**: 1583–7.

47 De Stefano, V, Martinelli I, Mannucci PM, *et al.* The risk of recurrent deep venous thrombosis among heterozygous

carriers of both factor V Leiden and the G20210A prothrombin mutation. *N Engl J Med* 1999; **341**: 801–6.

48   Marchetti M, Quaglini S, Barosi G. Cost-effectiveness of screening and extended anticoagulation for carriers of both factor V Leiden and prothrombin G20210A. *Q J Med* 2001; **94**: 365–72.

49   Yang Q, Khoury MJ, Botto L, *et al.* Improving the prediction of complex diseases by testing for multiple disease-susceptibility genes. *Am J Hum Genet* 2003; **72**: 636–49.

50   Sarasin FP, Bounameaux H. Decision analysis model of prolonged oral anticoagulant treatment in factor V Leiden carriers with first episode of deep vein thrombosis. *BMJ* 1998; **316**: 95–9.

51   Eckman MH, Singh SK, Erban JK, Kao G. Testing for factor V Leiden in patients with pulmonary or venous thromboembolism: a cost-effectiveness analysis. *Med Decis Making* 2002; **22**: 108–24.

52   Robertson L, Wu O, Langhorne P, *et al.* Thrombophilia in pregnancy: a systematic review. *Br J Haematol* 2006; **132**: 171–96.

53   Clark P, Twaddle S, Walker ID, *et al.* Cost-effectiveness of screening for the factor V Leiden mutation in pregnant women. *Lancet* 2002; **359**: 1919–20.

54   Di Castelnuovo A, D'Orazio A, Amore C, *et al.* Genetic modulation of coagulation factor VII plasma levels: contribution of different polymorphisms and gender-related effects. *Thromb Haemost* 1998; **80**: 592–7.

55   Rossouw JE. Hormones, genetic factors, and gender differences in cardiovascular disease. *Cardiovasc Res* 2002; **53**: 550–7.

56   Vandenbroucke JP, Koster T, Briet E, *et al.* Increased risk of venous thrombosis in oral-contraceptive users who are carriers of factor V Leiden mutation. *Lancet* 1994; **344**: 1453–7.

57   Lowe G, Woodward M, Vessey M, *et al.* Thrombotic variables and risk of idiopathic venous thromboembolism in women aged 45–64 years. Relationships to hormone replacement therapy. *Thromb Haemost* 2000; **83**: 530–5.

58   Glueck CJ, Wang P, Fontaine RN, *et al.* Interaction of estrogen replacement therapy with the thrombophilic 20210 G/A prothrombin gene mutation for atherothrombotic vascular disease: a cross-sectional study of 275 hyperlipidemic women. *Metabolism* 2001; **50**: 360–5.

59   Psaty BM, Smith NL, Lemaitre RN, *et al.* Hormone replacement therapy, prothrombotic mutations, and the risk of incident nonfatal myocardial infarction in postmenopausal women. *JAMA* 2001; **285**: 906–13.

60   Hulley S, Grady D, Bush T, *et al.* Randomized trial of estrogen plus progestin for secondary prevention of coronary heart disease in postmenopausal women. Heart and Estrogen/progestin Replacement Study (HERS) Research Group. *JAMA* 1998; **280**: 605–13.

61   Chesley LC, Annitto JE, Cosgrove RA. The familial factor in toxemia of pregnancy. *Obstet Gynecol* 1968; **32**: 303–11.

62   Cincotta RB, Brennecke SP. Family history of pre-eclampsia as a predictor for pre-eclampsia in primigravidas. *Int J Gynaecol Obstet* 1998; **60**: 23–7.

63   Dekker GA, Sibai BM. Etiology and pathogenesis of preeclampsia: current concepts. *Am J Obstet Gynecol* 1998; **179**: 1359–75.

64   Cnattingius S, Reilly M, Pawitan Y, Lichtenstein P. Maternal and fetal genetic factors account for most of familial aggregation of preeclampsia: a population-based Swedish cohort study. *Am J Med Genet A* 2004; **130**: 365–71.

65   Esplin MS, Fausett MB, Fraser A, *et al.* Paternal and maternal components of the predisposition to preeclampsia. *N Engl J Med* 2001; **344**: 867–72.

66   Nilsson E, Salonen RH, Cnattingius S, Lichtenstein P. The importance of genetic and environmental effects for pre-eclampsia and gestational hypertension: a family study. *Br J Obstet Gynaecol* 2004; **111**: 200–6.

67   Lin J, August P. Genetic thrombophilias and preeclampsia: a meta-analysis. *Obstet Gynecol* 2005; **105**: 182–92.

68   Kosmas IP, Tatsioni A, Ioannidis JP. Association of Leiden mutation in factor V gene with hypertension in pregnancy and pre-eclampsia: a meta-analysis. *J Hypertens* 2003; **21**: 1221–8.

69   Kosmas IP, Tatsioni A, Ioannidis JP. Association of C677T polymorphism in the methylenetetrahydrofolate reductase gene with hypertension in pregnancy and pre-eclampsia: a meta-analysis. *J Hypertens* 2004; **22**: 1655–62.

70   Zusterzeel PL, Visser W, Blom HJ, *et al.* Methylenetetrahydrofolate reductase polymorphisms in preeclampsia and the HELLP syndrome. *Hypertens Pregnancy* 2000; **19**: 299–307.

71   Disentangling Fetal and Maternal Susceptibility for Pre-Eclampsia: A British Multicenter Candidate-Gene Study. *Am J Hum Genet* 2005; **77**: 127–31.

5

Diabetes mellitus in women

ROBERT S LINDSAY

BACKGROUND

Diabetes describes a diverse range of conditions all of which result in hyperglycemia. In clinical terms the division between the two common forms – type 1 and type 2 – diabetes is familiar. Type 1 diabetes (previously insulin-dependent or juvenile-onset diabetes) comprises around 5–10 percent of European diabetic populations and has an autoimmune basis. People with type 2 diabetes (previously non-insulin-dependent or adult-onset diabetes) usually exhibit a combination of resistance to insulin action and reduced insulin secretion and this form accounts for 90 percent of cases. Increasingly the diversity and heterogeneity of diabetes are recognized – in part reflecting intense research efforts to understand the etiology of type 2 diabetes.

The latest classification of diabetes by the American Diabetes Association details not only type 1 and type 2 diabetes but also several other specific types with known etiology. These include diabetes secondary to endocrinopathies, diseases of the exocrine pancreas, and drugs, and also an array of rare forms of diabetes underpinned by genetic defects influencing insulin action, insulin secretion, or mitochondrial function.[1] In particular, recent progress has been made in describing the genetics of maturity-onset diabetes of the young – rare, monogenic, autosomal dominant forms of diabetes.[2] The cause of the majority of cases is now known to be mutation in one of six separate genes.[2]

There have been dramatic changes in the prevalence of diabetes in recent years. In the United States, the prevalence of diagnosed diabetes in adults (all those aged over 18 years) increased by 40 percent in the 1990s – from 4.9 percent in 1990 to 6.9 percent in 1999.[3,4] The incidence of both major forms of diabetes appears to be increasing. Incidence of type 1 diabetes has increased by up to 3 percent per year in many populations for reasons that are still debated.[5] The majority of the increase in diabetes prevalence noted in countries such as the United States, however, represents an increase in type 2 diabetes and, in turn, reflects major increases in adiposity in the population.[3] The prevalence of obesity (body mass index [BMI] $\geqslant 30\,\mathrm{kg/m^2}$) in adults in the United States rose from 11.1 percent in 1990 to 18.0 percent in 1998.[3] The 1988–94 National Health and Nutrition Examination Survey (NHANES) suggests that two-thirds of adult Americans are now either overweight (BMI $\geqslant 25\,\mathrm{kg/m^2}$) or obese.[6] In keeping with these marked secular changes, the projected lifetime risk of development of type 2 diabetes of children born in the United States in 2000 (based on data from the National Health Interview Survey 1984–2000) is calculated at 33 percent for males and 38 percent for females.[7] This is likely to have a large impact on health.

Diabetes results in a substantial effect on life expectancy: diagnosis of diabetes at age 40 is associated with loss of 11.6 life years (18.6 quality-adjusted life years) in men and 14.3 life years (22.0 quality adjusted life years) in women.[7] Given these data it is unsurprising that diabetes and its complications have a major economic impact on health-care systems. Total medical expenditures incurred by people with diabetes totaled $77.7 billion in 1997 in the United States and were almost four times those of people without diabetes per capita.[8] The importance and increasing prevalence of diabetes are by no means confined to the United States. Rising rates of obesity and type 2 diabetes are not only recorded in areas with economies and lifestyles similar to those in the United States, such as Western Europe, but also in countries undergoing economic transition, notably those in Asia and Latin America,[9] and a global 'epidemic' of obesity and diabetes has been described.[9,10]

The total prevalence of diabetes in adults worldwide is estimated at 4 percent (using 1995 figures) with more women than men having diabetes (73 vs. 62 million in 1995).[10] Although the prevalence of diabetes is higher in developed (5.9 percent) than developing (3.3 percent) countries, overall numbers, and therefore burden of disease, are greater in the developing countries and this is likely to worsen.[10] By 2025 an increase in the numbers of people with diabetes of 42 percent in the developed and 170 percent in the developing world is projected.[10] A further notable feature of these dramatic secular changes is the development of obesity and type 2 diabetes at younger ages. Thus, typical type 2 diabetes with onset in young adults and even children is increasingly recognized worldwide.[11]

Diabetes and its complications – retinopathy, nephropathy, neuropathy and vascular disease – create a large burden on individuals and healthcare systems. The purpose of this chapter is to highlight the impact of diabetes on women's health with particular focus on vascular disease and the interaction of diabetes and pregnancy.

VASCULAR RISK ASSOCIATED WITH DIABETES IN WOMEN

Vascular risk is of central importance to the management and public health importance of diabetes. Diabetes increases the risk of vascular disease including coronary heart disease and stroke.[12] This reflects an increased prevalence of several well-described vascular risk factors in people with type 2 diabetes (notably hypertension, dyslipidemia, and obesity), increased vascular risk associated with other complications of diabetes (most notably nephropathy), and association of diabetes with 'novel' vascular risk factors such as those marking inflammation and endothelial dysfunction as discussed below. Importantly, it is well described that the disadvantage of diabetes in terms of vascular risk is particularly marked in women.

Several large series have highlighted increased mortality in people with diabetes and emphasize vascular causes of death. In the recent World Health Organization (WHO) multinational study all-cause standardized mortality rates (SMRs) were increased by threefold to eightfold in type 1 diabetes and by 1.4-fold to fourfold in type 2 diabetes[12] – findings which are typical of previous studies.[13,14] A diverse range of populations was studied in the WHO multinational study and SMR increased in almost all populations (five European, Hong Kong, Cuban, and Native American), the single exception being Japan.[12] Diabetes (in the absence of prevalent cardiovascular disease at baseline) has been found to carry as great a risk of future coronary heart disease mortality as preexisting vascular disease,[15] although this has not been consistent in all populations.[16] Diabetes has a large impact on standardized mortality and the major part of this effect is due to vascular disease. Although diabetes is associated with a range of complications, the WHO study suggested that 44 percent of deaths in type 1 diabetes and

52 percent of deaths in type 2 diabetes were attributable to cardiovascular disease.[12]

The epidemiology of cardiovascular disease in women with diabetes is of particular interest. It has been noted for some time that the deleterious effect of diabetes on vascular disease appears to be greater in women. In the WHO study the proportion of men and women who died of cardiovascular causes were comparable in both type 1 (47 percent of men and 41 percent of women) and type 2 diabetes (54 percent of men and 49 percent of women). Although absolute rates of mortality in those with diabetes remained lower in women than in men, SMRs were higher compared with the nondiabetic population. Thus, the survival advantage of being female in terms of cardiovascular health is diminished or lost, as noted in other studies.[17,18] In keeping with this the relative risk of vascular disease in women with diabetes is increased by approximately twofold to fourfold in women as compared with twofold in men.[12]

Diabetes is associated with a range of other – particularly microvascular – complications and women appear to be at broadly similar risk of their development. Sex was not an independent risk factor for the development of retinopathy in the Diabetes Control and Complications Trial (DCCT).[19] The impact of sex on development of renal disease has received recent attention. Women appear to have at least a similar risk of diabetic nephropathy[20] and indeed some studies (notably the DCCT) have suggested that women are at greater risk of development of nephropathy after accounting for other risk factors.[21] This is of some interest as female sex may be protective against decline of renal function in nondiabetic renal disease[20] and suggests that a protective effect of female sex with regard to renal disease might be lost in women with diabetes in an analogous manner to the loss of survival advantage in vascular disease as noted above.[18] A number of mechanisms to account for sex differences in propensity to renal disease including effects on the renin–angiotensin system, nitric oxide production, inflammation, and proliferation of and collagen synthesis by mesangial cells have been proposed (reviewed in reference 21). Although intriguing it should be stressed that the basic epidemiology of sex differences in propensity to renal disease in diabetic and nondiabetic nephropathy remains controversial at present not least due to methodologic differences between studies.

Diabetes and vascular risk factors

As noted previously there are several potential reasons why diabetes in general is associated with an increase in vascular disease. There is a clear association of type 2 diabetes with a range of other traditional and nontraditional vascular risk factors. Type 2 diabetes is part of the 'metabolic syndrome'. It has been observed repeatedly that individuals tend to have multiple cardiovascular risk factors, including type 2 diabetes, more often than might be expected by chance. In the late 1980s and early 1990s, observations in large-scale epidemiologic series and careful investigation of insulin sensitivity – particularly in people with obesity, type 2 diabetes, and hypertension – led to more formal examination of these relations and eventually to the concept of the metabolic syndrome. Such associations were described under a variety of names including syndrome X, the insulin resistance syndrome, the deadly quartet and multiple metabolic syndrome among others (reviewed in reference 22; see also Chapter 3). Writing in 1988, Reaven described 'syndrome X' as the combination of insulin resistance, glucose intolerance, hyperinsulinemia, increased very-low-density lipoprotein, triglyceride, and hypertension.[23] He noted that resistance to insulin stimulated glucose uptake during euglycemic hyperinsulinemia clamp and hyperinsulinemia were associated with type 2 diabetes, cardiovascular disease, and hypertension, and he hypothesized that insulin or insulin action might be a common factor in the etiology of all of these conditions.[23] Thus in part the increase in vascular risk noted in diabetes acts through association with these other factors.

More recently a range of 'nontraditional' vascular risk factors have been described. Inflammation plays a key role in the development of atherosclerosis[24] being apparent at several levels of the cellular process.[24] Circulating markers, such as C-reactive protein (CRP), have proved effective measures of later risk in a number of large series.[25] Perhaps more surprisingly a number of recent studies have suggested that inflammation might also be involved in development of metabolic disease. It has been known for some time that a diverse range of markers of inflammation (for example tumor necrosis factor α, C reactive protein, interleukin-6, white cell count) were positively related to adiposity and higher in association with type 2 diabetes.[26] Further investigations suggest that several of these markers are also related to insulin resistance and indeed predict development of type 2 diabetes in diverse populations.[27,28] A proposed cellular mechanism to explain these findings is the nuclear factor (NF)-κB pathway – activated in inflammation and now shown to influence insulin sensitivity.[29]

In general this association of vascular risk factors has been apparent in both men and women.

Treatment of vascular risk in diabetes and the role of hormone replacement therapy

Our knowledge of increased vascular risk in women with diabetes means that this is a group of particular importance in cardiovascular prevention. Detailed examination of this is outwith the remit of this chapter, however, it is important to note that clinical management of women with diabetes has benefited in recent years from a number of large randomized trials which have included substantial numbers of women. The Heart Protection Study is of landmark importance in showing the benefits of cholesterol-lowering therapy. Some 5963 participants with diabetes at baseline were randomized of whom 30 percent (n = 1816)

were women.[30,31] In keeping with the overall results of the trial, cholesterol-lowering therapy was successful in reducing the incidence of first major vascular events in participants with diabetes, and more specifically women with diabetes.[31] Similarly, lowering of blood pressure is of clear benefit in reducing risk of both macrovascular and microvascular (retinopathy, nephropathy) complications of diabetes,[32,33] and women are well represented in such studies. The Hypertension Optimal Treatment trial included 1501 people with diabetes (47 percent women) and showed that the risk of major cardiovascular events could be halved by targeting diastolic blood pressure reduction to >80 mm Hg as opposed to >90 mm Hg.[32] The United Kingdom Prospective Diabetes Study Group, in a study population that was 45 percent female, demonstrated reduction in deaths attributable to diabetes, stroke and microvascular disease with tight blood pressure control.[33]

Given the large burden of vascular disease in women with diabetes it is not surprising that hormone replacement therapy (HRT) held great hope in prevention and delay of vascular disease specifically in women with diabetes. The place of hormone replacement in women with diabetes is now informed by a number of large multicenter randomized trials – most notably the Women's Health Initiative (WHI). As is now well known, many observational studies have shown that vascular disease is less prevalent in women who have taken HRT, usually in the form of estrogen alone. Further a range of short-term studies suggested important benefits in vascular risk factors. Despite this – and emphasizing the importance of randomized control trials – both combined and estrogen replacement alone have been shown to significantly increase the risk of vascular events in women and the role of HRT revised accordingly. The limb of the Women's Health Initiative examining combined estrogen and progestagen in women with a uterus showed an increase in incident coronary heart disease (hazard ratio [HR]1.29, 95 percent confidence interval [CI] 1.02 to 1.63), stroke (1.41, 1.07 to 1.85) and pulmonary embolism (2.13, 1.39 to 3.25) as well as breast cancer (1.26, 1.00 to 1.59]).[34] Estrogen and progestagen did not appear to influence incident peripheral vascular disease.[35] Benefits of HRT included a reduction in fractures (HR 0.76, 0.69 to 0.85).[34] Estrogen alone in women after hysterectomy was associated with an increase in stroke (HR 1.39, 1.10 to 1.77) with no significant effect on coronary heart disease.[36] Although these results are in some respects disappointing, the WHI is an important example of the importance of randomized control trials in guiding clinical practice.

Given the importance of vascular outcomes to women with diabetes, the failure of HRT to offer protection against vascular outcomes is unfortunate. The WHI included a reasonable proportion of women with diabetes (4.4 percent of the estrogen and progestagen limb and 7.7 percent of the estrogen alone limb) and subgroup analysis did not support a beneficial effect.[34] Advice on HRT for women with diabetes must now be similar to that of women without diabetes – that HRT may be beneficial for short-term control of menopausal symptoms but clearly cannot be prescribed for cardiovascular disease prevention. An interesting further observation arising from the WHI is a potential protective effect of HRT against the development of diabetes.[37] Clearly HRT will not be prescribed for this purpose, however, the reduction in type 2 diabetes incidence observed in these trials is impressive and the mechanism of the effect uncertain. Another intriguing aspect of this is the discordance between worsening of vascular disease and improvement in type 2 diabetes risk. Risk factors for type 2 diabetes and vascular disease are frequently shared but this is not the case in the case of estrogens. The mechanistic basis of this is not known at present.

DIABETES AND REPRODUCTION

Diabetes has a number of important effects on reproductive health. Most familiar are the influences of diabetes and its complications on pregnancy outcomes for mother and child and this section will concentrate on those aspects while dealing briefly with influences of diabetes on fertility.

Diabetes, fertility, and menstruation

Women with diabetes may experience reduced fertility for a variety of reasons. Polycystic ovary syndrome (PCOS) – characterized by increased androgen production, disordered gonadotrophin secretion, and chronic anovulation – has many associations with both type 2 diabetes and obesity. Obesity is an important risk factor for both PCOS and type 2 diabetes and the prevalence of abnormal glucose tolerance is increased in women with PCOS.[38–40] Long or highly irregular menstrual cycles in early adult life act as a risk factor for later development of type 2 diabetes.[41] More strikingly it is increasingly recognized that insensitivity to insulin action – a familiar feature of both type 2 diabetes and obesity – is a central feature of PCOS. Evidence of insulin resistance and raised insulin levels in women with PCOS dates back to 1980,[42] while recent studies suggest that ovulatory menstrual cycles can be stimulated in women with PCOS not only by weight reduction but also by pharmaceutical treatments designed to lower insulin levels,[39] notably agents commonly used in management of type 2 diabetes, such as metformin and the thiazolidinediones. These studies support a central role for insulin sensitivity in the pathogenesis of PCOS and suggest that the association of type 2 diabetes and PCOS may reflect shared etiological factors between the two conditions.[42] In practical terms this means that many women with type 2 diabetes will experience difficulty in conceiving secondary to PCOS.

Reports of menstrual disturbance in women with type 1 diabetes are more limited. Type 1 diabetes, particularly with onset in early childhood, has, however, been associated with later age at menarche,[43] whereas isolated reports suggest an increase in menstrual irregularity[43] and earlier

menopause.[44] The etiology and importance of these effects remain to be fully explored. Type 1 diabetes, however, exerts a major and undoubted effect on women's reproductive health by effects on pregnancy discussed in the next section.

Diabetes and pregnancy

Pregnancy in women with established diabetes remains a therapeutic challenge and, despite modern innovations in clinical management, a variety of adverse outcomes are seen in the child and mother. Disappointingly, even in recent series, higher rates of congenital malformation and perinatal mortality are found.[45,46] Management of blood glucose usually involves a multidisciplinary approach to care encouraging frequent home monitoring of blood glucose and insulin delivered either by multiple daily doses or by pump devices. Unfortunately such management is usually both intensive and burdensome to the mother and often limited by hypoglycemia. Gestational diabetes – glucose intolerance with first onset or recognition in pregnancy[1] – is the cause of several current controversies and is considered briefly at the end of this section.

Complications of maternal diabetes for the child

Genetic variation contributes to the risk of both type 1 and type 2 diabetes, and therefore offspring of mothers with diabetes are at an increased risk of diabetes compared with the general population. The main focus of this section are nongenetic complications related to being the offspring of a mother with diabetes. Complications seen during and shortly after pregnancy are most apparent but the potential for intrauterine effects to contribute to development of type 2 diabetes and obesity in the offspring will also be examined.

Diabetes is associated with a range of adverse outcomes most notably increase in congenital malformations, early pregnancy loss, and perinatal mortality. Many of these adverse effects relate clearly to levels of maternal glucose. A broad range of congenital abnormalities are noted, of which caudal regression syndromes are considered characteristic. Based on animal models, glycemia in early (that is, the first 6–8 weeks) of pregnancy would be predicted to lead to increases in congenital abnormalities. After some controversy, mainly attributable to small sample sizes in individual observational series, it is now clear that maternal glycemia in early pregnancy directly relates to the frequency of congenital abnormalities. In 1996, Kitzmiller et al. pooled data from seven series and showed that markedly raised HbA_{1c} – over 10 standard deviations (SD) above the mean for those without diabetes – was associated with a high risk (~27 percent) of congenital abnormality and HbA_{1c} between 6 and 10 SD was associated with a moderately increased risk (4–9 percent).[47] In contrast increased HbA_{1c} in early pregnancy less than 4 SD from the mean was not reliably associated with such adverse outcomes.[47] In keeping with this, examination of women taking part in the DCCT supported the view that tight glycemic control before and during pregnancy could substantially reduce rates of congenital malformation (and indeed spontaneous abortion) to rates similar to those in the nondiabetic population.[48] As participants in a randomized controlled trial, those taking part in the DCCT are, of course, a highly selected group. It is disappointing then that results in population-based series from a variety of European countries continue to show high rates of adverse outcomes which remain markedly different from those of the general population. Rates of congenital malformations are raised 2–10-fold compared with the background populations in series from France (2-fold increase[49]), the Netherlands (3.4-fold[50]), northwestern (10-fold[45]) and northeastern England (4-fold[46]). Similarly, rates of perinatal mortality are increased 3.5–6-fold in these various series,[46,49,50] all published in 1997 or later.

Offspring of mothers with diabetes also undergo characteristic overgrowth *in utero* along with biochemical complications in the newborn period such as hypocalcemia and hypoglycemia.[51,52] Increases in birthweight in turn reflect an increased supply of glucose and amino acids *in utero* with corresponding stimulation of the fetal pancreas and resulting hyperinsulinemia.[51] There is profound alteration of a number of fetal hormones in offspring of mothers with type 1 diabetes – median cord insulin is increased fourfold to fivefold and leptin threefold to fourfold over controls.[53] After adjustment for gestational age at delivery, birthweight is typically 1–1.5 SD above the average for offspring of mothers without diabetes.[45] In obstetric terms the most important immediate complication associated with fetal overgrowth is shoulder dystocia. Shoulder dystocia is more frequent in the presence of fetal overgrowth and is noted as a complication of type 1 diabetes and pregnancy in up to 14 percent of deliveries in some series.[50]

Interestingly the ill effects of being the offspring of a mother with diabetes may not be confined to the period *in utero* and the immediate postpartum period. Exposure to maternal diabetes *in utero* is associated with an increased risk of abnormal glucose tolerance[54–57] and obesity[56,58–60] in childhood. This is believed to be secondary to 'programming' of disease *in utero* – long-term alteration of physiology or disease risk due to early environmental exposure – and forms the most powerful example of programming in early life. The best-characterized studies of the influences of maternal diabetes on offspring obesity and glucose tolerance have been conducted in the Pima Indian population of Arizona. The presence of maternal diabetes during pregnancy is associated with an increase in both obesity[58] and type 2 diabetes[54] in their offspring. There is a large effect. Maternal diabetes increases risk of type 2 diabetes in childhood (up to 19 years) by 10-fold and is the most important risk factor for diabetes in childhood in this population.[61] A critical role of the intrauterine environment is supported by the lack of similar effects pertaining to paternal diabetes during pregnancy[54,58] and detailed studies of siblings before and after onset of maternal type 2 diabetes.[62]

The role of the intrauterine environment is also supported by studies examining metabolic outcomes in offspring of mothers with type 1 diabetes (either solely[59,56] or predominantly[57,60]) showing increases in adiposity[56,59,60] and abnormal glucose tolerance[55] in childhood.[56,57] Although relatively small (number of offspring 15–168[56,59,60,63]) these studies show high rates of impaired glucose tolerance (5 percent[57] to 17 percent[59]) in children aged between 5 and 9 years. A small study in young French adults (mean age 22 years) suggest rates of impaired glucose tolerance of up to 33 percent.[63] Notably, where available, hormonal markers highlight those most at risk. Amniotic fluid insulin (a marker of fetal insulin production induced by maternal hyperglycemia) is associated with obesity and impaired glucose tolerance.[56,57,60] Little is known about the intermediate mechanisms (apart from propensity to increased adiposity) which might cause predisposition to altered glucose tolerance in offspring of diabetic mothers, although two recent studies have suggested that insulin secretion may be reduced.[63,64] Other cardiovascular risk factors, usually associated with insulin resistance in adults, have been found to be higher in offspring of diabetic mothers including cholesterol[56,65] and blood pressure,[66] and a range of plasma measures related to endothelial dysfunction were also raised in a single study of 8-year-old children.[65] It should be noted that there are as yet no large series in Caucasian populations examining glucose tolerance in *adult* offspring of mothers with type 1 diabetes and so the long-term effects of maternal diabetes on offspring health remains to be fully elucidated in these groups.

Complications of pregnancy for mothers with diabetes

Pregnancy holds particular risks for women with diabetes especially if complications of diabetes are already present. Hemodynamic and hormonal changes in pregnancy hold potential for worsening of complications. In addition, there are special considerations in women with diabetes where improvement of metabolic control may paradoxically lead to short-term deterioration of microvascular disease. Further, mothers with diabetes are at increased risk of pregnancy-induced hypertension and preeclampsia. Risks for the mother are also influenced by preexisting complications of diabetes, most notably vascular disease, nephropathy, and retinopathy.

Some of the most extensive evidence with regard to the effect of pregnancy on diabetes complications comes from the DCCT. In the DCCT people with type 1 diabetes were randomized to either conventional or intensive diabetes control using multiple daily injections of insulin or insulin pumps.[67] Although not primarily designed to examine pregnancy outcomes, some 180 women became pregnant during the study with 270 pregnancies. This allowed valuable assessment of progression of microvascular complications comparing both those who did or did not become pregnant and those with conventional or intensive control of glycemia.[48] Pregnancy was associated with worsening of retinopathy, emphasizing the importance of careful retinal screening through pregnancy. This deterioration of retinal disease came from two sources. It had previously been demonstrated in the nonpregnant population of DCCT that there is a short-term worsening of retinopathy in the few months after improvement of glycemic control.[67] This early deterioration is more than compensated for in the longer term by benefits of improved glycemic control. In keeping with general guidelines all DCCT participants were encouraged to achieve tighter glycemic control before and during pregnancy and at least part of the short-term worsening of retinopathy in pregnancy can be associated with this fall in HbA$_{1c}$. Notably however, this did not explain all of the deterioration and there was an additional effect for pregnancy of itself to lead to worsening of retinopathy. This worsening of retinopathy was transient and in the longer term pregnancy was not associated with any deterioration of retinal outcomes.[48] Similarly, whereas the effect of pregnancy in more severe nephropathy remains controversial there was no long-term worsening of nephropathy in association with pregnancy in the DCCT.[48]

An increase in pregnancy-induced hypertension and preeclampsia has been noted in many previous series with rates of around 20–25 percent – some fourfold higher than the background population – being typical.[68] These findings are not universal, however, with some groups reporting no increase in preeclampsia in their diabetic populations.[69,70] The reasons for these discrepancies are not entirely clear. Interestingly differences in the frequency of preeclampsia have been related to poor glycemic control in early pregnancy,[68,71] and it is possible that differences in glycemia, underlying propensity to preeclampsia, or more prosaically study methods underpin the various findings.

As noted above diabetes increases the risk of vascular disease in women, nevertheless the presence of symptomatic cardiovascular disease during pregnancy is uncommon. In older series a markedly increased maternal and fetal mortality was noted if diabetes was complicated by cardiovascular disease.[72] This is believed to reflect the considerable hemodynamic stresses of pregnancy and labor on a compromised circulatory system. More recent literature is largely confined to individual case reports. In general maternal mortality during pregnancy appears rarer than in older reports, but it should be noted that the literature is sparse.[73] Improved results may reflect selection of women opting to become pregnant and reporting bias as well as improved management. Pregnancy in women with symptomatic vascular disease should only be undertaken after careful counseling and assessment.

Gestational diabetes

The American Diabetes Association defines gestational diabetes as glucose intolerance with first onset or recognition in pregnancy.[1] The diagnosis continues to be complicated by a variety of controversies leading to uncertainty as to the best mode of treatment and screening. Two major trials – the Australian Carbohydrate Intolerance Study (ACHOIS),[74] which reported in 2005, and Hyperglycaemia and Adverse Pregnancy Outcome (HAPO) study[75] which is due to report in the near future should help to clarify some of these controversies.

Gestational diabetes occurs in 2–9 percent of pregnancies.[1] In modern series perinatal mortality is not increased in association with gestational diabetes, however, the rate of macrosomia is increased.[76] In several series there is a clear relation between maternal glucose, as measured by an oral glucose tolerance test during pregnancy, and birthweight.[77] For the mother gestational diabetes is of prognostic importance. Women with gestational diabetes have an increased risk of development of type 2 diabetes. In keeping with this risk factors for gestational diabetes include ethnicity, obesity, and family history of type 2 diabetes.[1] The risk of later diabetes is considerable – Hispanic women with gestational diabetes but normal glucose tolerance postpartum have a 47 percent risk of development of type 2 diabetes by 5 years after pregnancy. Furthermore this risk is modifiable – the Troglitazone in the Prevention of Diabetes (TRIPOD) study indicated that treatment with troglitazone, a thiazolidinedione, reduces progression to type 2 diabetes in this group.[78] Detection of diabetes during pregnancy may also be of benefit to mothers if diabetes was present but undiagnosed before the pregnancy. Cundy et al. have described their extensive experience in Auckland with Maori and Pacific Island mothers – a population generally at high risk of type 2 diabetes. They have noted that the first diagnosis of type 2 diabetes is frequently during pregnancy.[79] Further, type 2 diabetes is associated with a poor pregnancy outcome, regardless of whether the diagnosis is made before or during pregnancy.[79]

Despite this, controversies remain. Until recently the evidence that management of gestational diabetes resulted in improved perinatal outcomes was not conclusive. Several trials had hinted that this might be the case. De Veciana et al. had shown that alteration of glycemic management resulted in significantly lower birthweight.[80] The trial was small, however, and blood glucose relatively high compared with the majority of women with gestational diabetes.[80] Similarly the Toronto tri-hospital series had shown normalization of birthweight in women treated for gestational diabetes compared with untreated 'borderline' cases, but rates of cesarean section were also much higher.[81] This was likely as a result of changes in clinical management consequent upon the diagnosis of gestational diabetes but raised concern that this might reduce the clinical benefits of screening and management of gestational diabetes.[81] Most recently the ACHOIS trial randomized women with gestational diabetes (in fact women with impaired glucose tolerance under WHO diagnostic criteria – 2 hour blood glucose 7.8–11.0 mmol/L 2 hours after a 75 g oral glucose tolerance test and fasting glucose <7.8 mmol/l.[74]) to either intervention or routine care. Intervention included dietary advice, blood glucose monitoring and insulin therapy as needed when capillary glucose exceeded 5.5 mmol/L fasting or 7.0 mmol/L 2 hours after meals. Serious perinatal outcomes (death, shoulder dystocia, bone fracture, or nerve palsy) were significantly reduced in the intervention group (4 percent routine to 1 percent intervention). Birthweight was significantly reduced (3.5 ± 0.7 kg routine vs. 3.3 ± 0.6 kg intervention) as was the rate of macrosomia (21 percent routine vs. 10 percent intervention). One critical and controversial feature of the study design of ACHOIS was that for the majority of women in the routine group the result of the oral glucose tolerance test was kept blinded – avoiding the diluting effect of intervention in the routine group. This important result supports efforts to detect and treat gestational diabetes. Questions remain. The level of glycemia for diagnosis at which diagnosis should be made will continue to be debated. The diagnostic criteria used by WHO were created for a nonpregnant population. It is clear that there is a continuum of risk and further critical information will come from the HAPO study. This international study of a planned 25 000 women in pregnancy is recording pregnancy outcomes in relation to a single 75 g oral glucose tolerance test at 24–32 weeks of pregnancy.[75] The results of HAPO should allow us to understand more clearly the relation of glycemia to adverse pregnancy outcomes. At the same time it is unlikely that a single test will satisfactorily predict adverse events. A number of groups have worked toward fetal-based strategies for management of gestational diabetes. Originally based on amniotic fluid measures of insulin, such strategies suggested that pregnancy management might be intensified in offspring showing evidence of excess insulin production.[82] More recently such strategies have been modified to use ultrasound measures in the second trimester to aid clinical decision making toward more or less intensive glucose control.[83–85] Such strategies offer some hope that therapy might be more efficiently targeted to women fulfilling glycemic criteria but in whom there is also evidence of adverse effects of maternal glucose on the fetus.

Finally, there are also newer therapeutic modalities that offer some hope that treatment of women with diabetes during pregnancy might be improved – and particularly that the burden of hypoglycemia might be reduced. In gestational diabetes the use of the sulfonylurea glyburide (known as glibenclamide in the United Kingdom) has shown promising results in a randomized controlled trial.[86] Glyburide does not cross the placenta but has been shown to be effective in reducing birthweight in women with gestational diabetes.[86] Novel short- and long-acting insulin analogs are also now available. Used out of pregnancy these agents are efficacious in reducing nocturnal hypoglycemia in patients with type 1 diabetes and may be more effective at controlling postprandial rises in blood sugar.[87] Hypoglycemia remains a major problem (although greater in management of type 1 diabetes in pregnancy) and use of these agents may offer an important benefit during pregnancy.[87] Although trial evidence is limited both of the available short-acting analogs have been used successfully in gestational diabetes.[88,89]

KEY LEARNING POINTS

- The prevalence of obesity and diabetes is increasing in most populations.
- Diabetes in women is associated with a twofold to fourfold increase in risk of vascular disease
- Recent landmark studies, including large numbers of female participants, show benefits of cholesterol and blood pressure management in lowering the incidence of vascular events in people with diabetes.
- Pregnancy complicated by preexisting diabetes is associated with a range of complications for child and mother that are partly modifiable by excellent glycemic control before and during pregnancy.
- Although controversies remain around the clinical diagnosis of gestational diabetes, important recent evidence suggests that perinatal outcomes are improved by diagnosis and glycemic management.

REFERENCES

1   Diagnosis and classification of diabetes mellitus. *Diabetes Care* 2004; **27**(Suppl 1): S5–S10.

2   Stride A, Hattersley AT. Different genes, different diabetes: lessons from maturity-onset diabetes of the young. *Ann Med* 2002; **34**: 207–16.

3   Mokdad AH, Ford ES, Bowman BA, *et al.* Diabetes trends in the US: 1990–1998. *Diabetes Care* 2000; **23**: 1278–83.

4   Mokdad AH, Ford ES, Bowman BA, *et al.* The continuing increase of diabetes in the US. *Diabetes Care* 2001; **24**: 412.

5   Gale EA. The rise of childhood type 1 diabetes in the 20th century. *Diabetes* 2002; **51**: 3353–61.

6   Harris MI, Flegal KM, Cowie CC, *et al.* Prevalence of diabetes, impaired fasting glucose, and impaired glucose tolerance in U.S. adults. The Third National Health and Nutrition Examination Survey, 1988–1994. *Diabetes Care* 1998; **21**: 518–24.

7   Narayan KM, Boyle JP, Thompson TJ, *et al.* Lifetime risk for diabetes mellitus in the United States. *JAMA* 2003; **290**: 1884–90.

8   Economic consequences of diabetes mellitus in the US in 1997. American Diabetes Association. *Diabetes Care* 1998; **21**: 296–309.

9   Seidell JC. Obesity, insulin resistance and diabetes – a worldwide epidemic. *Br J Nutr* 2000; **83**(Suppl 1): S5–8.

10 King H, Aubert RE, Herman WH. Global burden of diabetes, 1995–2025: prevalence, numerical estimates, and projections. *Diabetes Care* 1998; **21**: 1414–31.

11   Rosenbloom AL, Joe JR, Young RS, Winter WE. Emerging epidemic of type 2 diabetes in youth. *Diabetes Care* 1999; **22**: 345–54.

12   Morrish NJ, Wang SL, Stevens LK, *et al.* Mortality and causes of death in the WHO Multinational Study of Vascular Disease in Diabetes. *Diabetologia* 2001; **44**(Suppl 2): S14–21.

13   Nystrom L, Ostman J, Wall S, Wibell L. Mortality of all incident cases of diabetes mellitus in Sweden diagnosed 1983–1987 at age 15–34 years. Diabetes Incidence Study in Sweden (DISS) Group. *Diabet Med* 1992; **9**: 422–7.

14   Panzram G. Mortality and survival in type 2 (non-insulin-dependent) diabetes mellitus. *Diabetologia* 1987; **30**: 123–31.

15   Haffner SM, Lehto S, Ronnemaa T, *et al.* Mortality from coronary heart disease in subjects with type 2 diabetes and in nondiabetic subjects with and without prior myocardial infarction. *N Engl J Med* 1998; **339**: 229–34.

16   Evans JM, Wang J, Morris AD. Comparison of cardiovascular risk between patients with type 2 diabetes and those who had had a myocardial infarction: cross-sectional and cohort studies. *BMJ* 2002; **324**: 939–42.

17   Panzram G, Zabel-Langhennig R. Prognosis of diabetes mellitus in a geographically defined population. *Diabetologia* 1981; **20**: 587–91.

18   O'Sullivan JB, Mahan CM. Mortality related to diabetes and blood glucose levels in a community study. *Am J Epidemiol* 1982; **116**: 678–84.

19   Zhang L, Krzentowski G, Albert A, Lefebvre PJ. Risk of developing retinopathy in Diabetes Control and Complications Trial type 1 diabetic patients with good or poor metabolic control. *Diabetes Care* 2001; **24**: 1275–9.

20   Seliger SL, Davis C, Stehman-Breen C. Gender and the progression of renal disease. *Curr Opin Nephrol Hypertens* 2001; **10**: 219–25.

21   Zhang L, Krzentowski G, Albert A, Lefebvre PJ. Factors predictive of nephropathy in DCCT Type 1 diabetic patients with good or poor metabolic control. *Diabet Med* 2003; **20**: 580–5.

22   Liese AD, Mayer-Davis EJ, Haffner SM. Development of the multiple metabolic syndrome: an epidemiologic perspective. *Epidemiol Rev* 1998; **20**: 157–72.

23   Reaven GM. Banting lecture 1988. Role of insulin resistance in human disease. *Diabetes* 1988; **37**: 1595–607.

24   Ross R. Atherosclerosis – an inflammatory disease. *N Engl J Med* 1999; **340**: 115–26.

25   Ridker PM, Hennekens CH, Buring JE, Rifai N. C-reactive protein and other markers of inflammation in the prediction of cardiovascular disease in women. *N Engl J Med* 2000; **342**: 836–43.

26   Pickup JC, Crook MA. Is type II diabetes mellitus a disease of the innate immune system? *Diabetologia* 1998; **41**: 1241–8.

27   Schmidt MI, Duncan BB, Sharrett AR, *et al.* Markers of inflammation and prediction of diabetes mellitus in adults (Atherosclerosis Risk in Communities study): a cohort study. *Lancet* 1999; **353**: 1649–52.

28   Festa A, D'Agostino RB, Tracy RP, Haffner SM. Elevated levels of acute phase proteins and plasminogen activator inhibitor – 1 (PAI-1) predict the development of type 2 diabetes mellitus: the Insulin Resistance Atherosclerosis Study (IRAS). *Diabetes* 2002; **51**: 1131–7.

29   Hundal RS, Petersen KF, Mayerson AB, *et al.* Mechanism by which high-dose aspirin improves glucose metabolism in type 2 diabetes. *J Clin Invest* 2002; **109**: 1321–6.

30   MRC/BHF Heart Protection Study of cholesterol lowering with simvastatin in 20,536 high-risk individuals: a randomised placebo-controlled trial. *Lancet* 2002; **360**: 7–22.

31   Collins R, Armitage J, Parish S, *et al.* MRC/BHF Heart Protection Study of cholesterol-lowering with simvastatin in 5963 people with diabetes: a randomised placebo-controlled trial. *Lancet* 2003; **361**: 2005–16.

32   Hansson L, Zanchetti A, Carruthers SG, *et al.* Effects of intensive blood-pressure lowering and low-dose aspirin in patients with hypertension: principal results of the Hypertension Optimal Treatment (HOT) randomised trial. HOT Study Group. *Lancet* 1998; **351**: 1755–62.

33   Tight blood pressure control and risk of macrovascular and microvascular complications in type 2 diabetes: UKPDS 38. UK Prospective Diabetes Study Group. *BMJ* 1998; **317**: 703–13.

34   Rossouw JE, Anderson GL, Prentice RL, *et al.* Risks and benefits of estrogen plus progestin in healthy postmenopausal women: principal results from the Women's Health Initiative randomized controlled trial. *JAMA* 2002; **288**: 321–33.

35   Hsia J, Criqui MH, Rodabough RJ, *et al.* Estrogen plus progestin and the risk of peripheral arterial disease: the Women's Health Initiative. *Circulation* 2004; **109**: 620–6.

36   Anderson GL, Limacher M, Assaf AR, *et al.* Effects of conjugated equine estrogen in postmenopausal women with hysterectomy: the Women's Health Initiative randomized controlled trial. *JAMA* 2004; **291**: 1701–12.

37   Margolis KL, Bonds DE, Rodabough RJ, *et al.* Effect of oestrogen plus progestin on the incidence of diabetes in postmenopausal women: results from the Women's Health Initiative Hormone Trial. *Diabetologia* 2004; **47**: 1175–87.

38   Dunaif A. Hyperandrogenic anovulation (PCOS): a unique disorder of insulin action associated with an increased risk of non-insulin-dependent diabetes mellitus. *Am J Med* 1995; **98**: 33S–39S.

39   Dunaif A, Thomas A. Current concepts in the polycystic ovary syndrome. *Annu Rev Med* 2001; **52**: 401–19.

40   Ehrmann DA, Barnes RB, Rosenfield RL, *et al.* Prevalence of impaired glucose tolerance and diabetes in women with polycystic ovary syndrome. *Diabetes Care* 1999; **22**: 141–6.

41   Solomon CG, Hu FB, Dunaif A, *et al.* Long or highly irregular menstrual cycles as a marker for risk of type 2 diabetes mellitus. *JAMA* 2001; **286**: 2421–6.

42   Burghen GA, Givens JR, Kitabchi AE. Correlation of hyperandrogenism with hyperinsulinism in polycystic ovarian disease. *J Clin Endocrinol Metab* 1980; **50**: 113–16.

43 Strotmeyer ES, Steenkiste AR, Foley TP, Jr, *et al.* Menstrual cycle differences between women with type 1 diabetes and women without diabetes. *Diabetes Care* 2003; **26**: 1016–21.

44 Dorman JS, Steenkiste AR, Foley TP, *et al.* Menopause in type 1 diabetic women: is it premature? *Diabetes* 2001; **50**: 1857–62.

45 Casson IF, Clarke CA, Howard CV, *et al.* Outcomes of pregnancy in insulin-dependent diabetic women: results of a five year population cohort study. *BMJ* 1997; **315**: 275–8.

46 Hawthorne G, Robson S, Ryall EA, *et al.* Prospective population-based survey of outcome of pregnancy in diabetic women: results of the Northern Diabetic Pregnancy Audit, 1994. *BMJ* 1997; **315**: 279–81.

47 Kitzmiller JL, Buchanan TA, Kjos S, *et al.* Pre-conception care of diabetes, congenital malformations, and spontaneous abortions. *Diabetes Care* 1996; **19**: 514–41.

48 Pregnancy outcomes in the Diabetes Control and Complications Trial. *Am J Obstet Gynecol* 1996; **174**: 1343–53.

49 Boulot P, Chabbert-Buffet N, d'Ercole C, *et al.* French multicentric survey of outcome of pregnancy in women with pregestational diabetes. *Diabetes Care* 2003; **26**: 2990–3.

50 Evers IM, de Valk HW, Visser GH. Risk of complications of pregnancy in women with type 1 diabetes: nationwide prospective study in the Netherlands. *BMJ* 2004; **328**: 915.

51 Freinkel N. Banting Lecture 1980. Of pregnancy and progeny. *Diabetes* 1980; **29**: 1023–35.

52 Pedersen J. Weight and length at birth in infants of diabetic mothers. *Acta Endocrinol* 1954; **16**: 330–42.

53 Lindsay RS, Walker JD, Halsall I, *et al.* On behalf of The Scottish Multicentre Study of Diabetes in Pregnancy: Insulin and insulin propeptides at birth in offspring of diabetic mothers. *J Clin Endocrinol Metab* 2003; **88**: 1664–71.

54 Pettitt DJ, Aleck KA, Baird HR, *et al.* Congenital susceptibility to NIDDM. Role of intrauterine environment. *Diabetes* 1988; **37**: 622–8.

55 Plagemann A, Harder T, Kohlhoff R, *et al.* Glucose tolerance and insulin secretion in children of mothers with pregestational IDDM or gestational diabetes. *Diabetologia* 1997; **40**: 1094–100.

56 Weiss PA, Scholz HS, Haas J, *et al.* Long-term follow-up of infants of mothers with type 1 diabetes: evidence for hereditary and nonhereditary transmission of diabetes and precursors. *Diabetes Care* 2000; **23**: 905–11.

57 Silverman BL, Metzger BE, Cho NH, Loeb CA. Impaired glucose tolerance in adolescent offspring of diabetic mothers. Relationship to fetal hyperinsulinism. *Diabetes Care* 1995; **18**: 611–17.

58 Pettitt DJ, Baird HR, Aleck KA, *et al.* Excessive obesity in offspring of Pima Indian women with diabetes during pregnancy. *N Engl J Med* 1983; **308**: 242–5.

59 Plagemann A, Harder T, Kohlhoff R, *et al.* Overweight and obesity in infants of mothers with long-term insulin – dependent diabetes or gestational diabetes. *Int J Obes Relat Metab Disord* 1997; **21**: 451–6.

60 Silverman BL, Landsberg L, Metzger BE. Fetal hyperinsulinism in offspring of diabetic mothers. Association with the subsequent development of childhood obesity. *Ann N Y Acad Sci* 1993; **699**: 36–45.

61 Dabelea D, Hanson RL, Bennett PH, *et al.* Increasing prevalence of Type II diabetes in American Indian children. *Diabetologia* 1998; **41**: 904–10.

62 Dabelea D, Hanson RL, Bennett PH, *et al.* Intrauterine exposure to diabetes conveys risk for diabetes and obesity in offspring above that attributable to genetics. *Diabetes* 1999; **48**: A52.

63 Sobngwi E, Boudou P, Mauvais-Jarvis F, *et al.* Effect of a diabetic environment *in utero* on predisposition to type 2 diabetes. *Lancet* 2003; **361**: 1861–5.

64 Gautier JF, Wilson C, Weyer C, *et al.* Low acute insulin secretory responses in adult offspring of people with early onset type 2 diabetes. *Diabetes* 2001; **50**: 1828–33.

65 Manderson JG, Mullan B, Patterson CC, *et al.* Cardiovascular and metabolic abnormalities in the offspring of diabetic pregnancy. *Diabetologia* 2002; **45**: 991–6.

66 Cho NH, Silverman BL, Rizzo TA, Metzger BE. Correlations between the intrauterine metabolic environment and blood pressure in adolescent offspring of diabetic mothers. *J Pediatr* 2000; **136**: 587–92.

67 The effect of intensive treatment of diabetes on the development and progression of long-term complications in insulin-dependent diabetes mellitus. The Diabetes Control and Complications Trial Research Group. *N Engl J Med* 1993; **329**: 977–86.

68 Hanson U, Persson B. Epidemiology of pregnancy-induced hypertension and preeclampsia in type 1 (insulin-dependent) diabetic pregnancies in Sweden. *Acta Obstet Gynecol Scand* 1998; **77**: 620–4.

69 Gabbe SG, Mestman JH, Freeman RK, *et al.* Management and outcome of pregnancy in diabetes mellitus, classes B to R. *Am J Obstet Gynecol* 1977; **129**: 723–32.

70 Kitzmiller JL, Cloherty JP, Younger MD, *et al.* Diabetic pregnancy and perinatal morbidity. *Am J Obstet Gynecol* 1978; **131**: 560–80.

71 Hsu CD, Hong SF, Nickless NA, Copel JA. Glycosylated hemoglobin in insulin-dependent diabetes mellitus related to preeclampsia. *Am J Perinatol* 1998; **15**: 199–202.

72 Hare JW, White P. Pregnancy in diabetes complicated by vascular disease. *Diabetes* 1977; **26**: 953–5.

73 Leguizamon GF, Reece EA. Diabetic neuropathy and coronary heart disease. In: Reece EA, Coustan DR, Gabbe SG, eds. *Diabetes in Women*, 3rd ed. Philadelphia: Lippincott, Willliams & Wilkins, 2004: 425–32.

74 Crowther CA, Hiller JE, Moss JR, *et al.* Effect of treatment of gestational diabetes mellitus on pregnancy outcomes. *N Engl J Med* 2005; **352**: 2477–86.

75 The Hyperglycemia and Adverse Pregnancy Outcome (HAPO) Study. *Int J Gynaecol Obstet* 2002; **78**: 69–77.

76   Brody SC, Harris R, Lohr K. Screening for gestational diabetes: a summary of the evidence for the U.S. Preventive Services Task Force. *Obstet Gynecol* 2003; **101**: 380–92.

77   Sacks DA, Greenspoon JS, Abu-Fadil S, *et al.* Toward universal criteria for gestational diabetes: the 75-gram glucose tolerance test in pregnancy. *Am J Obstet Gynecol* 1995; **172**: 607–14.

78   Buchanan TA, Xiang AH, Peters RK, *et al.* Preservation of pancreatic beta-cell function and prevention of type 2 diabetes by pharmacological treatment of insulin resistance in high-risk Hispanic women. *Diabetes* 2002; **51**: 2796–803.

79   Cundy T, Gamble G, Townend K, *et al.* Perinatal mortality in type 2 diabetes mellitus. *Diabet Med* 2000; **17**: 33–9.

80   de Veciana M, Major CA, Morgan MA, *et al.* Postprandial versus preprandial blood glucose monitoring in women with gestational diabetes mellitus requiring insulin therapy. *N Engl J Med* 1995; **333**: 1237–41.

81   Naylor CD, Sermer M, Chen E, Sykora K. Cesarean delivery in relation to birth weight and gestational glucose tolerance: pathophysiology or practice style? Toronto Trihospital Gestational Diabetes Investigators. *JAMA* 1996; **275**: 1165–70.

82   Weiss PA. Diabetes in pregnancy: lessons from the fetus. In: Dornhorst A, Hadden DR, eds. *Diabetes and Pregnancy.* Chichester: Wiley, 2005: 221–240.

83   Buchanan TA, Kjos SL, Montoro MN, *et al.* Use of fetal ultrasound to select metabolic therapy for pregnancies complicated by mild gestational diabetes. *Diabetes Care* 1994; **17**: 275–83.

84   Kjos SL, Schaefer-Graf U, Sardesi S, *et al.* A randomized controlled trial using glycemic plus fetal ultrasound parameters versus glycemic parameters to determine insulin therapy in gestational diabetes with fasting hyperglycemia. *Diabetes Care* 2001; **24**: 1904–10.

85   Schaefer-Graf UM, Kjos SL, Fauzan OH, *et al.* A randomized trial evaluating a predominantly fetal growth-based strategy to guide management of gestational diabetes in Caucasian women. *Diabetes Care* 2004; **27**: 297–302.

86   Langer O, Conway DL, Berkus MD, *et al.* A comparison of glyburide and insulin in women with gestational diabetes mellitus. *N Engl J Med* 2000; **343**: 1134–8.

87   Hirsch IB. Insulin analogues. *N Engl J Med* 2005; **352**: 174–83.

88   Pettitt DJ, Ospina P, Kolaczynski JW, Jovanovic L. Comparison of an insulin analog, insulin aspart, and regular human insulin with no insulin in gestational diabetes mellitus. *Diabetes Care* 2003; **26**: 183–6.

89   Jovanovic L, Ilic S, Pettitt DJ, *et al.* Metabolic and immunologic effects of insulin lispro in gestational diabetes. *Diabetes Care* 1999; **22**: 1422–7.

6

Hemostatic factors in vascular disease

GORDON D O LOWE

INTRODUCTION

Hemostasis is the arrest of blood loss following blood vessel injury. Initial vasoconstriction is followed by formation of a platelet-fibrin hemostatic plug. Thrombosis has been described as 'hemostasis in the wrong place'.[1] Pathologic, pharmacologic, and epidemiologic studies have established that the interaction of blood platelets and coagulation factors with the blood vessel wall is important not only in hemostasis, but also in both arterial and venous thrombosis.[2–4] The aims of this chapter are to:

- outline the interactions of blood platelets and coagulation factors (and their inhibitors) with the blood vessel wall in hemostasis and thrombosis
- summarize epidemiologic studies of the associations of hemostatic variables with venous and arterial thrombosis
- to inform, and link to, subsequent chapters in this book on thrombophilias and hemophilias (Chapters 7–9), antithrombotic drugs (Chapters 11 and 12), hemostatic and thrombotic problems in reproduction (Section 2), and the thrombotic problems of oral contraceptives, hormone replacement therapy (HRT) and selective estrogen receptor modulators (SERMs) (Section 3).

PLATELETS

Platelets and hemostasis

Platelets are anuclear cell fragments, (1–3 μm in diameter), which are derived from bone marrow megakaryocytes, and circulate in human blood at a concentration of $150–450 \times 10^9$/L. They play a key role in hemostasis. Disruption of the vessel wall exposes circulating platelets to subendothelial collagen, and to products of cellular injury including adenosine diphosphate (ADP) and thrombin. These substances activate platelets through interaction with specific platelet membrane receptors, resulting in platelet activation through several biochemical pathways (Fig. 6.1). Activated platelets adhere to vascular subendothelium and aggregate, forming a hemostatic plug (Fig. 6.2). This is subsequently stabilized by strands of fibrin formed from circulating fibrinogen by thrombin, which is formed by the interaction of circulating coagulation factors upon the surface of activated platelets (Fig. 6.2).

Key cofactors in platelet aggregation include von Willebrand factor (vWF) and fibrinogen (which are present in plasma and in platelet granules); as well as shear rate and hematocrit. Von Willebrand factor binds to specific receptors on vascular endothelium and on platelet membranes (platelet glycoprotein Ib/IX), promoting both

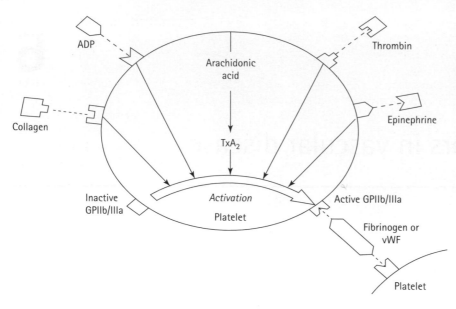

Figure 6.1 Platelet activation pathways. Platelets can be activated by collagen, adenosine diphosphate (ADP), thrombin or adrenaline; each of these agonists interacts with a specific platelet membrane receptor. Internal platelet activation pathways include the conversion of membrane-associated arachidonic acid to thromboxane A_2 (TxA_2). Platelet activation results in the activation of membrane glycoprotein (GP)IIb/IIIa receptors, which on adjacent platelets are then linked by fibrinogen or von Willebrand factor (vWF), resulting in platelet aggregation. (Redrawn from Lowe GD[5] with permission.)

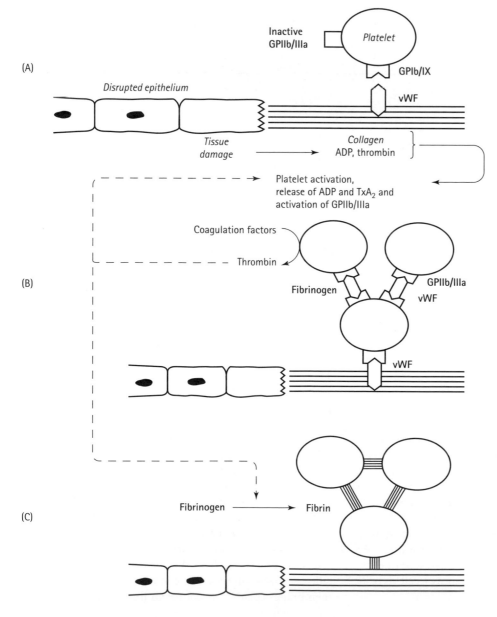

Figure 6.2 Platelet adhesion and activation, and fibrin formation. (A) Platelet adhesion. Activated platelets adhere to vascular subendothelium, especially subendothelial collagen which is linked by von Willebrand factor (vWF) to platelet membrane glycoprotein (GP)Ib/IX receptors. (B) Platelet aggregation, and interaction of coagulation factors on platelet surface, forming thrombin. Platelet activation results in their aggregation by fibrinogen or vWF, which link activated platelet membrane GPIIb/IIIa receptors. Plasma coagulation factors interact on the surfaces of activated platelets, forming thrombin. Thrombin further increases platelet activation. (C) Fibrin formation, stabilizing the hemostatic plug. Thrombin also converts circulating fibrinogen to fibrin, which stabilizes the hemostatic plug. TxA_2, thromboxane A_2. (Redrawn from Lowe GD[5] with permission.)

platelet adhesion to the vessel wall, and platelet aggregation (under high-shear conditions). Fibrinogen binds to platelet membrane glycoprotein IIb/IIIa, promoting platelet aggregation (under low-shear conditions). The functional significance of vWF is shown by the clinical bleeding tendency associated with congenital or acquired deficiency of vWD (von Willebrand disease); and the functional significance of fibrinogen is shown by the clinical bleeding tendency associated with congenital or acquired deficiency of fibrinogen (hypo- or dysfibrinogenemias).

Role of platelets in arterial thrombosis

Following arterial injury, activated platelets form a 'hemostatic plug', which may grow and either narrow or occlude the artery at the site of plaque rupture, or embolize resulting in distal arterial or microcirculatory occlusion (Fig. 6.3). Symptomatic ischemia may result from either type of occlusion. Alternatively, endothelial cells may grow over the thrombosed, ruptured arterial plaque, contributing to the development of atherosclerosis: the Rokitansky–Duguid

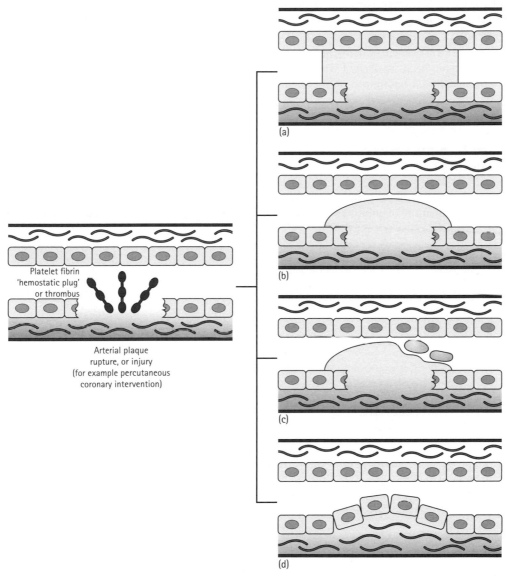

Figure 6.3   Arterial thrombosis and its consequences. Following spontaneous rupture of an arterial atherosclerotic plaque (or arterial injury, for example, percutaneous coronary intervention) a platelet-fibrin 'hemostatic plug' or thrombus forms, with four possible consequences. (A) Occlusive thrombus, for example, acute transmural/ST segment elevation myocardial infarction (STEMI), acute coronary syndromes including subendocardial myocardial infarction and unstable angina. (B) Partially occlusive thrombus, for example, non-STEMI acute coronary syndromes. (C) Embolism and distal arterial or microcirculatory occlusion, for example, sudden cardiac death (ventricular fibrillation) or transient cerebral ischemic attacks. (D) Further development of atherosclerosis. Endothelial cells grow over the mural thrombus, which is incorporated into the arterial wall, according to the Rokitansky–Duguid hypothesis. (Redrawn from Lowe GD[5] with permission.)

hypothesis (Fig. 6.3). Platelets release a variety of proinflammatory substances (for example, platelet derived growth factor [PDGF]) which may contribute to atherogenesis.[6]

Evidence for the role of platelets in arterial thrombosis and atherogenesis is partly based on pathologic and experimental studies.[7] There is also increasing evidence from prospective epidemiologic studies that blood levels of platelet activation markers or cofactors are associated with risk of ischemic cardiovascular events. Neither platelet count nor *ex vivo* platelet aggregation is associated with risk of myocardial infarction (MI) or stroke in samples of the general population.[8–10] However, mean platelet volume[11] and *ex vivo* platelet aggregation[12] have been associated with risk of recurrent MI, or of coronary occlusion after percutaneous coronary interventions (PCI), in patients with symptomatic coronary heart disease (CHD). Furthermore, platelet cofactors such as hematocrit,[13] fibrinogen,[14] and vWF[15] have been associated with risk of CHD in people with or without baseline clinical evidence of arterial disease.

Antiplatelet agents in prevention of cardiovascular events

Evidence for a possible causal role of platelets in arterial disease has led to the evaluation of inhibitors of platelet function in prevention of cardiovascular events (MI, stroke, cardiovascular death, arterial or graft occlusion, venous thromboembolism [VTE]). Several antiplatelet agents have been evaluated in randomized controlled trials.[2,16] Their mechanisms of action are summarized in Fig. 6.4.

The Antithrombotic Trialists' Collaboration[17] recently reported collaborative metaanalyses (systematic overviews) of the randomized trials of antiplatelet therapy in patients at high risk of occlusive vascular events (about 135 000 in comparisons of antiplatelet therapy versus control; and about 77 000 in comparisons of different antiplatelet regimens). The main outcome measure was 'serious vascular event': nonfatal MI, nonfatal stroke, or vascular death. Overall, antiplatelet therapy reduced this combined outcome by about a quarter, reflecting reductions in nonfatal MI of a third, in nonfatal stroke of a quarter, and in vascular mortality of a sixth. There was no significant adverse effect on other deaths, hence total deaths were also reduced by a sixth. In all common categories of vascular disease (acute or prior MI; acute or prior stroke; transient cerebral ischemic attack; stable or unstable angina; peripheral arterial disease; atrial fibrillation), the absolute benefits of antiplatelet therapy substantially outweighed the absolute risks of major bleeding. However, it should be noted that patients at high risk of bleeding were usually excluded from trials of antiplatelet therapy. The Antithrombotic Trialists' Collaboration[17,18] also reported that aspirin reduced the risk of symptomatic

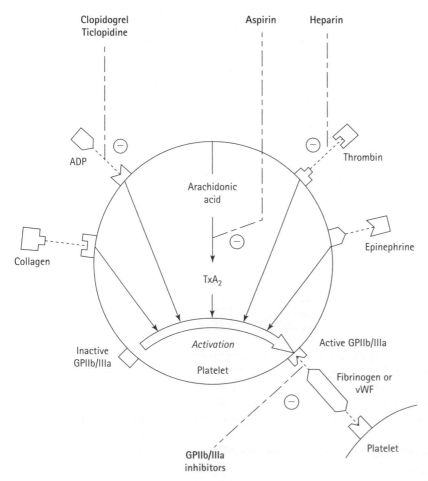

Figure 6.4 Mechanisms of action of antiplatelet agents. Clopidogrel and ticlopidine are inhibitors of one of the platelet adenosine diphosphate (ADP) receptors. Aspirin acetylates platelet cyclooxygenase, resulting in impaired production of thromboxane A_2 (TxA_2) and of proaggregatory prostaglandins. Heparin inhibits thrombin. Glycoprotein (GP)IIb/IIIa receptor blockers inhibit the platelet membrane GPIIb/IIIa receptor, preventing fibrinogen binding and platelet aggregation. vWF, von Willebrand factor. (Redrawn from Lowe GD[5] with permission.)

VTE which was confirmed in a recent large trial in patients undergoing orthopedic surgery.[19] Platelets therefore play an important role in VTE, and aspirin is recommended as prophylaxis in certain groups of at-risk hospitalized patients, (e.g. hip fracture patients).[20]

BLOOD COAGULATION

Blood coagulation and hemostasis

Figure 6.5 outlines blood coagulation pathways. Blood coagulation factors are given roman numerals: I (fibrinogen), II (prothrombin) and V–XIII (VI does not exist); the suffix 'a' denotes activation of the zymogen to the active enzyme. Blood coagulation is initiated through the tissue factor (extrinsic) pathway, when blood is exposed to tissue factor following tissue damage or inflammation. Tissue factor activates factor VII to factor VIIa, which in turn activates factors IX to IXa, and X to Xa. Factor Xa activates factor II (prothrombin) to IIa (thrombin), which in turn activates factor I (fibrinogen) to fibrin. Thrombin also activates factor XIII to XIIIa, which cross-links soluble fibrin to insoluble, cross-linked fibrin. Thrombin also activates blood platelets, promoting platelet adhesion to the damaged vessel wall and platelet aggregation, which together with insoluble,

cross-linked fibrin forms either a physiologic hemostatic plug or a pathologic venous or arterial thrombus (Fig. 6.5).

There are two self-amplification loops in this 'coagulation cascade'. First, factor Xa promotes further activation of the tissue factor–VIIa complex, amplifying the initial stage of thrombin and fibrin formation. Second, thrombin activates factor V to Va (which is the cofactor in the activation of factor X to Xa); activates factor VIII to VIIIa (which is the cofactor in the activation of factor IX to IXa); and finally activates factor XI to XIa, which activates factor IX to factor IXa (Fig. 6.5). Factor XI can also be activated to XIa by activated factor XII; however, the physiologic significance of factor XII in hemostasis is uncertain, because even total congenital deficiency of factor XII is not associated with increased risk of bleeding, in contrast to other congenital deficiencies of coagulation factors (hemophilias).

Unchecked activation of the coagulation system would rapidly lead to fatal disseminated intravascular coagulation or thrombosis; hence coagulation activation is controlled by three distinct pathways of coagulation inhibition (shown in gray in Fig. 6.5). Antithrombin is a direct inhibitor of thrombin, Xa and IXa; and is activated either by endogenous heparins or by therapeutic heparins. The protein C anticoagulant system is activated by thrombin, as a negative feedback loop controlling excessive thrombin formation. Thrombin acts with thrombomodulin on endothelial cells,

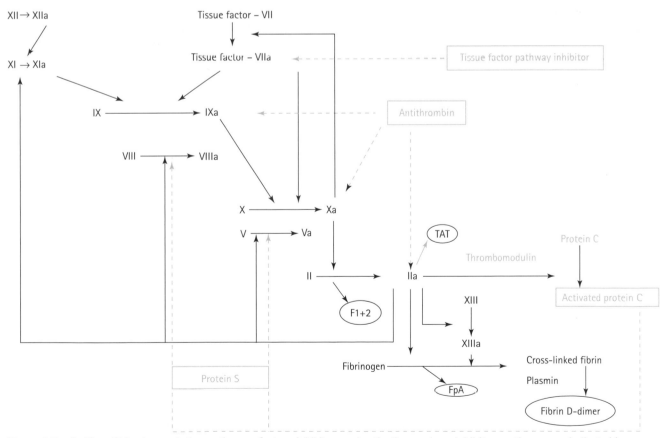

Figure 6.5   Outline of blood coagulation pathways: factors, inhibitors and activation markers. Inhibitory pathways are indicated in gray boxes and broken lines. Activation markers are indicated in the ovals.

and with the endothelial protein C receptor, to activate circulating protein C. Activated protein C, together with its cofactor protein S, inactivates factors Va and VIIIa. The third endogenous coagulation inhibitor, tissue factor pathway inhibitor (TFPI) inactivates the tissue factor–VII complex. As shown in Figure 6.5, these three coagulation inhibitors play complementary roles, each inhibiting different activated coagulation factors.

Although plasma levels of coagulation factors and of inhibitors indicate potential for coagulation activation, thrombin formation and thrombosis; plasma markers of coagulation activation (measured by sensitive immunoassays) are a measure of actual coagulation *in vivo*. Figure 6.5 shows (in ovals) three markers of thrombin activation: prothrombin fragment F1+2 (which is split from prothrombin when it is activated to thrombin by Xa); thrombin–antithrombin (TAT) complexes; and fibrinopeptide A (FpA) which is split from fibrinogen by thrombin. Each of these three activation markers is susceptible to artifactual elevation during venepuncture, especially FpA and TAT. In contrast, fibrin D-dimer is resistant to artifactual elevation, has a longer plasma half-life than the three markers of thrombin activity (days rather than minutes), and measures not only thrombin formation but also the formation of cross-linked fibrin, which is lysed to the D-dimer fragment by plasmin, generated by the endogenous fibrinolytic system (Fig. 6.5).

Blood coagulation and venous thromboembolism

If deficiency of physiologically important coagulation factors causes excessive bleeding (hemophilias), then high levels of coagulation factors and low levels of coagulation inhibitors might be expected to increase the risks of thrombosis (thrombophilias). This concept was supported in an epidemiologic study which showed that increasing plasma levels of F1+2 and TAT in a random sample of the general population were associated with increasing levels of factors VII, VIII and IX, and decreasing levels of protein C.[21] Levels of F1+2 and TAT also increased with age, which may partly reflect greater increases in coagulation factors compared to inhibitors with age; and may be relevant to the increased risk of thrombosis with age.[21] Currently recognized thrombophilias are summarized in Table 6.1.

Deficiencies of coagulation inhibition

Genetic deficiencies of coagulation inhibitors (antithrombin, protein C, and protein S) constitute the 'classical' thrombophilias, which were described between 1965 and 1983.[23] Homozygous antithrombin deficiency appears incompatible with life, and homozygous deficiency of protein C may be complicated by life-threatening skin necrosis in infancy[23] (now preventable or treatable by infusion of protein C concentrates). Table 6.1 shows that these three genetic coagulation deficiencies (whose inheritance is autosomal dominant) are uncommon in the general population (collectively comprising less than 1 percent) but comprise about 6 percent of consecutive patients with proved VTE (relative risk about 5–6) (see also Chapter 7).

OTHER DEFICIENCIES IN COAGULATION INHIBITION

In 1993–94, the discovery that many patients with proved VTE and a family history had a new phenotypic defect (resistance to activated protein C)[24,25] led to the discovery that this phenotype was commonly associated with a mutation in coagulation factor V (the Leiden mutation,[26]) which conferred resistance to its inactivation by activated protein C (Fig. 6.5). This mutation is common in the general populations of Western countries (prevalence 2–15 percent with marked geographic variation) and in consecutive patients with VTE (10–20 percent; relative risk about 4; Table 6.1). The prevalence is rare in populations at low risk of venous thromboembolism such as Africans, Chinese, Japanese, Indonesians, Aboriginals, South American Indians and the Inuit.[25] Another mutation, in the prothrombin gene (20210A), is also common in the general population (1–3 percent) and in consecutive patients with VTE (5–6 percent).[25,27] It is associated with increased plasma prothrombin levels,[27] but also with the phenotype of activated protein C resistance,[28] which may account for the supra-additive increase in risk of VTE when these two common mutations coincide.[29]

Table 6.1 Estimates of prevalences of thrombophilias in patients with confirmed venous thromboembolism (VTE) and in the general population; and of relative risks.

Thrombophilia	Patients with VTE (%)	General population (%)	Relative risk
Antithrombin deficiency	1	0.2	5
Protein C deficiency	2	0.3	6
Protein S deficiency	2	0.3	6
Factor V Leiden	10–20	2–15	4
Prothrombin 20210A	6	2	3
High factor VIII	20	10	2

Factor V Leiden and Prothrombin 20210A are also associated with arterial thrombosis.
See reference 22.

Although classic genetic thrombophilias are usually associated with extreme low values of coagulation inhibitors, case–control studies of VTE have also associated increased risk with relatively minor reductions in antithrombin[30,31] protein C,[30,31] and protein S.[32] The prospective Longitudinal Investigation of Thromboembolism Etiology (LITE) study has also associated VTE risk with low protein C levels.[33] Recently, deficiency of TFPI has been associated with risk of VTE in a case–control study[34] (see also Chapter 7).

Increases in coagulation factors

In recent years, the associations of plasma levels of coagulation factors with risk of VTE have been increasingly studied, as have functional genetic mutations which increase plasma levels. Prospective studies, such as the LITE study[33,35–38] of clinical VTE in two general population cohorts in the United States, and studies of the association of preoperative blood tests with asymptomatic postoperative deep vein thrombosis (DVT)[39] such as the European Concerted Action Against Thrombosis (ECAT) DVT study[40] are less subject to bias than case–control studies.

The association of fibrinogen (factor I) levels, or functional mutations, with VTE risk have been inconsistent in case–control studies[41,42] and generally nonsignificant in prospective studies.[35,39,40] However, extreme reduction in plasma fibrinogen levels by defibrination with the snake venom enzyme, ancrod, reduced the incidence of VTE in randomized, placebo-controlled trials,[43] possibly due to anticoagulation and reduction in blood viscosity. As discussed above, the associations of the functional prothrombin (factor II) mutation (20210A) with VTE risk are consistent with a role for this coagulation factor in pathogenesis of VTE. The associations of the factor V Leiden mutation with VTE risk are also consistent with a role for this coagulation factor in pathogenesis of VTE. Prospective studies have confirmed a significant association of VTE risk with this mutation, as well as with its associated phenotype: resistance to activated protein C.[36,40] Factor VII levels and functional polymorphisms have not shown consistent associations with VTE risk in case–control studies[30,41,42] or in prospective studies of postoperative DVT.[39,40] However, factor VII levels above the 95th percentile were associated with a relative VTE risk of 2.4, as compared with the lowest quartile in the LITE prospective study.[35]

Factor VIII levels have generally shown associations with VTE risk in several case–control studies[30,32,44–47] and in prospective studies of incidence[35,39,40] or recurrence.[48] The association was independent of acute-phase reactions.[35,45,49] The association of VTE risk with factor VIII was independent of levels of its carrier protein, von Willebrand factor, in the LETS case–control study,[44] but not in the prospective LITE study.[35] Factor VIII and von Willebrand factor levels are heritable[50] but no common functional gene polymorphisms have been reported to date. High factor VIII levels are also a common cause of activated protein C resistance.[25] Because high factor VIII levels are common, 20 percent of VTE might be attributable to elevated levels[25,35] (Table 6.1). The causal significance of high factor VIII levels is supported by their association with increasing levels of coagulation activation markers in the general population,[21,51] and is potentially testable by future randomized trials of antibodies which lower plasma factor VIII activity (D Collen, personal communication, 2003).

Factor IX levels have shown associations with VTE risk in two case–control studies[31,52] which require confirmation in prospective studies. Factor IX levels correlate strongly with levels of its cofactor, factor VIII,[21,53] and high levels of both factors VIII and IX appear to increase the risk of VTE.[52] Evidence that factor IX may play an important role in thrombosis has been reviewed recently.[53] With regard to factors X–XIII, reports from the LETS case–control study have reported that VTE risk is associated with increased levels of factors XI,[54] and X[55] but not XII.[56] A recent metaanalysis of case–control studies observed a weak protective effect of the factor XIII Val34 Leu polymorphism (which is associated with higher levels of factor XIII) on VTE risk.[57]

Increases in coagulation activation markers

Fibrin D-dimer levels have shown associations with VTE risk in two case–control studies,[31,58] and in prospective studies of incidence[37,39,40] or recurrence.[59] Although raised D-dimer levels may partly reflect other thrombophilias, such as factor V Leiden, the prothrombin 20210A mutation and possibly others,[31,37] it remained associated with incident or recurrent clinical VTE, independent of these factors.[37,58] D-dimer and other activation markers appear to have high heritability, supporting the hypothesis that they may reflect genetic factors.[60] It is likely that raised D-dimer levels reflect increased thrombin activity, rather than increased plasmin activity (Fig. 6.5), because anticoagulation with warfarin normalizes raised levels.[61,62] However there are no reported epidemiologic studies on the association of markers of thrombin activity with risk of VTE.

In conclusion, recent epidemiologic studies support the concept that VTE is a multicausal disease, resulting from interactions between multiple genetic and environmental variables, in which blood coagulation plays a central role[3] (see also Chapters 7 and 8).

Blood coagulation and arterial disease

DEFICIENCIES OF COAGULATION INHIBITION

As noted above, there is now strong evidence that deficiencies of coagulation inhibition are associated with increased risk of venous thromboembolism. Evidence for their associations with arterial thrombosis is generally weak. However, a recent metaanalysis of published studies of the factor V Leiden and prothrombin G20210A mutations observed modest, but statistically significant associations with coronary heart disease, stroke and peripheral arterial events, especially in younger people (age under 55 years) and in women.[22] These findings may be relevant to the increases in risk of myocardial infarction and stroke during pregnancy and use of combined oral contraceptives or oral HRT (see below).

FIBRINOGEN

Fibrinogen is the major plasma coagulation factor by weight (1.5–4 g/L). As noted above, fibrinogen is a major hemostatic factor (as a key mediator of platelet aggregation, and also the precursor of fibrin). It is also a major 'acute-phase reactant' protein, whose plasma concentration increases twofold to threefold as a response to tissue injury. Such increases lead to elevations in plasma viscosity and red cell aggregation (for example, as measured by the erythrocyte sedimentation rate [ESR]) and hence to increases in blood viscosity, especially under low-shear conditions. Finally, fibrinogen adheres to and infiltrates the vessel wall, and plays a role in leukocyte adhesion to the vessel wall. There are therefore several plausible mechanisms through which increased plasma fibrinogen levels might promote the risk of atherothrombosis.[63,64]

A recent literature-based metaanalysis[14] of prospective studies of fibrinogen and CHD risk reported that the relative risk of CHD for persons in the upper third of plasma fibrinogen level compared with those in the bottom third was 1.8 (95 percent confidence interval [CI] 1.5 to 2.0). This risk was similar in persons with and without baseline evidence of cardiovascular disease (Fig. 6.6). A further metaanalysis observed similar associations of plasma viscosity with risk of CHD.[13] The weaker association of the ESR with CHD risk[13] may be attributable to the association of hematocrit (which lowers ESR) with CHD risk.[13]

More reliable results on the individual predictive value of plasma fibrinogen for risk of CHD and stroke, over and above that of classic risk factors, has recently been reported from the Fibrinogen Studies Collaboration.[66,67] This collaborative metaanalysis of individual participants data from[39] prospective studies, involving over 150 000 people, confirmed that fibrinogen was an independent risk factor not only for CHD, but also for stroke.[67]

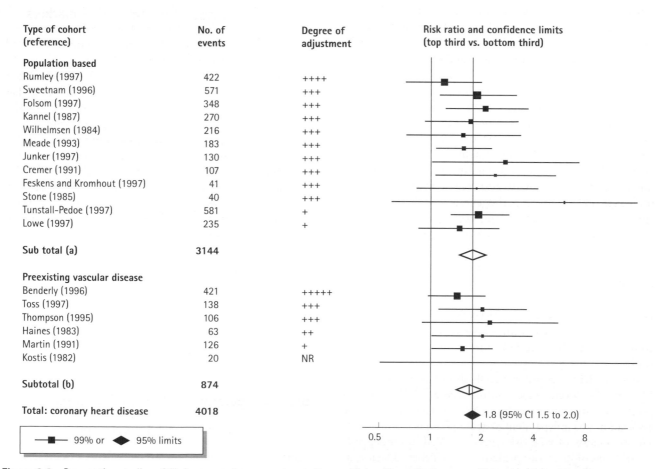

Figure 6.6   Prospective studies of fibrinogen and coronary heart disease. Risk ratios compare top and bottom thirds of baseline measurements. Degree of adjustment refers to adjustment for age and sex only (+), for these plus standard coronary heart disease (CHD) risk factors (++ and +++), chronic disease at baseline (++++) or not reported (NR). (Redrawn from Danesh J, Collins R, Appleby P, Peto R. Association of fibrinogen, C-reactive protein, albumin, or leukocyte count with coronary heart disease. Meta-analysis of prospective studies. *JAMA* 1998; **279**: 1477–82. Copyright © 1998, American Medical Association. All rights reserved with permission.)

Although there is a significant genetic component to variation in plasma fibrinogen, individual functional polymorphisms explain only a small percentage of such variation.[68,69] Such functional polymorphisms show little or no association with risk of CHD[64,68,69] which questions the causality of fibrinogen in pathogenesis of CHD, according to the hypothesis of 'Mendelian randomization'.[70] However, the effect of such polymorphisms on variation in plasma fibrinogen is weak; and a recent study suggests that CHD is associated not with plasma levels of 'intact' fibrinogen released from the liver under genetic control, nor with measures of acute-phase reactions (C-reactive protein, interleukin-6), but with 'hyperfunctional' plasma fibrinogen.[71] The relations of CHD with genetic and functional variations in fibrinogen require further study. Like the ESR, C-reactive protein is a relatively weak predictor of CHD events.[65]

As noted above, reducing plasma fibrinogen levels by ancrod reduced the incidence of VTE in randomized, placebo-controlled trials in patients with hip fractures, or with acute ischemic stroke.[43] The prognosis of stroke was also improved, perhaps due to reduction in blood viscosity which increases blood flow in the cerebral microcirculation and reduces the size of cerebral infarction.[41,72] Whether or not chronic reduction in plasma fibrinogen reduces the risk of CHD or stroke will require development of selective oral agents which can be taken safely for several years in randomized controlled trials (as statins have shown for chronic reduction in plasma low-density lipoprotein cholesterol).

THE FACTOR VIII–VON WILLEBRAND FACTOR COMPLEX

As noted above, vWF and factor VIII play, respectively, key roles in platelet adhesion and aggregation, and in thrombin formation. Measures of vWF antigen, vWF activity (platelet aggregation), and factor VIII activity are highly correlated in the general population ($r = 0.6$), and each predict risk of CHD in population cohorts.[73] A metaanalysis of prospective studies showed an odds ratio of about 1.5 (95 percent CI 1.1 to 2.0) for top versus bottom thirds of baseline measurements of vWF antigen.[15] A recent updated metaanalysis showed a lower odds ratio of 1.23 (95 percent CI 1.14 to 1.33).[65] Further studies are required before a reliable assessment of the predictive value of factor VIII can be made.

The importance of factor VIII (or factor IX) in CHD risk has recently been shown in an observational study from the Netherlands of female carriers of hemophilia A (who have low-normal plasma factor VIII levels) or hemophilia B (who have low-normal plasma factor IX levels).[74] Carriers had significantly lower risk of CHD than the age-matched female population. Because it had been previously reported that individuals with hemophilia (who have very low plasma levels of factor VIII or factor IX) had an even lower risk of CHD,[75] there appears to be a dose-dependent risk of CHD associated with plasma levels of factors VIII or IX. The results of this 'x-linked randomized trial' might be confirmed by future randomized controlled trials of lowering factor VIII levels, for example, by antibodies (D Collen, personal communication, 2003).

OTHER COAGULATION FACTORS

At present, there are insufficient data from prospective studies to establish whether or not there is an association of CHD risk with other coagulation factors, including factors VII,[76–82] XII,[82] or XIII.[83] On the other hand, the Thrombosis Prevention Trial showed that low-dose warfarin (which lowers plasma activity levels of factors II, VII, IX and X) reduced risk of CHD events in high-risk men.[84]

COAGULATION ACTIVATION MARKERS

As noted above, several studies have associated circulating levels of fibrin D-dimer with risk of venous thromboembolism. Fibrin D-dimer also predicts risk of CHD in population cohorts.[80,85,86] A recent metaanalysis[87] of prospective studies showed an odds ratio of 1.7 (95 percent CI

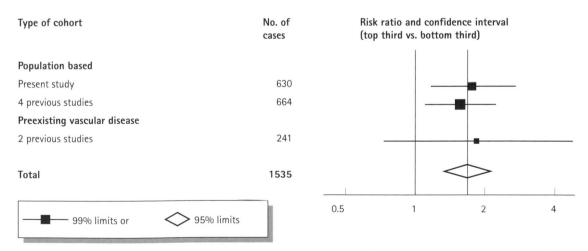

Figure 6.7   Prospective studies of fibrin D-dimer and coronary heart disease. Risk ratios compare top and bottom thirds of baseline measurements. (Redrawn from Danesh J, Whincup P, Walker M, *et al.* Fibrin D-dimer and coronary heart disease: prospective study and meta-analysis. *Circulation* 2001; **103**: 2323–7, with permission.)

1.3 to 2.2) for top versus bottom third of baseline D-dimer measurements (Fig. 6.7). There are insufficient data to establish whether or not other coagulation markers (for example, fibrinopeptide A, prothrombin fragment F1+2, TAT complexes) are also predictors of CHD.[81,82] The Thrombosis Prevention Trial showed that low-dose warfarin (which reduced risk of CHD events in high-risk men) also lowered plasma levels of prothrombin fragment F1+2 and D-dimer.[88] D-dimer levels are also raised in patients with nonrheumatic atrial fibrillation, and lowered by conventional-dose warfarin,[61,62] or cardioversion to sinus rhythm.[89] Two recent cohort studies have observed that D-dimer levels are associated with increased risk of stroke and CHD in patients with atrial fibrillation.[90,91]

THE FIBRINOLYTIC SYSTEM AND THROMBOSIS

A physiological balance between blood coagulation and fibrinolysis has been proposed, according to which relative increases in coagulation activation compared to fibrinolytic activation favor thrombosis.[51] However, there is little evidence that fibrinolytic variables such as plasminogen, tissue plasminogen activator (tPA) or plasminogen activator inhibitor type 1 (PAI-1) levels are related to risk of VTE.[38–40,92,93] Likewise, further studies are required to investigate the association of the thrombin-activatible fibrinolysis inhibitor and risk of VTE.[94]

Metaanalyses of prospective studies have shown that circulating tPA antigen (but not PAI-1) is associated with incident CHD in prospective studies of samples of general populations.[95] However, at least half of this association is accounted for by the association of tPA with confounding CHD risk factors; and further studies are required to assess the role of the endogenous fibrinolytic system in arterial disease and thrombosis.

EFFECT OF INCREASED ENDOGENOUS ESTROGENS (PREGNANCY) ON BLOOD COAGULATION AND THROMBOTIC RISK (SEE ALSO SECTION 2)

The relative risk of VTE in pregnancy and the puerperium increases approximately tenfold compared to nonpregnant women of similar age. This may be partly due to increases in coagulation factors (I, V, VII, VIII/vWF, IX, X, XII); decreased protein S, acquired resistance to activated protein C (which may be related to increases in factors V and VIII); decreased fibrinolytic activity (due to increases in both PAI-1 and the placenta-derived PAI-2); and changes in the deep venous system.[96] The risk is increased in congenital and acquired thrombophilias, and may require prophylaxis in women with such thrombophilias and/or previous VTE.

EFFECT OF EXOGENOUS ORAL ESTROGENS (COMBINED ORAL CONTRACEPTIVES AND HORMONE REPLACEMENT THERAPY) ON BLOOD COAGULATION AND THROMBOTIC RISK (SEE ALSO SECTION 3)

Since the first descriptions of increased risk of venous and arterial thrombosis with combined oral contraceptives (COC) in the 1960s, many studies have shown that COC use is associated with several prothrombotic changes in the blood coagulation system.[97,98] In contrast, progestin-only oral contraceptives have not been associated with these changes in blood coagulation, nor in risk of VTE.[20] The extent of such changes in blood coagulation, and of risk of VTE, are related to the dose of estrogen above $50\,\mu g$ ethinylestradiol, but not below.[98] The biochemical basis of these changes is probably stimulation of estrogen receptors in the liver, altering synthesis and release of coagulation proteins (and also lipoproteins, fibrinolytic and inflammatory proteins): the so-called 'first pass' effect of high doses of estrogens in the portal vein following oral ingestion.[97] In recent years, the higher risk of VTE with 'third-generation' COC (containing the progestin, desogestrel, or gestodene) compared with 'second-generation' COC (containing the progestin levonorgestrel) has been attributed to reduced compensation of estrogen-induced coagulation changes by desogestrel compared to levonorgestrel.[98,99]

It was believed for many years that oral HRT was not associated with increased risk of venous or arterial thrombosis, and possibly with reduced risks of CHD and stroke. These beliefs were partly based on the hypothesis that lower doses of more 'physiologic' estrogens in HRT preparations would have lesser effects on blood coagulation compared to COC preparations.[100] However, pharmacologic, epidemiologic, and randomized trial studies published over the past decade have shown that oral HRT (combined or unopposed) has very similar prothrombotic effects to COC (for example, increasing activated protein C resistance and factor IX levels; and decreasing antithrombin and protein S levels), and increases the relative risk of VTE and stroke to a similar extent.[100] Indeed, the absolute risk of VTE and stroke is tenfold higher in oral HRT users compared to COC users, due to their higher age and hence higher baseline risk of venous and arterial thrombosis.[100] The risk of VTE is increased in women with thrombophilias who use HRT.[31] Transdermal HRT has lesser prothrombotic effects on blood coagulation than oral HRT, and appears to have a lower risk of VTE.[31,100–102]

REFERENCES

1 Macfarlane RG. Haemostasis: introduction. *Br Med Bull* 1977; **33**: 183–5.
2 Verstraete M, Fuster V, Topol EJ, eds. *Cardiovascular Thrombosis*, 2nd edn. Philadelphia, PA: Lippincott-Raven, 1998.

◆ 3 Rosendaal FR. Venous thrombosis: a multicausal disease. *Lancet* 1999; **353**: 1167–73.

4 Lowe GDO, Rumley A, Whincup PH, Danesh J. Hemostatic and rheological variables and risk of cardiovascular disease. *Semin Vasc Med* 2002; **2**: 429–40.

5 Lowe GDO. Clopidogrel in prevention of cardiovascular events. *Rev Contemp Pharmacol* 2003; **12**: 265–98.

6 Ross R. Atherosclerosis – an inflammatory disease. *N Engl J Med* 1999; **340**: 115–26.

7 Woolf N. Thrombosis and atherosclerosis. In: Bloom AL, Thomas DP, eds. *Haemostasis and Thrombosis*, 2nd edn. Edinburgh: Churchill Livingstone, 1987: 651–78.

8 Meade TW. The epidemiology of atheroma, thrombosis and ischaemic heart disease. In: Bloom AL, Forbes CD, Thomas DP, Tuddenham EGD, eds. *Haemostasis and Thrombosis*, 3rd edn. Edinburgh: Churchill Livingstone, 1994: 1199–227.

9 Lowe GDO, Rumley A, Norrie J, *et al.*, on behalf of the West of Scotland Coronary Prevention Study Group. Blood rheology, cardiovascular risk factors, and cardiovascular disease. The West of Scotland coronary prevention study. *Thromb Haemost* 2000; **84**: 533–58.

10 Elwood PC, Beswick A, Pickering J, *et al.* Platelet tests in the prediction of myocardial infarction and ischaemic stroke: evidence from the Caerphilly prospective study. *Br J Haematol* 2001; **113**: 514–20.

11 Martin JF, Bath PMW, Burr ML. Influence of platelet size on outcome after myocardial infarction. *Lancet* 1991; **338**: 1409–11.

12 Trip MD, Cats VM, von Capelle FJL, Vreeken J. Platelet hyperactivity and prognosis in survivors of myocardial infarction. *N Engl J Med* 1990; **322**: 1549–54.

13 Danesh J, Collins R, Peto R, Lowe GDO. Haematocrit, viscosity, erythrocyte sedimentation rate: meta-analyses of prospective studies of coronary heart disease. *Eur Heart J* 2000; **21**: 515–20.

14 Danesh J, Collins R, Appleby P, Peto R. Association of fibrinogen, C-reactive protein, albumin, or leukocyte count with coronary heart disease. Meta-analyses of prospective studies. *JAMA* 1998; **279**: 1477–82.

15 Whincup P, Danesh J, Walker M, *et al.* Von Willebrand factor and coronary heart disease: new prospective study and meta-analysis. *Eur Heart J* 2002; **23**: 1764–70.

16 Patrono C, Coller B, Dalen JE, *et al.* Platelet-active drugs. The relationships among dose, effectiveness, and side effects. *Chest* 2001; **119**(Suppl): 39s–63s.

17 Antithrombotic Trialists' Collaboration Prevention of death, myocardial infarction and stroke by antiplatelet therapy: collaborative meta-analysis of 266 trials involving 200 000 patients at high risk of occlusive vascular disease. *BMJ* 2002; **325**: 71–86.

18 Antiplatelet Trialists Collaboration. Collaborative overview of randomised trials of antiplatelet therapy. III. Reductions in venous thrombosis and pulmonary embolism by antiplatelet prophylaxis among surgical and medical patients. *BMJ* 1994; **308**: 235–40.

19 Pulmonary Embolism Prevention (PEP) Trial Collaborative Group. Prevention of pulmonary embolism and deep vein thrombosis with low dose aspirin: pulmonary embolism prevention (PEP) trial. *Lancet* 2000; **355**: 1259–302.

★ 20 Scottish Intercollegiate Guidelines Network. *Prophylaxis of Venous Thromboembolism. A National Clinical Guideline.* (SIGN guideline 62). Edinburgh: Scottish Intercollegiate Guidelines Network, 2002.

21 Lowe GDO, Rumley A, Woodward M, *et al.* Epidemiology of coagulation factors, inhibitors and activation markers: The Third Glasgow MONICA Survey. I. Illustrative reference ranges by age, sex and hormone use. *Br J Haematol* 1997; **97**: 775–84.

22 Kim RJ, Becker RC. Association between factor V Leiden, prothrombin G20210A, and methylenetetrahydrofolate reductase C677T mutations and events of the arterial circulatory system: A meta-analysis of published studies. *Am Heart J* 2003; **146**: 948–57.

23 Lane DA, Mannucci PM, Bauer KA, *et al.* Inherited thrombophilia. *Thromb Haemost* 1996; **76**: 651–62 and 824–34.

24 Dahlback B, Carlsson M, Svenson PJ. Familial thrombophilia due to a previously unrecognised mechanism characterised by poor anticoagulant response to activated protein C. *Proc Natl Acad Sci U S A* 1993; **90**: 1004–8.

25 Nicolaes GAF, Dahlback B. Congenital and acquired activated protein C resistance. *Semin Vasc Med* 2003; **3**: 33–45.

26 Bertina RM, Koeleman BPC, Koster T, *et al.* Mutation in blood coagulation factor V associated with resistance to activated protein C. *Nature* 1994; **369**: 64–7.

27 Poort SR, Rosendaal FR, Reitsma PH, Bertina RM. A common genetic variant in the 3 – untranslated region of the prothrombin gene is associated with elevated plasma prothrombin levels and an increase in venous thrombosis. *Blood* 1996; **88**: 3698–703.

28 Castaman G, Tosetto A, Simioni M, *et al.* Phenotypic APC resistance in carriers of the A20210 prothrombin mutation is associated with an increased risk of venous thrombosis. *Thromb Haemost* 2001; **86**: 804–8.

29 Emmerich J, Rosendaal FR, Cattaneo M, *et al.* Combined effect of factor V Leiden and prothrombin 20210A on the risk of venous thromboembolism–pooled analysis of 8 case-control studies including 2310 cases and 3204 controls. *Thromb Haemost* 2001; **86**: 809–16.

30 Koster T. Deep-vein thrombosis. A population-based case-control study: Leiden Thrombophilia Study. MD Thesis, University of Leiden, 1995.

31 Lowe GDO, Woodward M, Vessey MP, *et al.* Thrombotic variables and risk of idiopathic venous thromboembolism in women aged 45–64 years: relationships to hormone replacement therapy. *Thromb Haemost* 2000; **83**: 530–5.

32 Balendra R. Deep vein thrombosis of the leg: natural history and haemostatic variables. MD Thesis, Queen's University of Belfast, 1991.

33   Folsom AR, Aleksic N, Wang L, *et al.* Protein C, antithrombin, and venous thromboembolism incidence. A prospective population-based study. *Arterioscler Thromb Vasc Biol* 2002; **22**: 1018–22.

34   Dahm A, van Hylckama Vlieg A, Bendz B, *et al.* Low levels of tissue factor pathway inhibitor (TFPI) increase the risk of venous thrombosis. *Blood* 2003; **101**: 4387–92.

35   Tsai AW, Cushman M, Rosamond WD, *et al.* Coagulation factors, inflammation markers, and venous H thromboembolism: the Longitudinal Investigation of Thromboembolism Etiology (LITE). *Am J Med* 2002; **113**: 636–42.

36   Folsom AR, Cushman M, Tsai MY, *et al.* A prospective study of venous thromboembolism in relation to factor V Leiden and related factors. *Blood* 2002; **99**: 2720–5.

37   Cushman M, Folsom AR, Wong L, *et al.* Fibrin fragment D-dimer and the risk of future venous thrombosis. *Blood* 2003; **101**: 1243–8.

38   Folsom AR, Cushman M, Heckbert SR, *et al.* A prospective study of fibrinolytic markers and venous thromboembolism. *J Clin Epidemiol* 2003; **56**: 598–603.

39   Lowe GDO. Prediction of postoperative deep vein thrombosis. *Thromb Haemost* 1997; **78**: 47–52.

40   Lowe GDO, Haverkate F, Thompson SG, *et al.*, on behalf of the ECAT DVT Study Group. Prediction of deep vein thrombosis after elective hip replacement surgery by preoperative clinical and haemostatic variables: the ECAT DVT Study. *Thromb Haemost* 1999; **81**: 879–86.

41   Koster T, Rosendaal FR, Reitsma PH, *et al.* Factor VII and fibrinogen levels as risk factors for venous thrombosis. A case-control study of plasma levels and DNA polymorphisms – the Leiden Thrombophilia Study (LETS). *Thromb Haemost* 1994; **71**: 719–22.

42   Austin H, Hooper WC, Lally C, *et al.* Venous thrombosis in relation to fibrinogen and factor VII genes among African-Americans. *J Clin Epidemiol* 2000; **53**: 997–1001.

43   Lowe GDO. Ancrod in treatment of acute ischaemic stroke. *Proc R Coll Phys Edinb* 2001; **31**(Suppl 8): 20–4.

44   Koster T, Blann AD, Briet E, *et al.* Role of clotting factor VIII in effect of von Willebrand factor on occurrence of deep-vein thrombosis. *Lancet* 1995; **345**: 152–5.

45   Kamphuisen PW, Eikenboom JC, Vos HL, *et al.* Increased levels of factor VIII and fibrinogen in patients with venous thrombosis are not caused by acute phase reactions. *Thromb Haemost* 1999; **81**: 680–3.

46   Kraajenhagen RA, in't Anker PS, Koopman MM, *et al.* High plasma concentration of factor VIIIc is a major risk factor for venous thromboembolism. *Thromb Haemost* 2000; **83**: 5–9.

47   Schambeck CM, Hinney K, Gleixner J, Keller F. Venous thromboembolism and associated high plasma factor VIII levels: linked to cytomegalovirus infection? *Thromb Haemost* 2000; **83**: 510–11.

48   Kyrle PA, Minar E, Hirschl M, *et al.* High plasma levels of factor VIII and the risk of recurrent venous thromboembolism. *N Engl J Med* 2000; **343**: 457–62.

49   O'Donnell J, Mumford AD, Manning RA, Laffan M. Elevation of FVIII: C in venous thromboembolism is persistent and independent of the acute phase response. *Thromb Haemost* 2000; **83**: 10–13.

50   Kamphuisen PW, Houwing-Duistermaat JJ, van Houwelingen HC, *et al.* Familial clustering of factor VIII and von Willebrand factor levels. *Thromb Haemost* 1998; **79**: 323–7.

51   Astrup T. The haemostatic balance. *Thromb Diath Haemorrh (Stutt)* 1958; **2**: 347–57.

52   van Hylckama Vleig A, van der Linden I, Bertina RM, Rosendaal FR. High levels of factor IX and venous thrombosis. *Blood* 2000; **95**: 3678–82.

53   Lowe GDO. Factor IX and thrombosis. *Br J Haematol* 2001, 115: 507–13.

54   Meijers JCM, Tekelenberg W, Bouma BN, *et al.* High levels of coagulation factor XI as a risk factor for venous thrombosis. *N Engl J Med* 1999; **342**: 696–701.

55   de Visser MCH, Poort SR, Vos HL, *et al.* Factor X levels, polymorphisms in the promoter region of factor X, and the risk of venous thrombosis. *Thromb Haemost* 2001; **85**: 1011–17.

56   Koster T, Rosendaal FR, Briet E, Vandenbroucke JP. John Hageman's factor and deep-vein thrombosis. Leiden Thrombophilia Study. *Br J Haematol* 1994; **87**: 422–4.

57   van Hylckama Vleig A, Komanasin N, Ariens RAS, *et al.* Factor XIII Val 34 Leu, factor XIII antigen levels and activity and the risk of deep vein thrombosis. *Br J Haematol* 2002; **119**: 169–75.

58   Andreescu ACM, Cushman M, Rosendaal FR. D-dimer as a risk factor for deep vein thrombosis: the Leiden Thrombophilia Study. *Thromb Haemost* 2002; **87**: 47–51.

59   Palareti G, Legnani C, Cosmi B, *et al.* Predictive value of D-dimer test for recurrent venous thromboembolism after anticoagulation withdrawal in subjects with a previous idiopathic event and in carriers of congenital thrombophilias. *Circulation* 2003; **108**: 313–18.

60   Ariens RAS, de Lange M, Freider H, *et al.* Activation markers of coagulation and fibrinolysis in twins: heritability of the pre-thrombotic state. *Lancet* 2002; **359**: 667–71.

61   Lip GYH, Lowe GDO, Rumley A, Dunn FG. Increased markers of thrombogenesis in chronic atrial fibrillation: effects of warfarin treatment. *Br Heart J* 1995; **73**: 527–33.

62   Lip GYH, Zafiris J, Watson RDS, *et al.* Fibrin D-dimer and beta-thromboglobulin as markers of thrombogenesis and platelet activation in atrial fibrillation. Effects of introducing ultra-low-dose warfarin and aspirin. *Circulation* 1996, **94**: 425–31.

63   Lowe GDO. Fibrinogen: an independent coronary heart disease risk factor. In: Betteridge DJ, ed. *Lipids and Vascular Disease*. London: Martin Dunitz 2000; 77–84.

64   Reinhart W. Fibrinogen-marker or mediator of vascular disease? *Vasc Med* 2003; **8**: 211–16.

65   Danesh J, Wheeler JG, Hirshfield GM, *et al.* C-reactive protein and other circulating markers of inflammation in the prediction of coronary heart disease. *N Engl J Med* 2004; **350**: 1387–97.

66   Fibrinogen Studies Collaboration. Collaborative meta-analysis of prospective observational studies of plasma fibrinogen and cardiovascular disease. *Eur J Cardiovasc Prev Rehabil* 2004; **11**: 9–11.

67 Fibrinogen Studies Collaboration. Plasma fibrinogen level and the risk of major cardiovascular diseases and non-vascular mortality. *JAMA* 2005; **294**: 1799–1809.

68 Simmonds RE, Hermida J, Rezende SM, Lane DA. Haemostatic genetic risk factors in arterial thrombosis. *Thromb Haemost* 2001; **86**: 374–85.

69 Lane DA, Grant PJ. Role of hemostatic gene polymorphisms in venous and arterial thrombosis. *Blood* 2000; **95**: 1517–32.

70 Davey-Smith G, Harbord R, Ebrahim S. Fibrinogen, C-reactive protein and coronary heart disease: does Mendelian randomisation suggest the associations are non-causal? *Q J Med* 2004; **97**: 163–6.

71 Lowe GDO, Woodward M, Rumley A, *et al.* Associations of plasma fibrinogen assays, C-reactive protein and interleukin-6 with previous myocardial infarction. *J Thromb Haemost* 2003; **1**: 2312–16.

72 Sherman DG, Atkinson RP, Chippendale T, *et al.* Intravenous ancrod for treatment of acute ischaemic stroke. *JAMA* 2000; **283**: 2395–403.

73 Rumley A, Lowe GDO, Sweetnam PM, *et al.* Factor VIII, von Willebrand factor and the risk of major ischaemic heart disease in the Caerphilly Study. *Br J Haematol* 1999; **105**: 110–16.

74 Sramek A, Kriek M, Rosendaal FR. Decreased mortality of ischaemic heart disease among carriers of haemophilia. *Lancet* 2003; **362**: 351–4.

75 Rosendaal FR, Briet E, Stibbe J, *et al.* Haemophilia protects against ischaemic heart disease: a study of risk factors. *Br J Haematol* 1990; **75**: 525–30.

76 Meade TW, North WRS, Chakrabarti R, *et al.* Haemostatic function and cardiovascular death; early results of a prospective study. *Lancet* 1980; i: 1050–4.

77 Smith FB, Lee AJ, Fowkes FGR, *et al.* Hemostatic factors as predictors of ischaemic heart disease and stroke in the Edinburgh Artery Study. *Arterioscler Thromb Vasc Biol* 1997; **17**: 3321–5.

78 Folsom AR, Wu KK, Rosamond WD, *et al.* Prospective study of hemostatic factors and incidence of coronary heart disease. The Atherosclerosis Risk in Comunities (ARIC) study. *Circulation* 1997; **96**: 1102–8.

79 Meade TW, Ruddock V, Stirling Y, *et al.* Fibrinolytic activity, clotting factors, and long-term incidence of ischaemic heart disease in the Northwick Park Heart Study. *Lancet* 1993; **342**: 1076–9.

80 Junker R, Heinrich J, Schulte H, *et al.* Coagulation factor VII and the risk of coronary heart disease in healthy men. *Arterioscler Thromb Vasc Biol* 1997; **17**: 1539–44.

81 Lowe GDO, Rumley A, Sweetnam P, *et al.* Fibrin D-dimer, markers of coagulation activation, and the risk of major ischaemic heart disease in the Caerphilly Study. *Thromb Haemost* 2001; **86**: 822–7.

82 Cooper JA, Miller GJ, Bauer KA, *et al.* Comparison of novel haemostatic factors and conventional risk factors for prediction of coronary heart disease. *Circulation* 102: 2816–22.

83 Reiner AP, Siscovick DS, Rosendaal FR. Hemostatic risk factors and arterial thrombotic disease. *Thromb Haemost* 2001; **85**: 584–95.

84 The Medical Research Council's General Practice Research Framework. Thrombosis Prevention Trial. *Lancet* 1998; **351**: 233–41.

85 Lowe GDO, Yarnell JWG, Sweetnam PM, *et al.* Fibrin D-dimer, tissue plasminogen activator, plasminogen activator inhibitor, and the risk of major ischaemic heart disease in the Caerphilly Study. *Thromb Haemostas* 1998; **79**: 129–33.

86 Lowe GDO, Yarnell JWG, Rumley A, *et al.* C-reactive protein, fibrin D-dimer, and incident ischemic heart disease in the Speedwell Study. Are inflammation and fibrin turnover linked in pathogenesis? *Arterioscler Thromb Vasc Biol* 2001; **21**: 603–10.

87 Danesh J, Whincup P, Walker M, *et al.* Fibrin D-dimer and coronary heart disease: prospective study and meta-analysis. *Circulation* 2001; **103**: 2323–7.

88 MacCallum PK, Rudnicka AR, Rumley A, *et al.* Warfarin reduces thrombin generation and fibrin turnover, but not low-grade inflammation, in men at risk of myocardial infarction. *Br J Haematol* 2004; **127**: 448–50.

89 Lip GYH, Rumley A, Dunn FG, Lowe GDO. Plasma fibrinogen and fibrin D-dimer in patients with atrial fibrillation: effects of cardioversion to sinus rhythm. *Int J Cardiol* 1995; **51**: 245–51.

90 Tait RC, Murdoch DL, O'Neill KF, *et al.* Fibrin D-dimer is an independent predictor of future stroke in patients with atrial fibrillation. *Circulation* 2003; **108**: 787.

91 Bozic M, Blinc A, Stegnar M. D-dimer, other markers of haemostasis activation and soluble adhesion molecules in patients with different clinical probabilities of deep vein thrombosis. *Thromb Res* 2002; **108**: 107–14.

92 Ridker PM, Vaughan DE, Stampfer MJ, *et al.* Baseline fibrinolytic state and the risk of future venous thrombosis. A prospective study of endogenous tissue-type plasminogen activator inhibitor. *Circulation* 1992; **85**: 1822–7.

93 Crowther MA, Roberts J, Roberts R, *et al.* Fibrinolytic variables in patients with recurrent venous thrombosis: a prospective cohort study. *Thromb Haemost* 2001; **85**: 390–4.

94 van Tilburg NH, Rosendaal FR, Bertina RM. Thrombin activatable fibrinolysis inhibitor and the risk for deep vein thrombosis. *Blood* 2000; **95**: 2855–9.

95 Lowe GDO, Danesh J, Lewington S, *et al.* Tissue plasminogen activator antigen and coronary heart disease: Prospective study and meta-analysis. *Eur Heart J* 2004; **25**: 252–9.

96 Greer IA. Epidemiology, risk factors and prophylaxis of venous thromboembolism in obstetrics and gynaecology. *Baillieres Clin Obstet Gynaecol* 1997; **11**: 403–30.

97 Kluft C, Lansink M. Effect of oral contraceptives on haemostasis variables. *Thromb Haemost* 1997; **78**: 315–26.

98 Rosendaal FR, Helmerhorst FM, Vandenbroucke JP. Oral contraceptives, hormone replacement therapy and thrombosis. *Thromb Haemost* 2001; **86**: 112–23.

99   Kemmeren JM, Algra A, Meijers JC, *et al.* Effects of
      second and third generation oral contraceptives and their
      respective progestogens on the coagulation system in the
      absence or presence of the factor V Leiden mutation.
      Thromb Haemost 2002; **87**: 199–205.

100   Lowe GDO. Hormone replacement therapy and cardio-
      vascular disease. *J Intern Med* 2004; **256**: 361–74.

101   Lowe GDO, Upton MN, Rumley A, *et al.* Different effects
      of oral and transdermal hormone replacement therapies

on Factor IX, APC resistance, t-PA, PAI and C-reactive
protein: a cross-sectional population survey. *Thromb
Haemost* 2001; **86**: 550–6.

102   Scarabin P-Y, Oger E, Plu-Bureau G. On behalf of the
      Estrogen and ThromboEmbolism Risk (ESTHER) Study
      Group. Differential association of oral and transdermal
      oestrogen-replacement therapy with venous
      thromboembolism risk. *Lancet* 2003; **362**: 428–32.

7

Congenital thrombophilia and venous disease

KENNETH A BAUER

INTRODUCTION

Improved understanding of the molecular basis of the coagulation mechanism coupled with clinical investigation has facilitated the identification of hemostatic risk factors in substantial numbers of patients presenting with venous thrombosis. Individuals with a tendency to thrombosis are defined as having thrombophilia, and the term congenital or inherited thrombophilia is applied to individuals with genetic defects that predispose them toward venous thromboembolism.

Until 1993, a genetic cause of thrombophilia was detectable in a relatively small percentage of patients with venous thrombosis. Hereditary abnormalities were found in only 5–15 percent of patients and were confined to deficiencies of antithrombin, protein C, and protein S. The discovery of two prothrombotic mutations prevalent in Caucasian populations, the factor V-Arg506Gln or factor V Leiden mutation and the prothrombin G20210A mutation, has greatly increased the percentage of patients in whom a hereditary risk factor is identifiable.[1] The pathogenesis of venous thromboembolism, however, is multifactorial and over 90 percent of individuals who carry the factor V Leiden or the prothrombin G20210A mutations will never sustain a venous thrombotic event during their lifetime. Acquired risk factors frequently precipitate symptomatic events for which patients with an identifiable genetic predisposition are more susceptible. Box 7.1 lists the major hereditary (primary) and acquired (secondary) hypercoagulable states along with several hematologic abnormalities of unknown etiology that have been reported to be risk factors for a first episode of venous thrombosis. Despite this expanding number of hemostatic risk factors, the available data do not indicate that the risk of recurrent venous thrombosis is greater in most patients with a single identifiable hereditary defect,[2] nor should the duration of anticoagulant therapy be altered in these patients; this has generated discussion regarding the clinical utility of thrombophilia screening.[3–5] This chapter will focus on the congenital thrombophilias and their role in the pathogenesis of venous thromboembolism.

CLINICAL APPROACH TO THE PATIENT WITH THROMBOSIS OR THROMBOPHILIA

When approaching patients suspected of having an active thrombotic process or a thrombotic diathesis, it is useful to place them in one of two major categories. The first group has characteristics that suggest the presence of an inherited thrombotic disorder or a primary hypercoagulable state (see Box 7.1). These disorders result from mutations in single genes encoding a plasma protein component of one of the major natural anticoagulant mechanisms. The anticoagulant systems most frequently involved in the inherited hypercoagulable states include antithrombin in the heparan sulfate–antithrombin mechanism and protein C, protein S, and factor V (substitution of the amino acid Gln for Arg at amino acid 506, termed factor V Leiden) in the protein C anticoagulant pathway. An elevation in the plasma prothrombin level in association with a G to A transversion at position 20210 in the 3′-untranslated region of the prothrombin gene is also a risk factor for venous thrombosis. The second category, the acquired or secondary hypercoagulable states, consist of transient and

---

Box 7.1 Disorders associated with hypercoagulability

Inherited (primary) hypercoagulable states
- Activated protein C resistance due to factor V Leiden mutation
- Prothrombin gene mutation (G to A transition at position 20210 in the 3'-untranslated region)
- Antithrombin III deficiency
- Protein C deficiency
- Protein S deficiency
- Dysfibrinogenemias (rare)

Acquired (secondary) hypercoagulable states
- In association with physiologic or thrombogenic stimuli
  - Pregnancy (especially the post-partum period)
  - Estrogen use (oral contraceptives, hormone replacement therapy)
  - Immobilization
  - Major trauma
  - Postoperative state
  - Advancing age
  - Obesity
  - Prolonged air travel
- Lupus anticoagulant or antiphospholipid antibody syndrome
- In association with other clinical disorders
  - Malignancy
  - Heparin-induced thrombocytopenia
  - Primary hematologic disorders (polycythemia vera, essential thrombocythemia, paroxysmal nocturnal hemoglobinuria)
  - Nephrotic syndrome
  - Inflammatory bowel disease

Mixed/unknown
- Hyperhomocysteinemia
- Activated protein C resistance in the absence of factor V Leiden
- Elevated factor VIII
- Elevated factor XI
- Elevated factor IX
- Elevated thrombin-activatable fibrinolysis inhibitor (TAFI)
- Decreased free tissue factor pathway inhibitor (TFPI)
- Decreased plasma fibrinolytic activity

---

permanent risk factors along with a heterogeneous group of disorders that are associated with an increased risk for developing thrombotic complications (see Box 7.1). Hyperhomocysteinemia is a common laboratory abnormality that results in an increased risk of venous as well as arterial thrombosis. Plasma homocysteine levels are determined by genetic as well as environmental factors, the latter including dietary intake of folic acid and vitamins B_{12} and B_6. It is listed separately from the inherited thrombotic disorders because it may result from defects in several genes encoding different enzymes involved in the metabolism of the amino acid or acquired factors.

The inherited thrombotic disorders have been almost exclusively associated with *venous thrombosis*. Although anecdotal reports suggest an association between arterial thrombosis and the inherited thrombotic disorders, it is generally not recommended to test for these defects in such patients. Hereditary deficiencies of antithrombin, protein C, or protein S are relatively infrequent and will be found in less than 5 percent of unselected individuals presenting with venous thromboembolism (Table 7.1). Resistance to activated protein C due to factor V Leiden, the prothrombin G20210A mutation, and hyperhomocysteinemia are more prevalent defects that can also be found in significant numbers of individuals with first episodes of idiopathic venous thrombosis (that is, no apparent precipitating factor such as recent surgery or active malignancy) after age 50 in the absence of a positive family history.[11–14]

Although the aforementioned classification of hereditary and acquired categories is useful in directing the laboratory evaluation for hypercoagulability, it is simplistic in the sense that thrombosis frequently results from an interplay of genetic and acquired factors. Patients with hereditary defects are at lifelong risk of developing thrombosis, and stimuli such as pregnancy, estrogen use, or surgery trigger thrombotic episodes in perhaps 50 percent of individuals. Also, defects in more than one coagulation protein are now being found in patients with venous thrombosis because of the high background frequency in the general population of abnormalities such as factor V Leiden (6 percent in US Caucasians)[6] and the prothrombin G20210A mutation.[15] Such individuals have a more severe thrombotic diathesis than those with a single identifiable mutation.[16–22] Thus, thrombosis can be viewed as a multigene disorder in which susceptible individuals will have one or more genetic mutations, with clinical events occurring

---

Table 7.1   Prevalence (%) of defects in patients with venous thrombosis

	Unselected	Selected
Activated Protein C resistance (factor V Leiden)*	12[6]	40[7]
Prothrombin gene mutation* (G to A transition at position 20210 in the 3'-untranslated region)	6[8]	18[8]
Deficiencies of antithrombin III, protein C, protein S	<5[9]	~15[10]

* Prevalence restricted to Caucasian populations.
Selected patients include patients with an initial venous thrombotic event before age 50, recurrent venous thrombosis, or a positive family history of venous thromboembolism in first-degree relatives.

when they are exposed to exogenous prothrombotic stimuli.[23] In many cases, however, the inciting precipitant to thrombosis is not reported by the patient and is therefore subclinical.

In the evaluation of patients with a recent or remote history of thrombosis, historical details should be obtained regarding the age of onset, location of prior thromboses, and results of objective diagnostic studies documenting thrombosis. The latter is critical, as the clinical diagnosis of deep vein thrombosis, in particular, is notoriously inaccurate. The patient should be carefully questioned about circumstances that were present proximate to the time of thrombosis that might have precipitated the event. These include surgical procedures, trauma, and immobility. Women should be questioned regarding pregnancy or fetal loss or intake of estrogens (that is, oral contraceptives, hormone replacement therapy). A family history is particularly important because a well-documented history of venous thrombosis in one or more first-degree relatives strongly suggests the presence of a hereditary defect.

A substantial proportion of women with thrombosis in association with oral contraceptive use or pregnancy will have an inherited disorder, especially the factor V Leiden[24,25] and prothrombin G20210A mutations.[26] The risk of venous thrombosis associated with oral contraceptives is related to the estrogen dose and most oral contraceptives prescribed today contain less than 50 µg of ethinylestradiol in combination with a progestational agent. The use of low-dose estrogen preparations containing older progestational agents (levonorgestrel, lynoestrenol, and norethisterone), however, still confers about a fourfold increased risk of venous thromboembolism as compared with nonusers. Unexpectedly, the newer progestagens (desogestrol, gestodene, and norgestimate) with less deleterious effects on lipid profiles carry a higher risk of venous thromboembolism than the previous generation of combined oral contraceptives.[27,28] This risk is particularly high among carriers of the factor V Leiden mutation.[29,30]

The puerperium, defined as the 6-week period following delivery, is associated with a higher rate of thrombosis than pregnancy itself. Risk factors such as older age, cesarean delivery, preeclampsia, obesity, and prior thromboembolism further increase the risk of venous thrombosis in pregnancy. The factor V Leiden and the prothrombin G20210A mutations individually are associated with an increased risk of venous thromboembolism during pregnancy and the puerperium, and the risk among women with both mutations is disproportionately higher than that among women with only one mutation.[31] Compression of the left iliac vein by the crossing right iliac artery is a local mechanical factor that is believed to underlie the threefold higher incidence of deep vein thrombosis in the left leg as compared with the right.

Venous thrombotic risk associated with hormone replacement therapy is increased twofold to fourfold, an effect that is similar in magnitude to oral contraceptives. However, the use of hormone replacement therapy leads to a considerably larger number of cases of thrombosis due to an overall age-related increase in the incidence of thrombosis. Carriers of the factor V Leiden mutation receiving hormone replacement therapy have a significantly increased risk of venous thromboembolism.[32,33] Data from the Heart and Estrogen Replacement Study (HERS) and the Estrogen Replacement and Atherosclerosis Trial indicate that heterozygous carriers of factor V Leiden on hormone replacement therapy had an odds ratio of 14.1 for venous thromboembolism as compared with noncarriers receiving placebo.[33]

The relation between prolonged air travel and venous thromboembolism has received considerable attention and a higher risk of pulmonary embolism has been found during or immediately after air travel of distances greater than approximately 4828 km (3000 miles) compared with lesser distances.[34–36] It has been suggested that the relevant risk factor may be prolonged sitting rather than air travel *per se* and the risk appears greatest among those with other risk factors for venous thromboembolism.[37] A case–control study carried out in the Netherlands, however, found no association of deep venous thrombosis with travel time of greater than 5 hours.[38]

Hereditary thrombophilia has also been identified as a risk factor in patients with venous thrombosis in uncommon sites such as the portal, hepatic, mesenteric, and cerebral veins. Interestingly, some studies indicate that individuals with axillary vein thrombosis appear to have a low prevalence of hereditary defects, even in the absence of triggering risk factors.[39] The presence of indwelling venous catheters is the most common risk factor today for upper extremity venous thrombosis, and patients with this complication generally do not warrant evaluation for an underlying hypercoagulable state.

In the general physical examination, special attention should be directed to the vascular system, extremities (looking for signs of superficial or deep venous thrombosis), chest, heart, abdominal organs, and skin (skin necrosis, livedo reticularis). The most common sites of thrombosis in patients with hereditary thrombophilia are the deep leg veins, iliac veins, and pulmonary arteries. Thrombosis in mesenteric, portal, and cerebral veins as well as superficial thrombophlebitis has been described in some series of patients with these disorders.

LABORATORY EVALUATION

Based on the history and physical examination, a decision must be made whether testing should be done to identify specific biologic risk factors predisposing to thrombosis. Clinical judgment must be exercised with regard to the scope of the evaluation as well as the optimal time for its performance. Historical features that increase the likelihood of identifying individuals with deficiencies of antithrombin III, protein C, and protein S include an initial venous thrombotic event before age 50, recurrent thrombosis, or positive family history.[10] These also increase the chances of identifying individuals with factor V Leiden and the prothrombin gene mutation, but these genetic defects can also frequently be identified in older individuals with an initial episode of deep venous thrombosis who do not have other acquired risk factors or a positive family history.

Some clinical features have been associated with individual hereditary thrombotic disorders. Approximately a third of individuals who sustain the rare complication of warfarin-induced skin necrosis will have underlying protein C deficiency; however, this syndrome has also been reported in patients with protein S deficiency[40] and factor V Leiden.[41] In neonates, the development of skin necrosis and visceral thrombosis (neonatal purpura fulminans) indicates a likely diagnosis of severe hereditary protein C deficiency, although cases have been reported in association with homozygous protein S deficiency as well. Both conditions require emergent therapy if major morbidity or mortality are to be averted. Although resistance to heparin's anticoagulant effect, as measured by the activated partial thromboplastin time (aPTT), often leads to consideration of antithrombin deficiency, congenital antithrombin III deficiency is infrequently diagnosed in such individuals.

Box 7.2 gives a list of tests useful in screening patients suspected of having a biologic defect predisposing to thrombosis. Coagulation assays with high sensitivity and specificity for the factor V Leiden mutation ('second generation' assays) are widely available and are based on the resistance of the mutant factor Va molecule to inactivation by activated protein C; positive results are confirmed by genetic testing of DNA obtained from peripheral blood mononuclear cells. Initial testing for the factor V Leiden mutation can also be done genetically; testing for the prothrombin G20210A mutation must be done genetically. Testing for hyperhomocysteinemia should be done after an overnight fast when the patient is on a normal diet. Homocysteine is measured using ion-exchange chromatography, gas chromatography-mass spectrometry, high performance liquid chromatography with electrochemical or fluorescent detection, or enzyme-linked immunosorbent assay.

The best screening tests for deficiencies of antithrombin, protein C, and protein S are functional assays that detect both quantitative and qualitative defects. Immunologic (antigenic) assays detect only quantitative deficiencies of these proteins. For plasma antithrombin, convenient functional assays are available that measure the heparin cofactor activity of the molecule. Among protein C assays, coagulation assays provide a more complete evaluation of the functional activity of the molecule than amidolytic assays. However, coagulation assays for protein C as well as protein S can give falsely low values if the factor V Leiden mutation is present, and reliable application of these assays requires initial assessment whether this mutation is present. To screen for a dysfibrinogenemia, the thrombin time is recommended along with measurements of plasma fibrinogen by clotting and immunologic assay.

An important consideration in the laboratory evaluation of patients with a suspected deficiency of antithrombin, protein C, or protein S is the timing of testing. Erroneous diagnoses can be made due to the influence of acute thrombosis,

---

Box 7.2 Screening laboratory evaluation for patients suspected of having a biologic defect predisposing to thrombosis

- Test for the presence of the factor V Leiden (factor V-Arg506Gln) mutation
  - Screen with clotting assay for resistance to activated protein C using factor V-deficient plasma* and confirm with genetic test

  or

  - Genetic test for factor V-Arg506Gln (factor V Leiden)
- Genetic test for prothrombin gene mutation (G to A transition at position 20210 in the 3′-untranslated region)
- Functional assay of antithrombin III (heparin-cofactor assay)*
- Functional assays of protein C*
- Functional assay of protein S/immunologic assays of total and free protein S*
- Screen for dysfibrinogenemias (immunologic and functional assays of fibrinogen, thrombin time)*

Measurement of fasting total plasma homocysteine level
Clotting assay for lupus anticoagulant*/serologic tests for antiphospholipid antibodies

*Coagulation assays are performed on platelet-poor plasma obtained from blood samples drawn into a solution containing 3.8 percent (weight/volume [vol]) sodium citrate. The ratio of anticoagulant to blood is 0.1:0.9 (vol/vol). In the absence of an accompanying clinical history for the individual, prothrombin time will help to exclude the ingestion of warfarin which will affect the measurements of protein C and protein S. Thrombin time as well as aPTT will help to exclude the administration of heparin.

---

comorbid illness, or anticoagulant therapy on the levels of these plasma proteins. Table 7.2 lists some of the common causes of acquired deficiencies of antithrombin III, protein C, and protein S.

Acute thrombosis by itself can result in transiently reduced levels of antithrombin and, occasionally, protein C and protein S. Heparin therapy can be associated with up to a 30 percent decline in plasma antithrombin levels over several days, whereas warfarin produces a marked drop in the functional activity of protein C and protein S and a lesser decline in immunologic levels. Warfarin has also been shown rarely to elevate antithrombin levels significantly, sometimes into the normal range, in patients with a hereditary deficiency of this inhibitor. For these reasons, it is optimal to test for these deficiency states at least 2 weeks after completing the initial 3–6-month course of oral anticoagulant therapy following a thrombotic event. If, however, levels of antithrombin, protein C, or protein S obtained on acute presentation are well within the normal range, these will effectively exclude the diagnosis of their deficiency states from consideration. However, the finding of a low

Table 7.2   Causes of acquired deficiencies in antithrombin III, protein C, or protein S

Antithrombin III	Protein C	Protein S
Neonatal period	Neonatal period	Neonatal period
Pregnancy		Pregnancy
Liver disease	Liver disease	Liver disease
DIC	DIC	DIC
Nephrotic syndrome	Chemotherapy (CMF)	
Major surgery		Inflammatory states
Acute thrombosis	Acute thrombosis	Acute thrombosis
Treatment with		
Heparin	Warfarin	Warfarin
L-asparaginase	L-asparaginase	L-asparaginase
Estrogens		Estrogens

CMF, cyclophosphamide, methotrexate, 5-fluorouracil; DIC, disseminated intravascular coagulation

Table 7.3   Assay measurements in heterozygous antithrombin (ATIII) deficiency

Type	Antigen	Activity Heparin cofactor	Activity Progressive ATIII
I	Low	Low	Low
II			
Active site defect	Normal	Low	Low
Heparin-binding site defect	Normal	Low	Normal

level during this period will need to be confirmed by repeat testing after anticoagulation is discontinued. The investigation of first-degree family members is useful to document the hereditary nature of the deficiency. Confirmation of a deficiency state in first-degree family members is particularly helpful diagnostically in patients in whom the risks of recurrent thrombosis are too great to temporarily discontinue anticoagulation. In such patients, a diagnosis of protein C or protein S deficiency can be confirmed by carrying out testing after warfarin has been discontinued for 2 weeks under the cover of heparin or low-molecular-weight heparin at therapeutic doses in order to minimize the risk of thrombosis and warfarin-induced skin necrosis when warfarin is reintroduced.

Elevations in the levels of several coagulation factors, including factor VIII,[42–44] factor XI,[45] factor IX,[46] TAFI,[47] decreased levels of free TFPI,[48] and decreased plasma fibrinolytic activity[49] have been implicated as risk factors for a first episode of venous thrombosis. The molecular basis for these abnormalities has not yet been elucidated. For factor VIII, high plasma activity levels cannot be attributed to overt inflammation because patients with levels greater than 150 percent did not have elevations in acute phase reactants such as C-reactive protein, fibrinogen, and erythrocyte sedimentation rate.[50] Austrian investigators found that the probability of recurrent venous thrombosis at 2 years in people with factor VIII levels >234 percent of normal (the 90th percentile of the values for the study sample) was 37 percent compared with 5 percent in patients with levels <120 percent of normal. Although a similar finding has been reported by an Italian group,[51] this was not corroborated by the Leiden Thrombophilia Study.[2]

There have been reports of thrombosis in association with abnormalities in other coagulation or fibrinolytic system proteins. These include heparin cofactor II deficiency, plasminogen deficiency (either hypo- or dysplasminogenemias),

factor XII deficiency, and elevations in plasminogen activator inhibitor-1. However causal associations between these abnormalities and an increased risk of thrombosis have not been clearly defined.

INHERITED HYPERCOAGULABLE DISORDERS

Antithrombin deficiency

In 1965, Egeberg[52] described a Norwegian family in which certain individuals who had a history of thrombosis had plasma concentrations of antithrombin that were 40–50 percent of normal. Subsequently, other investigators described additional families with a similar constellation of clinical and laboratory abnormalities.[53–55]

Antithrombin deficiency is usually inherited in an autosomal dominant fashion, and thus, affects both sexes equally. Two major types of inherited antithrombin deficiency have been delineated (Table 7.3). The type I deficiency state is a result of reduced synthesis of biologically normal protease inhibitor molecules.[56] In these cases, the antigenic and functional activity of antithrombin in the blood is reduced in parallel. The molecular basis of this disorder is either a deletion of a major segment of the antithrombin gene or, more commonly, the occurrence of small deletions/insertions, or single base substitutions. These mutations will introduce a frameshift, a direct termination codon, a change in mRNA processing, or unstable translation products. The antithrombin mutation database includes 80 distinct mutations in patients with a type I deficiency.[57] The second type of antithrombin deficiency is produced by a discrete molecular defect within the protease inhibitor (type II). The plasma levels of antithrombin are greatly reduced as judged by functional activity, whereas antithrombin immunologic activity is essentially normal.

The prevalence of type I antithrombin deficiency in the healthy population is estimated to be N1/2000. Studies of healthy blood donors employing functional assays that measure heparin cofactor activity have found that the prevalence of antithrombin deficiency in the general population is 1/250–500;[58–61] a substantial number, however, have a type II defect with mutations at the heparin-binding site which are associated with a lower risk of thrombosis.[59] The best single screening test for the disorder is the antithrombin III-heparin cofactor assay that measures factor Xa inhibition.

The thrombotic risk associated with antithrombin deficiency depends on population selection. In older reviews of antithrombin deficiency including families with a high penetrance of thrombosis, more than 50 percent of affected patients experience venous thrombotic episodes.[62,63] The initial clinical manifestations occur apparently spontaneously in about 42 percent of subjects, but are related to pregnancy, parturition, oral contraceptive ingestion, surgery, or trauma in the remaining 58 percent of patients.[62] The most common sites of disease are the deep veins of the leg and the mesenteric veins. Approximately 60 percent of individuals develop recurrent thrombotic episodes, and clinical signs of pulmonary embolism are evident in 40 percent.[62] Although cases have been reported in which antithrombin-deficient infants sustain cerebral venous thrombosis,[64-66] affected children rarely develop thrombotic episodes before puberty. At this time, thrombotic events start to occur with some frequency and the risk of thrombosis increases substantially with advancing age.[62] Recently published studies of the hereditary thrombophilias indicate that first-degree relatives of symptomatic individuals with antithrombin deficiency have an 8–10-fold increased risk of thrombosis as compared with noncarriers.[67,68] In the Leiden Thrombophilia Study, a case–control study of 474 consecutive patients following an initial episode of deep vein thrombosis,[9] the prevalence of antithrombin deficiency was only 1.1 percent and the odds ratio for thrombosis was only 5.0, although the confidence interval was relatively wide (95 percent confidence interval [CI] 0.7 to 34).[69]

The first family with type II antithrombin deficiency was reported in 1974.[70] Many families with this type of deficiency state have now been reported and they have been further subcategorized on the basis of two different functional assays of antithrombin III activity. The first is the antithrombin III-heparin cofactor assay, which measures the ability of heparin to bind to lysyl residues on the inhibitor and catalyze the neutralization of coagulation enzymes such as thrombin and factor Xa. This assay, based on factor Xa inhibition, is currently the most widely used functional antithrombin III assay. The second test is the progressive antithrombin activity assay, which quantifies the capacity of this inhibitor to neutralize the enzymatic activity of thrombin in the absence of heparin; this test is rarely done any more and is not widely available.

Many abnormal antithrombin molecules have been identified with reductions in heparin cofactor activity without a concordant reduction in progressive antithrombin activity.[57] These variants generally have mutations at a heparin-binding site at the amino-terminal end of the molecule. Variants with decreased activity in both antithrombin functional assays generally have mutations near the Arg393-Ser394 site at the carboxy-terminal end of the molecule. Another type of mutation has been described at the carboxy-terminal end of the antithrombin III molecule between

amino acids 402 and 429. These type II variants are termed pleiotropic as they exhibit multiple functional defects.[57] Mutations at positions 402–407 can lead to the presence of trace amounts of an electrophoretically and functionally abnormal antithrombin III molecule.[57] The similarity of the characteristics of these mutations indicates that the region of residues 402–407 is important for the maintenance of normal plasma levels of antithrombin antigen.[71]

The risk of thrombosis is substantially less in heterozygous patients with type II defects at the heparin binding site as compared to the thrombin binding site.[72] Individuals with plasma antithrombin-heparin cofactor activity measurements of ~50 percent and normal progressive antithrombin activity (heparin binding site defects) have infrequent thrombotic episodes.[73,74] Several of these cases were brought to clinical attention when young children of these heterozygous individuals developed severe venous or arterial thrombosis, or both, accompanied by plasma antithrombin-heparin cofactor levels below 10 percent.[75,76] There often was a history of parental consanguinity, and these children were homozygous for an antithrombin molecular defect. In contrast to this subgroup of patients, heterozygous type II patients with both diminished progressive antithrombin activity and antithrombin-heparin cofactor activity (thrombin-binding site defects) sustain venous thromboembolism as often as type I patients.

The mean concentration of antithrombin III in normal pooled plasma is ~140 μg/mL. Most laboratories report a normal range between 75 percent and 120 percent of normal pooled plasma for antithrombin-heparin cofactor determinations, and a somewhat wider range for immunoassay results.

Healthy neonates have about half the normal adult concentration of antithrombin[77] and gradually reach the adult level by 6 months of age.[78] The levels may be considerably lower in infants born after 30–36 weeks of gestation[78] and are even further reduced in infants with respiratory distress, necrotizing enterocolitis, sepsis, or disseminated intravascular coagulation (DIC). Thromboembolic events are rare in children with hereditary antithrombin deficiency. In the absence of heparin, antithrombin contributes ~80 percent of the thrombin-neutralizing capacity of normal adult plasma.[79,80] The levels of a second thrombin inhibitor, α_2-macroglobulin, are higher during the first two decades of life than in adults, and this may lessen the risk of thromboembolic complications in antithrombin-deficient patients during childhood.[81]

A variety of pathophysiologic conditions can reduce the concentration of antithrombin in the blood (see Table 7.2). Acute thrombosis infrequently lowers antithrombin levels substantially,[82] but DIC usually reduces the level of this inhibitor.[83] Lowered antithrombin concentrations occur in patients with liver disease due to decreased protein synthesis. Decreased antithrombin levels are also observed in individuals with the nephrotic syndrome as a consequence of urinary excretion.[84] Furthermore, modest reductions in plasma antithrombin concentration are found in users of oral contraceptives as well as in women receiving hormone replacement therapy.[62,85] The levels of antithrombin do not change substantially during normal pregnancy, but may decrease significantly in women with pregnancy-induced hypertension, preeclampsia, or eclampsia.[86] Infusions of L-asparaginase, a chemotherapeutic agent employed in the treatment of acute lymphocytic leukemia, can substantially lower the plasma concentration of this inhibitor. In addition, the administration of heparin decreases plasma antithrombin levels,[87] presumably on the basis of accelerated *in vivo* clearance. Evaluation of plasma samples from patients during a period of heparinization can therefore potentially lead to an erroneous diagnosis of antithrombin deficiency.

Due to the number of clinical disorders that can be associated with reductions in the plasma concentration of antithrombin, definitive diagnosis of the hereditary deficiency state is often difficult. Although an antithrombin III level in the normal range is usually sufficient to exclude the disorder, low levels should be confirmed by obtaining another sample at a subsequent time point. This determination is ideally performed when the patient is no longer receiving oral anticoagulants, as these medications have occasionally been reported to raise plasma antithrombin III concentrations into the normal range in patients with the hereditary deficiency state.[53] Confirmation of the hereditary nature of the disorder requires the investigation of other family members. Diagnosis of other affected family members also allows for appropriate counseling regarding the need for prophylaxis against venous thrombosis.

Protein C deficiency

In 1981, Griffin *et al.*[88] described the first kindred in which several individuals had plasma levels of protein C antigen of ∼50 percent of normal and a history of recurrent thrombotic events. Subsequently, other investigators[89–92] reported numerous other families with heterozygous protein C deficiency.

Heterozygous protein C deficiency is inherited in an autosomal dominant fashion; a more severe form of protein C deficiency is an autosomal recessive disorder. The phenotype of patients with heterozygous protein C deficiency is similar to hereditary antithrombin III deficiency. In severely affected families, ∼75 percent of protein C-deficient individuals experienced one or more thrombotic events. The initial episode occurs apparently spontaneously in ∼70 percent. The remaining 30 percent have the usual associated risk factors (pregnancy, parturition, contraceptive pill use, surgery, or trauma) at the time they develop acute thrombotic events. However, patients are infrequently symptomatic until their early twenties, with increasing numbers of individuals experiencing thrombotic events as they reach the age of 50. The most common sites of disease are the deep veins of the legs, the iliofemoral veins, the mesenteric veins, and the pulmonary arteries. Approximately 63 percent of affected patients develop recurrent venous thrombosis and

∼40 percent exhibit signs of pulmonary embolism.[93] Superficial thrombophlebitis of the leg veins as well as cerebral venous thrombosis can occur in protein C-deficient patients.[89,94] There have been reports of nonhemorrhagic arterial stroke in young adults with hereditary protein C deficiency,[95–97] but a causal relationship is uncertain.

The prevalence of protein C deficiency in outpatients presenting with an initial episode of venous thromboembolism ranges from 0.5 percent to 4 percent.[10,69,98] In earlier reports of more selected patient populations, protein C deficiency was more frequently identified, ranging from 2 percent to 9 percent.[90,99,100] Initial estimates placed the prevalence of protein C deficiency between 1 in 16 000 and 1 in 32 000 within the general population, based on the assumption that protein C was an autosomal dominant disorder with high penetrance and that at least half of the individuals with the deficiency would demonstrate symptomatic thrombosis. However, it was difficult to reconcile this with the infrequent history of thrombosis in parents of infants presenting with purpura fulminans, which is due to the homozygous or doubly heterozygous form of protein C deficiency (see below). This led to studies of healthy blood donors, which found a much higher prevalence of heterozygosity for protein C deficiency than was previously estimated, ranging from 1 in 200 to 1 in 500.[101,102]

The risk of thrombosis initially attributed to protein C deficiency was subject to selection bias, being overestimated from familial reports. Data from the Leiden Thrombophilia Study indicate that heterozygous protein C deficiency is associated with about a sevenfold increased risk for an initial episode of deep vein thrombosis as compared with normal individuals.[69] Among Italian patients, protein C deficiency is associated with a similar sevenfold increase in venous thrombotic risk.[67] In asymptomatic carriers of protein C deficiency, the incidence of thrombosis is fairly low at 0.4–1.0 percent annually.[68,103,104]

Two major subtypes of heterozygous protein C deficiency have been delineated using immunologic and functional assays (Table 7.4). The type I deficiency state is the most common form and is characterized by a reduction in both the immunologic and biologic activity of plasma protein C to ∼50 percent of normal. Studies of the genetic defects in patients with protein C deficiency have led to the identification of more than 160 different mutations.[105] In individuals with a type I deficiency, missense and nonsense mutations are most common. Other types of mutations resulting in type I protein C deficiency include promoter mutations, splice site abnormalities, in-frame deletions, frameshift deletions, in-frame insertions, and frameshift insertions. In families with a type II deficiency state, affected individuals have normal protein C levels on immunologic examination, yet possess lowered functional levels of the zymogen. Point mutations in the protein C gene result in the presence of dysfunctional protein C molecules in the affected patient's plasma.

Warfarin-induced skin necrosis has been associated with the presence of heterozygous protein C deficiency.[106,107]

Table 7.4 Assay measurements in heterozygous protein C deficiency

| Type | Antigen | Activity | |
		Amidolytic	Coagulant
I	Low	Low	Low
II	Normal	Low	Low
	Normal	Normal	Low

This syndrome typically occurs during the first several days of warfarin therapy, often in association with the administration of large loading doses of the medication. The skin lesions occur on the extremities, breasts, and trunk, as well as the penis and marginate over a period of hours from an initial central erythematous macule. If a product containing protein C is not rapidly administered, the affected cutaneous areas become edematous, develop central purpuric zones, and ultimately become necrotic. Biopsies demonstrate fibrin thrombi within cutaneous vessels with interstitial hemorrhage. The dermal manifestations of warfarin-induced skin necrosis are clinically and pathologically similar to those seen in infants with purpura fulminans due to severe protein C deficiency.

The pathogenesis of warfarin-induced skin necrosis is attributable to the emergence of a transient hypercoagulable state. The initiation of the drug at standard doses leads to a decrease in protein C anticoagulant activity levels to ~50 percent of normal within 1 day.[108] Although factor VII activity measurements follow a pattern similar to that of protein C, the levels of the other vitamin K-dependent factors decline at slower rates, consistent with their longer half-life. During this period, it therefore appears that the drug's suppressive effect on protein C has a greater influence on the hemostatic mechanism than its reduction in factor VII. These effects are augmented when more than 10 mg of warfarin daily is administered to initiate oral anticoagulation or the patient has an underlying hereditary deficiency of protein C. Only approximately a third of patients with warfarin-induced skin necrosis, however, have an inherited deficiency of protein C,[109] and this complication is only infrequently reported in individuals with the heterozygous deficiency state. A case report has also described this syndrome in association with an acquired functional deficiency of protein C.[110]

A rare disorder exists in which neonates develop a syndrome described as purpura fulminans and laboratory evidence of DIC in association with protein C antigen levels <1 percent of normal.[111–117] In some instances, there has been a history of consanguinity in the family, making it highly likely that the affected infants were homozygous for the deficiency state.[112,115,116] These newborns can also be double heterozygotes, as was demonstrated in a Chinese patient[117] who had a 5 nucleotide deletion in one protein C allele and a missense mutation in the other.[118] The heterozygous parents of these

infants only infrequently had thrombosis, in contrast with patients with thrombotic histories and a hereditary partial deficiency of protein C. There have also been a number of reports of older patients with homozygous or doubly heterozygous protein C deficiency who did not present with lesions resembling purpura fulminans. These individuals generally had protein C levels <20 percent of normal in the absence of oral anticoagulant therapy, and their clinical presentation was similar to that of severely affected subjects from thrombophilic kindreds with the heterozygous deficiency state.[119,120] Genotyping of such homozygous individuals identified several missense mutations in the protein C gene;[121–124] the variant protein C molecules produced by these individuals are either synthesized at a decreased rate or rapidly cleared from the circulation. The parents of these subjects and infants with purpura fulminans have a type I deficiency state.

The nature of the molecular defect in the protein C gene *per se* does not explain the marked phenotypic variability in heterozygous type I protein C deficiency. A mutation common among symptomatic Dutch patients has also been found in an asymptomatic Swedish person[125] and a parent of a doubly heterozygous child.[126] Also 4 of the 11 mutations observed in homozygotes, whose parents are frequently asymptomatic, have been found in symptomatic heterozygotes.[124] Similar to other inherited thrombotic disorders, the variable penetrance of thrombosis in heterozygous protein C deficiency reflects a complex interaction with other modulating factors.[127]

A variety of immunologic and functional techniques have been developed to measure protein C levels in plasma samples. The most common procedures for antigen determination are electroimmunoassay and enzyme-linked immunosorbent assay. Functional assays initially utilized either thrombin[128] or the thrombin-thrombomodulin complex[129,130] to activate protein C. Enzymatic activity is then assessed using either a chromogenic substrate[128–130] or by measuring its anticoagulant activity in a clotting assay.[108] The development of simpler functional assays has been facilitated by the observation that the venom of the Southern copperhead snake (*Agkistrodon contortix*) is able to activate protein C in plasma. After activation of protein C by this venom, the enzyme's amidolytic activity can be measured using a suitable chromogenic substrate, or its anticoagulant activity can be measured in a clotting assay.

Functional assays utilizing amidolytic and clotting endpoints may give useful information regarding the nature of the molecular defect in patients with type II protein C deficiency. Several individuals with normal protein C antigen measurements have been described who had substantial reductions in protein C anticoagulant activity, but normal or near normal amidolytic activity.[108] These defects potentially reflect a reduced ability of activated protein C to interact with platelet membranes, or its substrates such as factor V and factor VIII. Thus the protein C anticoagulant activity assay should have greater sensitivity than the amidolytic assay in screening for molecular defects resulting in type II protein C deficiency. Most clinical laboratories, however, prefer to use a chromogenic assay for initial screening as it is technically easier to perform and has a smaller coefficient of variation than the clotting assay. 'Global' coagulation assays are also being investigated as a means of screening for any major abnormality in the entire protein C pathway (for example, protein C deficiency, protein S deficiency, or the factor V Leiden mutation).[131] However, the utility of these assays has been limited by a poor sensitivity for protein S deficiency.

Protein C normally circulates in human plasma at an average concentration of 4 μg/mL. The levels of protein C antigen in healthy adults are log-normal distributed with 95 percent of the values ranging from 70 percent to 140 percent.[101] There is no significant sex dependence, but mean protein C concentrations increase by ~4 percent per decade. The relatively wide normal range of protein C measurements in the general population occasionally makes it difficult to identify a given individual as having heterozygous protein C deficiency.[132] If medical and pharmacologic causes of low levels are excluded (see below), patients with a protein C value of <55 percent of normal are very likely to have the genetic abnormality, whereas levels from 55 percent to 65 percent are consistent with either a deficiency state or the lower end of the normal distribution.[101] To document the presence of protein C deficiency with confidence, it is therefore useful to obtain repeat laboratory determinations as well as to perform family studies to identify an autosomal dominant inheritance pattern.

Protein C levels in neonates are 20–40 percent of normal adult levels.[133] Preterms have even lower levels,[134] and babies with significant perinatal thrombosis can have levels suggestive of the homozygous deficiency state.[135] Acquired protein C deficiency (see Table 7.2) occurs in liver disease,[133] severe infection and septic shock,[136] DIC,[133] adult respiratory distress syndrome,[133] the postoperative state,[133] breast cancer patients receiving cyclophosphamide, methotrexate, and 5-fluorouracil,[137] and in association with L-asparaginase.[138] A particularly severe form of acquired protein C deficiency has been reported in association with purpura fulminans and DIC in patients with acute viral or bacterial infections, in particular meningococcemia.[139,140] In contrast with antithrombin, the antigenic concentrations of vitamin K-dependent plasma proteins, including protein C, are often elevated in patients with the nephrotic syndrome.[141]

Warfarin therapy reduces functional[108,128] and, to a lesser extent, immunologic measurements of protein C,[88,142] making it difficult to diagnose heterozygous protein C deficiency in this setting. Several research laboratories have used a reduced ratio of protein C antigen to prothrombin or factor X antigen to identify patients with a type I deficiency state.[88,142] This approach, however, can only be used in individuals in a stable phase of oral anticoagulation, and the diagnostic criteria for the disorder vary with the intensity of warfarin therapy.[142] Other groups have successfully used protein C activity assays in conjunction with functional measurements of factor VII, a vitamin K-dependent

zymogen with a similar plasma half-life.[143,144] Therefore, in practice it is preferable to investigate patients suspected of having the deficiency state after oral anticoagulation has been discontinued for at least 2 weeks and to perform family studies. If it is not possible to discontinue warfarin because of the severity of the thrombotic diathesis, such individuals can be studied while receiving unfractionated or low-molecular-weight heparin therapy, which does not alter plasma protein C levels.

An acquired inhibitor of protein C has been documented in an Australian patient.[145] This individual had a bleeding diathesis for several years and developed purpura fulminans before his death. An autopsy showed arterial and venous thrombi in many organs. Laboratory evaluation demonstrated the presence of chronic DIC. The IgG fraction of the patient's plasma completely inhibited the functional anticoagulant activity of activated protein C.

Protein S deficiency

In 1984, members from several kindreds who exhibited reduced levels of protein S were described who had a striking history of recurrent venous thrombotic disease.[146,147] Subsequently, many additional families with this disorder have been reported.[148]

Heterozygous protein S deficiency is inherited in an autosomal dominant fashion with a reported frequency of ~10 percent in families with inherited thrombophilia.[67] However, the prevalence is less (between 1 percent and 7 percent) among consecutive outpatients with deep venous thrombosis.[10,69] Protein S deficiency is generally considered to confer a risk of thrombosis similar to protein C deficiency[149,150] although, as will be discussed, the association has been complicated by considerable phenotypic variability. A more severe form of protein S deficiency is an autosomal recessive disorder.

The clinical presentation of patients with heterozygous protein S deficiency is similar to that outlined for deficiencies of antithrombin III and protein C. Among 71 protein S-deficient members from 12 Dutch pedigrees,[151] 74 percent, 72 percent, and 38 percent of the individuals sustained deep venous thrombosis, superficial thrombophlebitis, and pulmonary emboli, respectively. The mean age of the first thrombotic event was 28 years with a range between 15 and 68; 56 percent of the episodes were apparently spontaneous and the remainder were precipitated by an identifiable factor. Thrombosis has also been reported in the axillary, mesenteric, and cerebral veins.

Several case reports have described young patients with arterial thrombosis and hereditary protein S deficiency.[152,153] In a cohort of 37 consecutive young adults (less than 45 years of age) presenting with arterial occlusive disease, three had hereditary protein S deficiency.[154] However, the occurrence of arterial thromboembolic events was not increased in protein S-deficient relatives of these people compared with their biochemically unaffected family members. Thus,

Table 7.5 Assay measurements in heterozygous protein S deficiency

| Type | Protein S antigen | | Protein S activity |
	Total	Free	
I ('classic')	Low	Low	Low
II	Normal	Normal	Low
III	Normal	Low	Low

current data do not support an association between hereditary protein S deficiency and an increased risk of arterial thrombosis.

Under normal conditions, ~60 percent of the total protein S antigen in plasma is complexed to a complement component, C4b-binding protein. Only the free 40 percent is functionally active as a cofactor in mediating the anticoagulant effects of activated protein C.[146] This observation has led to the development of methods for measuring total[147,155] and free protein S antigen.[156] Total protein S antigen can be reliably measured by enzyme-linked immunosorbent assay techniques, following dilution of plasma samples to allow dissociation of the protein S-C4b-binding protein complexes. After removing protein S-C4b-binding protein complexes from plasma by polyethylene glycol precipitation,[156] free protein S can be quantified by immunoassay of the supernatant fractions. It is also possible to measure free protein S specifically using a monoclonal antibody-based immunoenzymatic assay that uses antibodies specific for the free form.[157] Functional assay methods are based on the ability of protein S to serve as a cofactor for the anticoagulant effect of activated protein C. Some of the original coagulation assays developed to measure the functional activity of plasma protein S were later found to be sensitive to abnormalities associated with resistance to activated protein C (factor V Leiden),[158] which has led to the development of more accurate second generation assays.[159]

Three types of protein S deficiency states can be identified based on measurements of total and free antigen as well as functional activity (Table 7.5). Type I deficiency is associated with about 50 percent of the normal total protein S antigen level,[147,160] and decrements in free protein S antigen and protein S functional activity to less than about 40 percent of normal.[156] Another type of hereditary deficiency (type II) has been described in which the functional activity of protein S is decreased, but with normal total and free antigen levels. A type III deficiency state is characterized phenotypically by a decreased concentration of free and functional plasma protein S, but a normal total protein S antigen.

The analysis of mutations in patients with protein S deficiency was complicated by the presence of a protein S pseudogene.[161–163] Mutations, however, were subsequently identified in about 70 percent of thrombophilic families with protein S deficiency using mutation-screening strategies.[164] Type I deficiency is most often secondary to missense mutations, base pair insertions or deletions, premature stop

codons, or mutations affecting a splice site. There have been a few cases of large deletions of the gene. Of the more than 130 different mutations documented in patients with various types of protein S deficiency, only 7 different nucleotide substitutions have been identified with a type II deficiency.[165,166] Several of these mutations are located in the amino-terminal end of the protein S molecule, which includes the domains that interact with activated protein C.[167]

The biologic basis of type III protein S deficiency state is uncertain. Furthermore, the coexistence of the type I and type III deficiencies has been reported in some protein-S-deficient families, which has led to the proposal that the two types of protein S deficiency are phenotypic variants of the same genotype and are not the product of distinct genetic mutations.[168] In a follow-up analysis of one large family with a high prevalence of both type I and type III deficiencies, total protein S antigen, but not free protein S antigen levels, was shown to directly correlate with age.[169] These findings were independent of sex and also seen in nondeficient family members. The researchers concluded that a single point mutation in the protein S gene was responsible for the quantitative type I deficiency, but that the type III phenotype was actually due to an age-dependent free protein S deficiency; with increasing age, the relative concentrations of free protein S to total protein S decreased. Young patients with recurrent venous thromboembolic disease in association with doubly heterozygous or homozygous protein S deficiency have been identified.[146] The parents of the patients were asymptomatic and had laboratory studies consistent with type I protein S deficiency. Neonatal purpura fulminans has been described in association with homozygous protein S deficiency.[170,171]

The average concentration of total protein S antigen in normal adults is 23 μg/mL,[172] but there is considerable overlap between 'low normals' and individuals with heterozygous protein S deficiency. Levels increase with advancing age and are lower and more variable in females than males.[173,174] These factors have confounded the reliable estimation of the prevalence of heterozygous protein S deficiency in the normal population as well the relative risk for thrombosis conferred by the disorder.[69] Thus, it is difficult to make the diagnosis of heterozygous protein S deficiency by performing only a single assay; repeat sampling as well as family studies are usually required to establish the diagnosis firmly.

Acquired protein S deficiency occurs during pregnancy[175,176] and in association with the use of oral contraceptives.[173,177] Reduced protein S levels have also been noted in patients with DIC[178,179] and acute thromboembolic disease.[179] C4b-binding protein is an acute phase protein and the declines in protein S activity in the latter two conditions as well as in other inflammatory disorders is attributable to a shift of the protein to the complexed, inactive form.[179] The levels of total and especially free protein S are markedly reduced in men with human immunodeficiency virus (HIV) infection.[180] Total protein S antigen measurements are generally increased in patients with the nephrotic syndrome,[141] although functional assays give reduced values. This is, in part, due to the loss of free protein S in the urine and elevations in C4b-binding protein levels. Total and free protein S antigen levels are moderately decreased in liver disease[155,179] and in association with L-asparaginase chemotherapy.[138] An acquired severe deficiency of protein S has also been reported in association with cutaneous necrosis.[181] Several studies have noted an association between antiphospholipid antibodies and acquired protein S deficiency, especially in severe cases of varicella complicated by purpura fulminans.[182,183]

Interpretation of protein S measurements in individuals on oral anticoagulants is complicated inasmuch as the antigenic and functional levels of the protein drop substantially. A few groups have used reductions in the ratio of protein S antigen to prothrombin antigen to infer a diagnosis of the classic type of protein S deficient state; this is accomplished by employing a strategy similar to that described for protein C-deficient individuals.[147,160] Total protein S antigen values in healthy neonates at term are 15–30 percent of normal and C4b-binding protein is markedly reduced to <20 percent. Thus, the free form of the protein predominates in this setting and functional levels are only slightly reduced as compared with those in normal adults.[184,185]

Activated protein C resistance and the factor V Leiden mutation

In 1993, Dahlbäck et al.[186] identified a novel mechanism for familial thrombophilia; the plasma of individuals with unexplained personal and familial histories of venous thromboembolism exhibited a poor response to activated protein C (APC) in an aPTT assay. Dahlbäck's observations facilitated the development of an aPTT-based assay to screen for APC resistance, which demonstrated the abnormality in 33 percent of Swedish patients referred for evaluation of venous thrombosis (that is, defined as an anticoagulant response in the PTT-based assay below the 5th percentile of controls).[187] Precipitating factors for thrombosis, such as pregnancy and the use of oral contraceptives, were identified in 60 percent of their patients. Family studies revealed that relatives with APC resistance had a significantly higher frequency of thrombosis than relatives without the defect. In a US referral population of patients under age 50 with unexplained venous thromboembolic disease, it was found that ~50 percent had APC resistance.[7] Investigators in Italy and Austria confirmed that APC resistance was a frequent laboratory abnormality in patients with unexplained venous thrombosis.[158,189]

Major contributions to our understanding of the molecular basis and clinical relevance of APC resistance were made by Dutch investigators from Leiden. In 1987, they initiated the Leiden Thrombophilia Study, a large case–control study to investigate risk factors for first episodes of venous thrombosis in the general population of the Netherlands.[9] This effort grew from an attempt to define the true risk of venous thrombosis associated with protein

Table 7.6 The Leiden Thrombophilia Study data: relative and absolute risks of an initial episode of deep venous thrombosis in the general population due to common risk factors

	Risk	Incidence/ 100 person–years	Reference
Normal	–	0.008	
Hyperhomocysteinemia	2.5 × ↑	0.02	9
Prothrombin gene mutation	2.8 × ↑	0.022	8
Oral contraceptives	4 × ↑	0.03	29
Factor V Leiden heterozygotes	7 × ↑	0.057	11
Oral contraceptives + factor V Leiden	35 × ↑	0.285	29
Factor V Leiden homozygotes	80 × ↑	0.5–1	190

C deficiency. As noted above, there was a seeming paradox in that referred patients from families with protein C deficiency had a high frequency of venous thrombosis, but the deficiency state is present in 1/200–500 healthy blood donors. The criteria for accruing subjects into these studies were felt to a major factor underlying this difference.

Following Dahlbäck's initial observations, patients entering the Leiden Thrombophilia Study were screened for APC resistance following the completion of anticoagulant therapy.[11] Entry criteria were a first episode of deep venous thrombosis in outpatients under age 70 with the diagnosis having been confirmed by objective testing. Patients with malignancy were excluded. Each thrombosis patient was matched with a healthy age- and sex-matched control. APC resistance was found in 21 percent of thrombosis patients and 5 percent of controls. Patients with APC resistance were calculated to have a sevenfold increased risk of venous thrombosis as compared with controls (Table 7.6). The lower frequency of resistance to APC in this study as compared with other studies of referral populations cited earlier is attributable to different selection criteria for the thrombosis cohorts.

It was subsequently shown that a defect in factor V involving the mutation of arginine-506 to glutamine-506 (Arg506Gln or factor V Leiden) is most often the cause of APC resistance.[189–192] This is the site at which APC cleaves factor Va, and this sequence alteration makes the mutant factor Va molecule biochemically resistant to inactivation by the enzyme.[189,193,194] The Arg506Gln substitution was found to be the cause of APC resistance in about 90 percent of Dutch patients with APC resistance in the aPTT assay,[189] and the mutation was found in 2–4 percent of healthy Dutch controls. Most patients with APC resistance are heterozygous for the factor V Leiden mutation, but a number of homozygous patients with heightened APC resistance in aPTT assays have been identified.[189,192,195] Homozygotes are at higher thrombotic risk than heterozygotes (see Table 7.6)[190,192] as are patients with heterozygous resistance to APC combined with mutations in the genes for protein C, antithrombin, and probably protein S.[17–20,196] The genes for factor V and antithrombin are both located on the long arm of chromosome 1, thereby allowing for coinheritance of the factor V Leiden mutation and an antithrombin mutation within all affected members of a family. This situation is expected to lead to an even more severe thrombotic diathesis.[20] Although the factor V Leiden mutation is the dominant mechanism underlying APC resistance, factor V itself, but not purified factor Va, is able to enhance the inactivation of factor VIIIa by activated protein C.[197,198] Factor V Leiden is significantly less effective than normal factor V in mediating this effect.

The Physician's Health Study in the United States has also provided valuable data regarding factor V Leiden as a risk factor for venous as well as arterial thrombosis. In a retrospective case–control study of 14 916 healthy men over age 40 with a mean follow-up of 8.6 years, heterozygosity for the factor V Leiden mutation was identified in 12 percent of subjects (14/121) with a first episode of deep venous thrombosis or pulmonary embolism and 6 percent of controls.[6] The relative risk of venous thromboembolism was increased 3.5-fold in those individuals with no other concomitant risk factors, but surprisingly was reduced to 1.7-fold in those with preexistent cancer or recent surgery. This study also showed that elderly patients with venous thrombosis frequently have the mutation.[6,12] Among men over age 60 with initial episodes of venous thrombosis and no identifiable triggering factors, 26 percent (8/31) were heterozygotes for factor V Leiden.[6] Although factor V Leiden is not a major risk factor for thrombosis in patients with cancer, it has been reported that acquired APC resistance as determined by a 'first generation' assay is common in this population.[199]

A cohort study of over 9000 randomly selected adults in Denmark found that the simultaneous presence of smoking, obesity (body mass index $>30 \text{ kg/m}^2$), older age (>60 years), and the factor V Leiden mutation resulted in the highest risk of thromboembolism with absolute 10-year rates of 10 percent in heterozygotes and 51 percent in homozygotes.[200] A prospective cohort study determined the incidence of venous thromboembolism in asymptomatic carriers of the factor V Leiden mutation. Nine events occurred in 1564 observation-years resulting in an annual incidence of 0.58 percent. It was concluded that the absolute annual incidence of venous thromboembolism in asymptomatic carriers of the mutation is low.[201]

A number of studies have examined whether factor V Leiden, a prevalent abnormality in Caucasian populations, leads to an increased risk for arterial thrombotic events. There are no convincing data that other thrombophilic states such as deficiencies of antithrombin III, protein C, and protein S confer an increased risk of arterial thrombosis, but evaluation of these associations is complicated by the relative infrequency of these defects. In a cohort of men over age 40 in which there was a low prevalence of smoking, the US Physician's Health Study did not find an association between the factor V Leiden mutation and myocardial infarction or stroke.[6] In a younger cohort of Italian patients with myocardial infarction prior to age 45, an increased incidence of the factor V Leiden mutation also was not found *vis-à-vis* controls.[202] Furthermore, a report of 36 French homozygous patients with the mutation did not identify a tendency for the development of arterial thrombosis.[203]

However, data from a case–control study suggest that heterozygosity for factor V Leiden is a risk factor for a myocardial infarction in young women (18–44 years old) but only in the presence of other cardiac risk factors.[204] The presence of the factor V Leiden mutation was associated with a 2.4-fold increased risk of myocardial infarction after adjustment for age (8/79 or 9.5 percent of patients with myocardial infarction as compared to 4.1 percent in controls). The risk of myocardial infarction associated with factor V Leiden, however, was observed only among current cigarette smokers in whom the mutation conferred a three-fold increased risk. In comparison with women who did not smoke and did not carry factor V Leiden, women who smoked and carried the mutation had a 30-fold increased risk of myocardial infarction. Interestingly, whereas other cardiac risk factors such as older age, obesity, hypercholesterolemia, hypertension, diabetes, family history of ischemic heart disease, and postmenopausal status (surgically induced) were associated with cardiac events, the use of low-dose oral contraceptives was not. Data from this cohort indicate that the prothrombin gene mutation (see below) is also a risk factor for myocardial infarction, but again only in current cigarette smokers.[205]

Obstetric complications, such as severe preeclampsia, abruptio placentae, fetal growth retardation and stillbirth, are associated with intervillous or spiral artery thrombosis and consequent placental insufficiency. Factor V Leiden and the prothrombin gene mutation are associated with an approximate tripling of the risk of late fetal loss.[206,207] An increased incidence of factor V Leiden, as well as other thrombophilias, was also reported in women in association with other obstetric complications;[208] associations with preeclampsia and intrauterine growth retardation have, however, not been corroborated.[209,210]

The prevalence of heterozygosity for the factor V Leiden mutation in Caucasians, including European, Jewish, Israeli Arab, and Indian populations, ranges from 1 percent to 8.5 percent. The mutation is apparently not present in African black, Chinese, Japanese or native American populations.[211] In Europe, the mutation has been found to be more prevalent in northern countries such as Sweden as compared with southern countries such as Spain and Italy. Using dimorphic sites in the factor V gene to do haplotype analysis, data have been provided supporting the existence of a founder effect among Caucasians of differing ethnic backgrounds.[212] It was also estimated that the mutation originated $\sim$30 000 years ago, which came after the evolutionary divergence of Caucasian, African, and Oriental populations.

Two mutations at the Arg306 residue in factor V, the second APC cleavage site in the activated cofactor, have been described in patients with a history of thrombosis. These include replacement of Arg306 with threonine (factor V Cambridge),[213] or with glycine (in Hong Kong Chinese).[214] However, the latter mutation would not appear to have clinical relevance as it is not associated with APC resistance and the mutation is as common in healthy Chinese blood donors as in patients with thrombosis (4.5 percent and 4.7 percent, respectively).[215] The factor V Cambridge mutation is extremely rare among Caucasians with venous thromboembolic disease.

There have been reports of patients in which there is cosegregation of heterozygous APC resistance due to the factor V Leiden mutation and type I factor V deficiency.[216,217] The plasma of these individuals manifests severe APC resistance in aPTT assays similar to homozygous factor V Leiden patients (that is, they are pseudo-homozygous). These patients were seemingly more thrombosis prone than heterozygous relatives with factor V Leiden alone, suggesting that their clinical phenotype is similar to homozygous factor V Leiden patients.

Several polymorphisms are present in the factor V gene.[218,219] An extended factor V gene haplotype (HR2) containing the R2 polymorphism (His1299Arg) is associated with mild APC resistance and occurs with increased frequency in heterozygous patients with the factor V Leiden mutation with the lowest APC resistance ratios.[219] Although one case–control study found that the R2 allele was a risk factor for venous thromboembolism with an odds ratio of 2.0 after excluding subjects with genetic defects such as factor V Leiden,[220] another case–control study found no significant increase in risk.[221]

Dahlbäck's initial observations[186] facilitated the development of an aPTT-based assay that serves as a screening test for APC resistance. The aPTT is performed in the presence or absence of a standardized amount of APC, and the two clotting times are converted to an APC ratio. Results can be interpreted by comparing the ratio to the normal range, or by normalizing it to the APC resistance ratio obtained using normal pooled plasma. Although this 'first generation' APC resistance assay was conceptually quite simple and easy to perform in a coagulation laboratory, it required careful standardization and determination of the normal range in at least 50 controls. The level of APC, the aPTT reagent, and the instrumentation used for clot detection affected the performance characteristics of the assay. Some assays using this format, therefore, had inadequate sensitivity and specificity for the factor V Leiden mutation. Also, patients receiving anticoagulants or with an abnormal PTT due to other coagulation defects could not be investigated with this assay, and the test was not validated in patients with acute thrombotic events or pregnant women.

The discovery that factor V Leiden is the dominant genetic defect responsible for APC resistance facilitated

'second-generation' coagulation tests that with proper standardization can give nearly 100 percent sensitivity and 100 percent specificity for the mutation. This was achieved by diluting patient plasma in a sufficient volume of factor-V-deficient plasma and then performing an aPTT-based assay. This modification also permits the evaluation of plasma of patients receiving anticoagulants or with abnormal aPTT results due to coagulation factor deficiencies other than factor V.

The fact that the dominant mutation underlying APC resistance is factor V Leiden also makes it attractive to diagnose this defect by analyzing genomic DNA in peripheral blood mononuclear cells. This can be readily accomplished by amplifying a DNA fragment containing the factor V mutation site by polymerase chain reaction (PCR) and analyzing the cleavage products on ethidium bromide-stained agarose gels after restriction enzyme digestion with MnlI.[189] The substitution of an A for a G at nucleotide 1691 in the factor V cDNA (CGA to CAA) results in the Arg506Gln mutation and the loss of a MnlI cleavage site. Other diagnostic approaches include hybridization with allele-specific oligonucleotide probes. In most laboratories, the most cost-effective approach to diagnosing patients with factor V Leiden is to test for APC resistance using a 'second generation' coagulation assay. Patients with low APC resistance ratios should then be genotyped for the mutation though it can be argued that such confirmatory testing is unnecessary in laboratories that have perfect concordance between the results of their APC resistance assays and factor V Leiden genotype.

Using the 'first generation' PTT-based assay for APC resistance, some patients with APC resistance without the factor V Leiden mutation can be identified. The Leiden Thrombophilia Study demonstrated that this abnormality is a significant independent risk for an initial venous thrombotic event.[222] Performance of this assay is not recommended, however, as part of the routine laboratory evaluation since the commercially available APC resistance assays using undiluted plasma do not replicate the performance characteristics of the assay used in this study and the clinical implications of this type of APC resistance are uncertain. The use of such assays is therefore best restricted to thrombosis research centers. Two groups have reported individuals with cerebrovascular disease in association with APC resistance that is not due to the factor V Leiden mutation.[223,224] In one of the studies, the investigators divided patients into five categories of responsiveness to APC as opposed to the usual practice of using a cut-off value for optimal separation of carriers and noncarriers of the mutation.[224] Statistical analysis showed that a low response to APC was associated with an increased risk of cerebrovascular disease independent of the factor V Leiden mutation.

Prothrombin gene mutation

In 1996, investigators from Leiden reported that a G to A substitution at nucleotide 20210 in the 3′-untranslated region of the prothrombin gene is associated with elevated plasma prothrombin levels and an increased risk of venous thrombosis.[8] This mutation, which was discovered by directly sequencing the prothrombin gene of selected patients with venous thrombosis, is located at the last position of the 3'-untranslated region at the cleavage site for polyadenylation of prothrombin mRNA. A recent study indicates that the prothrombin 20210A mutation changes the position of the 3'-cleavage/polyadenylation reaction in prothrombin mRNA, thereby leading to increased prothrombin biosynthesis by the liver;[225] this is in contrast with previous data that the mutation changes mRNA stability by increasing mRNA 3'-end formation.[226]

Investigation of a referral population with a personal and family history of venous thrombosis demonstrated that 18 percent had the mutation in the 3'-untranslated region of the prothrombin gene but it was present in only 1 of 100 healthy controls.[8] Among these thrombosis patients, 40 percent also carried the factor V Leiden mutation, again emphasizing the current view of venous thrombosis as a multigene disorder.

In the Leiden Thrombophilia Study, 6.2 percent of venous thrombosis patients and 2.3 percent of healthy matched controls had the prothrombin gene mutation.[8] This mutation independently confers a 2.8-fold increased risk of venous thrombosis (see Table 7.6) and the effect is operative in both sexes and all age groups. Among heterozygotes with the prothrombin gene mutation, 87 percent of thrombosis patients and controls in the study had prothrombin activity levels that were >1.15 units/mL, whereas only 23 percent of those with a normal prothrombin genotype were elevated to this degree. In numerous subsequent studies, the prothrombin G20210A mutation was found at significantly higher frequency in patients with venous thrombosis than healthy controls.[227–229] Large population studies have shown that the prevalence of the mutation is ~2 percent in the general Caucasian population albeit with significant geographic variation. Among southern Europeans the prevalence was shown to be about 3 percent, but it was only rarely identified in individuals of Asian or African descent.

Polymerase chain reaction methods are used to detect the prothrombin G20210A mutation in genomic DNA[8] and methods are available to detect both the prothrombin G20210A mutation and factor V Leiden in the same reaction. Although plasma prothrombin activity and antigen levels are significantly higher in individuals with the prothrombin G20210A mutation, concentrations cannot be used to screen for the defect due to significant overlap with the normal population.[8,230]

Dysfibrinogenemias

Qualitative abnormalities of fibrinogen are usually inherited in an autosomal dominant manner. The dysfibrinogenemias are a heterogeneous group of disorders that may present with no clinical symptoms, or a bleeding diathesis, or a history of recurrent venous or arterial thromboembolism. A small number of variant fibrinogens have been reported to be associated with thrombotic complications. These defects can be detected with thrombin and reptilase times, which are often prolonged. Functional fibrinogen measurements are usually substantially lower than antigenic measurements in the plasma of these individuals. An occasional individual with a dysfibrinogenemia may have a prolonged prothrombin time or PTT, and the inability of some abnormal fibrinogens to clot completely *in vitro* can result in false-positive results in fibrin(ogen) degradation product tests.

The functional and biochemical defects of a number of abnormal fibrinogens associated with thromboembolic disease have been characterized.[231,232] The conversion of fibrinogen to fibrin by thrombin results in the proteolytic cleavage of fibrinopeptides A and B from the molecule. Defects in the release of these two peptides or abnormalities in fibrin polymerization have been reported. Such functional defects do not, however, offer a ready explanation for the thrombotic diathesis seen in these individuals. Abnormalities in the binding of thrombin to fibrin have also been found in some dysfibrinogenemias.[233,234] In one of these kindreds, three homozygous siblings with a Bβ chain substitution of Ala by Thr at position 68 had a severe clinical phenotype sustaining both arterial and venous thrombosis at a young age.[233] It has been suggested that decreased binding of thrombin by this mutant fibrinogen may lead to the presence of excessive thrombin in the circulation and the occurrence of thrombosis. Other fibrinogen mutants have been shown to cause abnormal fibrin polymerization. Some of the abnormal fibrinogens have been evaluated for their ability to resist or promote fibrinolysis on incorporation into a fibrin clot. The fibrin formed from fibrinogen 'Chapel Hill III' has been demonstrated to be abnormally resistant to lysis by plasmin.[235] Plasminogen activation is decreased in the presence of the fibrin formed from fibrinogen 'Dusart', despite normal tissue-type plasminogen activator binding to the substrate.[236] These abnormalities have the potential for decreasing fibrinolytic activity *in vivo*, which results in a familial thrombotic diathesis in biochemically affected persons.

A rare form of chronic conjunctivitis in young children, termed ligneous conjunctivitis, is characterized by fibrin-rich pseudomembranous lesions. Similar lesions may also occur on other mucous membranes of the body in some affected patients. Severe plasminogen deficiency has been found to be the cause of this disease; these patients were found to be homozygous or compound heterozygous for distinct mutations in the plasminogen gene.[237,238] One homozygous infant with severe ligneous conjunctivitis was treated successfully with a purified plasminogen concentrate.[239]

Inherited abnormalities of fibrinolysis

Although investigators have identified a few individuals with inherited abnormalities of the fibrinolytic mechanism and recurrent venous thromboembolism, the clinical association is considerably less striking than that in many kindreds with deficiencies of antithrombin III, protein C, or protein S, or with APC resistance due to the factor V Leiden mutation and the prothrombin gene mutation. Dysplasminogenemia or hypoplasminogenemia has been reported in a number of individuals with thromboembolic disease; the first case of an abnormal plasminogen was identified in Japan.[240] The propositus had a history of recurrent thrombosis and family studies demonstrated that the biochemical abnormality followed an autosomal dominant inheritance pattern. Despite the hereditary nature of the defect, none of the other biochemically affected members of the kindred had thrombotic events. Other Japanese pedigrees without thrombosis have since been described with the same biochemical defect and the gene frequency of this abnormality in Japan is 0.018.[241] Population studies in the United States have not uncovered any cases of this dysplasminogenemia. The non-Japanese cases of dysplasminogenemias and hypoplasminogenemias have also been remarkable for the lack of thrombotic episodes in biochemically affected family members other than the propositi.

A few reports documented the existence of thrombophilic families with other inherited abnormalities of fibrinolysis.[242,243] Individuals from these kindreds were initially observed to have reduced fibrinolytic potential after venous occlusion[242], and subsequently they were noted to have high levels of plasminogen activator inhibitor.[244,245] Reevaluation of two of these families[242,243] demonstrated the presence of hereditary protein S deficiency and no association between plasminogen activation inhibitor (PAI)-1 activity and a history of thrombosis.[246,247]

Immunochemical methods for the measurement of tissue-type plasminogen activator and functional assays for its inhibitors have been applied to the study of patients with documented venous thromboembolism. These studies suggested that defective synthesis or release of tissue-type plasminogen activator, as well as increased levels of PAI-1 may be important pathogenetic factors in as many as a third of these individuals.[248–250] Reduced fibrinolytic activity due to increased plasma levels of a rapid inhibitor of tissue-type plasminogen activator were also reported in young survivors of myocardial infarction.[251,252] The measurements of this inhibitor correlated strongly with serum concentrations of triglycerides. Subsequent studies, however, have not found a relation between impaired fibrinolytic activity and venous thromboembolism.[253–255]

MANAGEMENT

Treatment of acute thrombosis

The acute management of venous thrombosis or pulmonary embolism in individuals with biologic risk factors for thrombosis is generally not different from that of other individuals. Thrombolytic therapy should be seriously considered in individuals with massive acute venous thrombosis or pulmonary embolism. The usual treatment consists of unfractionated heparin or low-molecular-weight heparin followed by anticoagulation with warfarin (or other vitamin K antagonists). Warfarin can be started within the first 24 hours. Heparin or low-molecular-weight heparin is continued for at least 5 days or until the prothrombin time is in the therapeutic range, namely an international normalized ratio (INR) of 2.0–3.0. Special considerations may apply to selected patients with antithrombin III deficiency and hereditary protein C deficiency.

Antithrombin deficiency

Individuals with antithrombin deficiency can usually be treated successfully with intravenous heparin though in some situations higher than usual doses of the drug are required to achieve adequate anticoagulation. In antithrombin-deficient individuals receiving heparin for the treatment of acute thrombosis, the adjunctive role of antithrombin concentrate purified from human plasma is not clearly defined as controlled trials have not been performed. Antithrombin concentrate has been used safely and effectively in patients with antithrombin deficiency and acute venous thrombosis. It is recommended in those patients who have unusually severe thrombosis, have difficulty achieving adequate anticoagulation, or develop recurrent thrombosis despite adequate anticoagulation. It can also be used for antithrombotic prophylaxis in antithrombin-deficient patients in whom anticoagulation is contraindicated. The use of antithrombin concentrate as adjunctive therapy or as an alternative to heparin, however, has not been studied in a controlled trial.[256]

Antithrombin III concentrate is prepared from pooled normal human plasma. The manufacturing processes used to prepare antithrombin III concentrate result in a product that is greater than 95 percent pure; they also inactivate the hepatitis B virus and human immunodeficiency virus 1.[257] Hence, it is preferable to administer antithrombin concentrate rather than fresh frozen plasma. A human antithrombin concentrate has also been produced from the milk of transgenic goats using recombinant DNA technology[258] and is undergoing clinical trials in patients with hereditary antithrombin deficiency.

The infusion of 50 units of antithrombin concentrate per kilogram of body weight (one unit is defined as the amount of antithrombin in 1 mL of pooled normal human plasma) will usually raise the plasma antithrombin level to approximately 120 percent in a congenitally deficient individual with a baseline level of 50 percent.[259] Plasma levels should be monitored to ensure that they remain above 80 percent; the administration of 60 percent of the initial dose at 24-hour intervals is recommended to maintain inhibitor levels in the normal range.[259] Recovery of plasma-derived antithrombin concentrate *in vivo* in patients with antithrombin deficiency is 1.4–2.7 percent per unit per kg; recovery is lower in patients with acute thrombotic events and those receiving heparin therapy. The biologic half-life approximates 2.8–4.8 days.

Oral anticoagulants are highly effective in the management of patients with antithrombin III deficiency. Warfarin should be continued indefinitely in patients with recurrent venous thrombosis. Asymptomatic antithrombin individuals from thrombophilic kindreds are not generally anticoagulated prophylactically unless they are exposed to situations that predispose them to developing thrombosis (for example, prolonged immobilization, surgery, pregnancy).

Protein C deficiency

Hereditary protein C deficiency can rarely be associated with warfarin-induced skin necrosis due to a transient hypercoagulable state. Despite this risk, routine measurement of plasma protein C concentration in all individuals with thrombosis before the initiation of oral anticoagulants is not recommended. There are three observations underlying this conclusion: the infrequent occurrence of warfarin-induced skin necrosis even among patients with hereditary protein C deficiency; the frequency of asymptomatic hereditary protein C deficiency in the general population (1 in 200 to 500); and the diagnostic difficulty in making a rapid and definitive laboratory diagnosis of the deficiency state.

On the other hand, oral anticoagulation in a patient who is known or likely to be protein C deficient should be started under the cover of full heparinization. The dose of warfarin should be increased gradually, starting from a relatively low level (for example, 2 mg for the first 3 days and then in increasing amounts of 2–3 mg/day until therapeutic anticoagulation is achieved). Patients with heterozygous protein C deficiency and a history of warfarin-induced skin necrosis have been successfully re-treated with oral anticoagulants. Protein C administration, either in the form of fresh frozen plasma or protein C concentrate, can provide protection against recurrent skin necrosis until a stable level of anticoagulation is achieved.

Long-term therapy to prevent recurrent venous thromboembolism

After initial heparinization, standard therapy for patients with deep venous thrombosis or pulmonary embolism typically includes anticoagulation with warfarin for 3–12 months at a target INR between 2 and 3; this results in more than a 90 percent reduction in recurrence risk. In patients presenting with a first episode of symptomatic venous thromboembolism, Prandoni and colleagues[260] found the cumulative incidence of recurrent venous thrombosis after the cessation of anticoagulant therapy to be 24.8 percent at 5 years and 30.3 percent at 8 years. Other investigators have confirmed that this risk is about 5–15 percent per year for the first several years after a first or even a second episode of unprovoked venous thrombosis.[261–263] One trial found a much higher recurrence risk of 27 percent in the first year following 3 months of anticoagulation for a first unprovoked venous thrombotic episode.[264] In summary, the lowest recurrence risks after discontinuation of anticoagulant therapy have been found after 6–12 months of initial therapy. Recurrences are less common when the initial event is associated with a transient risk factor (for example, surgery, trauma). Despite this recurrence risk, there has not heretofore been an anticoagulant regimen available which has proved to have sufficient benefit as compared with the bleeding risk of chronic warfarin therapy at an INR of 2–3 to support long-term prophylaxis for all patients at substantial recurrence risk. For example, one controlled trial evaluated the efficacy of long-term warfarin therapy (INR 2–2.85) for 6 months or indefinitely in 227 patients with a second venous thrombotic episode, but not specifically inherited thrombophilia.[262] Long-term warfarin was highly effective in preventing recurrences as compared to 6 months of therapy (2.6 vs. 21 percent over 4 years); this benefit was partially counterbalanced by a trend toward an increased incidence of major hemorrhage (8.6 vs. 2.3 percent) and there was no difference in mortality between the two groups.

Due to the relatively high frequency of the factor V Leiden mutation (12–21 percent) in unselected patients with a first episode of venous thromboembolism, there are substantial data on the risk of recurrence. Although two groups initially reported that patients with factor V Leiden who had a first venous thrombotic event were more than twice as likely to have a recurrent episode than those without the mutation,[265,266] several other centers have not found that heterozygosity for this defect or the prothrombin G20210 mutation confers a higher recurrence risk.[21,264,267–271] Thus, the consensus view at present is that neither of these defects alone is predictive of recurrence, and several studies have argued against the use of long-term warfarin therapy after a first thromboembolic episode in these patient populations. As an example, the recurrence rate after discontinuation of oral anticoagulant therapy was assessed in 62 patients with factor V Leiden.[272] None of the patients had a recurrent event while taking warfarin. The median time to recurrence after stopping warfarin was 9 years; the period was shorter (3.5 years) among patients who experienced an idiopathic rather than precipitated first event. It was estimated that, even in the latter group, death from hemorrhage would probably exceed the number of fatal pulmonary emboli prevented with chronic warfarin therapy. A decision analysis model concerning the value of extended anticoagulation in patients with factor V Leiden who had a first deep vein thrombosis concluded that the number of major induced hemorrhages would exceed the number of clinical pulmonary emboli that would be prevented, and that extension of oral anticoagulation beyond 1 year would not produce clinical benefit.[273] There is no increase in mortality among patients with the factor V Leiden mutation,[274] further supporting the argument that the mortality risk of chronic warfarin therapy at a target INR of 2–3 in the average thrombophilic patient may exceed the potential benefit. The

Table 7.7 Long-term management of patients with venous thromboembolism

Risk classification	Management

High risk
   2 or more spontaneous events
   1 spontaneous life-threatening thrombosis
   1 spontaneous thrombosis at unusual sites (mesenteric or cerebral venous)
   1 spontaneous thrombosis in association with the antiphospholipid antibody
      syndrome* active cancer, antithrombin III deficiency, or more than one
      genetic or allelic abnormality
	Indefinite anticoagulation

Moderate risk 1 thrombosis with a known provocative stimulus Asymptomatic	Vigorous prophylaxis during high risk settings

recurrence risk appears to be significantly higher in the small subset of patients who are heterozygous for both mutations, homozygous for factor V Leiden, or have another thrombophilic defect.[17–22]

Due to the relatively low frequency of antithrombin, protein C, or protein S in unselected cohorts with an initial episode of venous thromboembolism, randomized clinical trials have included too few patients with these deficiencies to draw firm conclusions. A literature review and retrospective cohort study suggested that they have a high annual incidence of recurrent venous thromboembolism during the years immediately following a first episode and decline thereafter.[275] The application of decision analysis to this problem indicates that optimal anticoagulant treatment duration will vary, depending on the type of initial event (spontaneous or secondary; deep venous thrombosis or pulmonary embolism), patient age, and time passed since the initial thromboembolic episode.[276] Interestingly, retrospective studies are unable to demonstrate an increase in mortality in patients with antithrombin[277] or protein C deficiency.

For the individual patient, the decision to continue anticoagulation indefinitely requires estimation of the quantitative risk of recurrent thrombosis (including fatal pulmonary embolism) and major bleeding (including fatal bleeding) over time. Patient compliance has a major impact on the success of therapy, and patient preferences must be factored into the decision. Many clinicians with experience in managing these disorders recommend indefinite anticoagulation for patients with heterozygous antithrombin deficiency. Some also recommend such an approach for patients with heterozygous deficiencies of protein C and protein S. At present, the decision whether to undertake extended or indefinite anticoagulation must be tailored to the individual patient based on a number factors, and several criteria for long-term anticoagulation are outlined in Table 7.7.

Management of pregnancy

The management of pregnancy in women with thrombotic histories or hereditary thrombotic disorders poses special problems. The incidence of thrombotic complications during pregnancy and the postpartum period appears to be greater in women with antithrombin deficiency than in those with deficiencies of protein C or protein S.[278] During pregnancy, adjusted-dose unfractionated heparin or low-molecular-weight heparin administered by the subcutaneous route is the anticoagulant of choice because its efficacy and safety for the fetus are established. Low-molecular-weight heparin is an attractive alternative to unfractionated heparin in these individuals due to its better bioavailability and longer half-life. A recent study indicates a relatively low risk of venous thromboembolism antepartum without prophylactic anticoagulation in women with a history of thrombotic episodes;[279] the risk may be higher in women with the factor V Leiden mutation. Treatment, however, should be administered during the postpartum period. Affected women with antithrombin deficiency with or without previous thrombotic events should probably receive treatment. Treatment of asymptomatic women with other hereditary thrombotic disorders should be considered on an individual basis, but asymptomatic women with heterozygosity for factor V Leiden or the prothrombin G20210A mutation are at low risk and generally will not require prophylactic anticoagulation.

The dose and duration of heparin or low-molecular-weight heparin therapy in pregnancy are uncertain as appropriately designed clinical trials have not been performed. Individuals considered to be at high risk should receive therapeutic doses by subcutaneous injection every 12 hours for the duration of pregnancy. The dose of unfractionated heparin should be adjusted to maintain the 6-hour postinjection aPTT at 1.5 times the control value. In women considered to be at intermediate risk, lower doses of heparin (5000–10 000 units subcutaneously every 12 hours) or low-molecular-weight heparin can be used and therapy can be started during the second or third trimester and continued for approximately 6 weeks into the postpartum period. Low-risk individuals can be observed closely throughout the pregnancy.

In women who are planning pregnancy while under long-term oral anticoagulant therapy, several approaches can be taken to minimize the risk of both thrombotic complications and warfarin embryopathy. One is to stop warfarin and commence subcutaneous heparin or low-molecular-weight heparin therapy; this potentially exposes the patient to many months of heparin therapy while she is trying to conceive. Alternatively warfarin therapy could be continued with pregnancy tests on a frequent basis. As soon as pregnancy is confirmed and prior to the sixth week of gestation, oral anticoagulants must be discontinued and heparin therapy initiated. Although the risk of warfarin embryopathy appears to be quite small during the first 6 weeks of pregnancy,[280] even the small risk of this complication may make this a less preferable approach.

Management of warfarin-induced skin necrosis and neonatal purpura fulminans

As warfarin-induced skin necrosis is a rare complication, therapy has been guided primarily by knowledge regarding its pathogenesis. The diagnosis should be suspected in individuals with painful, red skin lesions developing within a few days after the initiation of the drug and immediate intervention is required to prevent rapid progression and reduce complications. Therapy should consist of immediate discontinuation of warfarin, administration of vitamin K, and infusion of heparin at therapeutic doses. Lesions, however, have been reported to progress despite adequate anticoagulation with heparin. In individuals with hereditary protein C deficiency, the administration of a source of protein C should be seriously considered, and it may also be appropriate in other individuals with warfarin-induced skin necrosis as they invariably have reduced plasma levels of functional protein C when the skin lesions first appear. Fresh frozen plasma has been used, but improved results can be expected with the administration of a highly purified protein C concentrate, which facilitates the rapid and complete normalization of plasma protein C levels.[281]

The management of neonatal purpura fulminans in association with homozygous or doubly heterozygous protein C deficiency is more complicated, and heparin therapy and antiplatelet agents have not been shown to be effective. The administration of a source of protein C appears to be critical in the initial treatment of these individuals. Fresh frozen plasma has been used with success to treat these babies. However, the half-life of protein C in the circulation is only about 6–16 hours, and the administration of plasma on a frequent basis is limited by the development of hyperproteinemia, hypertension, loss of venous access, and the potential for exposure to infectious viral agents. A highly purified concentrate of protein C has been developed and is efficacious in treating neonatal purpura fulminans.[282] Warfarin has been administered to these babies without the redevelopment of skin necrosis during the phased withdrawal of fresh frozen plasma infusions, and this medication has been used on a long term basis to control the thrombotic diathesis. Successful liver transplantation has been undertaken in a child with liver failure and homozygous protein C deficiency which resulted in normalization of the plasma protein C level and resolution of the thrombotic diathesis.[283]

KEY LEARNING POINTS

- The most common heritable risk factors for venous thromboembolism in Caucasian populations are the factor V Leiden and prothrombin G20210A mutations.
- Estrogen-containing oral contraceptives confer a fourfold increased relative risk for venous thromboembolism in women of childbearing age without heritable thrombophilia and a 35-fold increased risk in women who are heterozygous for the factor V Leiden mutation.
- Patients with venous thromboembolism associated with transient risk factors, such as oral contraceptives or pregnancy, are generally at low risk for recurrent venous thromboembolism.
- The risk for recurrent venous thrombosis in patients with the factor V Leiden or prothrombin G20210A mutation is not greater than in those without an underlying thrombophilic defect.
- Long-term oral anticoagulation should be considered for patients with major unprovoked venous thrombotic events whether or not they are found to have a thrombophilic defect.

REFERENCES

1 Crowther MA, Kelton JG. Congenital thrombophilic states associated with venous thrombosis: a qualitative overview and proposed classification system. *Ann Intern Med* 2003; **138**: 128–34.

2 Christiansen SC, Cannegieter SC, Koster T, *et al.* Thrombophilia, clinical factors, and recurrent venous thrombotic events. *JAMA* 2005; **293**: 2352–61.

3 Greaves M, Baglin T. Laboratory testing for heritable thrombophilia: impact on clinical management of thrombotic disease [annotation]. *Br J Haematol* 2000; **1094**: 699–703.

4 Bauer KA. The thrombophilias: well-defined risk factors with uncertain therapeutic implications. *Ann Intern Med* 2001; **135**: 367–73.

5 Walker ID, Greaves M, Preston FE. Investigation and management of heritable thrombophilia. *Br J Haematol* 2001; **1143**: 512–28.

6 Ridker PM, Hennekens CH, Lindpaintner K, *et al.* Mutation in the gene coding for coagulation factor V and the risk of myocardial infarction, stroke, and venous thrombosis in apparently healthy men. *N Engl J Med* 1995; **332**: 912–17.

7 Griffin JH, Evatt B, Wideman C, Fernandez JA. Anticoagulant protein C pathway defective in majority of thrombophilic patients. *Blood* 1993; **827**: 1989–93.

8 Poort SR, Rosendaal FR, Reitsma PH, Bertina RM. A common genetic variation in the 3′-untranslated region of the prothrombin gene is associated with elevated prothrombin levels and an increase in venous thrombosis. *Blood* 1996; **88**: 3698–703.

9 van der Meer FJM, Koster T, Vandenbroucke JP, *et al*. The Leiden Thrombophilia Study (LETS). *Thromb Haemost* 1997; **78**: 631–5.

10 Heijboer H, Brandjes DPM, Büller HR, *et al*. Deficiencies of coagulation-inhibiting and fibrinolytic proteins in outpatients with deep venous thrombosis. *N Engl J Med* 1990; **323**: 1512–16.

11 Koster T, Rosendaal FR, de Ronde H, Briët E, Vandenbroucke JP, Bertina RM. Venous thrombosis due to poor anticoagulant response to activated protein C: Leiden Thrombophilia Study. *Lancet* 1993; **342**: 1503–6.

12 Ridker PM, Glynn RJ, Miletich JP, *et al*. Age-specific incidence rates of venous thromboembolism among heterozygous carriers of factor V Leiden mutation. *Ann Intern Med* 1997; **126**: 528–31.

13 Selhub J, Jacques PF, Wilson PWF, *et al*. Vitamin status and intake as primary determinants of homocysteinemia in an elderly population. *JAMA* 1993; **270**: 2693–8.

14 Den Heijer M, Koster T, Blom HJ, *et al*. Hyperhomocysteinemia as a risk factor for deep-vein thrombosis. *N Engl J Med* 1996; **334**: 759–62.

15 Poort SR, Pabinger-Fasching I, Mannhalter C, *et al*. Twelve novel and two recurrent mutations in 14 Austrian families with hereditary protein C deficiency. *Blood Coagul Fibrinolysis* 1993; **42**: 273–80.

16 Ridker PM, Hennekens CH, Selhub J, *et al*. Interrelation of hyperhomocyst(e)inemia, factor V Leiden, and risk of future venous thromboembolism. *Circulation* 1997; **95**: 1777–82.

17 Koeleman BPC, Reitsma PH, Allaart CF, Bertina RM. Activated protein C resistance as an additional risk factor for thrombosis in protein C-deficient families. *Blood* 1994; **84**: 1031–5.

18 Gandrille S, Greengard JS, Alhenc-Gelas M, *et al*. Incidence of activated protein C resistance caused by ARG 506 GLN mutation in factor V in 113 unrelated symptomatic protein C-deficient patients. *Blood* 1995; **861**: 219–24.

19 Zöller B, Berntsdotter A, de Frutos GP, Dahlbäck B. Resistance to activated protein C as an additional risk factor in hereditary deficiency of protein S. *Blood* 1995; **12**: 3518–23.

20 van Boven HH, Reitsma PH, Rosendaal FR, *et al*. Factor V Leiden (R506Q) in families with inherited antithrombin deficiency. *Thromb Haemost* 1996; **75**: 417–21.

21 De Stefano V, Martinelli I, Mannucci PM, *et al*. The risk of recurrent deep venous thrombosis among heterozygous carriers of both factor V Leiden and the G20210A prothrombin mutation. *N Engl J Med* 1999; **341**: 801–6.

22 Emmerich J, Rosendaal FR, Cattaneo M, *et al*. Combined effect of factor V Leiden and prothrombin 20210A on the risk of venous thromboembolism – pooled analysis of 8 case-control studies including 2310 cases and 3204 controls. Study Group for Pooled-Analysis in Venous Thromboembolism. *Thromb Haemost* 2001; **863**: 809–16.

23 Schafer AI. Hypercoagulable states: molecular genetics to clinical practice. *Lancet* 1994; **344**: 1739–42.

24 Vandenbroucke JP, Rosing J, Bloemenkamp KWM, *et al*. Oral contraceptives and the risk of venous thrombosis. *N Engl J Med* 2001; **344**: 1527–35.

25 Press RD, Bauer KA, Kujovich JL, Heit JA. Clinical utility of factor V Leiden (R506Q) testing for the diagnosis and management of thromboembolic disorders. *Arch Pathol Lab Med* 2002; **126**: 1304–18.

26 Martinelli I, Sacchi E, Landi G, *et al*. High risk of cerebral-vein thrombosis in carriers of a prothrombin-gene mutation and in users of oral contraceptives. *N Engl J Med* 1998; **338**: 1793–7.

27 Jick H, Jick SS, Gurewich V, *et al*. Risk of idiopathic cardiovascular death and nonfatal venous thromboembolism in women using oral contraceptives with differing progestagen components. *Lancet* 1995; **346**: 1589–93.

28 Spitzer WO, Lewis MA, Heinemann LAJ, *et al*. Third-generation oral contraceptives and risk of venous thromboembolic disorders: an international case-control study. *BMJ* 1996; **312**: 83–8.

29 Vandenbroucke JP, Koster T, Briet E, *et al*. Increased risk of venous thrombosis in oral-contraceptive users who are carriers of factor V Leiden mutation. *Lancet* 1994; **344**: 1453–7.

30 Bloemenkamp KWM, Rosendaal FR, Helmerhorst FM, *et al*. Enhancement by factor V Leiden mutation of risk of deep-vein thrombosis associated with oral contraceptives containing a third-generation progestagen. *Lancet* 1995; **346**: 1593–6.

31 Gerhardt A, Scharf RE, Beckmann MW, *et al*. Prothrombin and factor V mutations in women with a history of thrombosis during pregnancy and the puerperium. *N Engl J Med* 2000; **342**: 374–80.

32 Rosendaal FR, Vessey M, Rumley A, *et al*. Hormonal replacement therapy, prothrombotic mutations and the risk of venous thrombosis. *Br J Haematol* 2002; **116**: 851–4.

33 Herrington DM, Vittinghoff E, Howard TD, *et al*. Factor V Leiden, hormone replacement therapy, and risk of venous thromboembolic events in women with coronary disease. *Arterioscler Thromb Vasc Biol* 2002; **226**: 1012–17.

34 Lapostolle F, Surget V, Borron SW, *et al*. Severe pulmonary embolism associated with air travel. *N Engl J Med* 2001; **345**: 779–83.

35 Perez-Rodriguez E, Jimenez D, Diaz G, *et al*. Incidence of air travel-related pulmonary embolism at the Madrid-Barajas airport. *Arch Intern Med* 2003; **163**: 2766–70.

36 Schwarz T, Siegert G, Oettler W, et al. Venous thrombosis after long-haul flights. Arch Intern Med 2003; 163: 2759–64.

37 Dalen JE. Economy class syndrome: too much flying or too much sitting? Arch Intern Med 2003; 163: 2674–6.

38 Kraaijenhagen RA, Haverkamp D, Koopman MMW, et al. Travel and risk of venous thrombosis. Lancet 2000; 356: 1492–3.

39 Martinelli I, Cattaneo M, Panzeri D, et al. Risk factors for deep venous thrombosis of the upper extremities. Ann Intern Med 1997; 126: 707–11.

40 Gailani D, Reese EP, Jr. Anticoagulant-induced skin necrosis in a patient with hereditary deficiency of protein S. Am J Hematol 1999; 60: 231–6.

41 Makris M, Bardhan G, Preston FE. Warfarin-induced skin necrosis associated with activated protein C resistance [letter]. Thromb Haemost 1996; 753: 523–4.

42 Koster T, Blann AD, Briët E, et al. Role of clotting factor VIII in effect of von Willebrand factor on occurrence of deep-vein thrombosis. Lancet 1995; 345: 152–5.

43 O'Donnell J, Tuddenham EGD, Manning R, et al. High prevalence of elevated factor VIII levels in patients referred for thrombophilia screening: role of increased synthesis and relationship to the acute phase reaction. Thromb Haemost 1997; 775: 825–8.

44 Kraaijenhagen RA, Anker PS, Koopman MMW, et al. High plasma concentration of factor VIIIc is a major risk factor for venous thromboembolism. Thromb Haemost 2000; 83: 5–9.

45 Meijers JCM, Tekelenberg W, Bouma BN, et al. High levels of coagulation factor XI as a risk factor for venous thrombosis. N Engl J Med 2000; 342: 696–701.

46 van Hylckama A, van der Linden IK, Bertina RM, Rosendaal FR. High levels of factor IX increase the risk of venous thrombosis. Blood 2000; 95: 3678–82.

47 van Tilburg NH, Rosendaal FR, Bertina RM. Thrombin activatable fibrinolysis inhibitor and the risk for deep vein thrombosis. Blood 2000; 95: 2855–9.

48 Dahm A, van Hylckama Vlieg A, Bendz B, et al. Low levels of tissue factor pathway inhibitor (TFPI) increase the risk of venous thrombosis. Blood 2003; 101: 4387–92.

49 Lisman T, de Groot PG, Meijers JC, Rosendaal FR. Reduced fibrinolytic potential is a risk factor for venous thrombosis. Blood 2005; 105: 1102–5.

50 Kamphuisen PW, Eikenboom JCJ, Vos HL, et al. Increased levels of factor VIII and fibrinogen in patients with venous thrombosis are not caused by acute phase reactions. Thromb Haemost 1999; 815: 680–3.

51 Legnani C, Cosmi B, Cini M, et al. High plasma levels of factor VIII and risk of recurrence of venous thromboembolism. Br J Haematol 2003; 124: 504–10.

52 Egeberg O. Inherited antithrombin deficiency causing thrombophilia. Thromb Diath Haemorrh 1965; 13: 516–30.

53 Marciniak E, Farley CH, DeSimone PA. Familial thrombosis due to antithrombin III deficiency. Blood 1974; 43: 219–31.

54 Gruenberg JC, Smallridge RC, Rosenberg RD. Inherited antithrombin-III deficiency causing mesenteric venous infarction: a new clinical entity. Ann Surg 1975; 181: 791–4.

55 Carvalho A, Ellman L. Hereditary antithrombin III deficiency: effect of antithrombin III deficiency on platelet function. Am J Med 1976; 61: 179–83.

56 Ambruso DR, Leonard BD, Bies RD, et al. Antithrombin III deficiency: decreased synthesis of a biochemically normal molecule. Blood 1982; 60: 78–83.

57 Lane DA, Bayston T, Olds RJ, et al. Antithrombin mutation database: 2nd (1997) update. Thromb Haemost 1997; 771: 197–211.

58 Wells PS, Blajchman MA, Henderson P, et al. Prevalence of antithrombin deficiency in healthy blood donors: a cross-sectional study. Am J Hematol 1994; 454: 321–4.

59 Tait RC, Walker ID, Perry DJ, et al. Prevalence of antithrombin deficiency in the healthy population. Br J Haematol 1994; 87: 106–12.

60 Meade TW, Dyer S, Howarth DJ, et al. Antithrombin III and procoagulant activity; sex differences and effects of the menopause. Br J Haematol 1990; 74: 77–81.

61 Tait RC, Walker ID, Davidson JF, et al. Antithrombin III activity in healthy blood donors: age and sex related changes and the prevalence of asymptomatic deficiency [letter]. Br J Haematol 1990; 751: 141–2.

62 Thaler E, Lechner K. Antithrombin III deficiency and thromboembolism. In: Prentice CRM, ed. Clinics in Haematology. London: Saunders, 1981: 369–80.

63 Demers C, Ginsberg JS, Hirsh J, et al. Thrombosis in antithrombin-III-deficient persons. Report of a large kindred and literature review. Ann Intern Med 1992; 1169: 754–61.

64 Ambruso DR, Jacobson LJ, Hathaway WE. Inherited antithrombin III deficiency and cerebral thrombosis in a child. Pediatrics 1980; 65: 125–31.

65 Winter JH, Bennett B, Watt JL, et al. Confirmation of linkage between antithrombin III and Duffy blood group and assignment of AT3 to 1q22-q25. Ann Hum Genet 1982; 46: 29–34.

66 Brenner B, Fishman A, Goldsher D, et al. Cerebral thrombosis in a newborn with a congenital deficiency of antithrombin III. Am J Hematol 1988; 27: 209–11.

67 Martinelli I, Mannucci PM, DeStefano V, et al. Different risks of thrombosis in four coagulation defects associated with inherited thrombophilia: a study of 150 families. Blood 1998; 927: 2353–8.

68 Simioni P, Sanson BJ, Prandoni P, et al. Incidence of venous thromboembolism in families with inherited thrombophilia. Thromb Haemost 1999; 812: 198–202.

69 Koster T, Rosendaal FR, Briët E, et al. Protein C deficiency in a controlled series of unselected outpatients: an infrequent but clear risk factor for venous thrombosis (Leiden Thrombophilia Study). Blood 1995; 85: 2756–61.

70 Sas G, Blasko G, Banhegyi D, et al. Abnormal antithrombin III (antithrombin III 'Budapest') as a cause of

familial thrombophilia. *Thromb Diath Haemorrh* 1974; **32**: 105–15.

71 Bock SC, Marrinan JA, Radziejewska E. Antithrombin III Utah: proline-407 to leucine mutation in a highly conserved region near the inhibitor reactive site. *Biochemistry* 1988; **27**: 6171–8.

72 Finazzi G, Caccia R, Barbui T. Different prevalance of thromboembolism in the subtypes of congenital antithrombin deficiency: review of 404 cases [letter]. *Thromb Haemost* 1987; **58**: 1094.

73 Owen MC, Borg JY, Soria J, *et al.* Heparin binding defect in a new antithrombin III variant: Rouen, 47 Arg to His. *Blood* 1987; **69**: 1275–9.

74 Borg JY, Owen MC, Soria C, *et al.* Proposed heparin binding site in antithrombin based on arginine 47. A new variant Rouen-II, 47 arg to ser. *J Clin Invest* 1988; **81**: 1292–6.

75 Brunel F, Duchange N, Fischer AM, *et al.* Antithrombin III Alger: a new case of Arg47-Cys mutation. *Am J Haematol* 1987; **25**: 223–4.

76 Ueyama H, Murakami T, Nishiguchi S, *et al.* Antithrombin III Kumamoto: identification of a point mutation and genotype analysis of the family. *Thromb Haemost* 1990; **63**: 231–4.

77 Andrew M, Paes B, Milner R, *et al.* Development of the human coagulation system in the full-term infant. *Blood* 1987; **70**: 165–72.

78 Andrew M, Paes B, Milner R, *et al.* Development of the human coagulation system in the healthy premature infant. *Blood* 1988; **72**: 1651–7.

79 Rosenberg RD, Damus PS. The purification and mechanism of action of human antithrombin-heparin cofactor. *J Biol Chem* 1973; **248**: 6490–505.

80 Downing MR, Bloom JW, Mann KG. Comparison of the inhibition of thrombin by three plasma protease inhibitors. *Biochemistry* 1978; **17**: 2649–53.

81 Mitchell L, Piovella F, Ofosu F, Andrew M. α_2-Macroglobulin may provide protection from thromboembolic events in antithrombin III-deficient children. *Blood* 1991; **789**: 2299–304.

82 de Boer AC, van Riel LAM, den Ottolander GJH. Measurement of antithrombin III, α_2-macroglobulin and α_1-antitrypsin in patients with deep venous thrombosis and pulmonary embolism. *Thromb Res* 1979; **15**: 17–25.

83 Damus PS, Wallace GA. Immunologic measurement of antithrombin III-heparin cofactor and α_2-macroglobulin in disseminated intravascular coagulation and hepatic failure coagulopathy. *Thromb Res* 1975; **6**: 27–38.

84 Kauffman RH, Veltkamp JJ, Van Tilburg NH, Van Es LA. Acquired antithrombin III deficiency and thrombosis in the nephrotic syndrome. *Am J Med* 1978; **65**: 607–13.

85 Caine YG, Bauer KA, Barzegar S, *et al.* Coagulation activation following estrogen administration to postmenopausal women. *Thromb Haemost* 1992; **68**: 392–5.

86 Weenink GH, Treffers PE, Vijn P, *et al.* Antithrombin III levels in preeclampsia correlate with maternal and fetal morbidity. *Am J Obstet Gynecol* 1984; **148**: 1092–7.

87 Marciniak E, Gockemen JP. Heparin-induced decrease in circulating antithrombin III. *Lancet* 1978; **2**: 581–4.

88 Griffin JH, Evatt B, Zimmerman TS, *et al.* Deficiency of protein C in congenital thrombotic disease. *J Clin Invest* 1981; **68**: 1370–3.

89 Broekmans AW, Veltkamp JJ, Bertina RM. Congenital protein C deficiency and venous thromboembolism: a study of three Dutch families. *N Engl J Med* 1983; **309**: 340–4.

90 Horellou MH, Conard J, Bertina RM, Samama M. Congenital protein C deficiency and thrombotic disease in nine French families. *Br Med J* 1984; **289**: 1285–7.

91 Pabinger-Fasching I, Bertina RM, Lechner K, *et al.* Protein C deficiency in two Austrian families. *Thromb Haemost* 1983; **50**: 810–13.

92 Bovill EG, Bauer KA, Dickerman JD, *et al.* The clinical spectrum of heterozygous protein C deficiency in a large New England kindred. *Blood* 1989; **73**: 712–17.

93 Broekmans AW, Bertina RM. Protein C. In: Poller L, ed. *Recent Advances in Blood Coagulation.* New York: Churchill Livingstone, 1985: 117–37.

94 Wintzen AR, Broekmans AW, Bertina RM, *et al.* Cerebral hemorrhagic infarction in young patients with hereditary protein C deficiency: evidence for 'spontaneous' cerebral venous thrombosis. *Br Med J* 1985; **290**: 350–2.

95 Kohler J, Kasper J, Witt I, Von Reuthern GM. Ischemic stroke due to protein C deficiency. *Stroke* 1990; **21**: 1077–80.

96 Grewal RP, Goldberg MA. Stroke in protein C deficiency. *Am J Med* 1990; **89**: 538–9.

97 Camerlingo M, Finazzi G, Casto L, *et al.* Inherited protein C deficiency and nonhemorrhagic arterial stroke in young adults. *Neurology* 1991; **41**: 1371–3.

98 Mateo J, Oliver A, Borrell M, *et al.* Laboratory evaluation and clinical characteristics of 2,132 consecutive unselected patients with venous thromboembolism – results of the Spanish multicentric study on thrombophilia (EMET Study). *Thromb Haemost* 1997; **77**: 444–51.

99 Gladson CL, Scharrer I, Hach V, *et al.* The frequency of type I heterozygous protein S and protein C deficiency in 141 unrelated patients with venous thrombosis. *Thromb Haemost* 1988; **59**: 18–22.

100 Ben-Tal O, Zivelin A, Seligsohn U. The relative frequency of hereditary thrombotic disorders among 107 patients with thrombophilia in Israel. *Thromb Haemost* 1989; **61**: 50–4.

101 Miletich JP, Sherman L, Broze GJ, Jr. Absence of thrombosis in subjects with heterozygous protein C deficiency. *N Engl J Med* 1987; **317**: 991–6.

102 Tait RC, Walker ID, Reitsma PH, *et al.* Prevalence of protein C deficiency in the healthy population. *Thromb Haemost* 1995; **73**: 87–93.

103   Bucciarelli P, Rosendaal FR, Tripodi A, et al. Risk of venous thromboembolism and clinical manifestations in carriers of antithrombin, protein C, protein S deficiency, or activated protein C resistance: a multicenter collaborative family study. Arterioscler Thromb Vasc Biol 1999; 19: 1026–33.

104   Sanson BJ, Simioni P, Tormene D, et al. The incidence of venous thromboembolism in asymptomatic carriers of a deficiency of antithrombin, protein C, or protein S: a prospective cohort study. Blood 1999; 94: 3702–6.

105   Reitsma PH, Bernardi F, Doig RG, et al. Protein C deficiency: a database of mutations, 1995 update. Thromb Haemost 1995; 73: 876–9.

106   McGehee WG, Klotz TA, Epstein DJ, Rapaport SI. Coumarin necrosis associated with hereditary protein C deficiency. Ann Intern Med 1984; 100: 59–60.

107   Zauber NP, Stark MW. Successful warfarin anticoagulation despite protein C deficiency and a history of warfarin necrosis. Ann Intern Med 1986; 104: 659–60.

108   D'Angelo SV, Comp PC, Esmon CT, D'Angelo A. Relationship between protein C antigen and anticoagulant activity during oral anticoagulation and in selected disease states. J Clin Invest 1986; 77: 416–25.

109   Broekmans AW, Teepe RGC, van der Meer FJM, et al. Protein C (PC) and coumarin-induced skin necrosis [abstract]. Thromb Res 1986; 6: 137.

110   Teepe RGC, Broekmans AW, Vermeer BJ, et al. Recurrent coumarin-induced skin necrosis in a patient with an acquired functional protein C deficiency. Arch Dermatol 1986; 122: 1408–22.

111   Branson HE, Katz J, Marble R, Griffin JH. Inherited protein C deficiency and coumarin-responsive chonic relapsing purpura fulminans in a newborn infant. Lancet 1983; 2: 1165–8.

112   Seligsohn U, Berger A, Abend M, et al. Homozygous protein C deficiency manifested by massive venous thrombosis in the newborn. N Engl J Med 1984; 310: 559–62.

113   Sills RH, Marlar RA, Montgomery RR, et al. Severe homozygous protein C deficiency. J Pediatr 1984; 105: 409–13.

114   Estelles A, Garcia-Plaza I, Dasi A, et al. Severe inherited 'homozygous' protein C deficiency in a newborn infant. Thromb Haemost 1984; 52:53–6.

115   Marciniak E, Wilson HD, Marlar RA. Neonatal purpura fulminans: a genetic disorder related to the absence of protein C in blood. Blood 1985; 65: 15–20.

116   Peters C, Casella JF, Marlar RA, et al. Homozygous protein C deficiency: observations on the nature of the molecular abnormality and the effectiveness of warfarin therapy. Pediatrics 1988; 81: 272–6.

117   Yuen P, Cheung A, Lin HJ, et al. Purpura fulminans in a Chinese boy with congenital protein C deficiency. Pediatrics 1986; 77: 670–6.

118   Sugahara Y, Miura O, Yuen P, Aoki N. Protein C deficiency Hong Kong 1 and 2: hereditary protein C deficiency caused by two mutant alleles, a 5-nucleotide deletion and a missense mutation. Blood 1992; 801: 126–33.

119   Bauer KA, Broekmans AW, Bertina RM, et al. Hemostatic enzyme generation in the blood of patients with hereditary protein C deficiency. Blood 1988; 71: 1418–26.

120   Melissari E, Kakkar VV. Congenital severe protein C deficiency in adults. Br J Haematol 1989; 72: 222–8.

121   Grundy C, Plendl H, Grote W, et al. A single base-pair deletion in the protein C gene causing recurrent thromboembolism. Thromb Res 1991; 613: 335–40.

122   Conard J, Horellou MH, van Dreden P, et al. Homozygous protein C deficiency with late onset and recurrent coumarin-induced skin necrosis [letter]. Lancet 1992; 339: 743–4.

123   Yamamoto K, Matsushita T, Sugiura I, et al. Homozygous protein C deficiency: identification of a novel missense mutation that causes impaired secretion of the mutant protein C. J Lab Clin Med 1992; 119: 682–9.

124   Aiach M, Gandrille S, Emmerich J. A review of mutations causing deficiencies of antithrombin, protein C and protein S. Thromb Haemost 1995; 741: 81–9.

125   Reitsma PH, Poort SR, Allaart CF, et al. The spectrum of genetic defects in a panel of 40 Dutch families with symptomatic protein C deficiency type I: heterogeneity and founder effects. Blood 1991; 784: 890–4.

126   Petrini P, Segnestam K, Ekelund H, Egberg N. Homozygous protein C deficiency in two siblings. Pediatr Hematol Oncol 1990; 72: 165–75.

127   Miletich JP, Prescott SM, White R, et al. Inherited predisposition to thrombosis. Cell 1993; 72: 477–80.

128   Bertina RM, Broekmans AW, Krommenhoek-van Es C, van Winhgaarden A. The use of a functional and immunologic assay for plasma protein C in the study of the heterogenecity of congenital protein C deficiency. Thromb Haemost 1984; 51: 1–5.

129   Sala N, Owen WG, Collen D. Functional assay for protein C in human plasma. Thromb Res 1984; 32: 605–13.

130   Comp PC, Nixon RR, Esmon CT. Determination of functional levels of protein C, an antithrombotic protein, using thrombin-thrombomodulin complex. Blood 1984; 63: 15–21.

131   Tripodi A, Akhavan S, Asti D, et al. Laboratory screening of thrombophilia. Evaluation of the diagnostic efficacy of a global test to detect congenital deficiencies of the protein C anticoagulant pathway. Blood Coagul Fibrinolysis 1998; 9: 485–9.

132   Pabinger I, Allaart CF, Hermans J, et al; the Protein C Transmitter Study Group. Hereditary protein C-deficiency: laboratory values in transmitters and guidelines for the diagnostic procedure. Report on a study of the SSC subcommittee on protein C and protein S. Thromb Haemost 1992; 684: 470–4.

133   Mannucci PM, Vigano S. Deficiencies of protein C, an inhibitor of blood coagulation. Lancet 1982; 2: 463–7.

134   Karpatkin M, Mannucci PM, Bhogal M, et al. Low protein C in the neonatal period. Br J Haematol 1986; 62: 137–42.

135 Manco-Johnson MJ, Marlar RA, Jacobson LJ, *et al.* Severe protein C deficiency in newborn infants. *J Pediatr* 1988; **113**: 359–63.

136 Hesselvik JF, Malm J, Dahlback B, Blomback M. Protein C, protein S and C4b-binding protein in severe infection and septic shock. *Thromb Haemost* 1991; **652**: 126–9.

137 Rogers JS, II, Murgo AJ, Fontana JA, Raich PC. Chemotherapy for breast cancer decreases plasma protein C and protein S. *J Clin Oncol* 1988; **6**: 276–81.

138 Pui CH, Chesney CM, Bergum PW, *et al.* Lack of pathogenic role of protein C and S in thrombosis associated with asparaginase-prednisone-vincristine therapy for leukemia. *Br J Haematol* 1986; **64**: 283–90.

139 Powars DR, Rogers ZR, Patch MJ, *et al.* Purpura fulminans in meningococcemia: association with acquired deficiencies of proteins C and S. *N Engl J Med* 1987; **317**: 571–2.

140 Gerson WT, Dickerman JD, Bovill EG, Golden E. Severe acquired protein C deficiency in purpura fulminans associated with disseminated intravascular coagulation: treatment with protein C concentrate. *Pediatrics* 1993; **912**: 418–22.

141 Vigano-D'Angelo S, D'Angelo A, Kaufman CE, Jr, *et al.* Protein S deficiency occurs in the nephrotic syndrome. *Ann Intern Med* 1987; **107**: 42–7.

142 Bertina RM, Broekmans AW, van der Linden IK, Mertens K. Protein C deficiency in a Dutch family with thrombotic disease. *Thromb Haemost* 1982; **45**: 237–41.

143 Pabinger I, Kyrle PA, Speiser W, *et al.* Diagnosis of protein C deficiency in patients on oral anticoagulant treatment: comparison of three different functional protein C assays. *Thromb Haemost* 1990; **633**: 407–12.

144 Jones DW, Mackie IJ, Winter M, *et al.* Detection of protein C deficiency during oral anticoagulant therapy-use of the protein C:factor VII ratio. *Blood Coagul Fibrinolysis*ysis 1991; **2**: 407–11.

145 Mitchell CA, Rowell JA, Hau L, Young JP, Salem HH. A fatal thrombotic disorder associated with an acquired inhibitor of protein C. *N Engl J Med* 1987; **317**: 1638–42.

146 Comp PC, Nixon RR, Cooper MR, Esmon CT. Familial protein S deficiency is associated with recurrent thrombosis. *J Clin Invest* 1984; **74**: 2082–8.

147 Schwarz HP, Fischer M, Hopmeier P, Batard MA, Griffin JH. Plasma protein S deficiency in familial thrombotic disease. *Blood* 1984; **64**: 1297–300.

148 Broekmans AW, van Rooyen W, Westerveld BD, Briet E, Bertina RM. Mesenteric vein thrombosis as presenting manifestation of hereditary protein S deficiency. *Gastroenterology* 1987; **92**: 240–2.

149 Faioni EM, Valsecchi C, Palla A, Taioli E, Razzari C, Mannucci PM. Free protein S deficiency is a risk factor for venous thrombosis. *Thromb Haemost* 1997; **78**: 1343–6.

150 Makris M, Leach M, Beauchamp NJ, *et al.* Genetic analysis, phenotypic diagnosis, and risk of venous thrombosis in families with inherited deficiencies of protein S. *Blood* 2000; **95**: 1935–41.

151 Engesser L, Broekmans AW, Briet E, Brommer EJP, Bertina RM. Hereditary protein S deficiency: clinical manifestations. *Ann Intern Med* 1987; **106**: 677–82.

152 Coller BS, Owen J, Jesty J, Horowitz D, Reitman MJ, Spear J, *et al.* Deficiency of plasma protein S, protein C or antithrombin III and arterial thrombosis. *Arteriosclerosis* 1987; **7**: 456–62.

153 Israels SJ, Seshia SS. Childhood stroke associated with protein C or protein S deficiency. *J Pediatr* 1987; **111**: 562–4.

154 Allaart CF, Aronson DC, Ruys T, Rosendaal FR, van Bockel JH, Bertina RM, *et al.* Hereditary protein S deficiency in young adults with arterial occlusive disease. *Thromb Haemost* 1990; **64**: 206–10.

155 Bertina RM, van Wijngaarden A, Reinalda-Poot J, Roort SR, Bom VJJ. Determination of plasma protein S – the protein factor of activated protein C. *Thromb Haemost* 1985; **53**: 268–72.

156 Comp PC, Doray D, Patton D, Esmon CT. An abnormal plasma distribution of protein S occurs in functional protein S deficiency. *Blood* 1986; **67**: 504–8.

157 Amiral J, Grosley B, Boyer-Neumann C, Marfaing-Koka A, Peynaud-Debayle E, Wolf M, *et al.* New direct assay of free protein S antigen using two distinct monoclonal antibodies specific for the free form. *Blood Coagul Fibrinolysis* 1994; **5**: 179–86.

158 Faioni EM, Franchi F, Asti D, *et al.* Resistance to activated protein C in nine thrombophilic families: interference in a protein S functional assay. *Thromb Haemost* 1993; **70**: 1067–71.

159 Brunet D, Barthet MC, Morange PE, *et al.* Protein S deficiency: different biological phenotypes according to the assays used. *Thromb Haemost* 1998; **79**: 446–7.

160 Broekmans AW, Bertina RM, Reinalda-Poot J, *et al.* Hereditary protein S deficiency and venous thrombo-embolism. A study in three Dutch families. *Thromb Haemost* 1985; **53**: 273–7.

161 Ploos van Amstel HK, van der Zanden AL, Bakker E, *et al.* Two genes homologous with protein S cDNA are located on chromosome 3. *Thromb Haemost* 1987; **58**: 982–7.

162 Schmidel DK, Tataro AV, Phelps LG, *et al.* Organization of the human protein S genes. *Biochemistry* 1990; **29**: 7845–52.

163 Ploos van Amstel HK, Reitsma PH, *et al.* Intron-exon organization of the active protein S gene PS alpha and its pseudogene PSb: duplication and silencing during primate evolution. *Biochemistry* 1990; **29**: 7853–61.

164 Borgel D, Gandrille S, Aiach M. Protein S deficiency. *Thromb Haemost* 1997; **78**: 351–6.

165 Gandrille S, Borgel D, Ireland H, *et al.* Protein S deficiency: a database of mutations. For the Plasma Coagulation Inhibitors Subcommittee of the Scientific and Standardization Committee of the International Society on Thrombosis and Haemostasis. *Thromb Haemost* 1997; **776**: 1201–14.

166　Gandrille S, Borgel D, Sala N, *et al.* Protein S deficiency: a database of mutations – summary of the first update. *Thromb Haemost* 2000; **84**: 918.

167　Dahlbäck B. Protein S and C4b-binding protein: components involved in the regulation of the protein C anticoagulant system. *Thromb Haemost* 1991; **66**: 49–61.

168　Zöller B, de Frutos PG, Dahlbäck B. Evaluation of the relationship between protein S and C4b-binding protein isoforms in hereditary protein S deficiency demonstrating type I and type III deficiencies to be phenotypic variants of the same genetic disease. *Blood* 1995; **85**: 3524–31.

169　Simmonds RE, Zöller B, Ireland H, *et al.* Genetic and phenotypic analysis of a large (122-member) protein S-deficient kindred provides an explanation for the familial coexistence of type I and type III plasma phenotypes. *Blood* 1997; **89**: 4364–70.

170　Mahasandana C, Suvatte V, Chuansumrit A, *et al.* Homozygous protein S deficiency in an infant with purpura fulminans. *J Pediatr* 1990; **117**: 750–3.

171　Pegelow CH, Ledford M, Young J, Zilleruelo G. Severe protein S deficiency in a newborn. *Pediatrics* 1992; **89**: 674–6.

172　Fair D, Revak DJ. Quantitation of human protein S in the plasma of normal and warfarin-treated individuals by radioimmunoassay. *Thromb Res* 1984; **36**: 527–35.

173　Boerger LM, Morris PC, Thurnau GR, *et al.* Oral contraceptives and gender affect protein S status. *Blood* 1987; **69**: 692–4.

174　Liberti G, Bertina RM, Rosendaal FR. Hormonal state rather than age influences cut-off values of protein S: reevaluation of the thrombotic risk associated with protein S deficiency. *Thromb Haemost* 1999; **82**: 1093–6.

175　Comp PC, Thurnau GR, Welsh J, Esmon CT. Functional and immunologic protein S levels are decreased during pregnancy. *Blood* 1986; **68**: 881–5.

176　Malm J, Laurell M, Dahlback B. Changes in the plasma levels of vitamin K-dependent proteins C and S and of C4B-binding protein during pregnancy and oral contraception. *Br J Haematol* 1988; **68**: 437–43.

177　Gilabert J, Fernandez JA, Espana F, *et al.* Physiological coagulation inhibitors (protein S, protein C and antithrombin III) in severe preeclamptic states and in users of oral contraceptives. *Thromb Res* 1988; **49**: 319–29.

178　Heeb MJ, Mosher D, Griffin JH. Activation and complexation of protein C and cleavage and decrease of protein S in plasma of patients with disseminated intravascular coagulation. *Blood* 1989; **73**: 455–61.

179　D'Angelo A, Vigano-D'Angelo S, Esmon CT, Comp PC. Acquired deficiencies of protein S. Protein S activity during oral anticoagulation, in liver disease, and in disseminated intravascular coagulation. *J Clin Invest* 1988; **81**: 1445–54.

180　Stahl CP, Wideman CS, Spira TJ, *et al.* Protein S deficiency in men with long-term human immunodeficiency virus infection. *Blood* 1993; **817**: 1801–7.

181　Alessi MC, Aillaud MF, Boyer-Neumann C, *et al.* Cutaneous necrosis associated with severe protein S deficiency. *Thromb Haemost* 1993; **695**: 524–6.

182　D'Angelo A, Valle PD, Crippa L, *et al.* Brief report: autoimmune protein S deficiency in a boy with severe thromboembolic disease. *N Engl J Med* 1993; **32824**: 1753–7.

183　Manco-Johnson MJ, Nuss R, Key N, *et al.* Lupus anticoagulant and protein S deficiency in children with post varicella purpura fulminans or thrombosis. *J Pediatr* 1996; **128**: 319–23.

184　Schwarz HP, Muntean W, Watzke H, *et al.* Low total protein antigen but high protein S activity due to decreased C4B-binding protein in neonates. *Blood* 1988; **71**: 562–5.

185　Malm J, Bennhagen R, Holmberg L, Dahlback B. Plasma concentrations of C4b-binding protein and vitamin K-dependent protein S in term and preterm infants: low levels of protein S-C4b-binding protein complexes. *Br J Haematol* 1988; **68**: 445–9.

186　Dahlbäck B, Carlsson M, Svensson PJ. Familial thrombophilia due to a previously unrecognized mechanism characterized by poor anticoagulant response to activated protein C: prediction of a cofactor to activated protein C. *Proc Natl Acad Sci U S A* 1993; **90**: 1004–8.

187　Svensson PJ, Dahlback B. Resistance to activated protein C as a basis for venous thrombosis. *N Engl J Med* 1994; **3308**: 517–22.

188　Halbmayer W-M, Haushofer A, Schon R, Fischer M. The prevalence of poor anticoagulant response to activated protein C (APC resistance) among patients suffering from stroke or venous thrombosis and among healthy subjects. *Blood Coagul Fibrinolysis* 1994; **5**: 51–7.

189　Bertina RM, Koeleman BPC, Koster T, *et al.* Mutation in blood coagulation factor V associated with resistance to activated protein C. *Nature* 1994; **369**: 64–7.

190　Voorberg J, Roelse J, Koopman R, *et al.* Association of idiopathic venous thromboembolism with single point-mutation at Arg^{506} of factor V. *Lancet* 1994; **343**: 1535–6.

191　Zöller B, Svensson PJ, He X, Dahlbäck B. Identification of the same factor V gene mutation in 47 out of 50 thrombosis-prone families with inherited resistance to activated protein C. *J Clin Invest* 1994; **94**: 2521–4.

192　Sun X, Evatt B, Griffin JH. Blood coagulation factor Va abnormality associated with resistance to activated protein C in venous thrombophilia. *Blood* 1994; **83**: 3120–5.

193　Kalafatis M, Bertina RM, Rand MD, Mann KG. Characterization of the molecular defect in Factor V^{R506Q}. *J Biol Chem* 1995; **270**: 4053–7.

194　Greengard JS, Sun X, Xu X, *et al.* Activated protein C resistance caused by Arg506Gln mutation in factor Va. *Lancet* 1994; **343**: 1361–2.

195　Rosendaal FR, Koster T, Vandenbroucke JP, Reitsma PH. High-risk of thrombosis in patients homozygous for factor V Leiden (APC-resistance). *Blood* 1995; **85**: 1504–8.

196 Koeleman BPC, van Rumpt D, Hamulyak K, *et al.* Factor V Leiden: An additional risk factor for thrombosis in protein S-deficient families? *Thromb Haemost* 1995; **74**: 580–3.

197 Shen L, Dahlback B. Factor V and protein S as synergistic cofactors to activated protein C in degradation of factor VIIIa. *J Biol Chem* 1994; **269**: 18735–8.

198 Lu D, Kalafatis M, Mann KG, Long GL. Comparison of activated protein C/protein S-mediated inactivation of human factor VIII and factor V. *Blood* 1996; **87**: 4708–817.

199 Haim N, Lanir N, Hoffman R, *et al.* Acquired activation protein C resistance is common in cancer patients and is associated with venous thromboembolism. *Am J Med* 2001; **110**: 91–6.

200 Juul K, Tybjaerg-Hansen A, Schnohr P, Nordestgaard BG. Factor V Leiden and the risk for venous thromboembolism in the adult Danish population. *Ann Intern Med* 2004; **140**: 330–7.

201 Middeldorp S, Meinardi JR, Koopman MM, *et al.* A prospective study of asymptomatic carriers of the factor V Leiden mutation to determine the incidence of venous thromboembolism. *Ann Intern Med* 2001; **135**: 322–7.

202 Ardissino D, Mannucci PM, Merlini PA, *et al.* Prothrombotic genetic risk factors in young survivors of myocardial infarction. *Blood* 1999; **941**: 46–51.

203 Emmerich J, Alhenc-Gelas M, Aillaud MF, *et al.* Clinical features in 36 patients homozygous for the ARG 506®GLN factor V mutation. *Thromb Haemost* 1997; **77**: 620–3.

204 Rosendaal FR, Siscovick DS, Schwartz SM, *et al.* Factor V Leiden (resistance to activated protein C) increases the risk of myocardial infarction in young women. *Blood* 1997; **898**: 2817–21.

205 Rosendaal FR, Siscovick DS, Schwartz SM, *et al.* A common prothrombin variant (20210 G to A) increases the risk of myocardial infarction in young women. *Blood* 1997; **905**: 1747–50.

206 Preston FE, Rosendaal FR, Walker ID, *et al.* Increased fetal loss in women with heritable thrombophilia. *Lancet* 1996; **348**: 913–16.

207 Martinelli I, Taioli E, Cetin I, *et al.* Mutations in coagulation factors in women with unexplained late fetal loss. *N Engl J Med* 2000; **343**: 1015–18.

208 Kupferminc MJ, Eldor A, Steinman N, *et al.* Increased frequency of genetic thrombophilia in women with complications of pregnancy. *N Engl J Med* 1999; **340**: 9–13.

209 de Groot CJ, Bloemenkamp KW, Duvekot EJ, *et al.* Preeclampsia and genetic risk factors for thrombosis: a case-control study. *Am J Obstet Gynecol* 1999; **181**: 975–80.

210 Infante-Rivard C, Rivard GE, Yotov WV, *et al.* Absence of association of thrombophilia polymorphisms with intrauterine growth restriction. *N Engl J Med* 2002; **347**: 19–25.

211 Rees DC, Cox M, Clegg JB. World distribution of factor V Leiden. *Lancet* 1995; **346**: 1133–4.

212 Zivelin A, Griffin JH, Xu X, *et al.* A single genetic origin for a common Caucasian risk factor for venous thrombosis. *Blood* 1997; **89**: 397–402.

213 Williamson D, Brown K, Luddington R, *et al.* Factor V Cambridge: A new mutation (Arg306®Thr) associated with resistance to activated protein C. *Blood* 1998; **91**: 1140–4.

214 Chan WP, Lee CK, Kwong YL, *et al.* A novel mutation of Arg306 of factor V gene in Hong Kong Chinese. *Blood* 1998; **91**: 1135–9.

215 Liang R, Lee CK, Wat MS, *et al.* Clinical significance of Arg306 mutations of factor V gene. *Blood* 1998; **92**: 2599.

216 Simione P, Soudeller A, Radossi P, *et al.* 'Pseudo homozygous' activated protein C resistance due to double heterozygous factor V defects (factor V Leiden mutation and type I quantitative factor V defect) associated with thrombosis: report of two cases belonging to two unrelated kindreds. *Thromb Haemost* 1996; **75**: 422–6.

217 Guasch JF, Lensen RPM, Bertina RM. Molecular characterization of a type I quantitative factor V deficiency in a thrombosis patient that is 'pseudo homozygous' for activated protein C resistance. *Thromb Haemost* 1996; **772**: 252–7.

218 Lunghi B, Iacoviello L, Gemmati D, *et al.* Detection of new polymorphic markers in the factor V gene: association with factor V levels in plasma. *Thromb Haemost* 1996; **75**: 45–8.

219 Bernardi F, Faioni EM, Castoldi E, *et al.* A factor V genetic component differing from factor V R506Q contributes to the activated protein C resistance phenotype. *Blood* 1997; **904**: 1552–7.

220 Alhenc-Gelas M, Nicaud V, Gandrille S, *et al.* The factor V gene A4070G mutation and the risk of venous thrombosis. *Thromb Haemost* 1999; **81**: 193–7.

221 Luddington R, Jackson A, Pannerselvam S, *et al.* The factor V R2 allele: risk of venous thromboembolism, factor V levels and resistance to activated protein C. *Thromb Haemost* 2000; **83**: 204.

222 de Visser MCH, Rosendaal FR, Bertina RM. A reduced sensitivity for activated protein C in the absence of factor V Leiden increases the risk of venous thrombosis. *Blood* 1999; **93**: 1271–6.

223 Fisher M, Fernández JA, Ameriso SF, *et al.* Activated protein C resistance in ischemic stroke not due to factor V arginine506 to glutamine mutation. *Stroke* 1996; **27**: 1163–6.

224 van der Bom JG, Bots M, Haverkate F, *et al.* Reduced response to activated protein C is associated with increased risk for cerebrovascular disease. *Ann Intern Med* 1996; **125**: 265–9.

225 Pollak ES, Lam H, Russell JE. The G20210A mutation does not affect the stability of prothrombin mRNA *in vivo*. *Blood* 2002; **100**: 359–62.

226 Gehring NH, Frede U, Neu-Yilik G, et al. Increased efficiency of mRNA 3' end formation: a new genetic mechanism contributing to hereditary thrombophilia. Nat Genet 2001; 28: 389–92.

227 Hillarp A, Zöller B, Svensson P, Dahlbäck B. The 20210 A allele of the prothrombin gene is a common risk factor among Swedish outpatients with verified deep vein thrombosis. Thromb Haemost 1997; 78: 990–2.

228 Kapur RK, Mills LA, Spitzer SG, Hultin MB. A prothrombin gene mutation is significantly associated with venous thrombosis. Arterioscler Thromb Vasc Biol 1997; 17: 2875–9.

229 Margaglione M, Brancaccio V, Giuliani N, et al. Increased risk for venous thrombosis in carriers of the prothrombin G→A20210 gene variant. Ann Intern Med 1998; 129: 89–93.

230 Soria J, Almasy L, Souto J, et al. Linkage analysis demonstrates that the prothrombin G21210A mutation jointly influences plasma prothrombin levels and risk of thrombosis. Blood 2000; 95: 2780–5.

231 Mossesson MW. Dysfibrinogenemia and thrombosis. Semin Thromb Hemost 1999; 25: 311–19.

232 Roberts HR, Stinchcombe TE, Gabriel DA. The dysfibrinogenemias. Br J Haematol 2001; 114: 249–57.

233 Haverkate F, Koopman J, Kluft C, et al. Fibrinogen Milano II: a congenital dysfibrinogenemia associated with juvenile arterial and venous thrombosis. Thromb Haemost 1986; 55: 131–5.

234 Marchi R, Lundberg U, Grimbergen J, et al. Fibrinogen Caracas V, an abnormal fibrinogen with an Alpha 532 Ser→Cys substitution associated with thrombosis. Thromb Haemost 2000; 84: 263–70.

235 Carrell N, Gabriel DA, Blatt PM, et al. Hereditary dysfibrinogenemia in a patient with thrombotic disease. Blood 1983; 62: 439–47.

236 Collet J-P, Soria J, Mirshahi M, et al. Dusart syndrome: a new concept of the relationship between fibrin clot architecture and fibrin clot degradability: hypofibrinolysis related to an abnormal clot structure. Blood 1993; 828: 2462–9.

237 Schuster V, Mingers AM, Seidenspinner S, et al. Homozygous mutations in the plasminogen gene of two unrelated girls with ligneous conjunctivitis. Blood 1997; 90: 958–66.

238 Schuster V, Seidenspinner S, Zeitler P, et al. Compound-heterozygous mutations in the plasminogen gene predispose to the development of ligneous conjunctivitis. Blood 1999; 93: 3457–66.

239 Schott D, Dempfle CE, Beck B, et al. Therapy with a purified plasminogen concentrate in an infant with ligneous conjuctivitis and homozygous plasminogen deficiency. N Engl J Med 1998; 339: 1679–86.

240 Aoki N, Moroi M, Sakata Y, et al. Abnormal plasminogen. A hereditary abnormality found in a patient with recurrent thrombosis. J Clin Invest 1978; 61: 1186–95.

241 Aoki N, Tateno K, Sakata Y. Differences of frequency distributions of plasminogen phenotypes between Japanese and American populations: new methods for the detection of plasminogen variants. Biochem Genet 1984; 22: 871–81.

242 Johansson L, Hedner U, Nilsson IM. A family with thromboembolic disease associated with deficient fibrinolytic activity in vessel wall. Acta Med Scand 1978; 203: 477–80.

243 Stead NW, Bauer KA, Kinney TR, et al. Venous thrombosis in a family with defective release of vascular plasminogen activator and elevated plasma factor VIII/von Willebrand factor. Am J Med 1983; 74: 33–9.

244 Nilsson IM, Tengborn L. Impaired fibrinolysis. New evidence in relation to thrombosis. In: Jespersen J, Kluft C, Korsgaard O, eds. Clinical Aspects of Fibrinolysis. Esberg: South Jutland University Press, 1983: 273–91.

245 Jorgensen M, Bonnevie-Nielsen V. Increased concentration of the fast-acting plasminogen activator inhibitor in plasma associated with familial thrombosis. Br J Haematol 1987; 65: 175–80.

246 Bolan CD, Krishnamurti C, Tang DB, et al. Association of protein S deficiency with thrombosis in a kindred with elevated levels of plasminogen activator-1. Ann Intern Med 1993; 119: 779–85.

247 Zöller B, Dahlbäck B. Protein S deficiency in a large family with thrombophilia previously characterized as having an inherited fibrinolytic defect [abstract]. Thromb Haemost 1993; 69: 1256.

248 Nilsson IM, Ljungner H, Tengborn L. Two different mechanisms in patients with venous thrombosis and defective fibrinolysis: low concentration of plasminogen activator or increased concentration of plasminogen activator inhibitor. Br Med J 1985; 290: 1453–6.

249 Wiman B, Ljungberg B, Chmielewska J, et al. The role of the fibrinolytic system in deep venous thrombosis. J Lab Clin Med 1985; 105: 265–70.

250 Juhan-Vague I, Valadier J, Alessi MC, et al. Deficient t-PA release and elevated PA inhibitor levels in patients with spontaneous or recurrent deep venous thrombosis. Thromb Haemost 1987; 57: 67–72.

251 Hamsten A, Wiman B, de Faire U, Blomback M. Increased plasma levels of a rapid inhibitor of tissue plasminogen activator in young survivors of myocardial infarction. N Engl J Med 1985; 313: 1557–63.

252 Hamsten A, Walldius G, Szamosi A, et al. Plasminogen activator inhibitor in plasma: risk factor for recurrent myocardial infarction. Lancet 1987; 2: 3–9.

253 Malm J, Laurell M, Nilsson IM, Dahlback B. Thromboembolic disease–critical evaluation of laboratory investigation. Thromb Haemost 1992; 681: 7–13.

254 Prins MH, Hirsh J. A critical review of the evidence supporting a relationship between impaired fibrinolytic activity and venous thromboembolism. Arch Intern Med 1991; 151: 1721–31.

255 Crowther MA, Roberts J, Roberts R, et al. Fibrinolytic variables in patients with recurrent venous thrombosis: a prospective cohort study. Thromb Haemost 2001; 85: 390–4.

256 Lechner K, Kyrle PA. Antithrombin III concentrates – are they clinically useful? *Thromb Haemost* 1995; **733**: 340–8.

257 Hoffman DL. Purification and large-scale preparation of antithrombin III. *Am J Med* 1989; **87**(Suppl 3B): 23S–26S.

258 Edmunds T, Van Patten SM, Pollock J, *et al.* Transgenically produced human antithrombin: structural and functional comparison to human plasma-derived antithrombin. *Blood* 1998; **91**: 4561–71.

259 Schwartz RS, Bauer KA, Rosenberg RD, *et al.* Clinical experience with antithrombin III concentrate in treatment to congenital and acquired deficiency of antithrombin. *Am J Med* 1989; **87**(Suppl 3B): 53S–60S.

260 Prandoni P, Lensing AWA, Cogo A, *et al.* The long-term clinical course of acute deep venous thrombosis. *Ann Intern Med* 1996; **125**: 1–7.

261 Schulman S, Rhedin AS, Lindmarker P, *et al.* A comparison of six weeks with six months of oral anticoagulation after a first episode of venous thromboembolism. *N Engl J Med* 1995; **332**: 1661–5.

262 Schulman S, Granqvist S, Holmström M, *et al.* The duration of oral anticoagulant therapy after a second episode of venous thromboembolism. *N Engl J Med* 1997; **3366**: 393–8.

263 Agnelli G, Prandoni P, Santamaria MG, *et al.* Three months versus one year of oral anticoagulant therapy for idiopathic deep venous thrombosis. *N Engl J Med* 2001; **345**: 165–9.

264 Kearon C, Gent M, Hirsh J, *et al.* A comparison of three months of anticoagulation with extended anticoagulation for a first episode of idiopathic venous thromboembolism. *N Engl J Med* 1999; **340**: 901–7.

265 Ridker PM, Miletich JP, Stampfer MJ, *et al.* Factor V Leiden and risks of recurrent idiopathic venous thromboembolism. *Circulation* 1995; **92**: 2800–2.

266 Simioni P, Prandoni P, Lensing AWA, *et al.* The risk of recurrent venous thromboembolism in patients with an Arg[506]→Gln mutation in the gene for factor V (factor V Leiden). *N Engl J Med* 1997; **336**: 399–403.

267 Eichinger S, Minar E, Hirschl M, *et al.* The risk of early recurrent venous thromboembolism after oral anticoagulant therapy in patients with the G20210A transition in the prothrombin gene. *Thromb Haemost* 1999; **811**: 14–17.

268 Eichinger S, Pabinger I, Schneider B, *et al.* The risk of recurrence of venous thromboembolism in patients with and without factor V Leiden. *Thromb Haemost* 1997; **774**: 624–8.

269 Lindmarker P, Schulman S, Sten-Linder M, *et al.* The risk of recurrent venous thromboembolism in carriers and non-carriers of the G1691A allele in the coagulation factor V gene and the G20210A allele in the prothrombin gene. *Thromb Haemost* 1999; **815**: 684–90.

270 Margaglione M, D'Andrea G, Colaizzo D, *et al.* Coexistence of factor V Leiden and factor II A20210

mutations and recurrent venous thromboembolism. *Thromb Haemost* 1999; **82**: 1583–7.

271 Baglin T, Luddington R, Brown K, Baglin C. Incidence of recurrent venous thromboembolism in relation to clinical and thrombophilic risk factors: prospective cohort study. *Lancet* 2003; **362**: 523–6.

272 Baglin C, Brown K, Luddington R, Baglin T. Risk of recurrent venous thromboembolism in patients with the factor V Leiden (FVR506Q) mutation: effect of warfarin and prediction by precipitating factors. East Anglian Thrombophilia Study Group. *Br J Haematol* 1998; **100**: 764–8.

273 Sarasin FP, Bounameaux H. Decision analysis model of prolonged oral anticoagulant treatment in factor V Leiden carriers with first episode of deep vein thrombosis. *BMJ* 1998; **316**: 95–9.

274 Hille ET, Westendorp RG, Vandenbroucke JP, Rosendaal FR. Mortality and causes of death in families with the factor V Leiden mutation (resistance to activated protein C). *Blood* 1997; **896**: 1963–7.

275 van den Belt AG, Sanson BJ, Simioni P, *et al.* Recurrence of venous thromboembolism in patients with familial thrombophilia. *Arch Intern Med* 1997; **157**: 2227–32.

276 van den Belt AG, Hutten BA, Prins MH, Bossuy PM. Duration of oral anticoagulant treatment in patients with venous thromboembolism and a deficiency of antithrombin, protein C or protein S – a decision analysis. *Thromb Haemost* 2000; **845**: 758–63.

277 van Boven HH, Vandenbroucke JP, Westendorp RG, Rosendaal FR. Mortality and causes of death in inherited antithrombin deficiency. *Thromb Haemost* 1997; **773**: 452–5.

278 Conard J, Horellou MH, Van Dreden P, *et al.* Thrombosis and pregnancy in congenital deficiencies in ATIII, protein C or protein S: study of 78 women [letter]. *Thromb Haemost* 1990; **63**: 319–20.

279 Brill-Edwards P, Ginsberg JS, Gent M, *et al.* Safety of withholding heparin in pregnant women with a history of venous thromboembolism. Recurrence of Clot in This Pregnancy Study Group. *N Engl J Med* 2000; **343**: 1439–44.

280 Iturbe-Alessio I, Fonseca MC, Mutchinik O, *et al.* Risks of anticoagulant therapy in pregnant women with artificial heart valves. *N Engl J Med* 1986; **315**: 1390–3.

281 Schramm W, Spannagl M, Bauer KA, *et al.* Treatment of coumarin-induced skin necrosis with a monoclonal antibody purified protein C concentrate. *Arch Dermatol* 1993; **129**: 753–6.

282 Dreyfus M, Magny JF, Bridey F, *et al.* Treatment of homozygous protein C deficiency and neonatal purpura fulminans with a purified protein C concentrate. *N Engl J Med* 1991; **325**: 1565–8.

283 Casella JF, Lewis JH, Bontempo FA, *et al.* Successful treatment of homozygous protein C deficiency by hepatic transplantation. *Lancet* 1988; **1**: 435–8.

8

Acquired thrombophilia

MICHAEL GREAVES

INTRODUCTION

A prothrombotic state or 'acquired thrombophilia' is a feature of a range of diseases and treatments. Well recognized examples are cancer and its treatment and use of the combined oral contraceptive, hormone replacement therapy, and ovarian stimulation therapy. These are considered elsewhere in this volume. This chapter focuses on antiphospholipid syndrome and the myeloproliferative disease essential thrombocythemia. In both conditions thrombosis is the principal clinical manifestation and there are special considerations in relation to pregnancy. Also, there is increasing evidence that increased plasma concentrations of several of the coagulation factors confer a risk of thrombosis. Although there appears to be a heritable component, environmental and lifestyle factors influence clotting factor levels and this type of heritable thrombophilia is also considered here.

ANTIPHOSPHOLIPID SYNDROME

Antiphospholipid syndrome is highly relevant to women's health because it is more prevalent in females than males and is a major cause of recurrent pregnancy failure and pregnancy complications, as well as systemic thrombosis.

Definition

Antiphospholipid syndrome is an acquired thrombophilia which appears to have an immune pathogenesis. The diagnosis requires the coexistence of clinical manifestations (thrombosis or recurrent pregnancy failure) and serologic or hematologic evidence of the presence of antiphospholipid antibodies. Because a range of less well-established additional clinical manifestations of the syndrome have been reported, and because antiphospholipid antibodies are not specific for the syndrome, internationally agreed diagnostic criteria have been established to better define the condition for the purposes of clinical research.[1] These are outlined in Box 8.1. It is important to recognize that in clinical practice there may be strong suspicion of the diagnosis even when these criteria are not met in full.

Antiphospholipid antibodies

The nomenclature employed to describe the relevant antibodies in antiphospholipid syndrome is a source of some confusion and is deserving of clarification. The development of antibodies which are apparently reactive with phospholipid, in association with disease, has been recognized for many decades. The so-called serologic false-positive test for syphilis is the earliest example. This was typically noted in individuals with systemic lupus erythematosus (SLE), in whom subsequent investigations demonstrated antibodies in serum that bind to negatively charged phospholipid. Cardiolipin, a phospholipid component of the mitochondrial membrane, was typically employed as antigen in assays for the presence of the antiphospholipid antibodies, giving rise to the terminology anticardiolipin antibodies. It was observed, also, that the plasma of some individuals with SLE has a prolonged clotting time, with no associated clinical bleeding diathesis. This was found to be due to the presence of a coagulation

Box 8.1 Diagnostic criteria of antiphospholipid syndrome

Clinical criteria
- Thrombosis – arterial, venous, or microvascular thrombosis in any tissue or organ
- Pregnancy complications:
  - Unexplained death of morphologically normal fetus at or after 10 weeks
  - Three or more unexplained consecutive abortions before 10 weeks
  - Premature birth before 34 weeks due to severe preeclampsia

Laboratory criteria
- IgG and/or IgM anticardiolipin antibodies at moderate or high concentration and/or
- Lupus anticoagulant

At least one clinical and at least one laboratory criterion must be present. The laboratory test must be consistently positive on at least two occasions 6 weeks apart as transient antibodies may occur, for example in infection. Such antibodies are not usually associated with clinical events.

There has been a recent revision of the criteria.[2] Antibodies to β_2 glycoprotein I have been included and repeat testing after 12 rather than 6 weeks recommended. Arbitrary definitions of medium/high titer antibodies have been given. Delivery before 34 weeks gestation due to placental insufficiency has been included among the clinical criteria.

instances the relevant antigenic sites do not reside on phospholipid. Since the early 1990s it has been recognized that at least some antiphospholipid antibodies bind to a protein, β_2 glycoprotein I. This is a protein that is present in high concentrations in normal plasma. Although its principal physiologic role is not known it is one of the family of complement control proteins (CCP) and it binds avidly to anionic phospholipids and has a weak anticoagulant effect. Indeed it has the alternative name of placental anticoagulant protein. It became apparent from additional investigations that some other plasma proteins can also serve as target antigens for antiphospholipid antibodies. These include the key zymogen in the coagulation mechanism, prothrombin, the physiologic anticoagulant protein C, and annexin V. They share the property of binding to anionic phospholipid. As a result of these observations it has been possible to conclude that the mechanism of apparent binding to phospholipid by antiphospholipid antibodies is through the clustering of antigenic sites on the target phospholipid binding protein when the latter binds to a negatively charged phospholipid surface. This facilitates bivalent antibody binding to epitopes on the bound protein. Indeed the situation can be replicated in the laboratory as an enzyme-linked immunoassay detection system for the antibodies, which utilizes the coating of plastic wells with β_2 glycoprotein I, prothrombin or other relevant protein, rather than cardiolipin.

Antiphospholipid antibodies and the lupus anticoagulant phenomenon

The recent insights into the true nature of so-called antiphospholipid antibodies have facilitated a better understanding of the lupus anticoagulant phenomenon. It is apparent that both antiprothrombin-type and anti-β_2 glycoprotein I-type antiphospholipid antibodies can prolong the clotting time of plasma. This can be explained by the dependence of efficient generation of thrombin on the interaction of coagulation enzymes and cofactors on a template of anionic phospholipid. *In vivo* this is supplied by the plasma membrane of activated platelets. For example, thrombin is generated by cleavage of peptides from the zymogen prothrombin by activated coagulation factor X and the cofactor-activated coagulation factor V brought together on anionic phospholipid in a complex referred to as prothrombinase. It seems likely that antiphospholipid antibody binding, through its protein cofactor, interferes with the construction of prothrombinase by reducing the sites available for binding of its components to the anionic phospholipid template.[3] This results in a slowing of the rate of thrombin generation, detected as a prolongation of clotting time in phospholipid-dependent tests of blood coagulation such as the activated partial thromboplastin time (aPTT).

Recently the properties of antibodies to β_2 glycoprotein I have been defined more clearly. β_2 glycoprotein I has five

inhibitor and the term lupus anticoagulant was applied to this phenomenon. The inhibitor causing the lupus anticoagulant phenomenon is an immunoglobulin and, in individuals with SLE, both anticardiolipin antibodies and lupus anticoagulant type inhibitor may be present.

It soon became apparent that, paradoxically, the presence of lupus anticoagulant is associated with an increased risk of thrombosis in SLE and subsequently the link with pregnancy failure was made. Even more importantly, it became apparent that antiphospholipid antibodies (both lupus anticoagulant and anticardiolipin) occur in individuals with recurrent thrombosis and/or recurrent pregnancy failure in whom the clinical and serologic features of SLE are not present. This gave rise to the concept of the acquired thrombophilia 'primary antiphospholipid syndrome', to distinguish it from 'secondary antiphospholipid syndrome' associated with SLE and occasionally other autoimmune conditions such as rheumatoid arthritis and Sjögren's syndrome. This chronology explains the misleading nomenclature employed: lupus anticoagulant is not restricted to SLE and is associated with a prothrombotic rather than an antithrombotic clinical state.

Recent observations on the true nature of antiphospholipid antibodies have demonstrated clearly that in many domains characterized by CCP repeats. The first four are regular repeats but the fifth is larger. It includes a cluster of positively charged amino acids and is the site responsible for binding to anionic phospholipids. There had been debate over which domains on β_2 glycoprotein I have epitopes for antiphospholipid antibody binding. Also, it has been unclear why only some antibodies are associated with thrombosis. It has been demonstrated that whereas antibodies may be directed against any of the five domains, it is only those which react with a specific epitope on domain I which have lupus anticoagulant activity. Also it is these latter antibodies which associate strongly with thrombotic manifestations.[4]

The reasons why antiphospholipid antibodies develop are becoming clearer. It has long been recognized that they are a frequent feature in chronic inflammatory diseases, especially SLE, and also in some acute and chronic infections, syphilis being the classic example. In these situations it is likely that there is increased exposure of negatively charged phospholipids, for example from apoptotic cells or invading microorganisms.[5] It has recently been demonstrated that β_2 glycoprotein I can be presented successfully to preexisting autoreactive T cell clones only when it is bound to phospholipids, for example the anionic phospholipids present in infection and inflammation.[6] This may be the mechanism underlying the generation of antibodies to β_2 glycoprotein I. Epitopes on domain V, the phospholipid-binding region of the protein, seem to be essential in this process; it is hypothesized that in some cases the phenomenon of epitope spreading leads to the generation of antibody to the specific epitope on domain I, which is pathogenic in antiphospholipid syndrome.[7]

Pathogenesis of thrombosis in antiphospholipid syndrome

Despite the paradoxical effects of antiphospholipid antibodies on coagulation *ex vivo*, blood vessel occlusion in antiphospholipid syndrome is due to thrombus formation and not to vasculitis. Therefore the condition is a true prothrombotic or hypercoagulable state. This observation has led to extensive research into the mechanism of thrombosis in antiphospholipid syndrome, and, in particular, into the direct role of antiphospholipid antibodies in the pathogenesis of thrombosis. No clearly defined, unique mechanism has been identified and it seems highly likely that thrombosis in the syndrome is multifactorial in pathogenesis.

The question whether antiphospholipid antibodies are themselves pathogenic in thrombosis or whether they merely represent a marker for some as yet unidentified process has been addressed in animal models.[8] In rodent thrombosis models it does appear that some purified human antiphospholipid antibodies are prothrombotic. In attempts to determine the mechanism for any prothrombotic property all aspects of the hemostatic process have been examined, including thrombin generation, physiologic anticoagulant

control mechanisms, platelet and endothelial activation, and fibrinolysis. Plausible evidence has been presented from *in vitro* experiments that antiphospholipid antibodies may, for example:

- stimulate tissue factor expression by monocytes
- bind to and activate vascular endothelial cells
- activate platelets via Fc receptors
- inhibit activated protein C and induce a state of acquired protein C resistance
- induce acquired protein S deficiency.

Which, if any of these or other prothrombotic mechanisms are important *in vivo* is not yet known.

Pathogenesis of pregnancy failure in antiphospholipid syndrome

Both mouse monoclonal and human polyclonal antiphospholipid antibodies have been shown to induce fetal death in mice, suggesting a pathogenetic role in pregnancy failure.[9] However the majority of human antiphospholipid antibodies have no such effect[10,11] and there is no clear relation with antibody titer, thus weakening the evidence for direct pathogenicity. By extrapolation from the apparent prothrombotic properties of antiphospholipid antibodies it has been inferred that placental ischemia underlies pregnancy failure in antiphospholipid syndrome. A potential mechanism has been proposed by Rand *et al*.[12,13] They demonstrated that binding of antiphospholipid antibodies to cultures of vascular endothelial cells or trophoblasts appeared to result in displacement of annexin V from the cell surface. It was postulated that this results in a procoagulant effect. However, others have demonstrated normal, or even increased, expression of annexin V in placenta from affected pregnancies in antiphospholipid syndrome.[14,15] Displacement of annexin V has not been found in other experiments.[16–18] The role of this mechanism in fetal loss is still not entirely clear.

Furthermore, although placental infarction has been reported in some cases it is not evident universally and many women have early first trimester losses which cannot easily be explained by placental thrombosis. However, the prothrombotic properties of antiphospholipid antibodies may be relevant even in early losses as there is evidence from gene knockout experiments that growth and survival of trophoblast cells is impaired by local thrombin formation.[19] Alternative nonthrombotic mechanisms have been postulated. For example, antiphospholipid antibodies have been reported to inhibit trophoblast proliferation[20] and human chorionic gonadotrophin production, as well as being capable of inhibition of trophoblast invasion of spiral arteries, in experiments *in vitro*.[21] Intriguingly early fetal loss has been linked to activation of complement, through the classical pathway, by antiphospholipid antibodies.[22]

Clinical features in antiphospholipid syndrome

As indicated in Box 8.1, the cardinal clinical features are thrombosis and/or pregnancy failure. Thrombosis can involve arteries, veins, or less commonly, the microvasculature. Limb deep vein thrombosis is a common manifestation of the syndrome, but thrombosis in intracranial veins, retinal veins, and visceral veins, including hepatic and portal vessels, is well recognized. Ischemic stroke and transient cerebral ischemic episodes are the most common arterial occlusive events. Women of child-bearing age may be affected, even in the absence of other risk factors, although these, such as smoking habit or use of hormonal contraception, are often present. Myocardial infarction occurs also, but is relatively uncommon, as is limb and visceral ischemia. Although arterial thrombus appears to form *in situ* in most cases, embolization from sterile endocardial and cardiac valve vegetations is also recognized in antiphospholipid syndrome. Indeed in some series, where transesophageal echocardiography has been used for screening, an extremely high prevalence of cardiac valve abnormality has been reported.

Microvascular thrombosis is a rare manifestation. In its most dramatic form there is multiorgan involvement with an acute onset. The term catastrophic antiphospholipid syndrome has been adopted to describe this phenomenon, in which renal, pulmonary, central nervous system, cardiac and skin involvement predominate. Catastrophic antiphospholipid syndrome may be the presenting illness or complicates the clinical course of otherwise typical antiphospholipid syndrome.[23]

Some women with thrombosis attributed to antiphospholipid syndrome also have a history of pregnancy failure and complicated pregnancies. However, a more common scenario is recurrent pregnancy failure and presence of antiphospholipid antibodies in a woman with no prior history of systemic thrombosis. Furthermore, in the experience of the author, pregnancy failure remains the only manifestation of the syndrome in the majority of such women: they do not progress to thrombotic complications in later life. Recurrent early losses are most common, but fetal death also occurs. The association between antiphospholipid antibody positivity and premature delivery due to placental insufficiency or severe preeclampsia is also sufficiently commonly encountered to be included in the diagnostic criteria for the syndrome (see Box 8.1).

Although thrombosis and pregnancy failure are the principal clinical features of antiphospholipid syndrome, a range of additional clinical relationships have been observed sufficiently frequently to suggest they are more than chance associations (Box 8.2). Although they are not included in the international criteria for diagnosis of antiphospholipid syndrome, the presence of one or more of these features in the face of antiphospholipid antibodies should certainly raise strong clinical suspicion of the diagnosis of antiphospholipid syndrome.

Thrombocytopenia is commonly present in antiphospholipid syndrome. It is usually moderate in degree,

---

Box 8.2 Conditions associated with antiphospholipid syndrome

Frequent associations
- Thrombocytopenia
- Livedo reticularis

Possible associations
- Transverse myelopathy
- Sensorineural deafness
- Chorea
- Cognitive deficit
- Multifocal central nervous system disease resembling multiple sclerosis
- Pulmonary hypertension
- Skin necrosis and ulceration
- Splinter hemorrhages
- Allograft failure

---

platelet counts of less than $50 \times 10^9/L$ being rare. Typically there is no increased bleeding tendency. To avoid diagnostic confusion it is important to understand that low titers of anticardiolipin antibodies are a feature of some cases of otherwise typical autoimmune thrombocytopenic purpura. In such cases the clinical course and response to therapy is generally no different from that of those without antiphospholipid antibodies. Such individuals do not have antiphospholipid syndrome. Livedo reticularis is due to dermal vessel thrombosis in some cases. It is not confined to antiphospholipid syndrome but when the typical skin lesions are present in an individual with thrombosis a diagnosis of antiphospholipid syndrome should be strongly considered.

The additional associations listed in Box 8.2 may have a thrombotic pathogenesis. Of particular interest is the suggestion that some patients diagnosed with multiple sclerosis have atypical clinical and neuroimaging features, and antiphospholipid antibodies are detectable in serum. It has been reported that some of these individuals respond to antithrombotic therapy.

Diagnosis of antiphospholipid syndrome

Although reaching a diagnosis of antiphospholipid syndrome is straightforward in a case with typical clinical features, such as premature ischemic stroke and high titer anticardiolipin antibodies which persist over time, there are numerous diagnostic pitfalls in clinical practice. These arise because:

- infection-related, often transient, antiphospholipid antibodies are common and not usually associated with a prothrombotic state
- tests for antiphospholipid antibodies may be positive in apparently healthy individuals

- assays for lupus anticoagulant are not completely specific
- assays for anticardiolipin antibody are incompletely standardized.

The agreed criteria for a confident diagnosis of antiphospholipid syndrome include demonstration of persistence of the antiphospholipid antibody over time (Box 8.1). This avoids overdiagnosis in the light of knowledge that some acute infections, often viral, result in transient antibody positivity, more commonly for anticardiolipin antibodies than lupus anticoagulant. Generally these antibodies are not associated with thrombosis, however. Exceptions occur. For example, severe thrombosis with purpura fulminans, antiphospholipid antibodies, and acquired protein S deficiency has been reported in acute viral infection in children.

In addition, persistently positive tests for antiphospholipid antibodies occur in association with some infections. These include syphilis, hepatitis C, infection with human immunodeficiency virus, leprosy, chronic malaria, and infection with *Helicobacter pylori*. Again, there does not appear to be any link to thrombosis. In some cases these antibodies seem to differ in their specificity from those in antiphospholipid syndrome. For example, they are generally not β_2 glycoprotein I dependent. However, there are exceptions, as in leprosy, where anti-β_2 glycoprotein I antibodies are seen. They have also been detected in individuals with syphilis, leptospirosis, and kala-azar.

The occurrence of antiphospholipid antibodies in apparently healthy individuals is another source of diagnostic confusion.[24] In some series up to 5 percent of control samples are positive, usually for anticardiolipin antibody rather than lupus anticoagulant. Asymptomatic positives appear to be most frequent among older people. Typically these are low titer antibodies, and the determination of the upper limit of normal in the assay employed is therefore of great importance if possibly irrelevant positives are to be avoided. This can be problematic as in most populations the range appears to be distributed in a non-Gaussian fashion. According to the internationally agreed diagnostic criteria the titer must be 'moderate' or 'high'. For example a titer of >40 GPL units may be considered moderate and >80 GPL units to be high. However, these are largely arbitrary definitions and despite attempts at standardization different assays are not directly comparable (see below).

Although incidental antiphospholipid antibodies have been considered to be of little clinical significance, this may not be true. For example, in the Physicians' Health Study, when stored serum from subjects who went on to have venous thrombosis was examined there was an excess of positive tests for anticardiolipin in that cohort compared with the remainder who did not develop venous thromboembolism.[25] Indeed, and rather curiously, in some cases the antibody test was no longer positive at the time of the thrombosis. Also, Vaarala et al.[26] found a relation between the highest titers of antiprothrombin antibodies in apparently healthy individuals and subsequent myocardial infarction. It appears from these data that these antiphospholipid antibodies may identify individuals at increased risk of vascular events.

Although the introduction of international standards for anticardiolipin and expression of results in standardized units (GPL for IgG and MPL for IgM antibodies) have improved assay performance, inter-assay comparability remains a problem. Gross discrepancies between eight commercial assay kits were highlighted by Reber et al. in 1995.[27] Disappointingly, the situation has not improved. For example in a recent report, the inter-laboratory coefficient of variation was >50 percent in 74 percent of tests in a quality assurance program. The authors had to conclude that 'in the majority of cases laboratories could not decide on whether a sample was positive or negative'.[28] It had been hoped that use of 'more specific' assays, for anti-β_2 glycoprotein I and antiprothrombin, might improve this situation, but this does not seem to be the case.[29] Some studies indicate that these assays do not seem to be more sensitive for the diagnosis of antiphospholipid syndrome than standard tests for anticardiolipin and lupus anticoagulant.[30] However, others disagree and anti-β_2 glycoprotein I is now included as a diagnostic criterion for clinical studies of antiphospholipid syndrome.[2]

Sadly, lupus anticoagulant assays do not perform very much better than immunoassays for anticardiolipin. It is important to note that these coagulation assays are not specific for antiphospholipid antibodies and are influenced by other factors. These include the presence of anticoagulant drugs or other inhibitors and raised or lowered levels of clotting factors. Guidelines for the standardization of diagnostic tests for lupus anticoagulant have been disseminated, for example those proposed by the British Committee for Standards in Haematology.[31] These deal with important issues of sample handling prior to testing, and methods to improve specificity. It is generally agreed that use of more than one type of coagulation assay is essential, as is the inclusion of a test to confirm phospholipid dependence of the antibody. The activated partial thromboplastin time and dilute Russell viper venom time with a phospholipid neutralization procedure are perhaps the most widely used assays. Although there is evidence that adoption of the United Kingdom guidelines drawn up by the British Committee for Standards in Haematology has improved diagnostic accuracy, over 10 percent of positive samples may be misclassified as negative for lupus anticoagulant.[32]

In summary there are significant diagnostic pitfalls and it is essential to consider the entire clinical history and have understanding of the limitations of the laboratory assays in order to minimize diagnostic error. Even when this approach is adopted there are extensive gray areas. For example:

- An asymptomatic subject with high titer anticardiolipin clearly does not fulfill the diagnostic criteria for the syndrome but may have a substantial risk of thrombosis.
- Neither a woman with two early miscarriages and moderate titer anticardiolipin nor one with three early

miscarriages who is positive for low titer anticardiolipin but negative for lupus anticoagulant fulfills the diagnostic criteria for antiphospholipid syndrome, but there should be substantial clinical suspicion about the diagnosis.

- An elderly smoker with longstanding hypertension, hypercholesterolemia, and obesity who has had myocardial infarction and is found to have moderate titer anticardiolipin fulfills the diagnostic criteria, but the relation of the antiphospholipid syndrome to the acute vascular event in the face of other major risk factors is far from clear.

Management of thrombosis in antiphospholipid syndrome

As already indicated, antiphospholipid syndrome is a pro-thrombotic rather than an inflammatory condition. It follows that antithrombotic therapy and attention to avoidable additional thrombosis risk factors are the mainstays of management.

The treatment of acute thrombosis is generally no different from that of thrombosis due to other causes. Depending on the clinical site, heparin, warfarin, or thrombolytics are given. However lupus anticoagulant may result in prolongation of the aPTT, rendering this test less appropriate for judgment of dose of unfractionated heparin. This can be overcome by employing standard, weight-adjusted doses of a low-molecular-weight heparin. Dose monitoring is not usually necessary when low-molecular-weight heparins are employed, but if it is, anti-Xa assay is appropriate. Rarely, the prothrombin time is prolonged in the presence of lupus anticoagulant, complicating warfarin dose monitoring using the international normalized ratio (INR). Usually this potential problem is circumvented by choosing a pro-thrombin time reagent with a low international sensitivity index. Such reagents are rarely sensitive to the lupus anti-coagulant effect and are ideal for warfarin monitoring.

Two important considerations arise in relation to antithrombotic management after the acute phase: first, whether the duration of therapy with warfarin should be any different from that employed in comparable cases without antiphospholipid antibody; and second, whether the intensity of warfarin therapy should be modified. In relation to the latter, retrospective observational studies suggested the need for an INR target of 3 to 4 in order to achieve optimal prevention of thrombosis recurrence, rather than the target of 2 to 3 which is most usually employed in both arterial and venous thrombosis. Indeed, high intensity warfarin anticoagulation combined with aspirin has been recommended.[33] However, both a higher target INR and combined therapy are associated with increased bleeding risk. This is an important consideration as the risk of life-threatening bleeding on standard intensity warfarin therapy is >1 percent per annum. Fortunately, two randomized clinical trials of target INR 3.5 versus 2.5 in patients with antiphospholipid syndrome

have indicated the lower-intensity treatment to be equivalent in relation to prevention of thrombosis recurrence.[34,35] It can reasonably be concluded that the target INR during warfarin therapy in antiphospholipid syndrome should be 2.5 in most cases, with an increase to 3.5 should there be a second thrombosis while in the lower target range. It should be noted, however, that these randomized trials included a preponderance of patients with venous thromboembolism. The evidence regarding the appropriate target INR in arterial thrombosis is less secure.

In relation to duration of anticoagulant therapy in antiphospholipid syndrome the concern is that large case series suggest a high rate of thrombosis recurrence if warfarin is discontinued. Hence, although warfarin is often discontinued after 3–6 months following a first episode of venous thromboembolism when antiphospholipid antibodies are not present, many clinicians recommend long-term treatment in antiphospholipid syndrome. Each case should be considered on an individual basis, however, taking account of risk factors for bleeding on warfarin (for example, old age, unstable gait), the severity and nature of the thrombotic event (for example, calf deep vein thrombosis vs. ischemic stroke) and whether there are any other risk factors present that can be addressed to reduce the risk of further thrombosis recurrence (for example, use of hormone replacement therapy or the combined oral contraceptive, smoking habit).

Whether aspirin alone has significant antithrombotic efficacy in antiphospholipid syndrome is not completely clear. However, observational data suggest a high rate of recurrent thrombosis when aspirin is used as sole therapy. Numerous other treatments have been employed in antiphospholipid syndrome (Box 8.3) but largely on pragmatic grounds. Evidence of efficacy is entirely anecdotal.

Recent observations indicate possible benefit from hydroxychloroquine.[36] Plasmapheresis to deplete antiphospholipid antibody and immunosuppressive therapies

---

Box 8.3 Treatments used in antiphospholipid syndrome

First line
- Anticoagulants
- Attention to additional risk factors

Other
- Aspirin
- Hydroxychloroquine
- Defibrotide
- Plasmapheresis
- Immunomodulatory
  - Intravenous human IgG
  - Corticosteroids
  - Rituximab
  - Cyclophosphamide
  - Azathioprine

should only be used in exceptional cases. Examples might be catastrophic antiphospholipid syndrome, where empirical therapy is justified in a life-threatening scenario. In the unusual situation of severe thrombocytopenia in antiphospholipid syndrome, corticosteroid or other immunosuppressive therapy may be indicated. Also, in exceptional cases antiprothrombin appears to be a neutralizing antibody which causes significant coagulopathy with prolongation of the prothrombin time. Plasmapheresis and immunomodulatory therapies have been used to manage hemorrhage in that situation.

Management of pregnancy in antiphospholipid syndrome

A significant proportion of women with recurrent (three or more consecutive) first trimester losses or an episode of fetal death in the second or third trimester are found to have persistent antiphospholipid antibodies. Bearing in mind the comments above on the poor performance of immunoassays and coagulation assays it is unsurprising that there is wide variation in this proportion between miscarriage clinics. Many of these women have low-titer anticardiolipin antibodies only, and do not fulfill the internationally agreed diagnostic criteria for the syndrome. However, in women with a clinical history of multiple pregnancy failures with no other cause identified, there is great pressure to offer treatment.

In the minority of cases in which there is fetal death with evidence of placental infarction, the use of antithrombotic therapy in any subsequent pregnancy is logical. In addition, as indicated above there are theoretical reasons for believing that a prothrombotic state might contribute to early losses. Weight is added to this argument from the results of epidemiologic studies which suggest that women with heritable thrombophilias may have an increased risk of failed pregnancies, including early losses. It is unsurprising, therefore, that treatment with heparin and aspirin is often offered to women with the appropriate obstetric history and persistent antiphospholipid antibodies. However,

the evidence base for the efficacy of this approach is controversial. Two studies comparing aspirin and heparin with aspirin alone suggested major benefit for the combined treatment and led to its adoption but a more recent study has cast doubt on these conclusions (Table 8.1). Of the three studies, Kutteh's[37] did not employ formal randomization, with the consequent potential for bias, and is not generalizable as the entry criteria included anticardiolipin positivity only. Women with lupus anticoagulant were excluded. Rai et al.[38] and Farquharson et al.[39] used largely comparable entry criteria. Rai et al. demonstrated a statistically significant advantage for the combined therapy whereas Farquharson et al. did not. In the former study prophylactic doses of unfractionated heparin were used and in the latter comparable doses of low-molecular-weight heparin. Whether the heparin formulation explains the discrepant results is not known.

Further doubt has been cast on the efficacy of antithrombotic treatment in this group of women by the results of a double-blind, randomized trial of low-dose aspirin versus supportive management only.[40] Forty women were randomized and the pregnancy failure rates were low in both groups (20 percent and 15 percent, respectively). Furthermore these proportions are comparable with those in both arms of Farquharson et al.'s study and the aspirin and heparin arms of Kutteh and Rai et al.'s studies. Large, randomized, placebo-controlled trials will be needed to resolve this question. However, the emotional issues surrounding this area make the conduct of such trials unusually difficult.

Other treatments have been given in an attempt to improve pregnancy outcome in antiphospholipid syndrome. In three randomized trials high-dose prednisolone was demonstrated to be no more effective than aspirin, heparin, or placebo.[41–43] Furthermore, use of prednisolone results in unacceptable maternal morbidity from hypertension, weight gain, and premature delivery.[43] Intravenous high-dose human IgG has also been employed. There are insufficient data to judge whether it is effective.

What approach to management should be adopted, based on current evidence? In women with repeated early

Table 8.1 Trials of aspirin alone vs. aspirin with heparin in antiphospholipid syndrome pregnancy failure

Study	Randomization (n)	Laboratory criteria	Treatment	Pregnancy failures (%)
Kutteh, 1996[37]	No (50)	Anticardiolipin only	Aspirin	56
			vs.	
			Aspirin + UFH	20
Rai et al., 1997[38]	Yes (90)	Anticardiolipin/ lupus anticoagulant	Aspirin	58
			vs.	
			Aspirin + UFH	29
Farquharson et al., 2002[39]	Yes (98)	Anticardiolipin/ lupus anticoagulant	Aspirin	28
			vs.	
			Aspirin + LMWH	22

LMWH, low-molecular-weight heparin; UFH, unfractionated heparin.

losses, clearly the usual nonpharmacologic methods for support through subsequent pregnancies should be adopted. The lack of definitive proof of efficacy of antithrombotics should be discussed. It is reasonable to offer supportive treatment only, or addition of low-dose aspirin on the grounds that it appears to be safe and is tolerated well. Although the main side effects of heparin (osteopenia and thrombocytopenia) are relatively uncommon, it is an inconvenient intervention because of the need for subcutaneous injection at least once daily. Heparin could be reasonably reserved for those women in whom there is failure with aspirin alone. However, many women will opt for the combined treatment, after counseling, despite the lack of firm proof of efficacy. The smaller number of women with a history of fetal death and evidence of placental infarction, or of early severe preeclampsia, will usually be offered combined low-dose aspirin and heparin in subsequent pregnancies, on pragmatic grounds. There is no place for treatment with corticosteroids in pregnancy failure due to antiphospholipid syndrome.

Finally, the question of risk of maternal thrombosis arises. As indicated above, the majority of women with antiphospholipid antibodies and pregnancy failure have no prior history of systemic thromboembolism. In the two randomized trials of aspirin with heparin the treatment was generally discontinued at or before full term. Therefore, there is no clear indication for pharmacologic thromboprophylaxis in the postpartum phase in a woman with no personal history of thrombosis and uncomplicated delivery.

MYELOPROLIFERATIVE DISEASE

The myeloproliferative diseases are generally clonal proliferations of the cells of the erythroid, myeloid, or megakaryocytic series. Although they are mainly disorders of middle and old age, women of childbearing age may be afflicted, with consequences in relation to pregnancy outcome as well as increased risk of systemic thrombosis. This is especially true of the myeloproliferative disease essential thrombocythemia.

Definitions

The principal features of the myeloproliferative diseases are described in Table 8.2. Progression to acute leukemia is a feature of all myeloproliferative diseases. Essential thrombocythemia and polycythemia rubra vera may progress to myelofibrosis after several years. Myelofibrosis is rare in women of childbearing age and is infrequently associated with vascular complications. Chronic myeloid leukemia occurs in all age groups. Again, thrombosis is uncommon. It is characterized by the presence in the malignant clone in most cases of a reciprocal translocation between chromosomes 9 and 22, the 'Philadelphia chromosome'. Progression to a terminal acute leukemia is typical. Polycythemia rubra vera has only rarely been reported in women of childbearing age,[44] and it is difficult to reach conclusions about its influence on pregnancy and optimal management. It is an important cause of vascular occlusion in older individuals. The diagnosis and management of this myeloproliferative disorder are not considered further here.

An acquired mutation in the gene for the tyrosine kinase (*JAK2*) has been identified recently in a high proportion of cases of myeloproliferative disease, including most cases of polycythemia rubra vera and around 50 percent of cases of essential thrombocythemia.[45] The resulting dysregulation of the kinase is likely to have a key role in pathogenesis, through increased sensitivity of hemopoietic precursors to growth factors resulting in unrestrained proliferation.

Essential thrombocythemia

Although classically associated with both thrombosis and hemorrhage many, if not most, cases present at a preclinical stage through the incidental finding of a thrombocytosis (platelets $>400 \times 10^9$/L and usually $>600 \times 10^9$/L) on a blood count carried out for an unrelated reason. This includes blood counts performed as a routine in the antenatal clinic. There may also be a neutrophilia but the

Table 8.2 Types of myeloproliferative disease

	Marrow cell types involved	Hematologic features	Principal clinical associations
Essential thrombocythemia	Megakaryocytes ± granulocyte series	Persistent and progressive thrombocytosis ± neutrophilia	Arterial, venous, and microvascular thrombosis
Polycythemia rubra vera	Erythroid series ± granulocyte series and megakaryocytes	Erythrocytosis ± neutrophilia and thrombocytosis	Hyperviscosity Arterial, venous, and microvascular thrombosis
Myelofibrosis	Megakaryocytes ± granulocyte series Reactive marrow fibroblast response	Anemia, often with thrombocytopenia	Symptoms of marrow failure and massive splenomegaly
Chronic myeloid leukaemia	Granulocyte series ± megakaryocytes	Neutrophilia with left shift ± thrombocytosis or thrombocytopenia	Symptoms of anemia and often massive splenomegaly

hemoglobin concentration and erythrocyte morphology are generally normal. The presence of erythrocytosis suggests polycythemia rubra vera rather than essential thrombocythemia. In the latter examination of the blood film may reveal an excess of unusually large platelets. At present there is no easily reproducible diagnostic test and the diagnosis of essential thrombocythemia is made by exclusion of causes of a reactive thrombocytosis and of other forms of myeloproliferative disease (Boxes 8.4 and 8.5).

SYMPTOMS AND SIGNS IN ESSENTIAL THROMBOCYTHEMIA

In symptomatic cases the predominant feature is vaso-occlusion. Microvascular occlusion is a common clinical presentation. This most frequently results in erythromelalgia: painful, dusky discoloration of digits. Peripheral pulses are typically normal. This symptom is often highly responsive to treatment with low-dose aspirin, indicating the importance of abnormal platelet interactions in its pathogenesis. Progression to digital gangrene may occur. There is an increased risk of ischemic stroke, transient cerebral ischemic episodes and myocardial infarction, especially when other risk factors for arterial disease are present, such as smoking. Ischemia affecting other organs, including the spleen and bowel, may be the presenting feature or may complicate the course of the disease. In the venous circulation limb deep vein thrombosis occurs, and also intracranial and visceral venous thrombosis, including mesenteric, portal, and hepatic venous thrombosis. Thrombosis may occur in essential thrombocythemia when the platelet count is only modestly raised, and there is no clear link with the degree of thrombocytosis. Paradoxically, in a small proportion of cases the principal clinical feature is bleeding rather than thrombosis. Skin bruising, mucosal bleeding, and excessive bleeding after surgical and other trauma are typical. There appears to be a relation between hemorrhagic manifestations and unusually high platelet counts ($>1500 \times 10^9$/L in essential thrombocythemia.

From personal experience it appears that most cases of essential thrombocythemia in nonpregnant women of childbearing age are asymptomatic, although exceptions certainly occur. However, the few significant case series reported suggest that the rate of pregnancy failure, especially first trimester abortion, is increased. Placental infarction has been reported, as well as fetal death and preeclampsia. Thirteen first trimester spontaneous abortions were noted in 40 pregnancies in one series.[46] At the Mayo clinic an incidence of miscarriage of 49 percent in 43 pregnancies in 20 women was reported by Wright and Tefferi.[47] Neither the pre-pregnancy platelet count nor presence or absence of prior symptoms appears to predict pregnancy outcome. Rarely, maternal hemorrhage has been attributed to essential thrombocythemia.

PATHOGENESIS OF BLEEDING AND THROMBOSIS IN ESSENTIAL THROMBOCYTHEMIA

Numerous studies of *ex vivo* platelet reactivity have been performed in individuals with essential thrombocythemia. Abnormally increased or decreased aggregation responses to agonists have been identified and spontaneous platelet aggregation *ex vivo* noted in some cases. A range of abnormalities in platelet surface receptors and mechanisms of cellular stimulus–response coupling have been reported, with no clear relation with the clinical thrombotic tendency in individual subjects. In some cases in which there is a bleeding tendency this appears to be secondary to an acquired von Willebrand disease. Plasma concentrations of von Willebrand factor and factor VIII are reduced.

Diagnosis

From the above it is apparent that the mainstay of diagnosis is the clinical history and physical examination, along with examination of the blood count and film, to determine supporting features for the diagnosis of essential thrombocythemia and to exclude other myeloproliferative disease and causes of reactive thrombocytosis. Supportive clinical findings are symptoms of erythromelalgia, generalized pruritus (which is exacerbated by bathing), and a degree of splenomegaly. Splenomegaly is detectable clinically in a minority of cases at presentation. In some cases

---

Box 8.4 Diagnostic criteria for essential thrombocythemia

- Platelets $>600 \times 10^9$/L*
- No cause for a reactive thrombocytosis
- No erythrocytosis/increased red cell mass
- No Philadelphia chromosome
- No overriding features to suggest myelofibrosis

*Because of the inexact upper limit of normal for platelet count, a cut-off of 600×10^9/L is generally used. However, this is arbitrary and the disorder presents with vessel occlusion before this level of thrombocytosis develops in some cases. Counts as high as 3000×10^9/L are seen on occasions.

Box 8.5 Causes of reactive thrombocytosis

- Acute hemorrhage
- Chronic iron deficiency
- Acute or chronic inflammatory disease
- Neoplasia
- Postoperative state and other tissue trauma
- Hyposplenism
- Transiently, after treatment of megaloblastic anemia or on recovery from marrow suppression

there is silent splenic infarction leading to features of hyposplenism on the blood film. This can lead to diagnostic uncertainty as a mild thrombocytosis is a feature of hyposplenism from other causes also. A history of thrombosis, especially in an unusual site, in an individual without additional risk factors or occurring at a young age (<45 years) favors a diagnosis of essential thrombocythemia, as reactive thrombocytosis does not appear to be associated with the same level of thrombotic risk. Assay of serum ferritin and of C-reactive protein may provide some useful information but examination of bone marrow is not generally helpful. Although the finding of clustering and abnormal location of megakaryocytes, sometimes with increased marrow reticulin in a bone marrow biopsy, is supportive of a diagnosis of essential thrombocythemia these morphologic features are often subtle or absent. Other tests such as bone marrow cell culture and clonal analysis are not readily available and are insufficiently sensitive and specific. In essence, the diagnosis is reached by exclusion. Indeed, in some asymptomatic cases with modest thrombocytosis it is prudent to refrain from making a firm diagnosis pending a period of observation to determine whether there is progression of the platelet count increase, or manifestation of a previously occult cause for reactive thrombocytosis. Identification of the role of the *JAK2* mutation is likely to improve diagnostic accuracy in essential thrombocythemia. It is not yet clear whether cases with the mutation behave differently from those without in relation to clinical manifestations, although suggestive data are beginning to emerge.[48]

Management

The platelet count may be rendered normal through the use of cytoreductive therapy, most commonly hydroxyurea. Historically, the alkylating agent busulfan or radioactive phosphorus (^{32}P) were employed but they are rarely given now, apart perhaps from elderly patients with short life expectancy, as their use is associated with a further enhancement of the risk of leukemic transformation. Hydroxyurea appears to be a safer option in this regard. The incidence of leukemic transformation with hydroxyurea is low and may be no higher than the background incidence in essential thrombocythemia.[49] In a study of high-risk patients there was an approximately sixfold reduction in thrombotic events with hydroxyurea.[50] Continuous daily dosing is required to maintain the target platelet count ($<400 \times 10^9$/L). Although usually well tolerated, a significant proportion of individuals receiving hydroxyurea develop a systemic illness with musculoskeletal pains, weight loss and raised erythrocyte sedimentation rate, necessitating discontinuation. Skin ulceration and gastrointestinal upset also occur occasionally.

Alternative therapies have been explored, including interferon α and anagrelide. The latter commonly causes fluid retention and concerns have been expressed regarding an increase in marrow fibrosis associated with its use. In the largest randomized trial to date anagrelide was associated with an excess of myelofibrosis, major hemorrhage, and arterial thrombosis as compared with hydroxyurea.[49] Headache is common on introduction of anagrelide therapy but resolves in 2–3 weeks. A significant proportion of patients cannot tolerate the drug in the long term and in a small proportion the thrombocytosis is resistant to the medication. Interferon α requires weekly injection and up to 50 percent of patients cannot tolerate the systemic side effects. Low-dose aspirin is often administered as an antithrombotic in essential thrombocythemia, if hemorrhagic symptoms are not present. Anecdotally it is effective for erythromelalgic symptoms and its use is justified on pragmatic grounds. However there are no randomized prospective data on the risk–benefit ratio of aspirin in essential thrombocythemia.

A difficult issue in the management of essential thrombocythemia is the appropriate timing of the introduction of chemotherapy. This is because survival is potentially long, with the risk of protracted exposure to cytoreductive agents. The degree of thrombocytosis gives little indication of thrombosis risk. Age and the presence of additional risk factors give some clue to the need for treatment. For example, the risk of vascular occlusion in asymptomatic individuals with essential thrombocythemia who are aged 60 years and greater is over 10 percent per annum. In those under 40 years it is 1–2 percent per annum and in those 40–60 years around 5 percent per annum. When there is presentation with vaso-occlusion or bleeding there is a clear need to control the elevated platelet count. It is prudent to do so also in older patients with symptoms of arterial disease, such as angina pectoris or claudication, and in asymptomatic subjects with additional risk factors, such as diabetes mellitus or hypertension.

MANAGEMENT OF ESSENTIAL THROMBOCYTHEMIA IN PREGNANCY

Because pregnant women with essential thrombocythemia have an apparent increased risk of first trimester loss and the potential additional thrombotic risk from the physiologic coagulation changes in pregnancy, a range of therapeutic approaches have been recommended (reviewed by Vantroyen and Vanstraelen[51]). However, these are based on case reports and small case series only and there has been no randomized controlled trial to guide therapy. Aspirin is generally administered as it is regarded as safe and potentially efficacious in reducing the risk of placental and maternal thrombosis. A dose of 150 mg daily is appropriate. Whether treatment should be given to reduce the platelet count is unclear. In many women this is unnecessary as uncomplicated pregnancy in the absence of intervention is certainly possible in essential thrombocythemia. Also, temporary spontaneous remission of the thrombocytosis during pregnancy occurs in some cases. In a primigravida or multigravida with no previous pregnancy failure, use of aspirin thromboprophylaxis alone seems to be a reasonable approach. When there has been recurrent pregnancy loss despite aspirin administration it is difficult to resist additional treatment. Combination antithrombotic therapy with aspirin and low dose heparin has been used. Whether there is benefit from rendering the blood platelet count normal is not known. Hydroxyurea has been administered in pregnancy, but many clinicians prefer to avoid cytotoxic therapy. There are reports of successful pregnancy outcomes in essential thrombocythemia treated with interferon α,[52] and this approach could be considered on pragmatic grounds in women with recurrent pregnancy failure. If treatment is given during pregnancy, it is prudent to continue therapy for at least 6 weeks after delivery in the hope that this might reduce the risk of maternal postpartum venous thromboembolism.

PLASMA COAGULATION FACTOR CONCENTRATIONS AND RISK OF THROMBOSIS

There is emerging evidence for a link between thrombosis and high plasma concentrations of factors VIII, IX, and XI, and fibrinogen. Environmental factors contribute to plasma concentrations of clotting factors in individual subjects. The strong link between inflammation and fibrinogen concentration is an obvious example and fibrinogen concentration is an independent risk factor for arterial and venous thrombosis in both sexes. There is particular relevance of this relation between thrombosis and coagulation factor concentration to women's health. The rise in concentrations of factor VIII and fibrinogen through normal pregnancy is well recognized. Also, in a study of induced thrombosis in a rodent model the factor VIII level in pregnancy correlated with thrombus formation in veins.[53] In humans the high factor VIII concentration contributes to the acquired relative resistance to protein C which is a feature of normal pregnancy.[54] Furthermore, women with the highest concentrations of factor VIII in pregnancy have an increased chance of venous thrombosis of around fourfold.[55] Finally, the acquired protein C resistance detected in some postmenopausal women is determined by increased plasma factor VIII concentration.[56] Although these observations cannot easily be used to stratify risk as a tool to guide targeted thromboprophylaxis, they provide insight into the pathogenesis of thrombosis at various stages of adult life and in association with other disease states.

KEY LEARNING POINTS

- Antiphospholipid syndrome is an important cause of pregnancy failure.
- The pathogenesis of pregnancy failure in antiphospholipid syndrome has not been fully defined.

- Although aspirin and heparin are commonly administered to women with antiphospholipid syndrome and pregnancy failure the efficacy of this treatment is disputed. Large randomized clinical trials are required.
- Pregnancy failure has been associated with essential thrombocythemia.
- Treatments given to women with essential thrombocythemia and pregnancy failure include aspirin and interferon α but there is no randomized trial to guide therapy.

REFERENCES

- 1 Wilson WA, Gharavi AE, Koike T, et al. International consensus statement on preliminary classification criteria for definite antiphospholipid syndrome: Report of an international workshop. Arthritis Rheum 1999; **42**: 1309–11.
- 2 Miyakis S, Lockshin MD, Atsumi T, et al. International consensus statement on an update of the classification criteria for definite antiphospholipid syndrome (APS). J Thromb Haemost 2005; **3**: 1–12.
- 3 Simmelink MJ, Horbach DA, Derksen RH, et al. Complexes of anti-prothrombin antibodies and prothrombin cause lupus anticoagulant activity by competing with the binding of clotting factors for catalytic phospholipid surfaces. Br J Haematol 2001; **113**: 621–9.
- 4 de Laat HB, Derksen RH, Urbanus RT, et al. β2-glycoprotein I-dependent lupus anticoagulant highly correlates with thrombosis in the antiphospholipid syndrome. Blood 2004; **104**: 3598–602.
- 5 Bengtsson AA, Sturfelt G, Gullstrand B, Truedsson L. Induction of apoptosis in monocytes and lymphocytes by serum from patients with systemic lupus erythematosus – an additional mechanism to increased autoantigen load? Clin Exp Immunol 2004; **135**: 535–43.
- 6 Kuwana M, Matsuura E, Kobayashi K, et al. Binding of beta 2-glycoprotein I to anionic phospholipids facilitates processing and presentation of a cryptic epitope that activates pathogenic autoreactive T cells. Blood 2005; **105**: 1552–7.
- 7 Vickers MA, Greaves M. The cryptic path from epitope to clot: A story of two domains. Blood 2005; **105**: 1371–2.
- 8 Blank M, Cohen J, Toder V, Shoenfeld Y. Induction of antiphospholipid syndrome in naive mice with mouse lupus monoclonal and human polyclonal anti-cardiolipin antibodies. Proc Natl Acad Sci U S A 1991; **88**: 3069–73.
- 9 Branch DW, Dudley DJ, Mitchell MD, et al. Immunoglobulin G fractions from patients with antiphospholipid antibodies cause fetal death in BALB/c mice: A model for autoimmune fetal loss. Am J Obstet Gynecol 1990; **163**: 210–16.
- 10 Silver RM, Pierangeli SS, Edwin SS, et al. Variable effects on murine pregnancy of immunoglobulin G fractions from

women with antiphospholipid antibodies. *Am J Obstet Gynecol* 1997; **176**: 628–33.

11 Chamley LW, Pattison NS, McKay EJ. The effect of human anticardiolipin antibodies on murine pregnancy. *J Rep Immunol* 1994; **27**: 123–34.

12 Rand JH, Wu XX, Andree HA, *et al.* Pregnancy loss in the antiphospholipid-antibody syndrome – a possible thrombogenic mechanism. *N Engl J Med* 1997; **337**: 154–60.

13 Rand JH, Wu XX, Andree HA, *et al.* Antiphospholipid antibodies accelerate plasma coagulation by inhibiting annexin-V binding to phospholipids: A 'lupus procoagulant' phenomenon. *Blood* 1998; **92**: 1652–60.

14 Lakasing L, Campa JS, Poston R, *et al.* Normal expression of tissue factor, thrombomodulin, and annexin V in placentas from women with antiphospholipid syndrome. *Am J Obstet Gynecol* 1999; **181**: 180–9.

15 Donohoe S, Kingdom JC, Mackie IJ, *et al.* Ontogeny of beta2 glycoprotein I and annexin V in villous placenta of normal and antiphospholipid syndrome pregnancies. *Thromb Haemost* 2000; **84**: 32–8.

16 Bevers EM, Janssen MP, Willems GM, Zwaal RF. No evidence for enhanced thrombin formation through displacement of annexin V by antiphospholipid antibodies. *Thromb Haemost* 2000; **83**: 792–4.

17 Willems GM, Janssen MP, Comfurius P, *et al.* Competition of annexin V and anticardiolipin antibodies for binding to phosphatidylserine containing membranes. *Biochemistry* 2000; **39**: 1982–9.

18 Patterson AM, Ford I, Graham A, *et al.* The influence of antiendothelial/antiphospholipid antibodies on fibrin formation and lysis on endothelial cells. *Br J Haematol* 2006; **133**: 323–30.

19 Isermann B, Sood R, Pawlinski R, *et al.* The thrombomodulin-protein C system is essential for the maintenance of pregnancy. *Nat Med* 2003; **9**: 331–7.

20 Chamley LW, Duncalf AM, Mitchell MD, Johnson PM. Action of anticardiolipin and antibodies to beta2-glycoprotein-I on trophoblast proliferation as a mechanism for fetal death. *Lancet* 1998; **352**: 1037–8.

21 Di Simone M, Meroni PL, del Papa N, *et al.* Antiphospholipid antibodies affect trophoblast gonadotrophin secretion and invasiveness by binding directly and through adhered beta2 glycoprotein I. *Arthritis Rheum* 2000; **43**: 140–50.

22 Girardi G, Redecha P, Salmon JE. Heparin prevents antiphospholipid antibody-induced fetal loss by inhibiting complement activation. *Nat Med* 2004; **10**: 1222–6.

23 Asherson RA, Cervera R, Piette JC, *et al.* Catastrophic antiphospholipid syndrome. Clinical and laboratory features of 50 patients. *Medicine* 1998; **77**: 195–20.

24 Petri M. Epidemiology of the antiphospholipid antibody syndrome. *J Autoimmun* 2000; **15**: 145–51.

25 Ginsburg KS, Liang MH, Newcomer L, *et al.* Anticardiolipin antibodies and the risk for ischemic stroke and venous thrombosis. *Ann Intern Med* 1992; **117**: 997–1002.

26 Vaarala O, Manttari M, Manninen V, *et al.* Anti-cardiolipin antibodies and risk of myocardial infarction in a prospective cohort of middle-aged men. *Circulation* 1995; **91**: 23–7.

27 Reber G, Arvieux J, Comby E, *et al.* Multicenter evaluation of nine commercial kits for the quantitation of anticardiolipin antibodies. The working group on methodologies in haemostasis from the GEHT (Groupe d'Etudes sur l'Hemostase et la Thrombose). *Thromb Haemost* 1995; **73**: 444–52.

28 Favaloro EJ, Silvestrini R. Assessing the usefulness of anticardiolipin antibody assays: A cautious approach is suggested by high variation and limited consensus in multilaboratory testing. *Am J Clin Pathol* 2002; **118**: 548–57.

29 Reber G, Schousboe I, Tincani A, *et al.* Inter-laboratory variability of anti-beta2-glycoprotein I measurement. A collaborative study in the frame of the European forum on antiphospholipid antibodies standardization group. *Thromb Haemost* 2002; **88**: 66–73.

30 Previtali S, Barbui T, Galli M. Anti-beta2 glycoprotein I and anti-prothrombin antibodies in antiphospholipid-negative patients with thrombosis. *Thromb Haemost* 2002; **88**: 729–32.

★ 31 Greaves M, Cohen H, MacHin SJ, Mackie I. Guidelines on the investigation and management of the antiphospholipid syndrome. *Br J Haematol* 2000; **109**: 704–15.

32 Jennings I, Greaves M, Mackie IJ, *et al.* Lupus anti-coagulant testing: Improvements in performance in a UK NEQAS proficiency testing exercise after dissemination of national guidelines on laboratory methods. *Br J Haematol* 2002; **119**: 364–9.

33 Khamashta MA, Cuadrado MJ, Mujic F, *et al.* The management of thrombosis in the antiphospholipid-antibody syndrome. *N Engl J Med* 1995; **332**: 993–7.

34 Crowther MA, Ginsberg JS, Julian J, *et al.* A comparison of two intensities of warfarin for the prevention of recurrent thrombosis in patients with the antiphospholipid antibody syndrome. *N Engl J Med* 2003; **349**: 1133–8.

35 Finazzi G, Marchioli R, Brancaccio V, *et al.* A randomized clinical trial of high-intensity warfarin vs. conventional antithrombotic therapy for the prevention of recurrent thrombosis in patients with the antiphospholipid syndrome (WAPS). *J Thromb Haemost* 2005; 3: 848–53.

36 Yoon KH. Sufficient evidence to consider hydroxychloroquine as an adjunct therapy in antiphospholipid antibody (Hughes') syndrome. *J Rheumatol* 2002; **29**: 1574–5.

37 Kutteh WH. Antiphospholipid antibody-associated recurrent pregnancy loss: treatment with heparin and low dose aspirin is superior to low dose aspirin alone. *Am J Obstet Gynecol* 1996; **174**: 1584–9.

38 Rai R, Cohen H, Dave M, Regan L. Randomised controlled trial of aspirin and aspirin plus heparin in pregnant women with recurrent miscarriage associated with phospholipid antibodies (or antiphospholipid antibodies). *BMJ* 1997; **314**: 253–7.

39   Farquharson RG, Quenby S, Greaves M. Antiphospholipid syndrome in pregnancy: A randomized, controlled trial of treatment. *Obstet Gynecol* 2002; **100**: 408–13.

40   Pattison NS, Chamley LW, Birdsall M, *et al.* Does aspirin have a role in improving pregnancy outcome for women with the antiphospholipid syndrome? A randomized controlled trial. *Am J Obstet Gynecol* 2000; **183**: 1008–12.

41   Cowchock FS, Reece EA, Balaban D, *et al.* Repeated fetal losses associated with antiphospholipid antibodies: A collaborative randomized trial comparing prednisone with low-dose heparin treatment. *Am J Obstet Gynecol* 1992; **166**: 1318–23.

42   Silver RK, MacGregor SN, Sholl JS, *et al.* Comparative trial of prednisone plus aspirin versus aspirin alone in the treatment of anticardiolipin antibody-positive obstetric patients. *Am J Obstet Gynecol* 1993; **169**: 1411–17.

43   Laskin CA, Bombardier C, Hannah ME, *et al.* Prednisone and aspirin in women with autoantibodies and unexplained recurrent fetal loss. *N Engl J Med* 1997; **337**: 148–53.

44   Subtil D, Deruelle P, Trillot N, Jude B. Preclinical phase of polycythaemia vera in pregnancy. *Obstet Gynecol* 2001; **98**: 945–7.

45   Baxter EJ, Scott LM, Campbell PJ, *et al.* Acquired mutation of the tyrosine kinase JAK2 in human myeloproliferative disorders. *Lancet* 2005; **365**: 1054–61.

46   Niittyvuopio R, Juvonen E, Kaaja R, *et al.* Pregnancy in essential thrombocythaemia: experience with 40 pregnancies. *Eur J Haematol* 2004; **73**: 431–6.

47   Wright CA, Tefferi A. A single institutional experience with 43 pregnancies in essential thrombocythemia. *Eur J Haematol* 2001; **66**: 152–9.

48   Campbell PJ, Scott LM, Buck G, *et al.* Definition of subtypes of essential thrombocythaemia and relation to polycythaemia vera based on JAK2 V617F mutation status: a prospective study. *Lancet* 2005; **366**: 1945–53.

49   Harrison CN. Essential thrombocythaemia: challenges and evidence-based management. *Br J Haematol* 2005; **130**: 153–65.

50   Cortelazzo S, Finazzi G, Ruggeri M, *et al.* Hydroxyurea for patients with essential thrombocythaemia and a high risk of thrombosis. *N Engl J Med* 1995; **332**: 1132–6.

51   Vantroyen B, Vanstraelen D. Management of essential thrombocythaemia during pregnancy with aspirin, interferon alpha-2a. *Acta Haematol* 2002; **107**: 158–69.

52   Delage R, Demers C, Cantin G, Roy J. Treatment of essential thrombocythaemia during pregnancy with interferon-alpha. *Obstet Gynecol* 1996; **87**: 814–17.

53   Iomhair MM, Lavelle SM. Quantitation of the thrombotic effects in artery and vein of the increase in coagulation factors during normal pregnancy in the rat. *Thromb Res* 1997; **87**: 359–62.

54   Walker MC, Garner PR, Keely EJ, *et al.* Changes in activated protein C resistance during normal pregnancy. *Am J Obstet Gynecol* 1997; **177**: 162–9.

55   Gerhardt A, Scharf RE, Zotz RB. Effect of hemostatic risk factors on the individual probability of thrombosis during pregnancy and the puerperium. *Thromb Haemost* 2003; **90**: 77–85.

56   Marcucci R, Abbate R, Fedi S, *et al.* Acquired activated protein C resistance in postmenopausal women is dependent on factor VIII levels. *Am J Clin Pathol* 1999;**111**;769–72.

9

Congenital and acquired hemorrhagic problems

ISOBEL D WALKER

INTRODUCTION

Menorrhagia and postpartum bleeding are important causes of morbidity in women. Although nowadays in the developed world, catastrophic maternal bleeding is rare, statistically hemorrhage remains a major cause of maternal mortality. Hemostasis is the result of complex interactions between the vascular endothelium, platelets, clotting factors and adhesive proteins, natural anticoagulants, and fibrinolysis. Normally these components of hemostasis acting in concert ensure a rapid and effective response to injury, preventing excessive bleeding while limiting the thrombogenic response to the site of injury and avoiding its persistence beyond the time for which it is required. Derangement, inherited or acquired, of any part of this complex mechanism may produce an imbalance with a resultant bleeding or thrombotic tendency.

INHERITED BLEEDING DISORDERS

The commonest inherited bleeding disorders are von Willebrand disease, hemophilia A (factor VIII deficiency), hemophilia B (factor IX deficiency), and factor XI deficiency. Deficiencies of other coagulation factors – fibrinogen and factors II, V, VII, X, XII, and XIII – are uncommon.

Hemophilia

Initially it was thought that hemophilia was a uniform entity but by the end of the 1940s it had been recognized that, in some cases, transfusion of blood from one hemophilic patient to another resulted in normalization of the recipient's coagulation abnormality. Now it is recognized that the more common form, hemophilia A, is due to a deficiency of coagulation factor VIII (FVIII) and a second form, hemophilia B, is due to deficiency of coagulation factor IX (FIX). The prevalence of hemophilia has been reported to be approximately 13–18 per 100 000 males[1] and the ratio of hemophilia A and hemophilia B about 4:1.[2] Both hemophilia A and hemophilia B are recessively inherited X-chromosome-linked disorders. Hemophilia in males can be readily detected with standard coagulation tests but the detection of carrier females is more difficult. Female carriers of hemophilia usually have intermediate levels of normal coagulation factor, lower than normal but adequate for hemostasis. Unless specifically sought, hemophilia carriers risk remaining undetected until they produce an affected son. Unexpectedly low levels of clotting factor activity occasionally occur in carriers and may be the result of extreme lyonization of the normal chromosome, of coincidental coinheritance of a variant von Willebrand factor allele, for example, a type 2N (*vide infra*), or, rarely, of coincidence with a chromosomal abnormality such as Turner syndrome (XO).

HEMOPHILIA SEVERITY CLASSIFICATION

In 2001 the Scientific and Standardisation Subcommittee of the International Society on Thrombosis and Hemostasis recommended that the plasma coagulation factor levels, rather than clinical bleeding symptoms, be used for the classification of the severity of hemophilia A or B.[3]

- Severe hemophilia – <0.01 IU/mL (<1 percent of normal)
- Moderate hemophilia – 0.01–0.05 IU/mL (1–5 percent of normal)
- Mild hemophilia – >0.05 IU/mL to <0.40 IU/mL (>5 percent to <40 percent of normal)

Symptoms of bleeding into joints and muscles correlate inversely and closely with the level of clotting factor activity. Bleeding may occur spontaneously in severe disease but usually only following trauma in patients with mild disease.

HEMOPHILIA GENETICS

The factor VIII gene is located at Xq28 and encompasses 186 kb of DNA.[4,5] Factor VIII is expressed predominantly in the liver, spleen, and lymph nodes.[6] In general, severe hemophilia A is the result of nonsense and frameshift mutations whereas missense change causes mild or moderate disease. About 50 percent of identified patients are severely affected, 10 percent moderately affected, and 30–40 percent mildly affected. The most common genetic abnormality in hemophilia A is the result of homologous intrachromosomal recombination of one of two repeats of a segment of intron 22.[7] It affects about 40 percent of patients with severe disease – around 20 percent of all patients with hemophilia A. Mutations in the other 80 percent of hemophilia A patients are predominantly single nucleotide changes, small deletions or insertions of one or a few base pairs. The factor IX gene is located on the long arm of the X chromosome at Xq27 and is 34 kb long. Factor IX mutations are of the same types as the noninversion mutations in the *FVIII* gene.

The diagnosis of hemophilia in affected males is usually readily made without the aid of genetic tests but identification of the specific mutation within a kindred may help predict the risk of complications, such as the development of coagulation factor inhibitors.

von Willebrand disease

von Willebrand disease (vWD) is the most commonly diagnosed inherited bleeding disorder. It has been suggested that the prevalence of vWD in various populations is approximately 1–2 percent.[8,9] von Willebrand disease is due to a quantitative or qualitative deficiency of von Willebrand factor (vWF) – a high-molecular-weight glycoprotein which carries factor VIII and protects it from proteolytic degradation. von Willebrand factor also plays an important role in platelet function, mediating the adhesion of platelets to the exposed vascular subendothelium and platelet–platelet aggregation in early thrombus formation.[10] von Willebrand factor is composed of homologous domains each with different functions and each repeated two to four times; A1

contains binding sites for platelet glycoprotein 1b (GP1b), collagen, and ristocetin; A2 contains the cleavage site for the vWF protease; A3 contains a second binding site for collagen; C1 contains a binding site for platelet glycoprotein IIb/IIIa (GPIIb/IIIa); D′ and part of D3 contain the binding site for factor VIII. Deficiency or qualitative abnormality of vWF results in a combined type of platelet and coagulation defect. Bleeding symptoms are predominantly mucocutaneous, including easy bruising, menorrhagia, post dental extraction bleeding, and epistaxis.

FORMATION OF VON WILLEBRAND FACTOR

In the majority of cases, vWD appears to be inherited as an autosomal dominant disorder but occasionally its inheritance appears to be autosomal recessive.[11] The *vWF* gene is located on chromosome 12 at p12-pter and comprises 52 exons spanning 178 kb of DNA. A partial pseudogene on chromosome 22 complicates the analysis of vWF. von Willebrand factor is synthesized by endothelial cells. The primary product undergoes considerable posttranslational modification resulting in the formation of dimers, tetramers, and ultimately large vWF multimers, which are stored in intracellular organelles known as Weibel–Palade bodies. Smaller multimers leave the cell constitutively. von Willebrand factor is also synthesized in megakaryocytes and stored in platelet alpha granules. Circulating vWF undergoes proteolytic cleavage under physiologic conditions. This is necessary for the regulation of the multimer size. Deficiency of a specific metalloproteinase leads to circulation of the supranormal-sized multimers seen in thrombotic thrombocytopenic purpura. In contrast, lack of large high-molecular-weight multimers results in excessive bleeding.

Inherited vWD has been divided into three subtypes (Box 9.1). Type 1 and type 3 vWD represent, respectively, a partial or virtually complete quantitative deficiency of qualitatively normal vWF. Type 2 vWD is the result of a

---

Box 9.1 Subtypes of von Willebrand disease

- Type 1 vWD – quantitative deficiency of vWF
- Type 2 vWD – qualitative deficiency of vWF
  - Type 2A vWD – qualitative variants with decreased platelet-dependent function due to absence of high-molecular-weight multimers
  - Type 2B vWD – qualitative variants with increased affinity for platelet GP1b
  - Type 2M vWD – qualitative variants with decreased platelet-dependent function not due to absence of high-molecular-weight multimers
  - Type 2N vWD – qualitative variants with markedly decreased affinity for factor VIII
- Type 3 vWD – virtually complete deficiency of vWF

qualitative defect in vWF. Type 2 vWD is divided into 4 subtypes (2A, 2B, 2M, and 2N) according to phenotypic features.[12] The bleeding severity is highly variable depending on the type and severity of vWD. Many patients with type 1 or type 2 vWD have mild or no bleeding tendency. Patients with type 3 vWD usually have a severe bleeding tendency. Type 1 vWD is the most prevalent with a frequency of 60–80 percent; type 2 variants have a frequency of 15–30 percent whereas type 3 is found in only 5–10 percent of patients.[13]

TYPE 1 VON WILLEBRAND DISEASE

The inheritance of type 1 vWD is usually autosomal dominant; rarely it may be autosomal recessive.[14–16] Type 1 vWD is characterized by concordantly reduced levels of vWF ristocetin cofactor activity and vWF antigen (the ratio of vWF ristocetin cofactor activity to vWF antigen being 0.7–1.2). There is also reduction in FVIII clotting activity (FVIII:C) and this reduction is concordant with the reduction in vWF antigen. Multimer studies reveal normal vWF multimers. The diagnosis of type 1 vWD is complicated by several factors. In particular, ABO blood groups[17] and exercise[18] modify vWF levels in plasma and vWF levels are influenced by estrogen and thyroid hormones – endogenous and exogenous. The clinical presentation is heterogeneous but the bleeding tendency is usually mild to moderate.

TYPE 2 VON WILLEBRAND DISEASE

With the exception of patients with type 2N vWD, patients with type 2 vWD have a discordantly severe reduction in vWF ristocetin cofactor activity with normal or only slightly reduced levels of vWF antigen (the ratio of plasma vWF ristocetin cofactor activity to vWF antigen being less than 0.7). Type 2A is the most prevalent type 2 subtype.[19] It is due to mutations in the A2 domain of vWF subunit. These mutations may cause impairment of the assembly and secretion of vWF multimers or may render multimers susceptible to proteolysis. Patients have an abnormal vWF multimer pattern with loss of high-molecular-weight multimers and display reduced ristocetin-induced platelet aggregation. Inheritance is generally autosomal dominant although a recessive pattern has been described.[20]

Type 2B vWD is characterized by an increased platelet aggregation response to ristocetin and an absence of large multimers from the plasma. The inheritance pattern is mainly autosomal dominant although recessive inheritance has been described.[21] Patients typically have mild thrombocytopenia with increased mean platelet volume, a prolonged bleeding time, and normal or low levels of FVIII:C. In some families, spontaneous platelet aggregation may occur. Thrombocytopenia may become more pronounced during pregnancy.[22,23] Type 2B vWD is due to mutations in the A1 domain of the vWF subunit which result in abnormal binding of vWF to platelet glycoprotein 1b.

Type 2M vWD includes variants with impaired platelet binding but normal vWF multimer distribution.

Investigations give results similar to those in type 2A but high-molecular-weight multimers are present. Mutations responsible for the type 2M phenotype occur in the A1 domain of the vWF subunit. The expressed mutants have reduced binding to platelet GP1b.

Type 2N vWD is characterized by normal levels of vWF antigen and vWF ristocetin cofactor activity and normal vWF multimers but a low level of FVIII:C. The phenotype therefore resembles hemophilia A, but it is autosomally transmitted. The low FVIII:C levels are not due to reduced FVIII:C production but to decreased plasma half-life as a consequence of impaired binding of FVIII:C to vWF.[24,25] Type 2N vWD may result from a variety of missense mutations localized in the D′ and D3 domains of the vWF subunit.

TYPE 3 VON WILLEBRAND DISEASE

Type 3 vWD is characterized by undetectable vWF antigen and vWF ristocetin activity in both plasma and platelets. Plasma FVIII:C levels are also significantly reduced (1–5 IU/dL). Affected patients therefore have a severe bleeding tendency with joint and muscle bleeding as well as mucocutaneous bleeding. Inheritance is autosomal recessive.

Factor XI deficiency

Inherited FXI deficiency is an uncommon autosomally transmitted abnormality. Approximately 40–50 percent of all individuals lacking FXI are of Ashkenazi Jewish extraction but it has been reported in individuals from all racial groups.[26] In homozygotes the FXI activity (FXI:C) levels are usually severely reduced but may be within the lower limits of the normal range in heterozygotes. The bleeding tendency is generally mild. Spontaneous bleeding is not a feature but affected patients may bleed following trauma or surgery. Bleeding risk correlates poorly with FXI:C levels.

DETECTION OF HEMOPHILIA CARRIERS AND WOMEN WITH OTHER HERITABLE BLEEDING DISORDERS

It is essential that, as far as possible, families with heritable bleeding disorders understand the genetic implications of their disease. In general, female carriers of hemophilia and women with vWD or other inherited bleeding disorders should be reviewed at regular intervals during their reproductive life, even if they remain asymptomatic. Review visits allow informal counseling and encourage women to take a positive attitude to carrier testing, family planning, and prenatal diagnosis.

Female carriers of hemophilia may feel isolated and under great stress. Usually their partner's family will have had no previous contact with inherited bleeding disorders and may find it difficult to come to terms with the possibility of having a child with a severe genetic disorder in the family. In general vWD and other inherited bleeding disorders are less severe than hemophilia but family planning advice and genetic counseling is important for these women. Counseling may allay previously unexpressed fears about the risks to themselves during pregnancy and delivery, and fears that their children may have a more severe bleeding disorder.

Hemophilia carriers

Hemophilia A and B are sex-linked recessive disorders. The daughters of affected men are obligate carriers who have a 50:50 chance of passing the disorder to a son and a 50:50 chance of passing the carrier state to a daughter (Fig. 9.1). Within any kindred the severity of the disorder remains constant. Knowledge of the specific mutation within a family is of paramount importance for carrier detection and may assist in reproductive decisions.

Ideally the carrier status of female relatives of known hemophilic individuals should be established prior to their first pregnancy to allow appropriate genetic counseling. Specific genetic testing is not necessary in women whose biologic father has hemophilia A or B – they are obligate carriers. However many hemophilia centers offer genetic testing to confirm carrier status in the daughters of patients with hemophilia. This policy has clear psychologic risks and invites ethical objection. If obligate carriers are to be offered confirmatory testing, the risks of uncovering nonpaternity and of genetic discrimination[27] should be discussed prior to blood sampling.

The status of women in the extended family is more difficult to establish. Potential carriers require genetic testing to confirm their status as a carrier or noncarrier but in practice this requires that the mutation within the family has been identified. Since genetic testing may take several weeks, potential carriers should be identified and offered testing to confirm their status if possible prior to becoming pregnant for the first time. Testing of minors raises specific ethical and legal problems. Education and counseling of potential carriers from early puberty is useful, but in general genetic testing should be delayed until the girl is able to understand the reasons for testing and is competent to give consent herself. Once the mutation within the family has been identified and carrier status confirmed, prenatal diagnosis becomes possible and selective termination of pregnancy an option. Some confirmed hemophilia carriers in whom the mutation has been identified may wish to consider *in vitro* fertilization with preimplantation genetic diagnosis (PGD) followed by the introduction of unaffected embryos. Where it has proved impossible to identify the mutation within a kindred, for example, where no informative blood samples are available, obligate carriers may choose to have female children only.

Genetic confirmation of von Willebrand disease

Genetic diagnosis of vWD involves either direct mutation detection or linkage analysis. Both are difficult and neither is at present considered a first-line investigation in the diagnosis of vWD. Clusters of mutations have been identified in type 2 vWD subtypes and in some centers it may be possible to screen for some of the commoner type 2 mutations. In most cases of type 1 and type 3 vWD, mutation detection involves sequencing the entire *vWF* gene. In these cases gene tracking by analysis of restriction fragment length polymorphisms or variable number of tandem repeat sequences of the *vWF* gene may be useful. Genetic tests may be considered in the prenatal diagnosis of severe vWD, to identify heterozygous carriers in recessive forms of vWD or in type 1 vWD families in which the phenotypic diagnosis is unclear.[28]

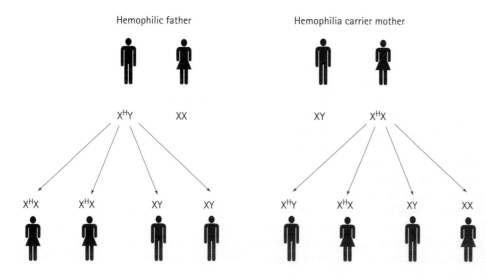

Figure 9.1   Inheritance of hemophilia. X^{H}Y, hemophilic male; X^{H}X, hemophilia carrier female; XY, normal male; XX, normal female.

Genetic testing for factor XI deficiency

A number of mutations have been described in individuals with FXI deficiency[26,29] but genetic testing to confirm FXI deficiency is not widely available.

TREATMENT OF HERITABLE BLEEDING DISORDERS

Plasma-derived clotting factors

Plasma-derived concentrates of FVIII and FIX are widely available and may be used for the treatment of patients with hemophilia A and B, respectively. When a patient with vWD is unresponsive to 1-deamino-8-D-arginine vasopressin (DDAVP) or when an immediate increase in vWF and FVIII:C is required, virus-inactivated intermediate purity plasma-derived FVIII concentrate or a highly purified, doubly virus-inactivated FVIII/vWF plasma concentrate[30] may be transfused. A lyophilized plasma-derived FXI concentrate is available for patients with FXI deficiency. This product is thrombogenic[31] and, if used, care should be taken to ensure that the patient's FXI:C activity does not exceed 100 IU/dL.

The safety of plasma-derived clotting factor concentrates has improved dramatically, and there is no longer significant risk of transmission of HIV or hepatitis agents.[32,33] However, the evidence that the highly thermoresistant B19 parvovirus may still be transmitted warns that other bloodborne viruses (other than hepatitis and human immunodeficiency virus [HIV]) may still be transmitted.[34] Parvovirus is a concern for pregnant women since it may cause fetal hydrops.[35] Recently fears that abnormal prion proteins associated with new variant Creuzfeldt–Jakob disease could be transmitted by plasma coagulation factors or albumin[36] have further increased pressures to minimize the use of plasma-derived products.

Recombinant clotting factor concentrates

Recombinant human FVIII (rhFVIII) and recombinant human FIX (rhFIX) are both available and widely used for the treatment of hemophilia A and B respectively.[37] Recombinant human vWF, which contains adequate levels of vWF activity and antigen, has been developed but is not currently available for use in humans.[38] No recombinant FXI product is available at present.

Over the past decade recombinant activated human factor VII (rhFVIIa) has been used widely for the treatment of patients with inhibitors to coagulation factors, but it has also been used for the management of severely bleeding patients without preexisting coagulopathy.[39,40] Infused as a bolus of 90–120 µg/kg to be repeated two to four times at 2–3-hour intervals, rhFVIIa is claimed to be useful in the management of major hemorrhage. Thromboembolic events have occurred in some patients give rhFVIIa and caution is advised in patients who have risk factors for

thrombosis.[40] Its use to prevent perinatal bleeding has been described but further studies are necessary.[41]

Desmopressin

Desmopressin (DDAVP) is a synthetic analogue of vasopressin. It increases the plasma levels of endogenous vWF and FVIII:C in patients with mild hemophilia A or type 1 vWD and in some patients with type 2A vWD. It is available in parenteral form for intravenous use and in a highly concentrated intranasal spray.[42] It appears to mediate the release of FVIII, vWF, and plasminogen activator from vascular endothelial cells and to shorten the bleeding time. When given for prophylaxis before invasive procedures or for acute bleeding episodes it is administered as a 30-minute intravenous infusion at a dose of 0.3 µg/kg (maximum 20 µg) diluted in 50 mL of saline.[42] Usually this dose increases FVIII:C and vWF threefold to fivefold within 30 minutes. The elevated levels of FVIII:C and vWF usually last for 6–8 hours. Depending on the type and severity of bleeding DDAVP infusions may be repeated every 12–24 hours. Most patients become less responsive with repeated DDAVP doses.

Intranasal administration may be preferable for patients who have less serious bleeding. It may be useful for some women with vWD to control excessive menstrual bleeding, for epistaxis or bleeding related to minor surgery or tooth extraction. It is administered in doses of 150 µg for patients weighing less than 50 kg and 300 µg for patients weighing 50 kg or more and is effective for 24–48 hours.[42,43] Following intranasal administration maximal plasma levels of vWF are noted 1–2 hours after the administration of the dose. In any one patient, the response to DDAVP is consistent. Thus it is usual to administer a test dose of DDAVP at the time of diagnosis to establish the individual's response pattern. There may be mild tachycardia, headache, and flushing due to DDAVP's vasomotor effect. It has been reported rarely to cause hyponatremia and volume overload due to its antidiuretic effect.[44]

In type 2 vWD, DDAVP corrects FVIII:C levels but the bleeding time usually remains prolonged. DDAVP is usually contraindicated in type 2B vWD because of the risk of promoting significant thrombocytopenia;[45] however, there are reports of its clinical usefulness in some patients with type 2BvWD.[46] In type 2N vWD relatively high levels of FVIII:C may be recorded after DDAVP infusion but the response is usually transient due to the lack of the stabilizing effect of normal vWF.[47] Patients with type 3 vWD are generally unresponsive to DDAVP.

Antifibrinolytic therapy

ε-Aminocaproic acid (EACA) and tranexamic acid may be used to prevent dissolution of the hemostatic plug and therefore reduce bleeding. They may be useful given during the first few days of menses to reduce menstrual bleeding. EACA is usually given four times daily in a dose of 50 mg/kg, and tranexamic acid is given three times daily in a dose of 25 mg/kg.

Estrogen

Estrogen results in increased plasma levels of FVIII:C and vWF, and estrogen therapy (with the combined oral contraceptive pill) may be used for the control of excessive bleeding in hemophilia A carriers and in some women with vWD.

MENSTRUAL PROBLEMS AND CONTRACEPTION IN WOMEN WITH CONGENITAL COAGULATION DEFECTS

Menorrhagia is a common problem in women with congenital bleeding disorders. It is frequently the presenting complaint and is often a problem from menarche.[48,49] Over 90 percent of women of reproductive age with diagnosed type 1 vWD complain of menorrhagia.[49] Often women with inherited bleeding disorders are misdiagnosed as having dysfunctional uterine bleeding and the underlying coagulopathy is missed.[50] In a series of women with objectively confirmed menorrhagia, carriership of hemophilia, vWD, and FXI deficiency was diagnosed in 57 percent, 73 percent and 59 percent, respectively.[51] Women with one of the less common coagulation factor deficiencies, including deficiencies of prothrombin, fibrinogen, or factors II, V, VII, X, or XIII, may also present with menorrhagia.[52]

For women with coagulopathy-related menorrhagia, there is no single best treatment. Local causes of bleeding should be excluded. Management depends on a wide range of factors, including the severity of the bleeding, the woman's age and her preferences.[53] Options include DDAVP in hemophilia A carriers, in women with type 1 vWd, and in some women with type 2A vWD,[42,50,54] antifibrinolytic agents such as tranexamic acid or EACA,[53] and the use of a combined oral contraceptive pill. Although there is no published study of its use specifically in women with coagulopathy-related bleeding, the levonorgestrel-releasing intrauterine device suppresses endometrial growth and has been shown to reduce menstrual blood loss in women with menorrhagia.[55,56] There are anecdotal reports of its usefulness in women with menorrhagia associated with a congenital or acquired bleeding disorder (secondary to oral anticoagulant use).

Women with inherited bleeding disorders may also have dysmenorrhea[51,57] and may bleed during intercourse. Rarely women with severe bleeding defects present with a broad ligament hematoma[57] or hemoperitoneum following rupture of a corpus luteum.[58] Any surgical intervention including gynecologic surgery may provoke excessive bleeding and may require clotting factor replacement, DDAVP, or other treatment. Liaison with a hematologist with expertise in managing patients with abnormalities of hemostasis is an essential step in planning surgery on these patients.

Contraception

Hemophilia carriers and women with other heritable bleeding disorders should be strongly encouraged to plan their families and avoid unplanned pregnancies where difficult decisions may have to be made under tight time constraints. The range of contraceptive methods available includes barrier methods, combined estrogen and progesterone pills, progesterone-only pills and depot preparations, intrauterine contraceptive devices, and male or female sterilization. No method is absolutely contraindicated. Where a patient may be a carrier of hepatitis B or HIV, the use of a barrier contraceptive should be strongly advised but where it is important to avoid pregnancy use of an additional contraceptive, such as a combined oral contraceptive may be prudent.

Apart from the progestin-impregnated intrauterine device, intrauterine contraceptive devices are unsuitable for women with vWD, FXI deficiency, or other significant clotting factor deficiency. Hemophilia A carriers and some women with vWD may benefit from the use of a combined estrogen and progesterone pill which offers not only contraception but also may reduce menstrual bleeding. Depot progesterone preparations may have a role to play in some carriers of hemophilia with virtually normal levels of clotting factors but, because of the risk of provoking large hematoma at injection or insertion sites, should usually be avoided in women with vWD or coagulation factor deficiency.

MANAGING PREGNANCY IN WOMEN WITH CONGENITAL COAGULATION DEFECTS

Management of pregnancy in women with a heritable bleeding disorder demands a multidisciplinary team approach involving not only obstetricians, midwives and anesthetists but also hematologists and neonatologists. Most affected women will be registered with a hemophilia center, and close liaison between the hemophilia center staff and the team delivering maternal and fetal care is essential.

Hemostasis in normal pregnancy

Fibrinogen concentration increases from early pregnancy to almost double prepregnancy levels at term. Both FVIII and vWF rise steadily from the end of the first trimester (Fig. 9.2). Factors VII and X also increase significantly during normal pregnancy but FIX, prothrombin, and factors V and XII show no or little increase and the levels of factors XI and XIII remain unchanged or fall slightly[59] (Fig. 9.3). The platelet count does not change significantly in normal pregnancies although some authors have reported a slight drop in the count in the third trimester. The activated partial

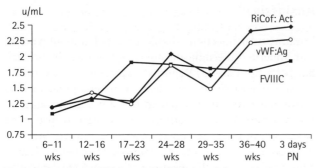

Figure 9.2   Factor VIII:C and von Willebrand factor during normal pregnancy.
FVII:C, factor VIII clotting activity; RiCof:Act, ristocetin cofactor activity; vWF:Ag, von Willebrand factor antigen.

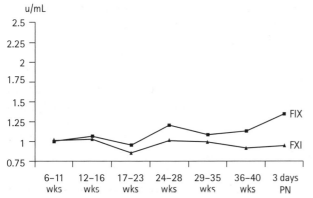

Figure 9.3   Factors IX:C (FIXC) and XI:C (FXIC) levels change little during normal pregnancy.

thromboplastin time (aPTT) and the prothrombin time (PT) usually remain within normal nonpregnancy adult ranges throughout pregnancy but during the third trimester they are shorter than earlier in pregnancy. Occasionally they fall below the lower limits of the nonpregnancy ranges for these tests.

Preconception counseling for women with inherited bleeding disorders

Pregnancy planning should be encouraged and women with inherited bleeding disorders should be offered the opportunity to discuss with their hematologist and an obstetrician experienced in the management of women with hemorrhagic disorders, all topics relevant to pregnancy. Those women who are not already immune, should be immunized against hepatitis B. Although immunization against hepatitis B is safe during pregnancy, immunization should, if possible, be completed prior to pregnancy.

Prenatal diagnosis of hemophilia

Several studies have suggested that the uptake of prenatal diagnostic testing may be around only a third of potential and confirmed hemophilia carriers.[60,61] Only a small minority of hemophilia carriers opt for termination of pregnancy if they are found to be carrying a child with hemophilia[61,62] and the number of boys born with hemophilia is not

falling.[63] Nonetheless, in couples where possible transmission of hemophilia is an issue, the availability of PGD or prenatal diagnosis, with or without selective termination of pregnancy, should be discussed.[64] The possibility of prenatal diagnosis may also be relevant to couples at risk of producing a child with type 3 vWD.

The procedures for obtaining samples for prenatal diagnoses of hemophilia and vWD are identical.[65,66] The most commonly used method is chorionic villous sampling but amniocentesis or fetal blood sampling may occasionally be used.[65,66] If genetic tests are not possible or produce noninformative results, fetal blood sampling from fetal umbilical vessels for measurement of clotting factors may be considered. This technique requires considerable expertise and is therefore not widely available. It is usually delayed until at least 18 weeks' gestation. Around 1 mL of fetal blood uncontaminated by maternal blood is need for clotting factor assay. At 19 weeks' gestation the levels of clotting factors VIII:C and IX:C in the normal fetus are 40 IU/dL (0.4 IU/mL) and 10 IU/dL (0.1 IU/mL), respectively.[67]

Management of pregnancy

Women with heritable bleeding disorders should be reviewed by a hemophilia center during pregnancy, usually in the first trimester at the time of booking antenatal care and in the third trimester to allow planning of delivery. Invasive procedures during early pregnancy need careful consideration on an individual patient basis. Spontaneous miscarriage, termination of pregnancy, or surgery during the first trimester may be complicated by serious maternal bleeding. Even chorionic villous sampling for prenatal diagnosis may be hazardous because of the risk of bleeding and it should be performed only after full discussion not only of the perceived benefits but also of the potential risks. Prior to any of these procedures maternal coagulation factor levels (as appropriate) must be checked and, if necessary, clotting factor replacement given to raise the level to at least 50 percent of normal (0.5 IU/mL). Knowledge of fetal sex is important in planning the management of labor and delivery in potential or confirmed hemophilia carriers. With modern ultrasound technology it is possible to diagnose the sex of the fetus accurately even in the first trimester.[68]

Hemophilia A carriers and most women with type 1 vWD show significant increases in the components of the FVIII complex during pregnancy – increasing sufficiently that the majority do not experience increased bleeding during pregnancy. When bleeding does occur in these women, it happens most frequently after delivery and usually only after operative delivery or if there has been significant trauma or tearing of the perineum or genital tract. Hemophilia A carriers seldom require treatment during normal pregnancy. In one study FVIII:C replacement was given in only 1 of 48 pregnancies in hemophilia A carriers;[62] in another review of 117 pregnancies in hemophilia A carriers coagulation factor replacement during pregnancy was required in none.[69]

Factor IX:C levels do not increase substantially during pregnancy. Carriers of hemophilia B have FIX:C levels significantly below normal even at the end of pregnancy. Similarly women with factor XI deficiency continue to have low FXI:C levels throughout pregnancy.

The bleeding time often shows little shortening during pregnancy and occasionally patients with vWD have a variable increase in the levels of the components of the FVIII complex (FVIII and vWF). Some women with type 2A vWD fail to demonstrate a significant increase in the levels of high-molecular-weight multimers. Women with type 2B vWD may develop increasing thrombocytopenia during pregnancy. Those with type 3 vWD have little or no increase in the FVIII complex levels and therefore remain at significant risk of bleeding during pregnancy and after delivery. Measurement of bleeding time, FVIII:C and vWF antigen or ristocetin cofactor activity during pregnancy may not predict the women who will bleed. In general women with type 1 vWD do not bleed excessively during pregnancy. On the other hand, women with type 2 or type 3 vWD have an increased tendency to bleed particularly following delivery.

Women with congenital bleeding disorders should be reviewed by a hemophilia center in their third trimester. Monitoring of coagulation factor activity, and vWF levels in women with vWD, usually around 34–35 weeks' gestation, allows discussion and planning of the management of their delivery.

Management of delivery

A planned delivery date may be considered if there are concerns about maternal hemostasis or about a potentially affected fetus. In the absence of an obstetric contraindication, vaginal delivery at term is usually preferred. The risk of serious fetal bleeding in conjunction with normal vaginal delivery is small, but vacuum extraction and rotational forceps delivery should be avoided. Application of fetal scalp electrodes and fetal blood sampling should also be avoided.

Clotting factor activity levels of 50 IU/dL (0.5 IU/mL) or greater are generally considered adequate. In women with type 1 vWD, FVIII:C activity is the best indicator of bleeding risk at delivery. If coagulation factor replacement is deemed necessary in carriers of hemophilia A or B, a recombinant product should be regarded as the product of choice. DDAVP is of potential value in hemophilia A carriers and in some women with vWD (type 1 and some type 2A vWD). It has been recommended that DDAVP should be used with caution in pregnant women because of a feared risk of premature labor or hyponatremia.[70] However, a growing experience of the use of DDAVP in pregnancy suggests that adverse events are rare.[71] In particular, DDAVP in now known not to stimulate uterine activity. Women with vWD unresponsive to DDAVP (including many women with type 2 and women with type 3 vWD) may require replacement therapy with plasma-derived clotting factor concentrate. Women with factor XI deficiency may require transfusion of plasma-derived FXI concentrate or of fresh frozen plasma.

Analgesia

Intramuscular injections should be avoided in all patients with inherited bleeding disorders unless their hemostasis has been normalized. Reported experience of the use of epidural anesthesia to cover delivery in hemophilia carriers or patients with vWD is limited but it has been suggested that providing the coagulation screen is normal, the platelet count 100×10^9/L or greater, and the Simplate bleeding time less than 10 minutes, there should be no hematological contraindication to the insertion of an epidural catheter.[72] Uncomplicated use of epidural anesthesia in type1 and type 2 vWD has been reported but each case must be considered individually and the benefits and risks carefully weighed in each case.[73,74] Before removing the epidural catheter, a repeat coagulation screen and platelet count would seem prudent. In the case of elective surgery, spinal anesthesia may offer a safer option.

Postpartum management

The risk of postpartum hemorrhage is significant in women with vWD. In one study the incidence of primary postpartum hemorrhage was 18.5 percent.[75] Careful clinical monitoring following delivery is advised. In general, coagulation factor activity levels should be monitored and maintained above 50 IU/dL (0.5 IU/mL) for 3–5 days following uncomplicated vaginal delivery and for around 7 days following cesarean section. DDAVP or clotting factor replacement should be given if necessary.

Care of the neonate

After delivery, a sample of the neonate's blood should be sent for coagulation factor assay. If an inherited bleeding defect is demonstrated, the pediatric hematologist should be notified. Intramuscular vitamin K should be avoided unless the neonate's clotting factor activity has been shown to be normal. Oral vitamin K should be used. Ultrasound scanning of the brain should be considered to confirm or exclude intracranial hemorrhage. Coagulation factor replacement is generally unnecessary unless there is evidence of bleeding.

RARE INHERITED BLEEDING DISORDERS

Afibrinogenemia has been associated with menorrhagia, recurrent fetal loss, and postpartum hemorrhage. Replacement treatment with a plasma-derived fibrinogen concentrate has been reported to allow successful pregnancy outcome.[76] Prothrombin deficiency[77,78] and deficiency of FV,[79] FVII,[80] or FX[81] have also been associated with menorrhagia and an increased risk of postpartum bleeding. Recombinant FVIIa has been used in the management of cesarean section in women with congenital FVII deficiency,[82,83] and may have a place in the management of women with other rare clotting factor deficiencies.

Factor XIII enhances fibrin clot stabilization. Deficiency of FXIII is associated with a severe bleeding tendency and defective wound healing. Women with FXIII deficiency are at increased risk of infertility and recurrent fetal loss. Factor XIII replacement, starting in childhood, aimed at maintaining the FXIII level above 1.5 percent (0.5 IU/mL) minimizes bleeding risk and may allow successful pregnancy outcome.[84]

ACQUIRED COAGULATION FACTOR DEFICIENCY

Compared with inherited bleeding disorders, acquired coagulation defects present different and often more challenging problems. Women with inherited disorders are usually already identified and investigated; with careful counseling, planning, and, if necessary, prophylaxis, they generally have few problems that are not predicted and treated early. Women who develop an acquired coagulopathy may be unwell and sometimes may be seriously ill.

Disseminated intravascular coagulation

Disseminated intravascular coagulation (DIC) is an acquired disorder secondary to underlying pathology[85] including a variety of obstetric complications. Its presence increases the risk of severe morbidity and mortality above the level associated with the underlying disorder.[86] Massive continuing activation of coagulation results in consumption of clotting factors and platelets. The clinical presentation may be anywhere in the spectrum from severe bleeding to thrombosis. There is no single test for DIC. Diagnosis depends on an awareness of the conditions, which may be complicated by DIC combined with a variety of laboratory tests.

The clinical presentation of disseminated intravascular coagulation is variable. In some cases coagulation activation may be detected only if sensitive assays of molecular markers of activation of clotting factors or pathways are performed. With more marked activation, routine coagulation screening tests become abnormal.[87] If the initiating event causes explosive activation of coagulation, the clinical picture is dominated by the effects of the rapid depletion of coagulation factors and platelets. Patients present with petechiae and bruising and there may be oozing from venepuncture sites and mucosal surfaces. If it involves the central nervous system, gastrointestinal tract, or placental bed or operative sites, the bleeding may become life-threatening. Intravascular deposition of fibrin leads to clinical organ dysfunction and contributes to the risk of multiorgan failure.[88] When activation of coagulation occurs more slowly, providing the liver can compensate for the consumption of clotting factors and the bone marrow maintains an adequate platelet count, severe bleeding is unlikely. Patients with chronic compensated DIC may be asymptomatic but some may have minor skin or mucosal bleeding.

Table 9.1 Obstetric complications predisposing to acute or chronic disseminated intravascular coagulation (DIC)

Acute DIC	Chronic DIC
Amniotic fluid embolism	Preeclampsia
Abruptio placentae	HELLP syndrome
Septic abortion	Retained dead fetus
Acute fatty liver	
Uterine rupture	
Extensive surgery	

Obstetric complications (Table 9.1) are frequently associated with clinically severe DIC.[89] Several obstetric complications such as placental abruption, amniotic fluid embolism and septic abortion are associated with acute decompensated DIC.[90] Placental abruption and amniotic fluid embolism probably result in the release of tissue factor and a direct activator of the prothrombinase complex into the maternal circulation.[91] About 10–20 percent of patients with Gram-negative bacteremia have evidence of DIC but other infections including Gram-positive bacteremia may also cause DIC.[92] Transfusion of ABO incompatible blood, although not strictly an obstetric complication does occasionally occur in the obstetric setting and can cause acute DIC. Other obstetric complications such as preeclampsia, the HELLP syndrome (*h*emolysis, *e*levated *l*iver enzymes, and *l*ow *p*latelet count), and retained dead fetus may cause chronic low-grade compensated DIC.

DIAGNOSIS OF DISSEMINATED INTRAVASCULAR COAGULATION

The basis of the diagnosis of DIC is an appreciation of the underlying disorders in which DIC can develop. Because acute DIC requires urgent intervention, DIC must always be considered where a complex coagulation disorder is noted in a woman with an underlying disorder which may be associated with DIC. Classically PT and aPTT are prolonged.[93] There is usually moderate to severe thrombocytopenia and evidence of red blood cell fragmentation on the peripheral blood film. Fibrinogen is reduced and levels of the products of fibrin breakdown, for example, D-dimers, are elevated.[94] Results within the normal ranges, however, do not exclude DIC, particularly in the acute phase and in pregnant women where the clotting times may be shortened and the fibrinogen level increased. These tests may be of limited value in patients with chronic compensated DIC in whom little abnormality may be observed (Box 9.2).

Identifying DIC at an early stage may be difficult if repeat testing is not performed. Detecting trends toward increasing prolongation of clotting tests, rising levels of D-dimers, and falling platelet counts and fibrinogen levels are practical markers of developing DIC. A scoring system that utilizes simple widely available laboratory tests, and for use

Box 9.2 Diagnosis of DIC

Early acute DIC or chronic DIC – activation of hemostasis compensated

- Frequently asymptomatic
- No measurable consumption of components – PT, aPTT within normal; platelet count within normal
- Activation markers increased – prothrombin fragment 1+2 (F1+2); thrombin antithrombin complex (TAT)
- Inhibitor levels may be reduced – antithrombin slightly reduced
- Peripheral blood film – occasional red blood cell (RBC) fragments

Acute DIC – activation of hemostasis decompensated

- Increased bleeding and decreased organ function (kidneys, lungs, liver)
- Consumption of coagulation factors – PT and aPTT prolonged; fibrinogen normal or reduced
- Consumption of platelets – platelet count reduced
- Activation markers increased – fibrin degradation products, F1+2, TAT, elevated; soluble fibrin increased
- Inhibitor levels reduced – antithrombin reduced
- Peripheral blood film – frequent RBC fragments

in situations where there is evidence of an underlying clinical condition predisposing to DIC, has been proposed.[85,95] Other trends such as falling levels of the natural anticoagulants, antithrombin, and protein C, may be helpful in confirming the diagnosis but, as they may not be immediately available in all hospitals, have limited use in the acute situation.

MANAGEMENT OF DISSEMINATED INTRAVASCULAR COAGULATION

Evidence on which to base guidance on the management of DIC is scant. Acute DIC is a serious complication which carries with it a high risk of mortality. It is generally accepted that the cornerstone of management of DIC is treatment of the underlying cause. In addition supportive therapies may be useful. Plasma and platelet replacement therapy should not be based on laboratory results but offered only to patients who are already bleeding or in danger of bleeding, for example at delivery or if an invasive procedure is planned. If replacement therapy is to be used, fresh frozen plasma at a dose of 15 mL/kg should be given. If fresh frozen plasma fails to maintain the fibrinogen level above 0.5 g/L, cryoprecipitate may be used in addition. Patients with a platelet count of less than 50×10^9/L may also benefit from administration of platelet concentrates in a dose of 1 donor unit/10 kg body weight.[92] In general, concentrates of coagulation factors should be avoided since they are potentially thrombogenic. Recombinant FVIIa has, however, been used

successfully and safely in a woman with DIC following cesarean section.[96]

The safety of heparin treatment in patients with DIC is debatable and a beneficial effect on clinical outcomes has never been demonstrated in a controlled trial.[97] The administration of unfractionated heparin or low-molecular-weight heparin is generally limited to patients with low-grade chronic compensated DIC who have predominantly thrombotic manifestations such as thrombophlebitis or who are at risk of venous thromboembolism. The use of antifibrinolytic agents is not recommended in patients with DIC.[98] A number of controlled trials using antithrombin concentrates in patients with DIC have been reported. In most of these trials, DIC has been associated with underlying sepsis or septic shock.[99,100] Some trials showed a modest reduction in DIC mortality in antithrombin treated patients but the effect did not reach statistical significance in individual trials. In a metaanalysis of the effect of antithrombin treatment on DIC mortality, Levi *et al.*[98] reported a statistically significant reduction in mortality.

Depression of the protein C system significantly contributes to the pathophysiology of DIC in some patients. There have been some reports of successful treatment with protein C concentrates in patients with DIC[101] but conversion to activated protein C requires adequate levels of the cell surface receptors thrombomodulin and endothelial protein C receptor and these may be significantly depleted in DIC. Activated protein C (aPC) has both anticoagulant and anti-inflammatory activities. In a randomized, double-blind trial of patients with severe sepsis, the mortality was 30.8 percent in the placebo-treated group (n = 840) compared with 24.7 percent in the group given recombinant aPC (n = 850).[102] The use of recombinant aPC was, however, associated with a significantly increased risk of bleeding (3.5 percent vs. 2 percent)[102] and caution is recommended in patients with platelet counts of less than 30×10^9/L.[86]

In animal studies, administration of tissue factor pathway inhibitor (TFPI) significantly reduces fibrin deposition in organs and prevents consumption of clotting factors.[103] However in a double-blind, placebo-controlled, clinical trial, treatment with recombinant TFPI had no effect on all-cause mortality in patients with severe sepsis and its administration was associated with an increase in risk of bleeding.[104]

ACQUIRED HEMOPHILIA

Acquired hemophilia usually occurs in elderly people but, rarely, acquired hemophilia A due to an inhibitor against FVIII presents in association with pregnancy in an otherwise healthy young woman.[105] Postpartum inhibitors of FVIII usually persist for a few months to several years.[106] Further pregnancies in women with prior postpartum inhibitor against FVIII do not provoke reappearance of the inhibitor.[106–108] The effectiveness of immunosuppressive therapy in patients with postpartum factor VIII inhibitors is debatable. In a review of 51 patients, corticosteroid therapy was not superior to no treatment and immunosuppression did not induce complete remission, although it may have shortened the time to remission (8 months) compared with steroid therapy (12 months) and no steroid or immunosuppressive therapy (16 months).[108] Treatment options include high-dose rhFVIII, FVIII inhibitor bypassing agent (FEIBA) or rhFVIIa.[109,110] DDAVP is of no clinical use because it induces no or little increase in factor VIII levels and what is produced is rapidly neutralized by the factor VIII inhibitor.

KEY LEARNING POINTS

- The most prevalent heritable bleeding disorder affecting women is von Willebrand disease but women with other heritable factor deficiencies, for example, FXI deficiency and carriers of hemophilia A or B may bleed excessively.
- Women with inherited abnormalities of coagulation frequently present with menorrhagia; often from menarche.
- As far as possible, women belonging to kindred with heritable bleeding problems should be identified and investigated to establish whether or not they are affected or carry the disorder, prior to their first pregnancy to enable them to make informed decisions about their reproductive choices.
- During pregnancy close liaison between the obstetric team and the hemophilia center is essential.
- Although most women with heritable bleeding disorders do not bleed spontaneously during pregnancy, invasive procedures, particularly during the first trimester may provoke excessive bleeding.
- Women with heritable bleeding disorders are at significant risk of postpartum hemorrhage and may require replacement clotting factors to reduce the risk of bleeding.
- Acute decompensated DIC may further complicate obstetric calamities. Management of the precipitating cause is the cornerstone of DIC treatment.

REFERENCES

1 Rosendaal FR, Smit C, Briet E. Hemophilia treatment in historical perspective: a review of medical and social developments. *Ann Hematol* 1991; **62**: 5–15.

2 Bauduer F, Degioanni A, Ducout L, *et al*. Distribution of haemophilia in the French Basque country. *Haemophilia* 2002; **8**: 735–9.

★ 3 White GC, Rosendaal F, Aledort LM, *et al*. Definitions in hemophilia. Recommendation of the scientific subcommittee on factor VIII and factor IX of the Scientific and Standardization Committee of the International Society on Thrombosis and Haemostasis. *Thromb Haemost* 2001; **85**: 560.

4 Theophilus BD, Enayat MS, Williams MD, Hill FG. Site and type of mutations in the factor VIII gene in patients and carriers of haemophilia A. *Haemophilia* 2001; **7**: 381–91.

5 Gitschier J, Wood WI, Goralka TM, *et al*. Characterization of the human factor VIII gene. 1984. *Biotechnology* 1992; **24**: 288–92.

6 Wion KL, Kelly D, Summerfield JA, *et al*. Distribution of factor VIII mRNA and antigen in human liver and other tissues. *Nature* 1985; **317**: 726–9.

7 Lakich D, Kazazian HH, Jr, Antonarakis SE, Gitschier J. Inversions disrupting the factor VIII gene are a common cause of severe haemophilia A [comment]. *Nat Genet* 1993; **5**: 236–41.

8 Werner EJ, Broxson EH, Tucker EL, *et al*. Prevalence of von Willebrand disease in children: a multiethnic study. *J Pediatr* 1993; **123**: 893–8.

9 Miller C, Lenzi R, Breen C. Prevalence of vWD among US adults [abstract]. *Blood* 1987; **70**(Suppl 1): 377.

10 Meyer D, Girma JP. von Willebrand factor: structure and function. *Thromb Haemost* 1993; **70**: 99–104.

11 Goodeve AC. Laboratory methods for the genetic diagnosis of bleeding disorders. *Clin Lab Haematol* 1998; **20**: 3–19.

★ 12 Sadler JE. A revised classification of von Willebrand disease. For the Subcommittee on von Willebrand Factor of the Scientific and Standardization Committee of the International Society on Thrombosis and Haemostasis. *Thromb Haemost* 1994; **71**: 520–5.

13 Tuddenham EG. von Willebrand factor and its disorders: an overview of recent molecular studies. *Blood Rev* 1989; **3**: 251–62.

14 Eikenboom JC, Reitsma PH, Peerlinck KM, Briet E. Recessive inheritance of von Willebrand's disease type I [comment]. *Lancet* 1993; **341**: 982–6.

15 Eikenboom JC, Castaman G, Vos HL, *et al*. Characterization of the genetic defects in recessive type 1 and type 3 von Willebrand disease patients of Italian origin. *Thromb Haemost* 1998; **79**: 709–17.

16 Federici AB, Mannucci PM, Bader R, *et al*. Heterogeneity in type IIB von Willebrand disease: two unrelated cases with no family history and mild abnormalities of ristocetin-induced interaction between von Willebrand factor and platelets. *Am J Hematol* 1986; **23**: 381–90.

17 Gill JC, Endres-Brooks J, Bauer PJ, *et al*. The effect of ABO blood group on the diagnosis of von Willebrand disease. *Blood* 1987; **69**: 1691–5.

18 Mohlke KL, Ginsburg D. von Willebrand disease and quantitative variation in von Willebrand factor [comment]. *J Lab Clin Med* 1997; **130**: 252–61.

19 Ruggeri ZM, Zimmerman TS. Variant von Willebrand's disease: characterization of two subtypes by analysis of multimeric composition of factor VIII/von Willebrand factor in plasma and platelets. *J Clin Invest* 1980; **65**: 1318–25.

20 Asakura A, Harrison J, Gomperts E, Abildgaard C. Type IIA von Willebrand disease with apparent recessive inheritance. *Blood* 1987; **69**: 1419–20.

21 Federici AB, Mannucci PM, Bader R. Heterogeneity in type IIB von Willebrand disease: Two unrelated cases with no family history and mild abnormalities of ristocetin-induced interaction between von Willebrand factor and platelets. *Am J Hematol* 1986; **23**: 381–90.

22 Rick ME, Williams SB, Sacher RA, McKeown LP. Thrombocytopenia associated with pregnancy in a patient with type IIB von Willebrand's disease. *Blood* 1987; **69**: 786–9.

23 Pareti FI, Federici AB, Cattaneo M, Mannucci PM. Spontaneous platelet aggregation during pregnancy in a patient with von Willebrand disease type IIB can be blocked by monoclonal antibodies to both platelet glycoproteins Ib and IIb/IIIa. *Br J Haematol* 1990; **75**: 86–91.

24 Mazurier C, Goudemand J, Hilbert L, *et al.* Type 2N von Willebrand disease: clinical manifestations, pathophysiology, laboratory diagnosis and molecular biology. *Baillieres Best Prac Clin Haematol* 2001; **14**: 337–47.

25 Mazurier C, Dieval J, Jorieux S, *et al.* A new von Willebrand factor (vWF) defect in a patient with factor VIII (FVIII) deficiency but with normal levels and multimeric patterns of both plasma and platelet vWF. Characterization of abnormal vWF/FVIII interaction. *Blood* 1990; **75**: 20–6.

◆ 26 Kitchens CS. Factor XI: a review of its biochemistry and deficiency. *Semin Thromb Hemost* 1991; **17**: 55–72.

27 Billings PR, Kohn MA, de Cuevas M, *et al.* Discrimination as a consequence of genetic testing [comment]. *Am J Hum Genet* 1992; **50**: 476–82.

28 Federici AB, Mannucci PM. Advances in the genetics and treatment of von Willebrand disease. *Curr Opin Pediatr* 2002; **14**: 23–33.

29 Ventura C, Santos AI, Tavares A, *et al.* Molecular genetic analysis of factor XI deficiency: identification of five novel gene alterations and the origin of type II mutation in Portuguese families. *Thromb Haemost* 2000; **84**: 833–40.

30 Federici AB, Baudo F, Caracciolo C, *et al.* Clinical efficacy of highly purified, doubly virus-inactivated factor VIII/von Willebrand factor concentrate (Fanhdi) in the treatment of von Willebrand disease: a retrospective clinical study. *Haemophilia* 2002; **8**: 761–7.

31 Richards EM, Makris MM, Cooper P, Preston FE. *In vivo* coagulation activation following infusion of highly purified factor XI concentrate. *Br J Haematol* 1997; **96**: 293–7.

◆ 32 Mannucci PM. Hemophilia: treatment options in the twenty-first century. *Thromb Haemost* 2003; **1**: 1349–55.

33 Tabor E. The epidemiology of virus transmission by plasma derivatives: clinical studies verifying the lack of

transmission of hepatitis B and C viruses and HIV type 1. *Transfusion* 1999; **39**: 1160–8.

34 Azzi A, Morfini M, Mannucci PM. The transfusion-associated transmission of parvovirus B19. *Transfus Med Rev* 1999; **13**: 194–204.

35 Tolfvenstam T, Papadogiannakis N, Norbeck O, *et al.* Frequency of human parvovirus B19 infection in intrauterine fetal death [comment]. *Lancet* 2001; **357**: 1494–7.

36 Ludlam CA. New-variant Creutzfeldt-Jakob disease and treatment of haemophilia. Executive Committee of the UKHCDO. United Kingdom Haemophilia Centre Directors' Organisation [comment]. *Lancet* 1997; **350**: 1704.

◆ 37 Lee C. Recombinant clotting factors in the treatment of hemophilia. *Thromb Haemost* 1999; **82**: 516–24.

38 Plaimauer B, Schlokat U, Turecek PL, *et al.* Recombinant von Willebrand factor: preclinical development. *Semin Thromb Hemost* 2001; **27**: 395–403.

39 Midathada MV, Mehta P, Waner M, Fink LM. Recombinant factor VIIa in the treatment of bleeding. *Am J Clin Pathol* 2004; **121**: 124–37.

40 O'Connell NM, Perry DJ, Hodgson AJ, *et al.* Recombinant FVIIa in the management of uncontrolled hemorrhage [see comment]. *Transfusion* 2003; **43**: 1711–16.

41 Bell JA, Savidge GF. Glanzmann's thrombasthenia proposed optimal management during surgery and delivery. *Clin Appl Thromb Hemost* 2003; **9**: 167–70.

42 Kadir RA, Lee CA, Sabin CA, *et al.* DDAVP nasal spray for treatment of menorrhagia in women with inherited bleeding disorders: a randomized placebo-controlled crossover study. *Haemophilia* 2002; **8**: 787–93.

43 Chuong CJ, Brenner PF. Management of abnormal uterine bleeding. *Am J Obstet Gynecol* 1996; **175**(3 Pt 2): 787–92.

44 Smith TJ, Gill JC, Ambruso DR, Hathaway WE. Hyponatremia and seizures in young children given DDAVP. *Am J Hematol* 1989; **31**: 199–202.

45 Holmberg L, Nilsson IM, Borge L, *et al.* Platelet aggregation induced by 1-desamino-8-D-arginine vasopressin (DDAVP) in Type IIB von Willebrand's disease. *N Engl J Med* 1983; **309**: 816–21.

46 Fowler WE, Berkowitz LR, Roberts HR. DDAVP for type IIB von Willebrand disease. *Blood* 1989; **74**: 1859–60.

47 Mazurier C, Gaucher C, Jorieux S, Goudemand M. Biological effect of desmopressin in eight patients with type 2N ('Normandy') von Willebrand disease. Collaborative Group. *Br J Haematol* 1994; **88**: 849–54.

48 Kadir RA, Economides DL, Sabin CA, *et al.* Frequency of inherited bleeding disorders in women with menorrhagia. *Lancet* 1998; **351**: 485–9.

49 Ragni MV, Bontempo FA, Cortese HA. On Willebrand disease and bleeding in women. *Haemophilia* 1999; 5.

50 Kouides PA. Menorrhagia from a haematologist's point of view. Part I: initial evaluation. *Haemophilia* 2002; **8**: 330–8.

51 Kadir RA, Economides DL, Sabin CA, *et al.* Assessment of menstrual blood loss and gynaecological problems in

patients with inherited bleeding disorders. *Haemophilia* 1999; **5**: 40–8.

◆ 52 Peyvandi F, Duga S, Akhavan S, Mannucci PM. Rare coagulation deficiencies. *Haemophilia* 2002; **8**: 308–21.

53 Siegel JE, Kouides PA. Menorrhagia from a haematologist's point of view. Part II: management. *Haemophilia* 2002; **8**: 339–47.

54 Leissinger C, Becton D, Cornell C, Jr, Cox GJ. High-dose DDAVP intranasal spray (Stimate) for the prevention and treatment of bleeding in patients with mild haemophilia A, mild or moderate type 1 von Willebrand disease and symptomatic carriers of haemophilia A. *Haemophilia* 2001; **7**: 258–66.

55 Lahteenmaki P, Haukkamaa M, Puolakka J, *et al*. Open randomised study of use of levonorgestrel releasing intrauterine system as alternative to hysterectomy [comment]. *BMJ* 1998; **316**: 1122–6.

56 Barrington JW, Bowen-Simpkins P. The levonorgestrel intrauterine system in the management of menorrhagia. *Br J Obstet Gyaenecol* 1997; **104**: 614–16.

57 Greer IA, Lowe GD, Walker JJ, Forbes CD. Haemorrhagic problems in obstetrics and gynaecology in patients with congenital coagulopathies. *Br J Obstet Gyaenecol* 1991; **98**: 909–18.

58 Gomez A, Lucia JF, Perella M, Aguilar C. Haemoperitoneum caused by haemorrhagic corpus luteum in a patient with type 3 von Willebrand's disease [see comment]. *Haemophilia* 1998; **4**: 60–2.

59 Clark P, Brennand J, Conkie JA, *et al*. Activated protein C sensitivity, protein C, protein S and coagulation in normal pregnancy. *Thromb Haemost* 1998; **79**: 1166–70.

60 Kadir RA, Sabin CA, Goldman E, *et al*. Reproductive choices of women in families with haemophilia. *Haemophilia* 2000; **6**: 33–40.

61 Varekamp I, Suurmeijer TP, Brocker-Vriends AH, *et al*. Carrier testing and prenatal diagnosis for hemophilia: experiences and attitudes of 549 potential and obligate carriers. *Am J Med Genet* 1990; **37**: 147–54.

62 Kadir RA, Economides DL, Braithwaite J, *et al*. The obstetric experience of carriers of haemophilia. *Br J Obstet Gyaenecol* 1997; **104**: 803–10.

63 Rizza CR, Spooner RJ, Giangrande PL. UK Haemophilia Centre Doctors' Organization. Treatment of haemophilia in the United Kingdom 1981–1996. *Haemophilia* 2001; **7**: 349–59.

64 Oyesiku JO, Turner CF. Reproductive choices for couples with haemophilia. *Haemophilia* 2002; **8**: 348–52.

★ 65 Peake IR, Lillicrap DP, Boulyjenkov V, *et al*. Haemophilia: strategies for carrier detection and prenatal diagnosis. *Bull World Health Organ* 1993; **71**: 429–58.

66 Peake IR, Lillicrap DP, Boulyjenkov V, *et al*. Report of a joint WHO/WFH meeting on the control of haemophilia: carrier detection and prenatal diagnosis. *Blood Coagul Fibrinolysis* 1993; **4**: 313–44 [erratum appears in *Blood Coagul Fibrinolysis* 1994 Feb; **5**: 148].

67 Forestier F, Daffos F, Galacteros F, *et al*. Hematological values of 163 normal fetuses between 18 and 30 weeks of gestation. *Pediatr Res* 1986; **20**: 342–6.

68 Bronshtein M, Rottem S, Yoffe N, *et al*. Early determination of fetal sex using transvaginal sonography: technique and pitfalls. *J Clin Ultrasound* 1990; **18**: 302–6.

69 Ljung R, Lindgren AC, Petrini P, Tengborn L. Normal vaginal delivery is to be recommended for haemophilia carrier gravidae. *Acta Paediatr* 1994; **83**: 609–11.

70 Chediak JR, Alban GM, Maxey B. von Willebrand's disease and pregnancy: management during delivery and outcome of offspring. *Am J Obstet Gynecol* 1986; **155**: 618–24.

71 Ray JG. DDAVP use during pregnancy: an analysis of its safety for mother and child. *Obstet Gynecol Surv* 1998; **53**: 450–5.

★ 72 Walker ID, Walker JJ, Colvin BT, *et al*. Investigation and management of haemorrhagic disorders in pregnancy. Haemostasis and Thrombosis Task Force [see comment]. *J Clin Pathol* 1994; **47**: 100–8.

73 Cohen S, Zada Y. Neuroaxial block for von Willebrand's disease [comment]. *Anaesthesia* 2001; **56**: 397.

74 Jones BP, Bell EA, Maroof M. Epidural labor analgesia in a parturient with von Willebrand's disease type IIA and severe preeclampsia. *Anesthesiology* 1999; **90**: 1219–20.

75 Kadir RA, Lee CA, Sabin CA, *et al*. Pregnancy in women with von Willebrand's disease or factor XI deficiency. *Br J Obstet Gyaenecol* 1998; **105**: 314–21.

76 Grech H, Majumdar G, Lawrie AS, Savidge GF. Pregnancy in congenital afibrinogenaemia: report of a successful case and review of the literature. *Br J Haematol* 1991; **78**: 571–2.

77 Catanzarite VA, Novotny WF, Cousins LM, Schneider JM. Pregnancies in a patient with congenital absence of prothrombin activity: case report. *Am J Perinatol* 1997; **14**: 135–8.

78 Girolami A. The hereditary transmission of congenital 'true' hypoprothrombinaemia. *Br J Haematol* 1971; **21**: 695–703.

79 Bennett K, Daley ML, Pike C. Factor V deficiency and menstruation: a gynecologic challenge. *Obstet Gynecol* 1997; **89**(5 Pt 2): 839–40.

80 Mariani G, Mazzucconi MG. Factor VII congenital deficiency. Clinical picture and classification of the variants. *Haemostasis* 1983; **13**: 169–77.

81 Knight RD, Barr CF, Alving BM. Replacement therapy for congenital Factor X deficiency. *Transfusion* 1985; **25**: 78–80.

82 Jimenez-Yuste V, Villar A, Morado M, *et al*. Continuous infusion of recombinant activated factor VII during caesarean section delivery in a patient with congenital factor VII deficiency. *Haemophilia* 2000; **6**: 588–90.

83 Eskandari N, Feldman N, Greenspoon JS. Factor VII deficiency in pregnancy treated with recombinant factor VIIa. *Obstet Gynecol* 2002; **99**(5 Pt 2): 935–7.

84 Burrows RF, Ray JG, Burrows EA. Bleeding risk and reproductive capacity among patients with factor XIII

deficiency: a case presentation and review of the literature. *Obstet Gynecol Surv* 2000; **55**: 103–8.

★ 85 Taylor FB, Jr., Toh CH, Hoots WK, Wada H, Levi M. Scientific Subcommittee on Disseminated Intravascular Coagulation (DIC) of the International Society on Thrombosis Haemostasis (ISTH). Towards definition, clinical and laboratory criteria, and a scoring system for disseminated intravascular coagulation. *Thromb Haemost* 2001; **86**: 1327–30.

86 Toh CH, Dennis M. Disseminated intravascular coagulation: old disease, new hope. *BMJ* 2003; **327**: 974–7.

87 Bauer KA, Rosenberg RD. The pathophysiology of the prethrombotic state in humans: insights gained from studies using markers of hemostatic system activation. *Blood* 1987; **70**: 343–50.

88 Wheeler AP, Bernard GR. Treating patients with severe sepsis [see comment]. *N Engl J Med* 1999; **340**: 207–14.

89 Letsky EA. Disseminated intravascular coagulation. *Best Pract Res Clin Obstet Gynaecol* 2001; **15**: 623–44.

90 Weiner CP. The obstetric patient and disseminated intravascular coagulation. *Clin Perinatol* 1986; **13**: 705–17.

91 Gordon SG, Hasiba U, Cross BA, *et al.* Cysteine proteinase procoagulant from amnion-chorion. *Blood* 1985; **66**: 1261–5.

◆ 92 Baglin T. Disseminated intravascular coagulation: Diagnosis and treatment. *BMJ* 1996; **312**: 683–7.

93 Spero JA, Lewis JH, Hasiba U. Disseminated intravascular coagulation. Findings in 346 patients. *Thromb Haemost* 1980; **43**: 28–33.

94 Lusher JM. Screening and diagnosis of coagulation disorders. *Am J Obstet Gynecol* 1996; **175**(3 Pt 2): 778–83.

◆ 95 Levi M. Current understanding of disseminated intravascular coagulation. *Br J Haematol* 2004; **124**: 567–76.

96 Moscardo F, Perez F, de la Rubia, *et al.* Successful treatment of severe intra-abdominal bleeding associated with disseminated intravascular coagulation using recombinant activated factor VII. *Br J Haematol* 2001; **114**: 174–6.

97 Feinstein DI. Diagnosis and management of disseminated intravascular coagulation: the role of heparin therapy. *Blood* 1982; **60**: 284–7.

98 Levi M, de Jonge E, van der PT, Ten Cate H. Disseminated intravascular coagulation. *Thromb Haemost* 1999; **82**: 695–705.

99 Harper PL. The clinical use of antithrombin concentrate in septicaemia. *Br J Hosp Medicine* 1994; **52**: 571–4.

100 Fourrier F, Chopin C, Huart JJ, *et al.* Double-blind, placebo-controlled trial of antithrombin III concentrates in septic shock with disseminated intravascular coagulation. *Chest* 1993; **104**: 882–8.

101 Smith OP, White B, Vaughan D, *et al.* Use of protein-C concentrate, heparin, and haemodiafiltration in meningococcus-induced purpura fulminans [see comment]. *Lancet* 1997; **350**: 1590–3.

102 Bernard GR, Vincent JL, Laterre PF, *et al.* Efficacy and safety of recombinant human activated protein C for severe sepsis [see comment]. *N Engl J Med* 2001; **344**: 699–709.

103 Creasey AA, Chang AC, Feigen L, *et al.* Tissue factor pathway inhibitor reduces mortality from *Escherichia coli* septic shock. *J Clin Invest* 1993; **91**: 2850–60.

104 Abraham E, Reinhart K, Opal S, *et al.* Efficacy and safety of tifacogin (recombinant tissue factor pathway inhibitor) in severe sepsis: a randomized controlled trial [see comment]. *JAMA* 2003; **290**: 238–47.

105 Green D, Lechner K. A survey of 215 non-hemophilic patients with inhibitors to Factor VIII. *Thromb Haemost* 1981; **45**: 200–3.

106 Michiels JJ, Hamulyak K, Nieuwenhuis HK, *et al.* Acquired haemophilia A in women postpartum: management of bleeding episodes and natural history of the factor VIII inhibitor. *Eur J Haematol* 1997; **59**: 105–9.

107 Coller BS, Hultin MB, Hoyer LW, *et al.* Normal pregnancy in a patient with a prior postpartum factor VIII inhibitor: with observations on pathogenesis and prognosis. *Blood* 1981; **58**: 619–24.

108 Hauser I, Schneider B, Lechner K. Post-partum factor VIII inhibitors. A review of the literature with special reference to the value of steroid and immunosuppressive treatment. *Thromb Haemost* 1995; **73**: 1–5.

109 Morrison AE, Ludlam CA, Kessler C. Use of porcine factor VIII in the treatment of patients with acquired hemophilia. *Blood* 1993; **81**: 1513–20.

110 Morrison AE, Ludlam CA. Acquired haemophilia and its management [comment]. *Br J Haematol* 1995; **89**: 231–6.

10

The vasculature in rheumatic disorders

RAVENDERA RAMACHANDRAN, KRISHNA DANI, HILARY A CAPELL, RAJAN MADHOK

INTRODUCTION

The vasculature has a fundamental role in both the pathogenesis and clinical manifestations of the autoimmune rheumatic disorders. It is also of interest because premature occlusive atheromatous disease (accelerated atherosclerosis) is now increasingly recognized as a cause of both morbidity and premature mortality in several of the autoimmune rheumatic disorders. A definite association with accelerated atherosclerosis has been noted particularly with rheumatoid arthritis (RA)[1] and systemic lupus erythematosus (SLE).[2] In addition in the small vessel vasculitides there is evidence of a generalized impairment of endothelial function at sites distant from clinical involvement. With better control of the inflammatory/immune processes characteristic of these disorders, understanding the mechanisms and addressing issues in the vasculature are now of equal priority.

This chapter provides the perspective of practicing rheumatologists with regard to the vasculature of two common autoimmune rheumatic diseases and primary vasculitis.

RHEUMATOID ARTHRITIS

Of the inflammatory joint disorders, RA is the most common. It is a systemic inflammatory disorder with major impact on synovial joints. Nonspecific features of inflammation are common in the majority of patients, but in a subset RA results in disease-specific extraarticular manifestations of which vasculitis is one.

The vasculature in rheumatoid arthritis

In RA vasculitis, inflammation resulting in fibrinoid necrosis in the vessel wall with thrombotic occlusion of the lumen is well documented. It can affect any part of the vasculature. Deposition of immune complexes leads to an inflammatory reaction in all layers of the vessel wall. Vasculitis occurs in 1 percent of RA patients and appears to be on the decline.[3] It is not clear why its presence is a marker of poorer outcome.

Men are more frequently affected; there is a positive association with both cigarette smoking and the possession of the human leukocyte antigen (HLA)-shared disease epitope encoded on the third hypervariable region of the DR1 from codons 67 to 74. The occurrence of vasculitis is independent of articular disease severity and rarely may precede its onset. It is more frequent in those with longer disease duration; median age of diagnosis is 60 years with disease duration between 10 and 13 years, often with evidence of other extraarticular complications such as rheumatoid nodules. Patients with vasculitis have more severe constitutional symptoms, such as fatigue, weight loss, and low-grade pyrexia. High titers of rheumatoid factor, evidence of complement consumption, and a marked acute phase response are characteristic laboratory findings.[4]

Vasculitis of the arterioles, capillaries, and venules is more frequent than that of small- to medium-sized arteries. The main clinical manifestations of microvasculature involvement are cutaneous lesions and sensorimotor peripheral neuropathies in a glove and stocking distribution. Clinical features of cutaneous vasculitis include nailfold infarcts, purpura, and punched out venous leg ulcers, and its presence is not always a harbinger of visceral vasculitis. Vasculitis has been proposed as a mechanism in nodule formation, but this is not proved.

When larger-caliber vessel involvement occurs it often results in a mononeuritis multiplex and digital gangrene. Vasculitis of the viscera is less common and has been particularly described in the kidney, lungs, heart, brain, and eye. Its presence invariably portends a grave outcome.

The vasculature in the pathogenesis of rheumatoid arthritis

The synovium in RA changes from a single layer of synovial cells supported by a network of capillaries and lymphatic vessels to an aggressive hyperplastic tissue comparable to tumor in areas infiltrated with activated inflammatory/immune cells, predominantly of the CD4[+] memory phenotype.[5] Within the joint space the synovial fluid contains primarily an acute inflammatory exudate. Changes in the vasculature that permit this include activation of the endothelium allowing for leukocyte trafficking and new blood vessel formation (angiogenesis).

LEUCOCYTE TRAFFICKING

Extravasation of leukocytes from blood to damaged tissue is essential to inflammation, and it is the result of a well-coordinated cascade of steps mediated by the expression of adhesion molecules on high endothelial venules and corresponding leukocyte ligands.[6] Normally, leukocytes roll over the endothelium tethered by the binding of L-selectin to endothelial ligands. On endothelial activation the expression of E-selectin slows leukocyte rolling and a more secure adherence is achieved via the two integrins expressed on leukocytes and intercellular adhesion molecule-1 on endothelial cells. The expression of vascular cell adhesion molecule-1 due to continued activation of endothelial cells facilitates leukocyte migration to the site of injury down the concentration gradient of chemoattractant molecules. Increased endothelial adhesion molecule expression has been documented in the RA synovium and correlates with the degree of joint inflammation. Therapies directed at inhibiting this process are an active area of investigation.

ANGIOGENESIS

The formation of new blood vessels is critical to perpetuating the inflammatory process, providing both a surface for leukocyte trafficking as well as a supply of nutrients to sustain the synovial hyperplasia. It has been proposed that the cartilage loss and bone erosion by pannus, so characteristic of RA, could not occur in the absence of angiogenesis.

The process of angiogenesis is the result of a complex and sequential change in endothelial cells and is precisely regulated by inhibitors and inducers.[7] The most potent promoter is vascular endothelial growth factor (VEGF), levels of which are elevated in the RA joint. Hypoxia can induce VEGF. In the rheumatoid joint intraarticular

pressure often exceeds capillary perfusion pressure[8] with resultant hypoxia. Cytokines that drive the inflammatory process in RA, such as interleukin-1, tumor necrosis factor (TNF), and CD40 ligand, also induce VEGF. Modulation of VEGF in murine arthritis models reduces arthritis severity and it has been proposed that one of the benefits of TNF antagonist therapy may be reduction in VEGF. Similarly, in vitro inhibition of endothelial cell proliferation is common to all conventional disease-modifying drugs such as sulfasalazine, methotrexate, and penicillamine, thus providing a unifying concept to their mode of action.[9]

ACCELERATED ATHEROGENESIS

Since the 1950s it has been known that RA reduces life expectancy. In one survey the median reduction in lifespan was 17 years.[10] However, despite many advances, a reduction in mortality has not been seen since the 1960s.[10] Most of the excess mortality can be attributed to cardiovascular events.[11] Unequivocal evidence supporting the association with premature cardiovascular disease comes from the Nurses' Health Study.[12] An 18-year analysis of a cohort of 114 342 nurses, who were free of cardiovascular and rheumatoid disease in 1976, showed that there were 527 incident cases of RA and 3622 myocardial infarctions. After correction for traditional risk factors, nonsteroidal anti-inflammatory agents (NSAIDs) and corticosteroid use, women with RA had double the risk for myocardial infarction and in those with disease duration greater than 10 years the risk was three times greater. However, this may be an underestimate as studies from our center and others show that the frequency of cardiovascular disease may be significantly higher with some groups finding that up to 50 percent of their patients have demonstrable evidence of ischemic heart disease.[13,14]

Recently much more has been understood about the underlying mechanisms. Surrogate markers of generalized atherosclerosis such as B mode ultrasound measurement of the carotid intima-media thickness show increments in RA equivalent to those in diabetes, which in longitudinal studies correlate with the extent of the inflammatory response.[15] Similarly, pulse wave analysis has shown reduced arterial compliance (which is another marker of vascular dysfunction) in RA patients with associations with markers of disease severity noted.[16] These and other data suggest that traditional risk factors cannot account for all the risk and as the inflammatory milieu characteristic of RA has many similarities to that in atheroma it has been proposed that the two may act in concert.

Risk factors for atheroma in rheumatoid arthritis

LIPIDS

The lipid profile in RA, like other chronic inflammatory diseases, results in a low total cholesterol and low-density lipoprotein and reduced high-density lipid cholesterol fraction thus giving an atherogenic lipid profile.[17] This not only parallels the acute phase response but also qualitatively minimizes the beneficial effect of high density lipoprotein by replacing its main anti-inflammatory protein apo-lipoprotein A1 with serum amyloid A, thus further reducing its cardio-protective effects.[18] Treatment with disease-modifying drugs seems to correct the ratio but the benefit is drug dependent, being most favorable with hydroxychloroquine and less so with intra-muscular gold.[19,20] Methotrexate use reduces the risk of cardiovascular events but the mechanism is not known.[21]

SMOKING

The link between smoking and RA is well documented but in studies of cardiovascular risk it has no additional influence.[22] It has been speculated that some of the adverse effects of smoking on connective tissue may be mediated by cytokines.

HYPERTENSION

Hypertension is the most common comorbid condition in RA, most often developing after disease onset; NSAID use may be contributory.[23] Most NSAIDs raise blood pressure by an average of 5 mm Hg, varying between NSAIDs, and is greatest with piroxicam, indometacin, ibuprofen, diclofenac, naproxen, and flurbiprofen but less so with sulindac.[24] The effect of cyclooxygenase-2 (COX-2) inhibitors on blood pressure is also well documented.[25] These drugs can also increase thrombotic risk by other mechanisms. Nonselective NSAIDs and aspirin share an active docking site on COX-1, raising the possibility of competition between the two.[26] This has been demonstrated in healthy volunteers with ibuprofen and seems also to be important in the clinic. The effect is not observed with diclofenac and may be due to different physical positioning of the molecule. Cyclooxygenase-2 inhibitors would not be expected to show such an effect but an increased risk of myocardial infarction has been observed with many of the COX inhibitors.[27] The mechanism is as yet not elucidated but some evidence suggests that temporary inhibition of prostacyclin may occur, an effect not seen with nonselective NSAIDs.[28]

OBESITY AND INSULIN RESISTANCE

Active RA in general results in weight loss, and in severe cases cachexia, which may promote insulin resistance. Insulin resistance has been demonstrated in RA correlating with inflammatory load and reversing with disease-modifying therapy.[29] As disability advances weight gain occurs because of reduced activity, which tends to be more centrally disturbed. This is a phenotype often associated with insulin resistance.

ENDOTHELIAL DYSFUNCTION

Altered function of the endothelium is an early event in the development of atheroma. An early measurable manifestation is an impaired ability of an artery to dilate in response to chemical or physical stimuli and is attributed to reduced nitric oxide bioavailability. Change in brachial artery diameter after occlusion measured by ultrasound is an accurate and reproducible noninvasive method for evaluating endothelial dysfunction.[30] In both active and quiescent RA endothelial dysfunction using this method has been found. It is reversed with disease-modifying therapy and is attributed by some to TNF, as improvements are seen with TNF antagonists.[31] However these preliminary observations are difficult to reconcile with studies which show that TNF is antithrombotic, an effect mediated via nitric oxide produced by the vessel to maintain patency so that leukocytes may transverse freely to sites of inflammation.[32]

In addition to control of risk factors, the suppression of inflammation is clearly important in reducing the cardiovascular morbidity of RA and in this regard the finding that statins have an anti-inflammatory effect in RA is of considerable interest.[33]

SYSTEMIC LUPUS ERYTHEMATOSUS

Systemic lupus erythematosus is a chronic disease predominantly affecting women in the prime of their life. It is a complex disorder characterized by the excessive production of autoantibodies, immune complex formation, and immunologically mediated injury.

The diagnosis requires a high index of suspicion and should only be made once the American College of Rheumatology criteria have been fulfilled.[34] With the availability of human cell substrates it would now be inappropriate to make the diagnosis in the absence of antinuclear antibodies. Such antibodies target intranuclear nucleic acids, proteins, and nucleoprotein complexes. The antibody profile can be helpful in predicting the nature of disease although it is not absolute. For example, lupus nephritis is invariably associated with double-stranded DNA antibodies, and antibody to the Ro and La particles has a high specificity for subacute cutaneous lupus, the sicca syndrome, and neonatal lupus syndrome.

The vasculature in systemic lupus erythematosus

The spectrum of damage to the vasculature in SLE is diverse and explains many but not all the clinical features. It may arise due to: immune complex deposition leading to vasculitis; a vasculopathy mediated by complement but in the absence of immune complex deposition; a thrombotic angiopathy due to anticardiolipin antibodies or rarely a hemolytic–uremic-like syndrome in association with antibody to the von Willebrand factor cleaving protease; and an increasingly recognized higher than expected incidence of atherosclerosis.

IMMUNE COMPLEX VASCULITIS

The binding of antibody to antigen in a soluble form is known as an immune complex. These are removed from the circulation by the reticuloendothelial system facilitated by complement. Immune complex clearance is slower in SLE, which in part is due to an acquired abnormality in red cell CR1 receptors.[35]

Immune complex size depends on the relative proportions of antigen and antibody and antibody class. In antibody excess the complexes are rapidly precipitated and localized to the site of antigen entry. In antigen excess the complexes are soluble and thus circulate and deposit on the basement membrane of small blood vessels and activate complement releasing C3a and C5a, which in turn attract neutrophils, mononuclear phagocytes, basophils, and mast cells. The subsequent binding of the immune complex to the Fc receptor stimulates phagocytic cells.

The site of deposition depends on many factors such as the amount of flow, local flow characteristics (turbulence, hydrostatic pressure), and the type of endothelium. Deposition of immune complexes is important in the pathogenesis of many lupus manifestations, in particular nephritis and some of the skin features.

NONIMMUNE COMPLEX COMPLEMENT–MEDIATED VASCULOPATHY

This is presumed to be important in the pathogenesis of central nervous system (CNS) disease in the absence of anticardiolipin antibody. Cytokine-mediated endothelial activation results in binding of neutrophils activated by complement, producing a leuko-occlusive vasculopathy.[36] In active systemic disease a syndrome similar to the systemic inflammatory response syndrome in sepsis may arise, initiated by the activation of complement.

ANTIPHOSPHOLIPID ANTIBODY SYNDROME

This syndrome is characterized by the presence of antiphospholipid antibodies and the presence of at least one clinical manifestation such as venous or arterial thrombosis or recurrent fetal loss. Criteria for classification of the diagnosis have been proposed.[37] The syndrome was first noted in patients with SLE in 1952 and occurs with other autoimmune rheumatic diseases as well as being a distinct clinical entity. Estimates of the frequency of lupus anticoagulant, antiphospholipid and anti β2 glycoprotein 1 antibodies in SLE have varied; these differences may be due to the sensitivities of the assays used and due to biases in patient selection. When associated with SLE the clinical manifestations of antiphospholipid antibody syndrome are independent of the severity of lupus and the two have no temporal relation. Management in SLE is similar to that of the primary syndrome. Antiphospholipid antibodies may also contribute to the premature atherosclerosis of SLE as the antibodies may cross-react with phospholipids in oxidized low-density lipoprotein (LDL), facilitating their uptake by macrophages.[38]

ACCELERATED ATHEROSCLEROSIS

The initial observation by Urowitz in 1967 of the death of a 30-year-old patient with SLE from premature coronary artery disease aroused curiosity rather than concern. On the basis of this observation Urowitz et al. found that mortality in lupus has a bimodal distribution, early death occurring due to disease exacerbations and infection and premature coronary artery disease accounting for later mortality.[39] As the management of SLE has improved the threat of early atheromatous vascular disease has emerged as a much more major source of concern with one estimate calculating the risk of myocardial infarction to be 50 times higher than expected.[2] Mortality studies indicate that the risk of death in lupus is now more likely from accelerated vascular disease than the disease itself or infection.[40] Similarly, surveys of morbidity due to atheromatous vascular disease (either ischemic heart disease or stroke) show a prevalence of between 6 percent and 15 percent.[41] Of greater concern is the finding of a much greater than expected prevalence of surrogates of atheromatous vascular disease, such as coronary artery calcification and carotid plaques on Doppler sonography suggesting that the risks are significantly greater than previously thought.[42,43]

Traditional risk factors

LIPIDS

As in RA the lipid profile in SLE is atherogenic despite low total levels of cholesterol.[42] Typically, triglyceride and lipoprotein(a) levels are elevated whereas high-density lipoprotein levels are reduced.[43] Such profiles could arise from the use of corticosteroids or the disease itself. Contributing to this risk may be impaired lipoprotein lipase activity, antibodies to which occur in up to 47 percent, and the inhibition of 27-hydroxycholesterol in the vessel due to complement fixing immune complexes, which in turn impair feedback inhibition and increase LDL receptor uptake.[44,45]

HYPERTENSION

Hypertension in SLE could arise due to underlying renal disease or use of NSAIDs and corticosteroids. Although blood pressure, compared with controls, is no different in those with carotid plaques there was a trend toward higher systolic and diastolic pressures but within the normal range.[25,42,43]

SMOKING

The prevalence of smoking is no different between lupus patients and controls when studied for cardiovascular risk factors.[42,43]

DIABETES

The prevalence is similar to controls but to date no studies of insulin resistance have been reported.

Nontraditional risk factors

Even when traditional risk factors are accounted for the rate of vascular events is seven times greater than expected, suggesting that disease- or treatment-related factors contribute. In a study of carotid artery plaques, patients with plaques were older, had longer disease duration, and more disease-related damage. In addition they were less likely to have been treated with prednisolone, cyclophosphamide, and hydroxychloroquine.[42] In other studies an association with antiphospholipid antibodies and a procoagulant profile with higher levels of fibrinogen, plasminogen activator inhibitor 1 and C-reactive protein was found.[45] It is thus likely that both traditional and as yet undefined SLE-related factors result in accelerated atheromatous disease. Management should be based on addressing traditional risk factors as well as prudent corticosteroid use; the judicious use of hydroxychloroquine may also be of benefit because of its known anti-inflammatory as well as antithrombotic profile.[46] The benefit of 'statins' is yet to be established but concerns of their use have been expressed as a drug-induced lupus-like syndrome has been described.[47]

VASCULITIS

Vasculitis describes a heterogeneous group of disorders in which there is inflammation of the blood vessel wall. The term is used irrespective of vessel size, or the etiology or pathogenesis of the inflammation. It may also arise in the context of a systemic disorder such as infection, malignancy, or an autoimmune rheumatic disease such as RA. Since vessels of any organ can be affected, the clinical manifestations are often diverse but certain patterns do emerge in the primary vasculitides which are helpful in their management. The classification of primary vasculitis has undergone many modifications but is achieving some consensus.[48] Most classifications consider blood vessel size, histology, etiology, and clinical manifestations (Fig. 10.1). The American College of Rheumatology has proposed classification criteria for seven vasculitic disorders (polyarteritis nodosa, Churg–Strauss syndrome, Wegener granulomatosis, Henoch–Schönlein purpura, hypersensitivity vasculitis, giant cell arteritis, and Takayasu arteritis) but this has limitations as overlaps occur.

A causative agent been identified in only a few of the primary vasculitides. For example, in some cases of classic polyarteritis nodosa the hepatitis B virus is responsible, and in mixed essential cryoglobulinemia hepatitis C is implicated in up to 40 percent.[49,50] The immune system has a fundamental role in the pathogenesis and there are

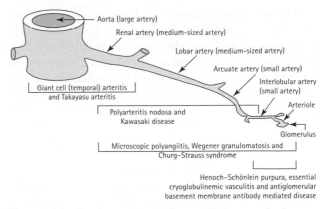

Figure 10.1   Spectrum of systemic vasculitides organized according to predominant size of vessel affected. (Adapted from Jennette *et al. Arthritis Rheum* 1994; **37**: 187–92 and redrawn with kind permission from Savage *et al. BMJ* 2000; **320**: 1325. Reproduced with permission from the BMJ Publishing Group.)

several potential mechanisms: deposition of immune complexes; antiendothelial cell antibodies; antibodies against exogenous antigens; endothelial damage by neutrophils or T cells. To understand some aspects of their pathogenesis the Gel and Coombs classification of hypersensitivity is a helpful albeit a loose framework.

TYPE 1 REACTIONS

Antigen attached to IgE bound to mast cells via Fc receptors results in release of preformed mediators of inflammation and the synthesis of metabolites of arachidonic acid via the cyclooxygenase and lipoxygenase pathways. The eosinophilia is the result of release of interleukins 4, 5, 9, and 13 produced by the T helper 2 (Th2) subclass of CD4 T cells. Urticarial vasculitis and the Churg–Strauss syndrome (also known as allergic granulomatosis and vasculitis) are examples.

TYPE 2 REACTIONS

The binding of circulating IgG or IgM antibody to an antigen on a cell membrane or on the extraarticular matrix can result in tissue damage by activating complement with phagocytosis of the antibody-bound cell by macrophages or by antibody-dependent cell-mediated cytotoxicity, mediated by killer cells. Alternatively, the antibody may activate the cell to which it is bound or it may bind to key molecules in blood, such as enzymes or enzyme inhibitors. The pauci-immune small vessel vasculitides in which antineutrophil cytoplasmic antibody (ANCA) is characteristic are examples. The ANCAs are directed against azurophilic granules, which contain mainly PR-3 and myeloperoxidase (MPO).[51] The ANCA-positive vasculitides are of four main types: Wegener granulomatosis, microscopic polyarteritis, Churg–Strauss syndrome, and idiopathic crescentic glomerulonephritis. They tend to be more common in men.

Wegener granulomatosis is characterized by chronic inflammation of the upper and lower respiratory tract, systemic necrotizing vasculitis, and a necrotizing crescentic glomerulonephritis. Forms of the disease limited to the respiratory tract are also described. It is typically associated with cytoplasmic staining ANCA pattern on immunofluorescence due to antibodies to PR-3, which is known to be proteolytic, microbicidal, can activate cytokines, and regulate hematopoiesis. Wegener granulomatosis appears to be more common in northern Europe and microscopic polyarteritis is more common in southern Europe.

Microscopic polyarteritis is associated with perinuclear ANCA staining pattern due to MPO antibodies. Myeloperoxidase is necessary to generate reactive oxygen species. Clinically it is characterized by lung and kidney disease but unlike Wegener granulomatosis in the lungs there is no granuloma formation but predominantly an alveolar capillaritis. Churg–Strauss syndrome is characterized initially by a history of asthma or allergy, an eosinophilia in blood and tissues and subsequently a systemic necrotizing vasculitis. Renal involvement is less common. The ANCAs are less frequent, occurring in 50–75 percent and when present are of anti-MPO specificity.

TYPE 3 REACTIONS

The presence of immune complexes deposited in the basement membrane of vessels mediates damage by activating complement and via the Fc receptor activating phagocytic cells. Henoch–Schönlein purpura, a small vessel vasculitis associated with IgA immune complexes, and the vasculitis associated with essential cryoglobulinemia often secondary to hepatitis C infection are examples.

TYPE 4 REACTIONS

Tissue injury resulting from sensitized T cells is the hallmark of type 4 hypersensitivity. The recognition that there are subsets of Th cells characterized by specific cytokine profiles provides a further understanding of how the immune system has evolved to deal with the variety of antigens it encounters. Granulomatous or cell-mediated immune responses are mediated by the cytokines interleukin-2, -3, TNF, and interferon, whereas if a predominantly humoral immune response is required the so-called Th2 cytokines, interleukin-4, -5, -10, and -13 operate. A predominant T cell infiltrate consisting of mainly CD4 positive cells is characteristic of giant cell arteritis and Takayasu arteritis, disorders primarily of the large arteries.[52]

Small–vessel vasculitis

Small-vessel vasculitis is defined as inflammation of vessels smaller than arteries – the arterioles, venules, and capillaries,

although involvement of the muscular arteries has been occasionally described.[53] It is often divided into ANCA-associated diseases (or pauci-immune vasculitis) of which microscopic polyarteritis or periarteritis (also referred to as microscopic polyangiitis) is the most frequent, and those due to immune complex deposition of which Henoch–Schönlein vasculitis and essential cryoglobulinemia are examples. The occurrence of multiorgan disease – most commonly skin, lung, renal, and neurologic disease – with marked constitutional features should lead to consideration of a small-vessel vasculitis.

The commonest skin manifestations are palpable purpura usually seen in the lower limbs, and urticaria. Vasculitic urticaria differs from the allergic form, tending to last longer than a day, can evolve into purpura, and there may be an associated hypocomplementemia. It is the result of immune complex deposition and complement activation. Small-vessel vasculitis may be confined to the skin when it characteristically involves the capillary venules and is referred to as a leuko-cytoclastic vasculitis. Drugs can be implicated in approximately 10 percent of such cases occurring between 7 and 21 days after exposure. In most, however, leuko-cytoclastic vasculitis usually heralds a systemic disorder – the presence of IgA immune complexes on biopsy suggests Henoch–Schönlein syndrome whereas ANCA in the serum suggests one of the three disorders associated with this antibody. A common neurologic feature is mononeuritis multiplex which is more frequent in the ANCA-related disorders; it is due to inflammation of the epineural arterioles resulting in nerve ischemia. Gastrointestinal features arise due to ischemic ulceration and are commoner in Henoch–Schönlein syndrome. Respiratory tract disease is a frequent manifestation of ANCA vasculitis and does not tend to occur in the immune complex disorders. Airway disease is a feature of Churg–Strauss syndrome and Wegener granulomatosis. Alveolar disease may present as fleeting infiltrates or less commonly interstitial fibrosis. Small vessel vasculitis and pulmonary hemorrhage are life-threatening features.

Medium–vessel vasculitis

Two disorders are included in this category: classic polyarteritis nodosa and Kawasaki disease. Classic polyarteritis nodosa is probably the disorder described by Kussmaul and Maier in 1866 – a seminal report in the study of vasculitis.[54] It is now recognized as a necrotizing inflammation of medium- and small-sized arteries without glomerulonephritis (but renal insufficiency or hypertension may occur due to renal infarcts due to vasculitis).[55] Clinical manifestations are similar to those of a small-vessel vasculitis but characteristically microaneurysms are found on angiography of the viscera. It is not associated with ANCAs but can be associated with hepatitis B infection although this association is on the decline. There is a rare variant confined to the skin.

Kawasaki disease was first described in 1967 in Japan.[56] It is disease predominantly of infants and children under 5 years of age, tending to be more common in boys. Although more common in children of oriental and Afro-Caribbean origin it has been described in most ethnic groups. An infective etiology is presumed. Histologically, inflammatory change is seen in large, medium and small arteries and there is an associated mucocutaneous syndrome. Cardiovascular complications occur in a third of children and coronary artery aneurysms are characteristic.

Large-vessel vasculitis

Two distinct clinical syndromes arise due to large vessel vasculitis – giant cell arteritis (temporal arteritis or granulomatous arteritis) and Takayasu disease. They differ from the other vasculitides not only in the size of vessel affected but more so because they are primarily T-cell-mediated diseases.[52] The infiltrate of macrophages and T cells affects all layers of the vessel wall but the initial site of injury seems to be the adventitia with primed T cells gaining access to the vessel through the vasa vasorum rather than the lumen.

Despite the similarities in the mechanism of damage between giant cell arteritis and Takayasu disease their manifestations differ. Giant cell arteritis is the most common primary vasculitis. It affects females more than males. In those over 50 years, the female to male ratio is 2:1. It is more common in those of northern European descent. Typical presentation is with symptoms in the distribution of one of the cranial arteries although internal and external carotid arteries can be affected. Characteristic symptoms are of headache with scalp tenderness, visual disturbance, and jaw claudication. An invariable feature of the disorder is a marked systemic inflammatory response characterized by constitutional symptoms and laboratory evidence of an acute phase response due to activation of both the innate and the adaptive immune response. Coexisting symptoms of polymyalgia rheumatica occur in between 40 percent and 50 percent.

In contrast Takayasu vasculitis (pulseless disease, aortic arch syndrome) affects a younger age group, classically women of oriental, African, Latin American and Eastern European extraction between the ages of 15 and 45.[57] The American College of Rheumatology classification criteria include: age of onset before the age of 40; upper and/or lower limb claudication; brachial artery pressure deficit of greater than 10 mm Hg; subclavian artery or aortic bruit and an abnormal or diagnostic angiogram. It is a chronic disease in which only small proportions achieve remission. The 15-year survival is 85 percent. The presence of retinopathy, hypertension, and aortic incompetence portend a poor prognosis. Four different variants of the disease are recognized: type I involves the ascending aorta, aortic arch, and arch vessels, with or without aneurysm formation; type II involves the thoracoabdominal aorta; type III involves the aortic arch and the thoracoabdominal aorta; and type IV involves the pulmonary arteries.

KEY LEARNING POINTS

- Vasculature in the autoimmune rheumatic disorders has a fundamental role in both pathogenesis and clinical presentation.
- Vasculitis presents in 1 percent of RA patients and is a marker of poorer outcome.
- In RA, vasculitis predominantly targets the microvasculature causing cutaneous and sensorimotor signs, but mononeuritis multiplex and less commonly visceral involvement can be seen.
- Rheumatoid arthritis may predispose to morbidity secondary to atheromatous disease by influencing traditional cardiovascular risk factors and also through more subtle mechanisms such as endothelial dysfunction.
- Better understanding of the molecular biology involved in leukocyte trafficking and angiogenesis may help to target therapies and RA.
- Systemic lupus erythematosus affects the vasculature in a number of ways: immune complex vasculitis, nonimmune complex complement-mediated vasculopathy, antiphospholipid antibody syndrome; and accelerated atherosclerosis.
- Of the primary vasculitides, each mediates damage via a characteristic mechanism (hypersensitivity class) and targets a particular vessel type.

REFERENCES

1 Van Doornum S, McColl G, Wicks IP. Accelerated atherosclerosis: an extraarticular feature of rheumatoid arthritis? *Arthritis Rheum* 2002; **46**: 862.

2 Manzi S, Meilahn EN, Rairie JE, *et al.* Age-specific incidence rates of myocardial infarction and angina in women with systemic lupus erythematosus: comparison with the Framingham study. *Am J Epidemiol* 1997; **145**: 408–15.

3 Watts RA, Lane SE, Bentham G, Scott DGI. Epidemiology of systemic rheumatoid vasculitis (SRV) – a ten year study. *Arthritis Rheum* 1999; **42**: S173–S174.

4 Older SA. The extra articular manifestations of rheumatoid arthritis. In: Fischbach M, ed. *Rheumatoid Arthritis*. New York: Churchill Livingstone,1991: 41–99.

5 Choy EH, Panayi GS. Cytokine pathways and joint inflammation in rheumatoid arthritis. *N Engl J Med* 2001; **344**: 907–16.

6 Frenette PS, Wagner DD. Adhesion molecules – Part II: Blood vessels and blood cells. *N Engl J Med* 1996; **335**: 43–5.

7 Koch AE. Angiogenesis as a target in rheumatoid arthritis. *Ann Rheum Dis* 2003; **62**: ii60–ii67.

8 Edwards JC. Synovial intimal fibroblasts. *Ann Rheum Dis* 1995; **54**: 395–7.

9 Madhok R, Wijelath E, Smith J, *et al.* Is the beneficial effect of sulfasalazine due to inhibition of synovial neovascularization? *J Rheumatol* 1999; **18**: 199–202.

10 Gabriel SE, Crowson CS, Kremers HM, *et al.* Survival in rheumatoid arthritis: a population-based analysis of trends over 40 years. *Arthritis Rheum* 2003; **48**: 54–8.

11 Wolfe F, Mitchell DM, Sibley JT, *et al.* The mortality of rheumatoid arthritis. *Arthritis Rheum* 1994; **37**: 481–94.

12 Solomon DH, Karlson EW, Rimm EB, *et al.* Cardiovascular mortality and mortality in women diagnosed with rheumatoid arthritis. *Circulation* 2003; **107**: 1303–7.

13 McEntegart A, Capell HA, Creran D, *et al.* Cardiovascular risk factors, including thrombotic variables, in a population with rheumatoid arthritis. *Rheumatology* 2001; **40**: 640–4.

14 Goodson N. Coronary artery disease and rheumatoid arthritis. *Curr Opin Rheumatol* 2002; **14**: 115–20.

15 Kumeda Y, Inaba M, Goto H, *et al.* Increased thickness of the arterial intima-media detected by ultrasonography in patients with rheumatoid arthritis. *Arthritis Rheum* 2002; **46**: 1489–97.

16 Wong M, Toh L, Wilson, A, *et al.* Arterial elasticity in rheumatoid arthritis and the relationship to vascular disease risk factors and inflammation. *Arthritis Rheum* 2003; **1**: 81–9.

17 Park YB, Lee SK, Lee WK, *et al.* Lipid profiles in untreated patients with rheumatoid arthritis. *J Rheumatol* 1999; **26**: 1701–4.

18 Hurt-Camejo E, Parades S, Masana L, *et al.* Elevated levels of small, low-density lipoprotein with high affinity for arterial matrix components in patients with rheumatoid arthritis: possible contribution of phospholipase A2 to this atherogenic profile. *Arthritis Rheum* 2001; **44**: 2761–7.

19 Wallace DJ, Metzger AL, Stecher VJ, *et al.* Cholesterol-lowering effect of hydroxychloroquine in patients with rheumatic disease: reversal of deleterious effects of steroids on lipids. *Am J Med* 1990; **89**: 322–6.

20 Munro R, Morrison E, McDonald, *et al.* Effect of disease-modifying agents on the lipid profiles of patients with rheumatoid arthritis. *Ann Rheum Dis* 1997; **56**:374–7.

21 Choi HK, Hernan MA, Seeger JD, *et al.* Methotrexate and mortality in patients with rheumatoid arthritis: a prospective study. *Lancet* 2002; **359**: 1173–7.

22 Harrison BJ. Influence of cigarette smoking on disease outcome in rheumatoid arthritis. *Curr Opin Rheumatol* 2002; **14**: 93–7.

23 Kroot EJ, van Gestel AM, Swinkels HL, *et al.* Chronic comorbidity in patients with early rheumatoid arthritis: a descriptive study. *J Rheumatol* 2001; **28**: 1511–17.

24 Johnson AG, Nguyen TV, Day RO. Do non-steroidal anti-inflammatory drugs affect blood pressure? A meta-analysis. *Ann Intern Med* 1994; **121**: 289–300.

25 Frishman WH. Effects of non-steroidal anti-inflammatory drug therapy on blood pressure and peripheral edema. *Am J Cardiol* 2002; **89**: 18D–25D.

26 Catella-Lawson F, Reilly MP, Kapoor SC, *et al.* Cyclooxygenase inhibitors and the antiplatelet effects of aspirin. *N Engl J Med* 2001; **345**: 1809–17.

27 Solomon DH. Selective cyclooxygenase 2 inhibitors and cardiovascular events. *Arthritis Rheum* 2005; **52**: 1968–78.

28 McAdam BF, Catella-Lawson F, Mardini IA, *et al.* Systemic biosynthesis of prostacyclin by cyclooxygenase (COX)-2: The human pharmacology of a selective inhibitor of COX-2. *Proc Natl Acad Sci U S A* 1999; **96**: 272–7.

29 Svenson KL, Pollare T, Lithell H, Hallgren, R. Impaired glucose handling in active rheumatoid arthritis: relationship to peripheral insulin resistance. *Metabolism* 1988; **7**: 125–30.

30 Corretti MC, Anderson TJ, Benjamin EJ, *et al.* Guidelines for the ultrasound assessment of endothelial-dependent flow-mediated vasodilation of the brachial artery: a report of the International Brachial Artery Reactivity Task Force. *J Am Coll Cardiol* 2003; **39**: 257–65.

31 Hurlimann D, Forster A, Noll G, *et al.* Anti-tumor necrosis factor-alpha treatment improves endothelial function in patients with rheumatoid arthritis. *Circulation* 2002; **106**: 2184–7.

32 Cambien B, Bergmeier W, Saffaripour S, *et al.* Antithrombotic activity of TNF-alpha. *J Clin Invest* 2002; **10**: 1589.

33 McCarey DW, McInnes IB, Madhok R, *et al.* Trial of Atorvastatin in Rheumatoid Arthritis (TARA): double-blind, randomised placebo-controlled trial. *Lancet* 2004; **363**: 2015–21.

34 Tan EM, Cohen AS, Fries JF, *et al.* The 1982 revised criteria for the classification of systemic lupus erythematosus. *Arthritis Rheum* 1982; **25**: 1271–7.

35 Walport MJ, Ross GD, Mackworth-Young C, *et al.* Family studies of erythrocyte complement receptor type 1 levels: reduced levels in patients with SLE are acquired, not inherited. *Clin Exp Immunol* 1985; **59**: 547–54.

36 Jacob HS, Craddock PR, Hammerschmidt DE, *et al.* Complement-induced granulocyte aggregation: an unsuspected mechanism of disease. *N Engl J Med* 1980; **302**: 789–94.

37 Wilson WA, Gharavi AE, Koike T, *et al.* International consensus statement on preliminary classification criteria for definite antiphospholipid syndrome: report of an international workshop. *Arthritis Rheum* 1999; **42**: 1309–11.

38 Svenungsson E, Jensen-Urstad K, Heimburger M. Risk factors for cardiovascular disease in systemic lupus erythematosus. *Circulation* 2001; **104**: 1887–93.

39 Urowitz MB, Bookman AA, Koehler BE, *et al.* The bimodal mortality pattern of systemic lupus erythematosus. *Am J Med* 1976; **60**: 221–5.

40 Ward MM, Pyun E, Studenski S. Causes of death in systemic lupus erythematosus. Long-term follow-up of an inception cohort. *Arthritis Rheum* 1995; **38**: 1492–9.

41 Sturfelt G, Eskilsson J, Nived O, *et al.* Cardiovascular disease in systemic lupus erythematosus. A study of 75

patients from a defined population. *Medicine (Baltimore)* 1992; **71**: 216–23.

42 Roman MJ, Shanker BA, David A, *et al.* Prevalence and correlates of accelerated atherosclerosis in systemic lupus erythematosus. *N Engl J Med* 2003; **349**: 2399–406.

43 Asanuma Y, Oeser A, Shintani AK, *et al.* Premature coronary-artery atherosclerosis in systemic lupus erythematosus. *N Engl J Med* 2003; **349**: 2407–15.

44 Reichlin M, Fesmire J, Quintero-Del-Rio AI, Wolfson-Reichlin M. Autoantibodies to lipoprotein lipase and dyslipidemia in systemic lupus erythematosus. *Arthritis Rheum* 2002; **46**: 2957–63.

45 Kao AH, Sabatine JM, Manzi, S. Update on vascular disease in systemic lupus erythematosus. *Curr Opin Rheumatol* 2003; **15**: 519–27.

46 Gallus AS, Hirsh, J. Antithrombotic drugs: part II. *Drugs* 1976; **12**: 132–57.

47 Antonov D, Kazandjieva J, Etugov D, *et al.* Drug-induced lupus erythematosus. *Clin Dermatol* 2004; **22**: 157–66.

48 Jennette JC, Falk RJ, Andrassy K. *et al.* Nomenclature of systemic vasculitides. Proposal of an international consensus conference. *Arthritis Rheum* 1994; **37**:187–92.

49 Guillevin L, Lhote F, Jarrousse, B, *et al.* Polyarteritis nodosa related to hepatitis B virus. A retrospective study of 66 patients. *Ann Med Interne (Paris)* 1992; **143**(Suppl 1): 63–74.

50 Pascual M, Perrin L, Giostra E, Schifferli JA. Hepatitis C virus in patients with cryoglobulinemia type II. *J Infect Dis* 1990; **162**: 569–70.

51 Gross WL. Antineutrophil cytoplasmic autoantibody testing in vasculitides. *Rheum Dis Clin North Am* 1995; **21**: 987.

52 Weyand CM, Goronzy JJ. Medium- and large-vessel vasculitis. *N Engl J Med* 2003; **349**: 160–9.

53 Jennette JC, Falk RJ. Small-vessel vasculitis. *N Engl J Med* 1997; **337**: 1512–23.

54 Kussmaul A, Maier K. Uber eine nicht bisher beschreibene eigenthumliche Arterienerkrankung (Periarteritis nodosa), die mit Morbus Brightii und rapid fortschreitender allgemeiner Muskelhamung einhergeht. *Dtsh Arch Klin Med* 1866; **1**: 484–518.

55 Stone JH. Polyarteritis nodosa. *JAMA* 2002; **288**: 1639.

56 Burns JC, Glode MP. Kawasaki syndrome. *Lancet* 2004; **364**: 533.

57 Johnston SL, Lock RJ, Gompels MM. Takayasu arteritis: a review. *J Clin Pathol* 2002; **55**: 481–6.

11

Anticoagulants in pregnancy

HUYEN TRAN, JEFFREY S GINSBERG

INTRODUCTION

Physiologic changes in hemostasis and fibrinolysis, altered blood flow, and venous stasis during pregnancy cause a hypercoagulable state. Venous thromboembolism (VTE), which includes pulmonary embolism (PE) and deep vein thrombosis (DVT), is a common cause of maternal morbidity and mortality in developed countries. Accordingly, the diagnosis, treatment, and prevention of VTE all pose clinically important challenges, because any intervention must take into account the potential for adverse experiences in both the mother and the fetus. Pregnant women with mechanical heart valves and native valvular heart disease can have systemic arterial thromboembolism, which can lead to a devastating outcome, such as a stroke. These women, particularly those with mechanical heart valves, are maintained on long-term warfarin therapy prior to conception, and throughout pregnancy they need effective, ongoing anticoagulation that will not adversely affect the fetus. Finally, antithrombotic therapy is indicated in some women with a past history of VTE to prevent recurrence and, more recently, for the prevention of recurrent pregnancy loss in some women with thrombophilia.

Morbidity and mortality resulting from arterial and venous thromboembolism can reduced by recognizing predisposing risk factors and selective use of antithrombotic therapy in high-risk patients. Although treatment of affected patients with anticoagulants is beneficial in preventing thromboembolism, all antithrombotic agents have the potential to cause bleeding, and individual agents have the potential to cause adverse effects that are drug or 'drug-class'

specific. In nonpregnant patients, anticoagulant therapy has been proved to be effective for the prevention of VTE, treatment of DVT, PE, and acute coronary syndromes; in patients undergoing cardiac surgery using cardiac bypass, vascular surgery, or coronary angioplasty; and in patients with mechanical heart valves or coronary stents. However, clinical trials examining the efficacy and safety of different anticoagulant drugs have excluded pregnant women. Therefore, recommendations regarding the use of anticoagulant therapy during pregnancy are largely based on extrapolation of data from nonpregnant patients, and from cohorts, case series and case reports of pregnant women. This chapter will provide an overview of the risks and benefits associated with the use of anticoagulants in pregnancy.

ANTICOAGULANT DRUGS

The antithrombotics *currently* available for the treatment and prevention of VTE and arterial thromboembolism during pregnancy include unfractionated heparin (UFH) and low-molecular-weight heparin (LMWH), heparinoids (danaparoid – no longer available in the UK and US), coumarin derivatives, and antiplatelet drugs, such as aspirin and clopidogrel.

Neither the catalytic factor Xa inhibitor, fondaparinux, nor the direct factor Xa, or direct thrombin inhibitors, such as hirudin, have been evaluated adequately in pregnancy. Hirudin crosses the placenta, has the potential to be teratogenic as well as anticoagulate the fetus, and fondaparinux may cross the placenta in small quantities.[1] Therefore, these drugs are not recommended for use during pregnancy, and will not be discussed further.

HEPARINS AND HEPARINOIDS

Because of their relatively large molecular size, their strong polarity and lipid insolubility, UFH,[2] LMWH, and danaparoid do not cross the placenta,[3–7] and therefore are safe for the fetus. However, the use of UFH and LMWH during pregnancy is problematic because it usually involves long-term parenteral administration of either of the two. LMWH is costly and both are inconvenient and painful, and are associated with bleeding, heparin-induced thrombocytopenia (HIT) and osteoporosis; the latter are less common with LMWH than UFH.

Heparins (UFH and LMWH) are the anticoagulants of choice during pregnancy for the treatment and prevention of VTE, as well as preventing recurrent fetal loss in women with thrombophilia. For an in-depth review on these topics, we direct the readers to Chapters 22 and 24.

Unfractionated heparin

Many studies of UFH in nonpregnant patients have elucidated concepts about the management of arterial and venous thrombosis. Although LMWH therapy has replaced UFH for many indications, it is still relevant to compare and contrast LMWH and UFH.

PHARMACOLOGY

Heparin is a heterogeneous group of molecules, which vary in molecular weight, anticoagulant activity, and pharmacokinetic properties. It is derived from porcine intestine and bovine lung.[8] The mean molecular weight of UFH is 15 000 D. Its anticoagulant activity varies because only approximately a third of heparin molecules contain the high-affinity pentasaccharide required for anticoagulant function.[9] It binds to heparin-neutralizing proteins, and its clearance is influenced by the chain length of the molecules; the higher molecular weight species are cleared from the circulation more rapidly than the lower molecular weight species.

The anticoagulant effect of heparin is mediated through binding of pentasaccharide-containing molecules to antithrombin, facilitating the inactivation of thrombin (factor IIa), and factors Xa, IXa, and XIIa. By inactivating thrombin, heparin not only prevents fibrin formation, but also inhibits thrombin-catalyzed activation of factors V and VIII.[10] At greater concentrations than those that are usually used clinically, UFH binds to heparin cofactor II, catalyzing its inactivation of thrombin. It also inhibits thrombin-related platelet function, contributing to its hemorrhagic potential.

Heparin clearance involves a combination of a rapid saturable and a much slower first order mechanism. The mechanism of the saturable phase of heparin clearance is through binding to receptors on endothelial cells and macrophages, where it is depolymerized, whereas the slower nonsaturable clearance mechanism is renal. When 'therapeutic' doses are given, heparin is cleared predominantly through the rapid, saturable dose-dependent mechanism and its anticoagulant effects are nonlinear with both the intensity and duration of effect rising disproportionately with increasing dose. With therapeutic intravenous (IV) doses of heparin, the half-life of UFH is approximately 60 minutes.

Unfractionated heparin should be administered parenterally, usually as a bolus IV dose followed by a continuous IV infusion. The efficacy of continuous IV heparin therapy depends on the starting dose; after an initial bolus dose of 5000 U, at least 30 000 U/day should be infused because lower doses result in higher recurrence rates.[11,12] The infusion should be adjusted to a therapeutic range using laboratory tests, because heparin has a narrow therapeutic window and patients vary in their responsiveness to it; some of the variability results from different plasma concentrations of heparin-binding proteins among patients, including histidine-rich glycoprotein, platelet factor 4, vitronectin, fibronectin, and von Willebrand factor.[13] These proteins bind to, and neutralize heparin. Chunilal and colleagues compared the anticoagulant response of UFH added *in vitro* to the plasma of pregnant women in the third trimester and nonpregnant women to determine if the measured activated partial thromboplastin time (aPTT) and anti-factor Xa levels were lower in pregnancy.[14] They reported that the aPTT response was attenuated in the plasma of pregnant women and was highly correlated with increased nonspecific plasma protein binding, as well as increased levels of factor VIII and fibrinogen. Therefore, in general, pregnant women need higher daily doses of UFH to achieve the same aPTT (and heparin level) as nonpregnant women; these higher doses might increase the risk of bleeding and osteoporosis if UFH dose adjustments during the third trimester are made utilizing a nonpregnant aPTT therapeutic range. Monitoring with anti-factor Xa heparin assays (target range 0.35–0.70 U/mL) results in less dose escalation than monitoring with aPTT.[15]

Provided sufficient starting doses are used (≥30 000 U/day) and therapeutic aPTT results are quickly achieved (within 48 hours), subcutaneous UFH administration is also effective.[16] A starting regimen of 17 500 IU 12 hourly is recommended with dose adjustments to maintain the aPTT within the therapeutic range.[17] Although effective, intermittent IV heparin causes excessive bleeding.[18]

MONITORING OF UFH IN PREGNANCY

Heparin should be monitored by measurement of the aPTT or heparin concentration, the latter measured using protamine sulfate titration assays or anti-factor Xa chromogenic assays. Plasma heparin concentrations of 0.2–0.4 U/mL by protamine sulfate titration are equivalent to concentrations of 0.35–0.70 U/mL by anti-factor Xa assays, both corresponding to the therapeutic range.[19] An aPTT ratio of 1.5–2.5 times control is often recommended as a target therapeutic range for UFH. The lower limit derives partly from results of a cohort study in which the recurrence rate was increased in UFH-treated patients with acute VTE whose aPTT results were below 1.5 times control compared with those whose aPTT results were above this cut-point.[19,20] However, over the past three decades, it has been shown that different aPTT reagents (and coagulometers) vary markedly in their sensitivities to UFH. Consequently, using fixed ratios of 1.5–2.5 times control reflects different plasma heparin concentrations from lab to lab.[21] Further, aPTT values of 1.5 times control consistently correspond to subtherapeutic heparin levels.[21] Ideally, to address this problem, the aPTT values equivalent to plasma heparin concentrations of 0.35–0.70 antifactor Xa units should be established for each reagent.

A subgroup analysis of a randomized controlled trial reported that patients with VTE who were treated with intravenous UFH and showed subtherapeutic aPTT values in the first 24 hours had a dramatic increase (15-fold) in recurrence rates.[19] However, since then, two overviews of clinical trials evaluating UFH regimens in patients with VTE in whom the starting infusion rates were over 30 000 U/day showed that the risk of recurrence was not significantly higher when the aPTT results were subtherapeutic in the first 24–48 hours than when they were not.[22,23] Therefore, the reported 15-fold increase in the risk of recurrence with early subtherapeutic results was undoubtedly an overestimate. Nevertheless, achieving therapeutic aPTT results quickly is desirable, because continual subtherapeutic results are likely to increase recurrence risk.

When initiating IV UFH, one of three approaches that simplify heparin administration by standardizing starting doses and using nomograms for dose adjustment should be used (Tables 11.1–11.3).[12,24,25]

Low-molecular-weight heparin

PHARMACOLOGY

The LMWHs are derived from heparin by enzymatic (for example, tinzaparin) or chemical (for example, dalteparin and enoxaparin) depolymerization of UFH. They have mean molecular weights of 4500–5000 D (range of 1000–10 000 D), one-third of the size of UFH. The pharmacokinetic, anticoagulant, and biologic differences between UFH and LMWH can be partly explained by a reduced interaction of LMWH with acute phase proteins in blood. Like UFH, LMWHs facilitate antithrombin's anticoagulant effect.[26] Compared with UFH, LMWH has reduced anti-factor IIa activity because the smaller fragments cannot bind simultaneously with antithrombin and thrombin to form ternary complexes, a necessary step in the efficient inhibition of thrombin by antithrombin. However, as bridging between antithrombin and factor Xa is not critical for anti-factor Xa activity, the smaller LMWH fragments inactivate factor Xa

Table 11.1 Published heparin dosing schemes 1: weight-based nomogram.[12] The initial dose was an 80 U/kg bolus followed by a starting infusion rate of 18 U/kg/h. aPTT was done every 6 hours and the heparin dose adjusted as shown

aPTT <35 s (<1.2 × control)	80 U/kg bolus, then increase infusion by 4 U/kg/h
aPTT 35–45 s (1.2 to 1.5 × control)	40 U/kg bolus, then increase infusion by 2 U/kg/h
aPTT 46–70 s (1.5 to 2.3 × control)	No change
aPTT 71–90 s (2.3 to 3 × control)	Decrease infusion rate by 2 U/kg/h
aPTT >90 s (>3 × control)	Hold infusion 1 h, then decrease infusion rate by 3 U/kg/h

aPTT, activated partial thromboplastin time.

Table 11.2 Published heparin dosing schemes 2: starting dose of 5000 U bolus followed by 1280 U/h[24]

aPTT	Bolus (U)	Hold (min)	Rate change (mL/h)*	Repeat aPTT
<50[†]	5000	0	+3	In 6 hours
50–59	0	0	+3	In 6 hours
60–85	0	0	0	Next morning
86–95	0	0	−2	Next morning
96–120	0	30	−2	In 6 hours
>120	0	60	−4	In 6 hours

*mL/h = 40 U/h
[†]If the aPTT (activated partial thromboplastin time) was subtherapeutic despite a heparin dose of 1440 U/h (36 mL/h) or greater at any time during the first 48 hours of therapy, the response to an aPTT of less than 50 seconds was a heparin bolus of 5000 U and a rate increase of 5 mL/h.

Table 11.3 Published heparin dosing schemes 3: intravenous heparin dose titration nomogram for aPTT starting dose = 5000 U bolus followed by 40 000 U/24 h (low bleeding risk) or 30 000 U/24 h (high bleeding risk)[25]

aPTT	Rate change (mL/h)	Dose change (U/24 h)	Additional action
IV infusion			
<45	+6	+5760	Repeat aPTT in 4–6 h
46–54	+3	+2880	Repeat aPTT in 4–6 h
55–85	0	0	None[†]
8–110	−3	−2880	Stop heparin for 1 h; repeat aPTT 4–6 h after restarting heparin treatment
>110	−6	−5760	Stop heparin for 1 h; repeat aPTT 4–6 h after restarting heparin treatment

*Heparin sodium concentration 20 000 U in 500 mL = 40 U/mL.
[†]During the first 24 hours, repeated aPTT 4–6 h. Thereafter, the aPTT will be determined once daily, unless therapeutic.

as well as larger molecules do. LMWH is cleared principally by the renal route, and its biologic half-life is prolonged in patients with renal failure.[27,28]

The LMWHs have several advantages over UFH during pregnancy. When given subcutaneously, their half-lives are longer and the antithrombotic dose responses are more predictable than UFH, allowing administration to patients in fixed, weight-adjusted doses without need for laboratory monitoring. They also cause less HIT and osteoporosis than UFH.[29,30] Several preparations of LMWH are available, and the use of any of them in weight-adjusted regimens is reasonable, as there is no convincing evidence that one is superior to another.[31] During pregnancy, the half-life of LMWH might be shorter compared with nonpregnant patients because of increased volume of distribution and increased renal blood flow which may lead to increased clearance of LMWH.[32] These physiologic changes are dynamic throughout pregnancy, and the pharmacokinetics might be trimester specific. Therefore, although once daily dosing is effective in nonpregnant patients, a twice-daily (12-hourly) dosage regimen might be preferred in pregnancy.[32,33]

In nonpregnant women, LMWH administered once or twice daily subcutaneously is at least as effective and safe as IV UFH for initial treatment of VTE.[28,34] A metaanalysis of trials, involving over 3000 nonpregnant patients, reported a risk reduction for recurrent VTE of about 15 percent in favor of LMWH and a risk reduction in major bleeding of about 40 percent ($P = 0.05$) also in favor of LMWH.[35] Similar studies comparing the efficacy and safety of twice-daily dosing regimens of LMWH with UFH in patients with unstable angina show short-term benefit.[36,37] Long-term LMWH therapy is as effective as warfarin in preventing recurrence following an acute episode of VTE.[38,39]

It is unknown if treatment doses of UFH and LMWH used in pregnant patients with VTE can be safely reduced following an initial period of full anticoagulation. In a randomized controlled trial of patients with VTE and contraindications to warfarin, enoxaparin, 5000 IU subcutaneously twice daily, was as effective as UFH, 10 000 IU subcutaneously twice daily in preventing recurrent VTE over 3–6 months of treatment.[30] In another randomized controlled trial of patients with cancer-related VTE, the dose of LMWH was safely reduced to 75 percent of the initial, weight-based dose after 1 month of treatment without an increased risk of recurrent VTE.[40] Since the risk of recurrent VTE among cancer patients likely outweighs that of pregnancy, adopting this strategy during pregnancy in patients with VTE on long-term anticoagulation seems reasonable, and might reduce the risk of bleeding. However, this regimen needs to be confirmed in a randomized clinical trial.

MONITORING OF LMWH IN PREGNANCY

Monitoring of LMWH therapy is usually unnecessary in nonpregnant patients, as several randomized trials have demonstrated their efficacy and safety when given in fixed weight-adjusted doses without monitoring.[34] However, pharmacokinetic studies and all randomized trials of LMWH have excluded pregnant patients (as well as morbidly obese patients [>130 kg], and patients with renal failure [or failed to specify whether such patients were recruited]). In pregnancy, the optimal dosing regimen of LMWH is a subject of debate.

Chromogenic anti-factor Xa assays are the most widely available and frequently used assays for LMWH monitoring. Although the anti-factor Xa level has shown to be inversely related to thrombus propagation in some studies,[41,42] the minimal therapeutic level has not been accurately defined. Similarly, anti-factor Xa level has not been demonstrated to be a good predictor of bleeding during treatment, although high anti-factor Xa levels at steady state in patients receiving therapeutic doses of LMWH have been associated with bleeding.[43,44] The usual time to measure the anti-factor Xa levels (if indicated) is 4 hours after subcutaneous injection of a weight-adjusted dose of LMWH. For twice-daily regimens, the current recommended therapeutic range in pregnancy is 0.5–1.0 IU/mL.[45,46] This is arbitrary and has been extrapolated from nonpregnant subjects. Some authorities consider an alternative range of 0.4–1.2 IU/mL during pregnancy appropriate.[47] In patients treated with LMWH once daily, the target range at 4 hours is less clear, but 1.0–2.0 IU/mL seems reasonable.[46] Although anti-factor Xa assays may provide some information about LMWH pharmacokinetics in individual patients, the above limitations of the information generated must be kept in mind. Nevertheless, when LMWH is administered to pregnant patients in therapeutic doses, it is prudent to monitor the anti-factor Xa levels periodically (monthly) to guide dosing, or change the dose intermittently according to weight.

Clinical observational studies have provided conflicting results.[48,49] Barbour and colleagues measured peak and trough levels of LMWH in 12 women who were receiving 'treatment' doses of dalteparin (100 U/kg) subcutaneously twice daily in 13 pregnancies at 2-weekly intervals.[48] Dosage adjustments were made to maintain peak anti-factor Xa levels between 0.5 IU/mL and 1.0 IU/mL. Eighty-five percent of pregnancies (11/13) required an upward dosage adjustment, and trough levels were in the 'therapeutic range' on only 9 percent of occasions; there were no bleeding complications or recurrent thromboembolic events. The authors concluded that twice-daily dalteparin dosing based on weight alone is inadequate to maintain most pregnant women in the therapeutic range during pregnancy as measured by anti-factor Xa levels. Contradicting these observations, Rodie and colleagues showed that no changes in the dosage of enoxaparin were needed when 'therapeutic' anticoagulation was given to 36 pregnant women with acute DVT based on early pregnancy weight.[49] In this study, no patients developed recurrent VTE. Therefore, until well-designed trials examining the impact of dose adjustment on clinical outcomes are performed, it is reasonable to dose LMWH during pregnancy according to weight, or anti-factor Xa levels can be measured periodically to guide dosing (see below).

There is concern regarding the effectiveness of heparin in preventing systemic embolism in pregnant women with mechanical heart valves. Treatment failures have been reported,[50–52] although many have been associated with inadequate dosing and/or use of an inappropriate therapeutic range.[53–56] Based on an undisclosed number of postmarketing reports of valvular thrombosis in patients receiving LMWH and the results of a very small randomized trial of pregnant women with mechanical heart valves, the manufacturer of enoxaparin has issued a warning about its safety in this clinical scenario.[57] This has led many to conclude that these agents should not be used in pregnant women with mechanical heart valves and has left clinicians in a quandary about what anticoagulant regimen is appropriate. However, given the inadequate doses and the small number of case reports, the true risk of failure with UFH and LMWH is unknown. Further, it is unclear if the risk is higher than that associated with warfarin adjusted to target an international normalized ratio (INR) between 2.5 and 3.5, especially if administered in high doses and aggressively monitored. A recent systematic review reported on 81 pregnancies in 75 women treated with LMWH for mechanical valves.[58] Valve thrombosis occurred in 8.64 percent (95 percent confidence interval [CI] 2.52 percent to 14.76 percent) and the overall thromboembolic complication rate was 12.35 percent (95 percent CI 5.19 percent to 19.51 percent). However, 9 of these 10 patients with thromboembolic complications had been treated with a fixed dose of LMWH and in 2 of these a fixed low dose of LMWH, suggesting that dosage may have been inadequate. In the 51 pregnancies where the anti-Xa levels were monitored and the LMWH dose adjusted, only one thromboembolic complication occurred. The frequency of live births was 87.65 percent (95 percent CI 80.49 percent to 94.81 percent).

Complications of heparin (UFH and LMWH) therapy in pregnancy

Maternal complications of heparin therapy in pregnancy include bleeding, HIT, and osteoporosis.

BLEEDING

Consistent with the rates of bleeding associated with heparin therapy in nonpregnant patients with DVT, a retrospective cohort study of 100 pregnant women receiving prophylactic or treatment doses of UFH reported a pooled major bleeding rate of 2 percent.[59] In a randomized controlled trial comparing adjusted-dose UFH and warfarin for prevention of recurrent VTE in patients with DVT, the major bleeding rate in patients receiving UFH was 1.8 percent.[60] A prospective cohort study of 33 pregnant women receiving enoxaparin as treatment for acute VTE reported no hemorrhagic complications,[49] while a retrospective study of 624 pregnant women receiving treatment or prophylactic doses of enoxaparin reported 1 case of major bleeding that was

attributed to anticoagulant therapy.[61] No bleeding was reported in a systematic review of 486 women receiving LMWH during pregnancy, although only 5 percent were receiving treatment doses.[3] A recent systematic review of over 2500 pregnancies treated with LMWH for prevention and treatment of thrombotic complications has also provided reassuring data with regard to bleeding risk.[62]

Reversal of anticoagulant effect of heparin

Protamine sulfate, a cationic protein derived from salmon sperm, can rapidly neutralize the anticoagulant effect of UFH. Protamine sulfate binds strongly to (anionic) heparin in a ratio of approximately 100 U UFH per mg; 50 mg is needed to counteract the anticoagulant effect of 5000 U of heparin given immediately as an intravenous bolus. When infused, only the heparin given during the preceding several hours should be included in the dose calculation since the half-life of heparin is approximately 60 minutes. About 30 mg of protamine sulfate is needed in a patient receiving an infusion of 1250 U/h. A prolonged infusion or repeated injections of protamine sulfate may be needed to neutralize a subcutaneous dose of heparin because plasma recovery of heparin following subcutaneous administration can be variable. A fall in aPTT can be used to confirm heparin neutralization. Protamine sulfate should be administered over 1–3 minutes to reduce the risk of severe adverse reactions, such as hypotension and bradycardia. Allergic reactions including anaphylaxis are associated with hypersensitivity to fish and previous exposure to protamine-sulfate-containing insulin. Protamine sulfate neutralizes the antithrombin activity of LMWH but incompletely neutralizes the anti-factor Xa activity.[63–65] The clinical impact of incomplete anti-factor Xa neutralization by protamine is unclear, and there have been no published studies, demonstrating or refuting a beneficial effect of protamine sulfate in patients with bleeding who have been treated with LMWH.

The American College of Chest Physicians (ACCP) guideline recommends the following when the antithrombotic effect of LMWH needs to be neutralized:[66]

- Within 8 hours of administration, protamine sulfate may be given in a dose of 1 mg per 100 anti-factor Xa units LMWH.
- If bleeding continues, a second dose of 0.5 mg protamine sulfate per 100 anti-factor Xa units may be given.
- Beyond 8 hours since the last injection of LMWH, smaller doses of protamine sulfate are needed.

HEPARIN–INDUCED THROMBOCYTOPENIA

Heparin-induced thrombocytopenia is an adverse reaction to heparin, which results in a transient hypercoagulable state and can cause venous and arterial thrombosis. The clinicopathologic syndrome of HIT is characterized usually by an unexplained fall in platelet count of greater than 50 percent (even if the nadir is $>150 \times 10^9$/L) with or without new thrombosis and a positive test for HIT antibodies. Heparin-induced thrombocytopenia occurs when heparin exposure causes formation of pathogenic antibodies (usually IgG class) that recognize multimolecular complexes of platelet factor 4 (PF-4) and heparin on platelet surfaces, and bind to platelet FcγIIa receptors, leading to *in vivo* platelet activation. Thrombin generation in patients with HIT results from procoagulant platelet-derived microparticles[67] and possibly by tissue factor exposed on endothelium and monocytes.[68] This explains the prothrombotic state that can be associated with venous and arterial thrombosis, and progression of DVT to gangrene in some patients with HIT who are treated with warfarin.[69] The frequency of HIT varies widely, depending on the type of heparin (UFH is more common than LMWH) and the patient population (surgical patients are more likely than medical and obstetric patients).[70] It has rarely been reported in pregnancy.[62,71] HIT antibodies are detected using either platelet 'activation' (functional) assays or PF-4 dependent 'antigen' assays,[72] including a rapid particle gel assay that utilizes PF-4 coated onto spheres.[73]

Isolated HIT has an unfavorable natural history; 25–50 percent of these patients develop thrombosis after stopping heparin (with or without warfarin replacement) and the risk of fatal thrombosis is 4–5 percent.[74–76] Therefore, in patients who are strongly suspected of having HIT, even when there is no clinically apparent thrombosis, all heparin therapy should be stopped and (usually) an alternative anticoagulant started and continued until the platelet count recovers. In pregnant women who develop HIT, danaparoid sodium (no longer available in the United States and United Kingdom) is recommended as it is an effective antithrombotic agent,[77,78] does not cross the placenta, and compared with LMWH has significantly less cross-reactivity with UFH[7] and therefore, is less likely to result in recurrent HIT. Fondaparinux, a novel anticoagulant with anti-factor Xa activity, is a potential alternative to danaparoid as treatment of HIT acquired in pregnancy, but more evidence is needed before definitive recommendations can be made. Lagrange and colleagues did not observe placental transfer of fondaparinux in an *ex vivo* model with the use of dually perfused human cotyledon.[79] However, a small (N = 5) case series reported that fondaparinux used in pregnant women who required ongoing anticoagulant therapy and were allergic to LMWH passed the placental barrier *in vivo*, resulting in measurable anti-factor Xa activity in the umbilical cord blood.[1]

HEPARIN–INDUCED OSTEOPOROSIS

Long-term (1 month or more) UFH therapy causes osteoporosis. Although the risk of fractures is low (2–3 percent),[80] a partially reversible reduction in bone density that might increase susceptibility to future fractures occurs in up to 30 percent of patients receiving long-term UFH.[81,82] There is accumulating evidence that the risk of osteoporosis is lower with LMWH than UFH.[30,83,84] In a randomized trial comparing UFH and dalteparin for thromboprophylaxis in pregnant women, bone mineral density in the lumbar spine for up to 3 years after delivery was measured. This was significantly lower in the UFH group when compared with both controls and dalteparin-treated women.[83] Density did not differ between healthy controls and the dalteparin group. Multiple logistic regression found that the type of heparin therapy was the only independent factor associated with reduced bone mass. A prospective cohort study involving 55 women treated with prophylactic dose LMWH throughout pregnancy reported that there was no significant difference in bone loss compared with physiologic loss in pregnancy.[85] In a systematic review of over 2500 women treated with LMWH during pregnancy there was only one case of osteoporotic fracture.[62] Therefore, it can be concluded that the risk of osteoporosis associated with prophylactic LMWH is negligible.

Danaparoid

Danaparoid is a low-molecular-weight heparinoid containing 84 percent heparan sulfate, 12 percent dermatan sulfate, and 4 percent chondroitin sulfate. It catalyzes the inactivation of factor Xa mediated by antithrombin and also exhibits some anti-factor IIa activity. Danaparoid does not cross the placenta,[6,7] nor is it secreted into breast milk.[86–88]

Danaparoid is given either subcutaneously or by continuous IV infusion. The peak anticoagulant effect after intravenous administration occurs within minutes; after subcutaneous injection, the peak anticoagulant effect is delayed and bioavailability is nearly 100 percent.[89] The half-life of the anti-factor Xa effect of danaparoid is 24.5 hours, whereas its antithrombin effect has a half-life of 4.3 hours.[89] Renal excretion accounts for 40–50 percent of plasma clearance of anti-factor Xa activity of danaparoid and hepatic disease does not affect its pharmacokinetics.[90] In nonpregnant patients, danaparoid significantly reduces the risk of both proximal DVT and total DVT when compared with UFH in patients with thrombotic stroke.[91] For treatment of patients with acute thrombosis, danaparoid was significantly more effective than IV UFH.[77] For therapy of isolated HIT with or without complicating thrombosis, an intravenous regimen has been used adjusted according to anti-factor Xa levels.[78] In pregnancy, danaparoid has been successfully used to manage women with HIT or allergies to UFH or LMWH.[7,87,88]

Laboratory monitoring is usually not necessary when danaparoid is administered subcutaneously, but its anticoagulant activity can be monitored using anti-factor Xa activity; a therapeutic level is similar to that required for LMWH (0.5–1.0 anti-factor Xa U/mL). Major or life-threatening bleeding in a patient who has received danaparoid is problematic because of its prolonged anti-factor Xa half-life. Protamine sulfate partially reverses the anti-factor IIa effect, but does not affect the anti-factor Xa anticoagulant activity.[92]

COUMARIN DERIVATIVES (WARFARIN)

The advantage of warfarin is that it can be taken orally. In nonpregnant patients, warfarin is highly effective in treating VTE (after an initial 5–10 days of UFH or LMWH) and is the drug of choice in patients with mechanical heart valves. However, in pregnancy, warfarin crosses the placenta, enters the fetal circulation and can cause teratogenicity and fetal bleeding (see below).[93] Warfarin has a prolonged anticoagulant effect, and its activity can only be rapidly reversed by using concentrates of clotting factors, although in nonpregnant women the administration of intravenous or oral vitamin K will achieve effective reversal within 24 hours.[94–100] Fresh frozen plasma can be given to rapidly restore the depleted clotting factors, especially in patients who bleed while receiving warfarin therapy, but is a blood product and carries some risk of viral transmission.[94,101] Recombinant activated Factor VII has been reported to stop life-threatening bleeding associated with oral anticoagulants in nonpregnant women, and it has been safely used in pregnant women with factor VII deficiency.[102–105]

Because of increasing blood volume and elevated levels of coagulation factors during pregnancy, warfarin requirements are likely to change constantly and more frequent INR monitoring and dose adjustments will be necessary compared with nonpregnant patients. Further, drugs which interact with warfarin will make its control more difficult and might increase the risk of bleeding in both mother and fetus.

Warfarin effects on the fetus

The effects on the fetus as a result of transplacental passage of warfarin in pregnancy include embryopathy, central nervous system (CNS) abnormalities, and fetal bleeding. Exposure to coumarin derivatives during the first trimester can result in chondrodysplasia punctata, a syndrome characterized by abnormal bone and cartilage formation, albeit warfarin is not the only cause. Skeletal abnormalities including skull abnormalities, radial deviation of the fingers, hypoplasia of terminal phalanges, and bradydactyly have been described with *in utero* warfarin exposure in the first trimester.[106] Warfarin-induced embryopathy consisting of nasal hypoplasia with or without epiphyseal stippling on radiography and hypertelorism can develop with warfarin exposure, although only between 6 and 12 weeks of gestation.[107,108] In a recent critical review of the literature, the estimated incidence of warfarin embryopathy associated with warfarin exposure between 6 and 12 weeks was less than 5 percent.[108] Further, follow-up studies of children born with warfarin embryopathy show that major morbidity was uncommon and most of these children developed normally[109,110] and the stippled epiphyses disappear with age.[111]

Abnormalities of the CNS (for example, eye abnormalities, agenesis of corpus callosum, and hydrocephalus) can develop after exposure during any trimester.[107,108] However, these outcomes are uncommon (<3 percent) and it is unknown if the incidence of CNS abnormalities is higher than in pregnancies not exposed to warfarin.[93,107] Numerous other associations have been reported including an increased risk of spontaneous abortion or prematurity, intrauterine growth restriction, transient hypotonia, seizures, persistent truncus arteriosus, hydrocephaly, macroglossia, Dandy–Walker malformation, abnormal urinary tract, and diaphragmatic hernia.[107,112] It remains to be seen whether warfarin causes any or these adverse experiences.

As coumarin derivatives cross the placenta, maternal use can cause an anticoagulant effect in the fetus and result in neonatal bleeding. Although this usually occurs when maternal warfarin control is poor, it has been described without apparent over-anticoagulation.[113] The concern about neonatal bleeding, which can be avoided by replacing warfarin with heparin in the last 2–4 weeks of pregnancy, is heightened during a traumatic delivery.

ANTIPLATELET DRUGS

Concerns regarding the use of aspirin during pregnancy include teratogenicity in the neonate and bleeding in the mother. In a metaanalysis and a large randomized controlled trial of pregnant women at high risk of pregnancy-induced hypertension or intrauterine growth retardation comparing low-dose aspirin (60–150 mg daily) with placebo, aspirin was safe for the fetus and mother if taken during the second and third trimesters. In particular, there were no significant effects on either fetal or maternal bleeding, or fetal ductus arteriosus flow.[114,115] The safety of use during the first trimester or of high-dose aspirin remains uncertain. The safety of clopidogrel in pregnancy is unknown. Although studies in rats and rabbits suggest no fetal toxicity, no human trials have been performed. We identified only a single case report of a patient with essential thrombocythemia who had a successful pregnancy outcome while taking clopidogrel.[116]

During pregnancy, aspirin can be combined with anticoagulant drugs to prevent pregnancy complications in women with antiphospholipid antibody syndrome[117] or other (inherited) thrombophilia with previous pregnancy complications, as well as to reduce the risk of thrombosis in high-risk women (for example, previous systemic embolism) with mechanical heart valves, bearing in mind the slight increase risk of bleeding.[118]

ANTICOAGULANT THERAPY AND BREASTFEEDING

The heparins, UFH and LMWH, can be safely prescribed to breastfeeding mothers since they cannot be absorbed via the gastrointestinal tract and they are not secreted into the breast milk.[119] Warfarin is also safe when taken by nursing mothers who require postpartum anticoagulation given that it does not induce an anticoagulant effect in the breastfed baby.[120–122]

PREGNANT WOMEN WITH MECHANICAL HEART VALVES

Anticoagulant therapy in women with mechanical heart valves during pregnancy remains controversial.[123] Some experts recommend the use of warfarin throughout pregnancy since they believe that the risk of warfarin-induced embryopathy is overstated, and in view of reported cases of valvular thrombosis associated with heparin use. From evidence outlined above, it is highly likely that warfarin therapy in pregnancy when used before 6 weeks of gestation and beyond 12 weeks until just before ($\geq$2 weeks) delivery is safe. However, these regimens are usually avoided in North America as the package insert indicates that warfarin is contraindicated in pregnancy.[124] All of these factors create a high-risk pregnancy, which is difficult to manage. In their reproductive years, women with mechanical heart valves should be intensively and explicitly educated about the potential dangers of their cardiac condition and possible risks of anticoagulation during pregnancy for themselves and their baby. Although it is hazardous and inconvenient for a woman to change to therapeutic heparin therapy prior to pregnancy while trying to conceive, the importance of early reporting of suspected pregnancy should be emphasized so that the switch from warfarin to therapeutic heparin can be made before 6 weeks of gestation to reduce the risk of warfarin-induced embryopathy. Some women might find this strategy unacceptable no matter how small the risk of warfarin-induced embryopathy and will prefer to have their warfarin treatment switched to heparin before attempting conception.

The ACCP guidelines suggest three strategies for women with mechanical heart valve who contemplate pregnancy:[33]

- Substitute warfarin with UFH or LMWH between 6 and 12 weeks, and at least 2 weeks before delivery, and use warfarin during the other times
- Adjusted-weight UFH, administered 12-hourly to maintain the mid interval aPTT at least two times control or anti-factor heparin Xa level between 0.35 IU/mL and 0.70 IU/mL
- Twice daily LMWH throughout pregnancy in doses adjusted according to weight or to keep a 4-hour postinjection anti-factor Xa heparin level at approximately 1.0–1.2 IU/mL

In women with mechanical heart valves at high risk of thromboembolism, low-dose aspirin, 75–162 mg, daily can be added. Long-term warfarin should be resumed postpartum with all regimens, and mothers can breastfeed as there is no hemostatic risk to the infant. For an in-depth review of women with heart disease and mechanical heart valves, we direct the reader to Chapter 25.

CONCLUSIONS

During pregnancy, anticoagulant therapy is indicated for a variety of conditions. Coumarin derivatives are teratogenic, although the true risk of embryopathy and CNS abnormalities is unknown, and probably low. The long-term risk of skeletal development in children born to mothers exposed to warfarin during pregnancy, particularly beyond the first trimester is low. It is most likely that warfarin exposure during pregnancy in the first 6 weeks, and beyond 12 weeks of gestation until just prior to delivery (2–4 weeks) is safe. Fetal and maternal perinatal hemorrhage can be avoided by substituting warfarin with heparin for at least 2 weeks before planned delivery. However, the use of warfarin during pregnancy can have medicolegal implications.

Although UFH and LMWH are the anticoagulants of choice to prevent and manage acute VTE during pregnancy, concerns regarding their effectiveness in preventing systemic embolization in pregnant women with mechanical heart valves have been raised, and might be attributed to insufficient dosing. Properly designed clinical trials to determine the optimal antithrombotic therapy in pregnant women with mechanical heart valves need to be performed before definitive recommendations can be made. Aspirin is safe during the second and third trimesters of pregnancy; clopidogrel has not been adequately studied in pregnancy.

KEY LEARNING POINTS

- Heparin derivatives can be used safely throughout pregnancy, with LMWH being the drug of choice in most women.
- Warfarin is teratogenic, although the true risk of embryopathy and CNS abnormalities is unknown, and probably low.
- The optimal anticoagulant therapy regimen in patients with mechanical heart valves during pregnancy remains controversial.
- Mothers can safely breastfeed while receiving heparin derivatives or warfarin.
- Aspirin can be safely used during the second and third trimester of pregnancy.

REFERENCES

1 Dempfle CE. Minor transplacental passage of fondaparinux in vivo. *N Engl J Med* 2004; **350**: 1914–15.
2 Flessa HC, Kapstrom AB, Glueck HI, Will JJ. Placental transport of heparin. *Am J Obstet Gynecol* 1965; **93**: 570–3.
3 Sanson BJ, Lensing AW, Prins MH, *et al.* Safety of low-molecular-weight heparin in pregnancy: a systematic review. *Thromb Haemost* 1999; **81**: 668–72.

4 Forestier F, Daffos F, Capella-Pavlovsky M. Low molecular weight heparin (PK 10169) does not cross the placenta during the second trimester of pregnancy study by direct fetal blood sampling under ultrasound. *Thromb Res* 1984; **34**: 557-60.

5 Forestier F, Daffos F, Rainaut M, Toulemonde F. Low molecular weight heparin (CY 216) does not cross the placenta during the third trimester of pregnancy. *Thromb Haemost* 1987; **57**: 234.

6 Greinacher A, Eckhardt T, Mussmann J, Mueller-Eckhardt C. Pregnancy complicated by heparin associated thrombo-cytopenia: management by a prospectively *in vitro* selected heparinoid (Org 10172). *Thromb Res* 1993; **71**: 123-6.

7 Magnani HN. Heparin-induced thrombocytopenia (HIT): an overview of 230 patients treated with orgaran (Org 10172). *Thromb Haemost* 1993; **70**: 554-61.

8 Warda M, Gouda EM, Toida T, *et al.* Isolation and characterization of raw heparin from dromedary intestine: evaluation of a new source of pharmaceutical heparin. *Comp Biochem Physiol C Toxicol Pharmacol* 2003; **136**: 357-65.

9 Anderson LO, Barrowcliffe TW, Holmer MK. Anticoagulant properties of heparin fractionated by affinity chromato-graphy on matrix-bound antithrombin III and by gel filtration. *Thromb Res* 1976; **9**: 575-83.

10 Ofosu FA, Sie P, Modi GJ, *et al.* The inhibition of thrombin-dependent positive-feedback reactions is critical to the expression of the anticoagulant effect of heparin. *Biochem J* 1987; **243**: 579-88.

11 Brandjes DP, Heijboer H, Buller HR, *et al.* Acenocoumarol and heparin compared with acenocoumarol alone in the initial treatment of proximal-vein thrombosis. *N Engl J Med* 1992; **327**: 1485-9.

12 Raschke RA, Reilly BM, Guidry JR, *et al.* The weight-based heparin dosing nomogram compared with a 'standard care' nomogram. A randomized controlled trial. *Ann Intern Med* 1993; **119**: 874-81.

13 Young E, Prins M, Levine MN, Hirsh J. Heparin binding to plasma proteins, an important mechanism for heparin resistance. *Thromb Haemost* 1992; **67**: 639-43.

14 Chunilal SD, Young E, Johnston MA, *et al.* The APTT response of pregnant plasma to unfractionated heparin. *Thromb Haemost* 2002; **87**: 92-7.

15 Levine MN, Hirsh J, Gent M, *et al.* A randomized trial comparing activated thromboplastin time with heparin assay in patients with acute venous thromboembolism requiring large daily doses of heparin. *Arch Intern Med* 1994; **154**: 49-56.

16 Hommes DW, Bura A, Mazzolai L, *et al.* Subcutaneous heparin compared with continuous intravenous heparin administration in the initial treatment of deep vein thrombosis. A meta-analysis. *Ann Intern Med* 1992; **116**: 279-84.

17 Buller HR, Agnelli G, Hull RD, *et al.* Antithrombotic therapy for venous thromboembolic disease: the Seventh ACCP Conference on Antithrombotic and Thrombolytic Therapy. *Chest* 2004; **126**(3 Suppl): 401S-428S.

18 Levine MN, Raskob G, Landefeld S, Hirsh J. Hemorrhagic complications of anticoagulant treatment. *Chest* 1995; **108**(4 Suppl): 276S-290S.

19 Hull RD, Raskob GE, Hirsh J, *et al.* Continuous intravenous heparin compared with intermittent subcutaneous heparin in the initial treatment of proximal-vein thrombosis. *N Engl J Med* 1986; **315**: 1109-14.

20 Basu D, Gallus A, Hirsh J, Cade J. A prospective study of the value of monitoring heparin treatment with the activated partial thromboplastin time. *N Engl J Med* 1972; **287**: 324-7.

21 Brill-Edwards P, Ginsberg JS, Johnston M, Hirsh J. Establishing a therapeutic range for heparin therapy. *Ann Intern Med* 1993; **119**: 104-9.

22 Anand S, Ginsberg JS, Kearon C, *et al.* The relation between the activated partial thromboplastin time response and recurrence in patients with venous thrombosis treated with continuous intravenous heparin. *Arch Intern Med* 1996; **156**: 1677-81.

23 Anand SS, Bates S, Ginsberg JS, *et al.* Recurrent venous thrombosis and heparin therapy: an evaluation of the importance of early activated partial thromboplastin times. *Arch Intern Med* 1999; **159**: 2029-32.

24 Cruickshank MK, Levine MN, Hirsh J, *et al.* A standard heparin nomogram for the management of heparin therapy. *Arch Intern Med* 1991; **151**: 333-7.

25 Hull RD, Raskob GE, Rosenbloom D, *et al.* Optimal therapeutic level of heparin therapy in patients with venous thrombosis. *Arch Intern Med* 1992; **152**: 1589-95.

26 Casu B, Oreste P, Torri G, *et al.* The structure of heparin oligosaccharide fragments with high anti-(factor Xa) activity containing the minimal antithrombin III-binding sequence. Chemical and 13C nuclear-magnetic-resonance studies. *Biochem J* 1981; **197**: 599-609.

27 Palm M, Mattsson C. Pharmacokinetics of heparin and low molecular weight heparin fragment (Fragmin) in rabbits with impaired renal or metabolic clearance. *Thromb Haemost* 1987; **58**: 932-5.

28 Siragusa S, Cosmi B, Piovella F, *et al.* Low-molecular-weight heparins and unfractionated heparin in the treatment of patients with acute venous thromboembolism: results of a meta-analysis. *Am J Med* 1996; **100**: 269-77.

29 Warkentin TE, Levine MN, Hirsh J, *et al.* Heparin-induced thrombocytopenia in patients treated with low-molecular-weight heparin or unfractionated heparin. *N Engl J Med* 1995; **332**: 1330-5.

30 Monreal M, Lafoz E, Olive A, *et al.* Comparison of subcutaneous unfractionated heparin with a low molecular weight heparin (Fragmin) in patients with venous thromboembolism and contraindications to coumarin. *Thromb Haemost* 1994; **71**: 7-11.

31 Dolovich LR, Ginsberg JS, Douketis JD, *et al.* A meta-analysis comparing low-molecular-weight heparins with unfractionated heparin in the treatment of venous thromboembolism: examining some unanswered questions regarding location of treatment, product type,

and dosing frequency. *Arch Intern Med* 2000; **160**: 181–8.

32 Casele HL, Laifer SA, Woelkers DA, Venkataramanan R. Changes in the pharmacokinetics of the low-molecular-weight heparin enoxaparin sodium during pregnancy. *Am J Obstet Gynecol* 1999; **181**(5 Pt 1): 1113–17.

33 Bates SM, Greer IA, Hirsh J, Ginsberg JS. Use of antithrombotic agents during pregnancy: the Seventh ACCP Conference on Antithrombotic and Thrombolytic Therapy. *Chest* 2004; **126**(3 Suppl): 627S–644S.

34 Lensing AW, Prins MH, Davidson BL, Hirsh J. Treatment of deep venous thrombosis with low-molecular-weight heparins. A meta-analysis. *Arch Intern Med* 1995; **155**: 601–7.

35 Gould MK, Dembitzer AD, Doyle RL, *et al.* Low-molecular-weight heparins compared with unfractionated heparin for treatment of acute deep venous thrombosis. A meta-analysis of randomized, controlled trials. *Ann Intern Med* 1999; **130**: 800–9.

36 Cohen M, Demers C, Gurfinkel EP, *et al.* A comparison of low-molecular-weight heparin with unfractionated heparin for unstable coronary artery disease. Efficacy and Safety of Subcutaneous Enoxaparin in Non-Q-Wave Coronary Events Study Group. *N Engl J Med* 1997; **337**: 447–52.

37 Klein W, Buchwald A, Hillis SE, *et al.* Comparison of low-molecular-weight heparin with unfractionated heparin acutely and with placebo for 6 weeks in the management of unstable coronary artery disease. Fragmin in unstable coronary artery disease study (FRIC). *Circulation* 1997; **96**: 61–8.

38 Pini M, Aiello S, Manotti C, *et al.* Low-molecular-weight heparin versus warfarin in the prevention of recurrences after deep vein thrombosis. *Thromb Haemost* 1994; **72**: 191–7.

39 Lopaciuk S, Bielska-Falda H, Noszczyk W, *et al.* Low-molecular-weight heparin versus acenocoumarol in the secondary prophylaxis of deep vein thrombosis. *Thromb Haemost* 1999; **81**: 26–31.

40 Lee AY, Levine MN, Baker RI, *et al.* Low-molecular-weight heparin versus a coumarin for the prevention of recurrent venous thromboembolism in patients with cancer. *N Engl J Med* 2003; **349**: 146–53.

41 Levine MN, Planes A, Hirsh J, *et al.* The relationship between anti-factor Xa level and clinical outcome in patients receiving enoxaparine low-molecular-weight heparin to prevent deep vein thrombosis after hip replacement. *Thromb Haemost* 1989; **62**: 940–4.

42 Alhenc-Gelas M, Jestin-Le Guernic C, Vitoux JF, *et al.* Adjusted versus fixed doses of the low-molecular-weight heparin fragmin in the treatment of deep vein thrombosis. Fragmin-Study Group. *Thromb Haemost* 1994; **71**: 698–702.

43 Albada J, Nieuwenhuis HK, Sixma JJ. Treatment of acute venous thromboembolism with low-molecular-weight heparin (Fragmin). Results of a double-blind randomized study. *Circulation* 1989; **80**: 935–40.

44 Nieuwenhuis HK, Albada J, Banga JD, Sixma JJ. Identification of risk factors for bleeding during treatment of acute venous thromboembolism with heparin or low-molecular-weight heparin. *Blood* 1991; **78**: 2337–43.

45 Abbate R, Gori AM, Farsi A, *et al.* Monitoring of low-molecular-weight heparins in cardiovascular disease. *Am J Cardiol* 1998; **82**(5B): 33L–36L.

46 Laposata M, Green D, Van Cott EM, *et al.* College of American Pathologists Conference XXXI on laboratory monitoring of anticoagulant therapy: the clinical use and laboratory monitoring of low-molecular-weight heparin, danaparoid, hirudin and related compounds, and argatroban. *Arch Pathol Lab Med* 1998; **122**: 799–807.

47 Thomson AJ, Greer IA. *Thromboembolic Disease in Pregnancy and the Puerperium: Acute Management.* London: RCOG Press, 2001.

48 Barbour LA, Oja JL, Schultz LK. A prospective trial that demonstrates that dalteparin requirements increase in pregnancy to maintain therapeutic levels of anticoagulation. *Am J Obstet Gynecol* 2004; **191**: 1024–9.

49 Rodie VA, Thomson AJ, Stewart FM, *et al.* Low-molecular-weight heparin for the treatment of venous thromboembolism in pregnancy: a case series. *Br J Obstet Gynaecol* 2002; **109**: 1020–4.

50 Roberts N, Ross D, Flint SK, *et al.* Thromboembolism in pregnant women with mechanical prosthetic heart valves anticoagulated with low-molecular-weight heparin. *Br J Obstet Gynaecol* 2001; **108**: 327–9.

51 Leyh RG, Fischer S, Ruhparwar A, Haverich A. Anticoagulation for prosthetic heart valves during pregnancy: is low-molecular-weight heparin an alternative? *Eur J Cardiothorac Surg* 2002; **21**: 577–9.

52 Mahesh B, Evans S, Bryan AJ. Failure of low-molecular-weight heparin in the prevention of prosthetic mitral valve thrombosis during pregnancy: case report and a review of options for anticoagulation. *J Heart Valve Dis* 2002; **11**: 745–50.

53 Sbarouni E, Oakley CM. Outcome of pregnancy in women with valve prostheses. *Br Heart J* 1994; **71**: 196–201.

54 Hurwitz A, Milwidsky A, Medina A, Yagel S. Failure of continuous intravenous heparinization to prevent stroke in a pregnant woman with a prosthetic valve and atrial fibrillation. A case report. *J Reprod Med* 1985; **30**: 618–20.

55 Watson WJ, Freeman J, O'Brien C, Benson M. Embolic stroke in a pregnant patient with a mechanical heart valve on optimal heparin therapy. *Am J Perinatol* 1996; **13**: 371–2.

56 Golby AJ, Bush EC, DeRook FA, Albers GW. Failure of high-dose heparin to prevent recurrent cardioembolic strokes in a pregnant patient with a mechanical heart valve. *Neurology* 1992; **42**: 2204–6.

57 Aventis Pharmaceuticals, assignee. Lovenox Injection (package insert), 2004.

58 Oran B, Lee-Parritz A, Ansell J. Low-molecular-weight heparin for the prophylaxis of thromboembolism in

women with prosthetic mechanical heart valves during pregnancy. *Thromb Haemost* 2004; **92**: 747–51.

59   Ginsberg JS, Kowalchuk G, Hirsh J, *et al.* Heparin therapy during pregnancy. Risks to the fetus and mother. *Arch Intern Med* 1989; **149**: 2233–6.

60   Hull R, Delmore T, Carter C, *et al.* Adjusted subcutaneous heparin versus warfarin sodium in the long-term treatment of venous thrombosis. *N Engl J Med* 1982; **306**: 189–94.

61   Lepercq J, Conard J, Borel-Derlon A, *et al.* Venous thromboembolism during pregnancy: a retrospective study of enoxaparin safety in 624 pregnancies. *Br J Obstet Gynaecol* 2001; **108**: 1134–40.

62   Greer IA, Nelson Piercy C. Low-molecular-weight heparins for thromboprophylaxis and treatment of venous thromboembolism in pregnancy: a systematic review of safety and efficacy. *Blood* 2005; **106**: 401–7.

63   Gram J, Mercker S, Bruhn HD. Does protamine chloride neutralize low molecular weight heparin sufficiently? *Thromb Res* 1988; **52**: 353–9.

64   Sugiyama T, Itoh M, Ohtawa M, Natsuga T. Study on neutralization of low-molecular-weight heparin (LHG) by protamine sulfate and its neutralization characteristics. *Thromb Res* 1992; **68**: 119–29.

65   Wolzt M, Weltermann A, Nieszpaur-Los M, *et al.* Studies on the neutralizing effects of protamine on unfractionated and low-molecular-weight heparin (Fragmin) at the site of activation of the coagulation system in man. *Thromb Haemost* 1995; **73**: 439–43.

66   Hirsh J, Raschke R. Heparin and low-molecular-weight heparin: the Seventh ACCP Conference on Antithrombotic and Thrombolytic Therapy. *Chest* 2004; **126** (3 Suppl): 188S–203S.

67   Warkentin TE, Sheppard JI. Generation of platelet-derived microparticles and procoagulant activity by heparin-induced thrombocytopenia IgG/serum and other IgG platelet agonists: a comparison with standard platelet agonists. *Platelets* 1999; **10**: 319–26.

68   Pouplard C, Iochmann S, Renard B, *et al.* Induction of monocyte tissue factor expression by antibodies to heparin-platelet factor 4 complexes developed in heparin-induced thrombocytopenia. *Blood* 2001; **97**: 3300–2.

69   Warkentin TE, Elavathil LJ, Hayward CP, *et al.* The pathogenesis of venous limb gangrene associated with heparin-induced thrombocytopenia. *Ann Intern Med* 1997; **127**: 804–12.

70   Warkentin TE, Sheppard JA, Horsewood P, *et al.* Impact of the patient population on the risk for heparin-induced thrombocytopenia. *Blood* 2000; **96**: 1703–8.

71   Warkentin TE, Greinacher A, eds. *Heparin-Induced Thrombocytopenia,* 2nd ed. New York: Marcel Dekker, 2001.

72   Warkentin TE. Platelet count monitoring and laboratory testing for heparin-induced thrombocytopenia. *Arch Pathol Lab Med* 2002; **126**: 1415–23.

73   Eichler P, Raschke R, Lubenow N, *et al.* The new ID-heparin/PF4 antibody test for rapid detection of

heparin-induced antibodies in comparison with functional and antigenic assays. *Br J Haematol* 2002; **116**: 887–91.

74   Warkentin TE. Heparin-induced thrombocytopenia: pathogenesis and management. *Br J Haematol* 2003; **121**: 535–55.

75   Warkentin TE, Kelton JG. A 14-year study of heparin-induced thrombocytopenia. *Am J Med* 1996; **101**: 502–7.

76   Wallis DE, Quintos R, Wehrmacher W, Messmore H. Safety of warfarin anticoagulation in patients with heparin-induced thrombocytopenia. *Chest* 1999; **116**: 1333–8.

77   de Valk HW, Banga JD, Wester JW, *et al.* Comparing subcutaneous danaparoid with intravenous unfractionated heparin for the treatment of venous thromboembolism. A randomized controlled trial. *Ann Intern Med* 1995; **123**: 1–9.

78   Farner B, Eichler P, Kroll H, Greinacher A. A comparison of danaparoid and lepirudin in heparin-induced thrombocytopenia. *Thromb Haemost* 2001; **85**: 950–7.

79   Lagrange F, Vergnes C, Brun JL, *et al.* Absence of placental transfer of pentasaccharide (Fondaparinux, Arixtra) in the dually perfused human cotyledon *in vitro. Thromb Haemost* 2002; **87**: 831–5.

80   Dahlman TC. Osteoporotic fractures and the recurrence of thromboembolism during pregnancy and the puerperium in 184 women undergoing thromboprophylaxis with heparin. *Am J Obstet Gynecol* 1993; **168**: 1265–70.

81   Douketis JD, Ginsberg JS, Burrows RF, *et al.* The effects of long-term heparin therapy during pregnancy on bone density. A prospective matched cohort study. *Thromb Haemost* 1996; **75**: 254–7.

82   Barbour LA, Kick SD, Steiner JF, *et al.* A prospective study of heparin-induced osteoporosis in pregnancy using bone densitometry. *Am J Obstet Gynecol* 1994; **170**: 862–9.

83   Pettila V, Leinonen P, Markkola A, *et al.* Postpartum bone mineral density in women treated for thromboprophylaxis with unfractionated heparin or LMW heparin. *Thromb Haemost* 2002; **87**: 182–6.

84   Muir JM, Hirsh J, Weitz JI, *et al.* A histomorphometric comparison of the effects of heparin and low-molecular-weight heparin on cancellous bone in rats. *Blood* 1997; **89**: 3236–42.

85   Carlin AJ, Farquharson RG, Quenby SM, *et al.* Prospective observational study of bone mineral density during pregnancy: low-molecular-weight heparin versus control. *Hum Reprod* 2004; **19**: 1211–14.

86   Schindewolf M, Mosch G, Bauersachs RM, Lindhoff-Last E. Safe anticoagulation with danaparoid in pregnancy and lactation. *Thromb Haemost* 2004; **92**: 211.

87   Harrison SJ, Rafferty I, McColl MD. Management of heparin allergy during pregnancy with danaparoid. *Blood Coagul Fibrinolysis* 2001; **12**: 157–9.

88   Lindhoff-Last E, Kreutzenbeck HJ, Magnani HN. Treatment of 51 pregnancies with danaparoid because of heparin intolerance. *Thromb Haemost* 2005; **93**: 63–9.

89   Danhof M, de Boer A, Magnani HN, Stiekema JC. Pharmacokinetic considerations on Orgaran (Org 10172) therapy. *Haemostasis* 1992; **22**: 73–84.

90 De Boer A, Stiekema JC, Danhof M, Breimer DD. The influence of Org 10172, a low molecular weight heparinoid, on antipyrine metabolism and the effect of enzyme induction on the response to Org 10172. *Br J Clin Pharmacol* 1991; **32**: 23–9.

91 Turpie AG, Levine MN, Hirsh J, *et al.* Double-blind randomised trial of Org 10172 low-molecular-weight heparinoid in prevention of deep-vein thrombosis in thrombotic stroke. *Lancet* 1987; **1**: 523–6.

92 Stiekema JC, Wijnand HP, ten Cate H, *et al.* Partial *in vivo* neutralisation of plasma anticoagulant effects of Lomoparan (Org 10172) by protamine chloride. *Thromb Res* 1991; **63**: 157–67.

93 Ginsberg JS, Hirsh J, Turner DC, *et al.* Risks to the fetus of anticoagulant therapy during pregnancy. *Thromb Haemost* 1989; **61**: 197–203.

94 Shetty HG, Backhouse G, Bentley DP, Routledge PA. Effective reversal of warfarin-induced excessive anticoagulation with low dose vitamin K1. *Thromb Haemost* 1992; **67**: 13–15.

95 Andersen P, Godal HC. Predictable reduction in anticoagulant activity of warfarin by small amounts of vitamin K. *Acta Med Scand* 1975; **198**: 269–70.

96 Crowther MA, Douketis JD, Schnurr T, *et al.* Oral vitamin K lowers the international normalized ratio more rapidly than subcutaneous vitamin K in the treatment of warfarin-associated coagulopathy. A randomized, controlled trial. *Ann Intern Med* 2002; **137**: 251–4.

97 Crowther MA, Donovan D, Harrison L, *et al.* Low-dose oral vitamin K reliably reverses over-anticoagulation due to warfarin. *Thromb Haemost* 1998; **79**: 1116–18.

98 Crowther MA, Julian J, McCarty D, *et al.* Treatment of warfarin-associated coagulopathy with oral vitamin K: a randomised controlled trial. *Lancet* 2000; **356**: 1551–3.

99 Duong TM, Plowman BK, Morreale AP, Janetzky K. Retrospective and prospective analyses of the treatment of overanticoagulated patients. *Pharmacotherapy* 1998; **18**: 1264–70.

100 Patel RJ, Witt DM, Saseen JJ, *et al.* Randomized, placebo-controlled trial of oral phytonadione for excessive anticoagulation. *Pharmacotherapy* 2000; **20**: 1159–66.

101 Makris M, Greaves M, Phillips WS, *et al.* Emergency oral anticoagulant reversal: the relative efficacy of infusions of fresh frozen plasma and clotting factor concentrate on correction of the coagulopathy. *Thromb Haemost* 1997; **77**: 477–80.

102 Deveras RA, Kessler CM. Reversal of warfarin-induced excessive anticoagulation with recombinant human factor VIIa concentrate. *Ann Intern Med* 2002; **137**: 884–8.

103 Lin J, Hanigan WC, Tarantino M, Wang J. The use of recombinant activated factor VII to reverse warfarin-induced anticoagulation in patients with hemorrhages in the central nervous system: preliminary findings. *J Neurosurg* 2003; **98**: 737–40.

104 Sorensen B, Johansen P, Nielsen GL, *et al.* Reversal of the International Normalized Ratio with recombinant activated factor VII in central nervous system bleeding during warfarin thromboprophylaxis: clinical and biochemical aspects. *Blood Coagul Fibrinolysis* 2003; **14**: 469–77.

105 Eskandari N, Feldman N, Greenspoon JS. Factor VII deficiency in pregnancy treated with recombinant factor VIIa. *Obstet Gynecol* 2002; **99**(5 Pt 2): 935–7.

106 Abbott A, Sibert JR, Weaver JB. Chondrodysplasia punctata and maternal warfarin treatment. *Br Med J* 1977; **1**: 1639–40.

107 Hall JG, Pauli RM, Wilson KM. Maternal and fetal sequelae of anticoagulation during pregnancy. *Am J Med* 1980; **68**: 122–40.

◆ 108 Chan WS, Anand S, Ginsberg JS. Anticoagulation of pregnant women with mechanical heart valves: a systematic review of the literature. *Arch Intern Med* 2000; **160**: 191–6.

109 Van Driel D, Wesseling J, Rosendaal FR, *et al.* Growth until puberty after *in utero* exposure to coumarins. *Am J Med Genet* 2000; **95**: 438–43.

110 Wesseling J, Van Driel D, Heymans HS, *et al.* Coumarins during pregnancy: long-term effects on growth and development of school-age children. *Thromb Haemost* 2001; **85**: 609–13.

111 Shaul WL, Hall JG. Multiple congenital anomalies associated with oral anticoagulants. *Am J Obstet Gynecol* 1977; **127**: 191–8.

112 Normann EK, Stray-Pedersen B. Warfarin-induced fetal diaphragmatic hernia. Case report. *Br J Obstet Gynaecol* 1989; **96**: 729–30.

113 Ville Y, Jenkins E, Shearer MJ, *et al.* Fetal intraventricular haemorrhage and maternal warfarin. *Lancet* 1993; **341**: 1211.

● 114 CLASP: a randomised trial of low-dose aspirin for the prevention and treatment of pre-eclampsia among 9364 pregnant women. CLASP (Collaborative Low-dose Aspirin Study in Pregnancy) Collaborative Group. *Lancet* 1994; **343**: 619–29.

◆ 115 Imperiale TF, Petrulis AS. A meta-analysis of low-dose aspirin for the prevention of pregnancy-induced hypertensive disease. *JAMA* 1991; **266**: 260–4.

116 Klinzing P, Markert UR, Liesaus K, Peiker G. Case report: successful pregnancy and delivery after myocardial infarction and essential thrombocythemia treated with clopidrogel. *Clin Exp Obstet Gynecol* 2001; **28**: 215–16.

117 Rai R, Cohen H, Dave M, Regan L. Randomised controlled trial of aspirin and aspirin plus heparin in pregnant women with recurrent miscarriage associated with phospholipid antibodies (or antiphospholipid antibodies). *BMJ* 1997; **314**: 253–7.

118 Turpie AG, Gent M, Laupacis A, *et al.* A comparison of aspirin with placebo in patients treated with warfarin after heart-valve replacement. *N Engl J Med* 1993; **329**: 524–9.

119 O'Reilly R. Anticoagulant, antithrombotic and thrombolytic drugs. In: Gilman AG, Goodman LS, Gilman A, eds. *The Pharmacologic Basis of Therapeutics*. 6th ed. New York: McMillan, 1980: 1347.

120   Orme ML, Lewis PJ, de Swiet M, *et al.* May mothers given warfarin breast-feed their infants? *Br Med J* 1977; **1**: 1564–5.

121   McKenna R, Cole ER, Vasan U. Is warfarin sodium contraindicated in the lactating mother? *J Pediatr* 1983; **103**: 325–7.

122   Brambel CE, Hunter RE. Effect of dicoumarol on the nursing infant. *Am J Obstet Gynecol* 1950; **59**: 1153–9.

◆ 123   Ginsberg JS, Chan WS, Bates SM, Kaatz S. Anticoagulation of pregnant women with mechanical heart valves. *Arch Intern Med* 2003; **163**: 694–8.

124   Bristol-Myers Squibb, assignee. Coumadin (Package Insert), 2004.

12

Antiplatelet agents

CARLO PATRONO, BIANCA ROCCA

INTRODUCTION

Platelets are vital components of normal hemostasis and key participants in pathologic thrombosis by virtue of their capacity to adhere to injured blood vessels and to accumulate at sites of injury.[1] Although platelet adhesion and activation can be viewed as a physiologic repair response to the sudden fissuring or rupture of an atherosclerotic plaque, uncontrolled progression of such a process through a series of self-sustaining amplification loops may lead to intraluminal thrombus formation, vascular occlusion, and transient ischemia or infarction. Currently available antiplatelet drugs interfere with some steps in the activation process, including adhesion, release, and/or aggregation,[1] and have a measurable impact on the risk of arterial thrombosis that cannot be dissociated from an increased risk of bleeding.[2]

In discussing antiplatelet agents, it is important to appreciate that approximately 10^{11} platelets are produced each day under physiologic circumstances, a level of production that can increase up to 10-fold at times of increased need.[3] Platelets form by fragmentation of megakaryocyte cytoplasm and have a maximum circulating lifespan of about 10 days in humans.[3] Thus, platelets are anucleate blood cells that provide a circulating source of chemokines, cytokines, and growth factors, which are preformed and packaged in storage granules. Moreover, activated platelets can synthesize prostanoids (primarily, thromboxane [TX] A_2) from arachidonic acid released from membrane phospholipids, through rapid coordinated activation of phospholipase(s), cyclooxygenase (COX)-1 and TX synthase (Fig. 12.1). Newly formed platelets also express the inducible isoforms of COX (COX-2) and prostaglandin (PG) E synthase, and this phenomenon is markedly amplified in association with

accelerated platelet regeneration.[4] Although activated platelets are not thought to synthesize proteins *de novo*, they can translate constitutive mRNAs into proteins, including interleukin-1β over several hours.[5] Thus, platelets may have previously unrecognized roles in inflammation and vascular injury, and antiplatelet strategies may be expected to impact on platelet-derived protein signals for inflammatory and/or proliferative responses (Fig. 12.2).

Negative modulation of platelet adhesion and aggregation is exerted by a variety of physiologic mechanisms, including endothelium-derived prostacyclin (PGI$_2$), nitric oxide, CD39/ecto-ADPase and platelet endothelial cell adhesion molecule-1. Some drugs may interfere with these regulatory pathways, as exemplified by the dose-dependent inhibition of PGI$_2$ production by aspirin and other COX inhibitors.[2]

MECHANISM OF ACTION AND CLINICAL EFFICACY OF ANTIPLATELET DRUGS

Aspirin

The best characterized mechanism of action of aspirin is related to permanent inactivation of the COX activity of prostaglandin H (PGH)-synthase 1 and PGH-synthase 2, also referred to as COX-1 and COX-2.[6] These isozymes catalyze the first committed step in prostanoid biosynthesis, that is, the conversion of arachidonic acid to PGH$_2$. PGH$_2$ is an unstable biosynthetic intermediate and a substrate for a number of downstream isomerases that generate at least five different bioactive prostanoids, including TXA$_2$ and prostacyclin (PGI$_2$). By diffusing through cell membranes,

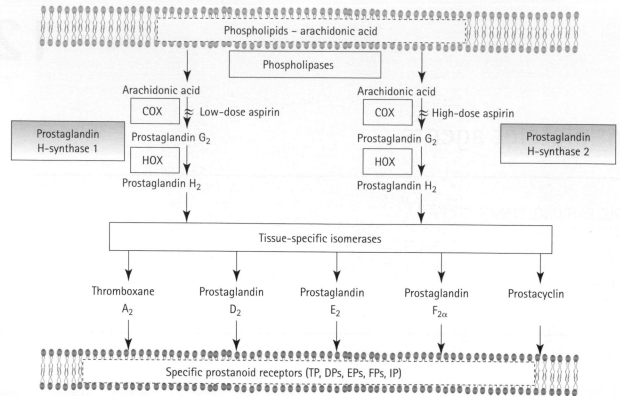

Figure 12.1 Arachidonic acid, a 20-carbon fatty acid containing four double bonds, is liberated from the sn2 position in membrane phospholipids by several forms of phospholipase A_2, which are activated by diverse stimuli. Arachidonic acid is converted by cytosolic prostaglandin H synthases, which have both cyclooxygenase (COX) and hydroperoxidase (HOX) activity, to the unstable intermediate prostaglandin H_2. The synthases are colloquially termed cyclooxygenases and exist in two forms, cyclooxygenase-1 and cyclooxygenase-2. Low-dose aspirin selectively inhibits cyclooxygenase-1, and high-dose aspirin inhibits both cyclooxygenase-1 and -2. Prostaglandin H_2 is converted by tissue-specific isomerases to multiple prostanoids. These bioactive lipids activate specific cell membrane receptors of the superfamily of G-protein-coupled receptors. DP, prostaglandin D_2 receptor; EP, prostaglandin E_2 receptor; FP, prostaglandin $F_{2\alpha}$ receptor; IP, prostacyclin receptor; TP, thromboxane receptor.

aspirin enters the COX channel, a narrow hydrophobic channel connecting the cell membrane to the catalytic pocket of the enzyme. Aspirin first binds to an arginine-120 residue, a common docking site for all nonsteroidal anti-inflammatory drugs (NSAIDs); then it acetylates a serine residue (serine-529 in human COX-1 and serine-516 in human COX-2) located in the narrowest section of the channel, thereby preventing access of arachidonic acid to the COX catalytic site of the enzyme (Fig. 12.3A). Aspirin inhibits COX-2 at higher concentrations than those required to inhibit COX-1. This may account, at least in part, for the different dose requirements for analgesic and anti-inflammatory versus antiplatelet effects of the drug.

A large database of randomized clinical trials now offers the most compelling evidence that prevention of myocardial infarction and ischemic stroke by aspirin is largely due to permanent inactivation of platelet COX-1.[6] These studies, which tested the efficacy and safety of the drug when given at daily doses ranging from as low as 30 mg to as high as 1500 mg, have established two important facts. First, the antithrombotic effect of aspirin is saturable at doses in the

range of 75–100 mg, as would be expected from human studies of platelet COX-1 inactivation (Fig. 12.3B). Second, despite a half-life of approximately 20 minutes in the human circulation, the antithrombotic effect of aspirin is observed with a dosing interval of 24 hours, reflecting the permanent nature of platelet COX-1 inactivation and the duration of TXA_2 suppression following oral dosing in humans (Fig. 12.3C). Other mechanisms of action that have been suggested to contribute to the antithrombotic effect of aspirin, such as an anti-inflammatory effect of the drug, are not compatible with these unique properties. Although sex-based differences in salicylate metabolism have been reported,[7] these do not appear to influence the pharmacodynamics of the antiplatelet effect of aspirin, which is virtually identical in men and women, both in terms of dose- and time-dependence.[6,8]

The search for the lowest effective dose of aspirin for platelet inhibition was largely driven by the explicit concern of concomitant inhibition of vascular PGI_2 production, yet it is still uncertain whether dose-dependent suppression of the latter attenuates the antithrombotic effect of aspirin in

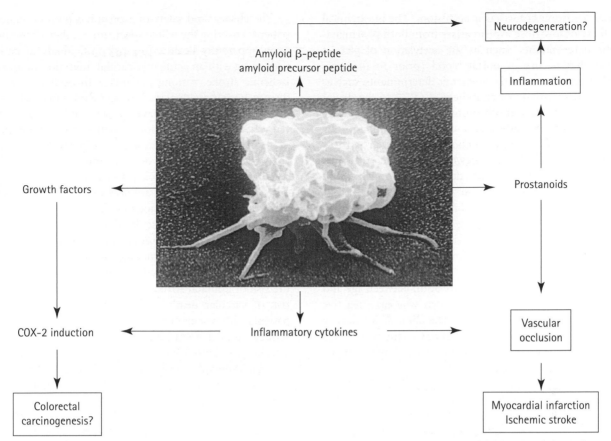

Figure 12.2 The activated human platelet: an anucleated repair machinery releasing a wide repertoire of lipid and protein mediators possibly contributing to several clinical syndromes responsive to low-dose aspirin therapy. Although the beneficial effects of aspirin in preventing myocardial infarction and stroke are firmly established, the effects on neurodegeneration and colorectal carcinogenesis are inconclusive. Modified from Ruggeri ZM. Platelets in atherothrombosis. *Nat Med* 2002; **8**: 1227–34. Reprinted with permission from Macmillan Publishers Ltd: Nature Medicine, Copyright 2002.

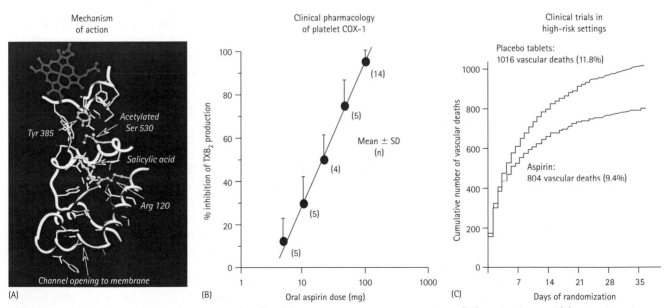

Figure 12.3 (A) Acetylation of cyclooxygenase (COX)-1, (B) inhibition of platelet thromboxane (TX) production, and (C) reduction of vascular death by aspirin. Inactivation of the enzyme, reduced product formation, and clinical efficacy display remarkable similarities in the required once-daily regimen and saturability of the effects at low doses. (Fig. 12.3A courtesy of Dr Patrick Loll; Fig. 12.3B redrawn from Patrignani *et al. J Clin Invest* 1982; **69**: 1366–72; Fig. 12.3C redrawn from the ISIS-2 Collaborative Group. *Lancet* 1988; **ii**: 349–60, Copyright 1998, with permission from Elsevier.)

clinical syndromes of vascular occlusion.[6] The biochemical selectivity of low-dose aspirin arises from both pharmacokinetic determinants, such as the acetylation of platelet COX-1 that occurs in portal blood (prior to first-pass metabolism), and pharmacodynamic determinants, such as the limited sensitivity of endothelial COX-2 to the drug.[6] Aspirin is an effective antithrombotic agent in a wide range of daily doses.[2] Whether dose-dependent inhibition by aspirin of a mediator of thromboresistance, such as PGI_2, may be responsible for a somewhat attenuated efficacy at high daily doses[9,10] remains to be demonstrated convincingly.

A sex-related difference in the production of 15-epi-lipoxin A_4 has been reported in healthy subjects treated with low-dose aspirin (81 mg daily for 8 weeks).[11] 15-Epi-lipoxin A_4 is synthesized via the transcellular metabolism of 15R-hydroxy-eicosatetraenoic acid (15R-HETE), which is produced by aspirin-acetylated COX-2.[12] In women treated with aspirin a positive correlation between age and 15-epi-lipoxin A_4 levels has been shown, whereas a negative correlation was observed in men. The clinical significance of this observation is presently unknown due to the lack of convincing evidence for a sex-based difference in the cardioprotective effect of aspirin.[6,13]

Aspirin's unique features in inhibiting platelet COX-1 – its ability to inactivate the enzyme permanently through a short-lived active moiety – are ideally suited to its role as an antiplatelet drug. This is because they severely limit the extent and duration of extraplatelet effects of the drug, including the inhibition of PGI_2. Moreover, the cumulative nature of platelet COX-1 acetylation by repeated low doses of aspirin[14] explains the clinical efficacy of doses as low as 30–50 mg daily,[2] the predictable high-grade inhibition of platelet TXA_2 biosynthesis, and the persistence of the drug's effect. These features, in turn, may limit the consequences of less-than-ideal compliance in a real world setting.

Permanent inactivation of platelet COX-1 by aspirin may lead to the prevention of thrombosis as well as to excess bleeding. At least two distinct COX-1-dependent mechanisms contribute to the increased risk of upper gastrointestinal bleeding associated with aspirin exposure: inhibition of TXA_2-mediated platelet function and impairment of PGE_2-mediated cytoprotection in the gastrointestinal mucosa.[2] Whereas the former effect is dose-independent, at least for daily doses in excess of 30 mg, the latter effect is clearly dose-dependent. Inhibition of platelet function is largely responsible for the twofold increase in the risk of upper gastrointestinal bleeding associated with daily doses of aspirin in the range of 75–100 mg, inasmuch as a similar relative risk is associated with other antiplatelet agents that do not act on COX and therefore do not affect PGE_2-mediated cytoprotection.[6] Inhibition of COX-1-dependent cytoprotection amplifies risk of bleeding/perforation by causing new mucosal lesions or aggravating existing ones, and is associated with a relative risk of 4–6 at the higher, analgesic, or anti-inflammatory doses of aspirin. Assessing the net effect of aspirin requires an estimation of the absolute risk of the individual patient for thrombotic and hemorrhagic complications.[6]

The efficacy and safety of aspirin has been evaluated in patients covering the whole spectrum of atherothrombosis, from apparently healthy low-risk individuals to patients presenting with an acute myocardial infarction or an acute ischemic stroke. Among patients with occlusive vascular disease, both individual studies[2] and a metaanalysis of trials of antiplatelet therapy[10] have shown that low-dose aspirin reduces the risk of a serious vascular event by approximately a quarter. This represents a composite of one-third reduction in nonfatal myocardial infarction, one-quarter reduction in nonfatal stroke, and one-sixth reduction in death from a vascular or unknown cause.[10] Since each of these proportional reductions applies similarly to all categories of patients with vascular disease, the absolute benefits of aspirin in the individual patient can be estimated by applying a one-third reduction to their absolute risk of nonfatal myocardial infarction, a one-quarter reduction to the risk of nonfatal stroke, and one-sixth reduction to the risk of vascular death.[10] Thus, among a wide range of patients with vascular disease, in whom the annual risk of a serious vascular event ranges from 4 percent to 8 percent, aspirin typically prevents at least 10–20 fatal and nonfatal vascular events for every 1000 patients treated for 1 year (number needed to treat: 50–100).[10] No appreciable sex- or age-related differences in the effects of aspirin were found in these analyses.[13]

Observational studies and a metaanalysis of trials[10] among high-risk patients have demonstrated that long-term therapy with low-dose aspirin is associated with around a twofold increased risk of major extracranial (mostly, upper gastrointestinal) bleeding, and this proportional excess hazard appears similar regardless of the variable underlying cardiovascular risk of the patient. In middle-aged patients, this corresponds to an estimated absolute excess of approximately 1–2 major bleeding complications per 1000 patients treated with low-dose aspirin for 1 year (number needed to harm: 500–1000).[6,10] Therefore, for most high-risk patients using low-dose aspirin, the expected number avoiding a serious vascular event clearly outweighs the number experiencing a major bleeding, unless there is some particular reason for an increased susceptibility to bleeding, such as advanced age, history of prior ulcer, or concomitant treatment with other drugs interfering with primary hemostasis. Such a favorable benefit/harm balance of low-dose aspirin in high-risk patients has resulted in consistent level 1 recommendations by both North American[2] and European[15] consensus documents and in regulatory approval by the Food and Drug Administration and European health authorities of practically all vascular indications except for peripheral arterial disease.

Thus, aspirin is recommended in all clinical conditions in which antiplatelet prophylaxis has a favorable benefit/risk profile. In consideration of dose-dependent gastrointestinal toxicity and its potential impact on compliance, physicians are encouraged to use the lowest dose of aspirin which was shown to be effective in each clinical setting (Table 12.1). The available evidence supports daily doses of

Table 12.1 High-risk disorders for which aspirin has been shown to be effective and lowest effective daily dose*

Disorder	Lowest effective daily dose (mg)
Chronic stable angina	75
Polycythemia vera	100
Unstable angina	75
Acute myocardial infarction	160
Transient ischemic attack and ischemic stroke	50
Severe carotid artery stenosis	75
Acute ischemic stroke	160
Atrial fibrillation	325

*The lowest daily aspirin dose for which direct randomized evidence of effectiveness is available.

aspirin in the range of 75–100 mg for the long-term prevention of serious vascular events in high-risk patients.[6] In clinical settings where an immediate antithrombotic effect is required (such as in acute coronary syndromes or in acute ischemic stroke), a loading dose of 160–200 mg should be given at diagnosis to ensure rapid and complete inhibition of TX-dependent platelet aggregation.[2]

Although the benefits of low-dose aspirin are clear among patients with vascular disease, the balance of benefit and harm of the same preventive strategy is uncertain in low-risk individuals with no clinically apparent vascular disease. The decision to prescribe low-dose aspirin in a person with no history of vascular disease must rely on an individual judgment that the likely benefits of aspirin will exceed any risks of bleeding. On the basis of the available evidence from six primary prevention trials, low-dose aspirin therapy for 4–10 years prevents nonfatal myocardial infarction by a quarter, but it has no clear protective effect against ischemic stroke or vascular death.[6] Therefore, assessing the benefits and risks of low-dose aspirin requires balancing any absolute reduction in nonfatal myocardial infarction (1–3 per 1000 treated for 1 year) against an increased risk of major gastrointestinal bleeding (1–2 per 1000) and hemorrhagic stroke (0.1–0.2 per 1000).[6]

At variance with the results of the first five primary prevention trials of low-dose aspirin, in which most or all randomized subjects were men, the recently reported Women's Health Study[16] found no evidence of a protective effect of aspirin 100 mg on alternate days against myocardial infarction but a marginally significant 17 percent reduction in the risk of stroke (relative risk, 0.83, 95 percent confidence interval [CI] 0.69 to 0.99; $P = 0.04$). It should be noted that stroke represented a secondary endpoint of the study and that the overall effects of 10-year prophylaxis with aspirin on the primary endpoint (a combination of nonfatal myocardial infarction, nonfatal stroke, and death from cardiovascular causes) failed to reach statistical significance (relative risk 0.91, 95 percent CI 0.80 to 1.03; $P = 0.13$). Despite the large

sample size of approximately 40 000 initially healthy women and the long duration of follow-up, the Women's Health Study was probably underpowered to detect a moderate treatment effect because of the lower than expected rate of vascular events (only 0.3 percent per year in the control group) and lower than expected relative risk reduction associated with aspirin (9 percent vs. 25 percent).[16] Thus, its results should be viewed within the context of all randomized evidence from aspirin trials.[6] However, the results of Ridker et al.'s sex-specific random effects metaanalysis[16] of the data from six primary prevention trials should be considered within the limitations of subgroup analysis.

It has been suggested that low-dose aspirin may be appropriate for individuals whose estimated annual risk of a coronary event, based on a risk prediction algorithm, exceeds a particular threshold. Various guidelines have adopted this approach using risk thresholds for coronary events ranging from 0.6 percent to 1.5 percent per year. In particular, the suggestion that aspirin therapy is safe and worthwhile at coronary event risk equal to or greater than 1.5 percent per year is potentially attractive.[17] However, there is inadequate information from randomized clinical trials assessing the efficacy and safety of low-dose aspirin in asymptomatic subjects at an estimated annual risk of 1.5–3.0 percent, and more evidence is clearly needed.[6] Women have a somewhat lower risk of arterial thrombosis as well as upper gastrointestinal bleeding than men, though both risks increase substantially in postmenopausal women.[18] Thus, it is not expected that the balance of benefits and risks of low-dose aspirin is importantly influenced by sex.

Finally, it should be emphasized that current estimates of the absolute excess of major bleeding complications associated with low-dose aspirin therapy are likely to underestimate the potential harm in individuals at increased risk of bleeding complications, who were typically excluded from aspirin trials. Thus, the number needed to harm may vary about 100-fold, as a function of age and prior history of gastrointestinal disturbances.[6]

Ticlopidine and clopidogrel

Ticlopidine and clopidogrel are structurally related thienopyridines with platelet inhibitory properties. Both drugs selectively inhibit ADP-induced platelet aggregation, with no direct effects on the metabolism of arachidonic acid.[2] Ticlopidine and clopidogrel also can inhibit platelet aggregation induced by collagen and thrombin, but these inhibitory effects are abolished by increasing the agonist concentration and, therefore, likely reflect blockade of ADP-mediated amplification of the response to other agonists.

Neither ticlopidine nor clopidogrel affects ADP-induced platelet aggregation when added in vitro up to 500 μmol/L, thus suggesting that in vivo hepatic transformation to an active metabolite(s) is necessary for their antiplatelet effects.[2] A short-lived, active metabolite of clopidogrel has been characterized.[19] Clopidogrel and, probably, ticlopidine induce irreversible alterations of the platelet ADP receptor P2Y12 mediating inhibition of stimulated adenylyl cyclase activity by ADP.[20] Inhibition of platelet function by clopidogrel is associated with a selective reduction in ADP-binding sites, with no consistent change in the binding affinity. Permanent modification of an ADP receptor by thienopyridines is consistent with time-dependent, cumulative inhibition of ADP-induced platelet aggregation on repeated daily dosing and with slow recovery of platelet function on drug withdrawal.[2]

After single oral doses of clopidogrel, ADP-induced platelet aggregation was inhibited in a dose-dependent fashion in healthy volunteers, with an apparent ceiling effect (that is, 40 percent inhibition) at 400 mg.[2] Inhibited platelet aggregation was detectable 2 hours after oral dosing of 400 mg, and it remained relatively stable up to 48 hours. With repeated daily dosing of 50–100 mg in healthy volunteers, ADP-induced platelet aggregation was inhibited from the second day of treatment (25–30 percent inhibition) and reached a steady state (50–60 percent inhibition) after 4–7 days. Such a ceiling effect is comparable to that achieved with ticlopidine (500 mg daily). Ticlopidine, however, is characterized by a slower onset of the antiplatelet effect as compared with clopidogrel.[2]

Thus, the active metabolite of clopidogrel has a pharmacodynamic pattern quite similar to that of aspirin in causing cumulative platelet inhibition on repeated daily low-dose administration.[2] As with aspirin, platelet function returned to normal 7 days after the last dose. Both the cumulative nature of the inhibitory effects and the slow recovery rate of platelet function are consistent with the active moieties of aspirin (that is, acetylsalicylic acid) and clopidogrel (that is, active metabolite) causing a permanent defect in a platelet protein that cannot be repaired during the 24-hour dosing interval and can be replaced only through platelet turnover.[2] This also justifies the once-daily regimen of both drugs despite their short half-life in the circulation. Bleeding times measured in the same multiple-dose study of clopidogrel described earlier showed a comparable prolongation (by 1.5–2.0-fold over controls) at 50–100 mg daily or ticlopidine at 500 mg daily.[2]

Clopidogrel has undergone an unusual clinical development, with limited phase II studies and a single large phase III trial (that is, Clopidogrel versus Aspirin in Patients at Risk of Ischaemic Events [CAPRIE]) to test its efficacy and safety at 75 mg daily compared with aspirin at 325 mg daily in 19 185 high-risk (28 percent female) patients.[21] Clopidogrel was slightly more effective than aspirin, and there was some suggestion from a marginally significant heterogeneity test that clopidogrel may be particularly effective in preventing vascular events in patients with symptomatic peripheral arterial disease. This interesting and unexpected finding suggests that the pathophysiologic importance of TXA_2 and ADP may vary in different clinical settings. In the CAPRIE trial, the frequency of severe rash was higher with clopidogrel than with aspirin (absolute excess approximately 1–2 per 1000),

as was the frequency of diarrhea, thus reproducing the characteristic side effects of ticlopidine. No excess neutropenia was associated with clopidogrel, however, the frequency of this serious complication was extremely low (0.05 percent) in this trial.[21] The Clopidogrel in Unstable angina to prevent Recurrent Events (CURE) trial[22] has demonstrated the efficacy and safety of adding clopidogrel (a loading dose of 300 mg, followed by 75 mg daily) to aspirin in the long-term management of patients with acute coronary syndromes without ST segment elevation. Moreover, the combination of aspirin and clopidogrel has become standard treatment for 1 month after coronary stent implantation.[23] The Clopidogrel for the Reduction of Events During Observation (CREDO) trial[24] has demonstrated that following percutaneous coronary interventions, long-term (1 year) clopidogrel therapy significantly reduces the risk of adverse ischemic events. The recently reported ClOpidogrel and Metoprolol in Myocardial Infarction Trial (COMMIT) trial[25] in 45 852 patients admitted to hospitals in China within 24 hours of suspected acute myocardial infarction demonstrated that adding a 2-week course of clopidogrel therapy (75 mg daily) on top of conventional treatments (including aspirin, 162 mg daily) produced a highly significant 9 percent proportional reduction in death, reinfarction or stroke, corresponding to 9 fewer events per 1000 patients. These effects of clopidogrel appeared consistent across a wide range of female (approximately 28 percent) and male patients and independent of other treatments being used. At variance with the CURE trial,[22] in which the additional benefit of clopidogrel was associated with enhanced risk of bleeding, no statistically significant excess risk (considering all fatal, transfused, or cerebral bleeds) was noted in the COMMIT trial, either overall or in patients aged over 70 years.[25]

Dipyridamole

The addition of dipyridamole to aspirin has not been shown clearly to produce additional reductions in serious vascular events in an overview of 25 trials in approximately 10 000 high-risk patients,[10] although two trials suggested that there may be a worthwhile further reduction in stroke.[26,27] The reasons for this effect of dipyridamole on stroke in the European Stroke Prevention Study (ESPS)-2 and European/Australasian Stroke Prevention in Reversible Ischaemia Trial (ESPRIT) study include the possibility that the newer formulation of the drug with improved oral bioavailability as well as the twofold higher daily dose (400 mg vs. 225 mg in previous studies) resulted in a clinically detectable antiplatelet effect of the drug.[2] Although the combination of low-dose aspirin and extended-release dipyridamole (200 mg twice daily) is considered an acceptable option for initial therapy of patients with noncardioembolic cerebral ischemic events,[28] there is no basis to recommend this combination in patients with ischemic heart disease.

Abciximab, eptifibatide, and tirofiban

The pharmacokinetics and pharmacodynamics of commercially available glycoprotein (GP)IIb/IIIa antagonists have been reviewed recently together with a detailed account of randomized clinical trial data that led to their regulatory approval.[2] Although abciximab currently has no place outside of the catheterization laboratory, the disappointing results of Global Utilization of Strategies To open Occluded coronary arteries trial IV in Acute Coronary Syndromes (GUSTO IV ACS)[29] are also causing reassessment of the role of eptifibatide and tirofiban in patients managed conservatively. A metaanalysis of all major randomized clinical trials of GPIIb/IIIa antagonists in 31 402 patients with acute coronary syndromes, who were not routinely scheduled to undergo early coronary revascularization, suggests a 9 percent reduction in the odds of death or myocardial infarction at 30 days.[30] However, the true size of the additional benefit resulting from short-term, high-grade blockade of GPIIb/IIIa combined with standard antithrombotic therapy is somewhat uncertain, since the 95 percent confidence interval ranged from 2 percent to 16 percent further reduction in serious vascular events.[30] Moreover, the 1 percent absolute difference in death or myocardial infarction was balanced by an absolute excess of 1 percent in major bleeding complications associated with GPIIb/IIIa antagonists versus control.[30] The Platelet IIb/IIIa Antagonism for the Reduction of Acute Coronary Syndrome Events in a Global Organization Network (PARAGON)-B investigators have reported that dose-titrated lamifiban had no significant effects on clinical outcomes in patients with non-ST-elevation acute coronary syndromes and yet caused excess bleeding,[31] thus reinforcing the uncertainty noted above.

No sex-related differences were observed for abciximab in different clinical trials in terms of efficacy or safety.[32,33] Thus, the benefit/risk profile of currently available GPIIb/IIIa antagonists is uncertain for patients with acute coronary syndromes who are not routinely scheduled for early revascularization. In contrast, for patients undergoing percutaneous coronary intervention, intensification of antiplatelet therapy by adding an intravenous GPIIb/IIIa blocker is an appropriate strategy to reduce the risk of procedure-related thrombotic complications.[2,15]

Reversible COX-1 inhibitors

A variety of non-selective NSAIDs can inhibit TXA_2-dependent platelet function through competitive, reversible inhibition of COX-1. When used at conventional antiinflammatory dosage, these drugs generally inhibit platelet COX-1 activity by only 70–90 percent. Such inhibition is insufficient to block platelet aggregation adequately *in vivo*, however, because of the substantial biosynthetic capacity of human platelets to produce TXA_2.[2] The only reversible COX-1 inhibitors that have been examined for

antithrombotic efficacy in relatively small randomized clinical trials are sulfinpyrazone, flurbiprofen, indobufen, and triflusal.[2] None of these reversible COX-1 inhibitors is approved as an antiplatelet drug in the United States, although they are available in a few European countries. Moreover, the randomized clinical trials comparing indobufen to aspirin and triflusal to aspirin largely lack adequate statistical power to test biologically plausible differences in efficacy, nor were they designed to establish therapeutic equivalence.[2]

Oral GPIIb/IIIa blockers

The success of short-term, high-grade blockade of platelet GPIIb/IIIa with intravenous agents[2] has led to the development of an array of oral GPIIb/IIIa antagonists in the hope of extending this benefit to the long-term management of patients with acute coronary syndromes. To date, five large-scale clinical trials have been completed[2] and a metaanalysis of four of these has been published.[34] The consistent finding of these large-scale trials involving over 40 000 patients is that oral GPIIb/IIIa antagonists (xemilofiban, orbofiban, sibrafiban and lotrafiban) are not more effective than aspirin or, when combined with aspirin, are not superior to placebo and may in fact increase mortality.[2,34] Several mechanisms have been put forward to explain these results. One is that the poor oral bioavailability of these compounds and the target of approximately 50 percent inhibition of platelet aggregation resulted in poor antiplatelet activity in many patients. This would explain a lack of clinical response, but not an increase in mortality. Indeed, overall there was an increase in the frequency of bleeding and a reduced requirement of urgent revascularization, suggesting some degree of clinical efficacy.[34]

An alternative explanation is that GPIIb/IIIa antagonists can activate platelets, at least in some individuals.[35,36] GPIIb/IIIa is not a passive receptor, rather like all integrins it responds to ligand binding by activating the cell. Thus, fibrinogen binding leads to signals that further activate platelets and are essential for platelet aggregation. Several studies suggest that ligands designed to bind to the receptor and prevent platelet aggregation may trigger some of these activating signals.[35,36] Moreover, the partial agonist activity may not be confined to oral drugs, as abciximab has been reported to activate platelets and promote procoagulant activity by promoting the shedding of CD40L.[2]

TP antagonists

The TXA_2/PGH_2 (TP) receptor is a G-protein–coupled receptor, which on ligand stimulation results in activation of phospholipase C and subsequent increase in inositol 1,4,5-triphosphate, diacylglycerol, and intracellular Ca^{2+}

concentrations.[2] Potent (K_d in the low nanomolar range) and long-lasting (half-life >20 hours) TP antagonists have been developed, including GR 32191, BMS180291 (ifetroban), and BM 13.177 (sulotroban). Despite the antithrombotic activity demonstrated in various animal species and the interesting 'cardioprotective' activity demonstrated in dogs and ferrets, these compounds have yielded disappointing results in phase II/III clinical trials.[2] Before drawing definitive conclusions on the apparent failure of this approach, however, it should be mentioned that these studies have severe limitations, including: (i) unrealistic hypotheses of risk reduction being tested (for example, a 50 percent reduction in the late clinical failure rate after successful coronary angioplasty); (ii) heterogeneous endpoints being pooled together, including 'clinically important restenosis', for which no evidence of TXA_2 dependence was obtained during earlier aspirin trials; and (iii) an anti-ischemic effect being tested in individuals with unstable coronary syndromes treated using standard therapy, including aspirin and heparin.[2]

Clinical development of GR 32191 and sulotroban has been discontinued because of these disappointing – though largely predictable – results. It would be interesting to see at least one such compound evaluated in phase III clinical trials with adequate endpoints and realistic sample sizes. The potential advantages of potent TP antagonists compared with low-dose aspirin are related to the discovery of aspirin-insensitive agonists of the platelet receptor, such as TXA_2 derived from the COX-2 pathway[37] and the F_2-isoprostane, 8-iso-$PGF_{2\alpha}$, which is a product of free-radical-catalyzed peroxidation of arachidonic acid.[38] The latter can synergize with subthreshold concentrations of other platelet agonists to evoke a full aggregatory response, thus amplifying platelet activation in those clinical settings associated with enhanced lipid peroxidation.[39] The TP antagonist, S-18886 (terutroban), has recently completed phase II clinical development and is currently being compared with low-dose aspirin in a large randomized trial (PERFORM) in patients with a recent cerebrovascular event.

Other P2Y12 antagonists

A new class of direct P2Y12 antagonists (for example, AZD6140)[40] and a novel thienopyridine (prasugrel)[41] are currently being developed that appear to block this ADP receptor more effectively than clopidogrel.

ACKNOWLEDGMENT

Supported by a grant form the Commission of the European Communities (EICOSANOX Project 005033). The expert editorial assistance of Ms Daniela Basilico is gratefully acknowledged.

KEY LEARNING POINTS

- Approximately 20 different agents have been shown to inhibit platelet aggregation through different mechanisms of action. However, inhibition of platelet aggregation as measured *ex vivo* does not necessarily translate into prevention of atherothrombosis.
- Antiplatelet drugs that have been successfully tested against placebo in adequately large randomized clinical trials include aspirin, ticlopidine, and clopidogrel for chronic oral dosing, and abciximab, tirofiban, and eptifibatide for short-term intravenous administration.
- Allocation of high-risk patients to a prolonged course of antiplatelet therapy reduced the combined outcome of nonfatal myocardial infarction, nonfatal stroke or vascular death ('serious vascular events') by about 25 percent.
- The absolute benefits of aspirin therapy substantially outweigh the absolute risks of major bleeding (particularly, gastrointestinal) complications in a variety of clinical settings characterized by moderate to high risk of occlusive vascular events. However, in low-risk individuals the benefit/risk profile of such a preventive strategy is substantially uncertain.

REFERENCES

1 Kroll MH, Sullivan R. Mechanisms of platelet activation. In: Loscalzo J, Schafer AI, ed. *Thrombosis and Hemorrhage.* Baltimore, MO: William & Wilkins, 1998: 261–91.

2 Patrono C, Coller B, FitzGerald GA, *et al.* Platelet-active drugs: The relationships among dose, effectiveness, and side effects. *Chest* 2004; **126**: 234S–64S.

3 Kaushansky K. Regulation of megakaryopoiesis. In: Loscalzo J, Schafer AI, ed. *Thrombosis and Hemorrhage.* Baltimore, MO: William & Wilkins, 1998: 173–93.

4 Rocca B, Secchiero P, Ciabattoni G, *et al.* Cyclooxygenase-2 expression is induced during human megakaryopoiesis and characterizes newly formed platelets. *Proc Natl Acad Sci U S A* 2002; **99**: 7634–9.

5 Lindemann S, Tolley ND, Dixon DA, *et al.* Activated platelets mediate inflammatory signaling by regulated interleukin 1β synthesis. *J Cell Biol* 2001; **154**: 485–90.

6 Patrono C, García Rodríguez LA, *et al.* Low-dose aspirin for the prevention of atherothrombosis. *N Engl J Med* 2005; **353**: 2373–83.

7 Montgomery PR, Berger LG, Mitenko PA, Sitar DS. Salicylate metabolism: effects of age and sex in adults. *Clin Pharmacol Ther* 1986; **39**: 571–6.

8 Ridker PM, Hennekens CH, Tokens GH, *et al.* Anti-platelet effects of 100 mg alternate day oral aspirin: a randomized, double-blind, placebo-controlled trial of regular and enteric coated formulations in men and women. *J Cardiovasc Risk* 1996; **3**: 209–212.

9 Taylor DW, Barnett HJ, Haynes RB, *et al.* Low-dose and high-dose acetylsalicylic acid for patients undergoing carotid endarterectomy: a randomised controlled trial. *Lancet* 1999; **355**: 1295–305.

10 Antithrombotic Trialists' Collaboration. Collaborative meta-analysis of randomised trials of antiplatelet therapy for prevention of death, myocardial infarction and stroke in high-risk patients. *BMJ* 2002; **324**: 71–86.

11 Chiang N, Hurwitz S, Ridker PM, Serhan CN. Aspirin has a gender-dependent impact on antiinflammatory 15-epi-lipoxin A4 formation. A randomized human trial. *Arterioscler Thromb Vasc Biol* 2006; **26**: e14–17.

12 Clària J, Serhan CN. Aspirin triggers previously undescribed bioactive eicosanoids by human endothelial cell-leukocyte interactions. *Proc Natl Acad Sci USA* 1995; **92**: 9475–9.

13 Antiplatelet Trialists' Collaboration. Collaborative overview of randomised trials of antiplatelet therapy-I: prevention of death, myocardial infarction, and stroke by prolonged antiplatelet therapy in various categories of patients. *BMJ* 1994; **308**: 81–106.

14 Patrignani P, Filabozzi P, Patrono C. Selective cumulative inhibition of platelet thromboxane production by low-dose aspirin in healthy subjects. *J Clin Invest* 1982; **69**: 1366–72.

15 Patrono C, Bachmann F, Baigent C, *et al.* Expert consensus document on the use of antiplatelet agents. *Eur Heart J* 2004; **25**: 166–81.

16 Ridker PM, Cook NR, Lee I-M, *et al.* A randomized trial of low-dose aspirin in the primary prevention of cardiovascular disease in women. *N Engl J Med* 2005; **352**: 1293–304.

17 Lauer M. Aspirin for primary prevention of coronary events. *N Engl J Med* 2002; **346**: 1468–74.

18 Barrett Connor E. Sex differences in coronary heart disease. Why are women so superior? *Circulation* 1997; **95**: 252–64.

19 Savi P, Pereillo JM, Uzabiaga MF, *et al.* Identification and biological activity of the active metabolite of clopidogrel. *Thromb Haemost* 2000; **84**: 891–6.

20 Hollopeter G, Jantzen HM, Vincent D, *et al.* Identification of the platelet ADP receptor targeted by antithrombotic drugs. *Nature* 2001; **409**: 202–7.

21 CAPRIE Steering Committee. A randomised, blinded trial of clopidogrel versus aspirin in patients at risk of ischaemic events (CAPRIE). *Lancet* 1996; **348**: 1329–39.

22 CURE Steering Committee. Effects of clopidogrel in addition to aspirin in patients with acute coronary syndromes without ST-segment elevation. *N Engl J Med* 2001; **345**: 494–502.

23 Bertrand ME, Rupprecht H-J, Urban P, Gershlick AH. Double-blind study of the safety of clopidogrel with and without a loading dose in combination with aspirin compared with ticlopidine in combination with aspirin after coronary stenting. The clopidogrel aspirin stent international cooperative study (CLASSICS). *Circulation* 2000; **102**: 624–9.

24 Steinhubl SR, Berger PB, Mann JT, 3rd, *et al.* Early and sustained dual oral antiplatelet therapy following percutaneous coronary intervention: a randomized controlled trial. *JAMA* 2002; **288**: 2411–20.

25 COMMIT Collaborative Group. Addition of clopidogrel to aspirin in 45 852 patients with acute myocardial infarction: randomised placebo-controlled trial. *Lancet* 2005; **366**: 1607–21.

26 Diener HC, Cunha L, Forbes C, *et al.* European Stroke Prevention Study II. Dipyridamole and acetylsalicylic acid in the secondary prevention of stroke. *J Neurol Sci* 1996; **143**: 1–13.

27 ESPRIT Study Group. Aspirin plus dipyridamole versus aspirin alone after cerebral ischaemia of arterial origin (ESPRIT): randomised controlled trial. *Lancet* 2006; **367**: 1665–73.

28 Albers GW, Amarenco P, Easton JD, *et al.* Antithrombotic and thrombolytic therapy for ischemic stroke. *Chest* 2004; **126**: 483S–512S.

29 The GUSTO IV-ACS Investigators. Effect of glycoprotein IIb/IIIa receptor blocker abciximab on outcome in patients with acute coronary syndromes without early coronary revascularisation: the GUSTO IV-ACS randomised trial. *Lancet* 2001; **357**: 1915–24.

30 Boersma E, Harrington RA, Moliterno DJ, *et al.* Platelet glycoprotein IIb/IIIa inhibitors in acute coronary syndromes: a meta-analysis of all major randomised clinical trials. *Lancet* 2002; **359**: 189–98.

31 The Platelet IIb/IIIa Antagonist for the Reduction of Acute coronary syndrome events in a Global Organization Network (PARAGON)-B Investigators. Randomized, placebo-controlled trial of titrated intravenous lamifiban for acute coronary syndromes. *Circulation* 2002; **105**: 316–21.

32 Cho L, Topol EJ, Balog C, *et al.* Clinical benefit of glycoprotein IIb/IIIa blockade with Abciximab is independent of gender: pooled analysis from EPIC, EPILOG and EPISTENT trials. Evaluation of 7E3 for the prevention of ischemic complications. Evaluation in percutaneous transluminal coronary angioplasty to improve long-term outcome with abciximab GP IIb/IIIa blockade. Evaluation of platelet IIb/IIIa inhibitor for Stent. *J Am Coll Cardiol* 2000; **36**: 381–6.

33 Lansky AJ, Pietras C, Costa RA, *et al.* Gender differences in outcomes after primary angioplasty versus primary stenting with and without abciximab for acute myocardial infarction: results of the Controlled Abciximab and Device Investigation to Lower Late Angioplasty Complications (CADILLAC) trial. *Circulation* 2005; **111**: 1611–18.

34 Chew DP, Bhatt DL, Sapp S, Topol EJ. Increased mortality with oral platelet glycoprotein IIb/IIIa antagonists: a meta-analysis of phase III multicenter randomized trials. *Circulation* 2001; **103**: 201–6.

35 Peter K, Schwarz M, Ylanne J, *et al.* Induction of fibrinogen binding and platelet aggregation as a potential intrinsic property of various glycoprotein

IIb/IIIa (alphaIIbbeta3) inhibitors. *Blood* 1998; **92**: 3240–9.

36 Cox D, Smith R, Quinn M, *et al.* Evidence of platelet activation during treatment with a GPIIb/IIIa antagonist in patients presenting with acute coronary syndromes. *J Am Coll Cardiol* 2000; **36**: 1514–19.

37 Maclouf J, Folco G, Patrono C. Eicosanoids and iso-eicosanoids: constitutive, inducible and transcellular biosynthesis in vascular disease. *Thromb Haemost* 1998; **79**: 691–705.

38 Patrono C, FitzGerald GA. Isoprostanes: potential markers of oxidant stress in atherothrombotic disease. *Arterioscler Thromb Vasc Biol* 1997; **17**: 2309–15.

39 Cipollone F, Ciabattoni G, Patrignani P, *et al.* Oxidant stress and aspirin-insensitive thromboxane biosynthesis

in severe unstable angina. *Circulation* 2000; **102**: 1007–13.

40 Husted S, Emanuelsson H, Heptinstall S, *et al.* Pharmacodynamics, pharmacokinetics, and safety of the oral reversible P2Y12 antagonist AZD6140 with aspirin in patients with atherosclerosis: a double-blind comparison to clopidogrel with aspirin. *Eur Heart J* 2006; **27**: 1038–47.

41 Wiviott SD, Antman EM, Winters KJ, *et al.* Randomized comparison of prasugrel (CS-747, LY640315), a novel thienopyridine P2Y12 antagonist, with clopidogrel in percutaneous coronary intervention: results of the Joint Utilization of Medications to Block Platelets Optimally (JUMBO)-TIMI 26 trial. *Circulation* 2005; **111**: 3366–73.

13

Prophylaxis for venous thrombosis in medical and surgical patients

GREGORY T GEROTZIAFAS, MEYER M SAMAMA

INTRODUCTION: THE BURDEN OF DISEASE

Venous thromboembolism (VTE) is one of the leading causes of death in industrial countries, killing more people than acquired immune deficiency syndrome (AIDS), breast cancer, and motor vehicle accidents combined.[1,2] In the United States, coronary heart disease is responsible for almost half a million deaths each year,[3] which compares with around 200 000 for pulmonary embolism (PE),[4] but this latter figure may be an underestimate because of the silent nature of VTE and the declining rate of autopsy. Of the 2 million Americans who have a deep vein thrombosis (DVT) each year, 600 000 subsequently develop PE, causing fatality in around 10 percent of cases.[5] Postthrombotic syndrome, a chronic, potentially disabling condition,[6,7] occurs in approximately 30–60 percent of patients with DVT, and a small proportion of patients develop pulmonary hypertension. A recent study has shown that in patients with an acute episode of PE but without prior VTE, the cumulative incidence of symptomatic chronic thromboembolic pulmonary hypertension is 3.8 percent at 2 years.[8] The estimated cost of care for VTE is estimated at US$1.5 billion each year.[9]

Epidemiologic data: women versus men

The association between sex and VTE is controversial, and there are a small number of studies on this topic. Two retrospective cohort studies and one case control study identified a slightly higher risk (odds ratio [OR] 1.2–1.7) of symptomatic VTE in males.[4,10,11] The Longitudinal Investigation of Thromboembolism Etiology (LITE) study identified an increased risk of VTE (OR 1.4, 95 percent confidence interval [CI] 1.1 to 1.9) among males.[12] In contrast, a French study identified a slightly higher incidence of VTE among females (OR 1.3) confined mainly to the age groups of 20–39 years and above 75 years,[13] and another study did not find a sex difference in the incidence of DVT.[14] Interestingly, a study conducted in 826 patients for an average of 36 months after a first episode of spontaneous VTE and the withdrawal of oral anticoagulants found that the risk of recurrent VTE was higher among men than women.[15] However, this observation was contradicted by Agnelli and Becattini who found no significant difference in the risk for recurrent VTE between men and women.[16]

Venous thromboembolism – a silent disease

Venous thromboembolism is often a silent disease and tends not to be suspected by physicians, especially in medical patients. In the Framingham study, which involved 3470 patients, autopsy results were available in 39 percent of 998 patients.[17] Overall, 16 percent of these patients were found to have had a fatal PE. Interestingly, in patients who had recently undergone surgery, a suspicion of PE before death was reported in nearly two-thirds of patients. In contrast, venous thrombosis was not suspected in almost three-quarters of medically ill patients who died of PE, highlighting the lack of awareness among physicians of the risk of VTE in this population. Autopsy studies conducted in Europe and the United States in the early 1980s and in the 1990s demonstrated that among medical patients who had a fatal PE, between 59 percent and 83 percent were not diagnosed with PE until autopsy.[18–20] A similar rate of fatal PE is observed in surgical patients.[21] Approximately 10 percent of hospital deaths are secondary to PE, although PE tends not to be recognized until autopsy. Of interest, 70 percent of these deaths occur in medical patients, with the remaining 30 percent occurring in surgical patients.[4,22]

Venous thromboembolism – a multifactorial disease

Venous thromboembolism is a multifactorial disease and patients may have multiple risk factors present simultaneously.[23,24] The more risk factors present in a patient the greater the risk of VTE. An essential step toward risk factor assessment is their classification into intrinsic or predisposing risk factors and extrinsic or triggering risk factors.[25] Patients can be stratified into risk groups (low risk, moderate risk, high risk, and very high risk[26–28]).

Awareness about venous thromboembolism

Venous thromboembolism remains an underestimated problem among clinicians, partly because it is often silent and partly because of its late occurrence following a surgical procedure. In two-thirds of patients undergoing major orthopaedic surgery, both DVT and PE occur following hospital discharge, which results in the surgeon not being aware of their occurrence.[29] A third important problem is that most of the trials that evaluated the efficacy and safety of prophylaxis, assessed the frequency of asymptomatic DVT (usually assessed by mandatory phlebography) as well as symptomatic VTE, but the former is much more common than the latter. The use of phlebography as a surrogate endpoint for clinically important DVT has been criticized, and it has not been readily accepted by clinicians.

METHODS OF PROPHYLAXIS FOR VENOUS THROMBOEMBOLISM

Prophylaxis for VTE can involve mechanical means or pharmacologic agents or both:

- Physical methods of prophylaxis are designed to reduce stasis in leg veins. Three types of physical method have been evaluated: graduated compression stockings (GCS), intermittent pneumatic compression (IPC) devices, and venous foot pumps. Physical methods of prophylaxis have not been systematically studied in medical patients but they have been extensively evaluated in surgical patients. They do not increase bleeding but they suffer from problems of compliance. Experience with these methods is limited and is much less than with pharmacologic agents. A combination of physical methods and pharmacologic agents is most often used in very-high-risk surgical patients.
- Low-molecular-weight heparins (LMWHs) are extensively used in prophylaxis of VTE in Europe, and unfractionated heparin (UFH) and warfarin are more frequently used in North America.
- Aspirin/other antiplatelet agents on their own are insufficient for prophylaxis of surgical patients since more effective agents are readily available.[30]
- Fondaparinux (Arixtra®), a synthetic indirect inhibitor of factor Xa (FXa)[31] and ximelagatran (Exanta®), a synthetic orally active direct thrombin inhibitor,[32] have been approved for prophylaxis against VTE in major orthopedic surgery in Europe and North America.

In this chapter we will discuss the critical trials carried out on prophylaxis for VTE in medical patients.

VENOUS THROMBOEMBOLISM PROPHYLAXIS IN MEDICAL PATIENTS: CLINICAL TRIALS

The average incidence of VTE disease among medical patients ranges from 18 percent to 23 percent.[33,34] In contrast with surgical patients clinical trials in nonsurgical patients are limited because the benefit is probably more difficult to demonstrate.[35] The MEDical patients with ENOXaparin (MEDENOX) trial, the Prospective Epidemiological Study of Myocardial Infarction (PRIME) study, the PRevention IN Cardiopulmonary Disease with Enoxaparin (PRINCE) study and the Prospective Randomized Evaluation of the Vascular Effects of Norvasc Trial (PREVENT) are considered to be more informative than previous studies. Thromboprophylaxis in nonsurgical cancer patients and in patients in intensive care medical units has not yet been adequately studied in controlled trials. Analysis of epidemiologic data and clinical outcomes does not show any sex-related differences in either the frequency of VTE or the efficacy and safety of the studied treatments.

Acutely ill medical patients

THE MEDENOX STUDY

The MEDENOX study[36] is considered to be a landmark trial in the prevention of VTE in medical patients because it assessed the efficacy and safety of two doses of enoxaparin (20 mg and 40 mg subcutaneously once daily) for

6–14 days compared with placebo in a large population of acutely ill medical patients, using systematic bilateral venography. The trial showed that the incidence of asymptomatic DVT in medical patients was 14.9 percent and that administration of 40 mg enoxaparin subcutaneously once daily reduces the frequency of asymptomatic DVT to 5.5 percent ($P < 0.001$) without any significant increase of the bleeding risk as compared with placebo. In contrast, the dose of 20 mg enoxaparin did not have any significant effect on the frequency of asymptomatic DVT (15 percent) as compared with placebo. Analytical data are presented in Table 13.1. The benefit observed with 40 mg of enoxaparin was maintained at 3 months. In addition, the MEDENOX trial showed that the presence of an acute infectious disease, in patients aged older than 75 years, with cancer, and a history of VTE, was independently associated with an increased VTE risk. The sex of the patient did not have any significant influence on the efficacy and safety profile of prevention with 40 mg of enoxaparin.[37]

THE PRIME STUDY

A multicenter, double-blind, randomized controlled trial compared enoxaparin (40 mg one subcutaneous injection per day) with UFH (5000 IU three subcutaneous injections daily) in DVT prophylaxis in a group of 959 hospitalized high-risk medical patients. The studied regimen was administered for 7 days. Ultrasonography was used for diagnosis of DVT. The incidence of DVT was 0.2 percent in the enoxaparin group and 0.82 in the UFH group ($P > 0.05$). A noteworthy reduction in PE was observed in the enoxaparin group as compared with the UFH group (0 percent and 0.8 percent, respectively). Major bleeding episodes were less frequent in the enoxaparin group (0.4 percent) than in the UFH group (1.8 percent). Prophylaxis with enoxaparin tended to reduce mortality as compared with UFH (1.46 percent and 2.28 percent, respectively). Enoxaparin was at least as efficacious as standard heparin, with fewer adverse events.[38] Summarized data are presented in Table 13.2.

Table 13.1   Efficacy and safety of prophylaxis with two doses of enoxaparin versus placebo in medical patients. The MEDENOX trial

	No. of patients	Diagnosis of VTE	Type of VTE	Placebo	Enoxaparin 2000 IU anti-Xa sc/day	Enoxaparin 4000 IU anti-Xa sc/day	Duration
MEDENOX[36] Randomized, multicenter, double-blind placebo-controlled (1999)	1102 acutely ill medical patients	Phlebography	Total VTE	14.9	15.0	5.5	6–14 days
			DVT	13.9	14.6	5.5	
			PE	0.7	0	0	
			DVT + PE	0.3	0.3	0	
			Proximal DVT	4.9	4.5	1.7	
			Distal DVT	9.4	10.5	3.8	
			Symptomatic DVT	0.7	1.0	0.3	

DVT, deep vein thrombosis; PE, pulmonary embolism; SC, subcutaneous; VTE, venous thromboembolism.

Table 13.2   Efficacy and safety of prophylaxis with LMWHs in medical patients

	No. of patients	Diagnosis of VTE	Type of VTE	Placebo	Enoxaparin 2000 IU anti-Xa sc/day	Enoxaparin 4000 IU anti-Xa sc/day	UFH 5000 IU × 3 sc/day	Duration
PRIME[38] Randomized double-blind (1996)	959 medical patients	Ultrasonography	DVT		0.2		0.82	7 days
			PE		0		0.8	
PRINCE[(39)] Randomized double-blind (1998)	451 patients with cardiopulmonary disease	Phlebography when D-Dimmer positive	DVT		7.9		10.3	10 days
			PE		0.4		0.4	

DVT, deep vein thrombosis; LMWH, low-molecular-weight heparin; PE, pulmonary embolism; SC, subcutaneous.

THE PRINCE STUDY

The efficacy and safety of enoxaparin was compared with UFH in 665 medical patients with severe cardiopulmonary disease (respiratory insufficiency or class III or IV heart failure); a population of patients comparable with that of MEDENOX study.[39] Patients were treated either with 40 mg enoxaparin subcutaneously once daily or UFH 5000 IU subcutaneously three times daily for 10 days. Systematic monitoring of D-dimer was performed, and bilateral phlebography was done if D-dimer levels were increased. Deep vein thrombosis was diagnosed in 7.9 percent of enoxaparin-treated patients and in 10.3 percent of UFH-treated patients ($P > 0.05$). Summarized data are presented in Table 13.2.

In both the PRIME and PRINCE studies enoxaparin 40 mg once daily was as effective and safe as UFH 5000 IU given subcutaneously three times daily. Interestingly, in North America most physicians are routinely using UFH 5000 IU twice daily, a dose that is not in accordance with the results of the previous trials.

THE PREVENT STUDY

The PREVENT study compared the efficacy and safety of dalteparin versus placebo in 3706 hospitalized, medically ill patients with moderate or high risk for VTE. The primary endpoint was symptomatic VTE, defined as fatal PE, sudden death, or asymptomatic proximal DVT at day 21. Asymptomatic proximal VTE was assessed with standardized bilateral compression ultrasound. Thus the PREVENT study was the first controlled trial to examine clinically important endpoints and in using compression ultrasound in evaluating the effect of a LMWH in hospitalized patients.[40] The trial demonstrated that the incidence of the primary outcome was 4.96 percent in the placebo group and 2.77 percent in the dalteparin group ($P = 0.0015$). Thus a daily dose of 5000 IU of dalteparin given for 21 days in medically ill patients with moderate or high risk for VTE reduces the relative risk of VTE by 45 percent as compared with placebo, with a low risk of bleeding.

Asymptomatic DVT as assessed by core laboratory compression ultrasonography accounted for the majority of the endpoints of the primary outcome (3.65 percent in the placebo group and 1.79 percent in the dalteparin group; relative risk reduction 52 percent in favor of dalteparin, $P = 0.003$).[41] At entry, 42 percent of all patients were receiving aspirin. In the placebo group, the incidence of the primary endpoint was 5.5 percent in patients who were not taking aspirin and 4.2 percent in those receiving aspirin. Comparing dalteparin with placebo for the patients not receiving aspirin, the relative risk of the primary endpoint was 0.42 (95 percent CI 0.25 to 0.70), whereas in patients receiving aspirin the relative risk was 0.81 (0.46 to 1.42). The combination of dalteparin with aspirin did not increase the bleeding risk since minor bleeds in patients not receiving aspirin were observed in 1.1 percent and 0.3 percent of the dalteparin and placebo group, respectively, whereas in the patients receiving aspirin the incidence was 0.9 percent in both groups.[42]

Extended venous thromboembolism prophylaxis in medical patients

THE EXCLAIM STUDY

Results of the MEDENOX trial showed that the risk for VTE extended beyond the 10-day period of prophylaxis with enoxaparin. Extended Prophylaxis for Venous Thrombo-Embolism (EXCLAIM) is a randomized, double-blind trial of 5800 patients considered at significant risk for VTE. The patients are given open-label prophylaxis with 40 mg of enoxaparin subcutaneously once daily until day 10 and are then randomized to receive either placebo or enoxaparin in the same dose for another 28 days. Follow-up will continue after the end of treatment out to 128 days. The primary endpoints are the rate of VTE and major bleeding with treatment in the period after randomization. Preliminary results of the EXCLAIM study showed that of patients enrolled that far, primary diagnoses were acute infection in 37 percent, respiratory insufficiency in 35 percent, and congestive heart failure in 13 percent, among other conditions. The final results of the EXCLAIM trial are expected in 2006/7.[43]

VENOUS THROMBOEMBOLISM PROPHYLAXIS IN NONSURGICAL CANCER PATIENTS

Active cancer is associated with a high risk of VTE and may be due to the hypercoagulable state of malignancy, or to its treatment including surgery, chemotherapy, radiotherapy, and central venous lines.[44,45] Advanced malignancies, renal carcinoma, and pancreatic, gastric, and brain tumors are independent variables strongly associated with the occurrence of venous thrombosis.[46] In addition active cancer is among the major risk factors for VTE.[47,48] In contrast with surgical cancer patients,[49] the efficacy and safety of antithrombotic prophylaxis in medical cancer patients has not been extensively evaluated. A randomized trial of 311 women with metastatic breast cancer receiving chemotherapy showed that low-dose warfarin (1 mg/day for 6 weeks) adjusted to maintain the international normalized ratio (INR) between 1.3 and 1.9 significantly reduced the frequency of symptomatic DVT (0.6 percent) as compared with placebo (4 percent; $P < 0.05$).[50] A recent survey reported that less than 5 percent of the medical oncologists surveyed use antithrombotic prophylaxis in nonsurgical cancer patients.[51] Analysis of trials assessing the efficacy of warfarin or heparins in the treatment and secondary prevention of VTE have generated the hypothesis that antithrombotic treatment prolongs the survival of cancer patients.[52–54] A prospective, randomized placebo-controlled trial conducted in 385 advanced cancer patients assessed the effect of a single daily subcutaneous injection of dalteparin (5000 IU) given for 1 year on the survival of patients at 1 year. This study showed that administration of dalteparin did not improve the 1-year survival in treated patients as compared with the placebo group. However, a *post hoc* analysis showed that dalteparin had a beneficial effect on the survival in a subgroup of patients with better prognosis and less advanced disease.[55]

Special attention has to be given to thrombosis related to central venous catheter use. The incidence of phlebographically detected asymptomatic upper limb DVT related to central venous catheters varies between 27 percent and 66 percent and that of symptomatic upper limb DVT related to central venous catheter has been reported to be between 0.3 percent and 28.3 percent.[56] In addition, the incidence of symptomatic PE in patients with a central venous catheter ranges from 15 percent to 25 percent, but an autopsy-proved PE rate of up to 50 percent has been reported.[56] Administration of low-dose warfarin or LMWH has been shown to reduce the risk of upper limb thrombosis related to central venous catheter in cancer patients.[57,58] However, these findings were not confirmed by more recent studies, which showed that low-dose warfarin increased the bleeding risk without a significant reduction of thrombosis related to central venous catheter in cancer patients.[59,60] In addition, trials with LMWH (dalteparin) failed to demonstrate efficacy of dalteparin (2500 IU subcutaneously once daily). Clinically relevant VTE occurred in 3.7 percent and 3.4 percent of the dalteparin and placebo recipients, respectively (reviewed in reference 32). Thus, the risk of clinically important VTE related to central venous catheters may be too low to warrant routine prophylaxis.[30] No significant difference in the frequency of VTE or major hemorrhage was found between women and men.

Venous thromboembolism prophylaxis with new antithrombotic agents (fondaparinux)

THE ARTEMIS TRIAL

Arixtra for ThromboEmbolism Prevention in a Medical Indications (ARTEMIS) was a study conducted in acutely ill elderly medical patients to assess the efficacy and safety of prophylaxis with fondaparinux (2.5 mg once daily for 6 to 14 days) versus placebo. The study design has been criticized for ethical reasons because of the use of placebo. In total, 849 patients were randomized, within 48 hours after hospital admission, to receive either fondaparinux or placebo. In the placebo group, the incidence of confirmed VTE was 10.5 percent, indicating a moderate VTE risk in the study population. Fondaparinux prophylaxis led to a significant decrease in VTE incidence – 5.6 percent ($P = 0.029$, odds reduction of 49.5 percent; 95 percent CI 72.1 percent to 8.6 percent). No symptomatic VTE occurred up to day 15 in the fondaparinux-treated patients compared with a 1.2 percent incidence of fatal PE in the placebo arm ($P = 0.029$). The rate of major bleeding was 0.2 percent in both groups. By day 32, the

mortality in the fondaparinux group was 3.3 percent compared with 6 percent in the placebo group ($P > 0.05$).[61]

VENOUS THROMBOEMBOLISM PROPHYLAXIS IN SURGICAL PATIENTS

The risk of postoperative VTE is well established in surgical patients. Prophylaxis with low-dose heparin has contributed significantly to the reduction in thromboembolic complications in surgery. Without prophylaxis, the rate of asymptomatic DVT is about 30 percent in patients undergoing general surgery, rising up to 70 percent in major orthopedic and trauma surgery. In reports by Collins *et al.*[62] and Clagett and Reisch,[63] heparin prevented at least 60 percent of DVTs. The efficacy of UFH treatment for the prevention of VTE in surgical and orthopedic patients is accepted worldwide and the data so far published do not show any significant influence of sex on the efficacy and safety of antithrombotic prophylaxis. During the past decade, a large number of clinical trials and several meta-analyses proved that the diverse preparations of LMWHs are, at least, as effective and safe as UFH in the prophylaxis of VTE in surgical patients.[64,65]

The LMWHs gained a predominant role in the prevention of VTE not only as a result of their proved efficacy and safety established by the above mentioned clinical trials and metaanalysis, but also as the consequence of their pharmacologic properties, their more predictable pharmacokinetics and pharmacodynamics, the reduced risk of heparin-induced thrombocytopenia, and more convenient use. The use of LMWHs in the prophylaxis of VTE in surgical patients is strongly recommended and is now included in the guidelines issued by the American College of Chest Physicians (ACCP) (2004 Consensus Guidelines on Antithrombotic Therapy).[30]

The 'new generation' of clinical trials in prophylaxis of VTE in surgical patients verify the efficacy and safety of LMWH. Some other important issues are also being more systematically approached. The most relevant topics of these recent clinical trials on the prevention of VTE in surgical patients are classification of surgical patients according to the risk for VTE based on either their disease or the type of the surgical procedure; the optimal duration and the optimal dosage of LMWH prophylactic regimen; and the need for adaptation of LMWH dosage according to the risk of thromboembolic risk.

Similar to medical patients, the incidence of VTE and the efficacy and safety of the prophylactic strategies is not different between men and women. Thus here both sexes will be treated in a pooled way. In this chapter we have classified the trials which will be presented in six categories: (i) low-risk patients; (ii) moderate-risk patients;(iii) high- and very-high-risk patients; (iv) patients undergoing specialized surgical procedures (neurosurgery); (v) long-term postoperative prophylaxis; and (vi) gynecologic surgery and VTE prophylaxis in pregnancy.

Low-risk surgical patients

In low-risk patients undergoing minimal surgical procedures the incidence of VTE is rather low and physical preventive measures are sufficient for the prophylaxis of VTE.

A prospective randomized controlled clinical trial of 718 selected low-risk patients who underwent laparoscopic cholecystectomy and other types of minimally invasive surgery and received graduated elastic stockings showed that the incidence of asymptomatic DVT diagnosed on duplex ultrasound was less than 0.2 percent in the whole population. The frequency of DVT was similar in the reviparin-treated group and in the placebo group.[66]

Moderate-risk surgical patients

Moreno Gonzalez et al.[67] carried out a prospective, multicenter, double-blind, randomized controlled trial in two groups of patients (n = 100 each) with a low/moderate risk of VTE, who underwent elective abdominal surgery. They evaluated the efficacy and safety of reviparin at a daily subcutaneous dose of 2500 IU anti-factor Xa, compared with UFH administered as subcutaneous injection of 5000 IU twice daily for 7 days. There were no cases of DVT, PE, or death in either group. The safety profile was similar in both groups.

An interesting prospective, double-blind, randomized, placebo-controlled study was carried out by Bergqvist et al.[68] on the efficacy of postoperative tinzaparin (once daily) in emergency abdominal surgery. The study enrolled 80 patients undergoing emergency abdominal surgery allocated to two groups. The fibrinogen uptake test was used for the diagnosis of VTE but because of withdrawal of the labeled fibrinogen from the market the target sample size was not reached. The frequency of DVT was reduced with prophylaxis from 22 percent in the placebo group (95 percent CI 11 percent to 38 percent) to 8 percent in the tinzaparin group (95 percent CI 2 percent to 21 percent), a risk reduction of 65 percent, which was not statistically significant in this underpowered study.

High- and very-high-risk surgical patients

Prophylaxis for VTE in patients undergoing major surgical procedures with either UFH or LWMH is widely used, and it is considered unethical not to give prophylaxis. Thus, there are few placebo-controlled trials in patients undergoing major surgery as reviewed by Bergqvist in 1994.[69] A placebo-controlled study demonstrated that the frequency of VTE was 15.9 percent in the placebo group and the administration of LMWH reduced the frequency of VTE to 4.2 percent. The subgroup analysis revealed that the frequency of VTE was even higher in patients operated for malignant disease, being rather low in noncancer patients. During the 1990s, the efficacy and safety of LMWHs in the prophylaxis of VTE in high-risk patients undergoing major surgery has been established by numerous trials reviewed by several authors. The use of LMWHs in the prophylaxis of VTE in high-risk surgical patients is a grade 1A recommendation of the ACCP 2004 Consensus Conference on Antithrombotic Therapy.[30]

Surgical cancer patients

The Enoxaparin and Cancer (ENOXACAN) study[49] and the study by von Tempelhoff et al.[70] demonstrated that enoxaparin 40 mg and certoparin 3000 IU anti-Xa, respectively, administered as once daily injections in cancer patients undergoing therapeutic surgical procedures, is as effective and safe as UFH administered three times daily for prevention of VTE. In the ENOXACAN trial the frequency of postoperative VTE was 18.2 percent in UFH-treated patients and 14.7 percent in the enoxaparin group. von Tempelhoff et al.[70] found the frequency of postoperative VTE was 0 percent in the UFH-treated group and 6.7 percent in the certoparin-treated group. The difference was not statistically significant, and only a small number of patients were included in the study and the diagnostic procedure for VTE was suboptimal (impedance plethysmography).

A third multicenter open randomized dose-finding trial[71] performed in lung cancer patients undergoing thoracic surgery demonstrated that administration of a single fixed dose of nadroparin (3075 IU anti-Xa, daily) is as effective as the administration of a single weight-adjusted dose (4100 IU–6150 IU anti-Xa, daily). Similarly, a low dose of reviparin (1750 IU anti-Xa, daily) is as effective as, and safer than UFH administered in high-risk surgical patients undergoing major abdominal surgery.[72] Low-dose enoxaparin (20 mg administered in a single daily injection) to surgical patients undergoing major abdominal surgery is as effective and slightly safer than low-dose UFH.[73] However, contradictory results were presented by Wiig et al.[74] In their study, the frequency of VTE in high-risk surgical patients undergoing elective gastrointestinal surgery receiving low-dose enoxaparin (20 mg daily) was rather high (33 percent) similar to that observed in high risk patients receiving prophylaxis with dextran (31 percent). In a third group of high-risk patients receiving enoxaparin, 40 mg daily, the frequency of VTE was significantly reduced (12 percent). Phlebography was used for the diagnosis of VTE. On the same lines, data from a trial carried out by Bergqvist et al.[75] on high-risk surgical patients demonstrated that a higher prophylactic dose of dalteparin (5000 IU anti-Xa, once daily) is more effective than a lower dose of dalteparin (2500 IU anti-Xa, once daily). The frequency of VTE was 6.8 percent in the former and 13.8 percent in the latter group. However, the frequency of important bleeding increases with high doses of LMWH.

Gynecologic surgery patients

Venous thromboembolism is an important and potentially preventable complication of major gynecologic surgery, with rates of DVT, PE, and fatal PE comparable to those seen after general surgical procedures. Several practice guidelines have addressed the issue of thromboprophylaxis in patients undergoing gynecologic surgery and specific recommendations have been formulated from the ACCP Consensus Conference on Antithrombotic therapy.[30] Women who are otherwise well and undergo brief procedures, typically defined as <30 minutes, do not require any specific prophylaxis but should be encouraged to mobilize early after surgery. Women having surgery for gynecologic cancers appear to derive less protection from twice daily dosing of low-dose UFH than those with benign disease. Either UFH, 5000 IU three times daily, or LMWH, at daily doses of at least 4000 IU, appears to be more effective in these cancer patients. An unresolved issue is the duration of antithrombotic prophylaxis following gynecologic surgery. One randomized, double-blind study compared 1 week with 1 month of LMWH prophylaxis in patients undergoing curative surgery for abdominal or pelvic malignancy (8 percent of the patients had a gynecologic oncology procedure). Extended prophylaxis conferred a relative risk reduction of 60 percent for both venographically screened DVT and proximal DVT. Although this trial suggested a potential advantage of post-hospital discharge prophylaxis in certain high-risk surgical oncology patients, the specific risk factors that warrant extended prophylaxis remain to be defined.

According to the ACCP Consensus Conference, thromboprophylaxis in all major gynecologic surgery patients is a Grade 1A recommendation. For patients undergoing major gynecologic surgery for benign disease, without additional risk factors, one of the following is recommended: low-dose UFH (5000 IU twice daily (Grade 1A); LMWH 3400 IU anti-Xa, once daily (Grade 1C+); or intermittent pneumatic compression started just before surgery and used continuously while the patient is not mobile (Grade 1B). For patients undergoing extensive surgery for malignancy, and for patients with additional VTE risk factors, the use of UFH 5000 IU three times daily (Grade 1A), or higher doses of LMWH (that is, >3400 IU anti-Xa, daily) (Grade 1A) are recommended. Alternative considerations include IPC on its own continued until hospital discharge (Grade 1A), or a combination of low-dose UFH or LMWH plus mechanical prophylaxis with GCS or IPC (all Grade 1C). For patients undergoing major gynecologic procedures, it is suggested that prophylaxis continue until discharge from the hospital (Grade 1C). For patients who are at particularly high risk, including those who have undergone cancer surgery and are >60 years of age or have previously experienced VTE, continuing prophylaxis for 2–4 weeks after hospital discharge is suggested (Grade 2C).

Neurosurgical patients

Although LMWHs have proved to be effective for prophylaxis of VTE when administered postoperatively, the perioperative anticoagulant prophylaxis for postoperative venous thromboembolism (VTE) in neurosurgical patients has not gained wide acceptance due to the high risk of intracranial bleeding. Physical methods such as GCS provide a worthwhile reduction of postoperative VTE but there still remains a substantial residual incidence.

In a multicenter, randomized, double-blind trial, Agnelli et al. assessed the efficacy and safety of enoxaparin (40 mg once daily) in conjunction with the use of compression stockings in the prevention of VTE in patients undergoing elective neurosurgery beginning within 24 hours after the completion of surgery.[76] Enoxaparin (or placebo) was given subcutaneously for not less than 7 days. The frequency of asymptomatic VTE was 32 percent in the placebo group and 17 percent in the enoxaparin group (relative risk in the enoxaparin group 0.52, 95 percent CI 0.33 to 0.82, $P = 0.004$). Major bleeding occurred in four patients receiving placebo (intracranial bleeding in all four) and four patients (intracranial bleeding in three) receiving enoxaparin (3 percent of each group). In a randomized controlled trial, Dickinson et al.[77] investigated the efficacy and safety of enoxaparin in preventing DVT in patients with brain tumors. The study was prematurely terminated because of the increased incidence of adverse events in the enoxaparin-treated groups. Nurmohamed et al.[78] performed a multicenter, randomized, double-blind trial in neurosurgical patients comparing nadroparin, initiated postoperatively, with GCS in the prevention of VTE. On the tenth postoperative day, the rates of asymptomatic VTE were 18.7 percent and 26.3 percent in patients receiving enoxaparin or GCS, respectively, and this difference remained until 56 days post operatively. Major bleeding complications during the treatment period occurred in six LMWH-treated patients (2.5 percent) and in two control patients (0.8 percent; $P = 0.87$). A higher mortality was observed in the LMWH-treated group over the 56-day follow-up period (22 vs. 10; $P = 0.026$), but none of the deaths in the enoxaparin group was attributed to the treatment.

Venous thromboembolism prophylaxis with new antithrombotic agents in surgical patients

FONDAPARINUX IN MAJOR ORTHOPEDIC SURGERY

Recent phase III clinical trials in the prevention of DVT in major orthopaedic surgery, as well as a meta-analysis, showed that prophylaxis with 2.5 mg of subcutaneous fondaparinux once daily for 10 days and started 6 hours post operatively, reduces the risk of venographically documented VTE by about 55 percent as compared with enoxaparin. The rate of major bleeding is somewhat higher than enoxaparin when the first injection of fondaparinux is given earlier than 6 hours after the operation but it is similar to enoxaparin when the first injection of fondaparinux is given 6 hours after the operation.[79–83]

The efficacy and safety of long-term prophylaxis with fondaparinux in major orthopedic surgery were studied in a double-blind, placebo controlled, multicenter study of 656 patients undergoing hip fracture surgery (PENTasaccharide in HIp-FRActure Surgery [PENTHIFRA]-plus trial). Patients were randomly assigned to receive prophylaxis with a once-daily subcutaneous injection of either 2.5 mg of fondaparinux sodium or placebo for 19–23 days. Before randomization, all patients had received fondaparinux for 6–8 days. The primary efficacy outcome was VTE occurring during the double-blind period (DVT detected by mandatory bilateral venography, or documented symptomatic DVT, or PE). The main safety outcome was major bleeding. The primary efficacy outcome was assessed in 428 patients. Fondaparinux reduced the incidence of VTE compared with placebo from 35 percent to 1.4 percent, a relative risk reduction of 95.9 percent ($P < 0.001$). Similarly, the incidence of symptomatic VTE was significantly lower with fondaparinux (0.3 percent) than with placebo (2.7 percent relative risk reduction 88.8 percent, $P < 0.05$). There was a trend toward more major bleeding in the fondaparinux group than in the placebo group, but there were no significant differences between the two groups.[84]

The clinical trials of fondaparinux in association with pharmacokinetics studies in healthy volunteers identified that during the first day of treatment, fondaparinux concentrations in plasma ranged from minimum 0.1 g/mL to a peak of 0.3 g/mL in prophylaxis and from 0.6 g/mL to a peak of 1.5 g/mL in treatment of VTE.

FONDAPARINUX IN GENERAL SURGERY

The results of a large multicenter, randomized, double-blind study of fondaparinux in abdominal surgery (PEntasaccharide in GenerAl SUrgery Study [PEGASUS] trial) have been recently presented. The primary efficacy outcome was the composite of asymptomatic DVT assessed by screening venography and symptomatic confirmed VTE. The main safety outcome was major bleeding. In the PEGASUS trial, the efficacy and safety of postoperative fondaparinux was compared with that of dalteparin started before surgery. Fondaparinux 2.5 mg was given once daily starting 6 hours after surgery. Dalteparin 5000 IU was given once daily, after a preoperative injection of 2500 IU 2 hours before surgery and a first postoperative injection of 2500 IU on the evening of the day of surgery. Both agents were given subcutaneously for 7 ± 2 days. Patients were eligible for inclusion if were classified as being at high or very high risk for VTE. Overall, 2927 patients were included and the primary efficacy outcome was assessed in 2048 patients. Fondaparinux was not inferior to dalteparin since it reduced the incidence of VTE compared with dalteparin from 6.1 percent to 4.6 percent, an odds reduction of 25.8 percent ($P > 0.05$). Among the 1408 very-high-risk patients (cancer patients) analyzed for efficacy, fondaparinux significantly reduced the incidence of VTE compared with dalteparin from 7.7 percent to 4.7 percent, an odds reduction of 40.5 percent ($P = 0.02$). In both groups the incidence of major bleeding and the mortality was similar.[85]

XIMELAGATRAN IN MAJOR ORTHOPEDIC SURGERY

Ximelagatran (Exanta), the first available oral direct thrombin inhibitor, and its active form, melagatran, have been evaluated in the prevention of VTE in patients undergoing hip or knee replacement surgery. After oral administration, ximelagatran is rapidly converted to melagatran. Melagatran inactivates both circulating and clot-bound thrombin by binding to the thrombin active site, thus inhibiting platelet activation and/or aggregation and reducing fibrinolysis time. The efficacy of subcutaneous melagatran followed by oral ximelagatran has been investigated in four European studies.

Two main dose-finding studies compared two different regimens of orally administered ximelagatran associated or not with melagatran versus enoxaparin or dalteparin in major orthopedic surgery.[86,87] The dose of 3 mg melagatran and 24 mg ximelagatran were chosen to be studied in a phase III trial in major orthopedic surgery (MElagatran for THRombin inhibition in Orthopaedic surgery [METHRO] III) where the first injection of melagatran was given 4–12 hours post operatively and this regimen was compared with prophylaxis with enoxaparin 40 mg started 12 hours preoperatively. Venous thromboembolism occurred in 31 percent and 27.3 percent of patients in the ximelagatran and enoxaparin group, respectively, a difference in risk of 3.7 percent in favour of enoxaparin ($P = 0.053$). Bleeding was comparable between the two groups.[88]

The series of METHRO trials was followed by the EXpanded PRophylaxis Evaluation Surgery Study (EXPRESS) trial in which the first subcutaneous injection of melagatran was given immediately before the operation, but the dose of melagatran was reduced to 2 mg and the subsequent dose given after the operation was 3 mg followed by 24 mg of oral ximelagatran twice daily beginning the next day. Enoxaparin 40 mg, administered subcutaneously once daily, was started 12 hours before surgery. The rates of major and total VTE were significantly lower in the melagatran/ximelagatran group compared with the enoxaparin group (2.3 percent vs. 6.3 percent, $P = 0.0000018$; and 20.3 percent vs. 26.6 percent, $P < 0.0004$, respectively). Fatal bleeding, critical site bleeding, and bleeding requiring reoperation did not differ between the two groups. Excessive bleeding as judged by the investigator was more frequent with melagatran/ximelagatran than with enoxaparin.[89] Finally, the efficacy and safety of 24 mg ximelagatran given orally twice daily in the prevention of VTE in major orthopedic patients was compared with enoxaparin given at 30 mg twice daily. Noninferiority of ximelagatran 24 mg twice daily based on a prespecified margin of 5 percent was not met, resulting in superiority of the enoxaparin regimen.[90]

As warfarin is a widely acceptable prophylactic regimen, especially in North America, the efficacy and safety of two doses of ximelagatran 24 mg or 36 mg twice daily, starting the morning after surgery, were compared with warfarin therapy started the evening of the day of surgery in the

EXanta Used to Lessen Thrombosis (EXULT) trial. The treatment was given for 7–12 days. Oral ximelagatran at a dose of 36 mg twice daily was superior to warfarin with respect to the primary composite endpoint (VTE and all-cause mortality) and both ximelagatran and warfarin were similar with respect to major bleeding.[91] Ximelagatran is the first orally active direct thrombin inhibitor which has been proved to be as effective as LMWHs in VTE prophylaxis in major orthopedic surgery, without increasing the bleeding risk. However, despite the antithrombotic efficacy and initial approval by some regulatory authorities, significant hepatic and cardiac side effects have led to this agent being withdrawn by the manufacturers.

THE TIMING OF THE FIRST DOSE OF ANTITHROMBOTIC PROPHYLAXIS

Clinical trial findings, together with the aggregate data from systematic reviews and emerging results of clinical trials with new anticoagulants, recently reviewed by Raskob and Hirsh,[92] support the following general conclusions about the relation between the timing of the first anticoagulant dose and the efficacy and safety of thromboprophylaxis after major orthopedic surgery of the legs:

- Preoperative administration is not required to achieve good efficacy, and when begun within 2 hours of surgery, increases major bleeding.
- Initiation between 6 and 9 hours post operatively is effective and not associated with increased major bleeding.
- initiation 6 hours post operatively increases major bleeding, without improved efficacy; therefore, 6 hours appears to be the threshold for early postoperative initiation.
- Initiation 12–24 hours postoperatively may be less effective than initiation at 6 hours.

However, these observations should not be extrapolated to all new antithrombotic agents.

Timing of the first anticoagulant dose and neuraxial anesthesia

Of special interest is the association between the timing of the first injection and the bleeding risk when regional or neuraxial anesthesia is used. In the same review (by Raskob and Hirsh) it is proposed that for once-daily regimens, the recommended timing of the first postoperative dose is 6–8 hours postoperatively, with the next dose to be given not sooner than 24 hours later.[93] Indwelling neuraxial catheters can be maintained. However, the catheter should be removed a minimum of 10–12 hours after the previous dose of LMWH, and subsequent doses of LMWH should be delayed until at least 2 hours after catheter removal. If a twice-daily regimen is used, such as enoxaparin 30 mg twice daily, the first dose should not be administered until 24 hours post operatively, and indwelling neuraxial catheters should be removed before the LMWH is commenced. The first dose should also be delayed until at least 24 hours if there is blood during needle or catheter placement (for once- or twice-daily regimens).

VENOUS THROMBOEMBOLISM PROPHYLAXIS IN INTENSIVE CARE UNITS

According to four prospective trials in critically ill patients not receiving prophylaxis, admitted in intensive care units,[94–97] recently reviewed by Geerts and Selby,[98] the asymptomatic DVT rates vary between 13 percent and 31 percent. Critically ill patients admitted in ICU, documented to have DVT detected by routine Doppler ultrasound, had a significantly greater frequency of subsequent pulmonary embolism during their hospitalization (11.5 percent versus 0 percent; $P = 0,01$).[98] Furthermore, even small pulmonary emboli may be poorly tolerated by critically ill patients, many of whom have reduced cardiorespiratory reserve.[96]

Three randomized thromboprophylaxis trials using routine screening with an objective diagnostic test for DVT in ICU patients[94,95,99] reviewed by Geerts and Selby,[98] suggest that both low-dose UFH (5000 IU subcutaneously twice daily) and LMWH are efficacious in reducing the relative risk of asymptomatic DVT by 45 percent to 65 percent, without any significant increase of the bleeding risk. A recently published Franco-Canadian cross-sectional observational study of medical ICU patients showed that 92 percent of eligible patients received either low-dose UFH or LWMH for VTE prophylaxis.[100] This trial confirms that critical care physicians consider thromboembolism to be an important problem worthy of preventive interventions.

VENOUS THROMBOEMBOLISM PROPHYLAXIS IN PREGNANCY

The existence of a physiologic hypercoagulable state in woman during pregnancy has been well documented but the risk of VTE in pregnant woman is low (1:10 000 pregnancies) although higher than in the control population. It is significantly increased in some special categories of pregnant women, such as those with a previous episode and/or with thrombophilia. The time of greatest risk is the puerperium. Pulmonary embolism remains the leading direct cause of maternal deaths in the United Kingdom. Additional risk factors for VTE in pregnancy and the puerperium include obesity, age over 35 years, thrombophilic states, cesarean section, and surgical procedures during pregnancy and the puerperium. The evaluation of the level of risk has been difficult. Several recommendations or suggestions regarding the pregnant woman at high risk of VTE have been made by the ACCP and by other scientific organizations, but their level of evidence is low.[101]

VENOUS THROMBOEMBOLISM PROPHYLAXIS IN GERIATRIC PATIENTS

The incidence of VTE increases steadily with age and reaches about 1 percent in patients aged 75 and older. Institutionalization has been found to be a significant risk factor.[4] In a recent prospective study in a geriatric university hospital with long-, intermediate-, and short-term facilities in 1096 patients aged 65 years and older,[102] among 23 potential risk factors, six were identified as being independently related to the development of DVT. Age older than 75 years was associated with an odds ratio of 15 per 10 years in a multivariate analysis. A score ranging from 8 to 16 was defined for the risk factor assessment. Interestingly, there was no significant difference between men and women. A reviewer operating characteristic curve for the risk score for symptomatic DVT showed a correlation between the score and the level of risk. These results extend and confirm previous studies.[103,104]

Due to the greater life expectancy, VTE prophylaxis in elderly patients has attracted greater attention and a review of the results has been published.[105] The efficacy and safety of LMWH and warfarin in elderly patients has been documented but heterogeneous populations have been studied. The prevention of symptomatic DVT in hospitalized elderly patients merits further revaluation. The problem of renal insufficiency appears as a frequent cause of minor and major bleeding episodes. Very close laboratory monitoring of plasma anti-Xa activity is recommended to reduce the risk of bleeding.[106] Fragile elderly patients may have a higher risk of side effects when LMWH is used and particular care should be taken in such patients. Interestingly, it has not been demonstrated that hereditary thrombophilia (that is, factor V Leiden and *FII* gene mutation) significantly increase the risk of VTE.

SIDE EFFECTS OF ANTITHROMBOTIC AGENTS USED IN PROPHYLAXIS OF VENOUS THROMBOEMBOLISM

There is a rather weak relation between the dose of injected LMWH and bleeding risk at the doses recommended in this population of patients. No correlation between anti-Xa activity and bleeding could be evidenced.[107] LMWHs administered at fixed doses and without monitoring show unpredictable anticoagulant effects in patients with chronic kidney disease (stages 4 and 5) leading to serious and even fatal hemorrhagic episodes.[108] A significant accumulation of anti-Xa activity has been observed in elderly patients and in patients with renal impairment treated with LMWH and monitoring of plasma levels of anti-Xa activity

has been suggested, although anti-Xa levels are not well correlated with the clinical outcome.[109]

Allergic reactions are rare as are reports of skin necrosis. Transient elevations of transaminases are seen after both UFH and LMWH administration. A significant increase of transaminase levels has been seen in about 6 percent of patients receiving long-term treatment with ximelagatran.[110] However, such an increase of transaminases has not been observed in patients receiving short-term prophylaxis with ximelagatran. Finally, heparin-induced thrombocytopenia type II, although less frequent with LMWH than with UFH, is potentially the most severe complication of heparin treatment. Thus, platelet count should be monitored regularly in LMWH-treated patients. The peak frequency of heparin-induced thrombocytopenia is between 5 and 21 days of treatment. This observation led to the recommendation of monitoring platelet count before the first injection, then 5 days later and twice a week until heparin interruption. Treatment with danaparoid or lepirudin is well tolerated and has been widely used. In rare cases, cross-reactivity danaparoid/heparin has been observed.[111] No case of heparin-induced thrombocytopenia or any other toxicity has been observed in patients treated with fondaparinux. In addition, it has been proposed to use fondaparinux as alternative antithrombotic treatment in patients with heparin-induced thrombocytopenia. However, health authorities recommend monitoring of platelet counts at the beginning and at the end of the treatment with fondaparinux. Thrombocytopenia is a serious adverse effect of LMWHs but thrombocytosis has been also observed in some patients treated with LMWHs.[112]

SUMMARY AND CONCLUSIONS

Until now, the risk of VTE has been poorly documented in medical patients and the necessity of preventive measures has not been established by large trials and metaanalyses. As a consequence, there are no well-accepted recommendations by any consensus conference in Europe or in America. The recently published studies confirm the notion that the risk of VTE in hospitalized medical patients is, at least, as high as in patients undergoing surgery who are at moderate risk for VTE.[113] According to the trials published so far the frequency of VTE and the efficacy and safety of the studied prophylactic methods is similar in women and men. The recently published studies demonstrate that acutely ill medical patients are at increased risk of VTE.

The discrepancies in the incidence of VTE in the studies presented in this chapter are mainly due to differences in the severity of the underlying diseases in the patients enrolled in each study. For example, the incidence of VTE was somewhat higher among the patients treated with 40 mg enoxaparin in the PRINCE study as compared with the respective patients in the MEDENOX trial, probably because the PRINCE study enrolled more severely ill patients with respiratory insufficiency or class III or IV heart failure. Moreover, the different methods used for the diagnosis of DVT further confound the discrepancies. It is well established, for example, that ultrasonography has a low sensitivity for diagnosis of DVT in asymptomatic patients undergoing medical treatment or orthopedic surgery.[114]

The MEDENOX study showed that a single daily subcutaneous injection of enoxaparin 40 mg reduces the risk of VTE by 63 percent in acutely ill hospitalized patients. The MEDENOX trial pivoted the investigation of the real prevalence of VTE in the medical patients. The most recent trials, ARTEMIS and PREVENT, demonstrate that prophylaxis with either a selective inhibitor of FXa (fondaparinux 2.5 mg subcutaneously once daily) or with dalteparin (5000 IU anti-Xa subcutaneously once daily) is effective and safe. The results of both studies are in good agreement with those from the MEDENOX trial. The findings of MEDENOX and PREVENT trials justified the approval of health authorities in the United States and in Europe for the prophylactic use of enoxaparin and dalteparin in the prevention of VTE in acutely ill medical patients. The LMWHs are now available for patients with medical illness, including cancer, respiratory failure, and congestive heart failure at risk of DVT or PE.

The optimal duration of the treatment has to be further investigated and probably should be adapted on an individual basis. The EXCLAIM study has been designed to evaluate the benefit risk of long-term prophylaxis with enoxaparin in acutely ill medical patients. Since severe heparin-induced thrombocytopenia may occur in patients treated with LMWH, monitoring of platelet count before treatment and regularly after its initiation, is important.[115] Due to the accumulation of anti-Xa activity and the increased bleeding risk, special attention has to be given when LMWHs are used in patients with renal insufficiency. In addition to the favorable benefit/risk ratio, thromboprophylaxis with LMWH is convenient for patients. The administration of the treatment is simple and easy (one subcutaneous injection daily) and is comfortable for both patients and nurses.

A stratification of surgical patients according to the risk for VTE allows a more beneficial outcome of the LMWH prophylactic regimen and may also improve the cost–benefit ratio. In low-risk patients, the use of physical preventive measures such as ECS and rapid mobilization is sufficient for the prevention of VTE. In this case, the LMWHs do not add anything other than an increased cost of hospitalization. In moderate-risk patients, a preventive regimen with LMWH seems to be beneficial for the patients. The efficacy and safety of LMWH are similar with UFH. A low dose of LMWH is proved to be sufficient for adequate prevention of VTE. In high-risk patients, prophylaxis with LMWH (administered as one subcutaneous injection per day) is, at least, as efficient and slightly safer that the regimen with UFH (in two or three injections per day). Higher doses of LMWH are required for adequate prevention. Another approach could be the development of computerized reminder systems as it has been recently proposed to be used in surgical patients.[116] The introduction of a computer-alert program increased physicians' use of prophylaxis and markedly reduced the rates of DVT and PE among hospitalized patients at risk.[117] In patients undergoing general surgical procedures, long-term prophylactic administration of LMWH does not seem to be beneficial as compared with the effect of the administration during the 7–10 postoperative days. However, long-term administration of LMWH is not associated with increased hemorrhagic risk. Still, the financial cost–benefit ratio is not favorable for long-term prophylaxis with LMWH. It is necessary to define which groups of patients need to receive prolonged prophylaxis with LMWH.

KEY LEARNING POINTS

- Considerable progress has been achieved in the past 20 years with increased information on the prophylaxis of venous thrombosis.
- Sex does not seem to influence the epidemiology and the clinical outcome of the preventive strategies of VTE.
- For prophylaxis of VTE, widely accepted guidelines recommend LMWH as the first line of pharmaceutical prophylaxis, and mechanical measures for inpatients requiring prophylaxis who have a high bleeding risk (that is, neurosurgical patients).
- It is clear that acutely ill medical patients have a significant risk of VTE and use of prophylaxis should be considered.
- Clinical judgment remains essential in the decision about prophylaxis for individual patients.

REFERENCES

1 National Highway Traffic Safety Association. *2002 Annual Report of Motor Vehicle Crashes*. University of North Carolina, 2002.

2 American Cancer Society. *Cancer Facts and Figures 2003*. Ohio: American Cancer Society, 2003.

3 American Heart Association. *Heart Disease and Stroke Statistics, 2003 Update*. Dallas, TX: American Heart Association, 2002.

4 Anderson FA Jr Wheeler HB, Goldberg RJ, *et al*. A population-based perspective of the hospital incidence and case-fatality rates of deep vein thrombosis and pulmonary embolism. The Worcester DVT Study. *Arch Intern Med* 1991; **151**: 933–8.

5 Hirsh J, Hoak J. Management of deep vein thrombosis and pulmonary embolism. A statement for healthcare professionals from the council on thrombosis (in consultation with the council on cardiovascular radiology), American Heart Association. *Circulation* 1996; **93**: 2212–45.

6   Brandjes DP, Buller HR, Heijboer H, *et al.* Randomised trial of effect of compression stockings in patients with symptomatic proximal-vein thrombosis. *Lancet* 1997; **349**: 759–62.

7   Kahn SR, Solymoss S, Lamping DL, Abenhaim L. Long-term outcomes after deep vein thrombosis: postphlebitic syndrome and quality of life. *J Gen Intern Med* 2000; **15**: 425–9.

8   Pengo V, Lensing AWA, Prins MH, *et al.*, for the Thromboembolic Pulmonary Hypertension Study Group. Incidence of chronic thromboembolic pulmonary hypertension after pulmonary embolism. *N Engl J Med* 2004; **350**: 2257–64.

9   Goldhaber SZ, Visani L, Rosa M. Acute pulmonary embolism: clinical outcomes in the International Cooperative Pulmonary Embolism Registry (ICOPER). *Lancet* 1999; **353**: 1386–9.

10 Silverstein MD, Heit JA, Mohr DN, *et al.* Trends in the incidence of venous thromboembolism and PE: a 25 year population-based study. *Arch Intern Med* 1998; **158**: 585–93.

11 Cogo A, Bernardi E, Prandoni P, *et al.* Acquired risk factors for DVT in symptomatic outpatients. *Arch Intern Med* 1994; **154**: 164–8.

12 Tsai AW, Cushman M, Rosamond WD, *et al.* Cardio-vascular risk factors and venous thromboembolism incidence. The Longitudinal Investigation of Thrombo-embolism Etiology. *Arch Intern Med* 2001; **162**: 1182–9.

13 Oger E. Incidence of venous thromboembolism: a community-based study in western France. EPI-GETBP Study Group. Groupe d'Etude de la Thrombose de Bretagne Occidentale. *Thromb Haemost* 2000; **83**: 557–60.

14 Nordsrom M, Lindblad B, Bergqvist D, Kjellstrom T. A prospective study of the incidence of DVT within a defined urban population. *J Intern Med* 1992; **232**: 155–60.

15 Kyrle PA, Minar E, Bialoncyk C, *et al.* The risk of recurrent venous thromboembolism in men and women. *N Engl J Med* 2004; **350**: 2558–63.

16 Agnelli G, Becattini C. Recurrent venous thrombo-embolism in men and women. *N Engl J Med* 2004; **351**: 2015–16.

17 Goldhaber SZ, Savage DD, Garrison RJ, *et al.* Risk factors for pulmonary embolism. The Framingham Study. *Am J Med* 1983; **74**: 1023–8.

18 Nielsen HK, Bechgaard P, Nielsen PF, *et al.* 178 fatal cases of pulmonary embolism in a medical department. *Acta Med Scand* 1981; **209**: 351–5.

19 Sperry KL, Key CR, Anderson RE. Toward a population-based assessment of death due to pulmonary embolism in New Mexico. *Hum Pathol* 1990; **21**: 159–65.

20 Cohen AT, Edmondson RA, Philis MJ, *et al.* The changing pattern of venous thromboembolic disease. *Haemostasis* 1996; **26**: 65–71.

21 Hauch O, Jorgensen LN, Khattar SC, *et al.* Fatal pulmonary embolism associated with surgery. An autopsy study. *Acta Chir Scand* 1990; **156**: 747–9.

22 Anderson FA, Jr, Wheeler HB. Venous thromboembolism. Risk factors and prophylaxis. *Clin Chest Med* 1995; **16**: 235–51.

23 Rosendaal FR. Venous thrombosis: a multicausal disease. *Lancet* 1999; **353**: 1167–73.

24 Heit JA, Silverstein MD, Mohr DN, *et al.* The epidemiology of venous thromboembolism in the community. *Thromb Haemost* 2001; **86**: 452–63.

25 Samama MM, Dahl OE, Quinlan DJ, *et al.* Quantification of risk factors for venous thromboembolism: a preliminary study for the development of a risk assessment tool. *Haematologica* 2003; **88**: 1410–21.

26 Heit JA, O'Fallon WM, Petterson TM, *et al.* Relative impact of risk factors for deep vein thrombosis and pulmonary embolism. *Arch Intern Med* 2002; **162**: 1245–8.

27 Nicolaides AN, Breddin HK, Fareed J, *et al.* Prevention of venous thromboembolism. International Consensus Statement. Guidelines compiled in accordance with the scientific evidence. *Int Angiol* 2001; **20**: 1–37.

28 Geerts WH, Heit Ja, Clagett P, *et al.* Prevention of venous thromboemblism. *Chest* 2001; **119**(Suppl. 1): 132S–175S.

29 Douketis JD, Eikelboom JW, Quinlan DJ, *et al.* Short-duration prophylaxis against venous thromboembolism after total hip or knee replacement: a meta-analysis of prospective studies investigating symptomatic outcomes. *Arch Intern Med* 2002; **162**: 1465–71.

30 Geerts W, Pineo GF, Hei JA, *et al.* Prevention of venous thromboembolism. The Seventh ACCP Conference on Antithrombotic and Thrombolytic Therapy. *Chest* 2004; **126**: 338S–400S.

31 Samama MM, Gerotziafas GT. Evaluation of the pharmacological properties and clinical results of the synthetic pentasaccharide (Fondaparinux). *Thromb Res* 2003; **109**: 1–11.

32 Gustafsson D. Oral direct thrombin inhibitors in clinical development. *J Intern Med* 2003; **254**: 322–34.

33 Gallus AS, Hirsh J, Tuttle RJ, *et al.* Small subcutaneous doses of heparin in prevention of venous thrombosis. *N Engl J Med* 1973; **288**: 545–51.

34 Warlow C, Terry G, Kenmure ACF, *et al.* A double-blind trial of low doses of subcutaneous heparin in the prevention of deep-vein thrombosis after myocardial infarction. *Lancet* 1973; **i**: 934–6.

35 Gallus AS, Nurmohammed M, Kearon C, Prins M. Thromboprophylaxis in non-surgical patients: who, when and how? *Haemostasis* 1998; **28**: 71–82.

36 Samama MM, Cohen AT, Darmon JY, *et al.* A comparison of enoxaparin with placebo for the prevention of venous thromboembolism in acutely ill medical patients. Prophylaxis in Medical Patients with Enoxaparin Study Group. *N Engl J Med* 1999; **341**: 793–800.

37 Alikhan R, Cohen AT, Combe S, *et al.* Risk factors for venous thromboembolism in hospitalized patients with acute medical illness. Analysis of the MEDENOX Study. *Arch Intern Med* 2004; **164**: 963–8.

38 Lechler E, Schramm W, Flosbach CW. The venous thrombotic risk in non-surgical patients: epidemiological

data and efficacy/safety profile of a low-molecular-weight heparin (enoxaparin). The Prime Study Group. *Haemostasis* 1996; **26**: 49–56.

39   Kleber FX, Witt C, Flosbach CW, *et al.*, PRINCE Study Group. Study to compare the efficacy and safety of the LMWH enoxaparin and standard heparin in the prevention of thromboembolic events in medical patients with cardiopulmonary diseases [abstract]. *Ann Hematol* 1998; **76**(Suppl I): A93.

40   Vaitkus PT, Leizorovicz A, Goldhaber SZ, PREVENT investigator Group. Rationale and design of a clinical trial of a low-molecular-weight heparin in preventing clinically important venous thromboembolism in medical patients: the prospective evaluation of dalteparin efficacy for prevention of venous thromboembolism in immobilized patients trial (the PREVENT study). *Vasc Med* 2002; **7**: 269–73.

41   Becker F, Leizorovicz A, Olsson CG, *et al.* Venous ultrasound: an alternative to venography fo evalluation of dalteparin prophylaxis in 3706 medically ill hospitalised patients. *Blood* 2003; **102**: abstract 1165.

42   Leizorovicz A, Cohen AT, Turpie AT, *et al.* Efficacy and safety of combining dalteparin with aspirin in preventing venous thromboembolism in medical patients. *Blood* 2003; **102**: abstract 1153.

43   Hull R, Schellong S, Tapson V, *et al.* Extended thromboprophylaxis with enoxaparin In acutely ill medical patients with prolonged periods of immobilization: the EXCLAIM study. *J Thromb Haemost* 2003; **1**(Suppl 1): abstract OC397.

44   Prandoni P, Piccioli A, Pagnan A. Recurrent thromboembolism in cancer patients: incidence and risk factors. *Semin Thromb Hemost* 2003; **29**: 3–9.

45   Duggan C, Marriott K, Edwards R, Cuzick J. Inherited and acquired risk factors for venous thromboembolic disease among women taking tamoxifen to prevent breast cancer. *J Clin Oncol* 2003; **21**: 3588–93.

46   Sallah S, Wan JY, Nguyen NP. Venous thrombosis in patients with solid tumors: determination of frequency and characteristics. *Thromb Haemost.* 2002; **87**: 575–9.

47   Samama MM, for the Sirus Study Group. An epidemiologic study on the risk factors for deep vein thrombosis in medical outpatients. *Arch Intern Med* 1994; **154**: 164–8.

48   Kearon C. Epidemiology of venous thromboembolism. *Semin Vasc Med* 2001; **1**: 7–25.

49   ENOXACAN Study Group. Efficacy and safety of enoxaparin versus unfractionated heparin for prevention of deep vein thrombosis in elective cancer surgery: a double-blind randomized multicentre trial with venographic assessment. *Br J Surg* 1997; **84**: 1099–103.

50   Levine M, Hirsh J, Gent M, *et al.* Double-blind randomised trial of very low dose warfarin for the prevention of thromboembolism in stage IV breast cancer. *Lancet* 1994; **343**: 886–9.

51   Kakkar AK, Levine M, Pinedo HM, *et al.* Venous thrombosis in cancer patients: insights from the FRONTLINE survey. *Oncologist* 2003; **8**: 381–8.

52   Zacharski LR, Henderson WG, Rickles FR, *et al.* Effect of warfarin anticoagulation on survival in carcinoma of the lung, colon, head and neck, and prostate: Final report of VA Cooperative Study. *Cancer* 1984; **53**: 2046–52.

53   Lebeau B, Chastang C, Brechot JM, *et al.* Subcutaneous heparin treatment increases survival in small cell lung cancer. 'Petites Cellules' Group. *Cancer* 1994; **74**: 38–45.

54   Siragusa S, Cosmi B, Piovella F, *et al.* Low-molecular-weight heparins and unfractionated heparin in the treatment of patients with acute venous thromboembolism: Results of a meta-analysis. *Am J Med* 1996; **100**: 269–77.

55   Kakkar AJ, Levine MN, Kadziola Z, *et al.* Low molecular weight heparin therapy with dalteparin and survival in advanced cancer: The Fragmin Advanced Malignancy Outcome Study (FAMOUS). *J Clin Oncol* 2004; **22**: 1944–48.

56   Verso M, Agnelli G. Venous thromboembolism associated with long-term use of central venous catheters in cancer patients. *J Clin Oncol* 2003; **21**: 3665–75.

57   Bern MM, Lokich JJ, Wallach SR, *et al.* Very low doses of warfarin can prevent thrombosis in central venous catheters: a randomised prospective trial. *Ann Intern Med* 1990; **112**: 423–28.

58   Monreal M, Alastrue A, Rull M, *et al.* Upper extremity deep vein thrombosis in cancer patients with venous access devices – prophylaxis with low-molecular-weight heparin (Fragmin). *Thromb Haemost* 1996; **75**: 251–3.

59   Couban S, Goodyear M, Burnell M. A randomized double-blind placebo-controlled study of low dose warfarin for the prevention of symptomatic central venous catheter-associated thrombosis in patients with cancer (abstract). *Blood* 2002; **100**(Suppl): 703a.

60   Heaton DC, Han DY, Inder A. Minidose (1 mg) warfarin as prophylaxis for central vein catheter thrombosis. *Intern Med* 2002; **32**: 84–8.

61   Cohen AT, Davidson BL, Gallus AS, *et al.* Fondaparinux for the prevention of VTE in acutely ill medical patients. *Blood* 2003; **102**: abstract 42.

62   Collins R, Scrimgeour A, Yusuf S, *et al.* Reduction in fatal pulmonary embolism and venous thrombosis by perioperative administration of subcutaneous heparin. Overview of results of randomised trials in general, orthopedic and urologic surgery. *N Engl J Med* 1988; **318**: 1162–72.

63   Clagett GP, Reisch JS. Prevention of venous thrombo-embolism in general surgical patients. Results of meta-analysis. *Ann Surg* 1988; **208**: 227–40.

64   Koch A, Bouges S, Ziegler S, *et al.* Low-molecular-weight heparin and unfractionated heparin in thrombosis prophylaxis after major surgical intervention: update of previous meta-analyses. *Br J Surg* 1997; **84**: 750–9.

65   Palmer AJ, Schramm W, Kirchhof B, Bergmann R. Low-molecular-weight heparin and unfractionated heparin for

prevention of thrombo-embolism in general surgery: a meta-analysis of randomised clinical trials. *Haemostasis* 1997; **27**: 65–74.

66 Baca I, Schneider B, Kohler T, *et al*. Prevention of thromboembolism in minimal invasive interventions and brief inpatient treatment. Results of a multicenter, prospective, randomized, controlled study with a low-molecular-weight heparin. *Chirurg* 1997; **68**: 1275–80.

67 Moreno Gonzalez E, Fontcuberta J, de la Llama F. Prophylaxis of thromboembolic disease with RO-11 (ROVI), during abdominal surgery. EMRO1 (Grupo Fstudio Multicintrico RO-11). *Hepatogastroenterology* 1996; **43**: 744–7.

68 Bergqvist D, Flordal PA, Friberg B, *et al*. Thrombo-prophylaxis with a low-molecular-weight heparin (tinzaparin) in emergency abdominal surgery. A double-blind multicenter trial. *Vasa* 1996; **25**: 156–60.

69 Bergqvist D. Low-molecular-weight heparins for prevention of venous thromboembolism following general surgery. In: Bounameaux, H ed. *Low Molecular Weight Heparins in Prophylaxis and Therapy of Thromboembolic Diseases*. New York: Marcel Dekker, 1994: 169–85.

70 von Tempelhoff GF, Dietrich M, Niemann F, *et al*. Blood coagulation and thrombosis in patients with ovarian malignancy. *Thromb Haemost* 1997; **77**: 456–61.

71 Azorin JF, Regnard JF, Dahan M, Pansart M. Efficacy and tolerability of fraxiparine in the prevention of thromboembolic complications in oncologic thoracic surgery. *Ann Cardiol Angiol* 1997; **46**: 341–7.

72 Kakkar VV, Boeckl O, Boneu B, *et al*. Efficacy and safety of a low-molecular-weight heparin and standard unfractionated heparin for prophylaxis of postoperative venous thromboembolism: European multicenter trial. *World J Surg* 1997; **21**: 2–8.

73 Nurmohamed MT, Verhaeghe R, Haas S, *et al*. A comparative trial of a low-molecular-weight heparin (enoxaparin) versus standard heparin for the prophylaxis of postoperative deep vein thrombosis in general surgery. *Am J Surg* 1995; **169**: 567–71.

74 Wiig JN, Solhaug JH, Bilberg T, *et al*. Prophylaxis of venographically diagnosed deep vein thrombosis in gastrointestinal surgery. Multicentre trials 20 mg and 40 mg enoxaparin versus dextran. *Eur J Surg* 1995; **161**: 663–8.

75 Bergqvist D, Burmark US, Flordal PA, *et al*. Low-molecular-weight heparin started before surgery as prophylaxis against deep vein thrombosis: 2500 versus 5000 XaI units in 2070 patients. *Br J Surg* 1995; **82**: 496–501.

76 Agnelli G, Piovella F, Buoncristiani P, *et al*. Enoxaparin plus compression stockings compared with compression stockings alone in the prevention of venous thromboembolism after elective neurosurgery. *N Engl J Med* 1998; **339**: 80–5.

77 Dickinson LD, Miller LD, Patel CP, Gupta SK. Enoxaparin increases the incidence of postoperative intracranial hemorrhage when initiated preoperatively for deep venous thrombosis prophylaxis in patients with brain tumors. *Neurosurgery* 1998; **43**: 1074–81.

78 Nurmohamed MT, van Riel AM, Henkens CM, *et al*. Low-molecular-weight heparin and compression stockings in the prevention of venous thromboembolism in neurosurgery. *Thromb Haemost* 1996; **75**: 233–8.

79 Lassen MR, Bauer KA, Eriksson BI, Turpie AG. Postoperative fondaparinux versus preoperative enoxaparin for prevention of venous thromboembolism in elective hip-replacement surgery: a randomised double-blind comparison. *Lancet.* 2002; **359**: 1715–20.

80 Turpie AG, Bauer KA, Eriksson BI, Lassen MR. Postoperative fondaparinux versus postoperative enoxaparin for prevention of venous thromboembolism after elective hip-replacement surgery: a randomised double-blind trial. *Lancet* 2002; **359**: 1721–26.

81 Bauer KA, Eriksson BI, Lassen MR, Turpie AG. Fondaparinux compared with enoxaparin for the prevention of venous thromboembolism after elective major knee surgery. *N Engl J Med* 2001; **345**: 1305–10.

82 Eriksson BI, Bauer KA, Lassen MR, Turpie AG. Fondaparinux compared with enoxaparin for the prevention of venous thromboembolism after hip-fracture surgery. *N Engl J Med* 2001; **345**: 1298–304.

83 Turpie AGG, Bauer KA, Eriksson BI, Lassen MR. Fondaparinux vs enoxaparin for the prevention of venous thromboembolism in major orthopedic surgery. A meta-analysis of 4 randomised double-blind studies. *Arch Intern Med* 2002; **162**: 1833–40.

84 Eriksson BI, Lassen MR, PENTasaccharide in HIp-FRActure Surgery Plus Investigators. Duration of prophylaxis against venous thromboembolism with fondaparinux after hip fracture surgery: a multicenter, randomized, placebo-controlled, double-blind study. *Arch Intern Med* 2003; **163**: 1337–42.

85 Agnelli G, Bergqvist D, Cohen AT, *et al.*, on behalf of the PEGASUS investigators. Randomized clinical trial of postoperative fondaparinux versus perioperative dalteparin for prevention of venous thromboembolism in high-risk abdominal surgery. *Br J Surg* 2005; **92**: 1212–20.

86 Heit JA, Colwell CW, Francis CW, *et al*. Comparison of the oral direct thrombin inhibitor ximelagatran with enoxaparin as prophylaxis against venous thromboembolism after total knee replacement. A phase 2 dose-finding study. *Arch Intern Med* 2001; **161**: 2215–21.

87 Eriksson BI, Arfwidsson AC, Frison L, *et al*. A dose-ranging study of the oral direct thrombin inhibitor, ximelagatran, and its subcutaneous form, melagatran, compared with dalteparin in the prophylaxis of thromboembolism after hip or knee replacement: METHRO I. MElagatran for THRombin inhibition in Orthopaedic surgery. *Thromb Haemost* 2002; **87**: 231–7.

88 Eriksson BI, Agnelli G, Cohen AT, *et al.*, METHRO III Study Group. Direct thrombin inhibitor melagatran followed by oral ximelagatran in comparison with enoxaparin for prevention of venous thromboembolism after total hip or knee replacement. *Thromb Haemost.* 2003; **89**: 288–96.

89 Eriksson BI, Agnelli G, Cohen AT, *et al.*, EXPRESS Study Group. The direct thrombin inhibitor melagatran followed by oral ximelagatran compared with enoxaparin for the prevention of venous thromboembolism after total hip or knee replacement: the EXPRESS study. *J Thromb Haemost* 2003; **1**: 2490–6.

90 Colwell CW, Jr, Berkowitz SD, Davidson BL, *et al.* Comparison of ximelagatran, an oral direct thrombin inhibitor, with enoxaparin for the prevention of venous thromboembolism following total hip replacement. A randomized, double-blind study. *J Thromb Haemost.* 2003; **1**: 2119–30.

91 Francis CW, Berkowitz SD, Comp PC, *et al.*, EXULT A Study Group. Comparison of ximelagatran with warfarin for the prevention of venous thromboembolism after total knee replacement. *N Engl J Med* 2003; **349**: 1703–12.

92 Raskob GE, Hirsh J. Controversies in timing of the first dose of anticoagulant prophylaxis against venous thromboembolism after major orthopedic surgery. *Chest* 2003; **124**: 379S–385S.

93 American Society of Regional Anesthesia and Pain Management. Regional anesthesia in the anticoagulated patient: defining the risks; anesthetic management of the patient receiving low-molecular-weight heparin (LMWH). Available at: http://www.asra.com (accessed November 17, 2003).

94 Moser KM, LeMoine JR, Nachtwey FJ, Spragg RG. Deep venous thrombosis and pulmonary embolism: frequency in a respiratory intensive care unit. *JAMA* 1981; **246**: 1422–4.

95 Fraisse F, Holzapfel L, Couland JM, *et al.* Nadroparin in the prevention of deep vein thrombosis in acute decompensated COPD. *Am J Respir Crit Care Med* 2000; **161**: 1109–14.

96 Cade JF. High risk of the critically ill for venous thromboembolism. *Crit Care Med* 1982; **10**: 448–50.

97 Kapoor M, Kupfer YY, Tessler S. Subcutaneous heparin prophylaxis significantly reduces the incidence of venous thromboembolic events in the critically ill. *Crit Care Med* 1999; **27**(Suppl): A69.

98 Geerts W, Selby R. Prevention of venous thromboembolism in the ICU. *Chest* 2003; **124**: 357s–363S.

99 Ibrahim EH, Iregui M, Prentice D, *et al.* Deep vein thrombosis during prolonged mechanical ventilation despite prophylaxis. *Crit Care Med* 2002; **30**: 771–4.

100 Lacherade JC, Cook D, Heyland D, *et al.*, French and Canadian ICU Directors Groups. Prevention of venous thromboembolism in critically ill medical patients: a Franco-Canadian cross-sectional study. *J Crit Care* 2003; **18**: 228–37.

101 Bates SM, Greer IA, Hirsh J, Ginsberg JS. Use of anti-thrombotic agents during pregnancy. The Seventh ACCP Conference on Antithrombotic and Thrombolytic Therapy. *Chest* 2004; **126**: 627S–644S.

102 Weill-Engerer S, Meaume S, Lahlou A, *et al.* Risk factors for deep vein thrombosis in inpatients aged 65 and older: A case-control multicenter study. *J Am Geriatr Soc* 2004; **52**: 1299–304.

103 Pineo GF, Hull R. Low-molecular-weight heparin for the treatment of venous thromboembolism in the elderly. *Clin Appl Thromb/Haemost* 2005; **11**: 15–23.

104 Couturaud F, Lacut K, Leroyer C, Mottier D. Assessment of the risk and prophylactic treatment of venous thromboembolism in the elderly. *Pathophysiol Haemost Thromb.* 2003; **33**: 362–5.

105 Farell SE. Special situations: pediatric, pregnant, and geriatric patients. *Emerg Med Clin North Am* 2001; **19**: 1013–23.

106 Siguret V, Gouin I, Debray M, *et al.* Initiation of wafarin therapy in elderly medical inpatients: a safe and accurate regimen. *Am J Med* 2005; **118**: 137–42.

107 Bara L, Planes A, Samama MM. Occurrence of thrombosis and haemorrhage, relationship with anti-Xa, anti-IIa activities, and D-dimmer plasma levels in patients receiving a low-molecular-weight heparin, enoxaparin or tinzaparin, to prevent deep vein thrombosis after hip surgery. *Br J Haematol* 1999; **104**: 230–40.

108 Farooq V, Hegarty J, Chandrasekar T, *et al.* Serious adverse incidents with the usage of low-molecular-weight heparins in patients with chronic kidney disease. *Am J Kidney Dis* 2004; **43**: 531–7.

109 Gouin-Thibault I, Pautas E, Sigutet V. Safety profile of different low-molecular-weight heparins used at thera-peutic dose. *Drug Saf* 2005; **28**: 333–49.

110 Petersen P, Grind M, Adler J, for the SPORTIF II Investi-gators. Ximelagatran versus warfarin for stroke prevention in patients with nonvalvular atrial fibrillation. *J Am Coll Cardiol* 2003; **41**: 1445–1.

111 Warkentin TE, Greinacher A. Heparin-induced thrombo-cytopenia: recognition, treatment, and prevention The Seventh ACCP Conference on Antithrombotic and Thrombolytic Therapy. *Chest* 2004; **126**: 311S–337S.

112 Liautard T. Low-molecular-weight heparins and thrombocytosis. *Ann Pharmacother* 2002; **36**: 1351–4.

113 Clagett G, Anderson FA, Geerts W, *et al.* Prevention of venous thromboembolism. *Chest* 1998; **114**: 531S–560S.

114 Wells PS, Lensing AWA, Davidson BL, *et al.* Accuracy of ultrasound for the diagnosis of deep venous thrombosis in asymptomatic patients after orthopedic surgery: a meta-analysis. *Ann Intern Med* 1995; **122**: 47–53.

115 Lecompte T, Luo SK, Stieljes N, *et al.* Thrombocytopenia associated with low-molecular-weight heparin. *Lancet* 1991; **338**: 1271.

116 Mosen D, Elliot CG, Egger MJ, *et al.* The effect of a com-puterised system on the prevention of venous thrombo-embolism. *Chest* 2004; **125**: 1635–41.

117 Kucher N, Koo S, Quiroz R, *et al.* Electronic alerts to prevent venous thromboembolism among hospitalized patients. *N Engl J Med* 2005; **352**: 969–77.

14

Coronary disease in women

GRAHAM JACKSON

INTRODUCTION

Cardiovascular disease respects no boundaries. Although still more common in men, it is the leading cause of death and disability in women in the developed and developing countries.[1–3] In Europe cardiovascular disease (CVD) is the cause of death in 43 percent of men and 55 percent of women. Stroke is more commonly fatal in women than men (18 percent vs. 11 percent, respectively) whereas coronary artery disease (CAD) death rates are similar (23 percent vs. 21 percent, respectively). Therefore, CVD causes more deaths than all cancers added together and clearly exceeds death from one of women's greatest fears, breast cancer, at 3 percent (Table 14.1). In the United Kingdom in 2002 CAD was the cause in 64 000 out of 288 000 deaths in men (22 percent or 1 in 5) and in 53 000 of 318 000 deaths in women (17 percent or 1:6).[4] In the United States CAD causes 240 000 deaths annually among women – 1:3 women.[5] Expressed in a tabloid but effective way – and the message needs to be expressed clearly – in the United Kingdom and Europe CVD causes 1 woman to die every 6 minutes and in the United States 1 every minute.

There is an increase in prevalence of CAD with age in men and women, but as life expectancy has increased more in women we can expect to see more women experiencing the consequences of CAD. It should therefore be a straightforward management issue – women and men need to be treated equally – unfortunately differences in presentation present problems for physicians in interpretation, and women themselves do not perceive CAD as their major threat and may ignore warning signs. In addition the concept of 'gender bias' in management has directed attention away from the need to put into context best practice which

Table 14.1 Causes of death in men and women*

Disease	Men (%)	Women (%)
CAD	21	23
Stroke	11	18
Other CVD	11	15
Cancer	21	18 (breast 3)
Respiratory	8	6
Injuries/poisoning	12	4
Other	16	16

World Health Organization figures for Europe 2004.[1]
CAD, coronary artery disease; CVD, cardiovascular disease.

may seem to be biased but could well be in the best interest of the individual (we treat people, not statistics). Focusing on perceived bias may be counterproductive whereas concentrating on educating women about the prevention and recognition of CAD is likely to achieve better care overall. Although women's awareness of the importance of CAD is increasing, they still believe it is predominantly a man's disease. It is important to educate healthcare professionals about CAD in women, but we need to communicate effectively with women themselves using the media so that women come forward for evaluation.

RISK FACTORS

The American Heart Association (AHA) has stratified women into the three risk categories of low, intermediate, or high risk (based on the Framingham risk score and clinical diagnosis) of developing a coronary event over 10 years

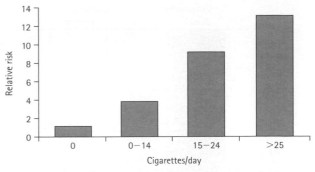

Figure 14.1   Relation between number of cigarettes smoked and myocardial infarction in women below 55 years of age. (Adapted from Bolego et al.[9] Copyright 2002, with permission from the European Society of Cardiology.)

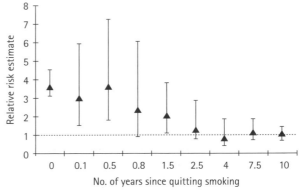

Figure 14.2   Rapid impact of smoking cessation on cardiac events in women. (From Rosenberg L, Palmer JR, Shapiro S. Decline in the risk of myocardial infarction among women who stop smoking. N Engl J Med 1990; **322**: 213–17, Copyright 1990. Massachusetts Medical Society. All rights reserved.)

(Box 14.1).[6] Intervention is then based on levels of evidence, class and the generalizability index whereby the results are extrapolated to women.

Risk factors are generally shared between men and women with the major differential being hormonal.[3,7] Nonmodifiable risk factors are age, sex and family history. The lifetime risk of developing CAD is about 40 percent for men and 30 percent for women with breast cancer in women much lower at 10 percent. Contrast this with 73 percent of Stanford University female graduates believing their CAD risk before 70 year of age to be less than 1 percent and 53 percent perceiving their breast cancer risk to be more than 10 percent.[8]

Cigarette smoking

Smoking is one of the principal risk factors for CAD in women.[9] Women under 55 years have a sevenfold increase in relative risk attributable to smoking and the increase in risk is dose dependent (Fig. 14.1). In addition, smoking multiplies deleteriously with other risk factors and is almost universally the cause of myocardial infarction in oral contraceptive users. Although smoking rates have declined in most groups they have done less so in women, and there is a disturbing rising trend in younger women perhaps related to the lower weight in smokers and the need to appear slim – clearly the wrong kind of weight control program.[10] It is hoped that banning smoking in public places will reverse this trend.

In general smoking trebles the risk of CAD but importantly the benefit from cessation is rapid (Fig. 14.2). Switching to filter or low-tar cigarettes is of no benefit.

Blood pressure

Hypertension significantly increases the risk of coronary disease and stroke. The increase in relative risk is approximately doubled for combined systolic and diastolic hypertension.

Isolated systolic hypertension which is more common in elderly people is also associated with similar increased risk. The evidence of benefit from treating hypertension has been demonstrated for men and women (Fig. 14.3) with women being well represented in the major studies (women live longer than men and have more hypertension so they have been recruited based on numbers rather than sex).[11]

Target blood pressures are 140/90 mm Hg or less in general and 130/80 mm Hg or less in those at high risk (diabetes, chronic renal disease) or with established CAD. The benefit curve extends down to 115/75 mm Hg with evidence that a more aggressive strategy confers increasing risk reduction. In the Comparison of AMlodipine vs. Enalapril to Limit Occurrences of Thrombosis (CAMELOT) trial patients with CAD had their systolic blood pressure lowered from a mean of about 130 mm Hg to 125 mm Hg which reduced their 2-year relative risk of cardiovascular events by 31 percent.[12] Women benefited to a similar degree to men. Unless specifically indicated, β-blockers and thiazides tend to be avoided because of their adverse metabolic/diabetogenic properties. It is important to emphasize the need for lifestyle changes as weight loss and salt reduction facilitate blood pressure control.[13]

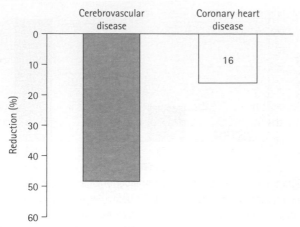

Figure 14.3   Effect of antihypertensive therapy on coronary disease and stroke. (Redrawn from MacMahon SW, Cutler JA, Furberg CD, Payne GH. The effects of drug treatment for hypertension on morbidity and mortality from cardiovascular disease: a review of randomized controlled trials. *Prog Cardiovasc Dis* 1986; **129**(Suppl 1): 99–118, Copyright 1986, with permission from Elsevier.)

Hyperlipidemia

In men and women an elevated cholesterol is associated with an increased risk factor for cardiovascular events. A cholesterol of 6.46 mmol/L (250 mg/dL) doubles and 7.75 mmol/L (300 mg/dL) trebles the risk of cardiac death compared with 5.17 mmol/L (200 mg/dL) in men and postmenopausal women.[14] The evidence for a single risk factor of hyperlipidemia prior to the menopause increasing risk is less clear, except for women with familial hypercholesterolemia. In women with established CAD, diabetes or at >20 percent risk over 10 years of developing CAD, total cholesterol and low-density lipoprotein (LDL)-cholesterol targets are equal to or less than 4.0 mmol/L and 2.0 mmol/L, respectively, and an LDL lowering of 30 percent from baseline.[15] For those not at risk a lifestyle guide of 5.0 mmol/L and 3.0 mmol/L, respectively, is advocated.

High-density lipoprotein (HDL)-cholesterol, which is protective for CAD, is typically higher in women. Thus the importance of always obtaining a full lipid profile when evaluating these patients. Although HDL levels are inversely predictive of CAD, unfortunately sex differences favoring women decline with age. Hypertriglyceridemia is a more potent risk factor for women with the CAD relative risk increased to 32 percent in men and 76 percent in women.[3] Whereas statins predominantly lower LDL-cholesterol and, to a variable degree, triglycerides, fibrates decrease triglycerides and increase HDL-cholesterol, suggesting women may need a combination strategy depending on their profile at baseline and its response to optimal dose statin therapy.

Diabetes

The prevalence of diabetes is increasing in men and women. Although CAD mortality appears to be higher in women

after adjusting for other risk factors, there is no difference. Diabetes is more common in the United Kingdom in women (17.7 percent) compared with men (13.4 percent) and it increases in ethnic groups, particularly Asians.[15] The risk of CAD is increased fourfold in women and 2.5-fold in men.[3,7] As obesity has increased, so has type 2 diabetes, so we are now faced with an ever-increasing problem. A woman with diabetes has a similar CAD risk as a woman who has had a myocardial infarction but is not diabetic. Diabetes is therefore considered to be a 'cardiovascular equivalent' and aggressive risk reduction advocated as if a coronary event has already occurred. Success has been reported in men and women with type 2 diabetes with the focus on lifestyle, setting a target HbA1c of less than 7 percent and controlling lipids (statins ± fibrates to target LDL-cholesterol <2 mmol/L, triglycerides <1.6 mmol/L and HDL-cholesterol >1.3 mmol/L), blood pressure (<130/80 mm Hg) and microalbuminuria (using angiotensin-converting [ACE] inhibitors and angiotensin II antagonists).[16]

It is essential that diabetic women do not smoke as the risk increases sevenfold in women who smoke over 15 cigarettes a day.

Metabolic syndrome

Unfortunately, the definition of the metabolic syndrome is not as precise as the name implies.[17] It is an umbrella term for a cluster of cardiovascular risk factors including type 2 diabetes, hyperlipidemia, abdominal obesity, and hypertension secondary to 'insulin resistance' and as a consequence, hyperinsulinemia. Umbrellas protect us from the elements and there is a danger that in using a unifying label we may not address each element of risk optimally. The definition itself has been challenged by the American Diabetes Association and the European Association for the Study of Diabetes.[17] In a joint statement they conclude that 'too much critically important information is missing to warrant its designation as a "syndrome"'. They encourage the treatment of all cardiovascular risk factors irrespective of whether the 'metabolic syndrome' has been diagnosed. Although the National Cholesterol Education Program's Adult Treatment Panel (ATP III), World Health Organization (WHO) and International Diabetes Federation (IDF) offer different definitions, there are similarities we can extract for day-to-day use.[18–20] The first is central obesity with a waist-to-hip ratio >0.90 in men and >0.85 in women, which translates to a waist circumference in European men of ≥94 cm and ≥80 cm in women. In addition, there should be any two of:

- raised triglycerides over 1.7 mmol/L
- reduced HDL-cholesterol of <1.0 mmol/L in men and <1.3 mmol/L in women
- blood pressure over 130/85 mm Hg *or* treated blood pressure *or* raised fasting glucose ≥6.1 mmol/L (and possibly 5.6 mmol/L).

Including those with diabetes and those with clinical CVD seems pointless as their risk status is known so that they add little to the understanding of risk for those otherwise having features of the 'metabolic syndrome'. Therefore, however we view these varying definitions, what we are talking about is increased vascular risk and in turn reducing it.

Women with the metabolic syndrome are at an intermediate risk compared with those with diabetes and those with a normal blood glucose. Their 4-year relative risk increases twofold compared with those with a normal metabolic status. Perhaps their abdominal obesity decreases their physical activity, perpetuating a vicious circle of risk. The link between depression and the metabolic syndrome is of interest because of the prevalence of depression in women (up to 70 percent) and the recognition that depression is a risk factor for CAD.[3]

Lifestyle factors

As body weight increases so does the risk of CAD.[3,21] The body mass index (BMI = weight in kg divided by height in m^2) has largely been replaced by waist circumference as an indication of obesity in clinical practice. Waist size is measured using a tape 1 cm above the navel or the midpoint between the lowest rib and the iliac crest. The patient should have breathed out and the abdomen should be relaxed. In the United Kingdom 43 percent of men and 34 percent of women are overweight and 22 percent of men and 23 percent of women are obese.[7] Central obesity as a risk factor is also a component of the metabolic syndrome.[22] A BMI of 25–30 kg/m^2 is classed as overweight and >30 kg/m^2 obese. Waist circumferences should be 80 cm or less (31.5 inches) in women with increased risk from 80 cm to 87 cm and a greater risk 88 cm and above. The ideal waist in a man is 94 cm (37 inches) or less but lower in Chinese, Japanese and South Asians (90 cm).

A weight loss program involves a long-term strategy of dietary modification combined with increased physical activity (a sedentary lifestyle increases CAD risk and reduces the effect of diet on weight).[23] Weight reduction reduces CAD risk, lowers blood pressure, LDL-cholesterol and triglycerides and increases HDL-cholesterol. Physical activity may, combined with other lifestyle changes, reduce cardiac mortality by 26 percent.[3] In the Women's Health Initiative (73 743 postmenopausal women aged 50–79 years) brisk walking for 30 minutes five times a week reduced CVD events by 30 percent over 3 years' follow-up.[24] The benefit was similar to those engaging in more strenuous activity, for example in a gymnasium, so all that is needed are good shoes, comfortable loose fitting clothes and commitment.

Alcohol in moderation lowers coronary mortality and there is no evidence that one form (for example, red wine) is better than another. Guidelines are 14 units or less per week for women and 21 for men. Alcohol is not a medication and does carry with it calories. Binge drinking increases the risk of sudden death and stroke.[15]

Hormones

When risk factors are considered the main difference between women and men, other than degree of risk, is their different hormonal status. The premenopausal lower risk in women has been linked to their higher endogenous estrogen levels and the subsequent postmenopausal increased risk to the decrease in endogenous estrogen.[25] Epidemiologic observational trials then indicated hormone replacement therapy (HRT) decreased CAD risk post menopause. Randomized trials failed to confirm this observation and a pattern of early harm, probably due to thrombogenesis, and later benefit due to improved risk factors was observed.[26] There are several forms of HRT with different hormone doses and different metabolic effects, with the differences not fully evaluated. However, at present HRT is not recommended (in any form) solely for the prevention and treatment of CAD. It significantly improves the quality of life of women who experience postmenopausal symptoms and is approved for this use (and osteoporosis reduction), but it seems wise for these women to minimize their conventional CAD risk factors while taking HRT (and preferably indefinitely) (see Chapters 32–34).

Risk factor recommendations

Although women have lower rates of CAD the classic risk factors are the same as in men and risk reduction advice is therefore the same. The hormone replacement story has further to go with the need to use low doses at the time of the menopause rather than high doses later but for now HRT cannot be recommended as primary or secondary prevention therapy.

PRESENTATION OF CARDIOVASCULAR DISEASE

Angina

Angina is more common as a presenting symptom in women, whereas sudden cardiac death and myocardial infarction are more common in men. However, 40 percent of initial cardiac events in women are fatal, emphasizing the importance of risk reduction and the early recognition of symptoms. Women more frequently present with atypical chest pain (Box 14.2). This may be due to the increased prevalence of less common causes of ischemia, such as cardiac syndrome X and nonischemic syndromes such as mitral valve prolapse, which is frequently associated with atypical pain after rather than during exercise.

The Coronary Artery Surgery Study (CASS) classified symptoms according to three criteria: (i) substernal chest discomfort, (ii) precipitated by effort, and (iii) relieved by rest or glyceryl trinitrate within 10 minutes.[27] Angina was considered typical if all three criteria were present, atypical

Box 14.2 Characteristics of chest pain

Typical
- Tightness
- Pressure
- Weight
- Constriction
- Ache
- Dull
- Squeezing feeling
- Crushing
- 'Like a band'
- Breathless (tightness)
- Retrosternal
- Precipitated by exertion or emotion
- Promptly relieved by rest or nitroglycerin

Atypical
- Sharp (not severe)
- Knife-like
- Stabbing
- 'Like a stitch'
- 'Like a needle'
- Pricking feeling
- Shooting
- Can walk around with it
- Continuous: 'It's there all day'
- Located in left chest, abdomen
- Back or arm in absence of mid-chest pain
- Unrelated to exercise
- Not relieved by rest or nitroglycerin
- Relieved by antacids; characterized by palpitations without chest pain

Women
- At rest
- During sleep
- Stress
- Jaw, teeth, arms, neck, shoulders, back, abdomen

Table 14.2   Chest pain characteristics and the prevalence of significant coronary heart disease in women and men

Angina	Women (%)	Men (%)
Definite	68	95
Possible/probable	30	71
Atypical	6	18

From Weiner et al.[27]

include the jaw, teeth, arms, neck and shoulders, back and abdomen.[28] The symptom itself may be different in women who more often complain of breathlessness, which is their perception of tightness, recent fatigue, perspiration, and palpitations.

It is important to remember that angina is a clinical diagnosis which is supported by further investigations. If a woman has a typical pain and an abnormal electrocardiogram (ECG) at rest, the diagnosis is straightforward. However, the resting ECG is usually normal or equivocal. A classic history and a normal resting ECG suggest good left ventricular function. A woman with atypical chest pain will be unlikely to have CAD in the absence of risk factors. In contrast, a woman with typical chest pain and one or two major risk factors will be more likely to have CAD. Where there are doubts regarding the diagnosis or when overall risk of a subsequent event has to be evaluated, non-invasive testing should be performed. However, as the prevalence of CAD in women is lower than in men, the value of noninvasive testing will be lower but a normal test at a good workload for the same reason will almost certainly rule out CAD.[29]

The exercise ECG is more accurate in detecting CAD when the prevalence is high, leading to a low false-positive rate for CAD but a higher false-negative rate. This means that, when compared with men, women will have a higher false-positive and lower false-negative rate because of their lower overall prevalence of CAD. However, the exercise ECG is widely available, inexpensive, and easy to perform. Interpretation should include exercise duration, hemodynamic response, symptoms at a given workload and ST-T changes. A normal test at less than 6 minutes of the Bruce treadmill protocol would be inconclusive, whereas a normal test at a good workload (over 9 minutes) rules out significant CAD. The sensitivity (positive for disease) averages 61 percent and specificity (excluding CAD) 70 percent.[30] If a test is inconclusive or when a woman cannot exercise adequately, stress echocardiography or nuclear imaging (single photon emission computed tomography [SPECT]) will provide diagnostic information and improve diagnostic accuracy. Stress echocardiography has a sensitivity of 86 percent and specificity of 79 percent and SPECT 78 percent and 64 percent, respectively.[30] In Figure 14.4 an approach to testing is summarized based on baseline risk.

Although angina may present differently, the disease process and risk factors are the same. Stable angina by

if any two, and nonanginal if only one criterion was present. Of interest, the probability of coronary disease prevalence could be predicted from age, sex, symptom characteristics and Framingham risk factors as accurately as from noninvasive testing. Women have a lower CAD incidence than men but symptoms still predict prevalence (Table 14.2). As women become older their CAD symptoms become more like those of men, so it is important in younger women to have a high index of suspicion and to be aware of the differences and difficulties in the interpretation of the history. To some extent the presentation may be influenced by a woman's incorrect perception of a reduced chance of CAD.

Women with chronic stable angina when compared with men are more likely to experience symptoms at rest, during sleep, and under emotional stress. Symptoms may be felt more outside the classic central chest location and

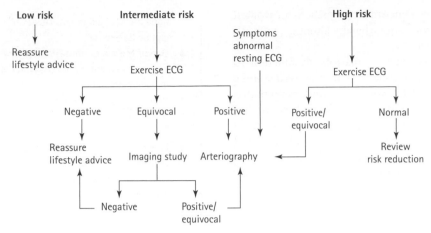

Figure 14.4   An approach to the management of coronary artery disease (CAD) in women. *Low risk*: the estimated risk of CAD is less than 10 percent; women are likely to be younger, with atypical pain and no risk factors of significance. *Intermediate risk*: risk is 10–20 percent; a mixture of typical and atypical pain; one major risk factor. *High risk*: More than 20 percent likelihood of CAD; typical pain; two major risk factors. see Box 14.1, p. 187.

definition is stable. At face value many might believe that a less aggressive approach results in sex bias in terms of investigation and treatment of CAD. However, when we consider age at presentation and extent of disease (women are generally older and have more extensive disease) plus other complicating factors (more women are diabetic) it may be that the management of women is being more carefully tailored to their clinical status at that time. Age is an important factor in management because women live longer than men and decision making for elderly people may be more focused on quality of life and the wish not to be a burden on others, rather than purely avoiding death as an endpoint and following any invasive option offered. However, different healthcare systems may differentially limit healthcare for elderly people, leading to a solely age-biased restriction, which is an unacceptable and unethical policy.

Women benefit as much as men from lipid-lowering therapy, aspirin and/or clopidogrel, ACE inhibitors or angiotensin II antagonists, percutaneous coronary intervention and coronary artery bypass surgery (CABG).[31] Increased interventional or surgical risks are related to small vessel size and disease extent (that is, they are lesion, not sex, specific) and comorbidities, such as diabetes. On the medical side women are more vulnerable to the ACE inhibitor cough (especially Chinese women) and cold extremities from β-blockers.

Women are less likely to attend cardiac rehabilitation programs, which offer valuable secondary prevention, post-CABG or post-percutaneous transluminal coronary angioplasty. Women who do attend have high dropout rates.[32] Women return to work less frequently and take longer to recover in general than men. This may reflect the lack of appropriate advice for women and begs the question whether rehabilitation tailored to women's needs may be more successful. As women live longer than men they more often live alone and may be afraid to venture out in large cities, particularly if rehabilitation classes or meetings take place outside daylight hours. The importance of social community support is self-evident and, if put in place, may help improve attendance rates.

Myocardial infarction

Women are older at presentation with an acute coronary syndrome (ACS) and have a high prevalence of risk factors such as diabetes, hypertension, and hyperlipidemia. Most studies identify delay in presentation and atypical symptoms influencing initial management and a higher rate of complications, such as cardiac failure, reinfarction, cardiogenic shock, and stroke.[33] Cerebral bleeding following thrombolysis is more common (twofold) perhaps highlighting the need for lower doses. The advent and superiority of primary angioplasty should minimize this risk and that has now been established with primary angioplasty now the therapy of choice. Sex does not appear to influence survival but the vascular characteristics do.

In unstable angina an early invasive strategy had no benefit in women with evidence of a worse outcome at 12 months (death 8.6 percent women, 5.1 percent men; myocardial infarction 10.1 percent women vs. 7.0 percent men).[33] In the presence of high risk, however (dynamic ST changes, positive troponin test), an early invasive strategy has been shown to benefit women as much as men.[34] The message is to treat women as aggressively as men but to be aware of the potential for increased risk due to the nature of their vascular disease.

Heart failure

Heart failure increases in prevalence with age and as women live longer and we are an aging population, the proportion of older women with heart failure will increase.[35] The mortality reduction achieved in the presence of systolic failure with ACE inhibitors and β-blockers is the same in women as men.[36] There is no evidence of lack of benefit for women from cardiac resynchronization therapy although, in trials, men outnumber women 3:1.

More women than men have diastolic dysfunction so that their heart failure is associated with preserved systolic function which may be why women are underrepresented in heart (systolic) failure studies. Diastolic dysfunction has a reduced life expectancy (independent of sex) with an annual mortality of 8.7 percent compared with age- and sex-matched controls at 3.0 percent. The management is symptomatic whereas with systolic failure it is both symptomatic and prognostic.

Cardiac syndrome X

Cardiac syndrome X is the association of typical exertional chest pain abnormal exercise electrocardiography with normal coronary arteries.[37] It is a disabling condition for some women and difficult to manage. It is important to rule out noncardiac causes of pain (for example, a hiatus hernia, esophageal pain). Studies revealing abnormal perfusion, myocardial lactate production, and endothelial dysfunction point toward microvascular abnormalities. Being more common in women peri-menopause, estrogen deficiency has been proposed as one of the mechanisms and HRT has been tried with varying degrees of success. The management is challenging and abnormally increased sensitivity to pain limits therapeutic success. Focus is mainly on vasodilators and attempts to improve endothelial dysfunction, for example with statins, but most women are given at some time all conventional antianginal agents, usually in combination. As cardiac syndrome X is associated with insulin resistance, insulin sensitizing agents such as metformin have been used effectively in preliminary studies and this may be a useful therapy in the future. It is not helpful to give the impression to women that the principal cause is psychologic, although the disabling symptoms often lead to depression. Most women with syndrome X have at sometime been dismissed because the prognosis is excellent. The problem is not a concern about longevity but the need to recognize the reality of the suffering and the need to be able to convey to the woman the fact that her condition is being taken seriously. It can be a nightmare to treat but there is no excuse for avoiding the challenge because it is difficult.

KEY LEARNING POINTS

- Coronary disease in women is their greatest medical enemy – not cancer.
- Differences exist in presentation and response to therapy, but overall women should receive the same advice on prevention and treatment as men.
- Sex bias needs to be dissociated from the possibility that management differences reflect individualized

good medical judgment. However, if it does occur there can be no excuse.
- One of the major limitations to optimal management is women's perception of risk, which does not necessarily include cardiac risk.
- Unless women recognize their cardiac risk and address the risk factors, they will always appear underprovided for.
- Importantly, women need to present earlier, which means there is a need to work with the media to educate women so that we can provide the evidence-based care they deserve.

REFERENCES

1 World Health Organization. Statistical Information System 2004 (www.who.int/whosis).
2 Bello N, Mosca L. Epidemiology of coronary heart disease in women. *Prog Cardiovasc Dis* 2004; **46**: 287–95.
3 Stramba-Badiale M, Fox KM, Priori SG, *et al.* Cardiovascular disease in women: a statement from the policy conference of the European Society of Cardiology. *Eur Heart J* 2006; **27**: 994–1005.
4 Shaw K-T. Epidemiology of coronary heart disease in women. *Heart* 2006; **92**(Suppl III): iii2–iii4.
5 American Heart Association. *Heart Disease and Stroke Statistics – 2004 Update 2*. Dallas, TX: American Heart Association, 2005.
6 Mosca L, Appel IJ, Benjamin EJ, *et al.* Evidence-based guidelines for cardiovascular disease prevention in women. *Arterioscler Thromb Vasc Biol* 2004; **24**: e29–50.
7 Collins P. Risk factors for cardiovascular disease and hormone therapy in women. *Heart* 2006; **92**(Suppl III): iii24–iii28.
8 Pilote L, Hlatky M. Attitudes of women toward hormone therapy and prevention of heart disease *Am Heart J* 1995; **129**: 1237–8.
9 Bolego C, Poli A, Paoletti R. Smoking and gender. *Cardiovasc Res* 2002; **53**: 568–76.
10 Califano JA. The wrong way to stay slim. *N Engl J Med* 1995; **333**: 1214–16.
11 Williams B. Recent hypertension trials: implications and controversies. *J Am Coll Cardiol* 2005; **45**: 813–27.
12 Nissen SE, Tuzcu EM, Libby P, *et al.* Effect of antihypertensive agents on cardiovascular events in patients with coronary disease and normal blood pressure. The CAMELOT Study: a randomised controlled trial. *JAMA* 2004; **292**: 2217–26.
13 Julios S, Kjeldsen SE, Weber M, *et al.* Outcomes in hypertensive patients at high cardiovascular risk treated with regimens based on Valsartan or Amlodipine: the VALUE randomised trial. *Lancet* 2004; **363**: 2022–31.
14 LaRosa JC, Hunninghake D, Bush D, *et al.* The cholesterol facts. A summary of the evidence relating dietary fats,

serum cholesterol, and coronary heart disease. A joint statement by the American Heart Association and the National Heart, Lung and Blood Institute. The task force on cholesterol issues, American Heart Association. *Circulation* 1990; **81**: 1721–33.

15 JBS2. Joint British Societies guidelines on prevention of cardiovascular disease in clinical practice. *Heart* 2005; **91**(Suppl V).

16 Gaede P, Vedel P, Larsen N, *et al.* Multifactorial intervention and cardiovascular disease in patients with type 2 diabetes. *N Engl J Med* 2003; **348**: 383–93.

17 Khan R, Buse J, Ferrannini E, Stern M. The metabolic syndrome: time for a critical appraisal. *Diabetes Care* 2005; **28**: 2289–304.

18 Grundy SM, Brewer HB Jr, Cleeman JI, *et al.* National Heart, Lung and Blood Institute. American Heart Association. Definition of metabolic syndrome: Report of the National Heart, Lung and Blood Institute/American Heart Association conference on scientific issues related to definition. *Circulation* 2004; **109**: 433–8.

19 World Health Organization: *Definition, Diagnosis and Classification of Diabetes Mellitus and its Complications: Report of a WHO Consultation.* Geneva, World Health Organization, 1999.

20 International Diabetes Federation. The IDF consensus worldwide definition of the metabolic syndrome. Available at: www.idf.org/webdata/docs/Metac_syndrome_def.pdf. (accessed March 6, 2006).

21 Allison DB, Fontaine KR, Manson JE, *et al.* Annual deaths attributable to obesity in the United States. *JAMA* 1999; **282**: 1530–8.

22 Grundy SM. Obesity, metabolic syndrome, and cardiovascular disease. *J Clin Endocrinol Metab* 2004; **89**: 2595–600.

23 Sesso HD, Paffenbarger RS, Ha T, *et al.* Physical activity and cardiovascular disease risk in middle-aged and older women. *Am J Epidemiol* 1999; **150**: 408–16.

24 Manson JE, Greenland P, LaCroix AZ, *et al.* Walking compared with vigorous exercise for the prevention of cardiovascular events in women. *N Engl J Med* 2002; **347**: 716–25.

25 Collins P. Clinical cardiovascular studies of hormone replacement therapy. *Am J Cardiol* 2002; **90**: F30–4.

26 Rossouw JE, Anderson GL, Prentice RL, *et al.* Risks and benefits of estrogen plus progestin in healthy postmenopausal women: principal results from the women's health initiative randomised controlled trial. *JAMA* 2002; **288**: 321–33.

27 Weiner DA, Ryan TJ, McCabe CH, *et al.* Exercise stress testing. Correlations among history of angina, ST-segment response and prevalence of coronary artery disease in the Coronary Artery Surgery Study (CASS). *N Engl J Med* 1979; **301**: 230–5.

28 Douglas PS, Ginsberg GS. The evaluation of chest pain in women. *N Engl J Med* 1996; **334**: 1311–15.

29 Redberg RF, Shaw LJ. Diagnosis of coronary artery disease in women. *Prog Cardiovasc Dis* 2003; **46**: 239–58.

30 Kwok Y, Kim C, Grady D, *et al.* Meta-analysis of exercise testing to detect coronary artery disease in women. *Am J Cardiol* 1999; **83**: 660–6.

31 Task Force of the European Society of Cardiology. Management of stable angina pectoris. *Eur Heart J* 1997; **18**: 394–413.

32 Gallagher R, McKinley S, Dracup K. Predictors of women's attendance at cardiac rehabilitation programmes. *Prog Cardiovasc Nurs* 2003; **18**: 121–6.

33 Fox KAA, Poole-Wilson PA, Henderson RA, *et al.* for the Randomized Intervention Trial of Unstable Angina (RITA) Investigators. Interventional versus conservative treatment for patients with unstable angina or non-ST-elevation myocardial infarction. The British Heart Foundation RITA 3 randomised trial. *Lancet* 2002; **360**: 743–51.

34 Glaser R, Hermann HC, Murphy SA, *et al.* Benefit of an early invasive management strategy in women with acute coronary syndromes. *JAMA* 2002; **288**: 3124–9.

35 Mehta PA, Cowie MR. Gender and heart failure: a population perspective. *Heart* 2006; **92**(Suppl III): iii14–iii18.

36 Ibrahim SA, Burant CJ, Kent KC. Elderly hospitalised patients with diastolic heart failure: lack of gender and ethnic differences in 18-month mortality rates. *J Gerontol A Biol Sci Med Sci* 2003; **58**: 56–9.

37 Kaski JC. Cardiac syndrome X in women: the role of oestrogen deficiency. *Heart* 2006; **92**(Suppl III): iii5–iii9.

15

Peripheral vascular disease

P SANJAY, GARETH GRIFFITHS

INTRODUCTION

This chapter examines aspects of peripheral vascular disease from a surgical viewpoint. There is generally little practical difference in everyday clinical practice between women and men in the surgical treatment of arterial disease, but where such differences exist they are commented upon. No attempt is made to be comprehensive in the space available. The emphasis is clinical, combining important but often forgotten aspects of patient presentation with background information and data from recent advances. For detailed discussion, the reader is referred to Rutherford's *Vascular Surgery*, from where some of the references in the current chapter were sourced.

ANATOMY

Arterial

Aortic arch branches

The ascending aorta originates immediately above the aortic valve, passes superiorly for a few centimeters then arches posterolaterally to the left as the aortic arch. The aorta then continues inferiorly through the thorax to the left of the vertebral column. The right and left coronary arteries are the first branches of the ascending aorta and originate immediately above the aortic valve. These arteries are unique in that they fill during diastole due to their being compressed in cardiac systole. The left main stem coronary artery is fairly short before it divides into the left anterior descending and circumflex arteries which between them

supply the bulk of the left ventricle. Disease in the left main stem therefore is particular significance as it is responsible for supplying the major proportion of cardiac muscle. The right coronary artery supplies the right ventricle and inferior surface of the heart.

The three branches of the aortic arch (the great vessels) are the innominate (often called the brachiocephalic in anatomy texts), the left common carotid, and the left subclavian arteries. These arise in sequence as the aortic arch passes posterolaterally to the left. Consequently, surgical exposure of the first two branches is best anteriorly via a median sternotomy, and the left subclavian is best exposed through an upper left thoracotomy. Occasionally two of the great vessels arise from a common origin on the aortic arch – the bovine variation.

CAROTID AND VERTEBRAL ARTERIES

The innominate artery passes upwards through the superior mediastinum and divides into the right subclavian and right common carotid arteries. The left common carotid artery follows a parallel course and both common carotids enter the base of the neck behind the origin of each sternomastoid. They pass up the neck on each side deep to sternomastoid and divide into the internal and external carotids at a variable point, but generally around the upper border of the thyroid cartilage. At this level the internal carotid lies lateral to the external carotid. The internal carotid continues to supply the ipsilateral cerebrum except the occipital cortex. Its first branch, however, is the ophthalmic artery which supplies the retina via the central retinal artery. This explains why emboli from a diseased carotid bifurcation may cause ipsilateral amaurosis fugax (caused by an embolus passing directly to the retina) or contralateral motor or sensory symptoms (caused by an embolus passing to the sensorimotor cortex).

The vertebral artery is the first branch of the subclavian artery and passes very quickly into the bony canal formed by the foramina within the transverse processes of the cervical vertebrae. As such it is only accessible surgically in the root of the neck for a short distance from its origin.

UPPER LIMB ARTERIES

Subclavian and axillary arteries

The subclavian artery on each side arches upwards and laterally to pass over the first rib. Surgical exposure involves an incision above the medial part of the clavicle which is then deepened through sternomastoid to expose scalenus anterior. The phrenic nerve is protected while scalenus anterior is divided to reveal the subclavian artery surrounded by the adjacent brachial plexus. Taking this dissection medially, the origin of the vertebral artery may be exposed, as may the common carotid.

The subclavian artery continues as the axillary artery as it passes over the lateral border of the first rib. Exposure of the axillary artery is through an infraclavicular incision deepened by splitting pectoralis major and dividing the origin of pectoralis minor. Arterial trauma in this region requires wide exposure to gain proximal control and this may involve incisions up to and including a median sternotomy extended laterally over the clavicle. A section of clavicle may need to be excised to expose the full length of the subclavian and axillary arteries.

Brachial, radial, and ulnar arteries

The axillary artery continues laterally through the axilla and enters the arm in the groove between biceps and brachialis. It continues in this line to the antecubital fossa where it lies just lateral to the median nerve. It divides into the larger ulnar and smaller radial and interosseous arteries. The radial and ulnar arteries enter the hand and communicate as the palmar arch from which arise the digital arteries. These divide to give one medial and one lateral artery to each finger. This anatomy can be variable and the palmar arch may not be complete. If this is the case, some or all of the fingers may be supplied by only the ulnar or radial artery.

AORTOILIAC SYSTEM

Abdominal aorta

The thoracic aorta enters the abdomen between the crura of the diaphragm. Its three anterior branches, the celiac axis, the superior mesenteric, and the inferior mesenteric, supply structures derived from the foregut, midgut, and hindgut, respectively. The celiac axis is short and gives rise to the hepatic artery, the left gastric artery, and the splenic artery. The splenic artery runs laterally in a tortuous course along the superior border of the pancreas before entering the hilum of the spleen. The renal arteries arise posterolaterally below the level of the superior mesenteric origin. Through the thorax and abdomen the aorta gives off intercostal and lumbar arteries, respectively, to supply the body wall.

Surgical access to the supraceliac aorta can be obtained anteriorly through a full length midline incision by reflecting the left lobe of the liver to the right, entering the lesser sac, and dividing the crura of the diaphragm. Better access to the whole length of the supra- and infrarenal aorta is obtained by the technique of medial visceral rotation in which the left colon, left kidney, spleen, and pancreas are lifted off the posterior abdominal wall and reflected medially to expose the aorta from its left lateral side.

The infrarenal aorta is usually exposed transperitoneally through either a full length midline incision or through a transverse incision at the level of the umbilicus. The small bowel is packed off to the right of the abdomen and the posterior peritoneum opened to expose the aorta.

Iliac arteries

The aorta divides at the level of the umbilicus into the common iliac arteries. These diverge and pass over the pelvic brim where they divide into the external and internal iliac arteries. At this point the ureters cross the iliac bifurcation. The internal iliac artery supplies the pelvic viscera, except the upper two-thirds of the rectum, and buttocks. The external iliac artery continues along psoas and passes under the inguinal ligament to become the common femoral artery.

Surgical exposure of the iliac arteries can be through a midline abdominal incision, extending the posterior peritoneal incision from where the aorta may already have been exposed. Alternatively, a completely retroperitoneal approach can be made through an iliac fossa incision.

LOWER LIMB ARTERIES

Femoral and popliteal

The common femoral artery is the continuation of the external iliac at it passes under the inguinal ligament. It can be exposed through either a vertical or a skin crease incision. The former offers better extensile exposure to a longer length, particularly distally, whereas the latter appears to heal better with possibly less risk of wound edge ischemia. About 5 cm below the inguinal ligament the common femoral divides into the superficial femoral and profunda femoris arteries.

The profunda supplies the thigh through many branches, and the superficial femoral artery passes through the thigh with no major branches. In its course the superficial femoral artery runs under the sartorius in Hunter's canal and then penetrates the adductor magnus through the adductor hiatus to become the popliteal artery. This continues through the popliteal fossa below the knee. A longitudinal incision anywhere along the length of the superficial femoral or popliteal artery can be used to expose the vessel.

Crural

The first major branch of the popliteal artery below the knee is the anterior tibial. This passes anterolaterally though the interosseous membrane of the calf to enter the anterior compartment. It then runs though this to enter the foot lateral to the tendon of flexor hallucis longus as the dorsalis pedis artery. Its origin can be exposed through the medial incision used to display the below-knee popliteal artery. It can then be exposed anywhere in the anterior compartment through an incision parallel and lateral to the lateral border of the tibia.

After giving off the anterior tibial artery, the popliteal continues as the tibioperoneal trunk for a few centimeters. This then divides into the posterior tibial which runs down the medial aspect of the calf and behind the medial malleolus. The peroneal artery runs on through the middle of the calf and divides into terminal branches above the ankle. The posterior tibial and peroneal arteries can be exposed surgically by continuing the dissection of the popliteal artery distally, along the tibioperoneal stem and under the soleal arch. Beyond their first few centimeters, they are more easily exposed through a medial incision centered 10 cm above the medial malleolus. Alternatively, the peroneal may be approached through a lateral incision excising a segment of fibula in the lower calf.

The anterior and posterior tibial arteries communicate in the foot through the superficial and deep plantar arches, from which arise the digital arteries in a similar manner to the hand.

SEX DIFFERENCES

Apart from the obvious anatomical differences, it is generally felt that women have smaller arteries than men. If true, this may lead to an increased rate of arterial disease as the arteries would thrombose, stenose, or occlude more rapidly for a given atherosclerotic load. Hormonal influences obviously affect this, however, and make the situation more complex. Furthermore, there is some evidence that the general view may not necessarily be correct. One study of patients undergoing carotid endarterectomy found no significant difference in the diameter of the internal carotid artery in women and men.[1]

Venous

UPPER LIMB, HEAD, AND NECK

The deep venous drainage of the upper limb follows the arterial supply as venae comitantes which join to form the major veins proximally. The superficial venous drainage of the arm is via the cephalic system laterally and the basilic medially. The cephalic vein passes in the deltopectoral groove and enters the axillary vein in the infraclavicular fossa, and the basilic vein runs deep to the deep fascia in the upper arm and joins the brachial vein below the axilla.

The internal jugular vein forms from the intracranial venous sinuses at the base of the skull and runs alongside the carotid system. It is joined by the subclavian vein on each side to form the right and left brachiocephalic veins. The left brachiocephalic vein passes transversely across the anterior part of the superior mediastinum and joins the right brachiocephalic vein which has simply continued the vertical course of the right internal jugular. The two brachiocephalic veins merge as the superior vena cava which drains into the right atrium.

LOWER LIMB

Deep

As in the upper limb, the deep venous drainage follows the arterial supply as venae comitantes which merge to form veins named to correspond to their accompanying arteries. This continues in the pelvis, with the two common iliac veins coming together as the inferior vena cava to the right of the aortic bifurcation. At this confluence the left common iliac vein passes behind the right common iliac artery and is prone to trauma during surgical dissection of this region. The lower limb veins below the inguinal ligament have valves, but the pelvic veins and inferior vena cava do not.

Superficial

The long saphenous vein runs up the medial side of the calf and thigh before joining the common femoral vein in the groin. The short saphenous vein runs in the posterior midline of the calf before perforating the deep fascia at a variable point and joining the popliteal vein just above the popliteal fossa.

The superficial and deep systems communicate through perforating veins which have valves which allow flow from the superficial to the deep systems.

VISCERAL

The inferior vena cava is joined by the renal and hepatic veins as it passes up through the abdomen. The inferior mesenteric vein (which often has to be divided to gain access to the infrarenal aorta) drains into the splenic vein which itself then joins the superior mesenteric vein to form the portal vein which enters the hilum of the liver. The ovarian veins pass up the posterior abdominal wall to drain into the renal vein on the left and into the inferior vena cava on the right.

PHYSIOLOGY

Arterial wall characteristics and pulse wave transmission

During cardiac systole about two-thirds of the left ventricular volume (about 80 mL, the left ventricular ejection fraction) is ejected into the ascending aorta. This volume is accommodated partially by forward propulsion of blood through the capillaries into the venous circulation and partially by expansion of the large elastic arteries. This expansion is in both the transverse and longitudinal directions and its extent depends on the stiffness of the arterial wall. A stiffer vessel will expand less and is said to be less compliant. The impact of reduced compliance is to increase blood pressure (because blood, being a liquid, is non-compressible) and so increase the strain on the left ventricle. Age and atherosclerosis both reduce arterial compliance.

The large proximal arteries have a more elastic wall than do the smaller, more distal muscular arteries. The muscular arteries are less compliant than the elastic arteries and so dilate less with cardiac systole. As they dilate less, there is less recoil and so diastolic pressure is maintained less well more distally. The opposite happens with systolic pressure; as the elastic arteries dilate the rise in systolic pressure is less than it is in the less compliant muscular arteries. The overall result of this is that pulse pressure increases with distance from the heart. Systolic pressure also increases more distally, so explaining why the ankle–brachial index is slightly greater than 1 in health.

Even though diastolic pressure falls with distance from the heart, it will still match the diastolic pressure in the more proximal arteries during the second half of diastole in many vascular beds. The result of this is that there is no flow of blood during this phase of the cardiac cycle. This is readily appreciated by the silence heard between each cycle when using a handheld Doppler.

Pulse palpation is an important part of vascular surgery, but its value depends on a number of factors. A normal femoral artery wall moves less than 0.5 mm with each pulse. This would obviously be impalpable, but the act of partially compressing the artery into an ellipse allows the wall to move much more because the energy need to distort an ellipse is less than that needed to distort a circle. Arteries therefore have to be slightly compressed to feel their pulse. A calcified artery is less compressible and its wall will move very little with each pulse wave, making it impossible to feel the pulse, even though there may be a good flow of blood through it.

Prosthetic arterial bypasses are less compliant than native arteries. They therefore resist deformation with each pulse wave and this has the flow dynamic effect of increasing the graft's resistance to pulsatile flow (known as impedance). Furthermore, at an anastomosis between a prosthesis and a native artery, the artery will move more with each pulse wave than will the prosthesis. This strains the suture line and is a factor in the formation of false aneurysms at these anastomoses[2] (along with low-grade infection which weakens the arterial wall).

Flow dynamics

Poiseuille's law describes the flow rate of fluid through a tube related to the pressure gradient and the resistance to flow. The resistance to flow is related to the viscosity of the fluid and to the diameter and the length of the tube. It is much easier to draw up a watery drink through a short wide straw than it is to draw up a thick milk shake through a long narrow straw. Mathematically, flow is directly proportional to the fourth power of the tube's radius and is inversely proportional to the tube's length and to the viscosity of the fluid. This has important implications when selecting bypass materials as the radius has by far the most effect on flow. The greater the flow, the less risk of thrombosis.

As atherosclerotic plaques progressively narrow the lumen of an artery, the artery compensates by dilation. The effect of this is that flow is not significantly affected until the lumen is narrowed by 50 percent or more.[3] Several stenoses along the length of an artery act in series, and although each individual stenosis may not be significant, the sum total of resistances has been shown to be greater than an equivalent single stenosis of the same total length.[4] The blood's viscosity can be an important factor in native vessel and bypass graft thrombosis. As the viscosity increases, flow reduces so making thrombosis more likely. Conditions such as polycythemia, myeloproliferative disorders, and malignancy are associated with excessive thrombosis, particularly in the presence of underlying arterial disease.

Normal flow within a normal artery is laminar, with the characteristic parabolic flow profile. In circumstances of very high flow, however, flow becomes turbulent. In health this generally only occurs in the ascending aorta at the peak of systole.[5] At a stenosis, however, the flow rate increases, often sufficiently for the flow to become turbulent. This is identified clinically as a bruit or thrill. It is important to realize that clinically significant stenoses are not always associated with bruits or thrills and conversely bruits or thrills may also occur in the absence of a significant stenosis.

A healthy artery is able to withstand the expansile forces of the pulse wave. In aneurysm formation, however, the vessel wall is weakened by a reduced production of elastin resulting in a relative excess of collagen. In these circumstances the arterial wall dilates.[6,7] Laplace's law is traditionally applied to aneurysms to explain their growth once dilation starts (the analogy is with inflating a balloon – it gets easier as the balloon gets larger). In such a biologic system it is difficult to strictly apply Laplace's law, but as the radius increases, the wall tension increases if blood pressure and wall thickness stay the same. This fact partly explains the increased risk of rupture in larger aneurysms. Rupture is also associated with further arterial wall weakening due to a reduction in collagen content over and above the previous weakening resulting from the reduction in elastin content.

Ischemia–reperfusion

Reperfusion of previously ischemic tissues can result in deleterious effects systemically and locally. During ischemia the metabolites of anaerobic metabolism, including lactic acid, build up. In severe ischemia, cell death releases intracellular substances, most notably potassium and myoglobin after muscle ischemia (rhabdomyolysis). When such tissues are reperfused, these accumulated substances are released into the general circulation, resulting in metabolic acidosis, hyperkalemia, and myoglobinemia. The myoglobin is precipitated in the renal tubules resulting in renal failure secondary to acute tubular necrosis. It is because of these consequences that careful thought is required before attempting revascularization of an ischemic limb with muscle tenderness suggesting muscle necrosis. In these circumstances, primary amputation may be the safer option. The reperfusion syndrome is also a major contributing factor to systemic upset after aortic aneurysm repair, particularly after rupture.

Locally, ischemia results in capillary damage and even necrosis. As a result, the capillaries loose their integrity and become more permeable. The effects of reperfusion amplify this[8] and as a result the reperfused limb becomes edematous. At one extreme, this results in post-reperfusion edema which settles with time. At the other extreme, edema within a tight fascial compartment increases intracompartment pressure and initially reduces venous return. This further exacerbates the edema and a vicious cycle results in compartment pressure increasing to levels which abolish tissue perfusion – a compartment syndrome. This is recognized by pain, paralysis of the affected muscle, and a tense swelling. Emergency decompression is required by fasciotomy. When a compartment syndrome is anticipated after surgical revascularization, prophylactic fasciotomy should be performed.[9]

CLINICAL SYNDROMES

Lower limb ischemia

Reduction in arterial blood flow may be either acute or chronic, and its severity either total or subtotal. The associated clinical syndromes are severe acute limb ischemia (no blood supply to the limb), less severe acute limb ischemia (some blood entering the limb), mild chronic ischemia (manifest only on exercise), and severe chronic limb ischemia (with rest pain or tissue loss). These conditions more commonly affect the lower limb than the upper limb, largely because of the distribution of atherosclerosis. However, the symptoms can present in either leg or arm.

CHRONIC LOWER LIMB ISCHEMIA

Clinical picture

- Claudication

As arterial stenoses exceed 50 percent of the vessel lumen, blood flow is increasingly reduced. This reduction is first manifest when metabolic demands are greatest as in exercise. When the supply of oxygen cannot match the demand of the tissues, anaerobic metabolism is used to provide the

additional energy. Lactic acid produced in this way directly stimulates nociceptors within skeletal muscle resulting in intermittent claudication. When the exercise stops, the metabolic demands reduce and anaerobic metabolism and lactic acid production cease. As residual lactic acid is carried away from the tissues the pain eases. This only takes a few minutes, corresponding to the length of time it takes for claudication to ease off on resting. Claudication is usually felt one segment beyond the level of arterial disease causing it. Aortic and proximal iliac disease cause buttock, thigh, and calf claudication. Distal iliac and proximal femoral disease cause thigh and calf pain, and superficial femoral and popliteal disease cause calf claudication. It is calf claudication which is most common because of the work done by the calf on walking and because of the common distribution of atherosclerosis.

It is important clinically to distinguish claudication from other causes of leg pain. One of the most common differential diagnoses is pain referred from the lumbar spine, often caused by pressure on the cauda equina (spinal stenosis) from chronic degenerative arthritic changes or disc prolapse. This pain tends to be postural and is most noticeable in the upright position, either walking or standing. Relief is obtained by sitting or lying down and often takes 20 minutes or more, in contrast with intermittent claudication which is relieved within a few minutes simply by standing still. The two conditions often coexist and features of both can be elicited in the patient's history.

The severity of claudication is difficult to determine objectively and often the patient's own perceptions are the best guide. Interestingly, this latter point, along with poorer cardiovascular fitness, has been found to be associated with a shorter treadmill claudication distance in women than in men.[10] There is generally little to find on clinical examination in patients with claudication. Absent pulses give an indication as to the anatomy of the atherosclerosis. The most important aspect here is the presence or absence of a femoral pulse. An absent femoral pulse suggests iliac disease which can often respond well to intervention. The more distal pulses are less reliably felt, but can sometimes distinguish between femoropopliteal and calf vessel disease.

- Critical ischemia

In the small number of patients in whom peripheral atherosclerosis progresses, critical ischemia will develop. The concept of critical ischemia implies that in the absence of revascularization, limb loss is the inevitable outcome. This immediately introduces the difficulty of balancing sensitivity against specificity. If a highly sensitive definition is chosen, everyone whose limb is truly at risk will be included; some patients, however, will be categorized as having critical ischemia even though their limbs are not at actually at risk. Conversely, if a highly specific definition is chosen, every patient who meets it will have a limb at risk; in this case, however, there will be patients who do not meet the criteria but whose limbs, nevertheless, are at risk. Against this background a number of attempts have been made to agree an international definition. These attempts have attempted to include pressure measurements as a diagnostic marker. This adds more difficulty because of variable results in the presence of arterial calcification. A generally agreed definition now simply states that the ischemia is critical if there is rest pain or tissue loss caused by arterial disease.[11]

Rest pain generally occurs in the forefoot where the circulation is most compromised. It may first be noticeable at night when cardiac output and blood pressure are lower, the hydrostatic advantage of the upright posture is lost and the tissues have a higher metabolic rate because of being warmer than during the day. In these circumstances the patient may obtain some relief by cooling the foot, sitting up or walking a few steps (which increases blood pressure and regains the hydrostatic benefit of standing up).

As the vascularity deteriorates further, the most precarious tissue (the toes, being most distal) may necrose and become gangrenous. Similarly, minor trauma elsewhere on the foot or lower calf may result in ulceration as the blood supply is insufficient to heal the wound, even though it had been enough to maintain the integrity of the skin previously

(intact skin has a lower metabolic requirement than a wound). A small wound becomes a larger ulcer as inflammatory edema compresses the precarious microcirculation, inducing ischemia around the originally wounded area. This process continues and the ulcer enlarges until tissue perfusion is sufficient to overcome the tissue pressure of edema. Infection will simply exacerbate this process. Deep tissue infection associated with ulceration or gangrene is particularly dangerous as it may spread rapidly along tissue planes in the presence of ischemia.

Epidemiology and natural history

The incidence and prevalence of atherosclerosis and claudication both increase with age (Figs 15.1 and 15.2). In postmenopausal women, there may be an association between atherosclerosis and the low bone mineral density of osteoporosis or osteopenia.[12] In keeping with atherosclerosis being a systemic disease, it is the cardiac, cerebral, and other vital organ manifestations which have the greatest impact on survival, even though from the patient's viewpoint it is often the claudication which is most noticeable. This point

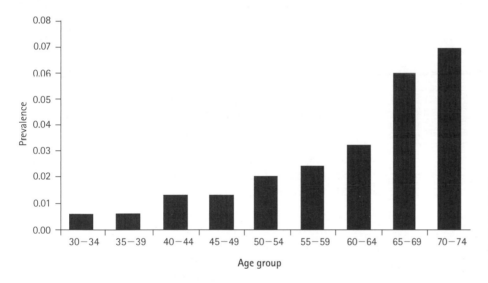

Figure 15.1 Prevalence of intermittent claudication by age. (Redrawn from *Eur J Vasc Endovasc Surg* 2000; **19**(Suppl A): S8–9, Copyright 2000, with permission from Elsevier.)

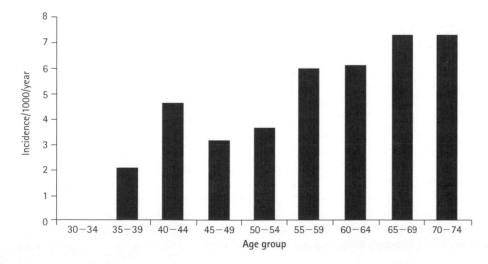

Figure 15.2 Incidence of intermittent claudication. (Redrawn from *Eur J Vasc Endovasc Surg* 2000; **19**(Suppl A): S8–9, Copyright 2000, with permission from Elsevier.)

is well illustrated by the schema in Figure 15.3. The causes of death in patients with claudication are vascular in about two-thirds compared with half in the general population over the age of 40 (Fig. 15.4). Another way of looking at this is to examine the 5-, 10- and 15-year survival figures after a diagnosis of claudication is made. Figure 15.5 shows this in comparison to the general population.

The important message here is that patients with claudication are best served by aggressive management of their medical risk factors in an attempt to prolong their survival. The outlook for the limb with claudication is benign, with reports showing a 1 percent limb loss rate at 5 years,[13] and consequently claudication is generally best treated with conservative measures in the majority of patients. Intervention is generally considered only if the symptoms are truly limiting. Reduction in functional capacity with time can occur but is most likely in patients with other comorbidities such as pulmonary disease and spinal stenosis.[14] Although male

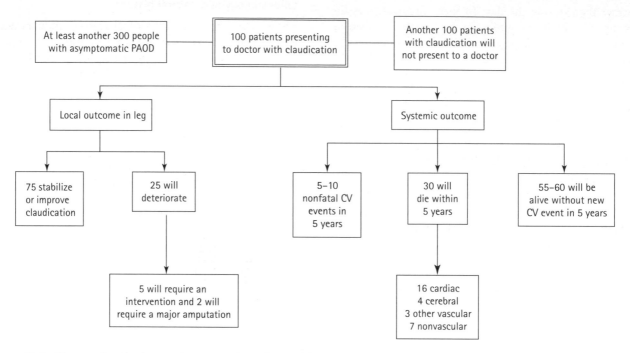

Figure 15.3 Five-year local and systemic outcome for patients with claudication. CV, cardiovascular; POAD, peripheral artery occlusive disease. (Redrawn from *Eur J Vasc Endovasc Surg* 2000; **19**(Suppl A): S19, Copyright 2000, with permission from Elsevier.)

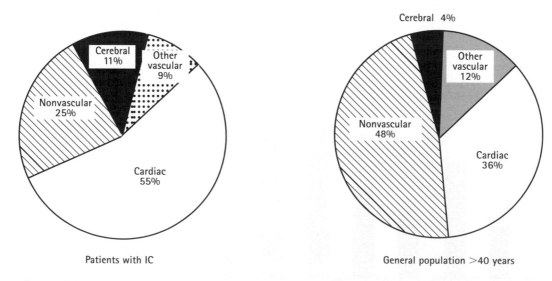

Patients with IC

General population >40 years

Figure 15.4 Causes of death in patients with claudication compared to the general population. IC, intermittent claudication. (Redrawn from *Eur J Vasc Endovasc Surg* 2000; **19**(Suppl A): S17, Copyright 2000, with permission from Elsevier.)

and female claudicants in one study showed no difference in objective function as measured by ankle–brachial index and walking distance, women were found to have poorer overall physical and mental function scores than men.[15]

The outlook for critical ischemia is poor both in terms of the limb and survival. It is becoming increasingly recognized that many of these patients have an underlying malignancy, with one recent report finding a frequency of 11.5 percent.[16] The overall 1-year survival following the diagnosis of critical ischemia is shown in Figure 15.6.

Investigation

Functional assessment by measurement of the ankle–brachial index can be helpful in making the diagnosis in those cases where the history is unclear. In milder cases, the ankle–brachial index may be normal at rest, but after exercise it will fall. Exercise induces a fall in peripheral vascular resistance through muscular vasodilation. If inflow is limited, then arterial pressure distal to the stenosis cannot be maintained in the face of this fall in resistance.[17]

Anatomical investigation is becoming increasingly noninvasive, with the traditional catheter angiogram being less commonly used. Duplex scanning in experienced hands gives an accurate picture of disease distribution, particularly in the infrainguinal segment,[18] although bowel gas can sometimes limit access to the aortoiliac segment. Duplex has the advantage of providing information on the effect a stenosis is having on flow. The other important noninvasive imaging modality is magnetic resonance angiography (MRA). This has progressed rapidly in the past few years and is now used, along with duplex scanning, as a first line of investigation in many centers.[19] A drawback is the underestimation of calf vessel disease in some patients, making it less useful for cases of severe ischemia. Nevertheless, the combination of duplex scanning and MRA allows procedure planning in those

patients deemed suitable for intervention. Digital subtraction catheter angiography still provides the most detailed anatomical images and will be required in some cases of claudication and almost all cases of critical ischemia. It is generally used to guide angioplasty, although in some centers this can be done by duplex scanning. Catheter angiography is conventionally performed using iodinated contrast media. These do carry the side effects of fluid overload, contrast nephropathy and, rarely, anaphylaxis. In selected cases and with appropriate equipment, these side effects may be overcome or reduced by the use of carbon dioxide gas[20] or gadolinium[21] as the contrast medium.

In all cases, the aim of investigation is to identify the segment or segments responsible for the ischemia, determine where flow into a potential reconstruction can come from (inflow) and where flow from the potential reconstruction

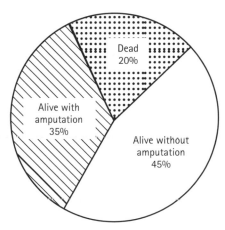

Figure 15.6 One year outcome for patients with critical limb ischemia. (Redrawn from *Eur J Vasc Endovasc Surg* 2000; **19**(Suppl A): S23, Copyright 2000, with permission from Elsevier.)

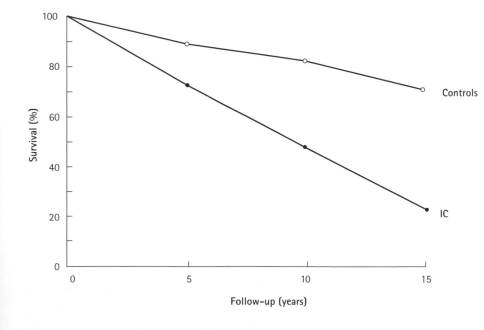

Figure 15.5 Five-, 10- and 15-year survival after diagnosis for patients with claudication (Redrawn from *Eur J Vasc Endovasc Surg* 2000; **19**(Suppl A): S17, Copyright 2000, with permission from Elsevier.)

can go to (outflow). It is these factors which determine which type of reconstruction (angioplasty or bypass) is possible. In critical ischemia, the outflow will be worse and more difficult to image than in claudication. It is important to use all possible modalities to identify outflow. Careful angiography and duplex are generally sufficient, but occasionally surgical exploration will reveal a useable outflow vessel which simply had too little blood flow to be demonstrable on imaging.

Treatment

- ### Claudication

Medical management is directed at appropriate drug therapy for associated conditions and arterial risk factors. It goes without saying that the most important intervention is the cessation of smoking. There is controversy regarding the value of supervised exercise classes for claudication. Whether or not the exercise is supervised, it can improve both the maximum walking distance and the distance to the onset of pain.

The most important aspect of radiological or surgical intervention is case selection. There are no rules here, but experience and informed discussion at multidisciplinary meetings form the basis of the decision-making process. An accurate diagnosis is essential. Particular emphasis is placed on what benefit the patient may expect from the proposed treatment bearing in mind the severity and nature of their symptoms in relation to their disease pattern. The risks of treatment are important to balance against the natural history of intermittent claudication. Surgery generally carries more risk than angioplasty and risk increases the more distal the reconstruction. In general, interventions for claudication are limited to the aortoiliac and femoropopliteal segments. Angioplasty has good results in the aortoiliac segment with low risk (69 percent 5-year patency for iliac angioplasty from pooled series[22]); below the groin, however, its longevity is much less predictable, with 5-year patency rates of 38 percent being reported in the femoropopliteal segment.[23] Surgery also has good results for aortoiliac disease but there is associated morbidity and mortality, especially for aortic surgery. Patency for aortobifemoral bypass is reported to be around 90 percent at 5 years[24] with operative mortality at around 3 percent. Femoropopliteal bypass has better long-term results than balloon angioplasty. Pooled data show 4-year patency rates of 69 percent in the above-knee position and 77 percent below the knee when using reversed long saphenous vein.[25]

Prosthetic conduits are now uncommonly used in this area because of poorer patency results, especially below the knee (40 percent 4 year patency),[25] and concerns about infection. Patency of below-knee prosthetic bypasses may be improved with the use of a vein cuff at the lower anastomosis.[26] Intervention on the infrageniculate segment is rarely carried out for claudication because of the risks of precipitating amputation should the procedure fail. When

used for critical ischemia, such infrageniculate bypasses may achieve patency rates of up to 62 percent at 4 years.[25]

- ### Critical ischemia

Treatment is directed at both limb salvage and the patient's comorbidity. Cardiac, respiratory, and renal disease are common in this patient group and any symptoms of a possible underlying malignancy should be pursued. The nutritional status of these patients is often poor,[27] further adding to their difficulties.

All reconstructive options are of potential value in critical ischemia. Depending on the anatomy of the arterial disease, some patients are best treated by angioplasty, others by surgery and yet more by a combination of both. Nevertheless, there are patients who are anatomically suitable for either angioplasty or surgery. In such cases, debate about whether an initial radiological approach is better than an initial surgical approach has been addressed recently.[28] Essentially 1-year amputation-free survival and mortality results were found to be similar in the two groups with a lower morbidity in the angioplasty first group. However, the early failure and reintervention rates were higher in the angioplasty group and beyond 2 years the bypass group had a more durable outcome. Essentially this trial suggested that angioplasty first is preferred in patients with limited life expectancy. In those expected to live longer, however, surgery would be the better option. Postoperative complications are common and need to be investigated and treated aggressively.

Women treated for critical ischemia by arterial bypass are thought generally to fare worse than men. There are some data to support this view, with one study showing that although operative mortality and limb salvage rates were similar between women and men, long-term survival and graft patency were lower in women.[29]

ACUTE LIMB ISCHEMIA

Clinical presentation

Acute limb ischemia is a surgical emergency. Depending on the degree of ischemia, as little as 6 hours or less may be available to restore a blood supply before irreversible changes occur. The traditional cause has been an embolus, originating from the heart in 90 percent of cases,[30] occluding a large proximal vessel. Because the embolus will generally lodge where the artery undergoes a sudden caliber change, the most common sites are the common femoral bifurcation, the aortic bifurcation (saddle embolus), and, less so, the popliteal bifurcation.[31] If the vascularity of the limb is otherwise normal, with no atherosclerosis, there will not be a developed collateral circulation. Occlusion of a major vessel, particularly the common femoral or aortic bifurcations, will then result in acute total ischemia of one or both limbs respectively. This results in the classic appearance of severe acute ischemia. The mnemonic commonly used to teach this ('6 Ps'– paralysis, pain, paresthesia, pulselessness, pallor, perishing cold) is a little misleading. In total ischemia, the paralysis, pallor, and coldness will be complete. The sensory changes and pulses need more explanation. A pulse may be felt in the common femoral, even if it is occluded by an embolus. The pulse wave can be propagated through embolus and thrombus before they become organized. In such a situation, however, there would be no pulses more distally in the leg. This serves as an example of the fact that the distribution of pulses is not directly related to the severity of the ischemia. A patient with claudication due to an iliac occlusion will have no pulses in the leg, yet the degree of ischemia may be mild because of the development of a good collateral circulation. The sensory changes of acute ischemia relate to the depth of ischemia and the modality being tested. Large nerve fibers are more susceptible to ischemia than small fibers. Light touch is carried by large fibers and so is often altered or abolished early in the course of acute ischemia resulting in paresthesia or anesthesia to light touch. Pain, however, is carried by smaller fibers, which are more resistant to ischemia. The pain of total acute ischemia is severe, but if the ischemia is so severe that small fibers cease to function then pain lessens. This is a poor prognostic sign.

In the past, total acute ischemia was most commonly due to emboli from atrial fibrillation secondary to mitral stenosis following rheumatic fever. These patients were generally young and had no arterial disease and so no collateral circulation. Nowadays, atrial fibrillation is more commonly secondary to ischemic heart disease and the patients have coexisting peripheral atherosclerosis with a collateral circulation developed to a greater or lesser degree. In these patients the cause of acute ischemia may still be embolic but may also be thrombosis *in situ* in major vessels affected by atherosclerosis. Occlusion of a major vessel in these circumstances results in less severe acute ischemia as the collateral circulation continues to provide some blood to the leg. In fact, the whole spectrum exists with some patients undergoing thrombotic occlusion of a major vessel (such as the superficial femoral artery) without any noticeable deterioration in their symptoms of claudication. Other patients, with a poorer collateral circulation, will experience subtotal acute ischemia in the same circumstances.

The clinical appearance of subtotal acute ischemia is a modulation of the classic appearance of total ischemia. Skin pallor may be evident, but more commonly there is mottling of the skin with areas appearing pale, cyanosed, or hyperemic as the dynamic microcirculation responds to no, sluggish, or improved blood supply, respectively. Such areas of skin remain viable if they blanch on pressure, but if the mottling becomes fixed then skin viability is lost. The sensory changes vary from no impairment through altered sensation to absence, depending on the degree of ischemia. Similarly muscle weakness may be absent in some cases, noticeable in others, and total in the most severe ischemia. If the calf muscle becomes tender to palpation with a 'doughy' feel, then there is probably muscle necrosis. If this is the case, revascularization would be contraindicated and primary amputation should be considered. It is these four features – appearance of the skin, sensory changes, muscle power, and muscle tenderness – which are used to determine the degree of severity of the ischemia, and hence the urgency of any revascularization that is needed. This may be classified according to the modified Rutherford criteria:[32]

- Grade 1 – viable limb with or without revascularization
- Grade 2A – threatened limb, but not requiring immediate revascularization
- Grade 2B – threatened limb requiring immediate revascularization
- Grade 3 – irreversible ischemia, salvage not possible

Management

The treatment of acute limb ischemia ranges from the most straightforward to the most complex. In milder cases with no limb threat, simple anticoagulation may be used initially. If embolic disease into an otherwise normal circulation is thought to be the cause of total acute ischemia (acute onset, identifiable source for an embolus, normal pulses in the contralateral leg and no chronic symptoms) then investigation should be limited to minimize the delay to treatment. All that is required is the identification of a suitable inflow source. Commonly this is provided by the palpation of a femoral pulse, even if this is only felt deeply above the inguinal ligament. In these cases simple femoral embolectomy restores the circulation. If this is not successful, on-table angiography may be required to confirm clearance distally. Distal thromboembolic occlusion may be treated by on-table thrombolysis, thromboembolectomy, clot aspiration, or bypass.

In the absence of a femoral pulse and if the degree of ischemia allows, an inflow source should be identified preoperatively by duplex scanning or catheter angiography. This is important because the acute occlusion may not be purely embolic and the inflow vessel may be occluded by underlying atherosclerosis with or without superadded embolus or thrombus. In these circumstances, simple embolectomy will not restore inflow and this has to be provided by bypass. Potential inflow sources are the proximal ipsilateral iliac system, the contralateral iliac or femoral arteries, the aorta, or the axillary artery.

Cases of subacute ischemia are more complex. These patients generally have underlying atherosclerosis, in which case thromboembolectomy is unlikely to clear the vessel and may even cause harm by traumatizing atherosclerotic plaques. Catheter angiography is useful here. Treatment is likely to require bypass surgery, but in some patients thrombolysis may be suitable. The usual contraindications apply to peripheral thrombolysis, even though the dose is lower and the drug is delivered directly into the thrombus by catheter. Thrombolysis should be viewed as a diagnostic adjunct as well as a therapeutic maneuver. After the lysis of propagated thrombus, the lesion responsible for the occlusion may be more clearly demonstrated on angiography. In this way treatment, either angioplasty or bypass, may be limited to dealing with the responsible lesion rather than having to deal with a longer segment of artery occluded only by propagated thrombus. In this way, initial thrombolysis may lower the initial morbidity and mortality of acute limb ischemia compared with immediate operative intervention.[33,34] It is fair to say, however, that outside the results of trials, the complications of thrombolysis in this elderly, frail population can be significant. There is a particular risk of hemorrhage and stroke and because of this the indications for lysis are still not entirely clear. A multidisciplinary approach is very useful here with input from radiologists, an interested physician as well as the surgeon. If lysis is contraindicated, inappropriate, or fails to make much impact on the occluded segment within a few hours, surgery to bypass the whole of the occluded segment will be required.[35]

Thromboangiitis obliterans (Buerger's disease)

The classic description of Buerger disease involves young, smoking men with an obliterative thrombotic process affecting distal, small arteries and veins in the arms and legs. However, there appears to have been an increased incidence in women over the past 20 years, possibly related to changes in smoking habits.[36] Clinical diagnostic criteria vary and a definitive diagnosis can only be made histologically.

Treatment requires the cessation of smoking. Measures to enhance vasodilation have been used but surgical bypass is rarely appropriate because of the distal nature of the disease. Amputation is required in significant number of cases.

Aneurysm

Collagen and elastin within the media of large- and medium-sized arteries resist the expansile force of each pulse wave and help maintain arterial wall integrity. Aneurysmal disease develops as a result of disordered elastin and collagen metabolism. An increase in the breakdown of elastin relative to its production reduces the amount of elastin in the arterial wall. This change weakens the wall and allows expansion.[6,7] As indicated previously, Laplace's law can be loosely applied to show that wall tension increases with diameter. If the tension exceeds the strength of the wall, rupture will occur. This event may be triggered by an increase in collagen breakdown within the aneurysm wall, weakening it further.

There is no precise definition of when an artery becomes aneurysmal, but this is generally taken to occur when the arterial diameter exceeds 1.5 times normal.[37] Affected sites include the aorta, iliac, popliteal, femoral, visceral, carotid, and subclavian arteries. Of these, aortoiliac aneurysms are the most common with popliteal aneurysms accounting for 70 percent of the remainder.[38]

AORTIC ANEURYSM

Any site along the whole length of the aorta may become aneurysmal, but that most commonly affected is the infrarenal aorta (65 percent of all aortoiliac aneurysms[39]). At this site the aneurysm may extend into one or both common iliac arteries or be limited to the aorta itself. The overall incidence of clinically apparent abdominal aortic aneurysm is 21 per 100 000 person years,[40] but this is increased in patients with arterial disease or hypertension. There is a further increase in incidence in patients with affected siblings.[41,42] The prevalence increases with age and with smoking and is certainly higher in men than in women.[43,44] In spite of this, the condition seems to follow a more aggressive course in women in terms of growth rate, rupture risk, outcome after surgery, and possibly the size at which rupture occurs.

The annual growth rate of aortic aneurysms is around 0.3–0.5 cm, although this can vary considerably both within individual patients and between patients. In women, there is emerging evidence that growth rates are independently and significantly higher than in men.[45] The UK Small Aneurysm Trial[46] showed that the risk of rupture in aneurysms less than 5.5 cm in diameter is less than 1 percent per year. Over this size the rupture risk increases and is higher in women than in men,[47] although precise figures obviously cannot be obtained. As a guide, the rupture risk is thought to increase to around 20 percent per year at 6.5 cm and to 30 percent per year at 7.5 cm with larger aneurysms being even more likely to rupture.[48] A national screening program for aortic aneurysms is currently being considered in the United Kingdom, based on a number of studies.[49] Whether such screening programs would include women is not yet decided. Because of the lower incidence of aneurysm in women, it would be more difficult to make an economic case for population screening.

Aortic aneurysms are generally clinically silent, although some patients experience abdominal pulsation or feel a mass. If a patient experiences back or abdominal pain (the symptomatic aneurysm) actual or threatened rupture should be considered seriously. Occasionally smaller aneurysms which contain a lot of mural thrombus may embolize distally.[50] These emboli tend to be small and may present as multiple pedal microinfarcts. Rupture generally presents with the well-known clinical picture, but occasionally the symptoms can be atypical. In such cases a high index of suspicion is needed with ready resort to computed tomography (CT). Infrequent presentations include an aortocaval fistula with high-output cardiac failure,[51] or a primary aortoenteric fistula[52] with gastrointestinal blood loss varying from minor low-grade iron deficiency anemia to catastrophic hemorrhage. Most aortoenteric fistulas arise after previous aortic surgery with duodenal adherence to an anastomotic suture line.

Plain abdominal or lumbar spine radiographs may reveal an aortic aneurysm, but cannot be used to measure it because of the magnification inherent in these studies.

Ultrasound has been shown to be the most reliable, cheap and safe method to diagnose and measure the size of aortic aneurysms. CT scanning gives more anatomic information, in particular the configuration and relation of the neck to the renal arteries and the degree of involvement of the iliac arteries. Angiography often does not demonstrate the dilation as the aneurysm wall is lined by laminated thrombus. The actual lumen in these cases may well be of a normal caliber.

Asymptomatic aneurysms less than 5.5 cm in diameter are simply kept under ultrasound surveillance. The UK Small Aneurysm Trial showed there was no survival benefit to early surgery in aneurysms less than this size. Even in this group, however, rupture is not impossible and repair would be recommended in fit patients if the aneurysm became symptomatic or grew by more than 1 cm in a year. Repair is generally recommended to patients with aneurysms over 5.5 cm, as long as the patient is considered fit enough. Mortality, which is generally related to cardiorespiratory complications, from open aneurysm repair in recent multicenter studies is around 3–8 percent[46,53] and tends to be higher in women than in men.[54,55] In contrast, endovascular repair (EVAR) of aortic aneurysm appears to have a similar mortality in women and men.[56,57]

The role of EVAR is now becoming established following publication of the EVAR trials 1 and 2. In EVAR, a two-piece modular bifurcated stent-graft combination is inserted via the femoral artery on each side. Anchorage between the infrarenal neck and the main body of the device, between the iliac arteries and device limbs, and between the main body and 'contralateral' limb is by radial force. The EVAR 1 Trial[53] randomized patients into either an open repair group or into an EVAR group. EVAR is less invasive than open repair and was shown to have a lower procedural mortality (2.3 percent compared to 5.3 percent in the open repair group). Although EVAR is associated with more postprocedural interventions than open repair, overall mortality at 4 years was the same for EVAR and open repair. For purely aneurysm-related death, however, EVAR retained its 30-day mortality advantage, suggesting that the comorbidity responsible for the higher mortality after open repair is also present in EVAR patients. As EVAR is less stressful, however, more patients survive the procedure only to succumb subsequently as their comorbid conditions deteriorate. Attention to these comorbidities may reduce subsequent EVAR mortality. The EVAR 2 Trial[58] studied patients unfit for open repair and compared best medical management with EVAR. Although some patients underwent open repair as their fitness improved over the trial period, EVAR 2 showed that EVAR did not improve survival in patients unfit to undergo open aneurysm repair.

Following rupture most patients are offered open repair unless their comorbidity or clinical status on presentation suggest that any attempt at repair would be futile. The role of EVAR for ruptures is being investigated in several centers and it would appear to hold some promise.[59] The true overall mortality from rupture, including those patients who die before reaching hospital, may well be as high as 95 percent. Operative mortality varies widely depending on case selection, but is generally around 40–60 percent with reports showing a higher mortality in women than in men.[55,60,61] Unoperated, aortic aneurysm ruptures carry a mortality of essentially 100 percent. In some cases, a retroperitoneal rupture becomes well contained and death is delayed by several days until more catastrophic rupture occurs. Rarely catastrophic rupture does not occur in such patients in which case survival may be more prolonged.

POPLITEAL ARTERY ANEURYSM

Popliteal aneurysms are the most common of the peripheral artery aneurysms accounting for 70 percent of all peripheral aneurysms. They most commonly occur in elderly men. A popliteal artery with a size of more than 1.5 cm is considered aneurysmal. Most popliteal artery aneurysms are fusiform and are bilateral in 25–70 percent of cases.[62] Popliteal artery aneurysms are associated with abdominal aortic aneurysms in 20–40 percent of cases, but only 7.5–10 percent of abdominal aortic aneurysms are associated with popliteal artery aneurysms.[63,64]

Most popliteal artery aneurysms are degenerative, although they can be associated with repetitive trauma from the popliteal entrapment syndrome. They are initially asymptomatic, but their significance lies in the fact that they tend to embolize distally from their contained thrombus. Over time this gradually occludes the calf vessels, to the extent that in some patients the aneurysm thromboses due to poor run off. Such patients may initially complain of claudication and when the aneurysm thromboses the presentation is one of acute ischemia. In these circumstances the outlook is poor because of the often occluded calf vessels.

The mainstay of elective and emergency treatment is bypass with ligation of the artery above and below the aneurysm. Results following surgery depend greatly on how many calf run off vessels have remained patent.[65] If no calf vessels are shown on angiography in emergency cases then catheter-directed thrombolysis into the distal popliteal artery may be used to clear a run off vessel to enable definitive bypass.[66] The limb loss risk of popliteal artery aneurysm thrombosis is high, at around 18 percent.[67]

VISCERAL ARTERY ANEURYSMS

Visceral artery aneurysms are an uncommon form of vascular disease whose pathogenesis and natural history remain incompletely characterized. Nonetheless, their importance to the practicing vascular surgeon lies in their potential for rupture or erosion into an adjacent viscus, resulting in life-threatening hemorrhage. Almost 22 percent of them present as emergencies with a mortality rate of 8.5 percent.[68] Visceral artery aneurysms are increasingly recognized because of greater availability of advanced imaging techniques: CT, MRI, MRA, and angiography.

The most common visceral artery affected by aneurysmal disease is the splenic artery (60 percent), although almost all the other named visceral arteries can also be affected. In keeping with aneurysmal disease elsewhere, patients with visceral aneurysms may have aneurysms at multiple sites.[69]

SPLENIC ARTERY ANEURYSM

Splenic artery aneurysms are often incidental findings, but have been reported in up to 10.4 percent of autopsies.[70] Most splenic artery aneurysms are small (less than 2.0 cm), saccular aneurysms, and more than 80 percent are located in the mid or distal splenic artery.[71] Splenic artery aneurysms are found in women four times more frequently than in men, with the mean age of presentation being 52 years (range 2–93 years). Abnormalities in vessel wall metabolism, portal hypertension, pancreatitis, and repeated pregnancy[72] are all implicated in the pathogenesis of splenic aneurysms. Symptoms are uncommon, but there may be chronic abdominal pain. Splenic aneurysms can rupture with predictably catastrophic consequences. Rupture of an aneurysm during pregnancy has high maternal and infant mortality. This may well be due to the condition mimicking more common complications of pregnancy.

Treatment is recommended for all patients who are found to have a 2 cm or greater aneurysm, particularly in women of childbearing age. Surgery may involve simple ligation of the splenic artery, bypass or more, recently, coil embolization.[73]

OTHER VISCERAL ARTERY ANEURYSMS

Of the other visceral arteries, hepatic artery aneurysms are the most common. They are generally asymptomatic and are found coincidentally. Once they are symptomatic, the risk of and mortality from rupture are significant. Treatment involves ligation with or without bypass or coil embolization.

Cerebrovascular disease

Stroke is the third commonest cause of death in the Western world and is a major cause of morbidity. The overall incidence is around 160 per 100 000 population per year. Women have a higher incidence of stroke than men but, as they tend to be older at presentation, this may only be due to the known increased frequency of stroke with age. The majority of cerebrovascular events are ischemic in origin rather than hemorrhagic, with the cause of ischemia being either embolic or thrombosis *in situ* on underlying disease. Thrombosis is most likely to occur in the intracerebral vessels and attention is currently being focused on the use of thrombolysis to minimize disability. Embolization occludes intracerebral vessels and in many cases originates from the surgically accessible carotid bifurcation. This discussion will concentrate on this aspect of cerebrovascular disease.

SPECTRUM OF PRESENTATION AND THE UNSTABLE PLAQUE

The carotid bifurcation is particularly prone to atherosclerotic stenosis and there appears to be some evidence that there is a sex difference in the plaque morphology. In a study examining patients from an atherosclerosis prevention clinic,[74] carotid plaque area and stenosis both increased with age. Women showed a greater degree of stenosis than men, whereas men had a larger area of plaque. The metabolic syndrome also appears to have a greater impact on early carotid atherosclerosis in women than in men.[75]

In the majority of cases, carotid plaque is clinically silent. A proportion of patients will embolize silently resulting in small infarcts, often lacunar, on CT scanning. The mildest form of symptomatic carotid disease is amaurosis fugax, caused by a platelet microembolus lodging in a branch of the ipsilateral central retinal artery. The transient loss of vision is limited to one eye, is ipsilateral to the source of the embolus, and is followed by full recovery. The classic description of a curtain lowering across the eye may vary with the visual loss starting in any quadrant and being complete or partial depending on the size and site of the retinal artery being occluded. It is important to distinguish amaurosis fugax from homonomous hemianopia. The latter affects the visual fields of both eyes, a fact which can often be elicited from the history, and is generally a feature of the posterior cerebral circulation. Only if there is an associated severe hemiplegic stroke implying middle cerebral artery occlusion would homonomous hemianopia be an anterior circulation phenomenon.

A cerebral transient ischemic attack is the next stage in this spectrum of presentation. A transient ischemic attack is a focal neurological deficit with a vascular cause lasting less than 24 hours and followed by full recovery. The important points here are that the deficit is focal with motor or sensory symptoms being precisely located to a region of the cerebral homunculus and with the symptomatic deficit being contralateral to the embolized cerebral hemisphere and hence contralateral to the embolizing carotid bifurcation. Crescendo transient ischemic attacks or amaurosis fugax represent the next stage of the spectrum of severity. Although there is no widely accepted definition of crescendo, in these circumstances it is generally taken to imply three or four attacks in as many days. A reversible ischemic neurologic deficit (RIND) arises following a larger embolus, but is nevertheless followed by full recovery within 1 week.

Stroke in evolution is defined as a neurological deficit in which the signs are progressing as the patient is being observed, suggesting possibly that there is continual or rapidly repeating embolization to the same cerebral territory. An established stroke is associated with a neurological deficit which persists beyond 1 week.

This spectrum of presentations and established knowledge about the role of carotid endarterectomy in symptomatic carotid disease provide a graphic example of the concept of the unstable atherosclerotic plaque. When a plaque becomes unstable, through ulceration of the fibrous cap, fissuring or hemorrhage into the plaque, thrombus is more likely to form on its surface and then to embolize. While the plaque remains unstable, repeated embolization is more likely. With time and appropriate treatment plaques can become stable again and are then less likely to embolize. The proved value of carotid endarterectomy is greatest early on after any embolic event.[76] As time passes the benefit of carotid endarterectomy falls off, correlating to the biologic process of plaque stabilization. The most unstable plaques cause more severe symptoms from this spectrum of presentations and are more likely to be associated with subsequent major stroke. This relates to the degree of clinical urgency in carrying out carotid endarterectomy. This is most urgent after a series of crescendo attacks or a RIND in order to prevent the significantly unstable plaque from throwing off a large embolus. The degree of operative urgency following a stroke with clinical recovery has to be carefully determined. Previous concerns about early endarterectomy after stroke centered on postoperative intracranial hemorrhage or ischemic stroke extension. The European and North American randomized trials (see below), however, both showed the risk of further stroke was highest in the first month after an event with a 30-day stroke risk of 4.9 percent in the medical arm. In neurologically stable patients, therefore, delay is now felt to be inappropriate.[77]

MANAGEMENT

All patients should be given best medical management and be encouraged to stop smoking. Antiplatelet therapy is central to this approach and along with the other aspects of medical treatment can help to stabilize plaque. In asymptomatic patients, it would appear that this medical approach carries a lower risk of subsequent cerebrovascular events in women than in men.[78] The role of surgery in symptomatic carotid disease is well established following the large European (European Carotid Surgery Trial [ECST][79]) and North American (North American Symptomatic Carotid Endarterectomy Trial, [NASCET][80]) trials of the late 1980s. Both demonstrated a lower risk of death or disabling stroke with carotid endarterectomy compared with medical management if surgery took place within three (North American) or six (European) months of the event in patients who had had amaurosis, a transient ischemic attack, or a stroke followed by recovery, and whose responsible internal carotid artery was 70–99 percent stenosed. Interesting controversy arises from the fact that these studies used a different method for calculating the degree of stenosis from a selective carotid angiogram. This investigation carries a stroke risk of about 1 percent in these patients and is now rarely carried out for this indication.

Using other imaging modalities, mainly duplex scanning but also CT or MR angiography, and using entirely different methods of stenosis calculation, the clinical results appear to be similar to the major trials although it is known that each imaging modality calculates a different result for any given stenosis. Biologically this probably correlates with the fact that the finding of a symptomatic, severe stenosis is a surrogate marker for an unstable plaque. Plaque surface irregularity as seen on angiography is one possible indicator of an unstable plaque and has been shown to be associated with an increased number of cardiovascular events.[81] Another suggested marker for the unstable plaque is the serum level of high sensitivity C-reactive protein. This has been shown to be associated with macrophage and T lymphocyte presence within plaque, cells which are known to increase plaque instability.[82] Microscopically, unstable plaques associated with symptomatic embolization have been shown to be associated with increased plaque vascularity and intraplaque hemorrhage[83] and with less fibrous tissue.[84] It is likely in the future that there will be a reliable indicator of the unstable plaque. These plaques have been shown to be associated with 'hyperintense white matter lesions'[85] which in turn can predict stroke.[86] Data such as these will allow more precise patient selection for carotid endarterectomy before any symptoms develop.

The duplex criteria for stenosis measurement have been correlated with angiography, but there is some evidence that carotid blood flow velocity is higher in women than in men.[87] This would affect the measurement of the degree of stenosis and as experience increases, different criteria for duplex measured stenoses in women and men may emerge.

Carotid endarterectomy for asymptomatic disease is now on a firmer foundation following publication of the Asymptomatic Carotid Surgery Trial (ACST).[88] This study showed a halving (from 12 percent to 5 percent, including the 3 percent operative risk) of 5-year stroke risk in asymptomatic patients under the age of 75 with a duplex measured 70 percent or greater carotid stenosis following surgery compared with best medical treatment. This benefit over medical treatment is smaller than for symptomatic disease, however, and only exists if the operative risk of stroke matches that of ACST. Practically speaking, the margin of benefit is generally viewed as being insufficient to recommend widespread carotid endarterectomy for all asymptomatic plaques. In those patients who find it difficult to live with the knowledge of having a tight stenosis and who request endarterectomy, however, there is now some evidence to support carrying out surgery.[89]

The details of surgery are beyond the scope of this section, but there remains debate on several aspects. Standard endarterectomy is slower than the eversion technique, but allows detailed inspection of the endarterectomized surface. Local anesthesia allows accurate functional cerebral monitoring and may reduce the myocardial risk compared with general anesthesia. The General Anaesthetic versus Local Anaesthetic for carotid surgery (GALA) trial[90] is currently examining whether either technique has an advantage over the other. When to use a shunt is clear with local anesthesia, but cannot be determined with certainty under general anesthesia despite a wide variety of cerebral monitoring devices. Shunt use has theoretical and practical disadvantages and one benefit of local anesthesia is to allow the safe avoidance of a shunt when neurologic function is not affected by carotid clamping. When to use patch closure after standard endarterectomy and what material to use is still debated, although there is some evidence that a patch does reduce early and late complications.

Whether women benefit as much as men from carotid endarterectomy and whether they have more or the same number of postoperative complications is uncertain.[91] The Asymptomatic Carotid Atherosclerosis Study[92] and the NASCET[80] both suggested that initial stroke risk reduction was less in women compared to men following carotid endarterectomy, largely due to a higher perioperative risk in women. Long-term benefit, however, in both NASCET and the ASA and Carotid Endarterectomy Trial was similar for both sexes.[93] Neither study, however, was designed to specifically answer this question. Other groups, however, have found no difference in outcome after surgery for symptomatic or asymptomatic disease.[94,95] There is a general feeling that the development of postoperative restenosis is more likely in women compared with men. Data which support this view[96] and other data which refute it[97] are available, but these studies were again not specifically designed to determine whether this is the case.

Mesenteric ischemia

Mesenteric ischemia is caused by an interruption in blood flow to all or part of the small intestine or colon. This disease represents a significant challenge because the diagnosis is frequently delayed and associated with a high mortality exceeding 60 percent.[98] Significant chronic ischemia usually only occurs when two or three of the mesenteric arteries are occluded or diseased. Acute ischemia may arise following embolic occlusion of one vessel, particularly the superior mesenteric artery (SMA).

ACUTE MESENTERIC ISCHEMIA

Acute mesenteric ischemia may result from several causes (Box 15.1). Embolization to the SMA (usually lodging at or just beyond its first major branch) accounts for 50 percent of all cases of acute mesenteric ischemia and 25 percent are secondary to thrombosis of preexisting atherosclerotic lesions at the origin of the vessel.[99] The majority of mesenteric arterial emboli originate from left atrial or ventricular mural thrombi or cardiac valvular lesions. They are often associated with cardiac arrhythmias such as atrial fibrillation or hypokinetic regions produced by previous myocardial infarctions. A substantial proportion of emboli are to the SMA and are associated with concurrent emboli to another part of mesenteric vasculature.[100]

Box 15.1 Causes of acute mesenteric ischemia

Arterial occlusion (50 percent)
- Emboli to superior mesenteric artery
  - Mural thrombi from cardiac hypokinesia or atrial fibrillation
  - Cardiac valvular lesions
  - Cholesterol embolization
- Thrombotic occlusion
  - Preexisting atherosclerotic vessel disease
  - Acute obstruction of chronic mesenteric ischemia
- Dissecting aortic aneurysm
- Vasculitis or arteritis
- Fibromuscular dysplasia
- Direct trauma
- Endotoxin shock

Nonocclusive mesenteric ischemia (20–30 percent)
- Systemic hypotension
- Cardiac failure
- Septic shock
- Mesenteric vasoconstriction (sympathetic response)

Venous occlusion (5–15 percent)
- Primary mesenteric vein thrombosis
  - Deficiency of proteins C and S, antithrombin III, factor V Leiden
  - Antiphospholipid syndrome
  - Paroxysmal nocturnal hemoglobinuria
- Secondary mesenteric vein thrombosis
  - Paraneoplastic
  - Pancreatitis
  - Inflammatory bowel disease
  - Cirrhosis and portal hypotension
  - Previous sclerotherapy of varices
  - Splenomegaly or splenectomy
  - Postoperative state
  - Trauma
  - Oral contraceptives

Extravascular sources
- Incarcerated hernia
- Volvulus
- Intussusception
- Adhesive bands

Acute mesenteric arterial thrombosis of the SMA or celiac axis is usually associated with preexisting critical stenosis. Patients with mesenteric arterial thrombosis have histories consistent with chronic mesenteric ischemia, including postprandial pain, weight loss, 'food fear', and early satiety. Nonocclusive mesenteric ischemia is the underlying cause at least 20 percent to 30 percent of cases of mesenteric ischemia and results in mortality in up to 70 percent of afflicted patients. Nonocclusive mesenteric ischemia, without anatomic arterial or venous obstruction, can occur during periods of relatively low mesenteric flow, especially if there is underlying atherosclerotic disease (see Box 15.1). A diagnosis of nonocclusive mesenteric ischemia usually requires a high index of suspicion because the majority of these patients may not present with the classic symptom complex of severe abdominal pain with disproportionately few abdominal signs.

Mesenteric venous thrombosis leading to mesenteric ischemia is usually secondary to hypercoagulable states (see Box 15.1). Venous thrombosis is usually induced by massive influx of fluid into the bowel wall and lumen, resulting in systemic hypovolemia and hemoconcentration. The resulting bowel wall edema, as well as the increased outflow resistance secondary to venous thrombosis and increased blood viscosity, can impede arterial flow, leading to submucosal hemorrhage, venous capillary congestion, and bowel infarction. Long-term mortality from mesenteric venous thrombosis can be as high as 83 percent.[101] Clinically, thrombosis can present acutely, subacutely, or chronically as a segmental disease, usually affecting the small intestine rather than the colon.

CHRONIC MESENTERIC ISCHEMIA

Chronic mesenteric ischemia, a disease more common in smokers, presents in patients with a mean age of about 58 years. In contrast with other vascular syndromes, approximately 60 percent of patients are female. More than a third of patients have hypertension, ischemic heart disease, and cerebrovascular disease. The importance of chronic mesenteric ischemia lies in the fact that most cases of acute mesenteric ischemia occur in patients with a history of chronic abdominal complaints, presumably due to undiagnosed chronic mesenteric ischemia.

CLINICAL PRESENTATION

Acute mesenteric ischemia can present can present precipitously with severe abdominal pain and decompensation over hours or insidiously with symptom progression over days. Mesenteric ischemia secondary to embolization presents as sudden abdominal pain. Classically the pain is disproportionately exaggerated relative to the unremarkable physical findings and persists beyond 2–3 hours. However, signs of an acute abdomen with distension, guarding (rigidity), and hypotension may also occur, particularly when diagnosis has been delayed.[102] Fever, diarrhea, nausea, and anorexia are all commonly reported. Melena or hematochezia occurs in 15 percent of cases, and occult blood is detected in at least half of patients. The subacute pattern of mesenteric ischemia is characterized by a more gradual development of nonspecific abdominal pain with nausea, vomiting, and changes in bowel habit. Signs of peritoneal irritation such as abdominal tenderness and guarding are absent. The majority of these patients test positive for fecal blood.

Postprandial abdominal pain is the pathognomonic symptom of chronic mesenteric ischemia. Typically, this pain occurs within the first hour after eating and diminishes 1–2 hours later. The postprandial timing of the pain is directly related to limitation in blood flow through celiac and SMA lesions in the face of increased metabolic demands after the meal. The most common physical sign of mesenteric ischemia is weight loss secondary to the patient's anticipation of postprandial pain leading to restriction of food intake ('food fear'). Severe stenosis or complete obstruction of at least two of the three major splanchnic arteries usually occurs before symptoms are evident, because of the formation of a rich collateral vascular supply. One of the most feared complications is acute thrombosis and the consequent development of bowel infarction.

DIAGNOSIS

The diagnosis of intestinal ischemia begins with the ability of the clinician to suspect and recognize it. The clinical history of abdominal pain and nonspecific findings may be misleading. However, common clinical conditions should be quickly excluded and mesenteric vascular disease aggressively pursued in patients with the risk factors mentioned above.

Metabolic acidosis from lactate production and a high white cell count may be clues to severe bowel ischemia. Findings on plain radiographs are usually nonspecific in acute mesenteric ischemia and are seen late in the course of illness; they include a nonspecific ileus pattern and mesenteric thickening. Classic thumbprinting, seen also on barium studies, indicates submucosal hemorrhage or edema resulting in focal mural thickening. Intramural pneumatosis and portal venous gas are also noted in acute mesenteric ischemia but usually in advanced stages of bowel infarction.[103] The role of plain films should be rapid identification of perforation or bowel obstruction to expedite surgical management. However, the clinician should also realize that findings might be nonspecific for up to 12–18 hours after the onset of symptoms.

Traditionally, conventional angiography has been regarded as the gold standard imaging method. This is accomplished by arterial injections into the superior mesenteric artery or celiac arteries and sometimes by direct transhepatic or transjugular portography for identification of venous thrombosis.[104] Disadvantages include the highly invasive nature of the investigation, with potential nephrotoxicity and increased exposure to radiation. Advantages of angiography include the ability for concomitant endovascular treatment as described below. Additionally, digital subtraction angiography allows the best visualization of peripheral splanchnic vessel disease.[105] Colour Doppler ultrasonography has been used because it is noninvasive and inexpensive. However, it is limited by overlying bowel gas, operator-dependent quality, and poor sensitivity for low flow vessel disease.

Axial CT is the test of choice in the diagnosis of acute mesenteric ischemia. Contrast-enhanced CT detects acute mesenteric ischemia with sensitivity rates exceeding 90 percent. Magnetic resonance imaging with angiography is another noninvasive modality that gives excellent visualization of the vascular anatomy. It is possible to assess portal venous patency, flow direction, splanchnic thrombosis, and changes suggestive of portal hypertension in mesenteric venous disease. Although MRI with angiography is an excellent tool for the evaluation of chronic mesenteric ischemia, it should not be the first technique used in the diagnosis of acute mesenteric ischemia, because of its potentially insufficient resolution to adequately identify nonocclusive low flow states or distal emboli.[106]

MANAGEMENT

The presence of peritoneal signs mandates surgical exploration, as bowel infarction has probably occurred. Resection of infarcted bowel as well as embolectomy can be accomplished during this process. In the absence of peritoneal signs, surgical embolectomy is still appropriate.[107] However, an interventional radiologic approach has been effectively used. Intraarterial infusion of thrombolytic agents such as streptokinase, urokinase, or recombinant tissue plasminogen activator has been shown to be effective when used within 12 hours of onset of symptoms.[108] Forgoing surgical embolectomy in favor of a less invasive approach may be appropriate in a patient with appreciable operative risk. In nonocclusive mesenteric ischemia, infusion of an intraarterial vasodilator such as papaverine into the SMA may be all that is needed to reverse vasoconstriction and prevent bowel infarction.[109]

In patients with mesenteric venous thrombosis, a search for an underlying hypercoagulable state is essential to prevent recurrent disease. The presence of peritoneal signs should prompt surgical exploration. In an asymptomatic patient, anticoagulation can be administered for 3–6 months followed by repeat evaluation. Several studies have shown that immediate heparinization followed by warfarin treatment improves survival. Patients with certain medical conditions such as coagulation disorders and atrial fibrillation may need lifelong anticoagulation.[110]

Surgical revascularization has been shown to give long-term symptom relief in up to 96 percent of patients with chronic mesenteric ischemia suitable for surgery.[111] The patency of the bypass graft, a more objective predictor of success, has been documented with rates of 78 percent at 5 years.[112] In the past decade, however, percutaneous transluminal mesenteric angioplasty with or without a stent has become a viable alternative for selected patients. Initial studies have shown angioplasty to have similar outcomes to surgical bypass and embolectomy but have included only small numbers of patients. This alternative has been used most often in patients who are at high risk for surgical revascularization.[113]

Renal artery stenosis

Renal artery stenosis (RAS) is a commonly overlooked condition that can cause uncontrolled hypertension and

---

> ### Box 15.2 Causes of renal artery stenosis
>
> - Atherosclerosis
> - Fibromuscular dysplasia
> - Nonspecific aortoarteritis (Takayasu arteritis)
> - Thrombotic or cholesterol embolization
> - Neurofibromatosis
> - Collagen vascular disease
> - Trauma
> - Posttransplant stenosis
> - Post radiation

lead to a progressive deterioration of renal function.[114] Though RAS is responsible for 2–5 percent of cases with hypertension, its importance lies in the fact that it is the most common curable form of hypertension. Several causes have been attributed to renal artery stenosis (Box 15.2) but the most common etiologies are atherosclerosis (70 percent) and fibromuscular dysplasia.[115] In 3–30 percent of patients with atherosclerotic RAS there is progressive loss of renal function over 3–5 years.[116] It is now recognized that 40–50 percent of patients with occlusive disease of lower limbs[117] and 15–30 percent of patients with coronary artery disease[118] have identifiable RAS.

CLINICAL FEATURES

The strong association of renovascular disease with generalized atherosclerosis indicates that any typical findings associated with cerebrovascular (for example, carotid bruits, old cerebrovascular accident, transient ischemic attack), cardiovascular, or peripheral vascular disease occur frequently in patients with RAS. Abdominal bruits are highly specific for RAS when heard over the flank.

The common clinical presentations of RAS include:

- renal failure
- sudden worsening of hypertension or renal function
- acute renal failure or decreased renal function after antihypertensive therapy, especially with angiotensin-converting enzyme inhibitors
- flash pulmonary edema in the presence of hypertension and normal left ventricular function.

DIAGNOSIS

A high index of clinical suspicion is paramount in the diagnosis of RAS. Patients with general hypertension have a low prevalence of renovascular hypertension. A careful review of medical history and thorough physical examination should be performed in all patients with hypertension to recognize important features suggestive of renovascular hypertension.

Several noninvasive and invasive tests are available to diagnose RAS. The commonly used noninvasive tests include Duplex ultrasound, captopril renography and MRI. Ultrasound gives an assessment of kidney size and structure while duplex adds a functional evaluation of the severity of stenosis. It is also useful for serial follow-up of patients following revascularization. Captopril renography is a highly sensitive and specific nuclear imaging test that can be used to identify critical RAS. However, the test lacks anatomic information about the renal arteries, and its accuracy is reduced in patients with impaired renal function. The sensitivity and specificity of MRI to diagnose RAS exceeds 90 percent.[119] Major disadvantages are related to costs, and false-positive artifacts related to respiration, peristalsis, and tortuous vessels. The commonly used invasive investigative technique for RAS is renal angiography. It is the gold standard investigative technique and provides information on the site and severity of stenosis, and appropriate revascularization strategies.

MANAGEMENT

The management of RAS is controversial, particularly with regard to timing and strategy of revascularization. In general, a stenosis becomes hemodynamically significant when it reaches 70 percent or more. Percutaneous transluminal angioplasty is currently the treatment of choice for fibromuscular dysplasia. Stenting is usually not necessary and recurrence rates are low, approximately 5 percent.[120] Atherosclerotic RAS usually involves the proximal renal artery, particularly around the ostium. Angioplasty in this group is associated with high rates of restenosis approaching almost 50 percent at 1 year. However stenting of atherosclerotic renal arteries has a high rate of procedural success and a low rate of restenosis. Results after stent placement have shown superior hemodynamic and angiographic outcomes when compared with balloon angioplasty alone, with a 6-month restenosis rate of 18.8 percent.[121]

Surgical revascularization is currently reserved for those patients with an occluded renal artery and a functional but ischemic kidney that is supplied via collateral blood flow or those associated with aortic aneurysm that require repair at the same time. It carries a mortality between 3 percent and 6 percent. Aggressive risk factor modification including lipid-lowering therapy forms the mainstay of medical management for RAS.

Takayasu disease

Inflammation of large arteries such as the aorta and its major branches occurs in a number of disorders, including Kawasaki syndrome, Behçet syndrome, rheumatoid arthritis, syphilis, and tuberculosis. Included in this list of arteritides are giant-cell (temporal) arteritis and Takayasu arteritis. These involve similar histologic abnormalities[122] but differ in the age of onset and the vascular structures that are targeted.[123,124] They share pathogenic pathways that distinguish them from other vasculitides. Cellular immune responses involving T cells, antigen-presenting cells, and macrophages are the main pathogenesis in giant-cell arteritis and Takayasu arteritis.

Takayasu arteritis is characterized by granulomatous inflammation of the aorta and its major branches. It results in a constellation of symptoms marked by weakening of upper extremity pulses secondary to fibrous thickening of the aortic arch with narrowing or complete obliteration of the origins of the great vessels arising from aorta. Although Takayasu arteritis is not uncommon, diagnosis is often missed or delayed resulting in clinical manifestations ranging from asymptomatic disease with impalpable pulses to catastrophic neurologic impairment.[125,126]

ETIOLOGY AND PATHOGENESIS

The disease is more common in women than men, occurring before the age of 40. Histologically, there is destruction of the elastic component of the media and fibrosis of medial smooth muscle, eventually all the layers of the arterial wall are involved.[127] There is further infiltration of lymphocytes, granulocytes and other inflammatory cells into the vessel wall suggesting an autoimmune etiology.

CLINICAL SYMPTOMS

The accepted sequence of general malaise, acute vessel wall inflammation and chronic fibrosis is not ubiquitous. Upper limb claudication is a common presentation, especially on the left due to subclavian involvement.[128] Because the lesion is often proximal to the vertebral artery origin, stoke can also be a presenting feature.[129]

INVESTIGATIONS AND MANAGEMENT

Catheter angiography is an important investigation particularly in patients who need intervention. Computed tomography and MRI can be used as screening tests during the early stages of the disease to identify vessel wall thickening. In addition to screening, CT and MRI are useful investigations to follow the response to treatment.[130] Duplex ultrasound may be useful in assessment of carotid arteries in patients with cerebral symptoms. Treatment during the early stages of the disease is directed towards controlling the inflammatory response. Steroid therapy forms the mainstay of treatment, with most patients responding favorably. However, cessation of steroid therapy in most patients results in disease recurrence. Methotrexate is shown to be effective in maintaining stable remission in patients unresponsive to steroids.[131]

Surgical intervention is recommended in patients with severe innominate and carotid stenosis, usually in the form of a bypass graft from the ascending aorta to the normal distal artery. Balloon angioplasty and stenting has been associated with high rates of restenosis in the cerebrovascular territory in comparison with patients with atherosclerotic disease.[132] Lower extremity symptoms secondary to descending aorta disease appear to respond favorably with radiological intervention.[133] Response to angioplasty in RAS has shown minimal restenosis rates compared with other territories.

Venous disease

A full discussion of the epidemiology, clinical features, and treatment of varicose veins and chronic venous insufficiency can be found elsewhere in this volume. The discussion here will be limited to vulval varicosities, phlegmasia, and interventional treatments for deep venous thrombosis.

VULVAL VARICOSITIES

Exactly how common these are is very difficult to determine. They present as clinically visually apparent varicose veins and may be a cause of dyspareunia. It is suggested that they may also be associated with pelvic pain.[134] Vulval varicosities may arise either from incompetent connections with the superficial venous system in the leg or from ovarian vein incompetence. Management is directed at diagnosing and correcting the source of incompetence. Ovarian vein reflux may be best demonstrated by venography and can be corrected by surgical resection or coil embolization. Duplex scanning will identify any incompetent connection with the superficial system of the leg and this can again be dealt with either surgically or by embolization. The vulval varicosities themselves may be treated by sclerotherapy. Using an approach which combines all these treatments, very acceptable symptomatic control can be achieved.[135]

PHLEGMASIA

An acute major proximal deep venous thrombosis usually of the iliofemoral segment will occasionally result in such a rapid increase in pressure in the leg that arterial inflow is prevented. The combination of a swollen, white leg which results is named phlegmasia alba dolens. It is an infrequent occurrence, but before more attention was paid to thromboprophylaxis it was known as the 'white leg of pregnancy'.

More commonly, a major proximal venous thrombosis results in a gradual increase in the pressure within the leg. In the great majority of cases this simply leads to the edema seen in patients with a deep venous thrombosis. Occasionally, however, the pressure increases sufficiently to impair capillary circulation. Under these circumstances, the capillaries thrombose and lose their integrity, resulting in tissue ischemia as well as edema. The foot and a variable part of the leg take on a confluent, purple discoloration – phlegmasia cerulea dolens. While this appearance superficially resembles acute arterial ischemia, it may be distinguished from the patient's history where swelling rather than pain is usually the first presenting symptom. On examination the swelling (which is generally absent in arterial ischemia) is apparent and the foot has the characteristic appearance.

Many of these patients have an underlying advanced malignancy and if this is the case then there is generally little

that can be done to improve the situation. Other patients should be treated by high elevation of the leg, anticoagulation, and observation. The alarming appearance of the foot and leg should not necessarily lead to early amputation as a remarkable degree of recovery sometimes occurs. In these patients a full search for a cause must be carried out.

Interventional treatment for phlegmasia

When a limb is threatened by phlegmasia, attempts may be made to improve venous drainage. Traditionally this was by surgical venous thrombectomy. This has very limited success due to the difficulty of mechanically removing thrombus which is often densely adherent to the vein wall. There is a high rate of re-thrombosis after such a procedure.

Better success can sometimes be achieved with venous thrombolysis, occasionally in combination with surgical thrombectomy.[136] Two approaches are used, sometimes in combination.[137] The first of these involves intraarterial delivery of the lytic agent into the affected limb.[138] This has the advantage of lysing thrombus in the peripheral microcirculation and improving tissue perfusion before progressing to lysing thrombus in the major draining veins. Paradoxically it works better in the more severely affected legs where there is little patent collateral venous drainage along which the lytic agent could leave the leg without lysing thrombus. The catheter is usually passed via the contralateral femoral artery over the aortic bifurcation and down into the affected leg. This avoids needle puncture through the edematous groin.

The second route of thrombolysis can augment the intraarterial route and involves direct, ultrasound guided cannulation of the popliteal or femoral vein. Lytic agent infused through a catheter placed in the major deep veins can then assist in the lysis of the major draining veins.[139]

Such treatment is a major intervention and should only be undertaken when the limb is threatened in a patient who may be otherwise expected to make a good recovery. Because of the risk of thromboembolization, a vena caval filter is generally placed before undertaking lysis to reduce the risk of pulmonary embolus. In all cases the prognosis has to be guarded and the risk of limb loss remains high.

KEY LEARNING POINTS

- There is generally little practical difference in everyday clinical practice between women and men in the surgical treatment of arterial disease.
- Reduction in arterial blood flow may be either acute or chronic, and its severity either total or subtotal.
- The associated clinical syndromes are: severe acute limb ischemia (no blood supply to the limb), less severe acute limb ischemia (some blood entering the limb), mild chronic ischemia (manifest only on exercise), and severe chronic limb ischemia (with rest pain or tissue loss).
- It is important clinically to distinguish claudication from other causes of leg pain.

- The outlook for the limb with claudication is benign, and consequently claudication is generally best treated with conservative measures in the majority of patients. The most important intervention is the cessation of smoking. Whether or not the exercise is supervised, it can improve both the maximum walking distance and the distance to the onset of pain.
- Ischemia is critical if there is rest pain or tissue loss caused by arterial disease. All reconstructive options are of potential value in critical ischemia. Depending on the anatomy of the arterial disease, some patients are best treated by angioplasty, others by surgery and yet more by a combination of both. Nevertheless, there are patients who are anatomically suitable for either angioplasty or surgery.
- Women treated for critical ischemia by arterial bypass are thought generally to fare worse than men.
- Four features – appearance of the skin, sensory changes, muscle power, and muscle tenderness – are used to determine the degree of severity of the ischemia, and hence the urgency of any revascularization that is needed.
- With regard to aneurysms, there is emerging evidence that growth rates are independently and significantly higher in women than in men.
- With regard to cerebrovascular disease, all patients should be given best medical management and be encouraged to stop smoking. Antiplatelet therapy is central to this approach and along with the other aspects of medical treatment can help to stabilize plaque. In asymptomatic patients, it would appear that this medical approach carries a lower risk of subsequent cerebrovascular events in women.
- Significant chronic ischemia usually only occurs when two or three of the mesenteric arteries are occluded or diseased.
- In contrast with other vascular syndromes, approximately 60 percent of patients with chronic mesenteric ischemia are female. The importance of chronic mesenteric ischemia lies in the fact that most cases of acute mesenteric ischemia occur in patients with a history of chronic abdominal complaints, presumably due to undiagnosed chronic mesenteric ischemia.

REFERENCES

1 Anderson A, Padayachee TS, Sandison AJP, et al. The results of routine primary closure in carotid endarterectomy. Cardiovasc Surg 1999; 7: 50–5.

2 Nichols WK, Stanton M, Silver D, et al. Anastomotic aneurysms following lower extremity revascularisation. Surgery 1980; 88: 366.

3 Moore WS, Malone JM. Effect of flow rate and vessel caliber on critical vessel stenosis. J Surg Res 1979; 26: 1.

4 Flanigan DP, Tullis JP, Streeter VL, et al. Multiple subcritical arterial stenoses: effect on poststenotic pressure and flow. Ann Surg 1977; 186: 663.

5 Schultz DL. Pressure and flow in large arteries. In: Bergel DH, ed. Cardiovascular Fluid Dynamics, Volume 1. New York: Academic Press, 1972: 287.

6 Keeling WB, Armstrong PA, Stone PA, et al. An overview of matrix metalloproteinases in the pathogenesis and treatment of abdominal aortic aneurysms. Vasc Endovasc Surg 2005; 39: 457–64.

7 Choke E, Cockerill G, Wilson WRW, et al. A review of biological factors implicated in abdominal aortic aneurysm rupture. Eur J Vasc Endovasc Surg 2005; 30: 227–44.

8 Walker P. Pathophysiology of acute arterial occlusion. Can J Surg 1986; 29: 340.

9 Perry M. Compartment syndromes and reperfusion injury. Surg Clin North Am 1988; 68: 853.

10 Gardner AW. Sex differences in claudication pain in subjects with peripheral arterial disease. Med Sci Sports Exerc 2002; 34: 1695–8.

11 Management of peripheral arterial disease (PAD): TransAtlantic Inter-Society Consensus (TASC). Section D: Chronic critical limb ischaemia. Eur J Vasc Endovasc Surg 2000;19 (Suppl A): S144–S243.

12 Gupta G, Aronow WS. Atherosclerotic vascular disease may be associated with osteoporosis or osteopenia in postmenopausal women: a preliminary study. Arch Geront Geriatr 2006; 17 Jan [epub ahead of print].

13 Dormandy JA, Murray GD. The fate of the claudicant – a prospective study of 1969 claudicants. Eur J Vasc Endovasc Surg 1991; 5: 131–3.

14 McDermott MM, Guralnik JM, Ferrucci L, et al. Functional decline in lower extremity peripheral arterial disease: associations with comorbidity, gender and race. J Vasc Surg 2005; 42: 1131–7.

15 Oka RK, Szuba A, Giacomini JC, Cooke JP. Gender differences in perception of PAS: a pilot study. Vasc Med 2003; 8: 89–94.

16 El Sakka K, Gambhir RPS, Halawa M, et al. Association of malignant disease with critical leg ischaemia. Br J Surg 2005; 92: 1498–501.

17 Carter SA. Response of ankle systolic pressure to leg exercise in mild or questionable arterial disease. N Engl J Med 1972; 287: 578.

18 Ligush J Jr, Reavis SW, Preisser JS, Jansen KJ. Duplex ultrasound scanning defines strategies for patients with limb-threatening ischaemia. J Vasc Surg 1998; 28: 482–91.

19 Konkus CJ, Czum JM, Jacobacci JT. Contrast enhanced MR angiography of the aorta and lower extremities with routine inclusion of the feet. Am J Roentgenol 2002; 179: 115–7.

20 Hawkins IF. Carbon dioxide digital subtraction angiography. Am J Roentgenol 1982; 139: 19–24.

21 Spinosa DJ, Angle JF, Hagspiel KD, et al. Feasibility of gadodiamide compared with dilute iodinated contrast

material for imaging the abdominal aorta and renal arteries. *J Vasc Interv Radiol* 2000; **11**: 733–7.

22 Rholl KS. Percutaneous aortoiliac intervention in vascular disease. In Baum S, Pentecost MJ, eds. *Abram's Angiography: Interventional Radiology.* Boston, MA: Little and Brown 1997: 225–61.

23 Johnston KW. Femoral and popliteal arteries: reanalysis of results of balloon angioplasty. *Radiology* 1992; **183**: 767–71.

24 Nevelsteen A, Wouters L, Suy R. Aortofemoral Dacron reconstruction for aorto-iliac occlusive disease: A 25 year survey. *Eur J Vasc Surg* 1991; **5**: 179.

25 Mills JL. Management of chronic ischaemia of the lower extremities. In Rutherford RB, ed. *Vascular Surgery.* Philadelphia, PA: Elsevier Saunders, 2005: 1154–74.

26 Stonebridge PA, Prescott RJ, Ruckley CV. Randomised trial comparing infrainguinal polytetrafluoroethylene bypass grafting with and without vein interposition cuff at the distal anastomosis. *J Vasc Surg* 1997; **26**: 543–50.

27 Spark JI, Robinson JM, Gallavin L, *et al.* Patients with chronic critical limb ischaemia have reduced total antioxidant capacity and impaired nutritional status. *Eur J Vasc Endovasc Surg* 2002; **24**: 535–9.

28 BASIL Trial Participants. Bypass versus angioplasty in severe ischaemia of the leg (BASIL): multicentre, randomised controlled trial. *Lancet* 2005; **366**: 1925–34.

29 Magnant JG, Cronenwett JL, Walsh DB, *et al.* Surgical treatment of infrainguinal arterial occlusive disease in women. *J Vasc Surg* 1993; **17**: 67–78.

30 Abbott WM, Maloney RD, McCabe CC. Arterial embolism: a 44 year perspective. *Am J Surg* 1982; **143**: 460–4.

31 Fecteau SR, Darling RC III, Roddy SP. Arterial thromboembolism. In: Rutherford RB, ed. *Vascular Surgery.* Philadelphia, PA: Elsevier Saunders, 2005: 974.

★ 32 Rutherford RB, Baker JD, Ernst C, *et al.* Recommended standards for reports dealing with lower extremity ischaemia: revised version. *J Vasc Surg* 1997; **26**: 517–38.

33 Ouriel K, Shortell CK, De Weese JA, *et al.* A comparison of thrombolytic therapy with operative revascularisation in the initial treatment of acute peripheral arterial ischaemia. *J Vasc Surg* 1994; **19**: 1021–30.

34 Anonymous. Results of a prospective randomised trial evaluating surgery versus thrombolysis for ischaemia of the lower extremity. The STILE trial. *Ann Surg* 1994; **220**: 251–66.

35 Dormandy JA, Rutherford RB. Management of peripheral arterial disease (PAD). TASC Working Group. TransAtlantic Inter-Society Consensus (TASC). *J Vasc Surg* 2000; **31**: S1–S296.

36 Olin JW, Childs MB, Bartholemew JR, *et al.* Anticardiolipin antibodies and homocysteine levels in patients with thromboangiitis obliterans. *Arthritis Rheum* 1996; **39**: S47.

★ 37 Johnston KW, Rutherford RB, Tilson MD, *et al.* Suggested standards for reporting on arterial aneurysms.

Subcommittee on reporting Standards for Arterial Aneurysms, Ad Hoc Committee on Reporting Standards, Society for Vascular Surgery and North American Chapter, International Society for Cardiovascular Surgery. *J Vasc Surg* 1991; **13**: 452.

38 Gaylis H. Popliteal arterial aneurysms: a review and analysis of fifty five cases. *S Afr Med J* 1974; **48**: 75.

39 Brunkwall J, Hauksson H, Bengtsson H, *et al.* Solitary aneurysms of the iliac arterial system: an estimate of their frequency of occurrence. *J Vasc Surg* 1989; **10**: 381.

40 Bickerstaff LK, Hollier L, Van Peenen HJ, *et al.* Abdominal aortic aneurysms: the changing natural history. *J Vasc Surg* 1984; **1**: 6.

41 Johansen K, Koepsell T. Familial tendency for abdominal aortic aneurysms. *JAMA* 1986; **256**: 1934.

42 Powell JT, Greenhalgh RM. Multifactorial inheritance of abdominal aortic aneurysm. *Eur J Vasc Surg* 1987; **1**: 29.

43 Scott RA, Ashton HA, Kay DN. Abdominal aortic aneurysm in 4237 screened patients: prevalence, development and management over 6 years. *Br J Surg* 1991; **78**: 1122–5.

44 Simoni G, Pastorino C, Perrone R, *et al.* Screening for abdominal aortic aneurysm and associated risk factors in a general population. *Eur J Vasc Endovasc Surg* 1995; **10**: 207–10.

45 Solberg S, Singh K, Wilsgaard, Jacobsen BK. Increased growth rate of abdominal aortic aneurysms in women. The Tromso study. *Eur J Vasc Endovasc Surg* 2005; **29**: 145–9.

46 UK Small Aneurysm Trial Participants. Mortality results for randomized controlled trial of early elective surgery or ultrasonographic surveillance for small abdominal aortic aneurysms. *Lancet* 1998; **352**: 1649.

47 Brown PM, Zelt DT, Sobolev B. The risk of rupture in untreated aneurysms: the impact of size gender and expansion rate. *J Vasc Surg* 2003; **37**: 280–4.

48 Lederle FA. Risk of rupture of large abdominal aortic aneurysms: disagreement among vascular surgeons. *Arch Intern Med* 1996; **156**: 1007.

49 Ashton HA, Buxton MJ, Day NE, *et al.* The Multicentre Aneurysm Screening Study (MASS) into the effect of abdominal aortic aneurysm screening on mortality rate in men. A randomised controlled trial. *Lancet* 2002; **360**: 1531.

50 Baxter BT, McGee GS, Flinn WR, *et al.* Distal embolisation as a presenting symptom of aortic aneurysms. *Am J Surg* 1990; **160**: 197.

51 Gilling-Smith GL, Mansfield AO. Spontaneous abdominal arteriovenous fistulae: report of eight cases and review of the literature. *Br J Surg* 1991; **78**: 421.

52 Wheeler WE, Hanks J, Raman VK. Primary aortoenteric fistulas. *Am Surg* 1992; **58**: 53.

53 EVAR Trial participants. Endovascular aneurysm repair versus open repair in patients with abdominal aortic aneurysm (EVAR trial 1): randomised controlled trial. *Lancet* 2005; **365**: 2179–86.

54 StenbaekJ, Granath F, Swedenborg J. Outcome after abdominal aortic aneurysm repair. Difference between

women and men. *Eur J Vasc Endovasc Surg* 2004; **28**: 47–51.

55 Dimick JB, Stanley JC, Axelrod DA, *et al.* Variation in death rate after abdominal aortic aneurysmectomy in the United States. *Ann Surg* 2002; **235**: 579–85.

56 Mathison M, Becker GJ, Katzen BT. The influence of female gender on the outcome of endovascular abdominal aortic aneurysm repair. *J Vasc Intervent Radiol* 2001; **12**: 1047–51.

57 Biebl M, Hakaim AG, Hugl B, *et al.* Endovascular aortic aneurysm repair with the Zenith AAA endovascular graft: does gender affect procedural success, postoperative morbidity or early survival? *Am Surg* 2005; **71**: 1001–8.

58 EVAR Trial participants. Endovascular aneurysm repair and outcome in patients unfit for open repair of abdominal aortic aneurysm (EVAR trial 2): randomised controlled trial. *Lancet* 2005; **365**: 2187–92.

59 Arya N, Lee B, Loan W, *et al.* Change in aneurysm diameter after stent-graft repair of ruptured abdominal aortic aneurysms. *J Endovasc Ther* 2004; **11**: 319–22.

60 Dillavou ED, Muluk SC, Makaroun MS. A decade of change in abdominal aortic aneurysm repair in the United States: have we improved outcomes equally between men and women? *J Vasc Surg* 2006; **43**: 230–8.

61 Semmens JB, Norman PE, Lawrence-Brown MMD, *et al.* Influence of gender on outcome from ruptured abdominal aortic aneurysm. *Br J Surg* 2000; **87**: 191–4.

62 Mitchell ME, Carpenter JP. *Popliteal Artery Aneurysm. Current Therapy in Vascular Surgery*, 4th ed. St. Louis, MO: Mosby, Inc. 2001: 341–5.

63 Diwan A, Sarkar A, Stanley JC. Incidence of femoral and popliteal artery aneurysms in patients with abdominal aortic aneurysms. *J Vasc Surg* 2000; **31**: 863–9.

64 Ebaugh JL, Matsumura JS, Morasch MD. Morphometric analysis of the popliteal artery for endovascular treatment. *Vasc Endovasc Surg* 2003; **37**: 23–6.

65 Lilly MP, Flinn WR, McCarthy WJ III, *et al.* The effect of distal arterial anatomy on the success of popliteal aneurysm repair. *J Vasc Surg* 1988; **7**: 653–60.

66 Thompson JF, Beard J Scott DJ, Earnshaw JJ. Intraoperative thrombolysis in the management of thrombosed popliteal aneurysm. *Br J Surg* 1993; **80**: 858–9.

67 Michaels JA, Galland RB. Management of asymptomatic popliteal aneurysms: the use of a Markov decision tree to determine the criteria for a conservative approach. *Eur J Vasc Surg* 1993; **7**: 136–43.

68 Stanley JC. Abdominal visceral aneurysms. In Haimovici H, ed. *Vascular Emergencies*. New York: Appleton-Century-Crofts, 1981: 387.

69 Carr SC, Mahvi DM, Hoch JR. Visceral artery aneurysm rupture. *J Vasc Surg* 2001; **33**: 806.

70 Stanley JC, Fry WJ. Pathogenesis and clinical significance of splenic artery aneurysms. *Surgery* 1974; **76**: 898.

71 Shanley CJ, Shah NL, Messina LM. Common splanchnic artery aneurysms: Splenic, hepatic, and celiac. *Ann Vasc Surg* 1996; **10**: 315.

72 Trastek VF, Pairolero PC, Joyce JW. Splenic artery aneurysms. *Surgery* 1982; **91**: 694.

73 McDermott VG, Shlansky-Goldberg R, Cope C. Endovascular management of splenic artery aneurysms and pseudoaneurysms. *Cardiovasc Intervent Radiol* 1994; **17**: 179.

74 Iemolo F, Martiniuk A, Steinman DA, *et al.* Sex differences in carotid plaque and stenosis. *Stroke* 2004; **35**: 477–81.

75 Iglseder B, Cip P, Malaimare L, *et al.* The metabolic syndrome is a stronger risk factor for early carotid atherosclerosis in women than in men. *Stroke* 2005; **36**: 1212–17.

76 Blaser T, Hofmann K, Buerger T, *et al.* Risk of stroke, transient ischaemic attack and vessel occlusion before endarterectomy in patients with symptomatic severe carotid stenosis. *Stroke* 2002; **33**: 1057–62.

77 Bettermann K, Toole JF. Diagnostic evaluation and medical management of patients with ischaemic cerebrovascular disease. In Rutherford RB, ed. *Vascular Surgery*. Philadelphia, PA: Elsevier Saunders, 2005: 1897–916.

78 Dick P, Sherif C, Sabeti S, *et al.* Gender differences in outcome of conservatively treated patients with asymptomatic high grade stenosis. *Stroke* 2005; **36**: 1178–83.

79 European Carotid Surgery Trialists' Collaborative Group (ECST): MRC European Carotid Surgery Trial. Interim results for symptomatic patients with severe (70–99%) or with mild (0–29%) carotid stenosis. *Lancet* 1991; **337**: 1235–43.

80 NASCET Collaborators. Beneficial effect of carotid endarterectomy in symptomatic patients with high grade carotid stenosis. *N Engl J Med* 1991; **325**: 445.

81 Rothwell PM, Villagra R, Gibson R, *et al.* Evidence of a chronic systemic cause of instability of atherosclerotic plaques. *Lancet* 2000; **355**: 19–24.

82 Garcia BA, Ruiz C, Chacon P, *et al.* High sensitivity C-reactive protein in high-grade carotid stenosis: risk marker for unstable carotid plaque. *J Vasc Surg* 2003; **38**: 1018–24.

83 Mofidi R, Crotty TB, McCarthy P, *et al.* Association between plaque instability, angiogenesis and symptomatic carotid occlusive disease. *Br J Surg* 2001; **88**: 945–50.

84 Verhoeven B, Hellings WE, Moll FL, *et al.* Carotid atherosclerotic plaques in patients with transient ischaemic attacks and stroke have unstable characteristics compared with plaques in asymptomatic and amaurosis fugax patients. *J Vasc Surg* 2005; **42**: 1077–81.

85 Altaf N, Daniels L, Morgan PS, *et al.* Cerebral white matter hyperintense lesions are associated with unstable carotid plaques. *Eur J Vasc Endovasc Surg* 2006; **31**: 8–13.

86 Henon H, Vroylandt P, Durieu I, *et al.* Leukoaraiosis more than dementia is a predictor of stroke recurrence. *Stroke* 2003; **34**: 2935–40.

87 Comerota AJ, Salles-Cunha SZ, Daoud Y, *et al.* Gender differences in blood velocities across carotid stenoses. *J Vasc Surg* 2004; **40**: 939–44.

88 Halliday A, Mansfield A, Marro J, *et al.* Prevention of disabling and fatal strokes by successful carotid endarterectomy in patients without recent neurological symptoms: randomised controlled trial. *Lancet* 2004; **363**: 1491–502.

89 Naylor AR. The Asymptomatic Carotid Surgery Trial: bigger study, better evidence. *Br J Surg* 2004; **91**: 787–9.

90 Rerkasem K, Bond R, Rothwell PM. Local versus general anaesthesia for carotid endarterectomy. *Cochrane Database Syst Rev* 2004; (2): CD000126.

91 Harthun NL, Cheanvechai V, Graham LM, *et al.* Outcome of carotid endarterectomy on the basis of patient sex: is there a difference? *J Thorac Cardiovasc Surg* 2004; **127**: 322–4.

92 Executive Committee for the Asymptomatic Carotid Atherosclerosis Study. Endarterectomy for asymptomatic carotid artery stenosis. *JAMA* 1995; **273**: 1421–8.

93 Alamowitch S, Eliasziw M, Barnett HJM, *et al.* The risk and benefit of endarterectomy in women with symptomatic internal carotid artery disease. *Stroke* 2005; **36**: 27–31.

94 Mattos MA, Summer DS, Bohannon WT, *et al.* Carotid endarterectomy in women: challenging the results from ACAS and NASCET. *Ann Surg* 2001; **234**: 438–46.

95 Rockman CB, Castillo J, Adelman MA, *et al.* Carotid endarterectomy in female patients: are the concerns of the asymptomatic carotid atherosclerosis study valid? *J Vasc Surg* 2001; **33**: 236–41.

96 Johnson CA, Tollefson DFJ, Olsen SB, *et al.* The natural history of early recurrent carotid stenosis. *Am J Surg* 1999; **177**: 433–6.

97 Ladowski JS, Sinabery LM, Peterson D, *et al.* Factors contributing to recurrent carotid disease following carotid endarterectomy. *Am J Surg* 1997; **174**: 118–20.

98 Heys SD, Brittenden J, Crofts TJ. Acute mesenteric ischaemia: The continuing difficulty in early diagnosis. *Postgrad Med J* 1993; **69**: 48–51.

99 Stoney RJ, Cunningham CG. Acute mesenteric ischaemia. *Surgery* 1993; **114**: 489–90.

100 Kaleya RN, Sammartano RJ, Boley SJ. Aggressive approach to acute mesenteric ischaemia. *Surg Clin North Am* 1002; **72**: 157–82.

101 Rhee RY, Mendonca CT. Mesenteric venous thrombosis: Still a lethal disease in the 1990's. *J Vasc Surg* 1994; **20**: 688–97.

102 Edwards MS, Cherr GS, Craven TE, Olsen AW, Plonk GW, Geary RL, *et al.* Acute occlusive mesenteric ischemia: surgical management and outcomes. *Ann Vasc Surg* 2003; **17**: 72–9.

103 Greenwald DA, Brandt LJ, Reinus JF. Ischemic bowel disease in the elderly. *Gastroenterol Clin North Am* 2001; **30**: 445–73.

104 Moawad J, Gewertz BL. Chronic mesenteric ischemia: clinical presentation and diagnosis. *Surg Clin North Am* 1997; **77**: 357–70.

105 Guttormson NL, Bubrick MP. Mortality from ischemic colitis. *Dis Colon Rectum* 1989; **32**: 469–72.

106 Laissy JP, Trillaud H, Douek P. MR angiography: noninvasive vascular imaging of the abdomen. *Abdom Imaging* 2002; **27**: 488–506.

107 Endean ED, Barnes SL, Kwolek CJ, *et al.* Surgical management of thrombotic acute intestinal ischemia. *Ann Surg* 2001; **233**: 801–8.

108 Simo G, Echenagusia AJ, Camunez F, *et al.* Superior mesenteric arterial embolism: local fibrinolytic treatment with urokinase. *Radiology* 1997; **20**: 775–9.

109 Rivitz SM, Geller SC, Hahn C. Treatment of acute mesenteric venous thrombosis with transjugular intramesenteric urokinase infusion. *J Vasc Intervent Radiol* 1995; **6**: 219–28.

110 Rhee RY, Gloviczki P. Mesenteric venous thrombosis. *Surg Clin North Am* 1997; **77**: 327–28.

111 Kihara TK, Blebea J, Anderson KM, *et al.* Risk factors and outcomes following revascularization for chronic mesenteric ischemia. *Ann Vasc Surg* 1999; **13**: 37–44.

112 Moaward J, McKinsey JF, Wyble CW, *et al.* Mesenteric arterial bypass grafts: early and late results and suggested surgical approach for chronic and acute mesenteric ischemia. *Arch Surg* 1997; **132**: 613–19.

113 Brown OJ, Schermerhorn ML, Powell RJ, *et al.* Mesenteric stenting for chronic mesentric ischaemia. *J Vasc Surg* 2005; **42**: 268–74.

114 Jacobson HR. Ischaemic renal disease: an overlooked entity? *Kidney Int* 1988; **34**: 729–43.

115 Renal artery stenosis: A cardiovascular perspective. *Am Heart J* 2002; **143**: 559–64.

116 Caps MT, Polissar NL. Risk of atrophy in kidneys with atherosclerotic renal artery stenosis. *Kidney Int* 1998; **53**: 735–42.

117 Choudri AH, Cleland JGF. Unsuspected renal artery stenosis in peripheral vascular disease. *BMJ* 1990; **301**: 1197–98.

118 Uzu T, Fujii T. Prevalence and predictors of renal artery stenosis in patients with myocardial infarction. *Am J Kidney Dis* 2000; **29**: 733–38.

119 Davidson RA, Wilcox CS. Predictors of cure of hypertension in fibromuscular renovascular disease. *Am J Kidney Dis* 1996; **28**: 334–8.

120 Hayes J, Risius B, Novick AC. Experience with percutaneous transluminal angioplasty for renal artery stenosis at the Cleveland clinic. *Clin J Urol* 1988; **139**: 488–92.

121 White CJ, Collins TJ. Renal artery stent placement: utility in lesions difficult to treat with balloon angioplasty. *J Am Coll Cardiol* 1997; **30**: 1445–50.

122 Bjornsson J. Histopathology of primary vasculitic disorders. In: Hoffman GS, Weyand CM, eds. *Inflammatory Diseases of Blood Vessels.* New York: Marcel Dekker, 2002: 255–65.

123 Johnston SL, Lock RJ, Gompels MM. Takayasu arteritis: a review. *J Clin Pathol* 2002; **55**: 481–6.

124 Salvarani C, Cantini F, Boiardi L, Hunder GG. Polymyalgia
rheumatica and giant-cell arteritis. *N Engl J Med* 2002;
347: 261–71.

125 Numano F, Okawara M, Inomata H, Kobayashi Y.
Takayasu's arteritis. *Lancet* 2000; **356**: 1023–5.

126 Kerr GS. Takayasu's arteritis. *Rheum Dis Clin North Am*
1995, 21:1041–58.

127 Sekiguchi M, Suzuki JI. An overview of Takayasu's
arteritis. *Heart Vessels Suppl* 1992; **7**: 6–10.

128 Angeli E, Angelo V, Massimo V. The role of radiology in
the diagnosis and management of Takayasu's arteritis.
J Nephrol 2001; **14**: 514–24.

129 Giordano JM. Surgical treatment of Takayasu's arteritis.
Int J Cardiol 2000; **75**: S123–S128.

130 Tanigawa K, Eguchi K, Kitamura Y. Magnetic resonance
imaging detection of aortic and pulmonary artery with CT
angiography. *Radiology* 1995; **196**: 89–93.

131 Sabbadini MG, Bozollo E, Baldissera E. Takayasu's arteritis.
Therapeutic strategies. *J Nephrol* 2001; **14**: 525–31.

132 Tyagi S, Verma PK, Gambhir DS, *et al*. Early and long term
results of subclavian angioplasty in aortoarteritis
(Takayasu's disease). Comparison with atherosclerosis.
Cardiovasc Intervent Radiol 1998; **21**: 219–24.

133 Sharma BK, Jain S, Bali HK. A follow-up study of balloon
angioplasty and de-novo stenting in Takayasu's arteritis.
Int J Cardiol 2000; **75**: S147–S152.

134 Hobbs JT. Varicose veins arising from the pelvis due to
ovarian vein incompetence. Int J Clin Pract 2005; **59**:
1195–203.

135 Scultetus AH, Villavicencio JL, Gillespie DL, *et al*. The
pelvic syndromes: analysis of our experience with 57
patients. *J Vasc Surg* 2002; **36**: 881–8.

136 Dayal R, Bernheim J, Clair DG, *et al*. Multimodal
percutaneous intervention for critical venous occlusive
disease. *Ann Vasc Surg* 2005; **19**: 235–40.

137 Chaer RA, Dayal R, Lin SC, *et al*. Multimodal therapy for
acute and chronic venous thrombotic and occlusive
disease. *Vasc Endovascular Surg* 2005; **39**: 375–80.

138 Wlodarczyk ZK, Gibson M, Dick R, Hamilton G. Low-dose
intra-arterial thrombolysis in the treatment of
phlegmasia caerulea dolens. *Br J Surg* 1994; **81**:
370–2.

139 Tardy B, Moulin N, Mismetti P, *et al*. Intravenous
thrombolytic therapy in patients with phlegmasia
caerulea dolens. *Haematologica* 2006; **91**: 281–2.

FURTHER READING

Rutherford RB, ed. Vascular Surgery. Philadelphia, PA: Elsevier
Saunders, 2005.

16

Cerebrovascular disease

PETER LANGHORNE, MORVEN M TAYLOR

INTRODUCTION

Cerebrovascular disease is the third leading cause of death in adult women in the United Kingdom and much of the developed world, exceeded only by ischemic heart disease and all causes of cancer.[1] Cerebrovascular disease is also the most important cause of serious disability in the adult population. This burden of disability in turn raises health service costs as well as causing impaired quality of life and substantial personal costs to patients and their carers.

Stroke is the main component of cerebrovascular disease with an annual incidence in women of between 47 and 198 per 100 000 in European populations.[2] The lifetime of risk of a woman having a stroke is 1 in 6.[3] Across all populations the incidence rates of stroke rise sharply with increasing age[4,5] (Fig. 16.1) and stroke severity is on average worse in women[6] possibly because of their higher average age at presentation. However, many stroke risk factors are potentially preventable and it is important to understand the causes of cerebrovascular disease and be aware of the appropriate risk factor management.

This chapter describes the causes of cerebrovascular disease in women. It then discusses the risk factors for the various types of cerebrovascular disease and the potential for modification of these risk factors. We recognize that many of the most important risk factors apply equally to both

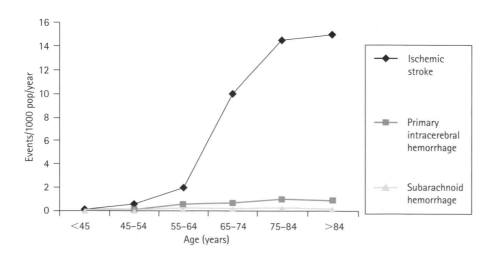

Figure 16.1 Incidence of the main causes of cerebrovascular events according to age.[5]

men and women and so we describe these first before covering sex-specific risk factors.

CAUSES OF CEREBROVASCULAR DISEASE

Although the full range of cerebrovascular diseases is mentioned here, we will focus on the most common manifestation, stroke. The most widely accepted definition of a stroke is that used by the World Health Organization:[6]

> A clinical syndrome characterised by rapidly developing clinical symptoms and/or signs of focal, and at times global (applied to patients in deep coma and those with subarachnoid hemorrhage), loss of cerebral function, the symptoms lasting more than 24 hours or leading to death, with no apparent cause other than of a vascular origin.

The range of cerebrovascular diseases can be divided into several categories, depending on etiology (Fig. 16.2).

Ischemic stroke and transient ischemic attacks

Ischemic stroke and transient ischemic attacks (TIAs) represent the most common type of cerebrovascular disease in women. The subdivision of ischemic stroke and TIA is arbitrarily made on the basis of the duration of symptoms. Transient ischemic attack has the same definition as stroke but the symptoms resolve within 24 hours; most TIAs last for a few hours only. These definitions are based on clinical symptoms; brain imaging demonstrates that as many as 20 percent of TIA patients will have a small infarct, especially if the symptoms persist for greater than half an hour.[7]

Atheromatous disease in large- and medium-sized arteries is believed to be the most common cause of ischemic stroke and TIA, accounting for about 50 percent of all events.[8,9] The clinical consequences of atheromatous lesions appear to be caused by the resultant thrombotic and embolic complications rather than the atheromatous lesions themselves. Atheromatous plaques can lead to direct obstruction

in the lumen of the artery through intramural thrombus. These thrombotic plaques can also embolize and obstruct narrower more distal arteries or be lysed and disperse into the microcirculation.[10]

Atheromatous lesions are especially prevalent at areas of arterial bending, convergence, and branching. Thus, atheroma is more likely to be found in the aortic arch, the basilar arteries, and the carotid bifurcations (Fig. 16.3).[10–15] People with atheroma involving one arterial territory are likely to have atheroma elsewhere.[16–20] Thus people with ischemic stroke or TIA commonly have or will acquire cardiovascular disease or peripheral vascular disease.

The remaining causes of ischemic cerebrovascular disease include small vessel disease and cardiac embolism (Fig. 16.4). Intracranial small-vessel disease affects the smaller arteries of the brain and is responsible for approximately 25 percent of ischemic strokes and TIAs. Small-vessel disease is more likely to lead to lacunar stroke events, which occur in the subcortical areas of the brain (involving the deep perforating arteries) and lead to subcortical symptoms such as motor or sensory loss or ataxia. There are probably several contributing factors to small-vessel disease including arteriosclerosis (the most common cause), atheroma, amyloid, vasculitis, and rarer inherited conditions such CADASIL (*C*erebral *A*utosominal *D*ominant, *A*rteriopathy with *S*ubcortical *I*nfarcts and *L*eukoencephalopathy).

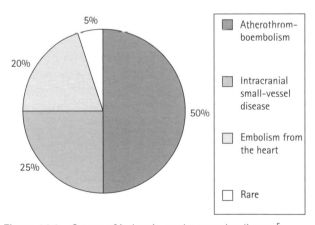

Figure 16.3 Causes of ischemic cerebrovascular disease.[5]

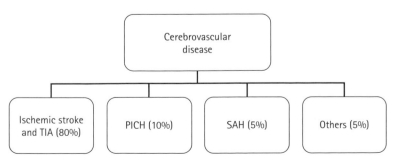

Figure 16.2 Causes of cerebrovascular disease. PICH, primary intracerebral hemorrhage; SAH, subarachnoid hemorrhage; TIA, transient ischemic attack.[5]

Embolism from the heart is believed to account for about 20 percent of ischemic strokes and TIAs. The most common sources of embolism are from left atrial thrombus in patients with atrial fibrillation, mural thrombus post myocardial infarction, mitral stenosis, prosthetic heart valves, bacterial endocarditis, atrial myxoma and during any invasive cardiac procedure such as angiography. Other causes of ischemic cerebrovascular events are rare. These include arterial trauma, arterial dissection, connective tissue diseases, and vasculopathies. An increasingly recognized risk factor in younger individuals is paradoxical embolism where a venous thrombus embolizes to the arterial circulation via a right to left cardiac shunt (for example, atrial septal defect, ventricular septal defect, patent foramen ovale). Factors which increase the risk of venous thrombosis are likely to be important in these individuals.

Primary intracerebral hemorrhage

Although there may be multiple contributing factors for primary intracerebral hemorrhages, the main risk factor is chronic hypertension. The final event is usually the rupture of small deep perforating arteries, secondary to degeneration of the vessel wall or microaneurysms.[22] These more frequent causes of primary intracerebral hemorrhage are commonly found in the basal ganglia, thalamus, brain stem, or cerebellum. In younger patients, abnormalities of the vascular system such as arteriovenous malformations and cavernomas are the most common causes of primary intracerebral hemorrhage.[23] In older age groups recurrent hemorrhage is more commonly observed in the cerebral white matter, often because of arterial degeneration (amyloid angiopathy).[24]

Subarachnoid hemorrhage

Subarachnoid hemorrhage accounts for about 5 percent of strokes and has high early mortality.[25] Most spontaneous subarachnoid hemorrhages (85 percent) occur as a result of rupture of a saccular aneurysm which is found at sites of arterial branching, either in the circle of Willis or nearby.[26,27] The remaining subarachnoid hemorrhages are nonaneurysmal and usually result from perimesencephalic hemorrhage.[28] Rare causes include arterial dissection and arteriovenous malformation of the cerebrum and spinal circulation. Arterial dissection as a cause of subarachnoid hemorrhage is found more frequently in the vertebral arteries than elsewhere and is usually as a result from extracranial injury to the vessel wall.[29,30]

Other causes of cerebrovascular disease

INTRACRANIAL VENOUS THROMBOSIS

Intracranial venous thrombosis is a rare condition caused by thrombosis of the intracranial venous system (venous sinuses, etc.). The superior sagittal sinus is affected in the majority (70–80 percent) of cases. Risk factors which predispose to deep venous thrombosis of the legs and pulmonary embolism, probably also contribute to intracranial venous thrombosis. The risk is increased with oral contraceptives, in pregnancy and the puerperium and with certain thrombophilias (for example, protein S and protein C deficiency, antithrombin III deficiency, and factor V Leiden mutations, etc.).[31,35,36]

SUBDURAL HEMATOMA

Subdural hematomas are usually associated with trauma resulting in hematoma formation in the subdural space. Risk factors include anticoagulant therapy and alcohol excess.[32] Subdural hematomas may mimic subarachnoid hemorrhage clinically but usually present with fluctuating or progressive neurological symptoms and signs.

RISK FACTORS FOR CEREBROVASCULAR DISEASE

Generic risk factors (relevant to both women and men)

Ischemic stroke is the most common type of stroke in most developed countries. We shall focus mainly on it. There are several known risk factors for ischemic stroke, most of which are relevant to both women and men.

AGE

Increasing age is the most powerful risk factor for ischemic stroke and TIA. This applies equally to both men and women and is probably associated with the fact that blood pressure levels tend to rise with age. One recent study has shown that women tend to present approximately 6 years later than men do with their first stroke.[5] This trend is borne out in other studies.[33,34]

BLOOD PRESSURE

Rising blood pressure increases the risk of not only an ischemic stroke but also primary intracerebral hemorrhage and subarachnoid hemorrhage. This is the main modifiable risk factor for the population as a whole as it carries both a high relative risk and is widely prevalent. The risk of a cerebrovascular event approximately doubles with every 7.5 mm Hg rise in diastolic blood pressure;[35,36] the pattern is similar with systolic blood pressure. The mechanism is believed to be the effect of hypertension on the extent and severity of atheromatous plaques (Fig. 16.5).

SMOKING

Cigarette smoking approximately doubles the risk of ischemic stroke in both men and women[37] and doubles or

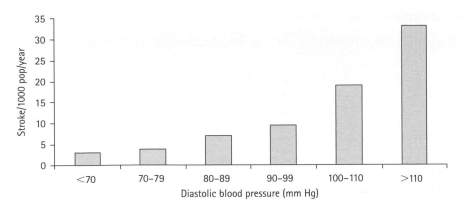

Figure 16.4 Diastolic blood pressure and incidence of stroke.[8]

trebles the risk of subarachnoid hemorrhage. There is a steady fall in risk on cessation.[38] Women who are current smokers are also at an increased risk of hemorrhagic stroke (intracranial and subarachnoid hemorrhages). The risk increases with the numbers of cigarettes smoked, for example smoking more than 15 cigarettes a day will double the risk of intracranial hemorrhage and result in a fourfold increase in the risk of subarachnoid hemorrhage.[39,40] Cigarette smokers also tend to have larger and often multiple saccular aneurysms. The association with increased risk of cerebrovascular disease and cigarette smoking is less apparent in older people than at younger ages.

DIABETES MELLITUS

People who are diabetic have approximately twice the risk of ischemic stroke.[41–43] In addition, those who are diabetic are more likely to die from their stroke event compared with the nondiabetic population.[44] The same pattern is seen in both men and women. One recent study has shown that women who have type 2 diabetes without overt cardiovascular risk factors have an increased risk of fatal stroke (similar to that of nondiabetic people who have a history of prior stroke).[45]

HYPERCHOLESTEROLEMIA

The association of cholesterol with ischemic stroke and TIA is less distinct than with cardiovascular disease. However a modest positive relationship is seen in both men and women and a reduction in cholesterol is associated with a reduction in ischemic stroke risk. This will be discussed later on in the chapter. One recent study has shown that to have a high total cholesterol to high-density lipoprotein (HDL) ratio also results in an increased risk in ischemic cerebrovascular events.[46]

ATRIAL FIBRILLATION

Atrial fibrillation is a common arrhythmia occurring in approximately 5–10 percent of people over 65 years of age and is the most common cause of stroke or TIA due to embolism from the heart to the brain. The absolute risk of first stroke in people with atrial fibrillation who are not anticoagulated is about 4 percent per year (four to six times greater than those in sinus rhythm) and increases in the presence of hypertension, cardiac failure, and a previous history of stroke.[47–49] In one study, the severity of stroke was worse in those with atrial fibrillation.[50]

RAISED PLASMA FIBRINOGEN

There is a positive relation between raised plasma fibrinogen and ischemic stroke. However, cigarette smoking is a confounding factor in that it increases plasma fibrinogen levels. Increasing age, high blood pressure, diabetes mellitus, and hypercholesterolemia are also associated with increased plasma fibrinogen levels.[51]

Sex-specific risk factors

SEX

Women appear to have a lower worldwide incidence of age-specific stroke than men, although this sex difference is less for ischemic stroke compared with other types of vascular disease. This pattern is not seen at the extremes of age (less than 45 years old and over 85 years old).[52] However as more women live to old age, a greater number of them will have a stroke. In contrast with ischemic stroke, subarachnoid hemorrhage is more common in women in whom there appears to be an association with increased risk of intracranial aneurysm formation and growth.[53–55]

MIGRAINE

Migraine has been reported to be a risk factor for ischemic stroke but not hemorrhagic stroke in young women. Such associations have not been reported in men and the mechanism for this is unclear. Cause and effect relations could be complex as migraine may also be caused by an arteriovenous malformation, which may independently precipitate migrainous attacks and lead to a hemorrhagic stroke.[56,57]

FEMALE SEX HORMONES

The association of female sex hormones with stroke is complex. Physiologic levels of estrogens appear to be protective

Table 16.1 Relative risk with oral contraceptive use for ischaemic stroke[67]

	Dose of estrogen	No. of studies	Relative risk of ischemic stroke (95% CI)
Low dose	<50 µg	7	2.08 (1.55 to 2.80)
Medium dose	50 µg	5	2.78 (2.00 to 3.85)
High dose	>50 µg	4	4.53 (2.17 to 9.50)
Total	All	16	2.75 (2.24 to 3.38)

in premenopausal women in whom bilateral oophorectomy without estrogen replacement roughly doubles the risk of vascular events.[58,59] However, exogenous estrogens may increase risks.

Oral contraceptives

The possibility that cerebrovascular events might be caused by oral contraceptive therapy was first raised by Lorentz in 1962.[60] Although the absolute risk of stroke is very low in young women, oral contraceptives are prescribed to millions of women per year[61] and any increased risk could have major cost implications. One recent metaanalysis showed that current oral contraceptive use with estrogen-containing preparations was associated with a tripling of the risk of ischemic stroke. However, there was a lesser risk with the lower estrogen-containing therapies in comparison with those containing over 50 µg of estrogen; the relative risk was 2.3 when taking tablets that contained less that 50 µg of estrogen compared with 4.5 with estrogen doses over 50 µg (Table 16.1). There is probably also an interaction with other risk factors such as hypertension, smoking and migraine.[62,63]

Hormone replacement therapy

Estrogens appear to be protective against stroke before the menopause (with benefits seen through both vascular and neuroprotective effects). However, after the menopause exogenous estrogens appear to increase stroke risks. In a trial of Premarin (0.625 mg of conjugated equine estrogen and 2.5 mg of medroxyprogesterone acetate) hormone replacement therapy did not reduce the risk of stroke in high-risk women with previous myocardial infarction.[68] In fact there was an increased risk of stroke and transient ischemic attack, with a relative risk of 1.13 (95% confidence interval [CI] 0.85 to 1.48). Similar results were seen in a trial of hormone replacement therapy given following a stroke or transient ischemic attack. The relative hazard of having a further stroke if taking hormone replacement therapy was 1.05 (0.79 to 1.40).

The role of hormone replacement therapy for primary prevention in women at relatively low risk of vascular disease was studied in the Women's Health Initiative Trial. The use of single-agent hormone replacement therapy (Premarin) was associated with an increased risk of both stroke (8 extra events per 10 000 person years) and coronary heart disease (7 extra events per 10 000 person years). This excess risk was not associated with age, ethnicity, or hypertension. It concluded that the combination hormone replacement therapy increases the risk of stroke events in apparently healthy women.[65] However, it is notable that a single combination preparation was used in this study.

The hormone replacement therapy studies outlined above suggested an initial excess risk of stroke events with possible later benefit. The cause of this apparent effect is unclear. Options for future research could include selective estrogen receptor modulators or the combination of hormone replacement therapy with vascular protection such as antiplatelet agents.[66]

Stroke and tamoxifen

Tamoxifen is known to increase the risk of venous thromboembolism in women with breast cancer. A recent meta-analysis of cerebrovascular outcomes in trials in women with breast cancer randomized to tamoxifen or placebo has shown a 40 percent increased risk of stroke in those on tamoxifen[67] although the absolute risk was relatively small (1.2 percent vs. 0.8 percent on placebo).

Pregnancy and puerperium

Cerebrovascular events in pregnancy and the puerperium are rare, with an approximate incidence in the developed world of 1–3/10 000 births.[68–70] The rates of both cerebral infarction and intracerebral hemorrhage are increased in incidence in the 6 weeks after delivery, but not during pregnancy itself.[71] It has been suggested that this increased risk is related to the large decrease in vascular volume or the rapid changes in hormonal status following delivery. One study did not identify factors that strongly predisposed women to stroke in pregnancy.[72] However, others have found certain characteristics that confer an increased risk of stroke in pregnancy, in particular: age over 35 years, multiparity, cigarette smoking, cesarean section and preeclampsia. The greatest relative risk was associated with preeclampsia.[73]

With regards to risk of recurrent stroke (in women who have a history of stroke or TIA), one study has shown an absolute risk of stroke of 1.8 percent in further pregnancies compared to a risk of 0.3 percent in women who have no further pregnancies.[74] The optimum secondary prevention in pregnancy is unclear. (Aspirin, heparin, and phased use of heparin and warfarin have all been advocated.)

Cerebral vein thrombosis in pregnancy

The risk of cerebral vein thrombosis is reported to be increased in pregnancy, particularly when associated with

Behçet disease and in the puerperium when associated with protein S deficiency. The risk also appears to increase with increasing maternal age and cesarean section. In studies of women with previous cerebral vein thrombosis who subsequently became pregnant, 3 percent had a recurrence of thrombosis[75–78] with the greatest risk seen in the peripartum period. Recommended management is to defer pregnancy for 2 years after a cerebral vein thrombosis event but there is no consensus on the role of anticoagulation.

Subarachnoid hemorrhage in pregnancy

One recent study has shown that increasing parity may confer a moderate long-term protective effect on the risk of subarachnoid hemorrhage. The mechanism underlying this association is unknown.[79]

MODIFYING THE RISK OF CEREBROVASCULAR DISEASE

Stroke disease is potentially preventable and there is a substantial evidence base for different strategies to reduce the risk of first and recurrent stroke. Secondary prevention measures should be commenced as soon as possible after the cerebrovascular event has occurred. In the UK Oxford Community Project the average risk of recurrence of a cerebrovascular event following the first stroke was 13 percent in the first year and 4 percent per year in the following years although recent analyses suggest the early risks may be higher. Modifying stroke risk can be considered in four stages: modifying vascular risk factors, treatment of specific medical problems, pharmacologic methods of prevention, and surgical methods of prevention.

Modifying vascular risk factors

LOWERING BLOOD PRESSURE

The most important treatable risk factor for cerebrovascular disease is elevated blood pressure. In primary prevention standard antihypertensive drugs can reduce the risk of first stroke by as much as 38 percent within 1 or 2 years of commencing therapy.[80] Secondary prevention trials have shown that blood pressure reduction with a combination of an angiotension-converting enzyme inhibitor and diuretic benefited all types of patients with recent cerebrovascular events irrespective of their baseline blood pressure. Blood pressure reduction lessened the risk of recurrent stroke after both ischemic and hemorrhagic strokes.[81]

SMOKING CESSATION

The cost to health of smoking is widely known. Smoking is a contributing factor to not only cerebrovascular disease but also other forms of other vascular disease and various cancers in both men and women. The risk of cerebrovascular

events declines within 2–5 years of stopping smoking. There are several nicotine replacement therapy options available and these have been shown to be effective in aiding smoking cessation.[82–84]

LOWERING CHOLESTEROL

Lowering cholesterol levels with statins reduces the risk of ischemic stroke as well as ischemic heart disease. The Heart Protection Study showed a 30 percent reduction in ischemic cerebrovascular events and 25 percent reduction in first stroke. The need for vascular surgical procedures such as coronary artery bypass grafting was also reduced by about 25 percent.[85] It is usual to give dietary instruction to reduce the cholesterol levels and prescribe a statin in patients with established ischemic cerebrovascular disease. The benefit in elderly people (over 80 years of age) is currently less clear.

DIABETES MELLITUS

Good glycemic control has been shown to improve microvascular outcomes although is less convincing for macrovascular outcomes such as stroke. In practice it is usual to try to optimize diabetic control. Good control of blood pressure is also important in people with diabetes. The United Kingdom Prospective Diabetes Trial (UKPDS)[86] in people with type 2 diabetes showed a 44 percent reduced risk of stroke with tight control of blood pressure (blood pressure of 144/82 mm Hg compared with 154/87 mm Hg).

DIET AND ALCOHOL

High fruit and vegetable intake appear to protect against cerebrovascular disease in both men and women.[87,88] Alcohol excess is associated with an increased risk hypertension and cerebrovascular disease. Therefore reducing alcohol consumption probably reduces the risk of cerebrovascular events.

EXERCISE

Increased regular aerobic exercise is associated with a lower instance of cerebrovascular events in both men and women and it is usual to advise regular aerobic activity.[89,90]

Treatment of specific medical problems

THROMBOPHILIAS

Spontaneous and recurrent venous thromboses are more likely to occur in people with thrombophilia (encompassing protein S and C deficiency, antithrombin III deficiency, and factor V Leiden mutations). Anticoagulation should be considered in patients in whom a venous thrombosis may pose a high risk, particularly in those with a history of paradoxical embolism or cerebral vein thrombosis.

Table 16.2 Annual risk of stroke on no treatment, aspirin or, warfarin in high-, moderate- or low-risk patients with nonvalvular atrial fibrillation. NNT denotes the number needed to treat with warfarin instead of aspirin for 1 year to prevent one event[96]

Risk group	Untreated (%)	Aspirin (%)	Warfarin (%)	NNT
Very High				
Previous ischemic stroke or TIA	12	10	5	13
High				
Age over 65 and one other risk factor:	5–8	4–6	2–3	22–47
Hypertension				
Diabetes mellitus				
Heart failure				
Left ventricular dysfunction				
Moderate				
Age over 65, no other risk factors	3–5	2–4	1–2	47–83
Age under 65, other risk factors				
Low				
Age under 65, no other risk factors	1.2	1	Approx 0.5	200

TIA, transient ischemic attack.

ANTIPHOSPHOLIPID SYNDROME

Antiphospholipid syndrome entails arterial and venous thrombosis, recurrent miscarriage, heart valve defects, thrombocytopenia, and migraine-like headaches, along with persistent positivity for antiphospholipid antibodies. Anticoagulation should be considered in these patients.

VASCULITIDES

Most of the vasculitides can present with cerebrovascular events, which result from embolism, aneurysm, dissection, or rupture. In elderly patients, cranial arteritis should be considered especially in those with general malaise, weight loss and raised erythrocyte sedimentation rate. If cranial arteritis is suspected steroid therapy should be commenced as soon as possible and arterial biopsy performed on the affected artery.

Pharmacologic methods for reducing cerebrovascular events

ANTIPLATELET MEDICATION

Platelets play an important role in the pathological pathway causing acute thrombosis in blood vessels and may also play a part in adhesion to vessel walls. Antiplatelet drugs such as aspirin reduce this effect and there is good evidence that long-term antiplatelet treatment reduces the risk of serious vascular events after transient ischemic attacks and minor strokes. A dose of 75 mg (81 mg in North America) aspirin a day is generally recommended. Other antiplatelet agents with evidence of benefit are clopidogrel, ticlopidine and dipyridamole. They are usually used as second-line therapy and in patients who cannot tolerate aspirin. Antiplatelet

medications are associated with a small excess of cerebral hemorrhagic events.[91,92]

ANTICOAGULANT MEDICATION

Anticoagulation is used for both primary and secondary prevention of ischemic cerebrovascular events in people with atrial fibrillation or valvular heart disease. In patients with atrial fibrillation who have had a previous ischemic stroke or transient ischemic attack, the annual risk of stroke on no treatment can be as high as 12 percent (Table 16.2). This risk of stroke can be greatly reduced by oral anticoagulation particularly in high-risk individuals (Table 16.2). For patients in sinus rhythm at present there is no evidence that anticoagulation offers any benefit over antiplatelet agents and it increases the risk of bleeding.[93–95]

Surgical methods of prevention

A proportion of stroke patients have a stenosis of the ipsilateral carotid artery. If this occludes more than 70 percent of the artery then surgical correction (carotid endarterectomy) largely eliminates the high risk of ipsilateral ischemic stroke over the following 2–3 years.[96] The effect lasts for at least 8 years. The procedure may confer less benefit in women and with increasing age (both indicating greater operative risk). In one collaborative study (European Carotid Surgery Trial) independent surgical risk factors were female sex, hypertension, and peripheral vascular disease.[97–99]

CAROTID ARTERY ANGIOPLASTY

Carotid angioplasty has been developed as an alternative to carotid surgery. One trial showed similar outcome to carotid endarterectomy but is currently in the experimental stages.[100,101] Trials of carotid angioplasty with stenting are also underway.

PREVENTIVE NEUROSURGERY

Recurrent subarachnoid and intracranial hemorrhages as a result of aneurysm or arteriovenous malformation may be prevented by neurosurgical interventions. With more readily available interventional radiology, coiling of aneurysms and injection of arterial venous malformations are now more frequently performed. A recent trial indicates that coiling of aneurysms may be the preferred option.[102]

KEY LEARNING POINTS

- Cerebrovascular disease in women is a common, potentially preventable condition.
- There are several types of cerebrovascular disease – ischemic stroke, primary intracerebral hemorrhage, subarachnoid hemorrhage, and intracranial venous thrombosis.
- Modification of risk factors in cerebrovascular disease is important from both a primary and secondary prevention perspective.
- Age, hypertension, smoking, diabetes mellitus, raised cholesterol, atrial fibrillation, and increased plasma fibrinogen are important risk factors for cerebrovascular disease in both sexes.
- There is a complex relation between female sex hormones and cerebrovascular disease with oral contraceptives with higher estrogen doses and hormone replacement therapy being risk factors.
- There is currently no evidence to support the use of hormone replacement therapy in the prevention of stroke.
- Risk factors for stroke in pregnancy in general are: age over 35, multiparity, cigarette smoking, cesarean section, and preeclampsia.
- Antithrombotic agents such as aspirin, dipyridamole, clopidogrel, and warfarin can reduce risk of cerebrovascular disease in appropriately selected individuals.
- Carotid endarterectomy can reduce risk of cerebrovascular disease in symptomatic patients. However, female sex is an independent surgical risk factor, and there may be less benefit to women and with increasing age.

REFERENCES

1 Department of Health. *Mortality Statistics.* London: Department of Health, 2001.

2 Thorvaldsen P, Asplund K, Kuulasmaa K, *et al.* Stroke incidence, case fatality and mortality in the World Health Organization MONICA Project. World Health Organization Monitoring Trends and Determinants in Cardiovascular Disease. *Stroke* 1995; **26**: 361–7. Errata in: *Stroke* 1995; **26**: 1504; 1995; **26**: 2376.

3 American Heart Association. *1997 Heart and Stroke Facts Statistical Update.* Dallas, TX: American Heart Association, 1996.

4 Bamford J, Sandercock P, Dennis M, *et al.* A prospective study of acute cerebrovascular disease in the community. The Oxfordshire Community Project 1981–86. 1. Methodology, demography and incident cases of first-ever stroke. *J Neurol Neurosurg Psychiatry* 1988; **51**: 1373–89.

5 Bamford J, Sandercock P, Dennis M, *et al.* A prospective study of acute cerebrovascular disease in the community: the Oxfordshire Community Stroke Project – 1981–86. 2. Incidence, case fatality rates and overall outcome at one year of cerebral infarction, primary intracerebral and subarachnoid haemorrhage. *J Neurol Neurosurg Psychiatry* 1990; **53**: 16–22.

6 Roquer J, Campello AR, Gomez M. Sex differences in first ever acute stroke. *Stroke* 2003; **34**: 1581–5.

7 Hatano S. Experience from a multicentre stroke register: a preliminary report. *Bull World Health Organ* 1976; **54**: 541–53.

8 Brown MM. Stroke: epidemiology and clinical features. *Medicine* 2003; **28**: 51–8.

9 Bamford J, Sandercock P, Dennis M, *et al.* Classification and natural history of clinically identifiable subtypes of cerebral infarction. *Lancet* 1991; **337**: 1521–6.

10 Sandercock PAG, Warlow CP, Jones LN, Stanley IR. Predisposing factors for cerebral infarction: the Oxford Community Stroke Project. *BMJ* 1989; **298**: 75–80.

11 Ware JA, Herstad DD. Platelet endothelium interactions. *N Engl J Med* 1993; **328**: 628–53.

12 Fisher CM. Occlusion of the internal carotid artery. *Arch Neurol Psychiatry* 1951; **65**: 628–35.

13 Fisher CM. Occlusion of the carotid arteries. *Arch Neurol Psychiatry* 1954; **72**: 187–204.

14 Hutchinson EC, Yates PO. Caratico-vertebral stenosis. *Lancet* 1957; **269**: 2–8.

15 Schwartz CJ, Mitchell JRA. Atheroma of the carotid and vertebral arterial systems. *Br Med J* 1961; **ii**: 1057–63.

16 Cornhill JF, Atkins D, Hutson M, Chandler AB. Localisation of atherosclerotic lesions in the human basilar arteries. *Atherosclerosis* 1980; **35**: 77–86.

17 Heinzlef O, Cohen A, Amarenco P. An update on aortic causes of ischaemic stroke. *Curr Opin Neurol* 1997; **10**: 64–72.

18 Mitchell JRA, Schwartz CJ. Relationship between arterial disease in different sites: a study of the aorta and coronary, carotid and iliac arteries. *BMJ* 1962; **i**: 1293–301.

19 Hertzer NR, Young JR, Beven EG, *et al.* Coronary angiography in 506 patients with extracranial cerebrovascular disease. *Archives of Internal Medicine* 1985; **145**: 849–52.

20 Craven TE, Ryu JE, Espelana MA, *et al.* Evaluation of the association between carotid artery atherosclerosis and coronary artery stenosis: case-control study. *Circulation* 1990; **82**: 1230–42.

21 Chimowitz MI, Poole RM, Starling MR, *et al.* Frequency and severity of asymptomatic coronary disease in patients with different causes of stroke. *Stroke* 1997; **28**: 941–5.

22 O'Leary DH, Polak JF, Kromal RA, *et al.* Carotid artery intima and media thickness as a risk factor for myocardial infarction and stroke in older adults for the cardiovascular health study collaborative research group. *N Engl J Med* 1999; **340**: 14–22.

23 Cole FM, Yates PO. The occurrence and significance of intracerebral microaneurysms; intracerebral microaneurysms and small cerebrovascular lesions; pseudoaneurysms in relation to massive cerebral haemorrhage. *Journal of Pathology and Bacteriology* 1967; **93**: 393–411.

24 Cole FM, Yates PO. Intracerebral microaneurysms and small cerebrovascular lesions. *Brain* 1967; **90**: 759–68.

25 Cole FM, Yates PO. Pseudoaneurysms in relation to massive cerebral haemorrhage. *J Neurol Neurosurg Psychiatry* 1967; **30**: 61–7.

26 Toffol GJ, Biller J, Adams Jr., P. Nontraumatic intracerebral haemorrhage in young adults. *Arch Neurol* 1987; **44**: 483–5.

27 Schutz H, Bodeker RH, Damian M, Dorndorf W. Age-related spontaneous intracerebral haematoma in a German community. *Stroke* 1990; **21**: 1412–18.

28 Hijdra A, Braakman R, van Gijn J, *et al.* Aneurysmal subarachnoid haemorrhage complications and outcome in a hospital population. *Stroke* 1987; **18**: 1061–7.

29 Fox JL, ed. *Intracranial Aneurysms, Volume 1.* New York: Springer-Verlag, 1983: 19–117.

30 Kassell NF, Tomer JC, Haley EC, *et al.* The international cooperative study in the timing of aneurismal surgery 1 overall management results. *J Neurosurg* 1990; **73**: 18–30.

31 Rinkel GJE, Wijdicks EF, Vermeulen M, *et al.* Nonaneurysmal perimesencephalic subarachnoid haemorrhage. CT, MR patterns that differ from aneurysmal rupture. *Am J Neuroradiol* 1991; **12**: 829–34.

32 Kaplan SS, Ogilvy CS, Gonzalez R, *et al.* Extracranial vertebral aneurysm presenting as subarachnoid haemorrhage. *Stroke* 1993; **24**: 1397–9.

33 Rinkel GJE, van Gijn J, Wijdicks EF. Subarachnoid haemorrhage without detectable aneurysm: a review of the causes. *Stroke* **24**: 1403–9.

♦ 34 Bouser MG, Ross Russell RW. *Cerebral Venous Thrombosis.* London: WB Saunders, 1997.

35 Sharshar T, Lamy C, Mas JL. for the stroke pregnancy group. Incidence and causes of strokes associated with the pregnancy and puerperium. A study in public hospitals of the Ile de France. *Stroke* 1995; **24**: 1403–09.

36 Cantu C, Bannaganementena F. Cerebral venous thrombosis associated with pregnancy and the puerperium: review of 67 cases. *Stroke* 1993; **24**: 1880–4.

37 Busch R, Ramm K. Clinical studies on chronic subdural haematomas in 140 adults. *Neurochirurgia* 1980; **23**: 224–8.

38 Arboix A, Oliveres M, Garcia-Eroles L, *et al.* Acute cerebrovascular disease in women. *Eur J Neurol* 2001; **45**: 199–205.

39 Moulin T, Tatu L, Vuillier F, *et al.* Role of a stroke data bank in evaluating cerebral infarction subtypes: patterns and outcome of 1776 consecutive patients from the Besancon stroke registry. *Cerebrovasc Dis* 2000; **10**: 261–71.

♦ 40 Whelton PK. Epidemiology of hypertension. *Lancet* **344**: 101–6.

41 Shinton R, Beevers G. Meta-analysis of relationship between cigarette smoking and stroke. *BMJ* 1989; **298**: 789–94.

42 Robbins A, Manson JE, Lee I, *et al.* Cigarette smoking and stroke in a cohort of US male physicians. *Ann Intern Med* 1994; **120**: 458–62.

43 Kurth T, Kase CS, Berger K, *et al.* Smoking and the risk of haemorrhagic stroke in men. *Stroke* 2003; **34**: 1151–5.

44 Kurth T, Kase CS, Berger K, *et al.* Smoking and the risk of haemorrhagic stroke in women. *Stroke* 2003; **34**: 2792–5.

45 Rosengren A, Welin L, Tsipogianni A, Wilhelmsen L. Impact of cardiovascular risk factors on coronary heart disease and mortality among middle-aged diabetic men: a general population study. *BMJ* 1989; **299**: 1127–31.

46 Manson JE, Colditz GA, Stampfer MJ, *et al.* A prospective study of maturity-onset diabetes and risk of coronary heart disease and stroke in men. *Arch Intern Med* 1991; **151**: 1141–7.

47 Quereshi AI, Giles WH, Croft JB. Impaired glucose tolerance and the likelihood of non-fatal stroke and myocardial infarction. The third national health and nutrition survey. *Stroke* 1998; **29**: 1329–32.

48 Jorgensen HS, Nakayama H, Raaschou HO, Olsen TS. Stroke in patients with diabetes. The Copenhagen heart study. *Stroke* 1994; **25**: 1977–84.

49 Ho JE, Paultre F, Mosca L. Is diabetes mellitus a cardio-vascular disease risk equivalent for fatal stroke in women? Data from the women's pooling project. *Stroke* 2003; **34**: 2812–16.

50 Bowman TS, Sesso HD, Ma J, *et al.* Cholesterol and the risk of ischaemic stroke. *Stroke* 2003; **34**: 2930–4.

51 Narayan SM, Cain ME, Smith JM. Atrial fibrillation. *Lancet* 1997; **350**: 943–50.

52 Anderson DC, Koller RL, Asinger RW, *et al.* Atrial fibrillation and stroke: epidemiology, pathophysiology and management. *Neurologist* 1998; **4**: 235–58.

♦ 53 Hart RG, Benavente O, McBride R, Pearce LA. Antithrombotic therapy to prevent stroke in patients with atrial fibrillation a meta analysis. *Ann Intern Med* 1999; **131**: 492–507.

54 Lin HJ, Wolf PA, Kelly-Hayes M, *et al.* Stroke severity in atrial fibrillation: the Framingham Study. *Stroke* 1996; **27**: 1760–4.

◆ 55 Ernst E, Resch KL. Fibrinogen as a cardiovascular risk factor: a meta analysis and review of the literature. *Ann Intern Med* 1993; **118**: 956–63.

56 Lerner DJ, Kannel WB. Patterns of coronary heart disease mortality and morbidity in the sexes: a 26 year follow-up of the Framingham population. *Am Heart J* 1986; **111**: 383–90.

57 Schievink WI. Intracranial aneurysms. *N Engl J Med* 1997; **336**: 28–40.

◆ 58 van Gijn J, Rinkel GJE. Subarachnoid haemorrhages: diagnosis, causes and management. *Brain* 2001; **124**: 249–78.

59 Juvela S, Poussa K, Porras M. Factors affecting formation and growth of intracranial aneurysms: a long term follow-up study. *Stroke* 2001; **32**: 485–91.

60 Becker WJ. Use of oral contraceptive pill in patients with migraine. *Neurology* 1999; **53**: S19–S25.

61 Chang CL, Donaghy M, Poulter N. World Health Organisation collaborative study of cerebrovascular disease and steroid hormone contraception: migraine and stroke in young women – case-control study. *BMJ* 1999; **318**: 13–18.

62 van der Schouw YT, van der Graaf Y, Steyberg, *et al.* Age at menopause as a risk factor for cardiovascular mortality. *Lancet* 1996; **347**: 714–18.

63 Hu FB, Goodstein F, Hennekens CH, *et al.* Age at natural menopause and risk of cardiovascular disease. *Arch Intern Med* 1999; **159**: 1061–6.

64 Lorentz IT. Parietal lesion and Enavid. *Br Med J* 1962; **2**: 1191.

65 United Nations. *World Contraceptive Use 1998.* New York: United Nations, 1999.

66 Siritho S, Thrift AG, McNeil J, *et al.* Risk of ischaemic stroke among users of the oral contraceptive pill. The Melbourne risk factor study group. *Stroke* 2003; **34**: 1575–80.

67 Gillum LA, Mamidipudi SK, Johnston SC, *et al.* Ischaemic stroke risk with oral contraceptives: a metaanalysis. *JAMA* 2000; **284**: 72–8.

68 Hulley S, Grady D, Bush T, *et al.* Randomized trail of estrogen plus progestin for secondary prevention of coronary heart disease in postmenopausal women. *JAMA* 1998; **280**: 605–13.

69 Writing Group for the Women's Health Initiative Investigators. Risks and benefits of estrogen plus progestin in healthy postmenopausal women: principal results from the women's health initiative randomised controlled trial. *JAMA* 2002; **288**: 321–33.

70 Barrett-Connor E, Grady D, Sashegyi A, *et al.* Raloxifene and cardiovascular events in osteoporotic postmenopausal women: four-year results from the MORE (multiple outcomes of raloxifene evaluation) randomised trial. *JAMA* 2002; **287**: 847–57.

71 Bushnell CD, Goldstein LB. Stroke risk is increased with tamoxifen treatment for breast cancer: a meta-analysis [abstract]. *Stroke* 2004; **35**: 244.

72 Grosset DG, Ebrahim S, Bone I, Warlow C. Stroke in pregnancy and puerperium: what magnitude of risk? *J Neurol Neurosurg Psychiatry* 1998; **58**: 129–31.

73 Mas JL, Lamy C. Stroke in pregnancy and the puerperium. *J Neurol* 1998; **245**: 305–13.

74 Kittner SJ, Stern BJ, Feeser BR, *et al.* Pregnancy and the risk of stroke. *N Engl J Med* 1996; **335**: 768–74.

75 Ros HS, Lichtenstein P, Bellocco R, *et al.* Increased risks of circulatory diseases in late pregnancy and puerperium. *Epidemiology* 2001; **12**: 456–60.

76 Ros HS, Lichtenstein P, Bellocco, *et al.* Pulmonary embolism and stroke in relation to pregnancy: how can high-risk women be identified? *Am J Obstet Gynecol* 2002; **186**: 198–203.

77 Lamy C, Hamon JB, Coste J, Mas JL. Ischaemic stroke in young women: risk of recurrence during subsequent pregnancies. *Neurology* 2000; **55**: 269–74.

78 Wechsler B, Genereau T, Biousse V, *et al.* Pregnancy complicated by cerebral venous thrombosis in Behçet's disease. *Am J Obstet Gynecol* 1995; **173**: 1627–9.

79 Galan HL, Mc Dowell AB, Johnson PR, *et al.* Puerperial cerebral venous thrombosis associated with decreased free protein S: a case report. *J Reprod Med* 1995; **40**: 859–62.

80 Mehraein S, Ortwein H, Busch M, *et al.* Risk or recurrence of cerebral venous and sinus thrombosis during subsequent pregnancy and puerperium. *J Neurol Neurosurg Psychiatry* 2003; **74**: 814–16.

81 Gaist D, Pedersen L, Cnattingius S, Sorensen HT. Parity and risk of subarachnoid haemorrhage in women: a nested case-control study based on the national Swedish Registries. *Stroke* 2004; **35**: 28–32.

82 Collins R, McMahon S. Blood pressure, antihypertensive drug treatment and the risks of stroke and coronary heart disease. *Br Medi Bull* 1994; **50**: 272–98.

● 83 PROGRESS Collaborative group. Randomised trial of a perindopril-based blood pressure lowering regime among 6105 individuals with previous stroke or transient ischaemic attack. *Lancet* 2001; **358**: 1033–41.

84 Peto R. Smoking and death: the past 40 years and the next 40. *BMJ* 1994; **309**: 937–9.

85 Foster C, Murphy M, Nicholas JJ, *et al.* Smoking cessation and primary prevention. In: *Clinical Evidence.* London: BMJ Publishing Group, 2004.

86 Pigone M, Rihal C, Bazian Ltd. Smoking cessation and secondary prevention. In: *Clinical Evidence.* London: BMJ Publishing Group, 2004.

● 87 Heart Protection Study of cholesterol lowering with simvastatin in 20536 high risk individuals: a randomised placebo controlled trial. *Lancet* 2002; **360**: 7–22.

● 88 UKPDS trial group. Intensive blood glucose control with sulphonylureas or insulin compared with conventional treatment and risks of complications in patients with type 2 diabetes. *Lancet* 1998; **352**: 837–53.

89 Gillman MW, Cupples A, Gagnon D, *et al.* Protective effect of fruits and vegetables on development of stroke in men *J Am Soc Med* 1995; **273**: 1113–17.

90   Gillum RF, Mussolino ME, Ingram DD. Physical activity and stroke incidence in women and men. *Am J Epidemiol* 1996; **143**: 860–9.

91   Wannamethee G, Shaper AG. Physical activity and stroke in British middle-aged men. *BMJ* 1992; **304**: 597–601.

92   Manson JE, Stampfer MJ, Willett WC, *et al*. Physical activity and incidence of coronary heart disease and stroke in women. *Circulation* 1995; **91**: 927.

◆ 93   Antithrombotic Trialists Collaboration. Collaborative meta-analysis of randomised trials of antiplatelet therapy for the prevention of death, myocardial infarction and stroke in high risk patients. *BMJ* 2002; **324**: 71–86.

94   Hankey GJ, Sudlow CL, Dunabin DW. Thienopyridines or aspirin to prevent stroke and other serious vascular events in patients at high risk of vascular disease? A systematic review of the evidence from randomised trials. *Stroke* 2000; **31**: 1779–84.

95   Algra A, De Schryver ELLM, van Gijn J, *et al*. Oral anticoagulants versus antiplatelet therapy for preventing further vascular events after transient ischaemic attack or minor stroke of presumed arterial origin. *Cochrane Library*, 2004.

★ 96   Scottish Intercollegiate Guidelines Network, *Antithrombotic Therapy*. Guideline no 36. Edinburgh: Royal College of Physicians, 1999.

◆ 97   Sandercock P. Anticoagulants for preventing recurrence following presumed non cardioembolic ischaemic stroke of transient ischaemic attack. Cochrane review. *Cochrane Library*, 2004.

98   Rothwell PM, Eliasziw M, Gutnikov SA, *et al*. The carotid endarterectomy trialists' collaboration. Analysis of pooled data from the randomised controlled trial of endarterectomy for symptomatic carotid stenosis. *Lancet* 2003; **361**: 107–16.

99   European Carotid Surgery Trialists' Collaborative Group. MRC European carotid surgery trail: interim results for symptomatic patients with severe (70–99%) or with mild (0–29%) carotid stenosis. *Lancet* 1991; **337**: 1235–43.

100   European Carotid Surgery Trialists' Collaborative Group. Randomised trial of endarterectomy for recently symptomatic carotid stenosis: final results of the MRC European Carotid Surgery Trial (ECST). *Lancet* 1998; **351**: 1379–87.

◆ 101   Rothwell PM, Slattery J, Warlow CP. Clinical and angiographic predictors of stroke and death from carotid endarterectomy: systematic review. *BMJ* 1997; **315**: 1571–7.

102   Brooks WH, McLure RR, Jones MR, *et al*. Carotid angioplasty and stenting versus carotid endarterectomy: randomized trial in a community hospital. *J Am Coll Cardiol* 2001; **38**: 1589–95.

103   Hobson RW and the CREST Executive Committee. Carotid stenting in the CREST lead-in phase: periprocedural stroke, myocardial infarction and death rates. *Stroke* 2003; **34**: 239.

◆ 104   Brilstra EH, Rinkel GJE, van der Graaf Y, *et al*. Treatment of intracranial aneurysms by embolisation with coils: a systematic review. *Stroke* 1999; **30**: 470–6.

17

Cancer and thrombosis in women

AGNES Y Y LEE

INTRODUCTION

Venous thromboembolism (VTE) is a common complication in patients with cancer. For women with cancer, the incidence of VTE is increased during treatment with chemotherapy, hormonal agents, as well as during exposure to the usual risk factors for VTE such as surgery and hospitalization. The development of VTE not only increases morbidity, but it is also associated with poorer survival compared with patients with cancer who do not have thrombotic complications. This chapter will review the pathogenesis, epidemiology, prevention and treatment of VTE in women with cancer. Aspects that are unique to women with breast cancer and gynecologic malignancies will be highlighted.

PATHOGENESIS OF THROMBOSIS IN CANCER

Virchow's triad

Virchow described three classic mechanisms that play a role in thrombogenesis: stasis, activation of blood coagulation, and vascular injury.[1] In patients with cancer, all three processes are involved as part of the complex interactions between the tumor, the patient, and the hemostatic system.

Stasis is an important contributing factor for deep vein thrombosis (DVT) and pulmonary embolism (PE) in patients with cancer. Many patients are often immobile and bedridden as a result of their malignancy or its complications (for example, infection, surgery, pain crisis). Also, extrinsic venous compression from tumor masses and lymphadenopathy can lead to stasis. This is particularly relevant for cancers in the pelvis and thoracic outlet where

there is limited space for tumor expansion. For example, women with axillary nodes from advanced breast cancer or large ovarian masses are at high risk for DVT in the upper and lower extremities, respectively.

Activation of coagulation in patients with cancer can result either directly from procoagulant molecules expressed by tumor cells or indirectly by initiating an inflammatory response in the patient. The best-characterized procoagulant associated with tumor cells is tissue factor (TF).[2] The human TF molecule is a single-chain 263 amino acid, 47 kDa transmembrane glycoprotein.[3] It acts as both a surface receptor and cofactor for activated coagulation protease factor VII (FVIIa). On binding of factor VIIa to TF, blood coagulation is initiated with downstream generation of activated coagulation serine proteases, factor Xa and factor IIa (thrombin). Therefore, tumors are capable of activating blood coagulation in the peritumoral environment through the expression of TF. Another cancer procoagulant has also been described but has yet remained uncharacterized. It is a cysteine protease that directly activates factor X and functions in the absence of factor VII.[4] It has been found almost exclusively on neoplastic tissue and its level correlates with disease status in acute promyelocytic leukemia.[5]

Host factors can also contribute to hypercoagulability in patients with cancer. Advanced age and obesity are well-recognized risk factors. Accumulating evidence also shows that the cytokine response to tumor cells contribute to the activation of coagulation through the enhancement of TF expression and downregulation of natural anticoagulants such as thrombomodulin.[6] In addition, studies have examined whether the presence of hereditary thrombophilia, for example, factor V Leiden, contributes to thrombosis in cancer patients. Some studies have reported an association between factor V Leiden and catheter-related thrombosis[7–9] but others have found no association with VTE.[10–13] One study has reported a higher risk of VTE associated with activated protein C resistance in the absence of factor V Leiden.[14] These conflicting findings are difficult to explain but it is possible that different interactions occur with different tumor types.

Vascular injury is a common occurrence in patients with cancer, as many of them undergo surgery, receive chemotherapeutic agents that are toxic to the endothelium, and have vascular catheters to facilitate venous access. Direct tumor invasion of the vasculature can also predispose to thrombus formation.

Mechanisms associated with tamoxifen

Thrombosis has been reported in patients receiving tamoxifen for breast cancer. A number of thrombotic mechanisms have been proposed for tamoxifen but none are well studied. The most widely accepted mechanism is tamoxifen's paradoxical estrogenic property, as estrogens are known to lower antithrombin and protein C levels.[15,16] Such changes in coagulation and hemostatic parameters have been documented in breast cancer patients on tamoxifen.[17–20] Although antithrombin levels have been shown consistently to decrease after tamoxifen therapy, it is difficult to rationalize that the observed 20–30 percent reductions are of any physiologic relevance.[17,18] There is also weak evidence that factor V Leiden significantly increases the risk of VTE in patients who receive tamoxifen therapy.[21] Since factor V Leiden acts synergistically with oral contraceptives to increase the risk of venous thrombosis, an interaction between this inherited thrombophilia and tamoxifen certainly is plausible.

Mechanisms associated with chemotherapy

The mechanism of chemotherapy-induced thrombosis is unclear but is likely to be multifactorial. Changes in the levels of pro- and anticoagulant proteins, endothelial cell damage and enhanced endothelial reactivity are possible mechanisms.[22,23] Rella et al. reported on the changes in coagulation and fibrinolytic markers in stage II breast cancer patients treated with cyclophosphamide, methotrexate, and 5-fluorouracil (CMF).[24] The only statistically significant changes before therapy and after each cycle of treatment were modest reductions in protein C and S antigen levels and activities (down to 70–90 percent), and a rise in plasminogen activator inhibitor-1 levels. There were no changes in prothrombin time (PT), partial prothrombin time (PPT), fibrinogen, antithrombin, D-dimer, thrombin-antithrombin III, and prothrombin fragment 1 + 2 levels. Others have also reported similar reductions in protein C and S activities in women receiving CMF.[25] Feffer et al. also prospectively followed platelet aggregation and coagulation parameters in women with localized or metastatic breast cancer while receiving CMF.[26] These investigators found a large decrease in protein C activity during treatment (down to 40–70 percent), but no changes in platelet aggregation, fibrin degradation products, D-dimer, antithrombin, or plasminogen levels; protein S activity was not specifically assayed. However, despite the consistent finding of CMF-related reductions in protein C activity, a link to clinical thrombotic events has not been demonstrated in any study.

Direct toxic effects on the endothelium have been reported with a number of chemotherapeutic agents.[23] Damage to the endothelium leads to activation of the coagulation system. Nicolson et al. found that doxorubicin, vincristine, and bleomycin cause endothelial retraction and increased platelet adhesion.[27] Ex vivo experiments also have suggested that enhanced endothelial cell reactivity to platelets may be a potential thrombogenic mechanism in women receiving cyclophosphamide, epirubicin, and 5-flurouracil for stage II breast cancer.[22] Chemotherapeutic agents may alter endothelial cell reactivity by inducing the release of interleukin-1, which, in turn facilitates adhesion molecule expression on the endothelial cell surface. In vitro studies have also shown that exposure of human umbilical vein endothelial cells to doxorubicin results in a dose- and time-dependent decrease in cell surface levels of endothelial cell protein C receptor, a key component of the anticoagulant protein C pathway that facilitates the binding and inactivation of thrombin on the endothelial surface.[28]

EPIDEMIOLOGY

Thrombosis in women with breast cancer

The incidence of VTE in women with breast cancer is best documented in clinical trials of systemic therapy in the 1990s (see Table 17.1 later). The rate of thrombosis over a 5-year period in women with axillary node-negative breast cancer on tamoxifen is approximately 0.9 percent,[29,30] representing a fourfold increased risk compared to women treated with placebo. In women with node-negative disease, the risk of VTE climbs to 4 percent when they are treated with tamoxifen and chemotherapy.[30] Consequently, tamoxifen is no longer given concurrently with chemotherapy and is relatively contraindicated in women with a prior history of VTE.

The thrombogenic effect of tamoxifen alone was clearly demonstrated in the Breast Cancer Prevention Trial conducted by the National Surgical Adjuvant Breast and Bowel Project (NSABP)[31] and the International Breast Cancer Intervention Study.[32] In these trials, healthy women at risk for developing breast cancer were randomized to either tamoxifen or placebo for 5 years. The tamoxifen group had an increased risk of DVT of 0.1–0.2 percent per year compared with the placebo group at 0.08–0.1 percent per year, representing an overall relative risk of about 2.0. In the

Table 17.1   Incidence of thrombosis in early-stage breast cancer

Study	Treatment	No. of patients	Patients with thrombosis (%)
Node-negative			
Fisher *et al.*, 1989[29]	T	1318	0.9
	Placebo	1326	0.15
Fisher *et al.*, 1997[30]	CMFT	768	4.2
	T	771	0.8
Node-positive			
Levine *et al.*, 1988[35]	CMFVP	102	8.8
	CMFVP + AT	103	4.9
Pritchard *et al.*, 1996[38]	CMF + T	353	9.6
	T	352	1.4
Clahsen *et al.*, 1994[37]	Perioperative FAC	1292	2.1
	No Rx	1332	0.8
Rivkin *et al.*, 1994[41]	CMFVP + T	303	3.6
	CMFVP	300	1.3
	T	295	0
Fisher *et al.*, 1990[36]	ACT	383	3.1
	T	367	1.6
Weiss *et al.*, 1981[34]	CMFVP	143	6.3
	CMF	144	3.5

A, adriamycin; C, cyclophosphamide; F, fluorouracil; M, methotrexate; P, prednisone; T, tamoxifen; V, vincristine.

NSABP trial, the highest rates of thrombosis associated with the use of tamoxifen were observed in women older than 50 years. Tamoxifen is also known to increase the incidence of superficial phlebitis, which can be bothersome but is not life threatening. All in all, the benefit of tamoxifen in preventing primary or recurrent breast cancer does outweigh the risk of venous thromboembolic complications.[33] In women with node-positive breast cancer on chemotherapy, the rate of thrombosis ranges between 1 percent and 9 percent, with the highest incidence observed in postmenopausal women (Table 17.1).[34–41] As seen in women with node-negative disease, chemotherapy plus tamoxifen increases the risk of thrombosis over either agent alone.

For women who are postmenopausal, aromatase inhibitors are now available as an alternative to tamoxifen. These agents block conversion of adrenal androgens to estrone and estradiol by inhibiting the cytochrome P450-dependent enzyme aromatase. As peripheral aromatization is the principal source of estrogen in men and postmenopausal women, blocking this activity effectively reduces systemic estrogen levels. In large randomized trials in advanced- and early-stage breast cancer, anastrozole is associated with approximately half the risk of thrombosis compared with tamoxifen.[42–44] However, anastrozole may have a higher risk of fracture compared with tamoxifen.[42,45] Trials in women with advanced or metastatic breast cancer have reported an incidence of 1.0 percent for venous thromboembolic events with an aromatase inhibitor, compared with 2.9 percent for those randomized to receive tamoxifen, over a median follow-up of 18 months.[44] The incidence in women with early-stage breast cancer is

2.8 percent and 4.5 percent, respectively, over a 5-year follow-up period.[42] Therefore, the risk of VTE associated with aromatase inhibitors is approximately 0.5–1 percent per year.

The rate of thrombosis in women with metastatic breast cancer is less certain. In a case series by Goodnough *et al.*, the rate of thrombosis in patients receiving chemotherapy for metastatic breast cancer was 17.5 percent.[46] However, in a randomized trial reported by Levine *et al.*, the rate was 4.5 percent.[47] Others have reported an average rate of 10 percent.[48] The use of high-dose medroxyprogesterone in patients with metastatic disease does not appear to increase the risk of VTE, but very limited data are available.[49,50]

Observational studies have shown that patients with cancer who develop VTE have a worse prognosis compared with those without thrombotic complications.[51,52] This association has been reported in a retrospective study specifically in women with breast cancer,[40] in which those with VTE had a 1.8-fold increased risk for subsequent cancer relapse and a fourfold increased risk of dying of cancer compared with those without VTE. The mechanisms are unknown, but the higher mortality may result from fatal pulmonary embolism, the aggressive nature of malignancies that are associated with VTE, or derailment of first-line cancer treatment because of the thrombotic event.

Thrombosis in other gynecologic malignancies

The incidence of VTE in women with specific gynecologic malignancies is not well documented. Few studies have been published and most of them included patients with different tumor types and stages and were small or retrospective. However, among solid tumors, it appears consistently that ovarian cancer is associated with one of the highest risks for VTE whereas breast cancer is associated with a relatively low risk for VTE. In a population-based study based on discharge records of over 7000 Medicare patients (>65 years of age) admitted to hospital with a diagnosis of both malignancy and DVT or PE,[52] the incidence of VTE per 10 000 patients was 120 for cancer of the ovary, 49 for cancer of the cervix, 44 for cancer of the uterus, and 22 for breast cancer. Another registry linkage study reported that the cumulative incidence of VTE in the first 6 months following a diagnosis of ovarian cancer is 32.6 per 1000 patients, 16.2 per 1000 patients diagnosed with cervical cancer, 10.5 per 1000 patients diagnosed with uterine cancer, and 8.0 per 1000 patients diagnosed with breast cancer.[53] In a retrospective review of 253 cases, the overall incidence of symptomatic VTE was 16.6 percent in women with epithelial ovarian cancer.[54] This is consistent with the finding in a small trial in which 10.6 percent of women with advanced ovarian cancer receiving chemotherapy developed VTE, despite prophylaxis with either low-molecular-weight heparin (LMWH) or unfractionated heparin (UFH) for thromboprophylaxis.[55]

Another group of women with a high risk of VTE appears to be those with cervical cancer who are receiving concurrent chemotherapy, radiation and recombinant erythropoietin. A risk of VTE as high as 23 percent has been reported in some series.[56,57] The use of erythropoietin was also reported to be associated with a high incidence of thrombosis in a trial in women with advanced breast cancer.[58] However, it remains uncertain whether erythropoietin is thrombogenic and the mechanisms of action have not been identified.

The incidence of postoperative VTE in women undergoing gynecologic procedures for malignant disease is higher than in those having benign gynecologic surgery. Based on a recent review using registry data from the California Patient Discharge Data Set from 1992 to 1996, the risk of symptomatic VTE within the 91 days after surgery was 2.3 percent for bilateral oophorectomy and 1.2 percent for total abdominal hysterectomy in women with a malignancy, whereas the respective risks for the same procedures in women without cancer were 0.3 percent each, respectively.[59] However, these numbers are likely to underestimate the true incidence of VTE. According to randomized trials and cohort studies performed in the 1980s and 1990s which used fibrinogen leg scanning for screening for DVT, the risk of DVT following surgery for pelvic malignancies ranged from 12 percent to 38 percent in women who did not receive prophylaxis and approximately 2 percent of women had PE.[60–66] Age above 60, obesity, advanced clinical stage, and previous history of thrombosis have been found to be associated with an increased risk of postoperative thrombosis.[67,68] The risk appears to be highest in patients undergoing surgery or radical surgery requiring pelvic lymphadenectomy and debulking ovarian cancer.[48,68] The

heightened risk with these procedures may be reflective of the extent of the cancer and the duration of general anesthesia.

PREVENTION OF THROMBOSIS

Surgical prophylaxis

Cancer patients undergoing surgery are at increased risk for postoperative thrombosis compared with patients undergoing surgery for benign conditions.[69] Clinical trials have demonstrated the efficacy of subcutaneous UFH in preventing DVT and PE in patients undergoing major surgery.[70,71] Recent studies, including a metaanalysis of randomized trials, have shown that once-daily injection of a LMWH and three-times-a-day dosing of UFH in high-risk major surgery are equally effective and safe in preventing postoperative thrombosis in both patients with and without cancer.[72] The once-per-day injection for LMWH administration is attractive because of the comfort for patients, convenience for medical staff, and the lower risk of drug error; LMWH is also associated with a lower risk of heparin-induced thrombocytopenia. A recent study has found that prophylaxis with LMWH in women undergoing gynecologic oncology surgery is cost-effective in terms of life years gained, even for patients with relatively short life expectancies.[73]

For gynecologic oncology surgery, randomized trials have reported that thromboprophylaxis with UFH, LMWH, or intermittent pneumatic compression is effective and safe.[60–66,74–77] With these regimens, the risk of symptomatic postoperative DVT is reduced by approximately 70 percent. However, there is no evidence to date that any of these regimens reduce the incidence of PE. Also, clinical trials that have compared these regimens directly have not found any significant differences in efficacy or safety, but the studies are small and lack the statistical power to detect small differences. Overall, the incidence of VTE with prophylaxis ranges from 2 percent in breast cancer and up to 20 percent in invasive pelvic surgery. In recent years, two trials have shown that the incidence of DVT detected on venography can be reduced with extended out-of-hospital prophylaxis with LMWH in patients undergoing major abdominal or pelvic surgery for cancer.[78,79] Women undergoing gynecologic oncology surgery represented only 8 percent of the study population in one of the trials.[78] Further research is required to show that continuing anticoagulant prophylaxis beyond hospitalization will reduce the risk of clinically important VTE.

Prophylaxis in the medical cancer patient

Only one randomized trial has studied primary prevention of VTE in ambulatory patients. In a double-blind randomized trial, Levine and colleagues showed that low dose warfarin is effective in reducing the incidence of symptomatic thrombosis during chemotherapy.[47] A statistically significant 85 percent risk reduction in the rate of VTE was found in women who received very-low-dose warfarin (1 mg for 6 weeks followed by adjusted dose to a target international normalized ratio [INR] of 1.3–1.9) compared with placebo. The average duration of therapy was 6 months. Increase in bleeding was not detected. Although these results are compelling, routine prophylaxis in ambulatory cancer patients receiving chemotherapy is not common practice. The most likely reasons are the concern for bleeding and the inconvenience of warfarin dose adjustment and laboratory monitoring. Prophylaxis for patients with a particularly high risk for VTE (for example, previous history of thrombosis or an obstructive pelvic mass) may be warranted, but each case must be assessed individually, taking into account the risks and benefits of prophylaxis and the patient's quality of life.

For cancer patients who are bedridden or hospitalized for acute medical complications, the risk for thrombosis is increased. Low-dose anticoagulation with UFH, LMWH, or fondaparinux has been found to be effective in patients hospitalized with acute medical illnesses.[80–82] It would seem reasonable, therefore, that patients with advanced malignancy who are bedridden would benefit from thromboprophylaxis.[83]

TREATMENT OF VENOUS THROMBOEMBOLISM

Treatment of cancer patients with VTE is difficult because these patients have an increased risk of recurrent VTE and anticoagulant-induced bleeding compared to patients without cancer.[84,85] The occurrence of thrombosis in patients with cancer not only has a negative impact on their quality of life but also increases mortality.[51,52]

Risk of recurrence and bleeding

Hutten et al. performed a retrospective analysis of the rates of recurrent thrombosis and bleeding for patients who received at least 3 months of vitamin K antagonist therapy in two large randomized clinical trials that compared LMWH with UFH for the initial therapy of acute VTE.[84] The incidence of recurrent thrombosis in patients with cancer was 27.1 per 100 patient years versus 9.0 per 100 patient years in those without cancer ($P = 0.003$). The risk of bleeding was approximately six times higher in cancer patients (13.3 per 100 patient-years) than in patients without cancer (2.1 per 100 patient-years) ($P = 0.002$).

Prandoni et al. confirmed these findings later in a prospective cohort study by following the outcomes of anticoagulant treatment in a cohort of 842 patients who received initial UFH or LMWH followed by vitamin K

antagonist for acute VTE.[85] The 12-month cumulative incidence of recurrent thromboembolism in the 181 cancer patients was 20.7 percent versus 6.8 percent in the 661 patients without cancer (hazard ratio 3.2). The 12-month cumulative incidence of major bleeding was 12.4 percent in patients with cancer compared to 4.9 percent in patients without cancer (hazard ratio 2.2). Recurrence and bleeding were both related to cancer severity and occurred predominantly during the first month of anticoagulant therapy. The incidence of recurrent VTE also directly correlates with the intensity of the INR but the risk of major bleeding appears to be independent of the anticoagulant effect.

Initial treatment of venous thromboembolism

In the majority of patients with acute VTE, LMWH has replaced UFH as the first line treatment. Large metaanalyses of clinical trials have shown that weight-adjusted subcutaneous LMWH is safer and more effective than UFH administered by continuous intravenous infusion and monitored by the activated partial thromboplastin time (aPTT).[86–89] Outpatient therapy with LMWH has also been shown to be effective and safe.[90–94] For cancer patients, home therapy is an important advantage for their quality of life.

One of the controversial areas in the initial treatment of acute VTE using LMWH is the optimal frequency of injections. Merli et al. compared UFH with once-a-day and twice-a-day dosing regimens of the LMWH enoxaparin.[95] In the subgroup of cancer patients, there was a suggestion that the rate of recurrent thromboembolism was twofold higher in the patients who received once-daily enoxaparin. Similar data for the LMWH reviparin have been reported.[96] It is conceivable that better antithrombotic efficacy might be achieved in the cancer patient with a twice-daily dosing, but this requires further research.

Few trials have compared LMWH with UFH in patients with acute PE. Simmoneau et al. compared the LMWH tinzaparin with intravenous UFH in hospitalized patients with PE, and no difference was detected in recurrent VTE and bleeding.[97] In the trial performed by the Columbus Investigators, which found no difference in these outcomes between the LMWH reviparin and UFH, the majority of patients were treated at home and 27 percent of all patients had PE.[92] In these two trials, 10 percent and 23 percent of patients had cancer, respectively. More recently, in a prospective cohort study, Kovacs et al. treated 108 patients with PE as outpatients with the LMWH dalteparin; 22 percent had cancer.[98] The rate of recurrent thrombosis was 5.6 percent, and major bleeding occurred in 2.9 percent of the patients. Hence, based on this evidence and the large experience with LMWHs in DVT, it seems reasonable to manage patients with acute PE who are hemodynamically stable by treating them with LMWH in the outpatient setting. However, patients with acute PE who are hemodynamically unstable should be admitted to hospital and treatment with intravenous UFH should be used because such patients were excluded from the clinical trials that compared LMWHs with UFH.

There is little evidence to support the routine insertion of inferior vena cava (IVC) filters in cancer patients with acute VTE. A large randomized trial has shown that filters will reduce the short-term risk of PE at the expense of an increased risk of recurrent DVT over the long term, despite concurrent oral anticoagulant therapy.[99] Other studies have also suggested that thrombosis at the insertion site is a common complication of filter placement.[100] Although patients with cancer have a higher risk of bleeding, particularly during periods of thrombocytopenia during chemotherapy, there is no evidence that filters should be used as first-line treatment of acute VTE in these patients. Filters should be reserved for patients who are actively bleeding and cannot receive anticoagulant therapy for acute VTE. Retrievable IVC filters can be inserted and then removed later once the bleeding has stopped, thus avoiding the long-term potential complications of IVC filters.[101,102] However, the results of additional studies in cancer patients are required.

Long-term anticoagulant therapy

Currently, oral coumarin derivatives are the standard for long-term anticoagulant therapy to prevent recurrent thrombosis. Warfarin, the most commonly used vitamin K antagonist, is commenced on the first or second day of treatment and the aim is to achieve an INR of 2.0–3.0.[103]

Maintenance of the anticoagulant effect within this therapeutic range requires frequent laboratory monitoring and dose adjustment. Because of its narrow therapeutic window, warfarin therapy is particularly complicated in patients with cancer. It is often difficult to maintain the INR within the therapeutic range because these patients often have anorexia, vomiting, and diarrhea. In addition, drug interactions can influence the anticoagulant effect of vitamin-K- dependent anticoagulants. Often it is necessary to interrupt anticoagulant therapy because of thrombocytopenia and invasive procedures, such as thoracentesis and abdominal paracentesis. This requires reversal of the anticoagulant effect with vitamin K. Subsequently, it takes several days to reestablish the targeted therapeutic range after reintroduction of warfarin. Finally, frequent blood sampling is required for the INR and this may be problematic in patients with difficult venous access.

Because LMWHs avoid many of the limitations of warfarin therapy, they have been investigated as an alternative for long-term treatment of VTE.[104–110] The majority of these trials have been relatively small and included few cancer patients. Several recent randomized trials, however, have provided new information concerning the long-term use of LMWHs in cancer patients with VTE (Table 17.2). In the trial reported by Meyer et al., cancer patients with acute VTE were randomized to 3 months of enoxaparin or warfarin at a targeted INR of 2.0–3.0.[111] The primary endpoint was a composite outcome consisting of major bleeding and recurrent VTE. In the 71 patients who received warfarin, the outcome event rate was 21 percent compared to 10.5 percent in the 67 patients who received LMWH

Table 17.2   Long-term treatment with low-molecular-weight heparin

Study	Treatment	Patient no.	Recurrent VTE (%)	Bleeding: major (%)
Meyer et al., 2002[111]	Enoxaparin 1.5 mg/kg for 3 months	67	3[†]	16.9[†]
	Warfarin INR 2.0–3.0 for 3 months	71	4.2	7.5
Deitcher et al., 2003[112]	Enoxaparin 1 mg/kg twice daily for at least 5 days followed by:			
	Enoxaparin 1 mg/kg once daily for 175 days	32	7.1	NR
	Enoxaparin 1.5 mg/kg once daily for 175 days	36	3.2	NR
	Warfarin target INR 2.5 for 175 days	24	10.3	NR
Lee et al., 2003[113]	Dalteparin 200 IU/kg daily for 1 month, followed by 75–80% of this dose for 5 months	336	8[††]	5.6*
	Dalteparin 200 IU/kg once daily for 5–7 days and warfarin or acenocoumarol at target INR 2.5 for 6 months	336	16	3.6
Hull et al., 2003[114]	Tinzaparin 175 IU/kg for 84 days	80	6.3	6.3
	IV unfractionated heparin followed by warfarin target INR 2.5 for 84 days	87	11.5	8.0

* $P = 0.27$
[†] P value for composite endpoint of VTE and bleeding = 0.09.
[††] P value for recurrent VTE = 0.002.
INR, international normalized ratio; IV, intravenous; NR, not reported; VTE, venous thromboembolism.

($P = 0.09$). This observed difference was mainly a result of the rates of major bleeding in the two groups; 16.9 percent in warfarin patients versus 7.5 percent in the LMWH patients. Overall, the underpowered study did not demonstrate any significant differences in efficacy and safety between enoxaparin and warfarin in patients with cancer. Another small study comparing two different doses of enoxaparin (1 mg/kg once daily or 1.5 mg/kg once daily) with warfarin also failed to show a difference in recurrent VTE, bleeding, or death.[112]

Using a randomized, open-label study design in the same patient population, Lee *et al.* conducted the Comparison of Low-molecular-weight heparin versus Oral anticoagulant Therapy for the prevention of recurrent venous thromboembolism in patients with cancer (CLOT) trial in which cancer patients with acute VTE and/or PE were randomized to long-term dalteparin versus long-term vitamin K antagonist therapy.[113] All patients received therapeutic doses of dalteparin for the first week. Those randomized to control therapy continued with a vitamin K antagonist at a target INR of 2.5, and those randomized to the experimental therapy continued with dalteparin at a therapeutic dose for the first month, followed by a reduced dose at 75–80 percent of the therapeutic dose for the next 5 months. Over the six-month study period, 27 of 336 patients in the dalteparin group compared with 53 of 336 patients in the oral anticoagulant group experienced recurrent VTE. The cumulative incidence of VTE at 6 months was reduced from 17.4 percent in the oral anticoagulant group to 8.8 percent in the dalteparin group, hazard ratio 0.48 ($P = 0.002$). No statistically significant difference was detected in major bleeding between groups (3.6 percent and 5.6 percent, respectively). The rate of any bleeding (major plus minor) was 18.5 percent in the oral anticoagulant group compared to 13.6 percent in the dalteparin group ($P = 0.09$). Finally, in a subgroup analysis of a trial that compared long-term tinzaparin LMWH with warfarin therapy both administered for 3 months, there was a reduction in recurrent VTE in the subgroup of cancer patients who received tinzaparin.[114]

On the basis of the results of these trials, long-term therapy with LMWH is now recommended as the treatment of choice in preventing recurrent VTE in patients with cancer.[115] It substantially reduces the rate of recurrent VTE without an increase in bleeding. The use of long-term LMWH also simplifies the management by avoiding the need for laboratory monitoring and allowing more flexibility to accommodate urgent invasive procedures.

In general the duration of long-term treatment of VTE is based on a patient's risk of recurrent thrombosis and bleeding. In patients with malignancy, the risk of recurrent thrombosis depends on the usual thrombotic risk factors (for example, surgery, bed rest) as well as factors specific to cancer, such as stage or activity of the cancer and the use of chemotherapy and hormonal agents. There are no trials evaluating the duration of anticoagulant therapy in cancer patients with VTE and data have to be extrapolated from trials in patients with idiopathic thrombosis.[116–118]

Currently, the recommendation from the ACCP Consensus Conference for Antithrombotic Therapy for patients with cancer who experience an acute thromboembolic event is to treat them indefinitely or until the active cancer is resolved.[115] However, as in patients without cancer, the exact duration of therapy should be tailored individually. In patients with metastatic disease, anticoagulant therapy should be continued indefinitely or until a contraindication to anticoagulation develops. In those who have active but not metastatic disease, anticoagulant therapy should be given for at least 6 months and as long as there is any evidence of cancer or while the patient is receiving chemotherapy. In cancer patients who have no evidence of active cancer and who developed the thrombotic event in association with a strong risk factor such as surgery, a minimum of 3 months of anticoagulant treatment may be reasonable, especially if there are relative contraindications for continuing anticoagulation.

KEY LEARNING POINTS

- Venous thromboembolism (VTE) is a common complication in women with cancer.
- Pathogenic mechanisms of thromboembolism involve the activation of coagulation, venous stasis, and vascular injury and are highly dependent on complex interactions between the tumor and the patient.
- Relative to other solid tumors, ovarian cancer is associated with a higher risk of VTE whereas breast cancer is associated with a lower risk of VTE.
- The major risk factors for VTE in women with cancer include: metastatic disease; anticancer therapy, including chemotherapy, hormonal therapy, particularly tamoxifen; supportive therapy, including growth factors and central venous catheters; surgery; high body mass index; and postmenopausal status or advanced age.
- Thromboprophylaxis is recommended for all women having surgery for cancer and during hospitalization for an acute medical illness.
- Anticoagulant therapy is the treatment of choice for women with acute VTE. Use of filters should be reserved only in patients with active bleeding.
- Risk of bleeding while on anticoagulant therapy and risk of recurrent VTE is higher in patients with cancer than without.
- Treatment with LMWH is the recommended treatment of choice for preventing recurrent VTE.
- Anticoagulant therapy should be continued for a minimum of 6 months and while the cancer is active or the patient is receiving systemic anticancer therapy.

REFERENCES

1 Virchow R. Gesammelt abhandlungen zur wissenchaftlichen medizin. *Meidinger Sohn* 1856: 219.

2 Ruf W. Molecular regulation of blood clotting in tumor biology. *Haemostasis* 2001; **31**(Suppl 1): 5–7.

3 Bazan JF. Structural design and molecular evolution of a cytokine receptor superfamily. *Proc Natl Acad Sci U S A* 1990; **87**: 6934–8.

4 Gale AJ, Gordon SG. Update on tumor cell procoagulant factors. *Acta Haematol* 2001; **106**: 25–32.

5 Falanga A, Consonni R, Marchetti M, *et al.* Cancer procoagulant and tissue factor are differently modulated by all-trans-retinoic acid in acute promyelocytic leukemia cells. *Blood* 1998; **92**: 143–51.

6 Lee AY. Cancer and thromboembolic disease: pathogenic mechanisms. *Cancer Treat Rev* 2002; **28**: 137–40.

7 Blom JW, Doggen CJ, Osanto S, Rosendaal FR. Malignancies, prothrombotic mutations, and the risk of venous thrombosis. *JAMA* 2005; **293**: 715–22.

8 Van Rooden CJ, Rosendaal FR, Meinders AE, *et al.* The contribution of factor V Leiden and prothrombin G20210A mutation to the risk of central venous catheter-related thrombosis. *Haematologica* 2004; **89**: 201–6.

9 Fijnheer R, Paijmans B, Verdonck LF, *et al.* Factor V Leiden in central venous catheter-associated thrombosis. *Br J Haematol* 2002; **118**: 267–70.

10 Kennedy M, Andreescu AC, Greenblatt MS, *et al.* Factor V Leiden, prothrombin 20210A and the risk of venous thrombosis among cancer patients. *Br J Haematol* 2005; **128**: 386–8.

11 Sifontes MT, Nuss R, Hunger SP, *et al.* The factor V Leiden mutation in children with cancer and thrombosis. *Br J Haematol* 1997; **96**: 484–9.

12 Ravin AJ, Edwards RP, Krohn A, *et al.* The factor V Leiden mutation and the risk of venous thromboembolism in gynecologic oncology patients. *Obstet Gynecol* 2002; **100**: 1285–9.

13 Otterson GA, Monahan BP, Harold N, *et al.* Clinical significance of the FV:Q506 mutation in unselected oncology patients. *Am J Med* 1996; **101**: 406–12.

14 Zangari M, Saghafifar F, Anaissie E, *et al.* Activated protein C resistance in the absence of factor V Leiden mutation is a common finding in multiple myeloma and is associated with an increased risk of thrombotic complications. *Blood Coagul Fibrinolysis* 2002; **13**: 187–92.

15 Caine YG, Bauer KA, Barzegar S, *et al.* Coagulation activation following estrogen administration to postmenopausal women. *Thromb Haemost* 1992; **68**: 392–5.

16 Nabulsi AA, Folsom AR, White A, *et al.* Association of hormone-replacement therapy with various cardiovascular risk factors in postmenopausal women. The Atherosclerosis Risk in Communities Study Investigators. *N Engl J Med* 1993; **328**: 1069–75.

17 Jordan VC, Fritz NF, Tormey DC. Long-term adjuvant therapy with tamoxifen: effects on sex hormone binding globulin and antithrombin III. *Cancer Res* 1987; **47**: 4517–19.

18 Love RR, Surawicz TS, Williams EC. Antithrombin III level, fibrinogen level, and platelet count changes with adjuvant tamoxifen therapy. *Arch Intern Med* 1992; **152**: 317–20.

19 Pemberton KD, Melissari E, Kakkar VV. The influence of tamoxifen *in vivo* on the main natural anticoagulants and fibrinolysis. *Blood Coagul Fibrinolysis* 1993; **4**: 935–42.

20 Auger MJ, Mackie MJ. Effects of tamoxifen on blood coagulation. *Cancer* 1988; **61**: 1316–19.

21 Weitz IC, Israel VK, Liebman HA. Tamoxifen-associated venous thrombosis and activated protein C resistance due to factor V Leiden. *Cancer* 1997; **79**: 2024–7.

22 Bertomeu MC, Gallo S, Lauri D, *et al.* Chemotherapy enhances endothelial cell reactivity to platelets. *Clin Exp Metastasis* 1990; **8**: 511–18.

23 Lazo JS. Endothelial injury caused by antineoplastic agents. *Biochem Pharmacol* 1986; **35**: 1919–23.

24 Rella C, Coviello M, Giotta F, *et al.* A prothrombotic state in breast cancer patients treated with adjuvant chemotherapy. *Breast Cancer Res Treat* 1996; **40**: 151–9.

25 Rogers JS, Murgo AJ, Fontana JA, Raich PC. Chemotherapy for breast cancer decreases plasma protein C and protein S. *J Clin Oncol* 1988; **6**: 276–81.

26 Feffer SE, Carmosino LS, Fox RL. Acquired protein C deficiency in patients with breast cancer receiving cyclophosphamide, methotrexate, and 5-fluorouracil. *Cancer* 1989; **63**: 1303–7.

27 Nicolson GL, Custead SE. Effects of chemotherapeutic drugs on platelet and metastatic tumor cell-endothelial cell interactions as a model for assessing vascular endothelial integrity. *Cancer Res* 1985; **45**: 331–6.

28 Shin LYY, Woodley-Cook J, Caruso S, *et al.* Effects of chemotherapeutic agents on the protein C anticoagulant pathway. Presented at the XXth Congress of the International Society for Thrombosis and Haemostasis, Sydney, Australia, August 6–12, 2005.

29 Fisher B, Costantino J, Redmond C, *et al.* A randomized clinical trial evaluating tamoxifen in the treatment of patients with node-negative breast cancer who have estrogen-receptor-positive tumors. *N Engl J Med* 1989; **320**: 479–84.

30 Fisher B, Dignam J, Wolmark N, *et al.* Tamoxifen and chemotherapy for lymph node-negative, estrogen receptor-positive breast cancer. *J Natl Cancer Inst* 1997; **89**: 1673–82.

31 Fisher B, Costantino JP, Wickerham DL, *et al.* Tamoxifen for prevention of breast cancer: report of the National Surgical Adjuvant Breast and Bowel Project P-1 Study. *J Natl Cancer Inst* 1998; **90**: 1371–88.

32 Cuzick J, Forbes J, Edwards R, *et al.* First results from the International Breast Cancer Intervention Study (IBIS-I): a randomised prevention trial. *Lancet* 2002; **360**: 817–24.

33 Goldhaber SZ. Tamoxifen: preventing breast cancer and placing the risk of deep vein thrombosis in perspective. *Circulation* 2005; **111**: 539–41.

34 Weiss RB, Tormey DC, Holland JF, Weinberg VE. Venous thrombosis during multimodal treatment of primary breast carcinoma. *Cancer Treat Rep* 1981; **65**: 677–9.

35 Levine MN, Gent M, Hirsh J, *et al.* The thrombogenic effect of anticancer drug therapy in women with stage II breast cancer. *N Engl J Med* 1988; **318**: 404–7.

36 Fisher B, Redmond C, Legault-Poisson S, *et al.* Postoperative chemotherapy and tamoxifen compared with tamoxifen alone in the treatment of positive-node breast cancer patients aged 50 years and older with tumors responsive to tamoxifen: results from the National Surgical Adjuvant Breast and Bowel Project B-16. *J Clin Oncol* 1990; **8**: 1005–18.

37 Clahsen PC, van de Velde CJ, Julien JP, *et al.* Thromboembolic complications after perioperative chemotherapy in women with early breast cancer: a European Organization for Research and Treatment of Cancer Breast Cancer Cooperative Group study. *J Clin Oncol* 1994; **12**: 1266–71.

38 Pritchard KI, Paterson AH, Paul NA, *et al.* Increased thromboembolic complications with concurrent tamoxifen and chemotherapy in a randomized trial of adjuvant therapy for women with breast cancer. National Cancer Institute of Canada Clinical Trials Group Breast Cancer Site Group. *J Clin Oncol* 1996; **14**: 2731–7.

39 Saphner T, Tormey DC, Gray R. Venous and arterial thrombosis in patients who received adjuvant therapy for breast cancer. *J Clin Oncol* 1991; **9**: 286–94.

40 von Tempelhoff GF, Schonmann N, Heilmann L. Thrombosis – a clue of poor prognosis in primary non-metastatic breast cancer? *Breast Cancer Res Treat* 2002; **73**: 275–7.

41 Rivkin SE, Green S, Metch B, *et al.* Adjuvant CMFVP versus tamoxifen versus concurrent CMFVP and tamoxifen for postmenopausal, node-positive, and estrogen receptor-positive breast cancer patients: a Southwest Oncology Group study. *J Clin Oncol* 1994; **12**: 2078–85.

42 Howell T, on behalf of the ATAC Trialists Group. The ATAC ('Arimidex', Tamoxifen, Alone or in Combination) trial in postmenopausal women with early breast cancer updated efficacy results based on median follow-up of 5 years. Presented at the 27th Annual San Antonio Breast Cancer Symposium, San Antonio, TX, December 8, 2004.

43 ATAC Trial. Anastrozole alone or in combination with tamoxifen versus tamoxifen alone for adjuvant treatment of postmenopausal women with early breast cancer: first results of the ATAC randomised trial. *Lancet* 2002; **359**: 2131–9.

44 Bonneterre J, Buzdar A, Nabholtz JM, *et al.* Anastrozole is superior to tamoxifen as first-line therapy in hormone receptor-positive advanced breast carcinoma. *Cancer* 2001; **92**: 2247–58.

45 Mortimer JE, Urban JH. Long-term toxicities of selective estrogen-receptor modulators and antiaromatase agents. *Oncology (Huntingt)* 2003; **17**: 652–9.

46 Goodnough LT, Saito H, Manni A, *et al.* Increased incidence of thromboembolism in stage IV breast cancer patients treated with a five-drug chemotherapy regimen. A study of 159 patients. *Cancer* 1984; **54**: 1264–8.

47 Levine M, Hirsh J, Gent M, *et al.* Double-blind randomised trial of a very-low-dose warfarin for prevention of thromboembolism in stage IV breast cancer. *Lancet* 1994; **343**: 886–9.

48 von Tempelhoff GF, Heilmann L. Antithrombotic therapy in gynecologic surgery and gynecologic oncology. *Hematol Oncol Clin North Am* 2000; **14**: 1151–69, ix.

49 Simons JP, Aaronson NK, Vansteenkiste JF, *et al.* Effects of medroxyprogesterone acetate on appetite, weight, and quality of life in advanced-stage non-hormone-sensitive cancer: a placebo-controlled multicenter study. *J Clin Oncol* 1996; **14**: 1077–84.

50 Anonymous. Protective effect of high-dose medroxyprogesterone acetate (HD-MPA) on hematological toxicity induced by chemotherapy for advanced solid tumors: a multicentric controlled clinical trial. *Chemiotherapia* 1986; **5**: 134–9.

51 Sorensen HT, Mellemkjaer L, Olsen JH, Baron JA. Prognosis of cancers associated with venous thromboembolism. *N Engl J Med* 2000; **343**: 1846–50.

52 Levitan N, Dowlati A, Remick SC, *et al.* Rates of initial and recurrent thromboembolic disease among patients with malignancy versus those without malignancy. Risk analysis using Medicare claims data. *Medicine (Baltimore)* 1999; **78**: 285–91.

53 Blom JW, Vanderschoot JP, Oostindier MJ, *et al.* Incidence of venous thrombosis in a large cohort of 66,329 cancer patients: results of a record linkage study. *J Thromb Haemost* 2006; **4**: 529–35.

54 Tateo S, Mereu L, Salamano S, *et al.* Ovarian cancer and venous thromboembolic risk. *Gynecol Oncol* 2005; **99**: 119–25.

55 von Tempelhoff GF, Dietrich M, Niemann F, *et al.* Blood coagulation and thrombosis in patients with ovarian malignancy. *Thromb Haemost* 1997; **77**: 456–61.

56 Wun T, Law L, Harvey D, *et al.* Increased incidence of symptomatic venous thrombosis in patients with cervical carcinoma treated with concurrent chemotherapy, radiation, and erythropoietin. *Cancer* 2003; **98**: 1514–20.

57 Lavey RS, Liu PY, Greer BE, *et al.* Recombinant human erythropoietin as an adjunct to radiation therapy and cisplatin for stage IIB-IVA carcinoma of the cervix: a Southwest Oncology Group study. *Gynecol Oncol* 2004; **95**: 145–51.

58 Rosenzweig MQ, Bender CM, Lucke JP, *et al.* The decision to prematurely terminate a trial of R-HuEPO due to thrombotic events. *J Pain Symptom Manage* 2004; **27**: 185–90.

59 White RH, Zhou H, Romano PS. Incidence of symptomatic venous thromboembolism after different elective or urgent surgical procedures. *Thromb Haemost* 2003; **90**: 446–55.

60 Clarke-Pearson DL, Synan IS, Creasman WT. Anticoagulation therapy for venous thromboembolism in patients with gynecologic malignancy. *Am J Obstet Gynecol* 1983; **147**: 369–75.

61 Clarke-Pearson DL, Creasman WT, Coleman RE, *et al.* Perioperative external pneumatic calf compression as thromboembolism prophylaxis in gynecologic

oncology: report of a randomized controlled trial. *Gynecol Oncol* 1984; **18**: 226–32.

62 Clarke-Pearson DL, Synan IS, Hinshaw WM, *et al.* Prevention of postoperative venous thromboembolism by external pneumatic calf compression in patients with gynecologic malignancy. *Obstet Gynecol* 1984; **63**: 92–8.

63 Clarke-Pearson DL, DeLong E, Synan IS, *et al.* A controlled trial of two low-dose heparin regimens for the prevention of postoperative deep vein thrombosis. *Obstet Gynecol* 1990; **75**: 684–9.

64 Clarke-Pearson DL, Synan IS, Colemen RE, *et al.* The natural history of postoperative venous thromboemboli in gynecologic oncology: a prospective study of 382 patients. *Am J Obstet Gynecol* 1984; **148**: 1051–4.

65 Crandon AJ, Koutts J. Incidence of post-operative deep vein thrombosis in gynaecological oncology. *Aust N Z J Obstet Gynaecol* 1983; **23**: 216–19.

66 Walsh JJ, Bonnar J, Wright FW. A study of pulmonary embolism and deep leg vein thrombosis after major gynaecological surgery using labelled fibrinogen-phlebography and lung scanning. *J Obstet Gynaecol Br Commonw* 1974; **81**: 311–16.

67 Clarke-Pearson DL, Jelovsek FR, Creasman WT. Thromboembolism complicating surgery for cervical and uterine malignancy: incidence, risk factors, and prophylaxis. *Obstet Gynecol* 1983; **61**: 87–94.

68 Clarke-Pearson DL, Dodge RK, Synan I, *et al.* Venous thromboembolism prophylaxis: patients at high risk to fail intermittent pneumatic compression. *Obstet Gynecol* 2003; **101**: 157–63.

69 Kakkar VV, Howe CT, Nicolaides AN, *et al.* Deep vein thrombosis of the leg. Is there a 'high risk' group? *Am J Surg* 1970; **120**: 527–30.

70 Kakkar AK, Williamson RC. Prevention of venous thromboembolism in cancer patients. *Semin Thromb Hemost* 1999; **25**: 239–43.

71 IMT. Prevention of fatal postoperative pulmonary embolism by low doses of heparin. An international multicentre trial. *Lancet* 1975; **2**: 45–51.

72 Mismetti P, Laporte S, Darmon JY, *et al.* Meta-analysis of low molecular weight heparin in the prevention of venous thromboembolism in general surgery. *Br J Surg* 2001; **88**: 913–30.

73 Maxwell GL, Myers ER, Clarke-Pearson DL. Cost-effectiveness of deep venous thrombosis prophylaxis in gynecologic oncology surgery. *Obstet Gynecol* 2000; **95**: 26–14.

74 Heilmann L, von Tempelhoff GF, Kirkpatrick C, *et al.* Comparison of unfractionated versus low molecular weight heparin for deep vein thrombosis prophylaxis during breast and pelvic cancer surgery: efficacy, safety, and follow-up. *Clin Appl Thromb Hemost* 1998; **4**: 268–73.

75 Fricker JP, Vergnes Y, Schach R, *et al.* Low dose heparin versus low molecular weight heparin (Kabi 2165, Fragmin) in the prophylaxis of thromboembolic complications of abdominal oncological surgery. *Eur J Clin Invest* 1988; **18**: 561–7.

76 Oates-Whitehead RM, D'Angelo A, Mol B. Anticoagulant and aspirin prophylaxis for preventing thromboembolism after major gynaecological surgery. *Cochrane Database Syst Rev* 2003: CD003679.

77 Ailawadi M, Del Priore G. A comparison of thromboembolic prophylaxis in gynecologic oncology patients. *Int J Gynecol Cancer* 2001; **11**: 354–8.

78 Bergqvist D, Agnelli G, Cohen AT, *et al.* Duration of prophylaxis against venous thromboembolism with enoxaparin after surgery for cancer. *N Engl J Med* 2002; **346**: 975–80.

79 Rasmussen MS. Preventing thromboembolic complications in cancer patients after surgery: a role for prolonged thromboprophylaxis. *Cancer Treat Rev* 2002; **28**: 141–4.

80 Samama MM, Cohen AT, Darmon JY, *et al.* A comparison of enoxaparin with placebo for the prevention of venous thromboembolism in acutely ill medical patients. Prophylaxis in Medical Patients with Enoxaparin Study Group. *N Engl J Med* 1999; **341**: 793–800.

81 Cohen AT, Davidson BL, Gallus AS, *et al.* Efficacy and safety of fondaparinux for the prevention of venous thromboembolism in older acute medical patients: randomised placebo controlled trial. *BMJ* 2006; **332**: 325–9.

82 Leizorovicz A, Cohen AT, Turpie AG, *et al.* Randomized, placebo-controlled trial of dalteparin for the prevention of venous thromboembolism in acutely ill medical patients. *Circulation* 2004; **110**: 174–9.

83 Geerts WH, Pineo GF, Heit JA, *et al.* Prevention of venous thromboembolism: the Seventh ACCP Conference on Antithrombotic and Thrombolytic Therapy. *Chest* 2004; **126**(3 Suppl): 338S-400S.

84 Hutten BA, Prins MH, Gent M, *et al.* Incidence of recurrent thromboembolic and bleeding complications among patients with venous thromboembolism in relation to both malignancy and achieved international normalized ratio: a retrospective analysis. *J Clin Oncol* 2000; **18**: 3078–83.

85 Prandoni P, Lensing AW, Piccioli A, *et al.* Recurrent venous thromboembolism and bleeding complications during anticoagulant treatment in patients with cancer and venous thrombosis. *Blood* 2002; **100**: 3484–8.

86 van Dongen CJ, van den Belt AG, Prins MH, Lensing AW. Fixed dose subcutaneous low molecular weight heparins versus adjusted dose unfractionated heparin for venous thromboembolism. *Cochrane Database Syst Rev* 2004: CD001100.

87 Hettiarachchi RJ, Prins MH, Lensing AW, Buller HR. Low molecular weight heparin versus unfractionated heparin in the initial treatment of venous thrombo-embolism. *Curr Opin Pulm Med* 1998; **4**: 220–5.

88 Gould MK, Dembitzer AD, Doyle RL, *et al.* Low-molecular-weight heparins compared with unfractionated heparin for treatment of acute deep venous thrombosis. A meta-analysis of randomized, controlled trials. *Ann Intern Med* 1999; **130**: 800–9.

89 Dolovich LR, Ginsberg JS, Douketis JD, *et al*. A meta-analysis comparing low-molecular-weight heparins with unfractionated heparin in the treatment of venous thromboembolism: examining some unanswered questions regarding location of treatment, product type, and dosing frequency. *Arch Intern Med* 2000; **160**: 181–8.

90 Levine M, Gent M, Hirsh J, *et al*. A comparison of low-molecular-weight heparin administered primarily at home with unfractionated heparin administered in the hospital for proximal deep-vein thrombosis. *N Engl J Med* 1996; **334**: 677–81.

91 Koopman MM, Prandoni P, Piovella F, Ockelford PA, Brandjes DP, van der MJ *et al*. Treatment of venous thrombosis with intravenous unfractionated heparin administered in the hospital as compared with subcutaneous low-molecular-weight heparin administered at home. The Tasman Study Group. *N Engl J Med* 1996; **334**: 682–7.

92 Columbus Investigators. Low-molecular-weight heparin in the treatment of patients with venous thromboembolism. The Columbus Investigators. *N Engl J Med* 1997; **337**: 657–62.

93 Harrison L, McGinnis J, Crowther M, *et al*. Assessment of outpatient treatment of deep-vein thrombosis with low-molecular-weight heparin [see comments]. *Arch Intern Med* 1998; **158**: 2001–3.

94 Wells PS, Kovacs MJ, Bormanis J, *et al*. Expanding eligibility for outpatient treatment of deep venous thrombosis and pulmonary embolism with low-molecular-weight heparin: a comparison of patient self-injection with homecare injection [see comments]. *Arch Intern Med* 1998; **158**: 1809–12.

95 Merli G, Spiro TE, Olsson CG, *et al*. Subcutaneous enoxaparin once or twice daily compared with intravenous unfractionated heparin for treatment of venous thromboembolic disease. *Ann Intern Med* 2001; **134**: 191–202.

96 Kakkar AK, Breddin HK, Kakkar VV, Kadziola ZA. Treatment of deep vein thrombosis in cancer: a comparison of unfractionated and low molecular weight heparin. *Blood* 2000; **96**: 449a.

97 Simonneau G, Sors H, Charbonnier B, *et al*. A comparison of low-molecular-weight heparin with unfractionated heparin for acute pulmonary embolism. The THESEE Study Group. Tinzaparine ou Heparine Standard: Evaluations dans l'Embolie Pulmonaire. *N Engl J Med* 1997; **337**: 663–9.

98 Kovacs MJ, Anderson D, Morrow B, *et al*. Outpatient treatment of pulmonary embolism with dalteparin. *Thromb Haemost* 2000; **83**: 209–11.

99 Decousus H, Leizorovicz A, Parent F, *et al*. A clinical trial of vena caval filters in the prevention of pulmonary embolism in patients with proximal deep-vein thrombosis. Prevention du Risque d'Embolie Pulmonaire par Interruption Cave Study Group. *N Engl J Med* 1998; **338**: 409–15.

♦ 100 Streiff MB. Vena caval filters: a comprehensive review. *Blood* 2000; **95**: 3669–77.

101 Hull RD. Changes in the technology of inferior vena cava filters promise improved benefits to the patient with less harm, but a paucity of evidence exists. *J Thromb Haemost* 2005; **3**: 1368–9.

102 Imberti D, Bianchi M, Farina A, *et al*. Clinical experience with retrievable vena cava filters: results of a prospective observational multicenter study. *J Thromb Haemost* 2005; **3**: 1370–5.

103 Ansell J, Hirsh J, Poller L, *et al*. The pharmacology and management of the vitamin K antagonists: the Seventh ACCP Conference on Antithrombotic and Thrombolytic Therapy. *Chest* 2004; **126**(3 Suppl): 204S–233S.

104 Pini M, Aiello S, Manotti C, *et al*. Low molecular weight heparin versus warfarin in the prevention of recurrences after deep vein thrombosis. *Thromb Haemost* 1994; **72**: 191–7.

105 Das SK, Cohen AT, Edmondson RA, *et al*. Low-molecular-weight heparin versus warfarin for prevention of recurrent venous thromboembolism: a randomized trial. *World J Surg* 1996; **20**: 521–6.

106 Lopaciuk S, Bielska-Falda H, Noszczyk W, *et al*. Low-molecular-weight heparin versus acenocoumarol in the secondary prophylaxis of deep vein thrombosis. *Thromb Haemost* 1999; **81**: 26–31.

107 Gonzalez-Fajardo JA, Arreba E, Castrodeza J, *et al*. Venographic comparison of subcutaneous low-molecular-weight heparin with oral anticoagulant therapy in the long-term treatment of deep venous thrombosis. *J Vasc Surg* 1999; **30**: 283–92.

108 Veiga F, Escriba A, Maluenda MP, *et al*. Low-molecular-weight heparin (enoxaparin) versus oral anticoagulant therapy (acenocoumarol) in the long-term treatment of deep venous thrombosis in the elderly: a randomized trial. *Thromb Haemost* 2000; **84**: 559–64.

109 Hull R, Pineo G, Mah A, Brant R, the LITE Investigators. Long-term low-molecular-weight heparin treatment versus oral anticoagulant therapy for proximal deep vein thrombosis. *Blood* 2000; **96**: 49a.

110 Iorio A, Guercini F, Pini M. Low-molecular-weight heparin for the long-term treatment of symptomatic venous thromboembolism: meta-analysis of the randomized comparisons with oral anticoagulants. *J Thromb Haemost* 2003; **1**: 1906–13.

111 Meyer G, Marjanovic Z, Valcke J, *et al*. Comparison of low-molecular-weight heparin and warfarin for the secondary prevention of venous thromboembolism in patients with cancer: a randomized controlled study. *Arch Intern Med* 2002; **162**: 1729–35.

112 Deitcher SR, Kessler CM, Merli G, *et al*. Secondary prevention of venous thromboembolic events (VTE) in patients with active malignancy: a randomized study of enoxaparin sodium alone vs. initial enoxaparin sodium followed by warfarin for a 180-day period. *J Thromb Haemost* 2003; **1**(Suppl 1): OC 194.

● 113   Lee AY, Levine MN, Baker RI, *et al.* Low-molecular-weight heparin versus a coumarin for the prevention of recurrent venous thromboembolism in patients with cancer. *N Engl J Med* 2003; **349**: 146–53.

114   Hull R, Pineo GF, Mah AF, Brant RF, for the LITE Investigators. A randomized trial evaluating long-term low-molecular-weight heparin therapy for three months vs. intravenous heparin followed by warfarin sodium in patients with current cancer. *J Thromb Haemost* 2003; **1**(Suppl 1): P1373.

★ 115   Buller HR, Agnelli G, Hull RD, *et al.* Antithrombotic therapy for venous thromboembolic disease: the Seventh ACCP Conference on Antithrombotic and Thrombolytic Therapy. *Chest* 2004; **126**(3 Suppl): 401S–428S.

116   Agnelli G, Prandoni P, Santamaria MG, *et al.* Three months versus one year of oral anticoagulant therapy for idiopathic deep venous thrombosis. Warfarin Optimal Duration Italian Trial Investigators. *N Engl J Med* 2001; **345**: 165–9.

117   Kearon C, Gent M, Hirsh J, *et al.* A comparison of three months of anticoagulation with extended anticoagulation for a first episode of idiopathic venous thromboembolism. *N Engl J Med* 1999; **340**: 901–7.

118   Schulman S, Rhedin AS, Lindmarker P, Carlsson A, Larfars G, Nicol P *et al.* A comparison of six weeks with six months of oral anticoagulant therapy after a first episode of venous thromboembolism. Duration of Anticoagulation Trial Study Group. *N Engl J Med* 1995; **332**: 1661–5.

18

Management of pulmonary embolism and deep vein thrombosis

BRUCE L DAVIDSON

INTRODUCTION

Pulmonary embolism (PE) is a common, life-threatening, yet still misdiagnosed and mistreated disease. Many aspects of the management of PE have changed significantly in recent years, whereas others have not. Deep vein thrombosis (DVT) is rarely life-threatening, but its management can have lasting consequences. Also, it is frequently associated with PE. This chapter summarizes key aspects of diagnosis and treatment of PE and DVT. Readers are referred to key texts and longer reviews for specific areas of interest.

PULMONARY EMBOLISM

Diagnosis

It is critical to understand that the vast majority of clinical studies of PE diagnosis have included symptomatic outpatients rather than inpatients. Inpatients have increased disease burden and more complicated illnesses. As predictive values of diagnostic tests depend to a great degree on the preexisting probability of having a PE, and this can be more difficult to estimate in complicated inpatients, it is understandable that the predictive values of diagnostic tests for PE may be lower for inpatients. In outpatients, the incidence of a proved PE with a 'negative' D-dimer accompanied by a 'low clinical probability' is ≤1 percent.[1] Two warnings pertain regarding using this information: (i) this does not apply to borderline D-dimer values; and (ii) inexperienced physicians should use a clinical scoring system

to arrive at their estimate of clinical probability. In outpatients, a management study of suspected PE has shown that no treatment is needed if the following three conditions pertain:[2]

- clinical suspicion is low or moderate
- duplex ultrasound of both proximal lower extremities (including the popliteal vein) is normal
- the contrast helical computed tomography (CT) pulmonary angiogram is truly negative (a CT that shows isolated subsegmental clot is considered indeterminate – not negative, not positive).

If clinical suspicion is high, further testing is required.

The usefulness of D-dimer testing remains controversial in inpatients, in part due to a high percentage of 'positive' D-dimer values consequent to a broad spectrum of diseases (other than PE) and procedures related to the hospitalization. Moreover, for inpatients, a negative D-dimer reduces suspicion but its sensitivity is only 89 percent, unsatisfactory to exclude PE.[3] If the helical contrast CT angiogram is negative and ultrasound is negative, there is still a 5 percent false-negative rate for inpatients.[2] There are no convincing data regarding a negative CT on its own for inpatients. Accordingly, CT and D-dimer evidence may add information but conventional pulmonary arteriography may still be required to make a secure diagnosis. In its absence, a 'clinical' decision to treat (and suspend treatment, if contraindications supervene) may be required. Fortunately, a 6-month course of treatment is usually safe. Multi-slice CT for confirmation and exclusion of pulmonary embolism appears to be more promising than prior CT technology but sensitivity was only 83 percent even after excluding indeterminate scans. Adding scanning of the pelvis and proximal lower extremity veins to the thorax scan only increased sensitivity to 90 percent.[4] The claim by some authors[5] that identification by CT of other pathology in the chest helps exclude PE and explains chest symptoms is not persuasive to this author, since occult pulmonary embolism can accompany many of these other diseases (lung cancer, pleural effusion, emphysema, etc.).

Special considerations apply to imaging tests of PE in pregnant and postpartum women. For many years it was recommended that pregnant women preferentially undergo radionuclide scanning (with half the usual dose of injected radioactivity compensated for by longer scan acquisition time) rather than radiographs because of the belief that the former exposed the mother and fetus to less radiation. Subsequently it has been proposed that CT scanning delivers less radiation to the gravid uterus than the radiolabeled technetium, which collects in the urinary bladder adjoining the uterus prior to urinary excretion.[6] Therefore, CT scanning with shielding below the diaphragm appears a safe method to use in pregnant women.

Additionally, there has been concern but little evidence regarding possible unsafe effects on neonatal thyroid function of breastfeeding infants when a mother is given intravenously administered radiocontrast for pulmonary embolism diagnosis. Updated European and North American recommendations differ somewhat. Currently, European experts recommend no interruption in breastfeeding;[7] North American experts recommend emptying the breast of milk prior to injection of radiocontrast for feeding of the baby, emptying and dumping breast milk 12 hours after radiocontrast injection, and resuming breastfeeding normally thereafter.

Oxygenation

A pulse oximeter should be employed on every encounter with the patient with PE and supplementary oxygen supplied as needed to keep the oxygen saturation >92 percent. Patients' oxygenation should be checked with activity (for example, stair-climbing), since most will do such minimal activity as outpatients. Supplemental oxygen, especially in patients with overload of the right ventricle and coexisting hypoxemia, is itself a pulmonary artery vasodilator which can decrease pulmonary artery pressure and vascular resistance elevated by pulmonary embolism and therefore improve right ventricular (and overall) cardiac output. Failure to maintain acceptable oxygen saturation during activity is an important finding requiring further close observation of the patient until cardiopulmonary hemodynamics improve. When patients can carry out activities of daily living without oxyhemoglobin desaturation, supplemental oxygen is no longer needed and may be discontinued.

Hemoptysis

Hemoptysis often accompanies PE sometime during its course and may be safely ignored most of the time – it is usually attributable to pulmonary infarction. Under these circumstances, it is not a contraindication to anticoagulation and patients may be reassured that it will stop soon. In rare instances, when persistent or of large volume, it may be a signal of an undiscovered bronchogenic tumor that warrants bronchoscopic airway examination when the patient stabilizes. Primary lung cancer or pulmonary metastases of various tumors can coexist with PE.

Pleuritic pain

Pleuritic-type pain, parasternal or in the back, and aggravated by coughing and deep breathing, is common with PE and is often a presenting symptom. It is easily relieved by indometacin[8] which we dose at 50 mg every 6–8 hours, or perhaps with another nonsteroidal anti-inflammatory drug prescribed at appropriate dosage and intervals. The author prophylactically administers 30 ml antacid with each dose to prevent dyspeptic distress. Pleuritic-type pain is reduced within 24 hours with this regimen and usually eliminated within 48 hours. There are no clinical reports to support the theoretical concern of increased bleeding risk due to possible platelet inhibition by short-term use of such nonsteroidal anti-inflammatory drugs. Moreover, there is usually no need for narcotic pain relief with its attendant constipation and sleepiness preventing ambulation.

Pleural effusion

Pleural effusion is common, is usually unilateral, an exudate, bloody a little less than half the time if it is sampled, and occupies <50 percent of the hemithorax.[9] Draining a pleural effusion secondary to pulmonary embolism is not necessary, but thoracentesis is sometimes done before the diagnosis is made or before anticoagulation is begun. If the patient is already anticoagulated, bleeding sites to which pressure cannot be directly applied should be minimized, precluding elective thoracentesis.

Low cardiac output

Low cardiac output frequently accompanies clinically significant PE. Clinical signs include tachycardia, weakness, and dyspnea with limited exertion. The pathophysiology is that obstructed pulmonary arteries and resulting hypoxia lead to increased pulmonary artery resistance and pressures and decreased delivery of oxygenated blood to the left heart. An enlarged right atrium and ventricle encroaches upon left ventricular filling. It is critical to recognize that these signs point to serious cardiopulmonary compromise, whatever the measured oxygen saturation at rest. Urine output should be monitored closely, oxygen administration and minimal exertion enforced, and the patient transferred to the intensive care unit and given pressor if required.[10]

Shock

Shock is considered present when there is underperfusion of vital tissues, usually accompanied by hypotension. Consider thrombolytic therapy if shock is due to PE and there is no contraindication. Drug choices include recombinant tissue plasminogen activator (r-tPA) (100 mg intravenously over 2 hours), streptokinase (1.5 million units infused over 1 hour [an unapproved regimen];[11] or 250 000 U as an intravenous bolus, followed by 100 000 U/h for 24 hours), and other drugs approved in various countries.[12] Other techniques, including pulmonary embolectomy, catheter clot fragmentation, pulmonary artery angioplasty, clot retrieval, and surgery on cardiopulmonary bypass have also been employed in selected patients.[13] For such therapy to be life-saving, it should, when possible, be given before the patient is in extremis and in a way that minimizes risk of subsequent complications (such as anticoagulant-induced bleeding). Different institutions will have different experience levels with these therapies.[14,15]

'Submassive pulmonary embolism'

Submassive PE is PE without shock but with echocardiographic evidence of right ventricular dysfunction. The argument for echocardiography in this setting is that echocardiography reveals many patients with right ventricular dysfunction (inconsistently defined) without overt shock, and that thrombolysis may save the lives of some such patients who would have a poor outcome. Of patients with acute PE, 31 percent have such findings without shock; this is 40 percent of the normotensive patients with PE.[16] Thrombolysis generally reduces pulmonary vascular obstruction when baseline and 24-hour perfusion lung scans or pulmonary arteriography have been employed for evaluation. Moreover, a recently published controlled, partially-blinded clinical trial[17] showed that if 'escalation of therapy' were the outcome, r-tPA followed by unfractionated heparin was superior to unfractionated heparin in such patients. The increased incidence of treatment escalation (25 percent in heparin vs. 11 percent in tPA recipients, $P = 0.006$) was due to a statistically significantly increased 'requirement' for thrombolysis (determined after unblinding) in the heparin recipients (23 percent vs. 8 percent in the tPA recipients). Moreover, the heparin recipients had a higher incidence of major bleeding (3.6 vs. 0.8 percent) and fatal bleeding, and no patients had hemorrhagic stroke. These safety results are quite contrary to prior reports. This study report prompted several published rebuttal letters.

The arguments against thrombolysis for submassive PE are that although it improves pulmonary perfusion at the end of day 1, day 7 perfusion is not changed and conflicting data exist about whether mortality is improved. Also, previous studies have shown intravenous thrombolysis increases the intracranial hemorrhage rate from 0.2 percent with heparin alone to around 2.2 percent, and the major bleeding rate from about 2 percent with heparin alone to 6–15 percent, depending on the study.[18] Modeling of thrombolysis use employing the incidence figures cited above (not those from the recently published Konstantinides study[17]) would lead to approximately 1800 excess hemorrhagic strokes per 300 000 incident patients with PE. This is a large safety cost, in addition to the economic cost. For these reasons, many experts recommend reserving thrombolysis for patients with shock.

One approach to the uncertainty regarding the best methodology for determining when to escalate therapy to thrombolysis (pharmacologic or mechanical) and how to determine if further escalation or repeat of therapy is required has been to monitor patients in ways that might be superior to echocardiography. Some experts consider echocardiography as imprecise and instead recommend sequential determinations of brain natriuretic peptide because it is short-lived in plasma and movement toward normal suggests reduction in cardiac wall strain.[19]

DEEP VEIN THROMBOSIS

Diagnosis

Compression ultrasound, usually augmented by evaluation of Doppler flow signals (therefore 'duplex' ultrasound, with or without the Doppler signal expressed as a color map) is the usual method of diagnosing DVT of the lower extremities. Ultrasound is highly accurate in the popliteal fossa and above, but less accurate below the trifurcation of calf veins (which is usually found 8–10 cm distal to the popliteal fossa crease). There are notable exceptions, that is, centers where management studies have validated accuracy of positive and negative ultrasound results in the calf.[20] Contrast venography, magnetic resonance imaging (MRI), and CT with radiocontrast evaluation of the pelvic and leg veins are alternative methods of evaluating veins of the lower extremities for clot. The key challenge in such imaging is distinguishing old from new clot, and although recommendations exist for doing this, experts acknowledge that it can be difficult in some cases.

D-dimer assay results and clinical presentation characteristics have been used separately and together to assist in deciding whom to image, and together with an imaging result to help decide whom to treat. As with diagnosis of PE, the evidence for the validity of these algorithms applies primarily to outpatients. D-dimer results, for example, are significantly less predictive of thromboembolism when studied in inpatients.

Pain, swelling, and bedrest

Pain and swelling are often presenting symptoms of DVT. Commonly they evolve over several days before the patient presents for diagnosis. Besides anticoagulation, treatment should be directed to the painful, swollen extremity. Some of the discomfort is due to tissue swelling and this can often be rapidly relieved by elevation above the heart (easiest for upper extremity DVT but can also be accomplished for lower extremity DVT). Cool compresses may help relieve skin discomfort. If there might be skin infection, bacteriologic culture followed by warm compresses may forestall the need for systemic antibiotics. There is no persuasive evidence for or against use of nonsteroidal anti-inflammatory medications as other than alternatives to analgesics, but they are often used. Compressive wrapping of the extremity with a bandage followed by ambulation has been shown superior to bedrest alone for pain relief and improving mobility in lower extremity DVT.[21] There was no difference in venous thromboembolism recurrence during follow-up. For this reason, compression of the affected extremity followed by its use unless discomfort is limiting is commonly recommended at present. There is no scientific evidence to support limiting ambulation because of worsening the involved extremity or dislodging clot and causing PE.

Extremity ischemia after deep vein thrombosis

Phlegmasia cerulea dolens is a syndrome in which venous hypertension of an extremity jeopardizes its tissue oxygenation. Proximal venous occlusion is the cause but initial thrombosis is not always the etiology: infection with fasciitis is a well-recognized cause. When extremity ischemia complicates DVT, careful weighing of approaches should ensue. If tissue oxygenation is previously and chronically impaired due to arterial insufficiency, occlusive DVT of the common femoral vein may seriously jeopardize distal tissue. Careful surveillance of the affected extremity, with ultrasound evaluation of arterial flow, measurement of plasma lactic acid levels, and surgical consultation may be required to optimize management of fragile patients.

When DVT appears to be the cause of important tissue hypoxia, a number of approaches might be taken.[22] Catheter-directed thrombolysis of such a clot distal to its site has been recommended and is under study in multiple sites. Different thrombolytic drugs are being used. Bleeding risks have been significant in prior published series, but it is believed that bleeding is reduced and efficacy improved with local installation of the thrombolytic drug, rather than systemic administration. Another alternative is surgical thrombectomy. A third alternative is surgical decompression of the extremity. Surgery in fully anticoagulated patients will lead to increased bleeding, and surgery in patients who have received thrombolytic therapy may lead to uncontrollable bleeding. There is no evidence that any of these approaches reduces the subsequent incidence of postthrombotic syndrome in survivors. Accordingly, patients presenting with DVT, in whom examination suggests there may be compromise of tissue oxygenation, should be hospitalized and receive more intensive surveillance than patients without such risks.

Hospitalization versus outpatient follow-up

Controlled studies in carefully selected patients comparing hospitalization with outpatient low-molecular-weight heparin treatment convincingly show similar efficacy and safety with respect to thromboembolism recurrence and bleeding risks. Outpatient treatment with subcutaneous anticoagulant injections followed by oral vitamin K antagonist with monitoring, along with office surveillance of treatment progress, will be more convenient for most patients and reduce healthcare costs in most instances. However, patients with complicated illness, inability to fully cooperate with all aspects of treatment, increased bleeding and/or thrombosis risks, and related problems should be hospitalized until these can be sorted out to assure successful continuation of therapy in the outpatient setting, if possible. Moreover, patients treated outside the hospital with worsening symptoms should be admitted, since this usually reflects incomplete adherence to therapy or alternative diagnoses.

Duration of pulmonary embolism treatment

Most commonly, patients receive a minimum of 6 months of treatment. Occasionally, some physicians will use 3 months of treatment after relief of a temporary risk factor. The British Thoracic Society[23] recently recommended 4–6 weeks of treatment in this latter circumstance, a recommendation with which this author cannot agree. There is renewed interest in re-imaging the pulmonary vasculature (for example, with a radionuclide perfusion scan or CT scan) when treatment cessation is considered, to confirm resolution or help decide, in conjunction with the patient, to continue therapy (see below, 'Chronic thromboembolic pulmonary hypertension').

Initial anticoagulant therapy

Initial anticoagulant therapy must be injected, concurrent for at least 5 days with oral anticoagulant often started the first day, and the patient must have an international normalized ratio (INR) >2.0 (target 2.5) for two consecutive days to assure it is safe to discontinue initial injected anticoagulant therapy.[12,24] Although sometimes this can be accomplished in 4–5 days, more often it takes 6–9 days in the setting of PE.[25] Since injected anticoagulants are more effective than oral anticoagulants, patients who are not recovering well from PE should remain on injected anticoagulant until they do improve substantially, even if the INR criterion is met earlier with an oral vitamin K antagonist. The latter patients can continue to receive both drugs together until their impairment from PE improves sufficiently that injected anticoagulant is judged no longer to be required.

There are several acceptable choices for injected initial anticoagulant therapy. They include unfractionated heparin, 80 U/kg intravenous bolus, then 18 U/kg per hour by continuous infusion in water with 5 percent dextrose. Patients are dosed by actual, rather than ideal body weight. This should be regulated with frequent monitoring of activated partial thromboplastin time (aPTT) (for example, every 6 hours at first, then as frequently as needed) to maintain the aPTT at 1.5–2.5 times the laboratory control value. Problems with this choice are: (i) the requirement for frequent monitoring and dose adjustment, (ii) the fact that evidence (Matisse investigators, unpublished data) suggests that if aPTT values fall below the target range, the risk of recurrence is increased, and (iii) the requirement for laboratories to determine the therapeutic range with each new batch of aPTT reagents and equipment changes, a requirement not commonly met. Advantages of this choice are the short half-life of infused heparin (60 minutes) and reversibility with protamine sulfate (1 mg per 100 U unfractionated heparin) if bleeding or bleeding risk requires cessation and reversal of anticoagulation.

Fondaparinux given subcutaneously once daily (5 mg for $<$50 kg, 7.5 mg for 50–100 kg, 10 mg for $>$100 kg)[25] is approved in the United States for treatment of PE and for DVT. The half-life of fondaparinux is 16 hours, allowing once-daily dosing. It does not require monitoring and was found to be comparable to intravenous heparin with respect to recurrence and bleeding in a large international clinical trial.[25] Advantages include minimal adjustment for weight, once-daily dosing (self-administered or with a health provider daily check-up), and the possibility of early discharge for selected patients at low risk for complications.

Several low-molecular-weight heparins have been studied for treatment in patients who have PE and concurrent DVT or DVT on its own.[26–30] Although some are approved for once-daily dosing, twice-daily dosing is preferred by some physicians, including this author, to increase the likelihood of maintaining adequate antithrombotic activity throughout a 24-hour period (these drugs have considerably shorter half-lives after subcutaneous injection than fondaparinux, for example, 6 hours). Like fondaparinux,[31] these do not require monitoring, and selected patients may be discharged early after observation.[25,30]

Patients with significant renal insufficiency have impaired hemostasis and may require downward adjustment of low-molecular-weight heparin or fondaparinux dosage. Regardless of the anticoagulant received, if patients with renal impairment bleed, hemostasis may require more attention than in other patients.

Special anticoagulation situations

OBESITY

Many patients with venous thromboembolism have a body mass index $>$25 (upper limit of normal) and some are quite obese. As dosages of intravenous unfractionated heparin

(for initial dosing prior to adjustments), low-molecular-weight heparins, and fondaparinux all depend upon the patient's weight, an area of uncertainty has been whether dosages should be 'capped' at some weight, such as 120 kg. For intravenous unfractionated heparin, the answer is no.[32] For the low-molecular-weight heparins, there is evidence that once-daily dalteparin[33] and tinzaparin[34] may be dosed by actual weight. There is no persuasive evidence that twice-daily enoxaparin dosages should have some upper limit, and no evidence to the contrary. There is evidence from clinical trials of fondaparinux for PE and DVT that patients weighing $>$100 kg (up to 176 kg) dosed with 10 mg subcutaneously once daily had recurrence and safety outcomes comparable to those weighing $<$100 kg and to the unfractionated heparin and enoxaparin patients enrolled in the studies. When these injectable drugs are chosen rather than vitamin K antagonists for subacute and stabilized patients (for example, after 2 weeks of treatment), this author recommends once daily dosing at actual body weight (low-molecular-weight heparins) or weight category (fondaparinux). If patient laboratory monitoring by anti-Xa assay is available, employing a standard curve created with the patient's specific anticoagulant, weekly checks of peak (4 h after dosing) and trough (just before the next dose) levels is recommended for a few weeks to assure stability. If bleeding or recurrent thrombosis supervene, obtaining a plasma anti-Xa level to later ascertain the anticoagulant level can be valuable in further management.

RENAL INSUFFICIENCY

Low-molecular-weight heparins and fondaparinux are primarily eliminated by renal excretion without prior metabolism. Therefore, if there is significant renal insufficiency, drug accumulation can be expected if usual dosages are employed. Moreover, since significant renal insufficiency is often associated with impaired hemostasis, care must be taken with extended dosing of these drugs to minimize bleeding risk. For these reasons, many physicians choose unfractionated heparin in these patients, with dose- rather than renal-function-dependent clearance, for acute treatment of PE, and vitamin K antagonists for continuing treatment.

Among the newer injected anticoagulants for acute treatment of PE and DVT, once daily subcutaneous fondaparinux was studied in patients with serum creatinine below 2 mg/dL (176 μmol/L); there is no significant experience for its use for treatment in renal insufficiency worse than this. Low-molecular-weight heparins have been studied in patients with a broad range of serum creatinine concentrations and estimated clearance. The conclusion of a recent thoughtful review is that although data are limited, the low-molecular-weight heparin tinzaparin can likely be dosed once daily at its usual treatment dosage of 175 U/kg once daily until the estimated creatinine clearance is below 20 mL/min.[35] Usual dosing of other low-molecular-weight heparins may lead to accumulation and bleeding risk when calculated creatinine clearance drops below 50 mL/min. Recently, the manufacturer of enoxaparin recommended reducing its daily treatment dosage by 50 percent, from 1 mg/kg every 12 hours to 1 mg/kg every 24 hours, in patients with calculated creatinine clearance <30 mL/min.

MEASURING INJECTED ANTICOAGULANT BLOOD LEVELS WITH ANTI-XA ASSAYS

Unlike unfractionated heparin, circulating low-molecular-weight heparins and fondaparinux levels cannot be reliably measured by the aPTT. The PT (INR) is similarly not predictive of the level of these drugs. For these reasons, measurement of activated factor X (anti-factor Xa, sometimes abbreviated aXa) level has become the prevalent measurement of these pharmacologic coagulation inhibitors in plasma. Most assays use a kit with an artificial substrate whose cleavage causes a color change, sufficient cofactors including antithrombin to facilitate inhibitor activity and factor Xa to enable the cleavage, and measure the reduction in substrate cleavage to calculate the concentration of factor Xa inhibitor (that is, drug level) in the plasma sample. Performance and interpretation of these assays is somewhat complex and dependent upon determining a standard curve with known concentrations of the same anticoagulant being assayed for in the patient's plasma. However, as the aPTT has been optimized to assay unfractionated heparin activity and INR to assay vitamin K antagonist effect, the anti-Xa assays have been optimized for low-molecular-weight heparins, and when 'pure' anti-Xa inhibitors like fondaparinux are assayed, aXa levels may overestimate the drug concentration. Moreover, 'therapeutic' and 'higher bleeding risk' aXa levels of fondaparinux and similar drugs in development may not be comparable to those estimated for low-molecular-weight heparins.

For low-molecular-weight heparins, treatment peak and trough levels (taken 4 and 12 [or 24] hours after a dose, respectively) should be in excess of 0.4 U/mL. Peak levels should be <1.5 (<1.0 is better) to reduce bleeding risk.

REVERSING ANTICOAGULANTS

Intravenous protamine sulfate, 1 mg/100 U unfractionated heparin, is used to reverse the latter's anticoagulant effect. Protamine administration may have to be repeated because it is cleared faster than heparin. If there is documented allergy to fish or NPH (neutral protamine Hagedorn) insulin, protamine should be given with caution. It is routinely used by many surgeons to reverse heparin effect as cardiac patients come off cardiopulmonary bypass. Unfractionated heparin is assumed to have a half-life after intravenous administration of 1 hour, and 4 hours after subcutaneous administration. Accordingly, an amount of residual heparin is estimated and protamine given.

Protamine is only partially effective in reversing biochemical activity of low-molecular-weight heparin (the anti-factor IIa [antithrombin] activity). Nonetheless, it can be part of a comprehensive effort to control and/or prevent bleeding in a patient given subcutaneous low-molecular-weight heparin. After a once-daily dose of low-molecular-weight heparin is given, protamine may need to be given several times, based on estimated residual activity (the half-life of subcutaneous low-molecular-weight heparin is approximately 6 hours). The protamine dosage is 1 mg/1 mg or 100 U of low-molecular-weight heparin. There is no evidence for protamine reversibility of fondaparinux.

Vitamin K antagonizes the anticoagulant effect of vitamin K antagonists but this takes approximately 12 hours. In patients with prothrombotic conditions after acute PE or DVT, care should be taken in administering vitamin K in high dosage, because thrombosis may extend. Because of the expected delay in vitamin K effect, fresh frozen plasma (which contains effective clotting factors missing endogenously after vitamin K antagonist administration) should also be administered when there is important bleeding and/or invasive procedures are required. Depending on seriousness of bleeding, partial or complete PT correction should be the goal.

Recombinant factor VIIa (NovoSeven), developed for hemophiliac patients with factor VIII inhibitors, has promise as a 'universal antidote' for bleeding. It acts rapidly after intravenous administration. The labeled dosage is 90 μg/kg per dose, but success has been reported with lower dosages (for example, 30 μg/kg per dose). Some authorities suggest giving more than 90 μg/kg per dose if bleeding is life-threatening and certain reversal is imperative (for example, for intracranial bleeding). Recently, one national group published guidelines for usage in life-threatening hemorrhage. Administration of 100–140 μg/kg body weight over 2–5 minutes was recommended; if hemorrhage persisted after 20 minutes, another 100 μg/kg was recommended.[36] Drawbacks of this drug include its high price and relatively short duration of activity (about 2 hours). Moreover, there is an ill-defined risk of increased arterial thrombotic events with its use.[37] However, there are numerous reports of hemostasis obtained after a single dose. The mechanism is presumed to be formation of a hemostatic plug for sufficient time to allow hemostasis that will persist even after the pharmacologic effect of the factor decays.

Essential for successful hemostasis in bleeding patients or those with trauma (surgical or otherwise) are adequate platelets and clotting factors, such as fibrinogen. Prothrombin may be reduced by 50 percent while the PT (INR) remains within the normal range. Accordingly, in anticoagulated patients who are bleeding, administration of fresh frozen plasma and other factors (platelet concentrates and packed red cells) as needed is as important as giving anticoagulant antidotes.

Vena cava interruption

Recently developed retrievable inferior vena cava filters (and permanent ones) should be used when a contraindication to injected anticoagulant is sufficiently grave to prevent its use. When the contraindication remits, anticoagulant therapy should be started. Implanted permanent vena cava filters significantly increase the rate of recurrent DVT at 2 years.[38]

Chronic anticoagulation therapy

Vitamin K antagonists (for example, warfarin, acenocoumarol) are begun orally, usually once daily, when patients are considered sufficiently stable that they will not require immediate reversal of anticoagulation, since reversal with vitamin K and fresh frozen plasma requires many hours. These drugs are begun with daily maintenance dosages (for example, 4 mg or 5 mg once daily of warfarin) rather than loading dosages, because the latter may unpredictably reduce protein C and protein S and risk the warfarin necrosis syndrome. They are continued until the INR is >2.0 for 2 consecutive days. After the criterion of 5 consecutive days of injected anticoagulant therapy has been met, the injected anticoagulant can be discontinued if other criteria are met. In community practice, the INR target of 2.5 is rarely consistently achieved.[39] The range of 2.0–3.0 is met approximately 50–60 percent of the time. In specialty clinics and studies, it is met approximately two-thirds of the time. Nonetheless, clinicians should keep trying to achieve excellence in oral anticoagulation despite the general challenges of monitoring and dosing and other challenges in specific patients. Some principles of anticoagulant adjustment include:

- make small changes up or down, equal to 15 percent of the total weekly dosage
- wait at least 5 days to see INR evidence of a changed dosage
- provide the patient a simple regimen. For example, if consistent daily dosage cannot be given provide a regimen for odd and even days, or certain days of the week (for example, Monday, Wednesday, Friday) rather than alternating dosage on alternate days, since patients tend to lose track with the lattermost approach.

Patients with cancer

Patients with cancer have higher risks of recurrence and bleeding than other patients when receiving acute and continued anticoagulant treatment for venous thromboembolism. Several studies suggest that prolonged injected anticoagulant (low-molecular-weight heparin) provides a better result. In some centers, unless there is no way to pay for prolonged injected anticoagulant, cancer patients with PE receive prolonged low-molecular-weight heparin (for example, dalteparin 200 U/kg once daily for one month, then 150–160 U/kg once daily;[40] or enoxaparin[41]) for 5 months or longer. Some centers use different low-molecular-weight heparins with supportive but less compelling data.

Chronic thromboembolic pulmonary hypertension

Recent data from the first published study[42] to follow the incidence of this disease in patients experiencing a first PE demonstrated it occurred in 4 percent of patients and was established by 2 years after the first event. A smaller study showed persistent measurable defects in cardiopulmonary function three years after an acute PE in patients who complied with usual therapy.[43] How to prevent this is uncertain at this time. Close attention to proper anticoagulation and sufficient oxygenation are reasonable suggestions while studies are developed. Some physicians, including the author, offer continued anticoagulant treatment if imaging studies show persistent clot at the time contemplated for anticoagulation to end. Patients with established thromboembolic pulmonary hypertension require therapeutic anticoagulation indefinitely, and possibly thromboendarterectomy.

KEY LEARNING POINTS

- Many aspects of the management of PE have changed significantly in recent years.
- Management of DVT can have lasting consequences.
- Predictive values of diagnostic tests for PE may be lower for inpatients. The usefulness of D-dimer testing remains controversial in inpatients, in part due to a high percentage of 'positive' D-dimer values consequent to a broad spectrum of diseases (other than PE) and procedures related to the hospitalization.
- A pulse oximeter should be employed on every encounter with the patient with PE and supplementary oxygen supplied as needed to keep the oxygen saturation >92 percent.
- The key challenge in imaging in DVT is distinguishing old from new clot, and it can be difficult in some cases. D-dimer results are significantly less predictive of thromboembolism when studied in inpatients.
- Outpatient treatment of DVT, with subcutaneous anticoagulant injections followed by oral vitamin K antagonist with monitoring, along with office surveillance of treatment progress, will be more convenient for most patients and reduce healthcare costs in most instances. If symptoms worsen these patients should be admitted to the hospital.
- Patients with complicated illness, inability to fully cooperate with all aspects of treatment, increased bleeding and/or thrombosis risks, and related problems should be hospitalized in the first instance.

REFERENCES

1   Kelly J, Hunt BJ. A clinical probability assessment and D-dimer measurement should be the initial step in the

investigation of suspected venous thromboembolism. *Chest* 2003; **124**: 1116–19.

2   Musset D, Parent F, Meyer G, *et al.* Diagnostic strategy for patients with suspected pulmonary embolism: a prospective multicentre outcome study. *Lancet* 2002; **360**: 1914–20.

3   Kuruvilla J, Wells PS, Morrow B, *et al.* Prospective assessment of the natural history of positive D-dimer results in persons with acute venous thromboembolism (DVT or PE). *Thromb Haemost* 2003; **89**: 284–7.

4   Stein PD, Fowler SE, Goodman LR et al. Multidetector computed tomography for acute pulmonary embolism. *N Engl J Med* 2006; **354**: 2317–27.

5   Marco JL, van Strijen MJL, Wouter de Monyé W, *et al.* Single-detector helical computed tomography as the primary diagnostic test in suspected pulmonary embolism: a multicenter clinical management study of 510 patients. *Ann Intern Med* 2003; **138**: 307–14.

6   Nijkeuter M, Geleijns J, De Roos A, *et al.* Diagnosing pulmonary embolism in pregnancy: rationalizing fetal radiation exposure in radiological procedures. *J Thromb Haemost* 2004; **2**: 1857–8.

7   Webb JAW, Thomsen HS, Morcos SK, and members of the Contrast Media Safety Committee of the European Society of Urogenital Radiology. Use of iodinated contrast and gadolinium contrast media during pregnancy and lactation. *Eur Radiol* 2005; **15**: 1234–40.

8   Sacks PV, Kanarek D. Treatment of acute pleuritic pain. *Am Rev Respir Dis* 1973; **108**: 666.

9   Bynum LK, Wilson JE III. Characteristics of pleural effusions associated with ulmonary embolism. *Arch Intern Med* 1976; **136**: 159.

10 Wood KE. Major pulmonary embolism: review of a pathophysiologic approach to the golden hour of hemodynamically significant pulmonary embolism. *Chest* 2002; **121**: 877–905.

11 Jerjes-Sanchez C, Ramirez-Rivera A, de Lourdes Garcia M, *et al.* Streptokinase and heparin versus heparin alone in massive pulmonary embolism: a randomized controlled trial. *J Thromb Thrombolysis* 1995; **2**: 227–9.

12 Buller HR, Agnelli G, Hull RD, *et al.* Antithrombotic therapy for venous thromboembolic disease: the seventh ACCP conference on anththrombotic and thrombolytic therapy. *Chest* 2004; **126**(Suppl): 401S–428S.

13 Aklog L, Wiliams CS, Byme JG, *et al.* Acute pulmonary embolectomy: a contemporary approach. *Circulation* 2002; **105**: 1416–19.

14 Meneveau N, Seronde M-F, Blonde M-C, *et al.* Management of unsuccessful thrombolysis in acute pulmonary embolism. *Chest* 2006; **129**: 1043–50.

15 Davidson BL, Karmy-Jones R. When pulmonary embolism treatment isn't working. *Chest* 2006; **129**: 839–40.

16 Grifoni S, Olivotto I, Cecchini P, *et al.* Short-term clinical outcome of patients with acute pulmonary embolism, normal blood pressure, and echocardiographic right ventricular dysfunction. *Circulation* 2000; **101**: 2817–22.

17 Konstantinides S, Geibel A, Heusel G, *et al.* Heparin plus alteplase compared with heparin alone in patients with submassive pulmonary embolism. *N Engl J Med* 2002; **347**: 1143–50.

18 Dalen JE. Thrombolysis in submassive pulmonary embolism? No. *J Thromb Haemost* 2003; **1**: 1130–2.

19 Torbicki A. Thrombolysis in submassive pulmonary embolism. *J Thromb Haemost* 2004; **2**: 1476.

20 Stevens SM, Elliott CG, Chan KJ, *et al.* Withholding anticoagulation after a negative result on duplex ultrasonography for suspected symptomatic deep venous thrombosis. *Ann Intern Med* 2004; **140**: 985–91.

21 Blattler W, Partsch H. Leg compression and ambulation is better than bedrest for the treatment of acute deep venous thrombosis. *Int Angiol* 2003; **22**: 393–400.

22 Dayal R, Bernheim J, Clair DG, *et al.* Multimodal percutaneous intervention for critical venous occlusive disease. *Ann Vasc Surg* 2005; **19**: 235–40.

23 British Thoracic Society guidelines for the management of suspected acute pulmonary embolism. *Thorax* 2003; **58**: 470–83.

24 Lensing AWA, Prandoni P, Prins MH, Buller HR. Deep-vein thrombosis. *Lancet* 1999; **353**: 479–85.

25 The Matisse Investigators. Subcutaneous fondaparinux versus intravenous unfractionated heparin in the initial treatment of pulmonary embolism. *N Engl J Med* 2004; **349**: 1695–702.

26 Merli G, Spiro TE, Olsson CG, *et al.* Subcutaneous enoxaparin once or twice daily compared with unfractionated heparin for treatment of venous thromboembolic disease. *Ann Intern Med* 2001; **143**: 191–202.

27 The Columbus Investigators. Low-molecular-weight heparin in the treatment of patients with venous thromboembolism. *N Engl J Med* 1997; **337**: 657–62.

28 Simonneau G, Sors H, Charbonnier B, *et al.* A comparison of low-molecular-weight heparin with unfractionated heparin for acute pulmonary embolism. *N Engl J Med* 1997; **337**: 663–9.

29 Breddin HK, Hach-Wunderle V, Nakov R, Kakkar VV, and CORTES investigators. Effects of a low-molecular-weight heparin on thrombus regression and recurrent thromboembolism in patients with deep-vein thrombosis. *N Engl J Med* 2001; **344**: 626–31.

30 Kovacs MJ, Anderson D, Morrow B, *et al.* Outpatient treatment of pulmonary embolism with dalteparin. *Thromb Haemost* 2000; **83**: 209–11.

31 Buller HR, Davidson BL, Decousus H, *et al.* Fondaparinux or enoxaparin for the initial treatment of symptomatic deep venous thrombosis: a randomized trial. *Ann Intern Med* 2004; **140**: 867–73.

32 Raschke RA, Gollihare B, Peirce JC. The effectiveness of implementing the weight-based heparin nomogram as a practice guideline. *Arch Intern Med* 1996; **156**: 1645–9.

33 Wilson SJ, Wilbur K, Burton E, Anderson DR. Effect of patient weight on the anticoagulant response to adjusted therapeutic dosage of low-molecular-weight heparin for

the treatment of venous thromboembolism. *Haemostasis* 2001; **31**: 42–8.

34 Hainer JW, Barrett JS, Assaid CA, *et al*. Dosing in heavy-weight/obese patients with the LMWH, tinzaparin: a pharmacodynamic study. *Thromb Haemost* 2002; **87**: 817–23.

35 Nagge J, Crowther M, Hirsh J. Is impaired renal function a contraindicaiton to the use of low-molecular-weight heparin? *Arch Intern Med* 2002; **162**: 2605–9.

36 Martinowitz U, Michaelson M for The Israeli Multi-disciplinary rFVIIa Task Force. Guidelines for the use of recombinant activated factor VII (rFVIIa) in uncontrolled bleeding: a report by the Israeli Multidisciplinary rFVIIa Task Force. *J Thromb Haemost* 2005; **3**: 640–8.

37 Mayer SA, Brun NC, Begtrup K, *et al*. Recombinant activated factor VII for acute intracerebral hemorrhage. *N Engl J Med* 2005; **352**: 777–85.

38 Decousus H, Leizorowicz A, Parent F, *et al*. A clinical trial of vena cava filters in the prevention of pulmonary embolism in patients with proximal deep-vein thrombosis. *N Engl J Med* 1998; **338**: 409–15.

39 Ansell J, Hirsh J, Dalen J, *et al*. Managing oral anticoagulant therapy. *Chest* 2001; **119**: 22S–38S.

40 Lee AY, Levine MN, Baker R, *et al*. Low-molecular-weight heparin versus coumarin for the prevention of recurrent venous thromboembolism in patients with cancer. *N Engl J Med* 2003; **345**: 146–53.

41 Meyer G, Marjanovic Z, Valcke J, *et al*. Comparison of low-molecular-weight heparin and warfarin for the secondary prevention of venous thromboembolism in patients with cancer: a randomized controlled study. *Arch Intern Med* 2002; **162**: 1729–35.

42 Pengo V, Lensing AW, Prins MH, *et al*.; Thromboembolic Pulmonary Hypertension Study Group. Incidence of chronic thromboemboilic pulmonary hypertension after pulmonary embolism. *N Engl J Med* 2004; **350**: 2257–64.

43 Ciurzynski M, Kurzyna M, Bochowicz A, *et al*. Long-term effects of acute pulmonary embolism on echocardiographic Doppler indices and functional capacity. *Clin Cardiol* 2004; 27: 693–7.

REPRODUCTIVE PROBLEMS

19

Irregular menstrual bleeding

SHARON CAMERON

INTRODUCTION

The endometrium consists of a basal layer and a superficial functional layer. In the absence of pregnancy, the corpus luteum undergoes regression with subsequent decline of progesterone. This results in shedding of the superficial layer of the endometrium known as menstruation. Repair and remodeling of the endometrium then begins in preparation for implantation of an embryo in a new cycle. Although the hormonal prerequisites for menstruation have been established, namely withdrawal of progesterone from an estrogen-progesterone primed endometrium, the factors responsible for inducing the vascular changes associated with menstruation have yet to be fully elucidated. Disorders of menstruation are of increasing importance in gynecology, since women in developed countries now experience 10-fold the number of menstrual periods (400 vs. 40) in their lifetime than their ancestors did 100 years ago.[1] This is likely to be due to an earlier menarche, fewer pregnancies, and reduced lactation.

In the United Kingdom, on average, 1 in 20 women of reproductive age consult their primary care physician due to a menstrual disorder.[2] By far the most common menstrual complaint is that of excessive menstrual blood loss or menorrhagia. Menorrhagia can be defined objectively or subjectively.[3] Objective menorrhagia is where menstrual blood loss exceeds 80 mL per menstruation. Population studies have shown that this amount of loss is present in 10 percent of the population.[4] Subjective menorrhagia is defined as a complaint of excessive menstrual blood loss occurring over several consecutive cycles in a woman of reproductive years.[3] Dysfunctional uterine bleeding, which accounts for the majority of cases of excessive menstrual blood loss, is the term used for menorrhagia in the absence of underlying pelvic pathology, systemic disease or complications of pregnancy. It has been reported that in United Kingdom, 20 percent of women had a hysterectomy for menstrual disorders by the age of 55 years.[5] Of those women who undergo hysterectomy for menorrhagia, the uterus is found to be normal in around half of the cases. Furthermore, hysterectomy is associated with a small risk of complications (3 percent).[6] In one study, minor pyrexial morbidity was found in 47 percent of women after abdominal hysterectomy.[7] Thus, menstrual disorders are an important cause of female morbidity, and place a significant burden on healthcare resources.

Recently, there have been advances in our understanding of endometrial physiology and putative mechanisms, which underlie menstruation. This has been combined with the development and availability of novel medical and surgical treatments to reduce heavy menstrual blood loss. However, the precise factors responsible for causing normal and abnormal menstruation are still to be elucidated. This chapter reviews the cellular and molecular mechanisms that are likely to be involved in the process of normal menstrual bleeding together with the evidence that exists for their role in abnormal bleeding including menorrhagia. It will also consider the assessment and treatment of heavy menstrual loss.

ENDOMETRIAL VASCULAR DEVELOPMENT

The uterus is supplied by branches of the uterine arteries, which anastomose with ovarian arteries bilaterally. The uterine arteries divide to form arcuate arteries within the myometrium, which subsequently give rise to radial arteries. These branch into basal arterioles which supply the basal

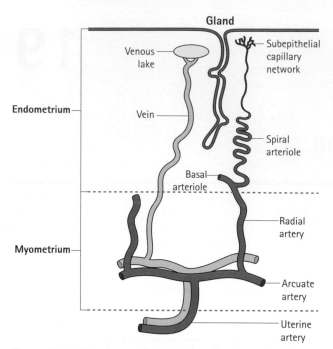

Figure 19.1 Vascular supply to uterus and endometrium.

layer of the endometrium. The superficial layer is supplied by the end arterioles, spiral arterioles, each supplying 4–7 mm^2 of the endometrial surface.[8] Spiral arterioles branch repeatedly to form a subepithelial vascular network beneath the surface, which drains into venous sinuses and larger veins toward the endomyometrial junction (Fig. 19.1).

The endometrial vasculature is unique in that it undergoes dynamic changes on a monthly basis. In the proliferative phase, under the influence of increasing levels of estradiol from growing follicles, there is growth of spiral arterioles together with glandular and stromal proliferation. Following ovulation, progesterone secretion from the corpus luteum induces secretory differentiation of glands, stromal edema, and coiling of terminal branches of spiral arterioles. Scanning electron microscopy has shown that there are small areas of tissue destruction within the endometrium at the end of the menstrual cycle.[9,10] There then follows rapid desquamation of the endometrial surface (within 24 hours of menstrual bleeding) exposing open vessels and glandular stumps. From these glandular stumps, new epithelial growth occurs over the following 2 days. By the fifth/sixth day of the cycle, the endometrium had been completely reepithelialized.[9,10] Mechanisms exist so that blood does not clot and that bleeding has ceased by the time that tissue destruction is complete.[11] Vasoactive agents such as prostaglandins and endothelins are believed to play important roles in regulating blood loss. There is also evidence that endometrial destruction is brought about by matrix-degrading enzymes, such as matrix metalloproteinases. Prolonged vasoconstriction of vessels, increasing estradiol levels, and release of local angiogenic factors are likely to be important in the endometrial repair process. The roles of each these putative mediators of importance in menstrual shedding and repair will be reviewed below.

Prostaglandins

In the classic studies by Markee, conducted in the rhesus monkey over 60 years ago, the vascular changes associated with menstruation were established.[8] Markee transplanted endometrium into the anterior chamber of the eye, and was thus able to visualize the vasodilatation and vasoconstriction of spiral arterioles and ensuing tissue necrosis and menstrual bleeding associated with progesterone withdrawal. Markee hypothesized that there must be release of vasoactive substances prior to menstruation, which were responsible for this change. There is now considerable evidence that prostaglandins are among the likely candidates that could induce such vascular changes.[12,13]

Prostaglandins are locally released fatty acids synthesized from precursors present as membrane-bound phospholipids. The enzyme responsible for the rate-limiting step in prostaglandin synthesis exists in three isoforms: cyclooxygenase (COX)-1, COX-2, and COX-3.[14,15] Cyclooxygenase-1 is constitutively expressed in most tissues, whereas COX-2 is the inducible form, and is particularly expressed in menstrual phase endometrium.[16] A functional role for COX-3 in human physiology and pathophysiology remains to be established. Arachidonic acid is converted to cyclic endoperoxidases (including prostaglandin PGE_2, $PGF_{2\alpha}$ and prostacyclin PGI_2) by the action of the enzyme cyclooxygenase. Specific synthases are then responsible for the conversion to various prostaglandins.[17] Prostaglandin E_2 and $PGF_{2\alpha}$ are present in high concentration in both endometrium and menstrual fluid, and it has been shown that both their synthesis and metabolism is influenced by estrogen and progesterone.[18–20] $PGF_{2\alpha}$ produces myometrial contractions and vasoconstriction whereas prostaglandins of the E series are vasodilators that work in synergy with other compounds such as bradykinin to increase pain and edema.[21,22] Although estradiol and progesterone increase the prostaglandin biosynthetic capacity of the endometrium, release occurs in response to progesterone withdrawal at demise of the corpus luteum. Furthermore, there is evidence to suggest that the prostaglandin metabolizing enzyme prostaglandin dehydrogenase (PGDH), which converts prostaglandins to inactive metabolites within secretory endometrium, is inhibited by progesterone.[23] Studies that have examined the endometrium of women who experience vaginal bleeding following mid-luteal phase administration of the progesterone antagonist mifepristone (Exelgyn, France), have demonstrated increased expression of COX-2 and reduced expression of PGDH.[24] This is further support for the hypothesis that an increase in local concentrations of prostaglandins in the endometrium is involved in the mechanism of menstrual bleeding, as a consequence of progesterone withdrawal.

It has been suggested that the relative balance of vasodilators to vasoconstrictors might impinge on menstrual loss. It has been shown that in women with excessive menstrual blood loss, PGE_2 synthesis in the uterus and the number of PGE binding sites are increased compared with those in women with normal menstrual loss.[25,26] Studies have also shown that expression and activity of the vasodilatory prostaglandin prostacyclin (PGI_2) is greatest in menstrual phase endometrium.[27] Furthermore synthesis of PGI_2 and the vasodilatory agent nitric oxide are raised in endometrium of women with menorrhagia, suggesting that heavy menstrual bleeding may be associated with an increase in vasodilatory factors.[28,29] The increased vasodilatory factors may further enhance menstrual blood loss by upregulation of the COX-PG biosynthetic pathway via a positive feedback loop, since prostaglandins are known to increase COX enzyme expression in several systems.[30,31]

Coagulation and fibrinolysis

The control of bleeding is dependent upon the functioning of the hemostatic system, namely blood vessels, platelets, coagulation, and fibrinolytic enzymes. Hemostatic events in the menstruating uterus are different from those elsewhere in the body. During menstruation, hemostatic platelet plugs are small and do not usually fully occlude the lumen of the vessels. Indeed, vasoconstriction is likely to be more important in securing hemostasis until endometrial repair is complete. Activation of both coagulation and fibrinolytic enzyme systems occur in the uterus during menstruation to prevent widespread clot formation with organization and development of intrauterine adhesions. Menstrual blood has been shown to contain only a fraction of the platelet and blood coagulation factor component of peripheral blood, no fibrinogen, and high levels of fibrin degradation products.[32,33] Coagulation and fibrinolysis have also been shown to play an important role in the pathophysiology of excessive menstrual blood loss. In women with dysfunctional uterine bleeding, both menstrual fluid and premenstrual phase endometrial biopsies have been demonstrated to have significantly higher levels of fibrinolytic pathway enzymes, such as tissue plasminogen activator (tPA), compared with those in women with normal volume loss.[32,34] This lends support for a role of increased fibrinolytic activators in the pathophysiology of heavy menstrual loss. Furthermore, the increased menstrual loss observed in users of a copper intrauterine contraceptive device (IUCD), has in part been attributed to a local effect of the IUCD on fibrinolysis.[35] Likewise, the reduced blood loss in women who use the combined oral contraceptive pill has been linked with the suppression of tPA in endometrium.[36]

Although heavy menstruation is a common symptom of women with hemostatic disorders, hematologic disorders have been estimated to account for only a small proportion of cases of menorrhagia.[37] The most common hemostatic disorder in women is von Willebrand disease (abnormal factor VIII molecule), in which both blood coagulation and platelet function are affected. von Willebrand factor plays an important role in hemostasis, acting as a bridge between platelets and exposed endothelium. The estimated prevalence in the general population is 0.8–1.3 percent.[38,39] A recent systematic review of 11 studies from Europe and the United States reported a prevalence of von Willebrand disease of around 13 percent in women attending for gynecologic investigation of menorrrhagia.[40] Menorrhagia has also been reported in women with less common blood coagulation abnormalities such as carriers of hemophilia A or B, deficiency of factors; cofactor V, VII, IX, X, XI, and prothrombin. Defects of platelet function or severe quantitative reduction of platelet count may also present with heavy menstrual blood loss.[41] Furthermore there are also reports that treatment with anticoagulants can result in heavy menstrual loss.[41]

Matrix metalloproteinases

Immediately prior to and during menstruation, there is an expression, secretion, and activation of matrix metalloproteinases (MMPs), enzymes which bring about degradation of the extracellular matrix (ECM).[42] MMPs are secreted in a latent form and activated by interactions with endometrial leukocytes, and stromal, vascular, and epithelial cells.[42] Natural tissue inhibitors of MMPs (TIMPs) which bind active forms are also present in the endometrium.[43] Thus, for tissue breakdown to occur there must be excess MMPs relative to TIMPs. Evidence supporting an important role for MMPs in menstruation comes from the increased activity of MMPs (gelatinase and collagenase) in menstrual endometrium, MMP upregulation in response to progesterone withdrawal, and from in vitro studies which have demonstrated that specific inhibitors of MMPs can prevent breakdown of endometrial explants in culture.[44,45]

Inflammatory mediators

The premenstrual withdrawal of progesterone is associated with an influx of leukocytes into the endometrium, consisting of neutrophils, macrophages, and other hemopoietic cells such as eosinophils.[46] For this reason menstruation has often been described as an inflammatory event. Furthermore, it has been demonstrated that mast cell activation/degranulation is a common feature of premenstrual endometrium.[46] Since both mast cells and eosinophils contain a variety of potent mediators that may activate precursor forms of MMPs it seems likely that both cell types play a functional role in tissue remodeling at menstruation.[46]

Two potential key inflammatory mediators in the endometrium which are chemotactic for leukocytes are interleukin (IL)-8 and monocyte chemotactic peptide (MCP)-1. Both cytokines are expressed in a perivascular location within the endometrium.[16,47,48] Using an *in vivo* model of progesterone withdrawal, it has been demonstrated that progesterone withdrawal results is an upregulation of IL-8, MCP-1 and COX-2.[48] Together with an inhibition of PGDH, this results in a local elevation of prostaglandins (PGE$_2$ and PGF$_{2\alpha}$). The consequence is an influx of leukocytes, which themselves are sources of cytokines that further enhance leukocyte entry. Both white cells and the endometrium release MMPs, resulting in tissue destruction and menstrual bleeding. In women who use an IUCD and who have excessive menstrual blood loss, it has been shown that there is an increase in leukocyte infiltration in the endometrium compared with nonusers with normal blood loss, supporting a role for inflammatory mediators in heavy menstrual loss.[49]

Endothelins

Endothelins are potent vasoactive agents (endothelin-1, -2 and -3), which have been proposed as potential candidates that could possibly mediate the vasoconstriction of spiral arterioles at menstruation. Endothelin immunoreactivity has been localized to vascular, glandular, and stromal compartments of the endometrium.[50,51] Furthermore the specific endothelin receptors (ET-A and ET-B) have been shown to be differentially expressed in endometrium across the menstrual cycle.[52] Endothelin expression varies across the menstrual cycle, reaching maximal levels in the premenstrual phase.[53] The activity of the endothelin metabolizing enzyme – neutral endopeptidase (NEP) 'enkephalinase' – has been shown to decline premenstrually, suggesting that endothelin activity is under indirect ovarian steroid control.[54] It has also been demonstrated that endothelins can induce PGF$_{2\alpha}$ and potentiate further endothelin release.[55] Thus, it is possible that these agents play a possible paracrine role in menstruation. In addition, ET-1 has been shown to have mitogenic actions on endometrial stromal cells. It has been proposed that, as a vasoconstrictor, endothelins may play a role in post menstrual vasoconstriction of basal blood vessels, to arrest bleeding, and then subsequent to this that they might act as a mitogen to aid reepithelialization.[56,57] Studies of endometrium from women with documented menorrhagia have shown that compared with normal endometrium there is reduced expression of endothelin and increased expression of NEP.[56,58] Thus in menorrhagia it has been hypothesized that the lack of endothelins may result in an endometrium that is fragile and susceptible to bleeding.

Vascular endothelial growth factor and angiopoietins

Vascular smooth muscle cell (VSMC) proliferation increases in spiral arterioles in the secretory phase.[59] However, in women with menorrhagia, it has been shown that VSMC proliferation in spiral arterioles is reduced, suggesting that underlying defects in angiogenesis may play a role in heavy menstrual loss.[60] Vasoconstriction of spiral arterioles is presumed to result in hypoxia of the uppermost zone of the endometrium. Vascular endothelial growth factor (VEGF) is a potent angiogenic growth factor that is present in endometrium and may be stimulated by hypoxia.[61] In addition to its angiogenic activity, it is a potent stimulator of microvascular permeability;[62] VEGF binds to its receptors, mainly in endothelial cells.[63] It has also been implicated in the modulation of MMPs in both VSMCs and endothelial cells.[64] It has been hypothesized therefore that via augmentation of MMPs in the superficial zone of the functional layer of the endometrium, it plays a role in the menstrual shedding process.[65]

There is also evidence that another family of angiogenic proteins 'angiopoietins', are key regulators of angiogenic steps including vessel branching, maturation, and vessel stabilization.[66] Angiopoietin-1 (Ang-1) promotes vascular integrity by optimizing the integration of the endothelial cells with the surrounding supporting cells. In contrast, Ang-2, which is a partial antagonist of Ang-1, enhances vascular permeability and branching, and thus may have a complementary role in vascular development and maintenance. Both proliferative and secretory endometrium exhibit immunoreactivity for Ang-1 and Ang-2, which is greatest in endothelium.[67] The role of angiopoietins in endometrium is unknown. It has, however, been hypothesized that they may play a role in the vascular remodeling at menstruation and that possible alterations in the balance of Ang-1 to Ang-2, in favor of Ang-2 could be linked with abnormal bleeding.[67] Support for this comes from recent studies which demonstrated increased expression of Ang-2 and its receptor in endometrium from women with menorrhagia compared with endometrium of women with normal menstrual loss.[68]

MODIFICATION OF MENSTRUAL LOSS BY DRUGS

The main classes of drugs used for the treatment of menorrhagia are prostaglandin synthesis inhibitors, antifibrinolytics, and hormonal therapies (progestogens, combined oral contraceptive pill, gonadotrophin hormone-releasing agonists). The effects of these will be considered below. Table 19.1 summarizes the approximate effectiveness of the main classes in women with dysfunctional uterine bleeding.

Prostaglandin synthesis inhibitors

The increased expression of prostaglandins in menstrual endometrium of women with menorrhagia has led to the administration of COX inhibitors, namely nonsteroidal anti-inflammatory drugs (NSAIDs) for treatment of heavy menstrual bleeding.[74] These drugs inhibit prostaglandin

Table 19.1 Effectiveness of first line medical treatments for dysfunctional uterine bleeding[69–73]

Treatment	Approximate percent reduction blood loss
Nonsteroidal anti-inflammatory drug	20
Antifibrinolytic	50
Combined oral contraceptive pill	50
Progestin (21 days)	80
Levonorgestrel intrauterine system	97 (at 1 year)

synthesis, thus reducing the concentrations of endometrial prostaglandins. Mefenamic acid, one of the most commonly used NSAIDs for menorrhagia, has been shown to inhibit both prostaglandin synthesis and binding of PGE_2 to its receptor.[3,75]

A recent Cochrane systematic review which examined 16 randomized controlled trials using NSAIDs supported their effectiveness in reducing heavy menstrual loss.[69] Generally, a reduction in the order of 20 percent blood loss is observed. These drugs have the advantage of requiring to be taken only during menses. Although NSAIDs may be associated with nausea, dizziness, headache and gastrointestinal upset, there is a low incidence of adverse effects in healthy women. Since the efficacy of mefenamic acid has been shown to be similar to naproxen, but with fewer gastrointestinal side effects, mefenamic acid would appear to be the preferred NSAID for treatment of menorrhagia.[69]

Antifibrinolytic therapy

The rationale for using antifibrinolytic agents to treat excessive menstrual blood loss is based upon the observation that fibrinolytic activity is greater in the endometrium of women with menorrhagia than in those with blood loss in the normal range. Evidence-based systemic reviews have shown that the antifibrinolytic agent tranexamic acid provides an effective treatment, reducing menstrual blood loss in the order of 50 percent.[70,76] Treatment also results in reduced endometrial levels of tPA.[77] Comparative studies have shown that measured blood loss is significantly less following treatment with tranexamic acid than following NSAIDs.[78] Tranexamic acid is administered orally during menstruation only. Side effects are mainly gastrointestinal and are dose related. Although there has been theoretical concern that antifibrinolytics may be implicated in the pathogenesis of thromboembolism, no increase in thromboembolic disease has been observed in epidemiologic studies conducted in Scandinavia, where antifibrinolytic treatments for menorrhagia have been popular since the 1970s.[79] In women with inherited bleeding disorders such as von Willebrand disease, tranexamic acid is effective in reducing menstrual loss. The combined contraceptive pill increases factor VIII and von Willebrand factor (vWF) levels and is also effective treat-

ment, as is intranasal desmopressin acetate, which also increases plasma factor VIII and vWF levels.[80]

Hormonal therapy

SYSTEMIC PROGESTOGEN

Use of progestogens to treat heavy menstrual loss is based upon the fact that progesterone inhibits endometrial proliferation. It has been shown that the synthetic progestogen norethisterone, taken orally, can reduce menstrual blood loss by around 80 percent, if given at a moderate dose for 21 days each month; days 5–25 inclusive of cycle.[71] In contrast, lower doses of progestogens, taken in the luteal phase only (for 5–10 days) are ineffective therapy for reducing blood loss.[81]

INTRAUTERINE PROGESTOGEN

The levonorgestrel intrauterine system (LNG-IUS) (Mirena, Schering Health Care), is an intrauterine device that releases 20 μg/day of the progestogen levonorgestrel into the uterus from a sustained released formulation that lasts for up to 5 years. There is little systemic absorption. Measured menstrual blood loss is reduced by around 86 percent at 6 months and 97 percent at 12 months of use.[72] In addition, it provides an effective reversible method of contraception, with an efficacy rate that rivals female sterilization.[82] Studies of endometrial morphology in users of the device show that the intrauterine progestogen results in a dramatic decidualization of the endometrium.[83] In one study of women who were invited to have the intrauterine system inserted, or to continue with current medical therapy prior to hysterectomy, 64 percent of those who agreed to have a LNG-IUS chose to remove themselves from the waiting list for hysterectomy, compared with 14 percent in the control group. This demonstrates that the LNG-IUS is an acceptable alternative to hysterectomy for some women.[84]

The main drawback of use of LNG-IUS is the high incidence of breakthrough bleeding that occurs, particularly within the initial months of use. Immunohistochemical studies have shown that there is an increase in immunoreactivity for potential local mediators of menstruation such as COX-2 and IL-8 in levonorgestrel-exposed endometrium in the initial months following insertion of the system.[83] Furthermore, there is a coexistent decrease in immunoreactivity for PGDH, implying that a local increase in concentration of prostaglandins might be associated with the observed breakthrough bleeding at this time.[83] The observation that there is an increase in MMP-9 (gelatinase-B) immunostaining in endometrium from women using a LNG-IUS, compared with that of women during a normal menstrual cycle, would also lend support for a role for MMPs in the pathogenesis of breakthrough bleeding.[85] Higher concentrations of VEGF have also been reported in endometrium from LNG-IUS users following insertion and particularly in those women who experience more bleeding with the device.[86] This may also give support to a role for aberrant angiogenesis in progestogen breakthrough bleeding. Aberrations in the distribution of the angiogenic protein Ang-1 have also been reported in endometrium from LNG-IUS users. In contrast to the even distribution of Ang-1 in normal endometrium, LNG-IUS-exposed endometrium has been reported to display patchy areas of Ang-1 staining, with most expression being in the stromal compartment rather than the endothelium.[67] No differences have been observed in terms of the pattern and distribution of immunostaining for Ang-2 in LNG-IUS and normal endometrium, suggesting that alteration in the balance of Ang-1 to Ang-2 might be associated with the irregular bleeding seen in users of the LNG-IUS.[67]

COMBINED ORAL CONTRACEPTIVE PILL

The combined oral contraceptive pill inhibits ovulation and suppresses endometrial development. It is associated with reduced blood loss in the majority of women by ~50 percent.[73] In low-risk women (healthy, normal weight, nonsmoking), there is no age restriction on use.

GONADOTROPHIN HORMONE-RELEASING ANALOGS

Gonadotrophin hormone-releasing analogs are derivatives of natural gonadotrophin-releasing hormone (GnRH), but peptide substitutions give the agonists greater potency and longer activity. Treatment results in pituitary downregulation and inhibition of ovarian activity, with resultant hypoestrogenism and amenorrhea. Women may experience problems of hypoestrogenism, such as hot flushes and vaginal dryness. With prolonged use, there is also the likelihood of loss of bone mineral density. GnRH analogs are thus usually reserved for short-term use only.[87]

ASSESSMENT OF HEAVY MENSTRUAL LOSS

Assessment of blood loss, based on history, examination and appropriate investigations, is important to determine the cause of menorrhagia (systemic, uterine pathology, dysfunctional) and in particular to exclude underlying endometrial cancer or hyperplasia. Furthermore, assessment of blood loss will help guide treatment. Assessment should include a full history and examination. Basic hematologic investigation (complete blood count) should be done, but other investigations are indicated on the basis of history and examination findings.[3]

History

A history of heavy cyclical menstrual bleeding over several cycles should be sought.[3] Although it has been a generally held belief that women themselves are poor judges of the degree of blood loss, a recent study that measured blood loss in women complaining of menorrhagia did show a correlation between number of sanitary products used, rate of

---

> **Box 19.1 Risk factors for endometrial cancer[90–96]**
>
> - Age
> - Nulliparity
> - Family history of colorectal/endometrial cancer
> - Tamoxifen
> - Unopposed estrogen therapy
> - Polycystic ovarian syndrome
> - Obesity

changing sanitary protection, and passage of clots with menstrual blood loss >80 mL.[88] Furthermore this study suggested that heaviness of menstrual flow may vary from month to month.[88] Complaints of 'flooding' or having to use double sanitary protection (towel and tampon) to prevent leakage of blood onto clothing are generally agreed to be indicative of heavy flow. Severity of bleeding may also be gauged from the impact that menstruation is having on the woman's quality of life, such as disability experienced, time lost from work, and social embarrassment. It should also be remembered, however, that in a recent study of women with objective menorrhagia, just over one third considered their menstrual disorder as a severe problem.[89] In addition, the patient should be questioned about symptoms suggestive of anemia. Symptoms suggestive of underlying pelvic pathology should also be sought such as irregular bleeding, intermenstrual bleeding, postcoital bleeding, dyspareunia, and pelvic pain. In addition, history taking should include details of any risk factors for endometrial cancer such as use of unopposed estrogen or the estrogen receptor antagonist tamoxifen, or coexisting medical problems such as polycystic ovarian syndrome, obesity, or family history of colorectal or endometrial cancer[90–96] (Box 19.1). Testing for bleeding disorders should be considered if the woman has a family history of hemostatic disease, or a personal history of menorrhagia since menarche, bleeding tendency post dental extraction, postoperative bleeding or postpartum hemorrhage.[40]

Examination

Guidelines from the Royal College of Obstetricians and Gynaecologists (RCOG) advise that an abdominal and pelvic examination should be conducted. A cervical smear should be taken if one is due. If the uterus is of normal size, the woman is <40 years of age and there are no suspicious findings on examination or symptoms suggestive of other pathology, a complete blood count is the only investigation that needs to be conducted at this stage (with iron supplementation if necessary). If treatment is required, then first-line medical management should be commenced, with prostaglandin synthesis inhibitors and/or antifibrinolytic therapy, before proceeding to hormonal therapy as above.[3]

If however, examination reveals an enlarged uterus, pelvic mass, or tenderness, or there are risk factors on history taking

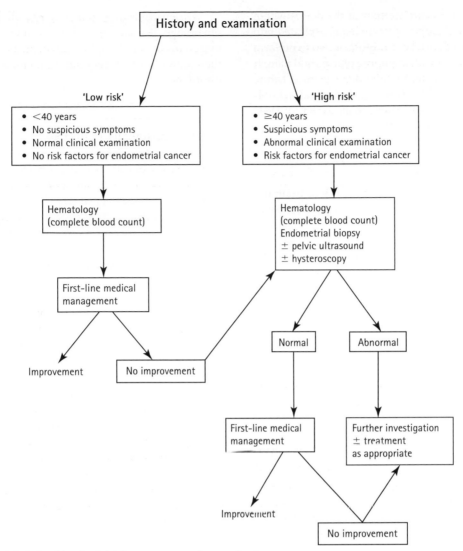

Figure 19.2   Simplified algorithm for initial management of menorrhagia.

for pelvic pathology, then further gynecological investigation should be performed. Based on the results of these investigations and presence or absence of pathology, further investigations and/or appropriate medical or surgical treatment can be instituted. A simplified algorithm for the initial management of menorrhagia is shown in Figure 19.2.

Investigations

A complete blood count to exclude anemia should be undertaken in all women complaining of excessive menstrual loss, but tests of thyroid function, other endocrine tests and tests of coagulation should be done only if there are features suggestive of this in the history.[3] Appropriate investigations include the following.

ENDOMETRIAL ASSESSMENT

In view of the low incidence of sinister pathology found in endometrial samples in women under 40 years (endometrial

cancer <7 in 100 000 women at age 40), the RCOG has recommended endometrial sampling should not be done routinely in women <40 years of age.[3,97] The RCOG suggest that endometrial assessment is justified in women ≥40 years and younger women with menorrhagia which fails to respond to first-line medical therapy, those with irregular bleeding or for whom there are risk factors for endometrial cancer.

Traditionally, the endometrium was assessed by dilatation and curettage (D&C), which required a short general anesthetic and in most cases was conducted as a day case procedure. It involves 'blind' curettage of the endometrium, and so the operator cannot assess whether lesions have been missed. In one study, which evaluated the completeness of endometrial sampling by D&C, less than half the cavity was sampled in 60 percent of cases.[98] With the advent of outpatient endometrial sampling devices, D&C has been largely superseded.

Most endometrial sampling devices (such as the Pipelle™, Eurosurgical, UK) consist of an outer plastic sheath with an aperture at its distal end and an inner piston.

Gentle forward and backward motion of the device within the uterus results in a sample of tissue being aspirated into the sheath. This procedure takes a minute or two to perform and is usually associated with cramping type period pain. It does have a procedure failure rate and tissue yield failure rate of around 10 percent.[99] It is an inexpensive and well-tolerated procedure, with a similar sensitivity to that of D&C for detecting endometrial cancer.[100,101]

ULTRASOUND

A pelvic ultrasound should be done if history or examination suggests structural pathology, or if it is not possible to assess the uterus clinically because of obesity. Ultrasound can assess endometrial thickness and morphology, the myometrium and adnexae. In situations where it is difficult to assess the endometrial thickness or there is suspicion of intracavity abnormality saline infusion sonography can be of value.[102] Saline infusion sonography involves the instillation of a few milliliters of sterile saline, through a fine catheter (such as those used in insemination techniques) into the uterus under real-time ultrasonography. Intracavity lesions may be observed to be more clearly defined against the sonolucent background of sterile saline.

HYSTEROSCOPY

Hysteroscopy allows direct visual examination of the uterine cavity. With the advent of fine (2–3 mm) hysteroscopes, this procedure is increasingly being done in the outpatient setting, with an accuracy and patient acceptability equivalent to inpatient hysteroscopy under general anesthetic.[103] Many newer generation hysteroscopes also have narrow operating channels, which enable one to resect intracavity lesions and biopsy focal areas of the endometrium at the same time.

ENDOMETRIAL CYTOLOGY

Endometrial cytological samples may be obtained by washing, aspiration or brushing (for example, Tao brush™ cook). The Tao brush method of endometrial assessment has been used in research studies which have shown that it is accurate in determining the presence of malignant cells.[104] It is not yet commonly used in clinical practice.

CONCLUSION

In conclusion, although the hormonal requirements for menstrual bleeding have been established, the precise mechanisms at cellular and at molecular level that are responsible for triggering menstrual shedding remain to be elucidated. There is good evidence that prostaglandins, fibrinolytic enzymes, endothelins, MMPs, inflammatory mediators, and angiogenic proteins are involved.

As science advances our understanding of endometrial physiology, it is anticipated that women will benefit with more effective and sophisticated medical treatments for the common, often debilitating conditions of menstrual disorders.

KEY LEARNING POINTS

- Precise molecular and cellular mechanisms responsible for menstruation are unknown.
- Hemostatic events that take place in the uterus at menstruation to arrest blood loss and bring about repair and regeneration are unique in the human body.
- Menstrual disorders are a common complaint of women of reproductive age, and place a significant burden on healthcare resources.
- Surgical hysterectomy is a common treatment for heavy menstruation and is associated with significant morbidity. In approximately half of cases, the removed uterus is normal.
- Disturbances in prostaglandin and fibrinolytic pathway have been demonstrated in the endometrium of women with excessive menstrual loss.
- There is growing evidence in support of a disturbance of angiogenesis in the endometrium of women with excess menstrual bleeding.
- Not all women with menorrhagia require endometrial assessment. In a woman <40 years, with no risk factors, and normal pelvic examination, first-line medical therapy can be instituted.

REFERENCES

1   Short RV. Oestrous and menstrual cycles. In: Austin CR, Short RV, eds. *Hormonal Control of Reproduction*, eds. Cambridge: Cambridge University Press, 1984: 115–52.

2   Royal College of General Practitioners and Department of Health. *Morbidity Statistics from General Practice, Fourth National Study 1991–1992*. London: HMSO, 1995.

3   Royal College of Obstetricians and Gynaecologists. *The Initial Management of Menorrhagia*. (Evidence-based guidelines No 1) London: RCOG, 1998.

4   Hallberg L, Hogdahl A, Nilsson L, Rybo G. Menstrual blood loss-a population based study: variation at different ages and attempts to define normality. *Acta Obstet Gynecol Scand* 1966; **43**: 320–51.

5   Vessey M, Villard-MacKintosh, McPherson K, *et al.* The epidemiology of hysterectomy: findings of a large cohort study. *Br J Obstet Gynaecol* 1992; **99**: 402–7.

6   McPherson K, Metcalfe MA, Herbert A, *et al.* Severe complications of hysterectomy: the VALUE study. *Br J Obstet Gynaecol* 2004; **111**: 688–94.

7   Pinion SB, Parkin DE, Abramovich DR, *et al.* Randomised trial of hysterectomy, endometrial laser ablation and transcervical resection for dysfunctional uterine bleeding. *BMJ* 1994; **309**: 979–83.

8   Markee JE. Menstruation in intraocular endometrial transplants in the rhesus monkey. *Contrib Embryol* 1940; **28**: 219–308.

9   Ludwig H, Metzger H, Fraull M. Endometrium, tissue remodelling and regeneration. In: d'Arcangues C, Fraser IS, Newton JR, Odlind V, eds. *Contraception and Mechanisms of Endometrial Bleeding.* Cambridge: Cambridge University Press, 1990: 441–66.

10 Ludwig H, Spornitz UM. Microarchitecture of the endometrium by scanning electron microscopy: menstrual desquamation and remodelling. *Ann N Y Acad Sci* 1991; **62**: 28–46.

11 Lockwood CJ, Schatz F. A biological model for the regulation of peri-implantational hemostasis and menstruation. *J Soc Gynecol Invest* 1996; **3**: 159–65.

12 Pickles VR. Plain muscle stimulant in the menstruum. *Nature* 1957; **180**: 1198–9.

13 Baird DT, Cameron ST, Critchley HOD, *et al.* Prostaglandins and menstruation. *Eur J Obstet Gynecol* 1996; **70**: 15–17.

14 Chandrasekharan NV, Dai H, Roos KL, *et al.* COX-3, a cyclooxygenase variant inhibited by acetaminophen and other analgesics/antipyretic drugs: cloning, structure and expression. *Proc Natl Acad Sci U S A* 2002; **99**: 13926–31.

15 Morita I. Distinct functions of COX-1 and COX-2. *Prostaglandins Other Lipid Mediat* 2002; **68–69**: 165–75.

16 Jones RL, Kelly RW, Critchley HOD. Chemokine and cyclooxygenase 2 expression in human endometrium coincides with leukocyte accumulation. *Hum Reprod* 1997; **12**: 1300–6.

17 Smith WS, Garavito RM, De Witt DL. Prostaglandin endoperoxidase H synthases (cyclo oxygenases -1 and -2). *J Biol Chem* 1996; **271**: 33157–60.

18 Downie J, Poyser NL, Wunderlich M. Levels of prostaglandins in human endometrium during the normal menstrual cycle. *J Physiol* 1974; **2365**: 465–72.

19 Abel MH, Baird DT. The effect of oestradiol-17β and progesterone on prostaglandin production by human endometrium maintained in organ culture. *Endocrinology* 1980; **106**: 1599–606.

20 Abel MH, Kelly RW. Metabolism of prostaglandins by the non pregnant human uterus. *J Clin Endocrinol Metab* 1983; **56**: 678–85.

21 Ylikorkala O, Makila U-M. Prostacyclin and thromboxane in gynecology and obstetrics. *Am J Obstet Gynecol* 1985; **152**: 318–29.

22 Williams TJ. Prostaglandin E2, prostaglandin I2 and the vascular changes of inflammation. *Br J Pharmacol* 1979; **65**: 517–24.

23 Cameron ST, Critchley HOD, Buckley HC, *et al.* Effect of two antiprogestins (mifepristone and onapristone) on endometrial factors of potential importance for implantation. *Fertil Steril* 1997; **67**: 1046–53.

24 Hapangama DK, Critchley HOD, Henderson TA, Baird DT. Mifepristone-induced vaginal bleeding is associated with increased immunostaining for cyclooxygenase-2 and decrease in prostaglandin dehydrogenase in luteal phase endometrium. *J Clin Endocrinol Metab* 2002; **87**: 5229–34.

25 Smith SK, Abel MH, Kelly RW, Baird DT. Prostaglandin synthesis in the endometrium of women with ovular dysfunctional uterine bleeding. *Br J Obstet Gynaecol* 1981; **88**: 434–42.

26 Rees MC, Anderson AB, Demers LM, Turnbull AC. Endometrial and myometrial prostaglandin release during the menstrual cycle in relation to menstrual blood loss. *J Clin Endocrinol Metab* 1984; **91**: 667–72.

27 Battersby S, Critchley HOD, de Brum-Fernades AJ, Jabbour H. Temporal expression and signalling of the prostacyclin receptor in human endometrium across the menstrual cycle. *Reproduction* 2004; **127**: 79–86.

28 Smith SK, Abel MH, Kelly RW, Baird DT. A role for prostacyclin in excessive menstrual bleeding. *Lancet* 1981; **i**: 522–4.

29 Makarainen L, Ylikorala O. Primary and myoma-associated role of prostaglandins and effect of ibuprofen. *Br J Obstet Gynaecol* 1986; **93**: 974–8.

30 Sales KJ, Katz AA, Howard B, *et al.* Cyclooxygenase-1 is up regulated in cervical carcinomas autocrine/paracrine regulation of cyclooxygenase-2, PGE receptors and angiogenic factors by cyclooxygenase-1. *Cancer Res* 2002; **62**: 424–32.

31 Clancy R, Vaernika B, Huang W, *et al.* Nitric oxide synthase/COX cross-talk nitric oxide activates COX-1 but inhibits COX-2 derived prostaglandin production. *J Immunol* 2000; **165**: 1582–7.

32 De Meere LJ, Moss JD, Pattison DS. The haematological study of menstrual discharge. *Obstet Gynecol* 1967; **30**: 830–3.

33 Hahn L. Composition of menstrual blood. In: Diczfalusy E, Fraser IS, Webb FTG, eds. *Endometrial Bleeding and Steroidal Contraception.* Bath: Pitman Press, 1980: 107–37.

34 Sheppard BL. Pathophysiology of dysfunctional uterine bleeding. In: Lowe D, Fox D, eds. *Advances in Gynaeco-logical Pathology.* Edinburgh: Churchill Livingstone, 1992: 191–204.

35 Antrade ATL, Orchard EP. Quantitative studies on menstrual blood loss in IUD users. *Contraception* 1987; **36**: 129–44.

36 Casslen B, Astedt B. Reduced plasminogen activator content of endometrium in oral contraceptive users. *Contraception* 1983; **27**: 131–40.

37 Kadir RA, Economides DL, Sabin CA, *et al.* Frequency of inherited bleeding disorders in women with menorrhagia. *Lancet* 1998; **351**: 485–9.

38 Rodeghiero F, Castaman G, Dini E. Epidemiological investigation of the prevalence of von Willebrand's disease. *Blood* 1987; **69**: 454–9.

39 Werner EJ, Broxon EH, TuckerEL, *et al.* Prevalence of von Willebrand's disease in children: a multiethnic study. *J Pediatr* 1993; **122**: 893–8.

40 Shankar M, Lee C, Sabin C, *et al.* von Willebrand disease in women with menorrhagia: a systematic review. *Br J Obstet Gynaecol* 2004; **111**: 734–40.

★ 41 Higham JM. Medical disease and menstrual disorders. In: *Disorders of the Menstrual Cycle.* London: RCOG Press, 2000: 214–26.

42 Salamonsen LA. Tissue injury and repair in the female reproductive tract. *Reproduction* 2003; **125**: 301–11.

43 Zhang J, Salamonsen LA. Tissue inhibitor of metalloproetinases (TIMP)-1,-2,-3 in human endometrium during the menstrual cycle. *Mol Hum Reprod* 1997; **3**: 735–41.

44 Zhang J, Salamonsen LA. *In vitro* evidence for active matrix metalloproetinases in human endometrium supports their role in tissue breakdown at menstruation. *J Clin Endocrinol Metab* 2002; **87**: 2346–51.

45 Marbaix E, Kokorine I, Moulin P, *et al.* Menstrual breakdown of human endometrium can be mimicked *in vitro* and is selectively and reversibly blocked by inhibitors of matrix metalloproteinases. *Proc Natl Acad Sci U S A* 1996; **93**: 9120–5.

46 Jezioska M, Salamonsen LA, Woolley DE. Mast cell and eosinophil distribution and activation in human endometrium throughout the menstrual cycle. *Biol Reprod* 1995; **53**: 312–20.

47 Critchley HOD, Kelly RW, Kooy J. Perivascular expression of chemokine interleukin-8 in human endometrium. *Hum Reprod* 1994; **9**: 1406–9.

48 Critchley HOD, Jones RL, Lea RG, *et al.* Role of inflammatory mediators in human endometrium during progesterone withdrawal and early pregnancy. *J Clin Endocrinol Metab* 1999; **84**: 240–8.

49 Wang IY, Russell P, Fraser IS. Endometrial morphometry in users of intrauterine contraceptive devices and women with ovulatory dysfunctional uterine bleeding: A comparison with normal endometrium. *Contraception* 1995; **51**: 243–8.

50 Cameron IT, Davenport AP, van Papendorp C, *et al.* Endothelin-like immunoreactivity in human endometrium. *J Reprod Fertil* 1992; **95**: 623–8.

51 Salamonsen LA, Butt AR, MacPherson AM, *et al.* Immunolocalization of the vasoconstrictor endothelin in human endometrium during the menstrual cycle and in the umbilical cord at birth. *Am J Obstet Gynecol* 1992; **167**: 163–7.

52 O'Reilly G, Charnock Jones DS, Davenport AP, *et al.* Presence of messenger ribonucleic acid for endothelin-1, endothelin-2 and endothelin-3 in human endometrium and a change in the ratio of ET-A and ET-B receptor subtype across the menstrual cycle. *J Clin Endocrinol Metab* 1992; **75**: 1545–9.

53 Marsh MM, Hampton AL, Riley SC, *et al.* Production and characterisation of endothelin by human endometrial epithelial cells in culture. *J Clin Endocrinol Metab* 1994; **79**: 1626–31.

54 Head JR, MacDonald PC, Casey ML. Cellular localisation of membrane metalloendopeptidase (endopeptidase) in human endometrium during the ovarian cycle. *J Clin Endocrinol Metab* 1993; **76**: 769–76.

55 Bacon CR, Morisson JJ, O'Reilly G, *et al.* ET-A and ET-B endothelin receptors in human myometrium characterised by selective ligands BQ123, BQ 3020, FR139317 and PD 151242. *J Endocrinol* 1995; **144**: 127–34.

56 Marsh MM, Findlay JK, Salamonsen LA. Endothelin and menstruation. *Hum Reprod* 1996; **11**: 83–9.

57 Salamonsen LA, Young RJ, Garcia S, Findlay JK. Mitogenic actions of endothelin and other growth factors in ovine endometrium. *J Endocrinol* 1997; **147**: 235–44.

★ 58 Salamonsen LA, Marsh MM, Findlay J. Endometrial endothelin: regulator of uterine bleeding and endometrial repair. *Clin Exper Pharmacol Physiol* 1999; **26**: 154–7.

59 Abberton KM, Taylor NH, Healy DL, Rogers PAW. Vascular smooth muscle cell proliferation in arterioles of the human endometrium. *Hum Reprod* 1999; **14**: 1072–9.

60 Rogers PA, Abberton KM. Endometrial arteriogenesis: vascular smooth muscle cell proliferation and differentiation during the menstrual cycle and changes associated with endometrial bleeding disorders. *Micros Res Tech* 2003; **60**: 412–19.

61 Sharkey AM, Day K, McPherson A, *et al.* Vascular endothelial growth factor expression in human endometrium is up regulated by hypoxia. *J Clin Endocrinol Metab* 2000; **85**: 402–9.

62 Ferrara N, Davis-Smyth T. The biology of vascular endothelial growth factor. *Endocr Rev* 1997; **18**: 4–25.

63 Skobe M, Rockwell P, Goldstein N, *et al.* Halting angiogenesis suppresses carcinoma cell invasion. *Nat Med* 1997; **3**: 1222–7.

64 Wang H, Keiser JA. Vascular endothelial growth factor upregulates the expression of matrix metalloproteinases in vascular smooth muscle cells. Role for flt-1. *Circulation Research* 1998; **83**: 832–40.

★ 65 Critchley HOD, Kelly RW, Brenner RM, Baird DT. The endocrinology of menstruation – a role for the immune system. *Clin Endocrinol* 2001; **55**: 701–10.

66 Yancopoulous GD, Davis S, Gale NW, *et al.* Vascular-specific growth factors and blood vessel. *Nature* 2000; **407**: 242–8.

67 Krikun G, Critchley H, Schatz F, *et al.* Abnormal uterine bleeding during progestin-only contraception may result from free radical-induced alterations in angiopoietin expression. *Am J Pathol* 2002; **161**: 979–86.

68 Blumenthal RD, Taylor AP, Goldman L, *et al.* Abnormal expression of the angiopoietins and Tie receptors in menorrhagic endometrium. *Fertil Steril* 2002; **78**: 1294–300.

69 Lethaby A, Allgood C, Duckitt K. NSAID drugs for heavy menstrual bleeding (systematic review). *Cochrane Database Syst Rev* 2004: 2.

70   Lethaby A, Farquhar C, Cooke I. Antibibrinolytics for heavy menstrual bleeding. *Cochrane Database Syst Rev* 2004: 2.

71   Irvine GA, Campbell-Brown M, Lumsden MA, *et al.* Randomised comaparative trial of the levonorgestrel intrauterine system and norethisterone for treatment of idiopathic menorrhagia. *Br J Obstet Gynaecol* 1998; **105**: 592–8.

72   Andersson K, Rybo G. Levonorgestrel-releasing intrauterine device in the treatment of menorrhagia. *Br J Obstet Gynaecol* 1990; **97**: 690–4.

73   Fraser IS, McCarron G. Randomised trial of two hormonal and two prostaglandin-inhibiting agents in women with a complaint of menorrhagia. *Aust N Z J Obstet Gynaecol* 1991; **149**: 788–93.

74   Stirrat GM. Choice of treatment for menorrhagia. *Lancet* 1999; **353**: 2175–6.

75   Rees MC, Canete-Soler R, Lopez Bernal A, Turnbull AC. Effect of fenamates on prostaglandin E receptor binding. *Lancet* 1988; **ii**: 541–2.

76   Bonnar J, Sheppard BL. Treatment of menorrhagia during menstruation randomised controlled trial of ethamsylate, mefenamic acid and tranexamic acid. *BMJ* 1996; **313**: 579–82.

77   Dockeray CJ, Sheppard BL, Daly L, Bonnar J. The fibrinolytic enzyme system in normal menstruation and excessive uterine bleeding and the effect of tranexamic acid. *Eur J Obstet Gynecol Reprod Biol* 1987; **24**: 309–18.

78   Ylikorkala O, Viinikka L. Comparison between antifibrinolytic and antiprostaglandin treatment in the reduction of increased menstrual blood loss in women with intrauterine contraceptive devices. *Br J Obstet Gynaecol* 1983; **90**: 78–83.

79   Rybo G. Tranexamic acid is effective treatment in heavy menstrual bleeding. *Clinical Update on Safety Therapeutic Advances* 1991; **4**: 1–8.

★ 80   Kadir RA, Lee CA, Economides DL. Reproduction and inherited bleeding disorders. *Contemp Rev Obstet Gynecol* 1998; **10**: 39–46.

81   Lethaby A, Irvine G, Cameron I. Cyclical progestogens for heavy menstrual bleeding. *Cochrane Database Syst Rev* 2004: 2.

82   Andersson K, Odlind V, Rybo G. Levonorgestrel-releasing and copper releasing (Nova-T) IUD's during five years of use: a randomised comparative trial. *Contraception* 1994; **49**: 56–72.

83   Jones RL, Critchley HO. Morphological and functional changes in human endometrium following intrauterine levonorgestrel delivery. *Hum Reprod* 2000; **15**: 162–72.

84   Lahteenmaki P, Haukkamaa M, Puolakka J, *et al.* Open randomised study of use of levonorgestrel-releasing intrauterine system as an alternative to hysterectomy. *BMJ* 1998; **316**: 1122–6.

85   Skinner JL, Riley SC, Gebbie AE, *et al.* Regulation of matrix metalloproteinase-9 in endometrium during the menstrual cycle and following administration of intrauterine levonorgestrel. *Hum Reprod* 1999; **14**: 793–9.

86   Roopa BA, Loganath A, Singh K. The effect of a levonorgestrel-releasing intrauterine system on angiogenic growth factors in the endometrium. *Hum Reprod* 2003; **18**: 1809–19.

87   Thomas EJ. Add-back therapy for long-term use in dysfunctional uterine bleeding and uterine fibroids. *Br J Obstet Gynaecol* 1996; **14**: 18–21.

88   Warner PE, Critchley HOD, Lumsden MA, *et al.* Menorrhagia I: Measured blood loss, clinical features, and outcome in women with heavy periods: A survey with follow-up data. *Am J Obstet Gynecol* 2004; **190**: 1216–23.

89   Warner P, Critchley HOD, Lumsden MA, *et al.* Referral for menstrual problems: cross-sectional survey of symptoms, reason for referral and management. *BMJ* 2001; **323**: 24–8.

90   Farquhar C, Lethaby A, Sowter M, *et al.* An evaluation of risk factors for endometrial hyperplasia in premenopausal women with abnormal menstrual bleeding. *Am J Obstet Gynecol* 1999; **181**: 525–9.

91   Neven P. Tamoxifen and endometrial lesions. *Lancet* 1993; **342**: 452.

92   Kedar R, Bourne T, Powles T, *et al.* Effects of tamoxifen on uterus and ovaries of postmenopausal women in a randomised breast cancer prevention trial. *Lancet* 1994; **343**: 1318–21.

93   Van Leeuwen F, Benraadt J, Coebergh JW, *et al.* Risk of endometrial cancer after tamoxifen treatment of breast cancer. *Lancet* 1994; **343**: 448–52.

94   Hulka B. Effect of exogenous estrogen on postmenopausal women: the epidemiologic evidence. *Obstet Gynecol Surv* 1980; **35**: 389–99.

95   Moller H, Mellemgaard A, Lindvig K, Olsen JH. Obesity and cancer risk: a Danish record linkage study. *Eur J Cancer* 1994; **30**: 344–50.

96   Dunlop MG, Farrington SM, Carothers AD, *et al.* Cancer risk associated with germline DNA mismatch repair gene mutations. *Hum Mol Genet* 1997; **6**: 105–10.

97   Sharp L, Black R, Harkness E, *et al. Cancer Registration Statistics Scotland, 1981–1990.* Edinburgh: ISD of the NHS in Scotland, 1993.

98   Stock RJ, Kanbour A. Prehysterecomy curettage. *Obstet Gynecol* 1975; **45**: 537–41.

99   Gordon SJ, Westgate J. The incidence and management of failed pipelle sampling in a general outpatient clinic. *Aust N Z J Obstet Gynaecol* 1999; **39**: 115–18.

100   Fothergill DJ, Brown VA, Hill AS. Histological sampling of the endometrium – a comparison between formal curettage and the pipelle sampler. *Br J Obstet Gynaecol* 1992; **99**: 779–80.

101   Ben-Baruch G, Seidman DS, Schiff E, *et al.* Outpatient endometrial sampling with the pipelle curette. *Gynecol Obstet Invest* 1994; **37**: 260–2.

102   Cameron ST, Walker J, Chambers S, Critchley HOD. Pilot study to compare transvaginal ultrasonography, saline

infusion sonography and hysteroscopy for investigating postmenopausal bleeding or unscheduled bleeding on HRT. *Aust N Z J of Obstet Gynaecol* 2001; **41**: 291–4.

103   Tahir MM, Bigrigg MA, Browning JJ, *et al*. A randomised controlled trial comparing transvaginal ultrasound, outpatient hysteroscopy and endometrial biopsy with inpatient hysteroscopy and curettage. *Br J Obstet Gynaecol* 1999; **106**: 1259–64.

104   Maksem JA, Knesel E. Liquid fixation of endometrial brush cytology endures a well-preserved representative cell sample with frequent tissue correlation. *Diagn Cytopathol* 1996; **14**: 367–73.

20

Polycystic ovarian syndrome: vascular and metabolic issues

NAVEED SATTAR

INTRODUCTION

Polycystic ovary syndrome (PCOS) is a common disorder of chronically abnormal ovarian function and hyperandrogenism affecting 5–10 percent of the female population of reproductive age.[1] The primary etiology remains unclear, and historically there has been no consensus on absolute defining features of the phenotype. At the National Institutes of Health conference in 1990, three key features of PCOS were generally agreed as oligomenorrhea, hyperandrogenism (clinical or laboratory evidence), and the absence of other endocrine disorders (congenital adrenal hyperplasia, hyperprolactinemia, thyroid dysfunction, and androgen-secreting tumors).[2] The presence of polycystic ovaries, determined by ultrasound evaluation, was not included at that stage as a definitive requirement. A more recent consensus statement (European Society of Human Reproduction and Embryology)[3] has revised the criteria for diagnosis of PCOS to include two from three of the following: oligomenorrhea/anovulation; clinical or biochemical evidence of hyperandrogenism; and polycystic ovaries. The inclusion of polycystic ovaries has been promoted by improvements in ultrasound technology and more robust criteria for diagnosis. Women with PCOS tend to present at clinics complaining of infertility, menstrual disturbance or hirsutism, with or

without acne. They are therefore seen by gynecologists, primary care physicians, endocrinologists, and dermatologists. It is noteworthy that it has been accepted for some years now that abnormal insulin metabolism is a major underlying feature of PCOS, but no aspect of it is included in the most recent definition.[3]

This chapter discusses the role of insulin resistance and obesity in PCOS and, arising from these features, will describe the range of metabolic perturbances that increase risk of future vascular disease. Finally, current evidence on the benefits of lifestyle intervention and insulin-sensitizing agents will be briefly overviewed.

INSULIN RESISTANCE IN POLYCYSTIC OVARIAN SYNDROME AND ITS ROLE IN REPRODUCTIVE ABNORMALITIES

A link between perturbed insulin action and PCOS was first highlighted in 1980[4] and subsequently confirmed by others.[5] Peripheral insulin resistance is most evident in overweight patients and previous researchers have noted that obesity and PCOS have separate and synergistic relations with insulin resistance (reviewed in reference 2) The etiological mechanism(s) underpinning insulin resistance and reproductive

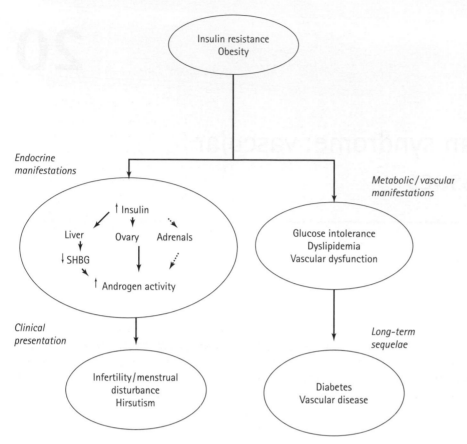

Figure 20.1 The postulated consequences linked to insulin resistance in women with polycystic ovarian syndrome. SHBG, sex-hormone-binding globulin.

abnormalities in women with PCOS are, as yet, unclear. Several factors have been potentially implicated including:

- genetic contributions to reproductive and metabolic features, with the possibility that the same genetic factor(s) are simultaneously responsible for both[2]
- defects in adipose tissue lipolytic cascades[6]
- inflammation mediators upstream to insulin resistance[7]
- fetal programming[8]
- primary ovarian hypersensitivity to insulin, leading firstly to altered hormonal milieu, and over time to alterations in body fat distribution (central > peripheral) with positive feedback toward greater insulin resistance.

Future research to clarify potential mechanisms requires larger studies than those published so far. This is particularly the case for genetic factors where they reduce the possibility of chance findings. The heterogeneity of PCOS also allows the possibility that differing factors underpin different phenotypes in women with PCOS.

Despite insulin resistance in adipose tissue and skeletal muscle, the ovary (and adrenals) may remain relatively sensitive to insulin, and both insulin and insulin-like growth factor 1 have stimulatory effects enhancing thecal and stromal androgen production within the ovary. This in turn leads to abnormal follicular development, which ultimately leads to dysfunctional ovarian and menstrual cyclicity. Androgens are carried in the circulation bound to

sex-hormone-binding globulin (SHBG) with high affinity. Conditions of increased androgen concentrations and hyperinsulinemia[9] are associated with reduced circulating SHBG, which results in high levels of free androgen activity. Thus, clinical manifestations of androgen activity (hirsutism, acne, and alopecia) depend upon the SHBG activity as well as the total circulating androgen concentrations (Fig. 20.1).

Despite the link between insulin resistance and PCOS, it should be recognized that many lean women with PCOS do not necessarily have rank insulin resistance, but may exhibit enhanced ovarian sensitivity to insulin or display insulin hypersecretion in the face of normal insulin sensitivity.[10] Thus, whereas many women with PCOS require a significant excursion into overweight/obesity ranges to manifest the syndrome, and may show distinct benefit from weight reduction, a minority (lean women) may have ovaries enduring excessive insulin exposure and/or are hyperresponsive to insulin leading to defects in ovarian or adrenal androgen production throughout all weight ranges (Fig. 20.2). This suggestion is speculative and requires further direct investigation.

INSULIN RESISTANCE AND METABOLIC FEATURES IN WOMEN WITH POLYCYSTIC OVARIAN SYNDROME

Insulin resistance is linked to a spectrum of metabolic abnormalities which can predate the onset of diabetes and

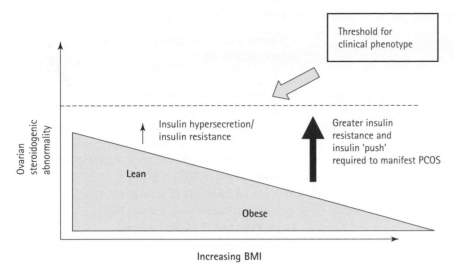

Figure 20.2   It is possible in broad terms that lean women with polycystic ovarian syndrome (PCOS) have either a greater basal steroidogenic abnormality which can manifest in the clinical phenotype with normal insulin levels or have insulin hypersecretion driving excess androgens, whereas women who are overweight or obese and diagnosed with PCOS required a far greater 'push' from insulin resistance and the associated hyperinsulinemia to reach the threshold for the clinical phenotype. BMI, body mass index.

cardiovascular disease by many years. Such abnormalities include lipid perturbances, hemostatic alterations, low-grade chronic inflammation, high blood pressure, endothelial dysfunction, body fat redistribution, and glucose intolerance. The evidence collated below (and summarized in Table 20.1) indicates that many such pathways are indeed altered in young women with PCOS.

Lipids and lipoproteins

The lipoprotein profile in obese women with PCOS is generally characterized by elevated plasma triglyccride, and reduced high-density lipoprotein (HDL)-cholesterol concentrations, which mirrors that seen in subjects with type 2 diabetes.[11–13] It is well recognized that insulin resistance can lead to elevations in triglyceride levels by promoting increased hepatic synthesis of very-low-density lipoprotein (VLDL) particles and by impairing triglyceride catabolism via a reduction in lipoprotein lipase activity. High VLDL and thus triglyceride concentrations can in turn reduce HDL-cholesterol concentrations via neutral lipid exchange. Low-density lipoprotein (LDL)-cholesterol is often only modestly elevated in PCOS. However, a simple quantitative measurement of LDL concentration may be misleading since LDL does not exist as homogeneous particles. Indeed, we and others[14,15] have demonstrated that women with PCOS have a preponderance of small, dense LDL particles, considered more atherogenic, relative to body mass index (BMI)-matched normal controls.

Despite the above evidence on the atherogenic direction of lipid profiles in overweight and obese women with PCOS, in terms of absolute CHD risk, the modest lipids levels – we recently reported a mean cholesterol to HDL-cholesterol ratio of around 4.2 in PCOS women[12] – when considered in conjunction with other risk factors (young age, blood pressure often not raised) result in a low 10-year risk for CHD events. Thus the vast majority of women with

PCOS are not eligible for primary prevention of CHD on current guideline thresholds in which a 20–30 percent event risk over 10 years is the cut-off for primary prevention (for example, with statin therapy) is considered. This factor must be kept in mind when debating whether to introduce mandatory lipid tests in women with PCOS. Our practice does not include routine lipids in all, but we restrict such measurements to women with PCOS who have other significant risk factors. This policy recognizes that in the majority of women, lipid measurements will not alter clinical practice.

Hemostatic factors

There is increasing evidence that elevated plasma levels of hemostatic factors (fibrinogen, factor VII, von Willebrand factor, fibrin D-dimer, and tissue plasminogen activator antigen [tPA]) are independently linked to risk for CHD. There is also increasing evidence that tPA antigen and plasminogen activator inhibitor (PAI)-1 are positively associated with insulin resistance in the general population.[14–18] Correspondingly, both PAI-1 and tPA have been shown to predict diabetes in the general population, independently of other known predictors.[19,20] Moreover, PAI-1 may be pathogenically linked to diabetes development.

Accumulated evidence suggests that circulating concentrations of factor VIIc, fibrinogen, D-dimer and von Willebrand factor are not different in women with PCOS.[21] In contrast, we and others have shown elevations in the PAI-1 and tPA in small cohorts of PCOS women.[21–23] Parallel elevations in both are predictable since tPA–PAI-1 complexes circulate in the plasma. In line with the non-PCOS population, tPA concentrations in women with PCOS correlated directly with the degree of obesity, and inversely with insulin sensitivity.[21] Of note, neither lipid abnormalities nor hemostatic perturbances correlate with total testosterone concentrations in women with PCOS.[14,21]

Table 20.1   Summary of evidence on risk factor abnormalities in PCOS and effects of insulin-sensitizing agents

Risk parameters	Consistency of evidence for abnormality in PCOS	Effects of insulin-sensitizing agents in women with PCOS
Adiposity/insulin resistance	Commonly obese, and evidence for greater central fat distribution or greater visceral fat context Greater insulin resistance for given BMI especially in overweight or obese women Perhaps insulin hypersecretion in lean women	Metformin associated with modest weight reduction (~4%) and insulin sensitization Glitazones tend to increase weight slightly but improve insulin resistance perhaps more than metformin. They do so largely by redistributing fat in diabetes patients. **Relevant studies in PCOS required**
Lipids	Generally raised triglyceride and lower HDL-cholesterol. Evidence of greater proportion and mass of small, dense LDL	Generally increased HDL-C, lowered LDL-C with metformin. Glitazones may increase HDL-C **Larger more robust studies required**
Blood pressure	Evidence conflicting – better studies required	No evidence of benefit with metformin
Inflammation	Several reports of elevated CRP, and one each of elevated white cell count and IL-18	Metformin reduced CRP in one study No data for glitazones but they lower CRP in type 2 diabetes. **More data needed**
Endothelial dysfunction	Majority of reports confirm impaired endothelial function	Troglitazone improved endothelial function in PCOS
Metabolic syndrome (ATP III criteria)	Twofold to fourfold higher prevalence of metabolic syndrome compared with controls with similar BMI Prevalence varies from 15% to 46% dependent on BMI of PCOS cohort studied	Reduction in several components of metabolic syndrome by combination of diet and metformin in women with PCOS fulfilling the ATP III defined metabolic syndrome
Glucose intolerance/type 2 diabetes	Up to 45% of women in some series have either IGT or type 2 diabetes Risk for IGT or type 2 diabetes around twofold to fourfold higher relative to age and BMI similar controls	Short-term studies suggest improvements in glucose tolerance **but currently lack prospective studies on incident diabetes**
Subclinical atherosclerosis	Evidence for greater carotid intima–media wall thickness, and coronary artery calcification	**Not examined**
CHD events	~50% increased risk of CHD events in women with very irregular cycles (majority of whom will have PCOS) independent of age and BMI	**Not examined**

ATP III, Adult Treatment Panel III; BMI, body mass index; C, cholesterol; CHD, coronary heart disease; CRP, C-reactive protein; HDL, high-density lipoprotein; IL, interleukin; LDL, low-density lipoprotein; PCOS, polycystic ovary syndrome.

Blood pressure

Patients with diabetes are at increased risk of hypertension and many already have hypertension by the time their diabetes is diagnosed. There are also plausible mechanistic links between insulin resistance and type 2 diabetes. It would be expected therefore that women with PCOS would have higher blood pressures than BMI-matched control women. However, in a recent excellent review,[16] Wild indicated that the current evidence on this concept is unconvincing. He also pointed out that current data are limited by small studies and weak methodology and suggested that much larger and robust studies are required before we can make any firm conclusions on blood pressure trends in women with PCOS.

Inflammation

Inflammation as a causal factor in the atherogenic process is currently a major topic of interest in the cardiovascular arena.[24] Surrogate markers of inflammation such as C-reactive protein (CRP) predict risk of CHD events in both men and women, independently of classic risk factors. However, the exact level of prediction afforded by elevated CRP is currently under debate.[25] At the cellular level, inflammation is involved in several stages of the atherosclerotic process. Moreover, many existing cardioprotective agents – aspirin, statins, and angiotensinogen-converting enzyme inhibitors – all possess anti-inflammatory properties.[26]

Our group has shown that women with PCOS had increased concentrations of circulating CRP[7] and that such elevations are independent of BMI and linked to greater insulin resistance. Indeed, there is now an expanding literature on the possible mechanistic links between inflammatory mediators/cells and the development of insulin resistance and type 2 diabetes.[26] For example, elevations in CRP levels have been shown by us[27] and others[28] to predict type 2 diabetes in men and in women. Thus, low-grade chronic inflammation might be another plausible mechanism contributing to increased risk of CHD and type 2 diabetes in women with PCOS.

Our observations on CRP in PCOS were confirmed by Boulman et al.[29] who showed a doubling of CRP (5.4 mg/L vs. 2.0 mg/L) in 116 PCOS patients compared with 94 similar-BMI controls. In addition, other markers linked to low-grade inflammation inclusive of white blood cell elevations,[30] and serum interleukin (IL)-18 levels[31] have been shown to be elevated in women with PCOS. At the genetic levels, preliminary evidence links common polymorphisms in the genes encoding tumor necrosis factor (TNF)-α, type 2 TNF receptor, IL-6, and the IL-6 signaling molecule gp130 with hyperandrogenism and PCOS.[32,33] Although these observations are of potential interest, much more work is required to dissect any pathogenic role of inflammation in PCOS. It should be remembered that insulin resistance could lead to low-grade inflammation rather than the reverse, and that obesity is a major factor promoting low-grade inflammation in general. Finally, whether inflammatory mediators (that is, CRP, IL-6, TNF-α) are truly causally related to diabetes and CHD remains to be proved.

Endothelial dysfunction in PCOS

Endothelial dysfunction is considered as both an early event in the atherogenic process and as a novel predictor of CHD events independent of traditional risk markers; recent longitudinal studies in the CHD arena provide some support for this proposition.[34] A number of studies have examined endothelial function in PCOS using differing techniques and most, but not all, report impaired function.[35–38] Of note, recent studies suggest impaired endothelial function even in young, normal weight women with PCOS which may be linked to both their relative greater insulin resistance and low-grade inflammation.[35,36] Despite such evidence, it should be recognized that endothelial dysfunction cannot be used as a surrogate for cardiovascular endpoints, and that improvements in endothelial function by any therapy does not guarantee clinical benefit.

Obesity and central body fat distribution

Obesity is common in PCOS with up to 50–60 percent of women having a BMI greater than 25 kg/m². It is well recognized that visceral distribution of body fat is of greater consequence to the metabolic effects of insulin resistance than obesity per se. Central obesity and insulin resistance lead to an altered lipolytic response to insulin, with impaired suppression of release of free fatty acids from adipose tissue. It is also speculated that an increased flux of free fatty acids from central sites enters the portal circulation, increasing the availability of substrate to the liver for triglyceride production, leading to greater hepatic fat accumulation and potentially provoking greater gluconeogenesis. There is some evidence of greater central fat accumulation in women with PCOS. For example, Holte and colleagues[39] noted a more pronounced truncal-abdominal fat distribution in 49 women with PCOS compared to 42 BMI-similar controls. Moreover, they noted that insulin resistance was seen only at higher BMI levels and was largely determined by the increased truncal-abdominal fat mass in PCOS. Similarly, others have shown greater waist circumference or waist-to-hip ratio in women with PCOS independent of BMI.[31] In a recent study, Yildrim and colleagues[40] measured intraabdominal, preperitoneal fat, and subcutaneous fat thickness by ultrasonography in 30 normal weight women with PCOS and healthy controls (average BMIs ∼20 kg/m²). They noted a near-twofold higher visceral and preperitoneal fat thickness in the women with PCOS despite near identical BMI and similar subcutaneous fat content. In addition, visceral fat thickness independently correlated with fasting insulin and triglyceride concentrations. Such findings concur with growing evidence for a potent role for visceral fat tissue in the genesis of metabolic syndrome and its related features. In contrast the lesser importance of the subcutaneous depot was elegantly demonstrated in a recent study revealing no metabolic benefit from liposuction of subcutaneous tissue.[41]

Metabolic syndrome criteria and prevalence in PCOS

There is considerable recent interest in metabolic syndrome criteria as a novel means to identify patients at elevated CHD risk. The criteria incorporate a series of cut-offs for risk parameters linked to insulin resistance including adiposity measures, lipid parameters, blood pressure, glucose levels, and in some cases estimates of insulin resistance. The World Health Organization (WHO) definition[42] focuses primarily on patients with existing evidence of glucose dysregulation, at which stage the risk of conversion to diabetes is already high. To identify patients without normal glucose levels with metabolic syndrome, the WHO criteria require at least a fasting insulin measurement. The difficulties involved in obtaining fasting insulin, and the lack of global standardization of insulin, preclude widespread clinical use of the WHO criteria in most subjects. Partly for this reason, in 2001 the Adult Treatment Panel (ATP) III of the National Cholesterol Education Program (NCEP)[43] proposed a new definition of the metabolic syndrome using thresholds for five easily measured variables linked to insulin resistance: waist circumference, triglyceride, HDL-cholesterol, fasting plasma glucose concentration, and blood pressure. Individuals have metabolic syndrome if predefined limits of any three criteria are exceeded and, therefore, many such individuals can have normal fasting glucose concentrations. This definition allows population data to be more easily gathered. Due to their simplicity, there is now a wealth of studies using the ATPIII criteria.[44–46] These demonstrate, unsurprisingly, that individuals with metabolic syndrome are at elevated risk for type 2 diabetes (severalfold higher) and CHD events (~70–200 percent higher). Whether ATPIII-defined metabolic syndrome predicts CHD events independent of traditional predictors remains contentious and requires more study.

Given that a large proportion of women with PCOS are overweight or obese, with a high incidence of rank insulin resistance with raised BMI, we would predict that women with PCOS show a high prevalence of metabolic syndrome. We noted previously that PCOS may be the gynecologic presentation of the metabolic syndrome in young women.[47] Using ATPIII criteria, Talbott and colleagues reported a 15 percent prevalence of metabolic syndrome in a cohort of PCOS women with a mean BMI of 25.8 kg/m^2 which compared to a 3.5 percent prevalence of healthy controls with a mean BMI of 24.6 kg/m^2.[48] Moreover, in the latter study, while more than one in three women with PCOS fulfilled two or more ATPIII criteria, fewer than one in 12 of the controls did. Recently, Apridonidze and colleagues in a retrospective observation reported a 46 percent incidence of metabolic syndrome (by modified ATPIII) in 106 mostly obese women referred to their clinics with PCOS over a 3-year period. This represents an incidence twice that of age-matched women in the general population.[49] Apridonidze *et al.* also noted that those with metabolic syndrome had, unsurprisingly, greater free testosterone, lower SHBG, and more acanthosis nigricans. Overall, these two reports confirm impressions from individual risk factor studies described above and demonstrate that both obesity and PCOS status separately influence the likelihood of having metabolic syndrome. In other words, women with PCOS accrue more metabolic abnormalities with increasing BMI compared with women without PCOS which is generally in keeping with greater increments in insulin resistance with increasing BMI (Fig. 20.3).

Should metabolic syndrome status be examined in PCOS?

Whether clinicians should routinely ascertain metabolic syndrome status in their patients with PCOS is currently debatable. A recent consensus statement suggested that features of metabolic syndrome (waist, triglyceride, HDL-cholesterol, blood pressure, fasting glucose) *should* be routinely recorded in women with PCOS, but it did not recommend measuring insulin.[3] However, consensus on treatment recommendations for non-PCOS subjects with metabolic syndrome is presently lacking, and there are no clear data to suggest metabolic syndrome or insulin resistance measures predict greater clinical benefit from metformin or

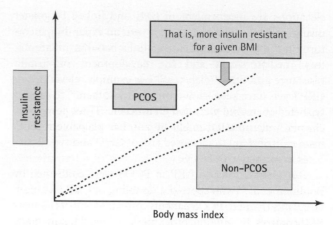

Figure 20.3   Women with polycystic ovarian syndrome (PCOS) are more insulin resistant and consistent with this, they have a greater prevalence of metabolic syndrome for a given body mass index (BMI).

other treatments in women with PCOS (reviewed in reference 50). The best use of metabolic syndrome criteria presently might be to facilitate targeting of more comprehensive lifestyle advice to those overweight or obese women with PCOS who also have elements of the metabolic syndrome. Future studies should address this issue.

Glucose intolerance and diabetes in PCOS

The excess risk of diabetes in women with PCOS compared with age-matched normal women is strongly contributed to by obesity, which remains one of the strongest predictors of type 2 diabetes. For example, in a recent 10-year follow-up of the Bruneck study, a population-based prospective study of 40–79-year-olds,[51] the relative risk for new-onset type 2 diabetes in non-diabetic individuals at baseline with BMI > 30 kg/m^2 was 9.9 (95 percent confidence interval [CI] 4.5 to 21.4) compared with similar subjects with BMI < 25 kg/m^2. In overweight subjects the relative risk for type 2 diabetes was 3.4-fold (95 percent CI 1.8 to 6.3). Individuals who also had impaired fasting glucose (>6.1 mmol/L) also showed an increased risk for developing new-onset diabetes. Yet, in line with greater insulin resistance for a given BMI, women with PCOS have an excess risk of diabetes even after accounting for total adiposity. Legro and colleagues[52] examined glucose tolerance in two large groups of women with PCOS (N = 254), and 80 control women of similar age, weight (generally obese) and ethnicity. The women with PCOS showed an incidence of impaired glucose intolerance (IGT) of 31.1 percent and diabetes of 7.5 percent, contrasting with 15.7 percent and 0 percent, respectively, in control women. Thus prevalence of glucose intolerance was significantly higher in PCOS vs. control women (odds ratio 2.76, 95 percent confidence interval 1.23 to 6.57). These data concur with smaller relevant studies (reviewed in reference 16). Variables associated with post oral glucose tolerance testing (OGTT) glucose levels in the study by Legro *et al.* included fasting glucose levels ($P < 0.0001$), PCOS status ($P = 0.002$), waist/hip ratio ($P = 0.01$), and BMI ($P = 0.021$). These investigators also noted that the American Diabetes Association criteria based on fasting glucose alone significantly underdiagnosed diabetes compared with the WHO criteria (3.2 percent vs. 7.5 percent; $P = 0.046$; odds ratio = 2.48, 95 percent confidence interval 1.01 to 6.69).

Overall, current evidence favors a twofold to fourfold increase risk of glucose intolerance/type 2 diabetes in women with PCOS over age- and weight-matched controls. Of course, this excess risk is consistent with the array of risk factors discussed previously and a greater prevalence of metabolic syndrome and visceral fat accumulation independent of total obesity. As a diagnosis of diabetes has clinical ramifications, all women with PCOS should have at least a fasting glucose done as part of their baseline tests and a selected subgroup should have a subsequent OGTT. Some groups perform OGTTs on all their patients with PCOS but the cost–benefit ratio of this approach has not been examined. We would suggest restricting OGTTs for PCOS women with another element such as obesity (BMI > 30 kg/m^2) or fasting glucose >5.5 mmol/L or a relevant family history; the vast majority of women with PCOS studied by different groups who had impaired glucose tolerance or frank diabetes had BMI > 30 kg/m^2, whereas frank diabetes by OGTT was rare if fasting glucose was less than 5.5 mmol/L in the series reported by Legro and colleagues.[52] Clearly, further research into glucose tolerance levels and the best screening methods and circumstances in PCOS is important.

Measures of atherosclerosis in women with polycystic ovarian syndrome

A number of studies have predicted an increased risk of vascular disease in women with PCOS based on surrogate endpoints including carotid intima–media wall thickness (IMT), coronary artery calcification, and angiography. Earlier angiographic studies linked androgenic and metabolic feature of PCOS as well as the presence of polycystic ovaries to greater likelihood of coronary lesions.[53,54] Talbott and coworkers determined carotid IMT in a series of PCOS cases and controls and noted among women aged $\geqslant 45$ years, women with a history of PCOS had significantly greater mean IMT than did control women (0.78 ± 0.03 vs. 0.70 ± 0.01 mm, $P = 0.005$).[55] This difference remained significant after adjustment for age and BMI ($P < 0.05$). Younger women showed no difference. The same group reported a lack of correlation of between higher CRP levels and elevated IMT in PCOS, a finding in keeping with data from the general population.[56] Talbott *et al.* stated that the effect of BMI on the PCOS–IMT relation is not completely determined by hyperinsulinemia or visceral fat, and might be mediated by other aspects of PCOS-related adiposity.

The findings of elevated IMT in PCOS are noteworthy since carotid IMT has recently been accepted by the United States Federal Drug Administration as a surrogate measure for CHD risk for the purposes of clinical trials.

There are now two studies reporting coronary calcification measurements assessed by electron beam computed tomography (EBCT) in women with PCOS.[48,57] Christian *et al.* examined women with PCOS, aged 30–45 years, control subjects matched by age and BMI. The prevalence of coronary artery calcification (CAC) in premenopausal women with PCOS was significantly greater than that of community-dwelling women (odds ratio 5.5) and similar to that of men of comparable age.[57] This finding was corroborated by Talbott *et al.*: PCOS status was a significant predictor of CAC (odds ratio 2.31; $P = 0.049$) even after accounting for age and BMI in their study.[48] However, CAC estimates imprecisely predict CHD events and many investigators remain concerned about the validity of the EBCT observations.

Coronary heart disease event risk in polycystic ovarian syndrome from observational and epidemiologic studies

Wild and colleagues examined the possibility of a link between PCOS and CHD in 2000 and examined women over a 31-year follow-up period.[58] A cohort of 786 women with PCOS before 1979 was traced and data obtained from death certificates for 70 women. Based on the relatively small number of CHD deaths (n = 15), they could not confirm an elevated CHD risk in women with PCOS relative to data from national statistics: odds ratio for CHD in PCOS was 1.5 (95 percent CI 0.7 to 2.9). The wide confidence interval reflects the study's modest sample size and it should be noted that PCOS diagnosis was based upon ovarian wedge resection, which may have limited extrapolation to the general PCOS population. Larger studies with better baseline phenotyping are clearly needed.

Perhaps the best indication of CHD risk in PCOS comes from a recent study by Solomon and colleagues.[59] In a prospective cohort of 82 439 female nurses they linked history on prior menstrual regularity (at ages 20–35 years) in 1982 to subsequent CHD endpoints over 14 years' follow-up. There were 1417 incident cases of CHD and 838 incident cases of stroke, including 471 cases of ischemic stroke. Compared with women reporting a history of very regular menstrual cycles (self-reported but with reasonable validation), women reporting usually irregular or very irregular cycles had an increased risk for nonfatal or fatal CHD (age-adjusted relative risks [RR] 1.25 and 1.67, respectively, 95 percent CI 1.07 to 1.47 and 1.35 to 2.06, respectively). Risk for stroke was nonsignificantly increased.[59] Importantly, the increased risk for CHD associated with very irregular cycle group remained significant (RR 1.53, 95 percent CI 1.24 to 1.90) after adjustment for BMI and several potential confounders inclusive of age, smoking, parity, and menopausal status. When investigators additionally controlled for

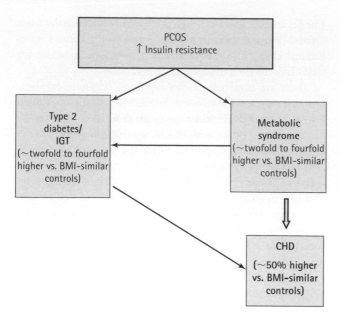

Figure 20.4   In line with greater insulin resistance, women with polycystic ovarian syndrome (PCOS) have greater prevalence of metabolic syndrome, and associated with this around a twofold to fourfold increased risk of impaired glucose tolerance (IGT)/type 2 diabetes relative to age and body mass index (BMI)-matched healthy controls. Data on risk for coronary heart disease (CHD) events is currently sparse but suggest around a 50% higher CHD risk relative to controls with adjustment for age, BMI, smoking, parity, and menopausal status. Whether adjustment for all traditional risk factors completely accounts for this excess risk remains to be determined.

some other conventional risk factors (diabetes, history of hypertension or hypercholesterolemia), the risk was attenuated to 1.34 (95 percent CI 1.08 to 1.66). This additional adjustment suggests traditional risk factors do at least partially account for greater CHD risk in PCOS. The lack of data on HDL-cholesterol was a notable omission and weakness. As up to 80–90 percent of women with very irregular cycles are likely to have PCOS, the data suggest PCOS is associated with a 50 percent increased risk for CHD compared to age, BMI-matched women without PCOS, a figure comparable with the odds ratio reported by Wild and colleagues.[58] This excess CHD risk is in keeping with greater prevalence of metabolic syndrome and IGT or type 2 diabetes in women with PCOS (Fig. 20.4). Future studies should address to what extent this excess risk is accounted for by a comprehensive panel of traditional risk factors including presence of diabetes, and direct measures of blood pressure, cholesterol, and especially HDL-cholesterol.

MECHANISMS TO REDUCE DIABETES AND VASCULAR RISK IN WOMEN WITH POLYCYSTIC OVARIAN SYNDROME (SUMMARIZED IN TABLE 20.2)

There is no long-term study examining effects of lifestyle or insulin-sensitizing agents on diabetes or CHD endpoints in women with PCOS. There are also sparse data about the effects of any intervention on surrogate vascular endpoints such as endothelial function measures or carotid IMT in PCOS. There are plentiful short-term data on changes in insulin measures and related reproductive hormonal changes, in particular with metformin. Only a minority of relevant, robustly designed studies have addressed changes in CHD risk factors with interventions, and further data are

required.[50] A summary of the evidence for changes effected with lifestyle changes, metformin and the thiazolidinediones (peroxisome proliferators-activated receptor [PPAR] agonists or 'glitazones') in women with PCOS are given below with a focus on metabolic changes associated with the metabolic syndrome.

Lifestyle modification

Mounting evidence demonstrates substantial metabolic and related benefits attainable by lifestyle improvements in the general population. In women with PCOS, a reduction in BMI of around 5–10 percent by dietary therapy has been shown to improve ovarian function and some metabolic risk factors.[60,61] This finding, allied to recent evidence demonstrating intensive lifestyle intervention, involving at least a 7 percent weight loss and at least 150 minutes of physical activity per week, can substantially reduce (by 58 percent) the development of diabetes in subjects at risk, provides compelling arguments to conduct more robust dietary and exercise intervention studies in women with PCOS.[62] These should include, where possible, a comprehensive panel of traditional and novel risk factors, direct measures of vascular function and quality of life measures. The much wider health benefits of physical activity and exercise should be noted in this context. Thus, achieving greater levels of physical activity in individuals at greater risk such as obese women with PCOS is rapidly becoming one of the major health goals in the United Kingdom and elsewhere. It could be argued that due to their greater accumulation of risk factors for similar weight gain, women with PCOS have more to gain from increasing physical activity levels than their non-PCOS counterparts. Finally, since many women with PCOS wish to improve fertility,

Table 20.2 Current practice and summaries of effects of interventions targeting weight/insulin resistance in women with PCOS. Indications for future research and evidence of long-term benefits of each intervention outwith PCOS are also given

	Demonstrable benefits in PCOS	Current practice in women with PCOS	Future areas for investigation	Diabetes and CHD endpoint benefits seen in non–PCOS
Lifestyle intervention	Improved fertility with weight loss, improved risk factor profile	Frequently inadequately addressed	More data, in particular on effects of increasing physical activity levels versus effects of insulin-sensitizing agents More research into mechanism to enhance and sustain higher levels of physical activity	Evidence for reduced diabetes in high-risk subjects with impaired glucose tolerance Consistent epidemiological evidence for reduced CHD events
Metformin	Modest effects on BMI, insulin resistance, lipids, ovulation and androgens Gestational diabetes	Commonly used to improve cycle regulation or fertility and occasionally used to treat hirsutism Continued through pregnancy in some centers	Larger randomized trials and effects of metformin in combination with lifestyle/physical activity Pregnancy safety data	Reduced diabetes risk Weight gain less than controls Reduced CHD event risk in type 2 diabetes
Glitazones	Possibly better improvements in insulin resistance independent of BMI, plus benefits on LH and SHBG/ androgens and mounting evidence of improved fertility Data on risk factor changes and body fat distribution presently limited	Recent introduction into PCOS armory in some centers but presently given with caution: women told not to become pregnant due to potential teratogenicity	Further larger trials with placebo control Effects of combined metformin and glitazones with adequate control Effects on surrogate markers of atherosclerosis Pregnancy safety data	Reduced risk for type 2 diabetes in women with prior gestational diabetes Endpoint CHD trials will report in near future
Xenical	Only one published study. Reduction in weight modest (~5%) but > metformin and equivalent effects of both in reducing testosterone No effects on other parameters but study was short and did not address ovulation potential		Randomized trial data required in larger numbers Combinations should also be explored	Reduced risk for type 2 diabetes in obese subjects

BMI, body mass index; CHD; coronary heart disease; LH, luteinizing hormone; PCOS, polycystic ovary syndrome; SHBG, sex-hormone-binding globulin.

lifestyle measures will be physiologically far better for subsequent pregnancy outcomes than approaches requiring medication.

Metformin

Metformin is an oral biguanide antihyperglycemic drug that has been used for many years in Europe and is now also widely used worldwide. Metformin is thought to have primary effects on increasing peripheral glucose uptake in response to insulin, with some reduction in basal hepatic glucose production. However, it also lowers adipose tissue lipolysis and improves insulin sensitivity in muscle. It does not provoke hyperinsulinemia and as such does not cause hypoglycemia. It is now recommended as first-line therapy in overweight patients with diabetes by most leading clinical associations (for example, Scottish Intercollegiate Guidelines Network guidelines, Diabetes UK). Most of the studies on metformin use in PCOS have addressed effects on ovulation rates, reproductive hormones and insulin metabolism. We and others[50,63] have recently reviewed the best studies in this area (Fig. 20.5 provides a summary of best evidence).

In terms of metabolic and anthropometric effects, current evidence supports a reduction in BMI by around 4 percent over a few months compared with placebo (representing ~2–3 kg reduction) in women with PCOS.[50] Clearly more data are required but a weight-reducing effect would be consistent with the documented effects of metformin in large

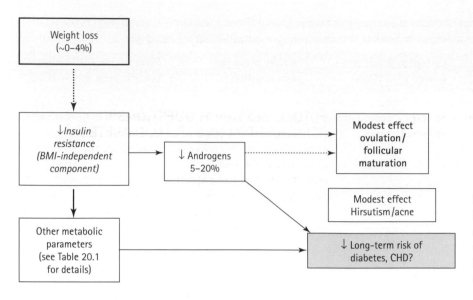

Figure 20.5   A summary of the proposed benefits including metabolic and vascular effects of metformin treatment in women with polycystic ovarian syndrome. BMI, body mass index; CHD, coronary heart disease.

prospective studies of patients at elevated risk for diabetes (~2 kg reduction relative to placebo at 6 months.[62] With respect to biochemical changes, total and free androgen levels decreased by ~20 percent relative to placebo with metformin[50] and fasting insulin levels declined by a mean of 5.4 mIU/L (95 percent CI −8.11 to −2.63) relative to placebo.[63] Reduction in LDL-cholesterol and tPA antigen and increases in HDL-cholesterol have been noted with metformin in PCOS but larger trials are required to confirm these effects.[64] More recently, a reduction in CRP with metformin use in PCOS has been noted by Morin-Papunen and colleagues, with waist-to-hip ratio ($P = 0.03$) and waist circumference ($P = 0.04$) the only significant determinants of the serum CRP decrease at 6 months of metformin treatment, explaining together about 20 percent of the overall effect.[65] Finally, a combination of diet and metformin for 6 months has been shown to lessen metabolic syndrome prevalence in women with PCOS.[66]

Thus, on balance the metabolic changes noted with metformin use in women with PCOS are consistent with its known effect in patients with type 2 diabetes. However, larger, longer duration and more comprehensive controlled studies on risk factor levels are required in women with PCOS receiving metformin. Ideally, these should include direct vascular measures and, if sufficiently powered, document risk reduction for development of diabetes. In the diabetes prevention program (DPP),[62] metformin treatment resulted in a 31 percent reduction in the incidence of diabetes, compared with placebo. The latter question may be difficult to address in the PCOS population since many women now seek metformin as a quick and easy 'cure' either for their impaired fertility/altered cyclicity or hirsutism and even to help them lose weight and, as a result few might be willing to take placebo or have no treatment for long periods. It is important to note, however, that metformin is not licensed for any of these indications and, from the evidence presented above it is certainly not a 'cure' for all reproductive and metabolic derangements in women with PCOS.

In view of metformin's modest benefits in women with PCOS, the relative merits of metformin combined to lifestyle changes, in particular exercise, would be very important to examine and such studies are being developed. It is interesting that both exercise and metformin upregulate adenosine monophosphate (AMP)-activated protein kinase activity, a metabolic switch regulating efficient glucose and fatty acid metabolism.[67] It should also be noted that lifestyle intervention was more successful than metformin alone in reducing risk of diabetes in DPP, once again emphasizing the critical role for lifestyle intervention.

Although studies in the nondiabetes population are lacking, an increasing body of evidence favors a reduction in CHD risk with metformin in patients with type 2 diabetes. For example, metformin treatment was more effective in reducing CHD risk than either insulin or sulfonylurea in the United Kingdom Prospective Diabetes Study.[68] In addition, follow-up in other cohorts suggests metformin lessens risk of vascular events by around a half compared with sulfonylurea therapy.[69]

Early trial evidence with peroxisome proliferators–activated receptor gamma agonists in polycystic ovarian syndrome

Despite the wealth of evidence for use of metformin in PCOS, data on other insulin sensitizers, in particular the PPAR-γ agonists are comparatively less. This is partly because the withdrawal of troglitazone in late 1990s (due to concerns over hepatotoxicity) led to a slower introduction of newer safer glitazones in to the diabetes field. Furthermore, the new glitazones (rosiglitazone and pioglitazone) are pregnancy class C drugs: there is evidence of teratogenicity in animal studies including lethality. Metformin is a class B drug (no evidence of teratogenicity). Despite these concerns, several relatively small studies reporting reproductive and metabolic benefits with rosiglitazone and pioglitazone in women with PCOS have now been published, including recent placebo-controlled reports.[70–76] The totality of data suggests that effects of glitazones on insulin resistance may be greater than with metformin. Consistent with the latter, preliminary evidence indicates that glitazones can improve reproductive and metabolic parameters and enhance menstrual cyclicity in women not optimally responsive to metformin,[76] although another recent report provided contradictory data.[71]

The metabolic benefits of glitazones in women with PCOS might be better than corresponding effects of metformin. Recent studies in patients with type 2 diabetes suggest more pronounced effects of glitazones compared with metformin on insulin resistance and endothelial function. For example, troglitazone therapy improved endothelial function to near normal levels in women with polycystic ovary syndrome[77] but similar observations for metformin in PCOS are conspicuously sparse. Glitazone effects on lipids in PCOS have been less well studied but of note, liver function tests improved (reduced γ-glutamyl transferase and alanine aminotransferase) in one study[73] consistent with data in non-PCOS subjects and a reduction in liver fat content.

Nevertheless, it should be remembered that although metformin often reduces weight by a few kilograms, glitazones can increase weight due in part to an expansion of the subcutaneous fat depot. The latter can be an unwelcome effect for many women, but thus far has not been widely reported as a reason for noncompliance in PCOS trials. Glitazones can also cause mild peripheral edema and in one recent randomized study, nearly 1 in 5 women receiving pioglitazone reported this side effect whereas none in the placebo group did so,[75] although other trials have reported fewer side effects. It should also be remembered that evidence for cardiovascular benefits of metformin are currently far more rigorous than those for glitazones. The major glitazones–CHD event trials are due to commence reporting in the near future and their evidence will determine the extent to which glitazones are used, both in the general population, and perhaps as longer-term treatment in women with PCOS. Of course neither metformin nor glitazones are currently licensed or recommended for the prevention of diabetes (or indeed CHD) in patients at elevated risk despite evidence of benefit in those with IGT[62] or post-gestational diabetes.[78]

Other modalities

A recent small study examined the effects of orlistat versus metformin on metabolic parameters in PCOS.[79] Orlistat is a lipase inhibitor which gives partial inhibition (approximately 30 percent) of dietary fat absorption and is licensed to aid weight reduction in conjunction with lifestyle changes in obese subjects. Orlistat has recently been shown to reduce risk for type 2 diabetes in obese subjects.[80] In women with PCOS, orlistat resulted in greater weight loss compared to metformin but equivalent effects in reducing

testosterone.[79] No effects on other parameters were noted including insulin and lipids and the size and length of study precluded examination of ovulation effects. Further studies are required before any conclusions can be reached.

FUTURE RESEARCH QUESTIONS IN RELATION TO LONG-TERM DIABETES AND VASCULAR RISK IN POLYCYSTIC OVARIAN SYNDROME

Several questions in relation to this topic remain uncertain or unanswered (see Table 20.2). First, despite the demonstrable array of risk factor abnormalities in women with PCOS, further larger, well-controlled studies addressing risk factors and clinical relevance in PCOS are required. In particular, large, perhaps multicenter longitudinal studies should address risk for vascular events in PCOS, and determine whether differing phenotypes, as would be predicted, are affected differently. Such studies should also determine whether traditional risk factors fully account for excess vascular risk in this patient group, and whether novel risk factors add predictive information. Large multicenter studies would also facilitate better genotype investigations and related work examining pathogenic pathways for insulin resistance/hypersecretion and steroid abnormalities in PCOS. One of the problems with these proposals is the way many with PCOS get metformin treatment on an *ad hoc* basis.

In terms of treatment, there is an urgent need for more robust lifestyle intervention studies, especially incorporating physical activity/exercise. There is a growing awareness in general of the substantial metabolic and wider health benefits of physical activity. The comparative metabolic and reproductive effects of metformin and the glitazones, as well as their combination, requires direct study. In addition, future studies employing other insulin-sensitizing or weight-losing modalities are needed. Finally, whether long-term treatment with metformin or other therapeutic interventions (for example, glitazones) lessen the risk for diabetes and vascular events in PCOS needs to be addressed. In the short term, such studies in PCOS could examine effects of treatment on surrogate atherosclerotic measures such as progression of carotid IMT thickness. In the longer term, event-driven trials would be the gold standard to test treatment effects but in reality such studies are unlikely to occur in the near future.

CONCLUSION

Insulin resistance is an important feature in many women with PCOS and insulin hypersecretion is potentially universal. It is clear that they have reproductive and metabolic consequences. Women with PCOS generally exhibit visceral adiposity, a dyslipidemia which mirrors the pattern in type 2 diabetes (elevated triglyceride, low HDL-cholesterol, small, dense LDL), low-grade inflammation, abnormalities in clotting and, in particular, glucose intolerance. They are therefore at elevated risk for type 2 diabetes or IGT (about twofold to fourfold relative to weight-matched controls) and CHD events. All women with PCOS should have at least a fasting glucose determination, with follow-up OGTT in those who have raised fasting glucose (>5.5 mmol/L) or are obese or have a relevant family history. The best estimates for increased CHD risk is currently around 50 percent higher risk relative to non-PCOS women of similar age and BMI. Since CHD risk is generally low in young women, absolute CHD risk in PCOS is likely low and thus the need for routine lipids or determination of metabolic syndrome status is not necessary in the absence of other significant risk factors.

In recognition of the role of insulin resistance in PCOS, use of metformin is increasingly undertaken, but its reproductive and metabolic effects are modest in the relatively short-term studies available. Although data are relatively sparse, metformin seems to achieve modest improvements in LDL-cholesterol, HDL-cholesterol, in tPA and CRP, at least in some circumstances. It is thus probable that longer-term treatment with metformin in PCOS will attenuate the progress to diabetes and perhaps vascular risk in PCOS, but prospective clinical trial data examining at least surrogate markers of atherosclerosis would be useful. Recent studies suggest at least equivalent and perhaps greater metabolic and reproductive benefits with glitazone therapy in women with PCOS but existing trial data are limited. The safety of these drugs with regard to ensuing pregnancy outcome also needs examination. Finally, the proved benefits of exercise in lowering diabetes and vascular risk, together with wider health benefits, suggest future studies should urgently address how best to enhance physical activity levels in women with PCOS. The latter approach has the potential to be the cheapest and physiologically best mechanism to lessen metabolic and vascular risk in this at-risk population.

KEY LEARNING POINTS

- Women with PCOS exhibit perturbations (albeit often modest) in many risk predictors for both type 2 diabetes and vascular disease.
- Many such risk factor abnormalities are linked to insulin resistance which is elevated in women with, compared to those without, PCOS.
- In general terms, relative risks for diabetes or IGT are about twofold to fourfold relative to weight-matched controls. All women with PCOS should therefore have at least a fasting glucose determination, with follow-up OGTT in those who have raised fasting glucose (>5.5 mmol/L), or are obese or have a relevant family history.
- The best estimate for increased CHD risk is currently around 50 percent higher *relative risk* to non-PCOS women of similar age and BMI.

- As CHD risk is generally low in young women, *absolute* CHD risk in PCOS is likely low or only minimally elevated and thus the need for routine lipids or determination of metabolic syndrome status is not necessary in the vast majority unless other significant risk factors, such as documented hypertension or family history of premature CHD, exist.
- Lifestyle factors leading to greater physical activity and weight loss are first priority in such women but there is increasing recognition of the benefits of insulin-sensitizing agents (in particular metformin) for reduction in risk of diabetes and potentially also CHD. However, long-term trials with such agents in PCOS are lacking and women considering long-term treatment for such purposes should be appropriately counseled.

REFERENCES

1 Franks S. Polycystic ovary syndrome. *N Engl J Med* 1995; 333: 853–61.
2 Dunaif A, Thomas A. Current concepts in the polycystic ovary syndrome. *Annu Rev Med* 2001; **52**: 401–19.
3 The Rotterdam ESHRE/ASRM-Sponsored PCOS consensus workshop group. Revised 2003 consensus on diagnostic criteria and long-term health risks related to polycystic ovary syndrome (PCOS). *Hum Reprod* 2004; **19**: 41–7.
4 Burghen GA, Givens JR, Kitabchi AE. Correlation of hyperandrogenism with hyperinsulinemia in polycystic ovarian disease. *J Clin Endocrinol Metab* 1980; **50**: 113–16.
5 Chang JR, Nakamura RM, Howard LJ, Kaplan SA. Insulin resistance in nonobese patients with polycystic ovarian disease. *J Clin Endocrinol Metab* 1983; **57**: 356–9.
6 Ek I, Arner P, Ryden M, *et al.* A unique defect in the regulation of visceral fat cell lipolysis in the polycystic ovary syndrome as an early link to insulin resistance. *Diabetes* 2002; **51**: 484–92.
7 Kelly CC, Lyall H, Petrie JR, *et al.* Low grade chronic inflammation in women with polycystic ovarian syndrome. *J Clin Endocrinol Metab* 2001; **86**: 2453–5.
8 Cresswell JL, Barker DJ, Osmond C, *et al.* Fetal growth, length of gestation, and polycystic ovaries in adult life. *Lancet* 1997; **350**: 1131–5.
9 Katsuki A, Sumida Y, Murashima S, *et al.* Acute and chronic regulation of serum sex hormone-binding globulin levels by plasma insulin concentrations in male non-insulin-dependent diabetes mellitus patients. *J Clin Endocrinol Metab* 1996; **81**: 2515–19.
10 Vrbikova J, Cibula D, Dvorakova K, *et al.* Insulin sensitivity in women with polycystic ovary syndrome. *J Clin Endocrinol Metab* 2004; **89**: 2942–5.
11 Wild RA, Alaupovic P, Parker IJ. Lipid and apolipoprotein abnormalities in hirsute women. I. The association with

insulin resistance. *Am J Obstet Gynecol* 1992; **166**: 1191–6.

12 Conway GS, Agrawal R, Betteridge DJ, Jacobs HS. Risk factors for coronary artery disease in lean and obese women with the polycystic ovary syndrome. *Clin Endocrinol (Oxf)* 1992; **37**: 119–25.

13 Rajkhowa M, Neary RH, Kumpatla P, *et al.* Altered composition of high density lipoproteins in women with the polycystic ovary syndrome. *J Clin Endocrinol Metab* 1997; **82**: 3389–94.

14 Pirwany IR, Fleming R, Greer IA, *et al.* Lipids and lipoprotein subfractions in women with PCOS: relationship to metabolic and endocrine parameters. *Clin Endocrinol (Oxf)* 2001; **54**: 447–53.

15 Dejager S, Pichard C, Giral P, *et al.* Smaller LDL particle size in women with polycystic ovary syndrome compared to controls. *Clin Endocrinol (Oxf)* 2001; **54**: 455–62.

16 Wild RA. Polycystic ovary syndrome: a risk for coronary artery disease? *Am J Obstet Gynecol* 2002; **186**: 35–43.

17 Meigs JB, Mittleman MA, Nathan DM, *et al.* Hyperinsulinemia, hyperglycemia, and impaired hemostasis the Framingham Offspring Study. *JAMA* 2000; **283**: 221–8.

18 Mennen LI, Balkau B, Charles MA, *et al.* Gender differences in the relation between fibrinogen, tissue-type plasminogen activator antigen and markers of insulin resistance: effects of smoking. D.E.S.I.R. Study Group. Data from an Epidemiological Study on Insulin Resistance Syndrome. *Thromb Haemost* 1999; **82**: 1106–11.

19 Festa A, D'Agostino R Jr, Tracy RP, Haffner SM; Insulin Resistance Atherosclerosis Study. Elevated levels of acute-phase proteins and plasminogen activator inhibitor-1 predict the development of type 2 diabetes: the insulin resistance atherosclerosis study. *Diabetes* 2002; **51**: 1131–7.

20 Eliasson MC, Jansson JH, Lindahl B, Stegmayr B. High levels of tissue plasminogen activator (tPA) antigen precede the development of type 2 diabetes in a longitudinal population study. The Northern Sweden MONICA Study. *Cardiovasc Diabetol* 2003; **2**: 19.

21 Kelly CJ, Lyall H, Petrie JR, *et al.* A specific elevation in tissue plasminogen activator antigen in women with polycystic ovarian syndrome. *J Clin Endocrinol Metab* 2002; **87**: 3287–90.

22 Atiomo WU, Bates SA, Condon JE, *et al.* The plasminogen activator system in women with polycystic ovary syndrome. *Fertil Steril* 1998; **69**: 236–41.

23 Sampson M, Kong C, Patel A, *et al.* Ambulatory blood pressure profiles and plasminogen activator inhibitor (PAI-1) activity in lean women with and without the polycystic ovary syndrome. *Clin Endocrinol* 1996; **45**: 623–9.

24 Ross R. Atherosclerosis – an inflammatory disease. *N Engl J Med* 1999; **340**: 115–26.

25 Danesh J, Wheeler JG, Hirschfield GM, *et al.* C-reactive protein and other circulating markers of inflammation in the prediction of coronary heart disease. *N Engl J Med* 2004; **350**: 1387–97.

26 Sattar N, Perry CG, Petrie JR. Type 2 diabetes as an inflammatory disorder. *Br J Diabetes Vasc Dis* 2003; **3**: 36–41.

27 Freeman DJ, Norrie J, Caslake MJ, *et al.* C-reactive protein is an independent predictor of risk for the development of diabetes in the West of Scotland Coronary Prevention Study. *Diabetes* 2002; **51**: 1596–600.

28 Pradhan AD, Manson JE, Rifai N, *et al.* C-reactive protein, interleukin 6, and risk of developing type 2 diabetes mellitus. *JAMA.* 2001; **286**: 327–34.

29 Boulman N, Levy Y, Leiba R, *et al.* Increased C-reactive protein levels in the polycystic ovary syndrome: a marker of cardiovascular disease. *J Clin Endocrinol Metab* 2004; **89**: 2160–5.

30 Orio F Jr, Palomba S, Cascella T, *et al.* The increase of leukocytes as a new putative marker of low-grade chronic inflammation and early cardiovascular risk in polycystic ovary syndrome. *J Clin Endocrinol Metab* 2005; **90**: 2–5.

31 Escobar-Morreale HF, Botella-Carretero JI, Villuendas G, *et al.* Serum interleukin-18 concentrations are increased in the polycystic ovary syndrome: relationship to insulin resistance and to obesity. *J Clin Endocrinol Metab* 2004; **89**: 806–11.

32 Peral B, San Millan JL, Castello R, *et al.* The methionine 196 arginine polymorphism in exon 6 of the TNF receptor 2 gene (TNFRSF1B) is associated with the polycystic ovary syndrome and hyperandrogenism. *J Clin Endocrinol Metab* 2002; **87**: 3977–83.

33 Escobar-Morreale HF, Calvo RM, Villuendas G, *et al.* Association of polymorphisms in the interleukin 6 receptor complex with obesity and with hyperandrogenism. *Obes Res* 2003; **11**: 987–96.

34 Widlansky ME, Gokce N, Keaney JF Jr, Vita JA. The clinical implications of endothelial dysfunction. *J Am Coll Cardiol* 2003; **42**: 1149–60.

35 Tarkun I, Arslan BC, Canturk Z, *et al.* Endothelial dysfunction in young women with polycystic ovary syndrome: relationship with insulin resistance and low-grade chronic inflammation. *J Clin Endocrinol Metab* 2004; **89**: 5592–6.

36 Orio F Jr, Palomba S, Cascella T, *et al.* Early impairment of endothelial structure and function in young normal-weight women with polycystic ovary syndrome. *J Clin Endocrinol Metab* 2004; **89**: 4588–93.

37 Paradisi G, Steinberg HO, Hempfling A, *et al.* Polycystic ovary syndrome is associated with endothelial dysfunction. *Circulation* 2001; **103**: 1410–15.

38 Mather KJ, Verma S, Corenblum B, Anderson TJ. Normal endothelial function despite insulin resistance in healthy women with the polycystic ovary syndrome. *J Clin Endocrinol Metab* 2000; **85**: 1851–6.

39 Holte J, Bergh T, Berne C, *et al.* Enhanced early insulin response to glucose in relation to insulin resistance in women with polycystic ovary syndrome and normal

glucose tolerance. *J Clin Endocrinol Metab* 1994; **78**: 1052–8.

40 Yildirim B, Sabir N, Kaleli B. Relation of intra-abdominal fat distribution to metabolic disorders in nonobese patients with polycystic ovary syndrome. *Fertil Steril* 2003; **79**: 1358–64.

41 Klein S, Fontana L, Young VL, *et al.* Absence of an effect of liposuction on insulin action and risk factors for coronary heart disease. *N Engl J Med* 2004; **350**: 2549–57.

42 Alberti KG, Zimmet PZ. Definition, diagnosis and classification of diabetes mellitus and its complications. Part 1: diagnosis and classification of diabetes mellitus provisional report of a WHO consultation. *Diabet Med* 1998; **15**: 539–53.

43 Expert Panel on detection, evaluation, and treatment of high blood cholesterol in adults. Executive Summary of The Third Report of The National Cholesterol Education Program (NCEP) Expert Panel on Detection, Evaluation, And Treatment of High Blood Cholesterol In Adults (Adult Treatment Panel III). *JAMA* 2001; **285**: 2486–97.

44 Sattar N, Gaw A, Scherbakova O, *et al.* Metabolic syndrome with and without C-reactive protein as a predictor of coronary heart disease and diabetes in the West of Scotland Coronary Prevention Study. *Circulation* 2003; **108**: 414–19.

45 Ridker PM, Buring JE, Cook NR, Rifai N. C-reactive protein, the metabolic syndrome, and risk of incident cardiovascular events: an 8-year follow-up of 14 719 initially healthy American women. *Circulation* 2003; **107**: 391–7.

46 Rutter MK, Meigs JB, Sullivan LM, *et al.* C-reactive protein, the metabolic syndrome, and prediction of cardiovascular events in the Framingham Offspring Study. *Circulation* 2004; **110**: 380–5.

47 Hopkinson ZE, Sattar N, Fleming R, Greer IA. Polycystic ovarian syndrome: the metabolic syndrome comes to gynaecology. *BMJ* 1998; **317**: 329–32.

48 Talbott EO, Zborowski JV, Rager JR, *et al.* Evidence for an association between metabolic cardiovascular syndrome and coronary and aortic calcification among women with polycystic ovary syndrome. *J Clin Endocrinol Metab* 2004; **89**: 5454–61.

49 Apridonidze T, Essah PA, Iuorno MJ, Nestler JE. Prevalence and characteristics of the metabolic syndrome in women with polycystic ovary syndrome. *J Clin Endocrinol Metab* 2005; **90**: 1929–35.

50 Harborne L, Fleming R, Lyall H, *et al.* Descriptive review of the evidence for the use of metformin in polycystic ovary syndrome. *Lancet* 2003; **361**: 1894–901.

51 Bonora E, Kiechl S, Willeit J, *et al.*; Bruneck study. Population-based incidence rates and risk factors for type 2 diabetes in white individuals: the Bruneck study. *Diabetes* 2004; **53**: 1782–9.

52 Legro RS, Kunselman AR, Dodson WC, Dunaif A. Prevalence and predictors of risk for type 2 diabetes mellitus and impaired glucose tolerance in polycystic

ovary syndrome: a prospective, controlled study in 254 affected women. *J Clin Endocrinol Metab* 1999; **84**: 165–9.

53 Wild RA, Grubb B, Hartz A, Van Nort JJ, *et al.* Clinical signs of androgen excess as risk factors for coronary artery disease. *Fertil Steril* 1990; **54**: 255–9.

54 Birdsall MA, Farquhar CM, White HD. Association between polycystic ovaries and extent of coronary artery disease in women having cardiac catheterization. *Ann Intern Med* 1997; **126**: 32–5.

55 Talbott EO, Guzick DS, Sutton-Tyrrell K, *et al.* Evidence for association between polycystic ovary syndrome and premature carotid atherosclerosis in middle-aged women. *Arterioscler Thromb Vasc Biol* 2000; **20**: 2414–21.

56 Talbott EO, Zborowski JV, Boudreaux MY, *et al.* The relationship between C-reactive protein and carotid intima-media wall thickness in middle-aged women with polycystic ovary syndrome. *J Clin Endocrinol Metab* 2004; **89**: 6061–7.

57 Christian RC, Dumesic DA, Behrenbeck T, *et al.* Prevalence and predictors of coronary artery calcification in women with polycystic ovary syndrome. *J Clin Endocrinol Metab* 2003; **88**: 2562–8.

58 Wild S, Pierpoint T, Jacobs H, McKeigue P. Long-term consequences of polycystic ovary syndrome: results of a 31 year follow-up study. *Hum Fertil (Camb)* 2000; **3**: 101–5.

59 Solomon CG, Hu FB, Dunaif A, *et al.* Menstrual cycle irregularity and risk for future cardiovascular disease. *J Clin Endocrinol Metab* 2002; **87**: 2013–17.

60 Kiddy DS, Hamilton-Fairley D, Bush A, *et al.* Improvement in endocrine and ovarian function during dietary treatment of obese women with polycystic ovary syndrome. *Clin Endocrinol* 1992; **36**: 105–11.

61 Clark AM, Thornley B, Tomlinson L, *et al.* Weight loss in obese infertile women results in improvement in the reproductive outcome for all forms of fertility treatment. *Hum Reprod* 1998; **13**: 1502–5.

62 Knowler WC, Barrett-Connor E, Fowler SE, *et al.* Reduction in the incidence of type 2 diabetes with lifestyle intervention or metformin. *N Engl J Med* 2002; **346**: 393–403.

63 Lord JM, Flight IH, Norman RJ. Metformin in polycystic ovary syndrome: systematic review and meta-analysis. *BMJ* 2003; **327**: 951–3.

64 Costello MF, Eden JA. A systematic review of the reproductive system effects of metformin in patients with polycystic ovary syndrome. *Fertil Steril* 2003; **79**: 1–13.

65 Morin-Papunen L, Rautio K, Ruokonen A, *et al.* Metformin reduces serum C-reactive protein levels in women with polycystic ovary syndrome. *J Clin Endocrinol Metab* 2003; **88**: 4649–54.

66 Glueck CJ, Papanna R, Wang P, *et al.* Incidence and treatment of metabolic syndrome in newly referred women with confirmed polycystic ovarian syndrome. *Metabolism* 2003; **52**: 908–15.

67   Hardie DG. Minireview: the AMP-activated protein kinase cascade: the key sensor of cellular energy status. *Endocrinology* 2003; **144**: 5179–83.

68   UK Prospective Diabetes Study (UKPDS) Group. Effect of intensive blood-glucose control with metformin on complications in overweight patients with type 2 diabetes (UKPDS 34). *Lancet* 1998; **352**: 854–65.

69   Johnson JA, Majumdar SR, Simpson SH, Toth EL. Decreased mortality associated with the use of metformin compared with sulfonylurea monotherapy in type 2 diabetes. *Diabetes Care* 2002; **25**: 2244–8.

70   Sepilian V, Nagamani M. Effects of rosiglitazone in obese women with polycystic ovary syndrome and severe insulin resistance. *J Clin Endocrinol Metab* 2005; **90**: 60–5.

71   Baillargeon JP, Jakubowicz DJ, Iuorno MJ, *et al.* Effects of metformin and rosiglitazone, alone and in combination, in nonobese women with polycystic ovary syndrome and normal indices of insulin sensitivity. *Fertil Steril* 2004; **82**: 893–902.

72   Belli SH, Graffigna MN, Oneto A, *et al.* Effect of rosiglitazone on insulin resistance, growth factors, and reproductive disturbances in women with polycystic ovary syndrome. *Fertil Steril* 2004; **81**: 624–9.

73   Ghazeeri G, Kutteh WH, Bryer-Ash M, *et al.* Effect of rosiglitazone on spontaneous and clomiphene citrate-induced ovulation in women with polycystic ovary syndrome. *Fertil Steril* 2003; **79**: 562–6.

74   Ortega-Gonzalez C, Luna S, Hernandez L, *et al.* Responses of serum androgen and insulin resistance to metformin and pioglitazone in obese, insulin-resistant women with polycystic ovary syndrome. *J Clin Endocrinol Metab* 2004; **90**: 1360–5.

75   Brettenthaler N, De Geyter C, Huber PR, Keller U. Effect of the insulin sensitizer pioglitazone on insulin resistance, hyperandrogenism, and ovulatory dysfunction in women with polycystic ovary syndrome. *J Clin Endocrinol Metab* 2004; **89**: 3835–40.

76   Glueck CJ, Moreira A, Goldenberg N, *et al.* Pioglitazone and metformin in obese women with polycystic ovary syndrome not optimally responsive to metformin. *Hum Reprod* 2003; **18**: 1618–25.

77   Paradisi G, Steinberg HO, Shepard MK, *et al.* Troglitazone therapy improves endothelial function to near normal levels in women with polycystic ovary syndrome. *J Clin Endocrinol Metab* 2003; **88**: 576–80.

78   Buchanan TA, Xiang AH, Peters RK, *et al.* Preservation of pancreatic beta-cell function and prevention of type 2 diabetes by pharmacological treatment of insulin resistance in high-risk hispanic women. *Diabetes* 2002; **51**: 2796–803.

79   Jayagopal V, Kilpatrick ES, Holding S, *et al.* Orlistat is as beneficial as metformin in the treatment of polycystic ovarian syndrome. *J Clin Endocrinol Metab* 2004; **90**: 729–33.

80   Torgerson JS, Hauptman J, Boldrin MN, Sjostrom L. XENical in the prevention of diabetes in obese subjects (XENDOS) study: a randomized study of orlistat as an adjunct to lifestyle changes for the prevention of type 2 diabetes in obese patients. *Diabetes Care* 2004; **27**: 155–61.

21

Effect of pregnancy on the hemostatic and metabolic systems

PETER CLARK

INTRODUCTION

Pregnancy is associated with significant changes in hemostasis, which prepare the mother for the hemostatic challenge of delivery. It is also likely that placental and maternal thrombin generation and fibrin formation are important in the developing feto/placental unit.[1] An excessive maternal coagulation response has been associated with pregnancy failure and thrombosis. Although the exact mechanism of the physiologic changes in hemostasis is unknown, as with maternal metabolism, it may relate to a number of factors, including alterations in: hormone-influenced factor synthesis; changes in the volume of distribution; coagulation–lipid interaction; and alterations in the catabolism of coagulation proteins. In particular, pregnancy is characterized by a progressive increase in maternal estrogen, which is capable of altering the uptake of coagulation proteins into the uterus,[2] and could increase uterine generation of tissue factor (TF).[3]

Normal fetal development also requires the transfer of carbohydrates, essential amino acids, and lipids across the placenta. This occurs essentially at the expense of the mother and as pregnancy progresses, this, along with nutritional support to the placenta, leads to striking change in maternal metabolism. Overall, maternal metabolism is initially anabolic, which in later pregnancy becomes catabolic with the utilization of energy stores. Like hemostasis, these processes appear to be influenced by a variety of maternal hormones, including estrogen, progesterone, and human placental lactogen.

A failure of placental or fetal development may place particular metabolic and hemostatic stress on the mother. Indeed, it has been suggested that pregnancy complications may alter the mother's future risk of vascular disease, perhaps as a result of an exaggeration of the physiologic metabolic response.

NORMAL LIPID METABOLISM

The major constituent of body fat is triglyceride, which is derived from the diet, or is synthesized by the liver. Such triglycerides consist of long-chain saturated or mono-unsaturated fatty acids which are esterified to glycerol. Cholesterol is derived from dietary sources or can be synthesized by a number of cell types. Cholesterol is important for cell membrane construction, as well as biliary acid and sterol formation. Triglycerides and cholesterols circulate as complex lipoprotein particles of variable size and density. Such particles consist of a lipid core and a phospholipid, apoprotein, and cholesterol shell. Classified by density, those lipoprotein particles with the lowest density have triglyceride as the principal lipid. With increasing density there is a reduction in the proportion of triglyceride and an increasing proportion of apoprotein and phospholipid. These apoproteins have a variety of functions which includes the presentation of lipoproteins to cell receptors. Such apoproteins can also be exchanged between different lipoprotein particles.

In addition, chylomicrons transport dietary lipid from the intestine to adipose tissue and other organs, where the triglyceride in the chylomicron is partially hydrolyzed by lipoprotein lipase (LPL). The fatty acid released from this hydrolysis is transported into the cell to be stored as triglyceride. The resulting chylomicron remnants are enriched with cholesterol from high-density lipoproteins (HDL) and are taken up by the liver where this cholesterol is released along with free fatty acids and glycerol. Similarly, very-low-density lipoprotein (VLDL) is also metabolized by tissue LPL to release triglyceride. On interaction with HDL, the VLDL remnants of this partial lipolysis are also enriched with cholesterol to form intermediate-density lipoproteins (IDLs). Much of the IDL is taken up by the liver, but some is converted to low-density lipoprotein (LDL) which is the major circulating source of cholesterol. Low-density lipoprotein (LDL) supplies cholesterol to the tissues via specific LDL receptors that recognize LDL apoproteins. As noted above, HDL particles facilitate the transport of lipids, including excess triglyceride to the liver and cholesterol to and from the peripheral tissues to the liver. One of the HDL apoproteins is also involved in the activation of LPL, thereby facilitating the hydrolysis of other lipoproteins. In addition there is a small circulating pool of free fatty acids bound to albumin. A small percentage of fatty acids cannot be synthesized by the body and are, therefore, 'essential' dietary components. These include polyunsaturated fatty acids that are required for membrane and prostaglandin synthesis.

A catabolic state, such as that which accompanies prolonged fasting, will result in glucose mobilization. This comes initially from hepatic glycogen and then from gluconeogenesis (via protein catabolism and glycerol release from fatty acid lipolysis) to maintain neurologic function. Fatty acids are released from stores to supply energy to muscle. This requires an upregulation of muscle LPL and a downregulation of adipose tissue LPL, to direct the fatty acid fuel source to muscles. The release of ketoacids leads to a tendency to metabolic acidosis and ketosis.

MATERNAL LIPID METABOLISM

The amount of triglyceride and cholesterol in all circulating lipid subfractions increases with increasing gestation,[4] with a 30–50 percent increase in total cholesterol and up to a threefold increase in triglyceride evident by the third trimester.[5,6] There is a rise in HDL-cholesterol with increasing gestation, peaking around 28 weeks' gestation,[5,7–9] with a slight fall evident in the latter stages of pregnancy. Although the level of LDL falls in the first trimester, it then progressively rises as pregnancy progresses,[10] reaching a peak in the third trimester.[9] Similarly, VLDL-cholesterol also rises with increasing gestation to a level ~2.5 times that of nonpregnant subjects by term. This is accompanied by a

comparable rise in VLDL-triglyceride.[7] Despite these alterations in VLDL composition, the triglyceride/cholesterol ratio remains stable with increasing gestation, whereas there is a progressive increase in the triglyceride/cholesterol ratio in both LDL and HDL moieties. By the first month of the puerperium, triglyceride levels have returned to nonpregnant levels, but serum cholesterol levels appear to normalize more slowly.[4,11]

In early pregnancy there is an increase in maternal lipogenesis[12] and an increase in food intake.[13,14] This leads to lipid deposition in maternal tissues. Whether this results from an increase in the activity of adipose tissue-LPL,[4,15,16] an increased sensitivity to insulin in early pregnancy, or combination of both mechanisms, is not yet resolved. The result, in any case, is the conversion of triglyceride from circulating maternal VLDL and chylomicrons to IDLs, which are incorporated into maternal adipose tissue along with glycerol and nonesterified fatty acids (NEFAs).

In the second and third trimesters there is an increase in lipolysis of maternal adipose tissue, leading to a release of NEFAs and glycerol into the circulation. The mechanism for this catabolism is not fully understood, although it could relate to: estrogen-enhanced hepatic synthesis of VLDL-triglycerides;[17] impaired removal of circulating lipoprotein triglycerides by an overall downregulation of LPL and/or hepatic lipase (HL)[4] or; a combination of both. The NEFAs derived from lipolysis can be converted by the maternal liver to acyl CoA which, along with glycerol 3-phosphate, can be converted to VLDL. The release of VLDL into the circulation in the latter stages of pregnancy may also be stimulated by increasing insulin resistance. Only a small amount of the glycerol released from these processes, however, can be transported to the fetus directly, but glycerol may be have a role as a fetal energy source via maternal gluconeogenesis.[18] Acetyl CoA, manufactured from NEFAs, can also form ketone bodies which, by crossing the placenta, can be used as a fetal energy source, or as a substrate for brain lipid synthesis. Triglyceride itself cannot directly cross the placenta. However, the placental trophoblast expresses a wide variety of lipolytic enzymes, as well as VLDL and LDL receptors, indicating that maternal triglycerides can be hydrolyzed by the placenta and passed to the fetus.[19] In the fetal circulation these metabolites can be taken up by the fetal liver and reconverted into essential triglycerides. The provision of an adequate supply of such essential fatty acids to the placenta may require the presence of the physiologic maternal hyperlipidemia. Essential fatty acids may also pass from the maternal to fetal circulation in the form of NEFAs, which can be transported across the placenta by an adenosine triphosphate (ATP) and sodium-dependent mechanism.

Lipoprotein (LP) (a) is a plasma lipoprotein which is closely related to plasma LDL. Although both lipoproteins are composed of apolipoprotein B-100 and lipid, Lp(a) contains a unique lipoprotein called apolipoprotein (a). The gene coding for this apolipoprotein is found on chromosome 6 close to the plasminogen gene. Indeed, Lp(a) appears to have plasminogen-like properties and may be capable of inhibiting fibrinolysis.[20] It has been implicated in atherosclerosis,[20] as well as venous thrombosis,[21] and acts as an acute phase reactant,[22] but its plasma levels appear to be insensitive to dietary manipulation. A variety of studies of normal pregnancy have shown either no,[23–25] or a twofold increase in Lp(a) levels with increasing gestation, with a maximum value evident in the third trimester.[26]

Cholesterol is an essential element in membrane development, cellular communication, bile acid metabolism, and steroid synthesis in the growing fetus.[27–31] Although there is some transport of maternal cholesterol to the fetus, its importance in man is not known[32] and it is likely that much of the required cholesterol is synthesized by the fetus.

MATERNAL CARBOHYDRATE AND INSULIN METABOLISM

Overall, pregnancy is associated with a reduction in plasma glucose levels, although 70 percent of the maternal glucose taken up by the placenta is used by placenta itself.[33] This tendency to maternal hypoglycemia during pregnancy predisposes the mother to ketosis.[34,35] In the latter stages of normal pregnancy there is also a twofold increase in the circulating level of insulin.[36] This is accompanied by maternal resistance to the effects of endogenous insulin, which preserve carbohydrate for the developing fetus. Insulin resistance may be a consequence of a number of influences including: progesterone (which enhances insulin secretion); estrogen (which enhances production of both insulin and the insulin antagonist, cortisol) and; human placental lactogen (which assists in the provision of alternative fuels to allow glucose sparing). Thus, increasing maternal energy requirements may need to be met by release of maternal free fatty acids from lipid stores. Maternal plasma glycerol levels are also elevated in late pregnancy but, as noted above, it is rapidly metabolized limiting transplacental passage.

MATERNAL PROTEIN METABOLISM

In pregnancy an overall reduction in maternal levels of serum proteins and amino acids occurs. This results from the increasing insulin levels, the use of amino acids for maternal gluconeogenesis, changes in the volume of distribution and the transfer of a number of amino acids, particularly alanine, glycine, and serine, to the fetus. The fetus uses such amino acids for protein manufacture and as a supply of carbon and nitrogen for conversion to other metabolic substrates. In addition, some amino acids that are not considered 'essential' in adult life, cannot be manufactured by the fetoplacental unit and are 'essential' to the developing fetus. Placental transfer of amino acids is an active process which requires adequate maternal stores. There is evidence, however, that some amino acids are used by the placenta, rather than directly transferred to the fetus.

In addition, there is the intriguing possibility of placental production of some amino acids from fetal substrates.

MATERNAL B$_{12}$, FOLATE, AND HOMOCYSTEINE LEVELS

Serum vitamin B$_{12}$ levels may fall by 30–50 percent during pregnancy, with reduced levels in the first trimester in some women.[37] This occurs despite a diet adequate in vitamin B$_{12}$ and is likely to be due to a combination of increasing maternal plasma volume, hormonal changes, increasing maternal requirement and transfer to the fetus. Despite this, it is not clear whether normal pregnancy is associated with a vitamin B$_{12}$-deficient state or not, and even if it is, whether this has any clinical significance.[38] In nonsupplemented pregnancies there is a progressive fall in serum folate with increasing gestation,[39] but pregnancy has a highly variable effect on red cell folate.[40,41] Overall, the bulk of evidence suggests that blood homocysteine levels fall with increasing gestation in most women.[39,42,43] The impact of folate repletion on these changes, however, requires further investigation.[39]

NORMAL HEMOSTASIS AND FIBRINOLYSIS

Normal coagulation is initiated by a combination of TF and activated factor VIIa (TF/FVIIa). In normal circumstances, the TF/FVIIa is rapidly inhibited by the specific inhibitor, tissue factor pathway inhibitor (TFPI). When required for hemostasis TF/FVIIa leads to a 'burst' of thrombin generation, which is capable of activating a number of other clotting factors, as well as platelets, monocytes, and the endothelium (Fig. 21.1). This results in the generation of fibrin and, via activation of FXIII, to the crosslinking and stabilization of the fibrin clot. The interaction of thrombin with endothelial thrombomodulin results in a loss of the fibrinogen-activating function of thrombin and leads to the activation of protein C. Activated protein C (APC), with its cofactor protein S inactivates activated FV and FVIII. This reduces further thrombin generation (Fig. 21.2). Activated protein C is also capable of neutralizing plasminogen activator inhibitor (PAI)-1, a reaction which can be accelerated by protein S *in vitro*.[44] Protein S can also inhibit thrombin activatable fibrinolysis inhibitor (TAFI),[45] and there is also a link between protein S and complement activation through the levels of its binding protein C4b. C4b can influence complement activation and also acts as an acute phase reactant.

Formed fibrin is rapidly broken down by plasmin. This generates fibrin degradation products, including dimers made from the D fragment of fibrin (D-dimers). There are a number of activators and inhibitors which influence the balance of fibrinolysis (Fig. 21.3). The principal physiological activator of plasminogen is tissue plasminogen activator (tPA)-1 which acts preferentially on plasminogen on the surface of fibrin. Urokinase (uPA) can also activate plasminogen whether or not it is fibrin-bound. Urokinase

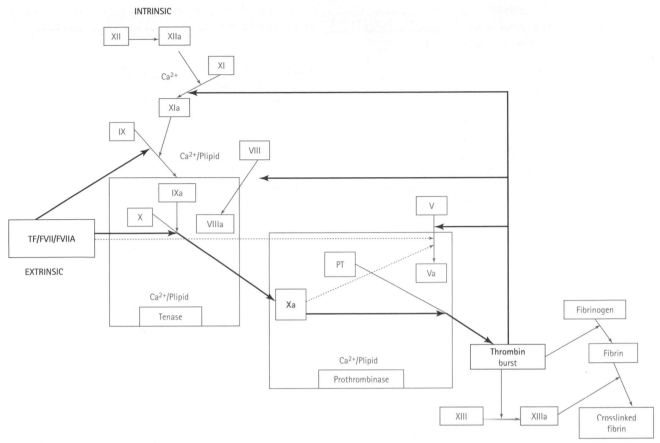

Figure 21.1 The coagulation cascade. The 'extrinsic' initiation of coagulation with a combination of tissue factor (TF), factor VII (FVII) and activated factor VII (FVIIa) is shown. Solid lines indicate activation and dotted lines indicate inhibition. The principal pathway is shown in thick black type. The FVII/FVIIa/TF complex activates factor X to Xa, as well as factor IX to IXa. This results in the activation of prothrombin (PT) in a prothrombinase complex of calcium (Ca^{2+}), phospholipid (Plipid) and activated factor V (Va), resulting in a burst of thrombin. This burst of thrombin activates factor V to Va, VIII to VIIIa, and XI to XIa. The combination of thrombin's action and activation of the 'intrinsic' coagulation pathway by exposure to damaged endothelium (via activation of factor XII to XIIa), results in activation of factor XI. This leads to activation of factor IX. The further activation of factor X in the tenase complex of factor IXa, factor VIIIa, Plipid, and Ca^{2+} amplifies the coagulation initiated by the thrombin burst. Thrombin also activates factor XIII, which crosslinks and stabilizes formed fibrin.

is formed from pro-uPA on limited hydrolysis by the action of either plasmin or kallikrein. The binding of plasmin to fibrin protects plasmin from rapid inhibition by α_2-antiplasmin. In human plasma PAI-1 is the principal inhibitor of tPA and uPA (Fig. 21.3). Although PAI-2, which is derived from the placenta, is capable of inhibiting tPA and uPA, it does not appear to be a major player in tPA regulation.[46,47]

MATERNAL ANTEPARTUM HEMOSTASIS

Changes in maternal coagulation factors in normal pregnancy

With increasing gestation there is a progressive rise in the plasma concentration of fibrinogen, FVII coagulation protein (c), FVIIIc, FXc, FXIIc, von Willebrand (vW) antigen

and vW ristocetin cofactor activity activity[48] (Table 21.1). There is no consistent change in FVc activity or FIXc, but a reduction in factor XIc has been noted in several studies[48] (Table 21.1). Despite the large number of studies of hemostasis in normal pregnancy, the mechanism and significance to the mother of these changes is poorly understood.

Changes in maternal protein C/protein S anticoagulants in normal pregnancy

Overall, there is no difference in protein C antigen levels when pregnant women are compared with nonpregnant subjects.[48] The bulk of evidence also shows no convincing effect of increasing gestation on the level of circulating protein C or antithrombin.[49–54] Pregnancy does, however, result in a fall in free and total protein S levels activity. Indeed, levels less than those of nonpregnant subjects may be observed

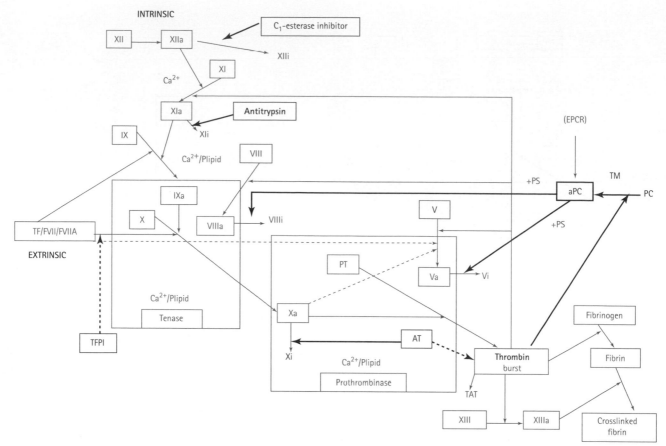

Figure 21.2 Coagulation control. The principal points of physiologic inhibition and downregulation of the coagulation cascade are shown. Solid lines indicate activation and dotted lines indicate inhibition. The main inhibitor is antithrombin (AT, previously called antithrombin III). It inhibits almost all of the coagulation factors, but its principal targets are FXa and thrombin. The interaction of AT with thrombin results in the formation of the thrombin–antithrombin complex (TAT). Thrombin, when it binds to endothelial thrombomodulin (TM), loses its procoagulant activity and activates protein C (PC) to activated protein C (APC). Activated protein C with its cofactor protein S (PS), cleaves activated factor V (Va) and factor VIII (VIIIa). Protein C can also be activated independently by the endothelial protein C receptor (EPCR). Other inhibitors of coagulation include tissue factor pathway inhibitor (TFPI) which rapidly inactivates the FVII/FVIIa/tissue factor (TF) complex. In addition, antitrypsin and C1-esterase inhibitor are capable of inhibiting XIa and XIIa, respectively.

as early as the first trimester, with levels less than 50 percent of nonpregnant values seen in the majority of women in the last weeks of pregnancy.[48]

The significance of resistance to the action of APC (APCR) was recognized by Dahlback and coworkers in 1993.[55] In the majority of subjects such resistance is inherited by a mutation in the gene coding for FV (commonly known as the factor V Leiden mutation – FVL[56]). This mutation results in a reduced sensitivity of activated FV (FVa) to proteolytic cleavage by APC. Pregnancy, however, can be associated with a progressive increase in 'acquired' APCR, which is independent of FVL.[51,57,58] Such resistance can be assessed by activated partial thromboplastin time (aPTT),[55] or TF-based assays.[59] Higher 'acquired' resistance occurs in association with oral contraceptive use, inflammation, hormone replacement therapy, and pregnancy.[60] Modification of the aPTT-based assay by predilution of the patient plasma with FV-deficient plasma renders the tests highly specific for inherited mutations in the factor V gene and insensitive to the effects of hormones or inflammation. In

pregnancy, the degree of resistance, assessed by the unmodified test, however, correlates positively with the plasma levels of FVIIIc (and perhaps FVc) and inversely with protein S.[60] In nonpregnant individuals, increasing resistance is also associated with higher antithrombin levels,[61,62] perhaps indicating compensation for a prothrombotic state. Both the unmodified aPTT and TF tests are influenced by the presence of a lupus inhibitor and are unreliable in the presence of anticoagulants.[59]

Changes in maternal thrombin and fibrin generation

The circulating levels of markers that are formed as a consequence of thrombin's formation or inactivation can be used to assess the amount of thrombin that has been generated. For example, as prothrombin is cleaved by FXa to form thrombin, a fragment is released. This fragment is called prothrombin fragment 1 + 2 (F1 + 2).[63] In addition,

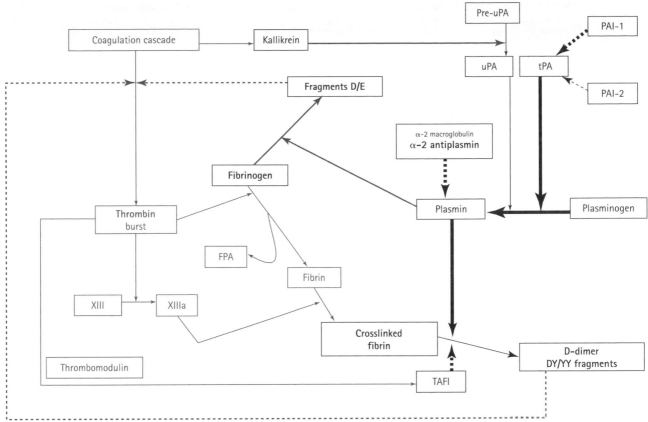

Figure 21.3 Fibrinolysis. The action and principal controls of fibrin breakdown (fibrinolysis) are shown. Solid lines indicate activation and dotted lines indicate inhibition. Tissue plasminogen activator (tPA) activates plasminogen to plasmin which can break down both fibrin and fibrinogen. This results in the generation of a number of fibrinogen and fibrin degradation products, which can have an overall inhibitory effect on further fibrin clot generation. Products released from fibrinogen include D and E fragments and products released from formed, crosslinked fibrin include D-dimer, Y-dimer, and DY fragments. Plasminogen activator inhibitor (PAI)-1 (PAI-1) in turn inhibits and controls tPA. In pregnancy the placenta produces PAI-2, although it does not have a major function in the control of fibrinolysis in the mother. Plasmin is principally inhibited by α-2 antiplasmin, although there is a contribution from α-2 macroglobulin. Thrombin is also capable of the activation of TAFI (thrombin activatable fibrinolysis inhibitor), which inhibits the action of plasmin on formed fibrin. In addition, urokinase (which is found in urine) can activate plasminogen. Urokinase (uPA), itself, is activated from pre-uPA after limited hydrolysis by kallikrein, which is derived from the intrinsic pathway of coagulation.

the circulating plasma level of the complex that thrombin forms with its principal inhibitor, antithrombin (the thrombin–antithrombin complex [TAT]) is also used to assess the amount of thrombin that has been formed.[63]

In normal pregnancy there is an increase in TAT levels, with concentrations higher than nonpregnant values evident in 50 percent of women in the first trimester.[48] In fact, almost all women show elevated levels in the second and third trimesters.[64] A significant positive correlation between gestation and F1 + 2 has also been shown, with elevated levels seen in early pregnancy[48]. As TAT complex formation occurs in the absence of an increase in antithrombin,[53,54] it is likely that heightened thrombin generation is a feature of normal pregnancy. Whether this physiologic generation indicates a prothrombotic state, requires consideration of the effect of pregnancy on the level of the anticoagulant activated protein C. It is possible to assess protein C activation by measuring the complex it forms with its inhibitor α1-antitrypsin.[65] By the third trimester there is ~twofold increase in the level

of APC/α1-antitrypsin without a comparable rise in α1-antitrypsin. This suggests that increasing gestation is associated with an increase in the activation of protein C and, therefore, an increase in antithrombotic activity. The overall thrombotic balance of pregnancy has not been clarified, but higher levels of fibrinopeptide A (a fragment released on the activation of fibrinogen) are also a feature of normal pregnancy, indicating that there is a progressive increase in fibrin generation.[66] This, along with the possibility of a reduction in fibrinolysis noted below, would support the clinical experience that the net effect of normal pregnancy is the induction of a prothrombotic state.

Changes in maternal fibrinolysis in normal pregnancy

The activation and inhibition of fibrinolysis occurs at a local level and study of plasma can only give a limited insight into

Table 21.1　Alterations in hemostasis from first trimester values in normal pregnancy (percent change)

Coagulation factor	Second trimester (%)	Third trimester (%)
Fibrinogen	↑ 11	↑ 31
FVIIc	↑ 16	↑ 42
FVIIIc	↑ 28	↑ 62
FXc	↑ 15	↑ 20
FXIIc	↑ 16	↑ 14
vW antigen	↑ 22	↑ 96
TAT	↑ 82	↑ 128
F1 + 2	↑ 80	↑ 140
FPA	↑ 83	↑ 80
Plasminogen activity	↑ 10	↑ 14
tPA antigen	↑ 17	↑ 92
PAI-1 antigen	↑ 120	↑ 400
PAI-2 antigen	↑ 160	↑ 500
TAFI	–	↑ 48
D–dimer	↑ 170	↑ 180
tPA activity	↓ 25	↓ 50
FXIc	↓ 5	↓ 5
Protein S total	↓ 9	↓ 15
Protein S free	↓ 20	↓ 30
APTT-APCR	↓ 13	↓ 20
Factor V depleted APTT-APCR		No change
Prothrombin		
FVc		
FIXc		
Protein C		
Antithrombin		

This table is a guide to the Expected percentage (%) rise (↑), or fall (↓) of coagulation, anticoagulant, and fibrinolytic factors from the first to the second or third trimester in normal pregnancy. This includes the levels of prothrombin Fragment 1+2 (F1+2), thrombin–antithrombin complexes (TAT), fibrinopeptide A (FPA), the levels of tissue plasminogen activator (tPA) antigen and activity, plasminogen activator inhibitor (PAI), thrombin activatable fibrinolysis inhibitor (TAFI), activated protein C resistance (APCR, when assessed by the activated partial thromboplastin time [aPTT]). In addition, some factors show no effect of gestation. These include the aPTT-APCR when the subject's sample is prediluted with factor FV depleted plasma (factor V depleted aPTT-APCR).

the balance of fibrinolysis. Increasing gestation is associated with a complex alteration in the plasma markers of plasminogen activation and inhibition. Plasminogen activity, PAI-1, and PAI-2 levels increase throughout pregnancy[48] (see Table 21.1). This rise is accompanied by an increase in the level of tissue plasminogen activator (tPA) antigen,[48] although there are reports of a reduction in tPA activity[52,67] and tPA release in response to venous occlusion.[68] No alteration in α_2-antiplasmin levels has been reported in normal pregnant subjects,[48] but TAFI levels also increase by 48 percent from the first to the third trimesters.[69]

A number of studies have concluded that increasing gestation is associated with an overall reduction in systemic fibrinolytic activity.[67,70,71] Despite this, pregnancy is associated with an increase in the levels of fibrin degradation products.[48] The reason for this apparent disparity is not known, although it may point to an increase in fibrin generation and degradation in the placenta (despite a

reduction in the fibrinolytic potential of the general circulation),[72] or to a reduction in the plasma clearance of these measurable products.[67]

MATERNAL POSTPARTUM HEMOSTASIS

Changes in maternal coagulation and fibrinolysis around delivery

On the limited information available[48] many factors show little change during labor. However, a fall in fibrinogen levels occurs, with a nadir evident at the delivery of the placenta. Levels then rise within hours of delivery. Fibrin degradation products are elevated in early labor, fall during placental delivery, but rise again immediately afterward. Whether there is an alteration in the overall fibrinolytic activity in the first few hours after delivery is unclear.[70,73]

There is no change in total protein S levels during delivery, but the effect of delivery on protein C is not fully understood. It appears that protein C levels fall during the delivery (prior to the clamping of the placental cord), rising again after clamping. Higher APCR has been reported at delivery[58] and a return toward nonpregnant values is seen in the first week of the puerperium activity.[48]

Changes in coagulation and fibrinolysis in the puerperium

In the first postpartum week, no reduction (and perhaps a further elevation) of fibrinogen levels has been reported in a number of longitudinal studies.[48] This may be accompanied by a slight rise from antenatal levels in FVc and FXIc. A fall, from antenatal levels, of FVIIIc and FVIIc is evident between day 1 and 7 post partum. In the first week of the puerperium, thrombin generation, soluble fibrin levels and D-dimer formation all remain higher than in early pregnancy. Increasing levels,[51,74] a fall,[75] and no change in protein C,[52] have all been reported in the first 3–5 days of the puerperium. A gradual return to nonpregnant levels of both free and total protein S becomes evident in the first week of the puerperium. The first postpartum week is also associated with a fall, from antenatal values, in plasma plasminogen and (consistent with a substantial placental origin) in overall PAI levels.[48]

LINKS BETWEEN MATERNAL HEMOSTASIS AND METABOLISM

The upregulation of coagulation in normal pregnancy mirrors, in part, the change in maternal metabolism and both may be influenced by the same stimuli. Whether changes in metabolism alter the risk of thrombotic disease in pregnancy is not fully understood, although there is a link between maternal obesity and a number of maternal thrombotic complications including preeclampsia.[76] In addition, maternal gestational hypercholesterolemia has also been linked with the progression of early atheromatous lesions in offspring, although whether this is due to a direct maternal effect, or to the sharing of similar genetic risk factors is not known.[77]

There are a number of recognized lipid-coagulation interactions evident both within and outwith pregnancy. In population studies, a positive correlation between plasma triglyceride and both FIXc and fibrinogen has been found.[78] Higher triglyceride levels are also associated with higher thrombin generation.[79] There is also an inverse relation between the level of the predominant polyunsaturated fatty acid, linoleic acid, with fibrinogen and plasminogen.[80] Cholesterol is positively correlated with acquired APCR (and therefore with thrombin generation[81]) both within and outwith pregnancy.[51,82] Despite this, in the general population there is also a positive correlation between

lipid levels and the level of the natural anticoagulants proteins C and S.[83] Overall, however, cholesterol and LDL-cholesterol appear to be positively related to FVIIc, fibrinogen levels, and thrombin generation.[79,84] In pregnancy the increasing levels of total cholesterol and triglyceride mirror the changes in FVIIc and PAI-1.[85] Both PAI-1 and triglyceride levels also relate to the degree of insulin resistance.[86] There is also an association between the change in triglyceride with tPA and D-dimer levels. There is no, however, no correlation between the change in lipids and the marked rise in von Willebrand factor which accompanies normal gestation.[85]

High maternal cholesterol levels could predispose to superoxide production[87] and oxidation of LDL is a prominent risk factor for arteriosclerosis.[88] There is also an association between higher levels of small dense LDL (which are more susceptible to oxidation) and the development of preeclampsia.[89] Furthermore, women with the greatest rise in plasma triglyceride during pregnancy have the most substantial reduction in the size of LDL particles.[90] The potential impact of LDL oxidation on coagulation has been investigated, indicating that oxidized LDL is capable of suppressing protein C activation[91] and may also reduce thrombomodulin expression on endothelial cells.[92] Oxidized LDL is also capable of inhibiting prostacyclin synthesis.[91] The presence of large triglyceride-rich VLDL can also promote the synthesis and release of PAI-1[93] and lipolysed remnants of such triglyceride-rich lipoproteins may increase the activation of circulating FVIIc to FVIIa.[94] It appears likely that any influence lipids have on coagulation is not the same in pregnancy as it is in nonpregnant subjects. Estrogen, in the form of hormone replacement therapy (HRT) can reduce Lp(a) levels,[95,96] but high endogenous estrogen in pregnancy does not have this effect. Similarly, unopposed estrogen HRT also reduces protein C and antithrombin levels,[97] but this does not occur in pregnancy.

The maternal alteration in coagulation is clearly a physiologic, rather than pathologic response. Although there is some evidence that the thrombotic/antithrombotic balance in early pregnancy may be a marker for the development of subsequent vascular disorders such preeclampsia,[98] a link between the physiologic alterations in coagulation and thrombosis remains unproved. Indeed, despite the progressive changes in coagulation and lipids with increasing gestation, the risk of venous thrombosis may be equal in the first and second trimesters.[99] It is conceivable that acquired or inherited thrombophilias could upset the delicate coagulation balance and increase the risk of thrombosis-linked disorders. Outwith pregnancy, the statin group of drugs reduce lipid levels and in one study a 21 percent reduction in serum total cholesterol with simvastatin therapy also resulted in a 36 percent reduction in thrombin generation.[79] Despite this, the statins appear to have no effect on either fibrinogen or homocysteine levels.[100] Whether any form of therapeutic lipid alteration in pregnancy would be safe, or could influence pregnancy failure (or indeed subsequent maternal thrombotic risk) is, at present, however, unknown.

KEY LEARNING POINTS

- The maternal metabolic response is initially anabolic, but becomes catabolic in the latter stages of pregnancy.
- Normal pregnancy leads to a physiologic upregulation of coagulation, which may be necessary for fetoplacental development and protection against delivery-associated bleeding.
- Normal pregnancy probably results in an overall reduction in fibrinolysis, which along with the changes in coagulation, most likely leads to a prothrombotic state.
- Although the changes in lipid metabolism may influence coagulation and fibrinolysis, it is not known whether therapeutic alteration of lipids in pregnancy would be safe, or beneficial in either preventing thrombosis-linked pregnancy disorders or in improving future maternal health.

REFERENCES

1 Bonnar J, Sheppard BL. The vascular supply of the placenta in normal and abnormal pregnancy. In: Baustein A, ed. *Pathology of the Female Genital Tract.* New York: Springer Verlag, 1977; 673–89.

2 Henrikson K. Thrombin as a hormonally regulated growth factor in oestrogen-responsive tissue. *Semin Thromb Hemost* 1992; **18**: 53–9.

3 Jazin EE, Dickerman HW, Henrikson KP. Estrogen regulation of a tissue factor-like procoagulant in the immature rat uterus. *Endocrinology* 1990; **126**: 176–85.

4 Alvarez JJ, Montelongo A, Iglesias A, *et al.* Longitudinal study of lipoprotein profile, high density lipoprotein subclass and post-heparin lipases during gestation in women. *J Lipid Res* 1996; **37**: 299–308.

5 Berge LN, Arnesen E, Forsdahl A. Pregnancy-related changes in some cardiovascular risk factors. *Acta Obstet Gynecol Scand* 1996; **75**: 439–42.

6 Ordovas J, Pocovi M, Grande F. Plasma lipids and cholesterol esterification rate during pregnancy. *Obstet Gynecol* 1984; **63**: 20–5.

7 Knopp RH, Warth MR, Charles D, *et al.* Lipoprotein metabolism in pregnancy, fat transport to the fetus and the effects of diabetes. *Biol Neonate* 1986; **50**: 297–317.

8 Desoye G, Schweditsch MO, Pfeiffer KP, *et al.* Correlation of hormones with lipid and lipoprotein levels during normal pregnancy and postpartum. *J Clin Endocrinol Metab* 1987; **64**: 704–12.

9 Jimenez DM, Pocovi M, Ramon-Cajal J, *et al.* Longitudinal study of plasma lipids and lipoprotein cholesterol in normal pregnancy and puerperium. *Gynecol Obstet Invest* 1988; **25**: 158–64.

10 Fahraeus L, Larsson-Cohn U, Wallentin L. Plasma lipoproteins including high density lipoprotein subfractions during normal pregnancy. *Obstet Gynecol* 1985; **66**: 468–72.

11 Montelongo A, Lasuncion M, Pallardo L, Herrera A. Longitudinal study of plasma lipoproteins and hormones during pregnancy in normal and diabetic women. *Diabetes* 1992; **41**: 1651–9.

12 Villar J, Cogswell M, Kestler E, *et al.* Effect of fat and fat-free mass deposition during pregnancy on birth weight. *Am J Obstet Gynecol* 1992; **167**: 1344–52.

13 Hytten F, Leitch I. *The Physiology of Human Pregnancy,* 2nd ed. Oxford: Blackwell Science, 1971.

14 Murphy S, Abrams B. Changes in energy intakes during pregnancy and lactation in a national sample of US women. *Am J Public Health* 1993; **83**: 1161–3.

15 Alsonso de la Torre SR, Serrano MA, Medina JM. Carrier-mediated beta-D-hydroxybutyrate transport in brush border membrane vesicles for the rat placenta. *Pediatr Res* 1992; **32**: 317–23.

16 Martin-Hidalgo A, Holm C, Belfrage P, *et al.* Lipoprotein lipase and hormone-sensitive lipase activity and mRNA in rat adipose tissue during pregnancy. *Am J Physiol* 1994; **266**: E930–5.

17 Walsh B, Sacks F. Effects of low dose oral contraceptives on very low- and low-density lipoprotein metabolism. *J Clin Invest* 1993; **91**: 2126–32.

18 Zorzano A, Lasuncion M, Herrera A. Role of the availability of substrates on hepatic and renal gluconeogenesis in the fasted pregnant rat. *Metab Clin Exp* 1986; **35**: 297–303.

19 Herrera A. Implications of dietary fatty acids during pregnancy in placental, fetal and posynatal development-A review. *Placenta* 2002; **23**: S9–19.

20 Scanu A, Fless G. Lipoprotein (a): heterogeneity and biological relevance. *J Clin Invest* 1990; **85**: 1709–15.

21 Bandello F, Vigano D, Parlavecchia M. Hypercoagulability and high lipoprotein (a) levels in patients with central retinal vein occlusion. *Thromb Haemost* 1994; **72**: 39–43.

22 Maeda S, Abe A, Seishima M, *et al.* Transient changes of serum lipoprotein (a) as an acute phase protein. *Atherosclerosis* 1989; **78**: 145–50.

23 Zechner R, Desoye G, Schweditsch MO, *et al.* Fluctuations of plasma lipoprotein-A concentrations during pregnancy and post partum. *Metab Clin Exp* 1986; **35**: 333–6.

24 Cachia O, Legger C, Boulet P, *et al.* Red blood cell vitamin E concentration in fetuses are related to, but lower than those in mothers during gestation. *Am J Obstet Gynecol* 1995; **173**: 42–51.

25 Wang J, Mimuro S, Lahoud R, *et al.* Elevated levels of lipoprotein (a) in women with pre-eclampsia. *Am J Obstet Gynecol* 1998; **178**: 146–9.

26 Sattar N, Clark P, Greer I, *et al.* Lipoprotein (a) levels in normal pregnancy and in pregnancy complicated with pre-eclampsia. *Atherosclerosis* 2000; **148**: 407–11.

27 Ohvo-Rekila H, Ramstedt B, Leppimaki P, Slotte JP. Total cholesterol interaction with phospholipids in membranes. *Prog Lipid Res* 2002; **41**: 66–97.

28 Martinez-Botas J, Suarez Y, Ferruelo AJ, *et al.* Cholesterol starvation decreases p34 (cdc2) kinase activity and arrests the cell cycle at G2. *FASEB J* 1999; **13**: 1359–70.

29 Suarez Y, Fernandez C, Ledo B, *et al.* Differential effects of ergosterol and cholesterol on cell activation and SRE0 driven transcription. *Eur J Biochem* 2002; **269**: 1761–71.

30 Mauch DH, Nagler K, Schumacher S, *et al.* CNS synaptogenesis is promoted by glia-derived cholesterol. *Science* 2001; **294**: 1354–57.

31 Woollett L. The origins and roles of cholesterol and fatty acids in the fetus. *Curr Opin Lipidol* 2001; **12**: 305–12.

32 Parker CR, Deahl T, Drewery P, Hankins G. Analysis of the potential for transfer of lipoprotein-cholesterol across the human placenta. *Early Hum Dev* 1983; **8**: 289–95.

33 Hay W, Saprks J, Battaglia F. Maternal-fetal glucose exchange: necessity of a three pool model. *Am J Physiol* 1984; **246**: E528–34.

34 Baird J. Some aspects of the metabolic and hormonal adaptation to pregnancy. *Acta Endocrinologica Suppl (Copenhagen)* 1986; **112**: 11–18.

35 Waisman H, Kerr G. Amino acid and protein metabolism in the developing fetus and newborn infant. *Pediatr Clin North Am* 1965; **12**: 551–72.

36 Hare J. *Diabetes complicating pregnancy: The Joslin Clinic Method.* New York: Alan R Liss, 1989.

37 Koebnik C, Heins U, Dagnelie P, *et al.* Longitudinal concentrations of vitamin B_{12} and vitamin B_{12}-binding proteins during uncomplicated pregnancy. *Clin Chem* 2002; **48**: 928–33.

38 Parrdo J, Peled Y, Bar, J. *et al.* Evaluation of low serum vitamin B_{12} in the non-anaemic pregnant patient. *Hum Reprod* 2000; **15**: 224–6.

39 Ellison J, Clark P, Walker I, Greer I. Effect of supplementation with folic acid throughout pregnancy on plasma homocysteine concentration. *Thromb Res* 2004; **114**: 25–7.

40 Zamorano A, Arnalich F, Sanchez, *et al.* Levels of iron, vitamin B12, folic acid and their binding proteins during pregnancy. *Acta Haematol* 1985; **74**: 92–6.

41 Qvist I, Abdulla M, Jagerstad M, Svensson S. Iron, zinc and folate status during pregnancy and two months after delivery. *Acta Obstet Gynecol Scand* 1986; **65**: 15–22.

42 Andersson A, Hultberg B, Brattstrom L, Isaksson A. Decreased serum homocysteine in pregnancy. *Eur J Clin Chem Clin Biochem* 1992; **30**: 377–9.

43 Steegers-Theunissen RP, Wathen NC, *et al.* Maternal and fetal levels of methionine and homocysteine in early human pregnancy. *Br J Obstet Gynaecol* 1997; **104**: 20–4.

44 de Fouw N, Haverkate F, Bertina R, *et al.* The cofactor role of protein S in the acceleration of whole blood clot lysis by activated protein C *in vitro. Blood* 1986; **67**: 1189–92.

45 Mosnier L, Meijers J, Bouma B. The role of protein S in the activation of thrombin activatable fibrinolysis inhibitor (TAFI) and regulation of fibrinolysis. *Thromb Haemost* 2001; **86**: 1040–6.

46 Kruithof E, Chien T, Gundinchet A. Fibrinolysis in pregnancy: a study of plasminogen activation inhibitors. *Blood* 1987; **69**: 460–6.

47 Thorsen S, Philipds M, Selmer J, *et al.* Kinetics of inhibition of tissue-type and urokinase-type plasminogen activator by plasminogen activator inhibitor type 1 and type 2. *Eur J Biochem* 1988; **175**: 33–9.

48 Clark P. Changes of haemostasis variables in pregnancy. *Semin Vasc Med* 2003; **3**: 13–24.

49 Gatti L, Tenconi PM, Guarneri D, *et al.* Hemostatic parameters and platelet activation by flow-cytometry in normal pregnancy: a longitudinal study. *Int J Clin Lab Res* 1994; **24**: 217–19.

50 Faught W, Garner P, Jones G, Ivey B. Changes in protein C and protein S levels in normal pregnancy. *Am J Obstet Gynecol* 1995; **172**: 147–50.

51 Clark P, Brennand J, Conkie JA, *et al.* Activated protein C sensitivity, protein C, protein S and coagulation in normal pregnancy. *Thromb Haemost* 1998; **79**: 1166–70.

52 Kjellberg U, Andersson N, Rosen S, *et al.* APC resistance and other haemostatic variables during pregnancy and puerperium. *Thromb Haemost* 1999; **81**: 527–31.

53 Weenink GH, Treffers PE, Kahle LH, ten Cate JW. Antithrombin III in normal pregnancy. *Thromb Res* 1982; **26**: 281–7.

54 Ramalakshmi BA, Raju LA, Raman L. Antithrombin III levels in pregnancy induced hypertension. *Natl Med J India* 1995; **8**: 61–2.

55 Dahlback B, Carlsson M, Svensson PJ. Familial thrombophilia due to a previously unrecognized mechanism characterized by poor anticoagulant response to activated protein C: prediction of a cofactor to activated protein C. *Proc Natl Acad Sci U S A* 1993; **90**: 1004–8.

56 Bertina R, Koeleman B, Koster T, *et al.* Mutation in blood-coagulation factor-V associated with resistance to activated protein-C. *Nature* 1994; **369**: 64–7.

57 Cumming AM, Tait RC, Fildes S, *et al.* Development of resistance to activated protein C during pregnancy. *Br J Haematol* 1995; **90**: 725–7.

58 Mathonet F, de Mazancourt P, Bastenaire B, *et al.* Activated protein C sensitivity ratio in pregnant women at delivery. *Br J Haematol* 1996; **92**: 244–6.

59 Nicolaes GAF, Thomassen M, Tans G, *et al.* Effect of activated protein C on thrombin generation and on the thrombin potential in plasma of normal and APC-resistant individuals. *Blood Coagul Fibrinolysis* 1997; **8**: 28–38.

60 Clark P, Walker ID. The phenomenon known as acquired activated protein C resistance. *Br J Haematol* 2001; **115**: 1–8.

61 Freyburger G, Javorschi S, Labrouche S, Bernard P. Proposal for objective evaluation of the performance of various functional APC-resistance tests in genotyped patients. *Thromb Haemost* 1997; **78**: 1360–5.

62   Lowe G, Rumley A, Woodward M, *et al.* Activated protein C resistance and the FV:R506Q mutation in a random population sample – associations with cardiovascular risk factors and coagulation variables. *Thromb Haemost* 1999; **81**: 918–24.

63   Bauer KA, Rosenberg RD. The pathophysiology of the prethrombotic state in humans: insights gained from studies using markers of hemostatic system activation. *Blood* 1987; **70**: 343–50.

64   Bremme K, Ostlund E, Almqvist I, *et al.* Enhanced thrombin generation and fibrinolytic activity in normal pregnancy and the puerperium. *Obstet Gynecol* 1992; **80**: 132–7.

65   Heeb MJ, Espana F, Griffin JH. Inhibition and complexation of activated protein C by two major inhibitors in plasma. *Blood* 1989; **73**: 446–54.

66   Gerbasi F, Bottoms S, Farag A, *et al.* Increased intravascular coagulation associated with pregnancy. *Obstet Gynecol* 1990; **75**: 385–9.

67   Wright J, Cooper P, Astedt B, *et al.* Fibrinolysis during normal human pregnancy: complex inter-relationships between plasma levels of tissue plasminogen activator and inhibitors and the euglobulin clot lysis time. *Br J Haematol* 1988; **69**: 253–8.

68   Ballegeer V, Mombaerts P, Declerck P, *et al.* Fibrinolytic response to venous occlusion and fibrin fragment D-dimer levels in normal and complicated pregnancy. *Thromb Haemost* 1987; **58**: 1030–2.

69   Ku D-HW, Arkel Y, Paidas M, Lockwood C. Circulating levels of inflammatory cytokines, (IL-1 beta and TNF alpha), resistance to activated protein C, thrombin and fibrin generation in uncomplicated pregnancies. *Thromb Haemost* 2003; **90**: 1074–9.

70   Condie RG, Ogston D. Sequential studies on components of the haemostatic mechanism in pregnancy with particular reference to the development of pre-eclampsia. *Br J Obstet Gynaecol* 1976; **83**: 938–42.

71   Stirling Y, Woolf L, North WRS, *et al.* Haemostasis in normal pregnancy. *Thromb Haemost* 1984; **52**: 176–82.

72   Bonnar J, Prentice C, McNicol G, Douglas A. Haemostatic mechanism in the uterine circulation during placental separation. *Br Med J* 1970; **2**: 564–7.

73   Nilsson I, Kullander S. Coagulation and fibrinolytic studies during pregnancy. *Acta Obstet Gynecol Scand* 1967; **46**: 273–85.

74   Mannucci P, Vigano S, Botasso B, *et al.* Protein C antigen during pregnancy, delivery and the puerperium. *Thromb Haemost* 1984; **52**: 217–19.

75   Malm J, Laurell M, Dalhback B. Changes in the plasma levels of vitamin K-dependent proteins C and S and of C4b-binding protein during pregnancy and oral contraception. *Br J Haematol* 1988; **68**: 437–43.

76   Sattar N, Clark P, Holmes A, *et al.* Antenatal waist circumference and hypertension risk. *Obstet Gynecol* 2001; **97**: 268–71.

77   Palinski W, Glass C, Witztum J, *et al.* Influence of maternal hypercholesterolaemia during pregnancy on progression of early atherosclerotic lesions in childhood: Fate of early lesions in children (FELIC) study. *Lancet* 1999; **354**: 1234–41.

78   Woodward M, Lowe GDO, Rumley A, *et al.* Epidemiology of coagulation factors, inhibitors and activation markers: the Third Glasgow MONICA Survey II. Relationships to cardiovascular risk factors and prevalent cardiovascular disease. *Br J Haematol* 1997; **97**: 785–97.

79   Alessandri C, Basili S, Maurelli M, *et al.* Relationship between prothrombin activation fragment F1 + 2 and serum cholesterol. *Haemostasis* 1996; **26**: 214–19.

80   Salomaa V, Salminen I, Rasi V, *et al.* Association of the fatty acid composition of serum phospholipids with haemostatic factors. *Arterioscl Thromb Vasc Biol* 1996; **17**: 809–13.

81   Clark P, Walker I, Greer I. Acquired activated protein-C resistance in pregnancy and association with increased thrombin generation and fetal weight. *Lancet* 1999; **353**: 292–3.

82   Tosetto AM, E. Gatto, E. Rodeghiero, F. The VITA project: phenotypic resistance to activated protein C and FV Leiden mutation in the general population. *Thromb Haemost* 1997; **78**: 859–63.

83   MacCallum P, Cooper J, Martin J, *et al.* Associations of protein C and protein S with serum lipid concentrations. *Br J Haematol* 1998; **102**: 609–15.

84   MacCallum P, Cooper J, Martin J, *et al.* Haemostatic and lipid determinants of prothrombin fragment F1.2 and D-dimer in plasma. *Thromb Haemost* 2000; **83**: 421–6.

85   Sattar N, Greer I, Rumley A, *et al.* A longitudinal study of the relationship between haemostatic, lipid and oestradiol changes during normal human pregnancy. *Thromb Haemost* 1999; **81**: 71–5.

86   Juhan-Vague I, Alessi M. Plasminogen activatior inhibitor-1 and atherothrombosis. *Thromb Haemost* 1993; **70**: 138–43.

87   Ohara Y, Peterson T, Harrison T. Hypercholesterolaemia increases endothelial superoxide anion production. *J Clin Invest* 1993; **91**: 2546–51.

88   Napoli C, d'Armiento FP, Mancini FP, *et al.* Fatty streak formation occurs in human fetal aortas and is greatly enhanced by maternal hypercholesterolaemia. Intimal accumulation of LDL and its oxidation precede monocyte recruitment into early atherosclerotic lesions. *J Clin Invest* 1997; **100**: 2680–90.

89   Sattar N, Greer IA, Louden J, *et al.* Lipoprotein subfraction changes in normal pregnancy: threshold effect of plasma triglyceride on appearance of small dense low-density lipoprotein. *J Clin Endocrinol Metab* 1997; **82**: 2483–91.

90   Silliman K, Shore V, Forte T. Hypertriglyceridaemia during late pregnancy is associated with the formation of small dense low-density lipoproteins and the presence of large buoyant high-density lipoproteins. *Metabolism* 1994; **8**: 1035–41.

91   Sattar N, Gaw A, Packard C, Greer I. Potential pathogenic roles of aberrant lipoprotein and fatty acid metabolism in pre-eclampsia. *Br J Obstet Gynaecol* 1996; **103**: 614–20.

92   Oida K, Tohda G, Ishii H, *et al.* Effect of oxidized low density lipoprotein on thrombomodulin expression by THP-1 cells. *Thromb Haemost* 1997; **78**: 1228–33.

93   Stewart DJ, Monge JC. Hyperlipidaemia and endothelial dysfunction. *Curr Opin Lipidol* 1993; **4**: 319–24.

94   Mitropoulos K, Reeves B, Miller G. The activation of factor VII in citrated plasma by charged long-chain fatty acids at the interface of triglyceride-rich lipoproteins. *Blood Coagul Fibrinolysis* 1993; **4**: 943–51.

95   Sebire N, Jolly M, Harris J. Maternal obesity and pregnancy outcome: a study of 287213 pregnancies in London. *Int J Obes* 2001; **25**: 1175–82.

96   Kumari A. Pregnancy outcome in women with morbid obesity. *Int J Obstet Gynecol* 2001; **73**: 101–7.

97   Kessler CM, Szymanski LM, Shamsipour Z, *et al.* Estrogen replacement therapy and coagulation: relationship to lipid and lipoprotein changes. *Obstet Gynecol* 1997; **89**: 326–31.

98   Clark P, Sattar N, Walker I, Greer I. The Glasgow Outcome, APCR and Lipid (GOAL) Pregnancy Study: significance of pregnancy-associated activated protein C resistance. *Thromb Haemost* 2001; **85**: 30–5.

99   McColl MD, Ramsay JE, Tait RC, *et al.* Risk factors for pregnancy-associated venous thromboembolism. *Thromb Haemost* 1997; **78**: 1183–8.

100 Balk E, Lau J, Goudas L, *et al.* Effect of statins on non-lipid serum markers associated with cardiovascular disease. *Ann Intern Med* 2003; **139**: 670–82.

22

Venous thrombosis in pregnancy

SIMON J MCRAE, JEFFREY S GINSBERG

INTRODUCTION

Venous thromboembolism (VTE), consisting of deep vein thrombosis (DVT) and pulmonary embolism (PE), is a potentially fatal disease with an estimated annual incidence of 0.1 percent in Caucasian populations.[1] Long-term sequelae, in particular postphlebitic syndrome (PPS), are frequent and can be disabling. Pregnancy has long been recognized as a risk factor for VTE, with the importance of this relation underlined by the fact that at the end of the twenty-first century, PE remains a leading cause of maternal mortality in developed countries. This chapter covers several aspects of pregnancy-related VTE including epidemiology, etiology, and the unique challenges in diagnosis and management presented by both changes in maternal physiology and the need to include an assessment of fetal risk in any decision-making process.

EPIDEMIOLOGY

Incidence of fatal venous thromboembolism associated with pregnancy

The most comprehensive data on pregnancy-related fatal VTE come from the Confidential Enquiries into Maternal Deaths, established in the United Kingdom in 1952.[2] Health professionals in the UK are required to provide a full account of all maternal deaths to the enquiry, and, as a result, accurate data on incidence and cause of death are available. The incidence of fatal PE during pregnancy fell progressively from approximately 7 deaths in 100 000 maternities in the 1950s to 1.3 deaths per 100 000 maternities for the triennium 1991–93,[3] with the main reason for the reduction being a fall in deaths following vaginal delivery. In the triennial report for 1997–99, the reported incidence of fatal PE was 1.45 per 100 000 maternities, and PE remained the most common direct cause of maternal death in the United Kingdom, constituting 33 percent of maternal mortality.[4] Of note, the fall in deaths from thromboembolism following cesarean section published in this report followed the introduction of the United Kingdom guidelines for thromboprophylaxis post-cesarean section. In the most recent report for the triennium 2000–02, published in 2004, thromboembolic disease remained the leading cause of direct maternal mortality. The mortality rate for PE was 1.2 per 100 000 maternities with the reduction being in the number of women dying in the antenatal period compared with the previous triennium.[5]

Although a mandatory reporting system for maternal deaths does not exist in the United States, studies using largely retrospective data derived from death certification have documented a fall in the rate of fatal PE in the two decades leading up to 1990.[6–8] In 1987, the Centers for Disease Control and Prevention established the Pregnancy Mortality Surveillance System (PMSS) to prospectively collect maternal mortality data using information from state maternal mortality review committees, the media, and individual reports, in addition to that from death certification nationwide.[8] The PMSS reported rates of fatal PE during pregnancy of 1.8 and 2.3 per 100 000 live deliveries for the periods 1987–90 and 1991–99, respectively.[8,9] In the latter study, PE was the most frequent cause of maternal death after a live birth, being responsible for 21 percent of fatalities. A higher rate of fatal PE of 4.5 per 100 000 live births was found in a prospective survey of maternal deaths in a single perinatal network, which may have reflected more accurate data collection or a high-risk obstetric population.[10]

In the UK Confidential Enquiry report for the triennium 1997–99, 42 percent of fatal embolic events occurred antepartum, with nearly two-thirds of these occurring in the first trimester.[4] Identifiable risk factors for VTE were present in 25 of 31 women, with increased maternal weight in particular identified. In the report for 2000–02 identifiable and specific risk factors were present in almost 80 percent of women dying from PE (information on specific risk factors was not available for the remainder). At least 50 percent of those dying post partum were obese. Substandard care, such as delay in diagnosis, failure to identify risk and provide prophylaxis was found in 57 percent of cases.[5] Increasing maternal age has been reported as a risk factor for fatal PE during pregnancy, with one retrospective study reporting the risk in women over the age of 40 to be 10-fold that of women under 25.[6] A smaller twofold increase in the incidence of fatal PE associated with maternal age over 35 years has been reported in a subsequent Confidential Enquiry.[3] In the United States the rate of fatal PE, like all cause maternal mortality, has been consistently found to be twofold to threefold higher in black women in comparison to white women, a ratio maintained despite reductions in the overall incidence of VTE.[6,9] Whether this relates to differences in severity of disease, diagnostic methods, or treatment remains unclear.

Incidence of nonfatal pregnancy–associated venous thromboembolism

The incidence of nonfatal venous thromboembolic events during pregnancy or the puerperium is less certain.[11] Studies designed to accurately determine the rate of asymptomatic

VTE during pregnancy have not been performed, and, as sensitive tests for asymptomatic VTE are invasive and involve exposure to radiation, are unlikely to occur. In a small trial using radiolabeled fibrinogen to screen for DVT in the puerperium, calf vein thrombosis was detected in three of 100 women by the seventh day post partum, with all events resolving without anticoagulation.[12] In another study, in which 140 unselected women were screened on day 4 post partum for proximal DVT using duplex ultrasonography, no thrombotic events were detected.[13] Unfortunately, the small size of the studies precludes any firm conclusion concerning the incidence of VTE following delivery.

In nonpregnant women of childbearing age, studies from both the United States and Sweden have reported the annual incidence of symptomatic VTE to be approximately 1 in 10 000 individuals.[14–16] Considerable variability has been seen in estimates of the incidence of nonfatal symptomatic VTE during pregnancy over the years, likely due to differences in the methods used to diagnose VTE. Early studies,[17–19] in which the diagnosis of acute thrombosis was made entirely on clinical grounds, are likely to have overestimated the incidence of VTE, as the majority of women with suspected DVT or PE during pregnancy did not have the diagnosis confirmed by objective testing.[20,21] The results from more recent studies (Table 22.1), in which the majority or all patients underwent objective testing for suspected VTE, are more likely to reflect true disease incidence. Most studies are retrospective, and use national,[22,23] regional,[16,24] or institutional[25–29] discharge and birth data to determine incidence, with rates ranging from 0.6 to 1.3 episodes per 1000 deliveries, that is, 5–10-fold that reported for nonpregnant women of reproductive age. Some of these studies only included patients with DVT.

INCIDENCE OF DVT IN COMPARISON TO PE

As shown in Table 22.2, the majority of individuals with VTE during pregnancy are diagnosed with DVT rather than PE, with DVT constituting approximately 85 percent of

Table 22.1   Incidence of nonfatal pregnancy-related venous thromboembolism

Study	Design	Incidence/1000 pregnancies
Bergqvist et al.[30]	Prospective, antepartum DVT only	0.7
Kierkegaard[25]	Retrospective, DVT only	0.7
Polak and Wilkinson[29]	Prospective, antepartum DVT only	0.7
Macklon and Greer[22]	Retrospective, DVT and PE	1.1
Lindqvist et al.[23]	Retrospective, DVT and PE	1.3
Anderson et al.[24]	Retrospective, DVT and PE	0.85
Gherman et al.[27]	Retrospective, DVT and PE	0.6
McColl et al.[26]	Retrospective, DVT and PE	0.86
Simpson et al.[28]	Retrospective, DVT and PE	0.85
Samuelsson and Hagg[16]	Retrospective, DVT and PE	0.95

DVT, deep vein thrombosis; PE, pulmonary embolism.

Table 22.2 Relative incidence of antepartum deep vein thrombosis (DVT) and pulmonary embolism (PE)

Study	Pregnancies n	Episodes DVT n (%)*	Episodes PE n (%)*	Incidence DVT/1000 pregnancies	Incidence PE/1000 pregnancies
Lindqvist et al.[23]	479 422	518 (85.2)	90 (14.8)	1.1	0.2
Anderson et al.[24]	63 319	52 (96.3)	2 (3.7)	0.8	0.03
Gherman et al.[27]	268 525	127 (78.1)	38 (21.9)	0.5	0.1
McColl et al.[26]	72 201	51 (82.3)	11 (17.7)	0.7	0.2
Simpson et al.[28]	395 335	317 (88.3)	42 (11.7)	0.8	0.1
Total	1 278 802	1 065 (85.3)	183 (14.7)	0.8	0.1

*Represents percentage of overall episodes of antepartum venous thromboembolism.

thrombotic events. This compares with a figure of approximately 70 percent in nonpregnant patients with VTE, derived from clinical studies that did not include autopsy data.[1] Younger age and better cardiorespiratory reserve may account for the reduced likelihood of clinical symptoms of PE in pregnancy-related VTE. In nonpregnant patients with DVT, up to 50 percent of individuals will be shown to have asymptomatic PE if routine ventilation–perfusion (V/Q) lung scanning is performed.[31] This is also likely to be true for patients with DVT during pregnancy, particularly given, as will be discussed, the increased frequency of iliofemoral DVT in this patient group.

TIMING OF PRESENTATION WITH PREGNANCY–RELATED VTE

The distribution of episodes of DVT throughout pregnancy and the puerperium has been examined in a metaanalysis.[32] Pooling the results from studies in which objective methods were used to diagnose DVT, 65.5 percent of events occurred ante partum and 34.5 percent post partum. The antepartum events were distributed throughout pregnancy, with 21.9 percent occurring in the first trimester, 33.7 percent in the second, and 47.6 percent in the third. Because the puerperal period lasts only 6 weeks in comparison with the 38 weeks of an average pregnancy, the daily risk of DVT during the puerperium is almost fourfold that during pregnancy.[32] With one exception,[28] studies published subsequent to the above metaanalysis have reported a similar distribution of events ante partum and post partum.[16,24,27] In comparison to DVT, a higher proportion of pregnancy-related episodes of PE occur after delivery, with 43–60 percent of events occurring post partum.[26–28] Based on these results, the daily risk of PE is substantially higher following delivery than during the antepartum period.

Anatomic distribution of pregnancy–related deep vein thrombosis

In nonpregnant patients with symptomatic DVT, the majority of individuals will have femoropopliteal thrombus,[33] whereas isolated calf vein thrombus is the most frequent finding when venographic screening is performed in asymptomatic postoperative patients.[34,35] Isolated iliofemoral vein thrombosis is an uncommon finding in the above patient groups, occurring in less than 2 percent of such patients.[35] This contrasts sharply with the anatomic distribution of pregnancy-related DVT, during which iliofemoral vein thrombosis without popliteal involvement is common, making up between 45 percent and 70 percent of cases.[29,30] The contrast in distribution of DVT between nonpregnant and pregnant patients suggests that the natural history of the disease in the two groups differs. Whereas symptomatic DVT in nonpregnant patients is usually a result of proximal extension of calf vein thrombosis,[34] it appears that pregnancy-related DVT often results from distal extension of an initial pelvic vein thrombosis.

A preponderance of left-leg over right-leg DVT during pregnancy was initially noted over 20 years ago.[30] This observation was confirmed in subsequent larger cohort studies,[29,36] one of which reported 58 of 60 episodes of confirmed episodes of DVT to involve the left leg, with the other two patients having bilateral DVT.[36] A metaanalysis pooling data from 12 studies that documented the side of objectively confirmed pregnancy-related DVT reported that 82.2 percent of episodes were left-sided, a small proportion of which had bilateral DVT.[32] As almost equal proportions of patients with suspected DVT during pregnancy present with symptoms isolated to either the left or right leg,[20] a higher proportion of individuals with left-sided symptoms will have the diagnosis confirmed. A much smaller predominance of left-leg DVT is seen in nonpregnant patients.[29,35]

The mechanism of this propensity for DVT to be left-sided during pregnancy is unclear. In nonpregnant patients, anatomic abnormalities or 'spurs' producing abnormal narrowing of the common iliac vein are more frequently found in the left side.[37] These 'spurs', combined with direct compression of the left common iliac vein where it crosses the right common iliac artery have been alleged to contribute to the development of left-sided iliofemoral DVT,[38,39] and that the degree of left iliac vein compression can be exaggerated by pregnancy.[36] Although this phenomenon has not been directly demonstrated, venous flow velocity as measured by Doppler ultrasonography is reduced in the left leg in comparison to the right leg during pregnancy,[40] and this difference persists up to 6 weeks post partum.[41] A similar left-sided predominance has been observed for DVT associated with use of the oral contraceptive, suggesting a hormonal influence on the unequal distribution of events.[42]

Clinical risk factors for pregnancy–associated VTE

Evidence for an association between clinical factors and an increased rate of VTE during pregnancy is almost entirely derived from case–control studies, with conflicting data existing for many characteristics. Increased maternal age (often defined as >35 years),[3,19,22,43] increased body mass index (BMI),[3,28] a history of smoking,[23,44] and for postpartum VTE, delivery by cesarean section,[19,23,27,43] have been most consistently identified as risk factors for VTE, although contradictory results have been reported.[23,44] Prior superficial thrombophlebitis,[44] a family history of VTE,[26] blood group A[28,30] and post-partum hemorrhage[44] have also been identified as markers of increased risk. Contradictory results have been reported for increased parity[28,44] and preeclampsia.[23,28,44] None of the above individual risk factors, with the possible exception of delivery by cesarean section, are strong enough predictors of VTE to enable management decisions about anticoagulant prophylaxis during pregnancy and the puerperium to be determined. The influence of a past personal history of VTE on the risk of further thrombotic events in subsequent pregnancies, and therefore, the need for prophylactic therapy, will be discussed below.

PATHOGENESIS

Venous thromboembolism is now recognized as a multifactorial disease, with thrombosis resulting from the interplay between separate predisposing conditions.[45] The same is likely to be true in pregnancy-related VTE, with all three of Virchow's triad of risk factors, namely hypercoagulability, venous stasis and vascular damage, potentially present. The changes in endogenous procoagulant, anticoagulant, and fibrinolytic factors that occur during normal pregnancy, resulting in a net prothrombotic state in preparation for delivery, are considered in detail in Chapter 3, and will not be discussed further. Vascular damage, particularly to the pelvic veins, may occur as a direct result of trauma during normal vaginal or operative delivery.[11] It has also been suggested that venous distension associated with pregnancy may lead to endothelial injury,[46] resulting in prothrombotic changes on the endothelial surface.[40] The effect of pregnancy on venous hemodynamics, and the role of inherited and acquired thrombophilia in pregnancy-related VTE is discussed in more detail.

Changes in venous hemodynamics during pregnancy

Venous stasis is felt to be a significant contributing factor to the development of DVT, in both pregnant and nonpregnant patients. Flow in the deep leg veins during pregnancy was initially studied by the intravenous injection of radioactive sodium,[47] with decreased flow starting early in the second trimester and continuing to fall until delivery. This finding has been supported by subsequent studies using standard[48,49] or impedance plethysmography,[50] and Doppler ultrasonography,[40,51] although a single study using plethysmography had contradictory results.[52] Flow is maximally decreased in the third trimester,[40,50] and improves upon moving from the supine to the left lateral position,[40,50] presumably due to increased flow in the inferior vena cava which, when lying supine, may be completely compressed by the gravid uterus in late pregnancy.[53]

Direct mechanical obstruction of the pelvic veins, by both the gravid uterus and fetal head, is likely to play a major role in the reduction in deep venous flow, a theory supported by the rapid return to normal of flow rates of radioactive sodium following delivery.[47] A persistent increase in distensibility or capacitance of the deep leg veins,[48,49,54] a well-documented phenomenon during pregnancy attributed to hormonal effects on vascular smooth muscle,[41] has been suggested as an explanation for the ongoing reduction in flow rates post delivery.[49] Whatever the cause, the persistent venous stasis is likely to contribute to the ongoing risk of VTE during the puerperium.[11]

Thrombophilia and pregnancy-related VTE

Thrombophilia can be defined as an increased tendency to develop thrombosis, which may be either acquired or inherited.[55] Thrombophilic conditions predisposing to venous thrombosis vary both in prevalence, and in the magnitude of the associated increase in risk of VTE (Table 22.3). The risk of pregnancy-related VTE associated with individual thrombophilic states is discussed below. The relation between thrombophilia and adverse pregnancy outcome will not be discussed here, but it is the focus of Chapter 7.

ANTITHROMBIN DEFICIENCY, PROTEIN C DEFICIENCY, AND PROTEIN S DEFICIENCY

Antithrombin is a single-chain plasma glycoprotein belonging to the serine protease inhibitor superfamily (serpins). It is a physiologic inhibitor of thrombin and other activated coagulation factors (factors Xa, IXa, XIa, XIIa).[56] Thrombin inhibition by antithrombin is potentiated more than 1000-fold by heparin, due to conformational change of the antithrombin molecule on heparin binding.[57] Familial antithrombin deficiency, described in 1965, was the first identified inherited thrombophilia.[58] Individuals with type I deficiency typically have antithrombin levels of 40–60 percent, and

Table 22.3 Thrombophilic conditions predisposing to venous thromboembolism (VTE)

Thrombophilic condition	Population prevalence (%)	Prevalence (%) in unselected patients with VTE	Associated increase in risk of VTE
Antithrombin deficiency	0.02[59,60]	0.5–2.0[61–64]	5–50-fold[55,62,65–67]
Protein C deficiency	0.2–0.4[74,75]	1–3[61–64]	6–11-fold[62,65–67,76,77]
Protein S deficiency	Unknown	1–7[61–64]	8–32-fold[65,67]
Factor V Leiden	3–7[92,93]	12–20[94,95]	3–7-fold[66,94,95,97]
Prothrombin gene mutation	2[117,119]	4–7[117,119]	2–5-fold[117,119,121,122]
Elevated factor VIII levels*	10[130]	18.4[130]	4.8-fold[130]

*Odds ratio for individuals with factor VIII level 175–200 IU/dL in comparison to level <100 IU/dL.

constitute 0.02 percent of the general population.[59,60] Type II antithrombin deficiency, with functional antithrombin levels often between 60 percent and 80 percent, may be more prevalent than type I deficiency with community rates of up to 0.15 percent reported.[59] Approximately 0.5–2 percent of unselected individuals with VTE will have antithrombin deficiency.[61–64] Estimates of the increase in risk of VTE associated with antithrombin deficiency vary from fivefold to 50-fold.[55,62,65–67]

Protein C (PC) and protein S (PS) are both vitamin-K-dependent plasma glycoproteins synthesized in the liver.[55] When activated by thrombin, a process potentiated by the binding of thrombin to thrombomodulin, PC is converted to the active serine protease, activated protein C (APC).[68] In combination with its cofactor, PS, APC inactivates both factor Va and VIIIa, with the later process also enhanced by factor V. This protein C pathway plays a central role in controlling the thrombotic process.[69] As well as having a role as a cofactor for PC, PS also has direct anticoagulant activity.[70] In plasma, PS circulates both free (40 percent) and bound to the C4b-binding protein (60 percent). It is the free form of PS that has cofactor activity.[55]

Inherited PC deficiency was first described as a cause of venous thrombosis in 1981,[71] whereas PS deficiency was initially described as a cause of venous thrombosis in 1984.[72] Protein C and S deficiency both have type I and type II subgroups, and in addition a type III PS deficiency state with normal total circulating but reduced free levels can occur.[55,73] The estimated prevalence of heterozygous PC deficiency in the general population is between 0.2 percent and 0.4 percent,[74,75] with many of these individuals having no history of thrombosis. The community prevalence of PS deficiency is unknown. Protein C deficiency is found in 1–3 percent, and PS deficiency in 1–7 percent of unselected patients diagnosed with VTE.[61–64] Estimates from case–control and family cohort studies of the increase in risk of VTE associated with PC deficiency range from 6.4 to 11.3,[62,65–67,76,77] and 8.5–32-fold for PS deficiency.[65–67]

There is significant variation in estimates of the risk of pregnancy-related VTE in women with inherited deficiencies of the natural anticoagulants, likely due to differences in inclusion criteria between studies (Table 22.4). In early retrospective family cohort studies, the estimated risk of developing VTE during pregnancy and the puerperium ranged from 35 percent to 70 percent for women with antithrombin deficiency, 13 percent to 20 percent for PC deficiency, and 13 percent to 27 percent for PS deficiency.[78–81] However, the inclusion in these studies of propositi and individuals with VTE prior to pregnancy, and the common failure to diagnose VTE using accurate testing makes it likely these figures are overestimates of the risk of VTE, particularly for previously asymptomatic women. In a subsequent study, in which propositi and women with a prior personal history of VTE were excluded, the rates of pregnancy-related VTE were 3 percent, 2 percent, and 7 percent, for women with AT, PC, and PS deficiency, respectively.[82] The influence of prior history was confirmed by a study in which the rate of pregnancy-related VTE in women with antithrombin deficiency and no previous thrombosis was 14 percent (all post partum) in comparison to a rate of 60 percent in those with a prior episode of VTE.[83]

It is likely that women with a natural coagulation inhibitor deficiency and a personal history of VTE have a high risk of developing VTE during pregnancy, likely greater than 30 percent for antithrombin-deficient women and 10–30 percent for PC or PS deficiency. The risk in the same women without a past history of thrombosis is less well defined, and appears to be substantially lower but still increased above that of the general population.

The above-mentioned data are derived from family cohort studies, which will be relevant to most clinical situations, as the majority of women will be identified through symptomatic siblings. Attempts have also been made to estimate the risk associated with AT, PC, and PS deficiency in unselected women, although, due to the low population prevalence of these conditions, accurate estimates are difficult to obtain. In a case–control study enrolling unselected patients, Martinelli *et al.* found the relative risk of a first episode of VTE during pregnancy for women with antithrombin, PC, or PS deficiency grouped together to be 13.1 (95 percent confidence interval [CI] 5.0 to 34.2).[84] Using the observed prevalence of antithrombin deficiency in women with pregnancy-related VTE, and the known community prevalence of antithrombin deficiency, McColl and

Table 22.4 Cohort studies examining venous thromboembolism (VTE) risk during pregnancy in patients with inherited natural anticoagulant deficiency states

Study	Study characteristics	Antithrombin deficiency*	Protein C deficiency*	Protein S deficiency*
Hellgren et al.[78]	Propositi and relatives Prior VTE included	32/47 (66), 24/8	–	–
Conard et al.[79]	Propositi and relatives Prior VTE included	18/50 (36), 7/11	15/74 (20), 3/12	4/31 (13), 0/4
De Stefano et al.[80]	Propositi and relatives Prior VTE included	21/54 (39), 6/13[†]	6/48 (13), 1/5	3/22 (14), 0/3
Pabinger and Schneider[81]	Propositi and relatives Prior VTE included	21/45 (46), 18/3	9/60 (15), 6/3	19/71 (27), 4/15
Friederich et al.[82]	Relatives only No prior VTE	1/33 (3.0), 1/0	1/60 (2.0), 1/0	5/76 (7), 0/5
van Boven et al.[83]	Relatives only			
	No prior event	4/28 (14), 0/4	–	–
	Prior event	6/10 (60), 2/4	–	–

* VTE n/pregnancies n (%), antepartum VTE n/postpartum VTE n.

† The timing of two episodes of VTE was unknown.

colleagues[85] calculated odds ratios of 282 (95 percent CI 31 to 2532) for type I antithrombin deficiency, and 28 (95 percent CI 5.5 to 142) for type II deficiency.[86] Women with VTE prior to pregnancy were included in the analysis. Finally, in a case–control study involving 119 women with pregnancy-related VTE and 233 controls, Gerhardt et al. found the adjusted relative risk for AT deficiency (defined as levels <80 percent) to be 10.4 (95 percent CI 2.2 to 62.5), and did not find PC deficiency (defined as levels <75 percent) to be a statistically significant risk factor (relative risk 2.2, 95 percent CI 0.8 to 6.1).[87] It is not clear that low antithrombin or PC results were confirmed by repeat testing in the later studies, and, as many individuals with low antithrombin, PC, and PS levels in population studies will demonstrate normalization of results if follow-up testing is performed;[59,62] this effects the interpretation of their findings, since some of the 'thrombophilic' patients were probably misclassified.

FACTOR V LEIDEN

In 1993, Dahlback and colleagues noted that plasma taken from a family with a strong history of venous thrombosis was resistant to the anticoagulant effect of APC.[88] This phenotype became known as APC resistance and a point mutation in the factor V gene (G1691A), characterized by a single amino acid change (Arg[506] to Gly) at a site where activated factor V (fVa) is cleaved by APC, was identified as the cause in more than 90 percent of individuals.[89–91] The mutation results in resistance of fVa to inactivation by APC, and reduced cofactor activity of factor V in the inactivation of fVIIIa by APC.[69]

The common underlying genotype is known as FV Leiden (FVL), and has a high community prevalence with 3–7 percent of Caucasians being heterozygous for the mutation, although a lower incidence is found in other ethnic groups.[92,93] It is the most commonly identified cause of inherited thrombophilia, being present in 12–20 percent of unselected patients with VTE,[94,95] and up to 50 percent of individuals from thrombophilic families presenting with venous thrombosis.[96] The heterozygous state is a relatively low-risk thrombophilia being associated with a threefold to sevenfold increase in risk of VTE,[66,94,95,97] with one study finding greater than 90 percent of individuals remaining event free by the age of 65.[97] Unlike individuals homozygous for natural anticoagulant deficiency states, homozygosity for FVL does not result in a catastrophic thrombotic state early in life, and it is estimated that 0.1 percent of the population are FVL homozygotes.[92] The risk of VTE, however, in homozygotes for FVL is greater than that in heterozygotes,[98] with estimates of the magnitude of risk ranging from 25-fold to 80-fold that of the healthy controls.[99,100]

In an early study, 59 percent of women with a history of pregnancy-related VTE had abnormal APC resistance.[101] Subsequent case-series of similar individuals found the prevalence of heterozygosity for the FVL mutation, confirmed by genotyping, to range from 20 percent to 78 percent,[102–104] although the highest estimate comes from a study of only nine women. Estimates of the magnitude of the increase in risk of pregnancy-related VTE associated with the FVL mutation have been obtained from a number of case–control studies. Most studied age-matched women with a history of uneventful pregnancy as controls,[84,105,106] although nulliparous women were included as controls in one study,[87] and the odds ratio was calculated from the known population prevalence of the FVL mutation in another.[85] Calculated odds ratios range from 4.5 to 16.3 (Table 22.5). Given an estimated population incidence of one episode of VTE in 1000 pregnancies, this calculated risk correlates well with data from retrospective population

Table 22.5 Case–control studies examining risk of pregnancy-related venous thromboembolism (VTE) associated with the factor V Leiden and prothrombin gene mutations

Thrombophilia study	Cases (VTE in pregnancy) Carriers n/total n (%)	Controls Carriers n/total n (%)	Odds ratio (95%CI)
Factor V Leiden			
Grandone et al.[105]	10/42 (23.8)	4/213 (1.9)	16.3 (4.8 to 54.9)
Gerhardt et al.[87]	52/119 (43.7)	18/233 (7.7)	9.0 (4.7 to 17.4)
McColl et al.[85]	7/75 (9.3)	5/224 (2.2)	4.5 (2.1 to 14.5)
Martinelli et al.[84]	22/119 (18.5)	6/232 (2.6)	10.6 (5.6 to 20.4)
Yilmazer et al.[106]	7/35 (20)	0/32	–
Prothrombin gene			
Grandone et al.[105]	13/42 (31.0)	9/213 (4.2)	10.2 (4.0 to 25.9)
Gerhardt et al.[87]	20/118 (16.9)	3/226 (1.3)	10.8 (2.9 to 40.3)
McColl et al.[85]	5/55 (9.1)	5/224 (2.2)	4.4 (1.2 to 16)
Martinelli et al.[84]	7/119 (5.9)	7/232 (3.0)	2.9 (1.0 to 8.6)
Yilmazer et al.[106]	2/35 (5.7)	0/32	–

Table 22.6 Cohort studies examining venous thromboembolism (VTE) risk during pregnancy in women with the factor V Leiden (FVL) mutation

Study	Study characteristics	FVL + Women VTE n/pregnancies n (%)	Controls VTE n/pregnancies n (%)
Heterozygotes			
Middeldorp et al.[108]	Retrospective, family cohort	5/235 (2.1)	0/188 (0)
Simioni et al.[65]	Retrospective, family cohort	3/157 (1.9)	0/93 (0)
Tormene et al.[109]	Retrospective, family cohort	6/242 (2.5)	1/215 (0.46)
Lindqvist et al.[116]	Prospective, population based	3/270 (1.1)	3/2210 (0.14)
Middledorp et al.[110]	Prospective, family cohort	0/17 (0.0)	–
Simioni et al.[111]	Prospective, family cohort	2/12 (17)	0/3 (0)
Murphy et al.[112]	Prospective, population based	0/16 (0)	0/572 (0)
Homozygotes			
Lindqvist et al.[116]	Prospective, population based	0/18 (0)	3/2210 (0.14)
Middeldorp et al.[114]	Retrospective, family cohort	4/24 (17)	–
Martinelli et al.[113]	Retrospective, family cohort	3/19 (16)	1/182 (0.5)
Tormene et al.[109]	Retrospective, family cohort	1/14 (7.1)	–
Procare Group[115]	Retrospective cohort	(12)	–

or family cohort studies, with observed rates of VTE in FVL heterozygotes ranging from 1 percent to 3 percent (Table 22.6).[65,107–109] To date prospective studies have included only small numbers of pregnancies, and report incidences of between 0 percent and 17 percent.[110–112]

FACTOR V LEIDEN HOMOZYGOTES

Fewer studies have examined the risk of pregnancy-related VTE in women homozygous for the FVL mutation. In studies in which FVL homozygotes were identified either due to symptomatic relatives or a personal history of thrombosis, the incidence of pregnancy-related VTE ranges from 7 percent to 17 percent,[109,113–115] although due to the small number

of individuals the confidence intervals of these estimates are wide. Most studies excluded propositi and pregnancies that followed an initial episode of VTE. In a prospective study of 18 homozygotes, identified by population screening rather than due to a family or personal history, no episodes of VTE were documented during pregnancy or the postpartum period.[116] Based on the results of all studies, the risk of pregnancy-related VTE in FVL homozygous women with either a personal or family history of VTE, is approximately 10 percent, whereas the risk is probably lower in women identified incidentally. Pooling data from a number of studies, Martinelli and colleagues found episodes to be equally divided between the antepartum and postpartum periods, resulting in a higher daily risk in the postpartum period.[113]

THE PROTHROMBIN (G20210A) GENE MUTATION

In 1996, Poort and colleagues described a common mutation (G20210) of the prothrombin gene, which has become known as the prothrombin gene mutation (PGM).[117] Located in the 3′ untranslated region of the gene, the mutation is associated with increased mean plasma prothrombin levels due to increased efficiency of 3′ end processing of the gene resulting in accumulation of the encoded mRNA.[118] The prevalence of the mutation in Caucasian populations is approximately 2 percent,[117,119–122] and it is rare in Asian and African populations.[120] In unselected patients with venous thrombosis the mutation has been found in between 4.0 percent and 7.1 percent of individuals,[117,119,121,122] and 18 percent of individuals with a strong family history of VTE.[117] The PGM is therefore a relatively weak risk factor for VTE, being associated with a twofold to fivefold increase in risk.

Although there have been no prospective studies examining the incidence of pregnancy-related VTE in women carrying the PGM mutation, a number of case–control studies have provided estimates of the increase in risk associated with the mutation (see Table 22.5). In these studies, the calculated odds ratios for the risk of VTE in heterozygous women range from 2.9 to 10.8, with differences in selection criteria and control populations among studies likely accounting for the range in estimates.[84,87,105,106] Taking these data and the community incidence of VTE in 1 per 1000 pregnancies into account, it can be conservatively estimated that the incidence of pregnancy related VTE in PGM heterozygotes is of the magnitude of 0.5–1 percent.

FVL/PGM COMPOUND HETEROZYGOTES

Given the high community prevalence of both the FVL and PGM mutations it is not uncommon for individuals to be heterozygous for both conditions, with an expected prevalence of 1 per 1000 in Caucasian populations.[123] In a pooled analysis of case–control studies, double heterozygotes were estimated to have a 20-fold increase in risk of VTE in comparison to healthy controls.[123] Two retrospective cohort studies of double heterozygotes have reported the incidence of pregnancy-related VTE to be 4 percent and 13.5 percent in women without VTE prior to pregnancy,[113,124] whereas the estimated risk from a case–control study was 5 percent.[125] The majority of events in the cohort studies occurred post partum, making a strong case for prophylaxis during this period whereas the need for antepartum therapy is less clear.

OTHER INHERITED CONDITIONS

An association has been sought between a number of other postulated inherited thrombophilic conditions and an increased risk of VTE during pregnancy. Homozygosity for the C667T mutation in the methylenetetrahydrofolate reductase (MTHFR) gene, producing a thermolabile gene product with reduced function, is the commonest inherited cause of raised homocysteine levels.[126] C667T homozygosity is only weakly associated with an increased risk of venous thrombosis,[127] and although there are conflicting data,[105] the majority of studies have shown no association with an increase in risk of pregnancy-related VTE.[85,87,112,125,128,129] Elevated factor VIII levels have been shown to be associated with increased VTE risk,[130] and although a specific genetic defect is yet to be identified, familial clustering of raised FVIII levels suggests an underlying inherited cause.[131] In a single case–control study, FVIII levels of greater than 172 percent were associated with an increased risk of pregnancy-related VTE (odds ratio 3.2, 95 percent CI 1.1 to 9.7).[125] Small case–control studies have shown no association between the plasminogen activator inhibitor gene 4G/5G polymorphism[129] and pregnancy-related VTE. Finally, evidence supporting an increased risk of VTE in women carrying the I allele of the tissue plasminogen activator Alu I/D polymorphism has been reported,[132] although the small size of the study precludes firm conclusions.

ACQUIRED THROMBOPHILIA

The antiphospholipid antibody syndrome is defined by the combination of the presence of antiphospholipid antibodies (APLA, either a lupus anticoagulant or anticardiolipin antibody) and a characteristic clinical feature, such as venous thrombosis.[133] On screening approximately 1–5 percent of healthy control subjects will be found to have APLA,[133] whereas in the general obstetric population the prevalence has been reported to be between 1 percent and 4 percent of women,[134–136] with the majority of these being anticardiolipin antibodies. The risk of an initial thrombotic event in APLA-positive individuals, either during or outside pregnancy, is unknown, but is likely to be low. As such, prophylaxis is not recommended in this population. In contrast, the presence of APLA, in particular a positive test for a lupus anticoagulant, is associated with a high risk of recurrent VTE in patients who cease anticoagulation after an initial event, and most such patients receive long-term anticoagulation.[137] Therefore, despite a lack of data on the risk of recurrent VTE during pregnancy in the absence of prophylaxis, most such individuals receive treatment during the antepartum and postpartum periods.

Risk of pregnancy-related VTE in women with previous venous thrombosis

Individuals with a history of prior VTE have an increased risk of future episodes of venous thrombosis, when compared with individuals lacking such a history. The magnitude of the increase in risk is influenced by whether the initial episode was associated with an identifiable transient or permanent risk factor.[138] Until recently, controversy has existed with regard to the magnitude of the risk of VTE during pregnancy in women with a prior episode of VTE, with estimates from early studies ranging from 0 percent to 13 percent.[139–142] These studies, however, had methodologic limitations, including patient selection, a lack of objective diagnosis of thrombotic events, and small sample sizes. Estimates from the two small prospective trials[139,141] were lower than those derived from retrospective studies.

In an attempt to provide a more accurate estimate of risk, Brill-Edwards and colleagues performed a prospective trial enrolling 125 women with a prior single episode of VTE. All women had antepartum prophylaxis withheld and then received postpartum prophylaxis for 4–6 weeks (predominantly initial unfractionated heparin [UFH] or low-molecular-weight heparin [LMWH] followed by warfarin with a target international normalized ratio [INR] of 2.0–3.0).[143] Three women had a recurrent event antepartum (2.4 percent, 95 percent CI 0.2 to 6.9 percent), and a further three women were diagnosed with recurrent VTE postpartum. Ninety-five of the women enrolled in the study underwent thrombophilia testing. When subgroup data were analyzed, it was found that there were no recurrent events in 44 women with negative thrombophilia testing and a temporary risk factor, including pregnancy, at the time of the initial event (0 percent, 95 percent CI 0.0 to 8.0 percent). In comparison, women with abnormal thrombophilia testing and/or a prior idiopathic event had an antepartum risk of recurrent VTE of 5.9 percent (95 percent CI 1.2 to 16 percent). A subsequently published retrospective series of women with prior VTE and various thrombophilic conditions reported antepartum recurrence in 25 percent of pregnancies during which anticoagulant prophylaxis was not given.[144]

Thus, although it appears that women with prior VTE have a higher risk of recurrence during pregnancy than outside pregnancy,[145] the magnitude of the risk in women without thrombophilia and with an initial temporary risk factor does not justify routine administration of antepartum prophylaxis. The presence of other risk factors as well as underlying cardiovascular status (influencing the patients' ability to tolerate a PE) and patient preference, need to be taken into consideration in making this decision.

DIAGNOSIS OF VENOUS THROMBOEMBOLISM DURING PREGNANCY

In both pregnant and nonpregnant patients, the diagnosis of both DVT and PE is complicated by the fact that no individual symptom or sign is unique to either disorder, nor invariably found in the presence of confirmed disease.[146,147] This is reflected by the low incidence of confirmed VTE in patients in whom it is clinically suspected, with the rates of proved DVT and PE being as low as 16 percent and 10 percent, respectively, in recent studies involving nonpregnant individuals.[148–150] The prevalence of confirmed disease has been found to be even lower in two cohort studies of pregnant women; 8 percent of women having confirmed DVT in one study,[151] and 5 percent confirmed PE in another.[21] A possible explanation is that symptoms of leg swelling, chest pain and shortness of breath, not due to underlying thrombosis are more common throughout pregnancy.

Due to the difficulty in clinical diagnosis of VTE, accurate diagnostic testing is required to confirm or refute a suspected diagnosis. The gold standards for diagnosis of DVT and PE, venography, and pulmonary angiography, are both invasive and expensive. Noninvasive diagnostic strategies utilizing different diagnostic tests in combination have been validated in nonpregnant individuals, and been shown both to be safe and accurate.[152,153] To date, these diagnostic strategies, which incorporate clinical assessment, diagnostic imaging, and laboratory testing have not been validated in pregnant women. Therefore, although there are concerns with regard to the effect of alterations in venous hemodynamics and the higher rate of isolated ilio femoral vein thrombosis on the sensitivity and specificity of diagnostic tests during pregnancy, most recommendations in pregnant women are based on the results of trials involving nonpregnant patients.

Fetal risk associated with diagnostic imaging

An additional concern, when performing diagnostic tests on pregnant women, is the risk associated with the exposure of the fetus to ionizing radiation. Ginsberg and colleagues calculated the level of fetal radiation exposure likely to occur occurring during common diagnostic procedures for VTE, and then comprehensively reviewed the literature on the degree of associated risk.[154] If maximal precautions were taken, calculated fetal exposure was <0.0005 Gy (0.05 rad) for limited venography, and pulmonary angiography by the brachial route, and <0.00012 Gy (0.012 rad) with low-dose perfusion scanning. The review concluded that radiation exposure *in utero* of up to 0.05 Gy (5 rad) was associated with up to a twofold increase in risk of childhood malignancy (baseline incidence in the general community of approximately 0.1 percent up to 10 years of age), and a slight increase in minor congenital eye abnormalities. Therefore, the fetal risk associated with the above diagnostic imaging tests, with appropriate precautions such as fetal shielding, and reduction of radioisotope dose, was felt to be minimal. Against this should be balanced the risk of significant maternal and fetal morbidity or even mortality from a missed diagnosis of venous thrombosis, and the potential side effects of unnecessary anticoagulant therapy if empiric treatment is given in the absence of VTE. The study did not examine the radiation exposure associated with spiral computed tomography (CT), which has become a frequently used investigation in the diagnosis of PE, despite ongoing debate over the exact role it should play in the diagnostic workup.[152,155] A recent study, using maternal-fetal geometry and dose modeling techniques, found the mean fetal dose exposure with a modern helical CT scanner to depend on which trimester of pregnancy the scan was performed in, but to between 3.3 μGy and 130 μGy, a level lower than that related to V/Q lung scanning.[156]

D-dimer

D-dimer is a plasma protein specifically produced after lysis of cross-linked fibrin by plasmin. Levels are elevated up to eightfold above normal in the presence of acute VTE, and a normal D-dimer result has been shown to exclude DVT or PE in nonpregnant individuals.[157] D-dimer assays vary in diagnostic accuracy. Currently available tests can be divided into highly sensitive assays, with sensitivities of 95–100 percent for acute VTE, and moderately sensitive tests, with sensitivities of 80–95 percent.[153] As well as being elevated with acute VTE, plasma D-dimer levels are also raised in a number of other nonthrombotic conditions, including normal pregnancy.[158] D-dimer levels rise progressively from the second trimester of pregnancy onwards,[159–163] with higher levels seen in patients with complications of pregnancy, such as placental abruption and preeclampsia.[160,161] Therefore, although a negative result is still likely to be helpful in excluding VTE, an increased rate of false-positive results will limit the clinical utility of D-dimer testing during pregnancy. It is possible that establishment of different cutpoints specific for pregnancy may reduce this problem.[163] At present, D-dimer testing has not been validated for use in the pregnant population.

Diagnosis of deep vein thrombosis during pregnancy

Typical symptoms of DVT in nonpregnant patients include leg discomfort (often located in the calf), leg swelling, discoloration, and warmth. The same symptoms were also common in a large series of women with pregnancy-associated DVT.[27] In women diagnosed with iliofemoral DVT during pregnancy, lower abdominal and inguinal discomfort have been reported as presenting features.[30] Although, as mentioned, individual symptoms and signs lack sensitivity and specificity for diagnosing DVT,[146] prediction rules incorporating (i) the presence of symptoms and signs (ii) the presence of recognized risk factors, and (iii) the presence of an alternative likely diagnosis, have enabled nonpregnant patients to be accurately stratified as having a low, moderate or high pretest probability of disease, optimizing choice and interpretation of further diagnostic tests.[148,164] Clinical prediction rules for DVT have not as yet been validated in pregnant women, and there are theoretical reasons why their predictive accuracy may be reduced during pregnancy.[165] These include younger age with differing risk factor profile, different baseline risk during pregnancy, and failure to include the left-leg predisposition of DVT during pregnancy into the model, which is likely to improve the accuracy of pretest probability assessment.

ULTRASONOGRAPHY

Venous compression ultrasonography (CUS) has become the most frequently used first-line investigation for suspected

DVT in the nonpregnant population.[166] Within this patient group, CUS has a sensitivity of 95 percent and a specificity of 96 percent for symptomatic proximal vein thrombosis.[167] It is less accurate for the diagnosis of distal calf vein thrombosis (approximate sensitivity and specificity of 70–80 percent),[168] which accounts for approximately 20 percent of confirmed cases of DVT in symptomatic patients.[169] Isolated calf vein thrombosis, however, rarely causes PE unless there is extension of thrombus into the proximal veins. This will develop in 20–30 percent of cases, normally within the first week.[170] Knowledge of this natural history of calf vein thrombosis led to a diagnostic strategy of serial CUS of the proximal veins for suspected DVT, with CUS performed on day 1 and 7. This allows immediate detection in patients with proximal DVT, and subsequent detection of extending calf vein DVT. This strategy has been validated in management studies of nonpregnant patients,[171,172] however, there are limited published data on the accuracy and safety of CUS for diagnosis of DVT during pregnancy. Changes in venous hemodynamics resulting in increased venous distension, a higher incidence of isolated iliac vein thrombosis, and possibly altered rates of extension of calf vein thrombosis all have the potential to limit the safety of CUS during pregnancy. In a pilot study involving 53 consecutive women with suspected DVT during pregnancy, individuals with a negative initial CUS had D-dimer testing performed using the Simpli-Red D-dimer assay. Patients with a positive D-dimer result then underwent serial CUS, and patients with a negative D-dimer test had no further investigations. Fourteen women with negative serial CUS and 31 women with a negative SimpliRed D-dimer test and a single negative CUS had no evidence of VTE occurring during clinical follow-up, making it possible that the above concerns are theoretical.[173] Ongoing studies are addressing this issue.

ILIAC VEIN THROMBOSIS

As noted isolated iliac DVT is more common during pregnancy and is poorly detected by CUS. Symptoms suggestive of thrombosis limited to the pelvis include swelling of the entire leg, and prominent back or lower abdominal pain. The use of pulsed Doppler may improve the diagnosis of iliac vein thrombosis,[174] and this, along with direct visualization of the iliac vein, should be attempted if the clinical suspicion of iliac DVT exists. Impedance plethysmography has been validated as a tool to exclude DVT during pregnancy,[20] but is no longer widely available. Magnetic resonance (MR) venography, which utilizes the difference in MR signal between flowing blood and stationary clot, is emerging as a diagnostic tool for DVT, with one study reporting 100 percent sensitivity and 93 percent specificity for proximal DVT in comparison with contrast venography.[175] It has the potential advantages of detecting isolated iliac DVT and not being associated with radiation exposure, but its use is currently limited by availability and a lack of data from management trials. Due to the above limitations

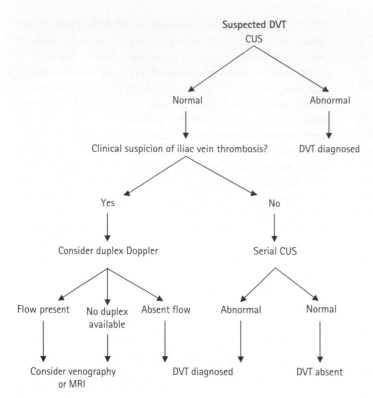

Figure 22.1   Algorithm for a clinical suspicion of DVT in pregnancy. CUS, compression ultrasonography; DVT, deep vein thrombosis; MRI, magnetic resonance imaging.

of alternative tests, venography is often the investigation of choice when iliac vein thrombosis is suspected.

PROPOSED DIAGNOSTIC ALGORITHM FOR DVT

Acknowledging the above limitations, a suggested algorithm for investigation of suspected DVT during pregnancy is shown in Figure 22.1. Women with a clinical suspicion of DVT should initially undergo CUS of the proximal leg veins. An abnormal proximal ultrasound justifies antithrombotic treatment. Women with an initial normal CUS, and in whom isolated iliac vein thrombosis is not suspected should have follow-up testing performed on days 2–3 and days 6–8. If calf vein thrombosis is strongly suspected, consideration should be given to venography or MR venography. The findings of either a very small area of noncompressibility of a proximal vein or noncompressibility of a calf vein on CUS should be considered equivocal, due to a reduced specificity of these results for DVT. To avoid unnecessary treatment and therapeutic implications for future pregnancies, limited venography is recommended to confirm the diagnosis when these findings are present on CUS.

Diagnosis of pulmonary embolism during pregnancy

As is the case in nonpregnant patients, acute onset or progressive shortness of breath, hemoptysis, or pleuritic chest pain should lead to a clinical suspicion of PE. Shortness of breath and chest pain are, however, common symptoms in pregnant women,[176] and although clinical prediction rules for stratifying pretest probability of PE have been validated in nonpregnant individuals,[149,177] neither empiric nor structured assessment of pretest probability has been evaluated in pregnant women with suspected PE. Accurate diagnostic testing is therefore mandatory in pregnant women with suspected PE, due to the inconvenience of treatment and potential catastrophic consequences of a missed diagnosis.

VENTILATION–PERFUSION LUNG SCANNING

Ventilation–perfusion lung scanning remains widely used in the diagnosis of PE in nonpregnant patients, although use of spiral CT as the primary diagnostic test is increasing.[165] A normal perfusion pattern on V/Q scanning has been shown to safely exclude a diagnosis of PE in nonpregnant individuals,[178] whereas a high probability V/Q scan, defined by the presence of a segmental or greater perfusion defect with normal ventilation, has sufficient specificity for PE to justify commencing anticoagulant therapy,[179,180] provided the pretest probability is moderate or high. The diagnostic utility of V/Q scanning is limited by the high rate of scans showing nondiagnostic perfusion defects, and as PE will be proved angiographically in approximately 25 percent of these patients, further investigation is required before treatment can be either instituted or withheld.[179,180] Pulmonary angiography, the gold standard investigation in this situation, is invasive with a procedure-related fatality rate of 0.2 percent, and expertise in performing the procedure is declining.[181] This has led to the validation of diagnostic strategies in which either normal serial bilateral leg CUS over a 2-week period (based on the common coexistence of PE and DVT),[182,183] or a low pretest probability and a negative moderately sensitive D-dimer result,[149] allow PE to be safely excluded in nonpregnant patients with a nondiagnostic V/Q scan without resorting to angiography. As patients with a low pretest probability and a high-probability lung scan will have angiographic evidence of PE in only 50 percent of cases,[180] they should also undergo further diagnostic testing as outlined below.

The performance of V/Q scanning for diagnosis of PE during pregnancy has been examined in a retrospective cohort study involving 120 women.[21] The distribution of lung scan patterns differed in comparison with nonpregnant patients, with high probability scans seen in less than 2 percent of pregnant women (compared with 10–15 percent in nonpregnant populations), nondiagnostic scans in 20 percent of pregnant women (in comparison with 50–70 percent), and normal scans present in nearly 75 percent (as opposed to 10–30 percent in nonpregnant individuals).[21,179,180] No woman with either normal or nondiagnostic scan results was reported to have venous thromboembolic events during a mean follow-up period of 26 months. In addition, no increase in the rates of congenital or developmental anomalies was observed in the 110 live offspring delivered by the women included in the study. V/Q scanning, therefore, will be normal in a large proportion of pregnant women in whom it is suspected, and although the data are retrospective, it appears that anticoagulation can be safely withheld in these women. Despite this fact, and the above theoretical and observed data suggesting no significant threat to the fetus, a significant proportion of physicians remain reluctant to perform V/Q scanning in pregnancy.[184]

COMPUTED TOMOGRAPHY

The introduction and refinement of helical (or spiral) CT has resulted in widespread use of this test as the primary diagnostic test for PE.[166] Although the presence of an intraluminal filling defect within a segmental or more proximal pulmonary artery is diagnostic of PE, current evidence does not support the use of helical CT as a standalone test, with reported sensitivity for PE ranging from 53 percent to 100 percent, and specificity from 81 percent to 100 percent. In addition, many published studies have methodological flaws, which limit the reliability of their findings.[185,186] Although three recent studies have validated the safety of withholding anticoagulants in patients with non-high pretest probability, negative helical CT, and normal bilateral CUS, pregnant women were excluded from these studies.[187–189] In the absence of either retrospective or prospective supportive data, and despite evidence that it is already commonplace,[190] it is suggested that helical CT should only be used to diagnose PE during pregnancy in the context of a clinical trial, or where alternative diagnostic tests are not available.

PROPOSED ALGORITHM FOR DIAGNOSIS OF PE

A proposed algorithm for diagnosis of PE during pregnancy, adapted from previous guidelines,[191] is presented in Figure 22.2. A careful initial clinical assessment and a chest radiograph should be done to help exclude alternative diagnoses. Although structured clinical prediction rules have not been formally validated during pregnancy, it is likely that experienced clinicians' gestalt provides a reasonable assessment pretest probability in pregnant women, as it does in nonpregnant individuals.[192] Therefore, some assessment of pretest probability should be performed which might guide diagnostic testing, and then V/Q scanning done. In women with a normal lung scan, PE can be excluded. Women with a high probability lung scan and high or intermediate pretest probability should be treated for PE. If a high probability scan occurs in combination with a low pretest probability, due to a moderate rate of proved PE in nonpregnant individuals with these findings, further investigation is suggested. In women with a nondiagnostic V/Q scan and a normal initial CUS, either serial CUS repeated on days 3–4, 6–8, and 12–14 (an approach that has been validated in nonpregnant subjects, but not pregnant women), helical CT or pulmonary angiography is recommended in the absence of good evidence. The choice between the three options will be guided by pretest probability and an open discussion should be undertaken with individual patients. Although not validated in this population, a normal D-dimer result is likely to be useful in limiting the need for further investigation by excluding PE.

TREATMENT OF VENOUS THROMBOEMBOLISM DURING PREGNANCY

In nonpregnant patients, anticoagulant therapy has proved to be effective for the prevention of initial VTE in high-risk situations,[193] the recurrence or extension of thrombus in patients with established DVT,[194] and death in patients with clinically diagnosed PE.[195] Randomized controlled trials examining the efficacy and safety of various anticoagulants for the treatment and prevention of VTE, have, as a rule, excluded pregnant women. As a result, much of the data presented below are either extrapolated from trials of nonpregnant patients, or are derived from small observational studies in pregnant women. Drugs studied for the management of VTE include UFH, LMWH and its derivative fondaparinux, the heparinoid drug danaparoid, warfarin and related drugs, and, more recently, direct thrombin inhibitors such as ximelagatran. Direct thrombin inhibitors, which cross the placenta, and fondaparinux, which has not been adequately assessed in pregnant patients and may cross the placenta in small amounts,[196] will not be discussed

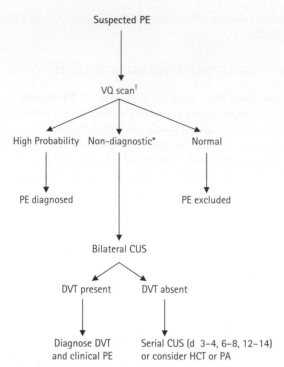

Figure 22.2 Algorithms for a clinical suspicion of PE in pregnancy.
†If hCT is used as the first line investigation for PE, in the event of a normal scan bilateral proximal CUS should also be performed before, and, if normal, PE can then be excluded. *Nondiagnostic: no high-probability or no normal result on VQ scan. CUS, compression ultrasonography; DVT, deep vein thrombosis; hCT, helical computed tomography; PA, pulmonary angiography; PE, pulmonary embolism; VQ scan, ventilation–perfusion scan.

further. For a more complete discussion with regards to pharmacology and mechanism of action see Chapter 11.

Fetal complications of anticoagulant therapy during pregnancy

Both UFH[197] and LMWH[198,199] have been shown not to cross the placenta during pregnancy. Therefore, neither agent has the ability to cause teratogenicity or fetal bleeding, although fetal compromise due to uteroplacental hemorrhage is a potential risk. Both a retrospective cohort study[200] and a comprehensive literature review[201] have reported no significant increase in risk of serious adverse fetal outcomes following maternal treatment with UFH during pregnancy. Similarly, a systematic review in 1999 reported the rate of adverse fetal outcomes in women exposed to LMWH during pregnancy, after exclusion of women with significant comorbid disease, to be the same as that in the general population.[202] This is supported by accumulating data from subsequent observational studies, and a recent systematic review in which treatment with either prophylactic or therapeutic dose LMWH during pregnancy did not appear to increase the rate of adverse fetal outcomes.[203–209]

In contrast, coumarin derivatives cross the placenta and are known to be teratogenic.[210] Warfarin exposure during the

first trimester can result in a characteristic embryopathy, with clinical features of nasal hypoplasia, stippled epiphyses, and extremity shortening.[211] In a recent systematic review, the prevalence of congenital fetal anomalies in live births was found to be 11.1 percent when warfarin exposure had occurred between weeks 6 and 12 of pregnancy, in comparison with 0 percent if it had not.[212] This suggests that the risk of embryopathy is minimal if warfarin is stopped prior to 6 weeks of gestation. Central nervous system abnormalities, although rare, have been reported with warfarin exposure in the second and third trimesters.[211] Increased rates of spontaneous miscarriage have also been reported with warfarin,[211,212] and neonatal hemorrhage may complicate warfarin exposure close to the time of delivery.[213] Due to the above safety issues, either UFH or LMWH should be used for the treatment and prevention of VTE during pregnancy wherever possible, and warfarin exposure avoided, particularly between 6 and 12 weeks of gestation and close to term.[214] None of these anticoagulants appear to be secreted in breast milk, and therefore, warfarin or heparin-related anticoagulants are safe for the breastfed baby of nursing mothers during the postpartum period.[214–216]

Maternal complications of anticoagulant therapy during pregnancy

Maternal risks of anticoagulant therapy consist of hemorrhagic and nonhemorrhagic complications. Discussion will be limited to complications associated with use of either UFH or LMWH.

HEMORRHAGIC COMPLICATIONS

In a retrospective cohort study of 100 pregnant women receiving prophylactic or therapeutic dose UFH, the reported rate of significant bleeding was 2 percent.[200] This is similar to that seen in nonpregnant patients receiving long-term adjusted dose UFH for treatment of acute VTE.[217] In a systematic review of 486 pregnancies during which LMWH was administered, no episodes of clinically important bleeding were recorded, although only 5 percent of these patients received full-dose anticoagulation.[202] No hemorrhagic complications were reported in a prospective cohort study of 33 pregnant women receiving enoxaparin for treatment of VTE,[203] whereas 11 episodes of serious bleeding occurred in 624 pregnancies during which either prophylactic or treatment dose enoxaparin was used (1.8 percent); only one episode was judged to be related to anticoagulant therapy,[208] with similar findings from a large systematic review of LMWH in pregnancy.[209] Therefore, from the limited data available, the risk of maternal bleeding during pregnancy appears to be low with LMWH and UFH therapy.[218]

NONHEMORRHAGIC COMPLICATIONS

Long-term UFH is associated with a risk of loss of bone density when administered for longer than 1 month, due to decreased rates of bone formation accompanied by increased bone resorption.[219] Significantly reduced lumbar spine bone mineral density has been reported in up to 30 percent of women receiving long-term UFH during pregnancy,[220,221] with symptomatic vertebral fracture occurring in 2.2 percent of a series of 184 women receiving heparin twice daily throughout pregnancy.[222] There is accumulating evidence that the risk of osteoporosis is minimal and much lower with LMWH than UFH therapy.[209] Monreal and colleagues found that nonpregnant patients treated with LMWH had a lower rate of fracture than those receiving UFH.[223] Another study reported identified lumbosacral fracture in 2 of 36 women treated with UFH during pregnancy, and none of 39 with LMWH.[224] Follow up at 52 weeks post delivery found lumbar spine bone mineral density to be significantly reduced in the UFH group, but did not differ from normal controls in the LMWH group.[225] Finally, in a prospective study involving 55 patients treated with low-dose LMWH throughout pregnancy, bone loss was not significantly different from the physiologic losses seen in normal pregnancy.[226] It is highly likely that bone loss associated with 'prolonged prophylactic' dose LMWH is negligible.[209]

Heparin-induced thrombocytopenia (HIT) is a rare but serious syndrome, consisting of characteristic clinical events and concurrent detection of heparin antibodies, in the setting of recent heparin therapy.[227] A fall in platelet count is usually the first clue that HIT might be present, and HIT should be suspected if the platelet count falls to less than 50 percent baseline or absolute levels of less than $100 \times 10^9/L$ within 5–15 days of commencing heparin. Extension of venous thrombosis or the development of new arterial thrombosis is a common complication.[227] Approximately 3 percent of nonpregnant patients receiving UFH will develop HIT, with the frequency varying in different clinical settings. The incidence of HIT with LMWH therapy appears to be less than that with UFH,[209,228] however accurate estimates of the frequency of HIT with the use of either agent during pregnancy are not available. Use of the heparinoid, danaparoid sodium, is recommended for treatment of HIT during pregnancy as it is an effective antithrombotic that does not cross the placenta,[229] and, unlike LMWH, has low cross-reactivity with UFH.[214]

Recommended treatment of acute venous thromboembolism during pregnancy

Based on the above safety data, either LMWH or UFH should be used for treatment of VTE during pregnancy. Evidence for the efficacy of either agent for treating VTE during pregnancy is largely extrapolated from trials in nonpregnant patients. Analysis of pooled data from such trials has found LMWH to be at least as effective and safe as UFH in the initial treatment of VTE.[218,230] Studies have also shown that long-term LMWH or UFH is comparable with warfarin for secondary prophylaxis following an episode of VTE.[217,231,232] Therefore two regimens for treatment of

acute VTE during pregnancy have been suggested in recent guidelines: (i) intravenous UFH followed by either subcutaneous LMWH or adjusted-dose UFH; and (ii) adjusted-dose subcutaneous UFH or LMWH for both initial and long-term treatment.[214]

The preferred therapeutic option in most patients with VTE during pregnancy is LMWH, due to a more predictable anticoagulant response to weight-based therapy,[57] likely lower rates of associated HIT and osteoporosis, and the inconvenience of frequent activated partial thromboplastin time (aPTT) monitoring with UFH. Although there has been debate,[233] the data discussed above support this approach as safe for both mother and fetus. Several LMWH preparations are available, and although there is insufficient data to firmly conclude equivalent efficacy and safety,[209,218] use of any of the weight-adjusted regimens shown in Table 22.7 is reasonable. Although once-daily dosing has been shown to be effective in nonpregnant patients, due to increased clearance of LMWH, twice-daily dosing is recommended in pregnant women.[214,234] The majority of women will gain weight throughout the course of pregnancy, and the associated change in volume of drug distribution may alter plasma drug levels. Pharmacokinetic studies have shown LMWH activity, as measured by an anti-Xa assay, to decrease during pregnancy if a fixed dose of LMWH is used;[235] the clinical importance of this is unclear. Nonetheless, it has been suggested that when LMWH is used, either the dose should be changed intermittently according to weight, or that regular (monthly) anti-factor Xa levels are performed, with the sample taken 4–6 hours after the morning dose, and the dose of LMWH adjusted to maintain an anti-Xa level of between 0.5 U/mL and 1.2 U/mL if a twice-daily dosing regimen is being used, or 1.0–2.0 U/mL if a once-daily regimen is adopted.[191,214] At present, there are insufficient published data to provide firm recommendations about dosing of LMWH during pregnancy.[203,236]

In women with extensive iliofemoral VTE, or with a high risk of bleeding, initial use of adjusted-dose intravenous UFH may be preferred. In nonpregnant patients, evidence suggests a minimum threshold dose of heparin is required to achieve therapeutic efficacy, with a pooled data metaanalysis supporting a starting dose of at least 30 000 U per 24 hours.[237] Although there is debate about an association between the time taken to achieve a minimum aPTT and therapeutic efficacy,[237,238] the dose of intravenous UFH is routinely adjusted to maintain the aPTT within a therapeutic range corresponding to a plasma heparin level of 0.3–0.7 IU/mL anti-Xa activity.[57] The response of the aPTT to UFH in pregnancy is attenuated, due to increased factor VIII and heparin-binding-protein levels, with higher plasma heparin levels required to obtain therapeutic aPTT levels.[239] Although this has not translated into reported rates of increased bleeding, if large doses of UFH are required to obtain 'therapeutic' aPTT results, adjustment of UFH dose according to anti-Xa heparin levels is appropriate. When subcutaneous UFH is used, either acutely or long term, a starting regimen of at least 17 500 U 12 hourly is recommended, with dose adjustment to maintain the aPTT taken 6 hours post dose at therapeutic levels.[240] The mid-interval aPTT should be used to adjust the dose of UFH every 1–2 weeks.

Management of pregnant women with an increased risk of venous thromboembolism

As previously discussed, individual women who have an increased risk of pregnancy-related VTE can be identified due either to a personal history of thrombosis, or the presence of an inherited or acquired thrombophilia. In such women the decision to use prophylactic anticoagulant therapy, either ante partum and post partum, or post partum alone, is a balance between the estimated magnitude of the risk of VTE, and the potential side effects of anticoagulant therapy including the inconvenience and anxiety associated with long-term subcutaneous injections of LMWH. The threshold for recommending postpartum prophylaxis is lower than that for antepartum therapy due to the low bleeding risk associated with the shorter length of required treatment, the increased average daily risk of VTE during the postpartum period, and the suitability of warfarin therapy for oral administration, and its safety for mother and breastfed babies. LMWH is usually the anticoagulant of choice for antepartum prophylaxis. Suggested regimens, which have been associated with low rates of thrombosis in uncontrolled trials, are shown in Table 22.7. Routine screening with CUS is not recommended. The following recommendations on prophylaxis are similar to those from recent guidelines of the American College of Chest Physicians on anticoagulation during pregnancy.[214] Postpartum prophylaxis is given for 6 weeks, and consists of either LMWH or warfarin with a target INR of 2–3.

Table 22.7 Therapeutic and prophylactic low-molecular-weight heparin regimens

Drug*	Regimen†
Therapeutic regimens	
Dalteparin	100 U/kg every 12 hours
Enoxaparin	1 mg/kg every 12 hours
Tinzaparin	175 U/kg once daily
Prophylactic regimens	
Dalteparin	5000 U once daily
Enoxaparin	40 mg once daily or 30 mg twice daily
Tinzaparin	4500 U once daily

*There are fewer published data on tinzaparin's safety and efficacy in pregnancy compared with dalteparin and enoxaparin.
†All regimens are administered by subcutaneous injection.

WOMEN WITH A PRIOR EPISODE OF VTE

As previously discussed, the thrombotic risk, and therefore, the need for prophylaxis, can be stratified by determining whether the prior episode of VTE was unprovoked or associated with a transient risk factor, and the presence or absence of an inherited thrombophilia. Based on these circumstances, the following recommendations are made:

- **Prior VTE with transient risk factor, inherited thrombophilia is absent.** Antepartum clinical surveillance, postpartum anticoagulation. Consider antepartum prophylaxis if the transient risk factor was pregnancy or estrogen-containing medication, or if additional risk factors are present (such as obesity).
- **Prior VTE unprovoked in nature and/or inherited thrombophilia is present.** In those women not receiving long-term anticoagulants, antepartum prophylaxis with LMWH followed by postpartum anticoagulation is recommended. In women with antithrombin deficiency, FVL homozygotes, FVL/PGM compound heterozygotes, or prior multiple episodes of VTE, an intermediate-dose LMWH regimen is suggested (examples of intermediate-dose LMWH regimens are dalteparin 5000 U subcutaneously 12 hourly, or enoxaparin 40 mg subcutaneously 12 hourly).
- **Prior VTE in the setting of the antiphospholipid antibody syndrome.** Most women in this category will be receiving long-term anticoagulation, and should be treated with full-dose anticoagulation.

WOMEN WITH INHERITED THROMBOPHILIA AND NO PRIOR HISTORY OF VTE

As previously discussed, women with inherited thrombophilia have an increased risk of pregnancy-related VTE, with the degree of risk dependent on the type of thrombophilia, whether the woman is heterozygous or homozygous. Inherited conditions include antithrombin, PC and PS deficiency, as well as *FVL* and *PGM* gene mutations. A history of prior adverse pregnancy outcomes also influences decision making on the use of prophylactic anticoagulation in these women. This issue is discussed further in Chapter 24.

- **Antithrombin-deficient women, FVL/PGM compound heterozygotes, FVL homozygotes.** Antepartum prophylaxis with LMWH, postpartum anticoagulation. In FVL homozygotes who lack a personal or family history of VTE, based on the absence of thrombotic episodes during pregnancy in a small series of such women,[116] postpartum prophylaxis alone may be reasonable after consideration of other individual risk factors and patient preference.
- **Heterozygous FVL, PGM, PC, and PS deficiency with no prior VTE.** Antepartum clinical surveillance, postpartum anticoagulation. This recommendation is based on the low rate of antepartum VTE without

prophylaxis in such women, resulting in the risks and inconvenience of antepartum prophylaxis outweighing the potential benefit.

MANAGEMENT OF WOMEN ON LONG-TERM ANTICOAGULANT THERAPY PRIOR TO PREGNANCY

As discussed, the risk of fetal complications appears to be minimal with warfarin exposure prior to 6 weeks' gestation. Given this fact, and as it may take some time before couples conceive, continued use of warfarin until a positive pregnancy test occurs is reasonable, provided testing is done frequently. Some women are unwilling to accept any risk, no matter how small, of embryopathy, and prefer to switch from warfarin to LMWH prior to attempting conception. Women receiving long-term anticoagulation with coumarin derivatives can therefore be reasonably offered two options:

- Frequent pregnancy tests and substitution of LMWH for warfarin as soon as pregnancy occurs.
- Replacement of warfarin with LMWH as soon as conception is attempted.

The potential limitations of either approach should be discussed openly with patients.

WOMEN POST CESAREAN SECTION

Minimal data are available about the benefits of individual interventions to prevent VTE following cesarean section. Guidelines established by the Royal College of Obstetricians and Gynaecologists, recommending low-dose UFH administration commencing preoperatively and continuing for a further 5 days post delivery, were based on expert consensus opinion.[241] At present, it is suggested that all patients wear graduated compression stockings before and after surgery, and women judged as being at 'high risk' (for example, other risk factors such as age greater than 35, obesity, or prolonged bed rest) receive LMWH or UFH.

Management of anticoagulant therapy at the time of delivery

Women who are receiving anticoagulant therapy should ideally undergo elective induction of labor, so as to minimize the risk of spontaneous delivery whilst anticoagulated, including the risk associated with neuroaxial anesthesia, and minimizing the duration of time during which anticoagulation is stopped. Extended prolongation of the aPTT has been documented with use of subcutaneous UFH in pregnancy, and it is therefore recommended that subcutaneous UFH is discontinued 24 hours prior to induction of labor. The same approach should be taken with women receiving therapeutic LMWH. In women who develop VTE within 2–4 weeks of term, the risk of recurrent VTE is high.

Therefore, therapeutic intravenous UFH can be commenced in place of LMWH and ceased 4–6 hours prior to the expected time of delivery, or a temporary inferior vena-cava filter can be inserted. As long as the delivery is uncomplicated, UFH or LMWH can usually be restarted in prophylactic doses, along with warfarin, the same evening or the day following delivery. Anticoagulation should not be restarted within 3 hours of epidural removal. Anticoagulant therapy is normally continued for at least 6 weeks following delivery, or for at least 3 months total when VTE occurs late in pregnancy.

THE POSTTHROMBOTIC SYNDROME AND PREGNANCY-RELATED DEEP VEIN THROMBOSIS

The postthrombotic syndrome (PTS) is a frequent and potentially debilitating long-term complication of DVT, characterized by chronic pain and swelling in the affected limb.[242] Depending on the criteria used for diagnosis, PTS develops in 20–50 percent of nonpregnant individuals with proximal DVT.[242] In a study of 23 women with a history of pregnancy-related DVT, 35 percent had clinical signs or symptoms of PTS and 65 percent had objective evidence of venous valvular insufficiency in the affected leg.[243] Graduated compression stockings remain the mainstay of treatment, and there is a need for new and effective treatment strategies for patients in whom stockings are ineffective.

CEREBRAL VENOUS SINUS THROMBOSIS

Cerebral venous sinus thrombosis is a potentially devastating illness, and presents with symptoms ranging from headache to loss of consciousness.[244] It is felt to be more common during pregnancy and the postpartum period,[244,245] with pregnancy-related events having a more acute presentation, but also an improved chance of successful outcome.[246] Magnetic resonance angiography is considered the gold standard for diagnosing cerebral venous sinus thrombosis. Intravenous UFH is normally used for initial treatment, followed by extended therapy with either LMWH or warfarin, with the optimal duration being unclear.[244] Local thrombolytic therapy should be considered in cases where clinical improvement is not seen with standard anticoagulants.[247] Successful outcomes, with or without prophylaxis, have been reported in pregnancies following previous cerebral venous sinus thrombosis.[248]

CONCLUSIONS AND FUTURE DIRECTIONS

Continued effort is needed in the prevention of pregnancy-related VTE. The recent discovery of novel thrombophilic conditions as risk factors for VTE during pregnancy brings with it the need for properly designed prospective trials to determine optimum management of both previously symptomatic and asymptomatic women with thrombophilia both ante partum and post partum. International collaboration is likely to be required to make such trials feasible. Continued improvement in diagnostic tools such as CT and MR venography are likely to impact on strategies used for VTE diagnosis, and new diagnostic algorithms should be adequately assessed in the pregnant population. Finally, alternative anticoagulant agents are likely to become available over the next 10 years, and, it is hoped, may be suitable for use during pregnancy.

KEY LEARNING POINTS

- Pulmonary embolism remains a leading cause of maternal mortality in developed countries.
- The incidence of pregnancy-related VTE is approximately 1 per 1000 pregnancies, 5–10-fold that of nonpregnant women of similar age, with the daily risk of VTE being higher in the postpartum rather than the antepartum period.
- Inherited thrombophilic conditions and clinical risk factors including a prior history of VTE increase the risk of VTE during pregnancy.
- The risks of diagnostic testing to mother or fetus are minimal, and objective testing should be performed in pregnant women with suspected VTE.
- Unlike warfarin, heparin derivatives can be safely used throughout pregnancy, with LMWH being the drug of choice in most women.
- The decision to use anticoagulant prophylaxis in individual women is determined by the presence or absence of an underlying thrombophilic condition, prior history of VTE and patient preference.

REFERENCES

1   White RH. The epidemiology of venous thromboembolism. *Circulation* 2003; **107**: 14–18.

2   Weindling AM. The confidential enquiry into maternal and child health (CEMACH). *Arch Dis Child* 2003; **88**: 1034–7.

3   Department of Health, Welsh Office, Scottish Home and Health Department and Department of Health and Social Services Northern Ireland. *Confidential Enquiries into Maternal Deaths in the United Kingdom 1994–1997*. London: The Stationery Office, 1998.

4   The National Institute for Clinical Excellence, Scottish Executive Health Department and Department of Health, Social Services and Public Safety: Northern Ireland. *Confidential Enquiries into Maternal Deaths in the United Kingdom 1997–1999*. London: The Stationery Office, 2001.

5   Royal College of Obstetricians and Gynaecologists. *Confidential Enquiries into Maternal and Child Health. Why Mothers Die 2000–2002.* London: RCOG Press, 2004. (Chapter 2 available at: www.cemach.org.uk/publications/WMD2000_2002/wmd-02.htm; accessed January 2005).

6   Franks AL, Atrash HK, Lawson HW, Colberg KS. Obstetrical pulmonary embolism mortality, United States, 1970–1985. *Am J Public Health* 1990; **80**: 720–2.

7   Atrash HK, Koonin LM, Lawson HW, *et al.* Maternal mortality in the United States, 1979–1986. *Obstet Gynecol* 1990; **76**: 1055–60.

8   Berg CJ, Atrash HK, Koonin LM, Tucker M. Pregnancy-related mortality in the United States, 1987–1990. *Obstet Gynecol* 1996; **88**: 161–7.

9   Chang J, Elam-Evans LD, Berg CJ, *et al.* Pregnancy-related mortality surveillance – United States, 1991–1999. *MMWR Surveill Summ* 2003; **52**: 1–8.

10 Panting-Kemp A, Geller SE, Nguyen T, *et al.* Maternal deaths in an urban perinatal network, 1992–1998. *Am J Obstet Gynecol* 2000; **183**: 1207–12.

11 Greer IA. Thrombosis in pregnancy: maternal and fetal issues. *Lancet* 1999; **353**: 1258–65.

12 Friend JR, Kakkar VV. The diagnosis of deep vein thrombosis in the puerperium. *J Obstet Gynaecol Br Commonw* 1970; **77**: 820–3.

13 Macklon NS, Barry J, Greer IA. Duplex ultrasound screening for deep venous thrombosis in the puerperium. *Br J Obstet Gynaecol* 1995; **102**: 255–6.

14 Anderson FA, Jr, Wheeler HB, Goldberg RJ, *et al.* A population-based perspective of the hospital incidence and case-fatality rates of deep vein thrombosis and pulmonary embolism. The Worcester DVT Study. *Arch Intern Med* 1991; **151**: 933–8.

15 Nordstrom M, Lindblad B, Bergqvist D, Kjellstrom T. A prospective study of the incidence of deep-vein thrombosis within a defined urban population. *J Intern Med* 1992; **232**: 155–60.

16 Samuelsson E, Hagg S. Incidence of venous thromboembolism in young Swedish women and possibly preventable cases among combined oral contraceptive users. *Acta Obstet Gynecol Scand* 2004; **83**: 674–81.

17 Aaro LA, Johnson TR, Juergens JL. Acute deep venous thrombosis associated with pregnancy. *Obstet Gynecol* 1966; **28**: 553–8.

18 Solomons E. Puerperal thrombophlebitis: prevention and treatment. *Postgrad Med* 1963; **34**: 105–11.

19 Treffers PE, Huidekoper BL, Weenink GH, Kloosterman GJ. Epidemiological observations of thrombo-embolic disease during pregnancy and in the puerperium, in 56,022 women. *Int J Gynaecol Obstet* 1983; **21**: 327–31.

20 Hull RD, Raskob GE, Carter CJ. Serial impedance plethysmography in pregnant patients with clinically suspected deep-vein thrombosis. Clinical validity of negative findings. *Ann Intern Med* 1990; **112**: 663–7.

21 Chan WS, Ray JG, Murray S, *et al.* Suspected pulmonary embolism in pregnancy: clinical presentation, results of

lung scanning, and subsequent maternal and pediatric outcomes. *Arch Intern Med* 2002; **162**: 1170–5.

22 Macklon NS, Greer IA. Venous thromboembolic disease in obstetrics and gynaecology: the Scottish experience. *Scott Med J* 1996; **41**: 83–6.

23 Lindqvist P, Dahlback B, Marsal K. Thrombotic risk during pregnancy: a population study. *Obstet Gynecol* 1999; **94**: 595–9.

24 Andersen BS, Steffensen FH, Sorensen HT, *et al.* The cumulative incidence of venous thromboembolism during pregnancy and puerperium – an 11 year Danish population-based study of 63,300 pregnancies. *Acta Obstet Gynecol Scand* 1998; **77**: 170–3.

25 Kierkegaard A. Incidence and diagnosis of deep vein thrombosis associated with pregnancy. *Acta Obstet Gynecol Scand* 1983; **62**: 239–43.

26 McColl MD, Ramsay JE, Tait RC, *et al.* Risk factors for pregnancy associated venous thromboembolism. *Thromb Haemost* 1997; **78**: 1183–8.

27 Gherman RB, Goodwin TM, Leung B, *et al.* Incidence, clinical characteristics, and timing of objectively diagnosed venous thromboembolism during pregnancy. *Obstet Gynecol* 1999; **94**: 730–4.

28 Simpson EL, Lawrenson RA, Nightingale AL, Farmer RD. Venous thromboembolism in pregnancy and the puerperium: incidence and additional risk factors from a London perinatal database. *Br J Obstet Gynaecol* 2001; **108**: 56–60.

29 Polak JF, Wilkinson DL. Ultrasonographic diagnosis of symptomatic deep venous thrombosis in pregnancy. *Am J Obstet Gynecol* 1991; **165**: 625–9.

30 Bergqvist A, Bergqvist D, Hallbook T. Deep vein thrombosis during pregnancy. A prospective study. *Acta Obstet Gynecol Scand* 1983; **62**: 443–8.

31 Huisman MV, Buller HR, ten Cate JW, *et al.* Unexpected high prevalence of silent pulmonary embolism in patients with deep venous thrombosis. *Chest* 1989; **95**: 498–502.

32 Ray JG, Chan WS. Deep vein thrombosis during pregnancy and the puerperium: a meta-analysis of the period of risk and the leg of presentation. *Obstet Gynecol Surv* 1999; **54**: 265–71.

33 Cogo A, Lensing AW, Prandoni P, Hirsh J. Distribution of thrombosis in patients with symptomatic deep vein thrombosis. Implications for simplifying the diagnostic process with compression ultrasound. *Arch Intern Med* 1993; **153**: 2777–80.

34 Kearon C. Natural history of venous thromboembolism. *Circulation* 2003; **107**: 122–30.

35 Ouriel K, Green RM, Greenberg RK, Clair DG. The anatomy of deep venous thrombosis of the lower extremity. *J Vasc Surg* 2000; **31**: 895–900.

36 Ginsberg JS, Brill-Edwards P, Burrows RF, *et al.* Venous thrombosis during pregnancy: leg and trimester of presentation. *Thromb Haemost* 1992; **67**: 519–20.

37 May R, Thurner J. The cause of the predominantly sinistral occurrence of thrombosis of the pelvic veins. *Angiology* 1957; **8**: 419–27.

38 Cockett FB, Thomas ML, Negus D. Iliac vein compression. Its relation to iliofemoral thrombosis and the post-thrombotic syndrome. *Br Med J* 1967; **ii**: 14–9.

39 Chung JW, Yoon CJ, Jung SI, *et al.* Acute iliofemoral deep vein thrombosis: evaluation of underlying anatomic abnormalities by spiral CT venography. *J Vasc Interv Radiol* 2004; **15**: 249–56.

40 Macklon NS, Greer IA, Bowman AW. An ultrasound study of gestational and postural changes in the deep venous system of the leg in pregnancy. *Br J Obstet Gynaecol* 1997; **104**: 191–7.

41 Macklon NS, Greer IA. The deep venous system in the puerperium: an ultrasound study. *Br J Obstet Gynaecol* 1997; **104**: 198–200.

42 Bergqvist A, Bergqvist D, Hedner U. Oral contraceptives and venous thromboembolism. *Br J Obstet Gynaecol* 1982; **89**: 381–6.

43 Stein PD, Hull RD, Kayali F, *et al.* Venous thromboembolism in pregnancy: 21-year trends. *Am J Med* 2004; **117**: 121–5.

44 Danilenko-Dixon DR, Heit JA, Silverstein MD, *et al.* Risk factors for deep vein thrombosis and pulmonary embolism during pregnancy or post partum: a population-based, case-control study. *Am J Obstet Gynecol* 2001; **184**: 104–10.

45 Rosendaal FR. Venous thrombosis: a multicausal disease. *Lancet* 1999; **353**: 1167–73.

46 Stewart GJ, Lachman JW, Alburger PD, *et al.* Venodilation and development of deep vein thrombosis in total hip and knee replacement patients. *Thromb Haemost* 1987; **58**: 242–5.

47 Wright HP, Osborn SB, Edmonds DG. Changes in the rate of flow of venous blood in the leg during pregnancy, measured with radioactive sodium. *Surg Gynecol Obstet* 1950; **90**: 481–5.

48 Goodrich SM, Wood JE. Peripheral venous distensibility and velocity of venous blood flow during pregnancy or during oral contraceptive therapy. *Am J Obstet Gynecol* 1964; **90**: 740–4.

49 Skudder PA, Jr, Farrington DT, Weld E, Putman C. Venous dysfunction of late pregnancy persists after delivery. *J Cardiovasc Surg (Torino)* 1990; **31**: 748–52.

50 Clarke-Pearson DL, Jelovsek FR. Alterations of occlusive cuff impedance plethysmography results in the obstetric patient. *Surgery* 1981; **89**: 594–8.

51 Ikard RW, Ueland K, Folse R. Lower limb venous dynamics in pregnant women. *Surg Gynecol Obstet* 1971; **132**: 483–8.

52 Sandstrom B. Plethysmographic studies of venous volume in the lower legs during normal primipregnancy. *Acta Obstet Gynecol Scand* 1974; **53**: 97–101.

53 Kerr MG, Scott DB, Samuel E. Studies of the inferior vena cava in late pregnancy. *Br Med J* 1964; **Feb 29**: 532–3.

54 McCausland AM, Hyman C, Winsor T, Trotter AD, Jr. Venous distensibility during pregnancy. *Am J Obstet Gynecol* 1961; **81**: 472–9.

◆ 55 Lane DA, Mannucci PM, Bauer KA, *et al.* Inherited thrombophilia: Part 1. *Thromb Haemost* 1996; **76**: 651–62.

56 Bayston TA, Lane DA. Antithrombin: molecular basis of deficiency. *Thromb Haemost* 1997; **78**: 339–43.

◆ 57 Hirsh J, Raschke R. Heparin and low-molecular-weight heparin: the Seventh ACCP Conference on Antithrombotic and Thrombolytic Therapy. *Chest* 2004; **126**: 188S–203S.

58 Egeberg O. Inherited antithrombin deficiency causing thrombophilia. *Thromb Diath Haemorrh* 1965; **13**: 516–30.

59 Tait RC, Walker ID, Perry DJ, *et al.* Prevalence of antithrombin deficiency in the healthy population. *Br J Haematol* 1994; **87**: 106–12.

60 Wells PS, Blajchman MA, Henderson P, *et al.* Prevalence of antithrombin deficiency in healthy blood donors: a cross-sectional study. *Am J Hematol* 1994; **45**: 321–4.

61 Heijboer H, Brandjes DP, Buller HR, *et al.* Deficiencies of coagulation-inhibiting and fibrinolytic proteins in outpatients with deep-vein thrombosis. *N Engl J Med* 1990; **323**: 1512–16.

62 Koster T, Rosendaal FR, Briet E, *et al.* Protein C deficiency in a controlled series of unselected outpatients: an infrequent but clear risk factor for venous thrombosis (Leiden Thrombophilia Study). *Blood* 1995; **85**: 2756–61.

63 Baglin T, Luddington R, Brown K, Baglin C. Incidence of recurrent venous thromboembolism in relation to clinical and thrombophilic risk factors: prospective cohort study. *Lancet* 2003; **362**: 523–6.

64 Mateo J, Oliver A, Borrell M, *et al.* Laboratory evaluation and clinical characteristics of 2,132 consecutive unselected patients with venous thromboembolism – results of the Spanish Multicentric Study on Thrombophilia (EMET-Study). *Thromb Haemost* 1997; **77**: 444–51.

65 Simioni P, Sanson BJ, Prandoni P, *et al.* Incidence of venous thromboembolism in families with inherited thrombophilia. *Thromb Haemost* 1999; **81**: 198–202.

66 Vossen CY, Conard J, Fontcuberta J, *et al.* Familial thrombophilia and lifetime risk of venous thrombosis. *J Thromb Haemost* 2004; **2**: 1526–32.

● 67 Martinelli I, Mannucci PM, De Stefano V, *et al.* Different risks of thrombosis in four coagulation defects associated with inherited thrombophilia: a study of 150 families. *Blood* 1998; **92**: 2353–8.

68 Esmon CT. The protein C pathway. *Chest* 2003; **124**: 26S–32S.

69 Mann KG, Kalafatis M. Factor V: a combination of Dr Jekyll and Mr Hyde. *Blood* 2003; **101**: 20–30.

70 Heeb MJ, Mesters RM, Tans G, *et al.* Binding of protein S to factor Va associated with inhibition of prothrombinase that is independent of activated protein C. *J Biol Chem* 1993; **268**: 2872–7.

71 Griffin JH, Evatt B, Zimmerman TS, *et al.* Deficiency of protein C in congenital thrombotic disease. *J Clin Invest* 1981; **68**: 1370–3.

72 Comp PC, Esmon CT. Recurrent venous thromboembolism in patients with a partial deficiency of protein S. *N Engl J Med* 1984; **311**: 1525–8.

73 Reitsma PH, Bernardi F, Doig RG, *et al.* Protein C deficiency: a database of mutations, 1995 update. On behalf of the Subcommittee on Plasma Coagulation Inhibitors of the Scientific and Standardization Committee of the ISTH. *Thromb Haemost* 1995; **73**: 876–89.

74 Tait RC, Walker ID, Reitsma PH, *et al.* Prevalence of protein C deficiency in the healthy population. *Thromb Haemost* 1995; **73**: 87–93.

75 Miletich J, Sherman L, Broze G, Jr. Absence of thrombosis in subjects with heterozygous protein C deficiency. *N Engl J Med* 1987; **317**: 991–6.

76 Bovill EG, Bauer KA, Dickerman JD, *et al.* The clinical spectrum of heterozygous protein C deficiency in a large New England kindred. *Blood* 1989; **73**: 712–17.

77 Allaart CF, Poort SR, Rosendaal FR, *et al.* Increased risk of venous thrombosis in carriers of hereditary protein C deficiency defect. *Lancet* 1993; **341**: 134–8.

78 Hellgren M, Tengborn L, Abildgaard U. Pregnancy in women with congenital antithrombin III deficiency: experience of treatment with heparin and antithrombin. *Gynecol Obstet Invest* 1982; **14**: 127–41.

79 Conard J, Horellou MH, Van Dreden P, *et al.* Thrombosis and pregnancy in congenital deficiencies in AT III, protein C or protein S: study of 78 women. *Thromb Haemost* 1990; **63**: 319–20.

80 De Stefano V, Leone G, Mastrangelo S, *et al.* Thrombosis during pregnancy and surgery in patients with congenital deficiency of antithrombin III, protein C, protein S. *Thromb Haemost* 1994; **71**: 799–800.

81 Pabinger I, Schneider B. Thrombotic risk in hereditary antithrombin III, protein C, or protein S deficiency. A cooperative, retrospective study. Gesellschaft fur Thrombose- und Hamostaseforschung (GTH) Study Group on Natural Inhibitors. *Arterioscler Thromb Vasc Biol* 1996; **16**: 742–8.

● 82 Friederich PW, Sanson BJ, Simioni P, *et al.* Frequency of pregnancy-related venous thromboembolism in anticoagulant factor-deficient women: implications for prophylaxis. *Ann Intern Med* 1996; **125**: 955–60.

83 van Boven HH, Vandenbroucke JP, Briet E, Rosendaal FR. Gene–gene and gene–environment interactions determine risk of thrombosis in families with inherited antithrombin deficiency. *Blood* 1999; **94**: 2590–4.

● 84 Martinelli I, De Stefano V, Taioli E, *et al.* Inherited thrombophilia and first venous thromboembolism during pregnancy and puerperium. *Thromb Haemost* 2002; **87**: 791–5.

85 McColl MD, Ellison J, Reid F, *et al.* Prothrombin 20210 G→A, MTHFR C677T mutations in women with venous thromboembolism associated with pregnancy. *Br J Obstet Gynaecol* 2000; **107**: 565–9.

86 Greer IA. Inherited thrombophilia and venous thromboembolism. *Best Pract Res Clin Obstet Gynaecol* 2003; **17**: 413–25.

87 Gerhardt A, Scharf RE, Beckmann MW, *et al*. Prothrombin and factor V mutations in women with a history of thrombosis during pregnancy and the puerperium. *N Engl J Med* 2000; **342**: 374–80.

88 Dahlback B, Carlsson M, Svensson PJ. Familial thrombophilia due to a previously unrecognized mechanism characterized by poor anticoagulant response to activated protein C: prediction of a cofactor to activated protein C. *Proc Natl Acad Sci U S A* 1993; **90**: 1004–8.

89 Bertina RM, Koeleman BP, Koster T, *et al*. Mutation in blood coagulation factor V associated with resistance to activated protein C. *Nature* 1994; **369**: 64–7.

90 Greengard JS, Sun X, Xu X, *et al*. Activated protein C resistance caused by Arg506Gln mutation in factor Va. *Lancet* 1994; **343**: 1361–2.

91 Voorberg J, Roelse J, Koopman R, *et al*. Association of idiopathic venous thromboembolism with single point-mutation at Arg506 of factor V. *Lancet* 1994; **343**: 1535–6.

92 Ridker PM, Miletich JP, Hennekens CH, Buring JE. Ethnic distribution of factor V Leiden in 4047 men and women. Implications for venous thromboembolism screening. *JAMA* 1997; **277**: 1305–7.

93 Press RD, Bauer KA, Kujovich JL, Heit JA. Clinical utility of factor V Leiden (R506Q) testing for the diagnosis and management of thromboembolic disorders. *Arch Pathol Lab Med* 2002; **126**: 1304–18.

94 Koster T, Rosendaal FR, de Ronde H, *et al*. Venous thrombosis due to poor anticoagulant response to activated protein C: Leiden Thrombophilia Study. *Lancet* 1993; **342**: 1503–6.

95 Ridker PM, Hennekens CH, Lindpaintner K, *et al*. Mutation in the gene coding for coagulation factor V and the risk of myocardial infarction, stroke, and venous thrombosis in apparently healthy men. *N Engl J Med* 1995; **332**: 912–17.

96 Griffin JH, Evatt B, Wideman C, Fernandez JA. Anticoagulant protein C pathway defective in majority of thrombophilic patients. *Blood* 1993; **82**: 1989–93.

97 Rodeghiero F, Tosetto A. Activated protein C resistance and factor V Leiden mutation are independent risk factors for venous thromboembolism. *Ann Intern Med* 1999; **130**: 643–50.

98 The Procare Group. Comparison of thrombotic risk between 85 homozygotes and 481 heterozygotes carriers of the factor V Leiden mutation: retrospective analysis from the Procare Study. *Blood Coagul Fibrinolysis* 2000; **11**: 511–18.

99 Rosendaal FR, Koster T, Vandenbroucke JP, Reitsma PH. High risk of thrombosis in patients homozygous for factor V Leiden (activated protein C resistance). *Blood* 1995; **85**: 1504–8.

100 Folsom AR, Cushman M, Tsai MY, *et al*. A prospective study of venous thromboembolism in relation to factor V Leiden and related factors. *Blood* 2002; **99**: 2720–5.

101 Hellgren M, Svensson PJ, Dahlback B. Resistance to activated protein C as a basis for venous thromboembolism associated with pregnancy and oral contraceptives. *Am J Obstet Gynecol* 1995; **173**: 210–13.

102 Hirsch DR, Mikkola KM, Marks PW, *et al*. Pulmonary embolism and deep venous thrombosis during pregnancy or oral contraceptive use: prevalence of factor V Leiden. *Am Heart J* 1996; **131**: 1145–8.

103 Bokarewa MI, Bremme K, Blomback M. Arg506-Gln mutation in factor V and risk of thrombosis during pregnancy. *Br J Haematol* 1996; **92**: 473–8.

104 Hallak M, Senderowicz J, Cassel A, *et al*. Activated protein C resistance (factor V Leiden) associated with thrombosis in pregnancy. *Am J Obstet Gynecol* 1997; **176**: 889–93.

105 Grandone E, Margaglione M, Colaizzo D, *et al*. Genetic susceptibility to pregnancy-related venous thromboembolism: roles of factor V Leiden, prothrombin G20210A, and methylenetetrahydrofolate reductase C677T mutations. *Am J Obstet Gynecol* 1998; **179**: 1324–8.

106 Yilmazer M, Kurtay G, Sonmezer M, Akar N. Factor V Leiden and prothrombin 20210 G-A mutations in controls and in patients with thromboembolic events during pregnancy or the puerperium. *Arch Gynecol Obstet* 2003; **268**: 304–8.

107 Lensen RP, Bertina RM, de Ronde H, *et al*. Venous thrombotic risk in family members of unselected individuals with factor V Leiden. *Thromb Haemost* 2000; **83**: 817–21.

108 Middeldorp S, Henkens CM, Koopman MM, *et al*. The incidence of venous thromboembolism in family members of patients with factor V Leiden mutation and venous thrombosis. *Ann Intern Med* 1998; **128**: 15–20.

109 Tormene D, Simioni P, Prandoni P, *et al*. Factor V Leiden mutation and the risk of venous thromboembolism in pregnant women. *Haematologica* 2001; **86**: 1305–9.

110 Middeldorp S, Meinardi JR, Koopman MM, *et al*. A prospective study of asymptomatic carriers of the factor V Leiden mutation to determine the incidence of venous thromboembolism. *Ann Intern Med* 2001; **135**: 322–7.

111 Simioni P, Tormene D, Prandoni P, *et al*. Incidence of venous thromboembolism in asymptomatic family members who are carriers of factor V Leiden: a prospective cohort study. *Blood* 2002; **99**: 1938–42.

112 Murphy RP, Donoghue C, Nallen RJ, *et al*. Prospective evaluation of the risk conferred by factor V Leiden and thermolabile methylenetetrahydrofolate reductase polymorphisms in pregnancy. *Arterioscler Thromb Vasc Biol* 2000; **20**: 266–70.

113 Martinelli I, Legnani C, Bucciarelli P, *et al*. Risk of pregnancy-related venous thrombosis in carriers of

severe inherited thrombophilia. *Thromb Haemost* 2001; **86**: 800–3.

● 114 Middeldorp S, Libourel EJ, Hamulyak K, *et al.* The risk of pregnancy-related venous thromboembolism in women who are homozygous for factor V Leiden. *Br J Haematol* 2001; **113**: 553–5.

115 The Procare Group. Risk of venous thromboembolism during pregnancy in homozygous carriers of the factor V Leiden mutation: are there any predictive factors? *J Thromb Haemost* 2004; **2**: 359–60.

● 116 Lindqvist PG, Svensson PJ, Marsaal K, *et al.* Activated protein C resistance (FV:Q506) and pregnancy. *Thromb Haemost* 1999; **81**: 532–7.

● 117 Poort SR, Rosendaal FR, Reitsma PH, Bertina RM. A common genetic variation in the 3′-untranslated region of the prothrombin gene is associated with elevated plasma prothrombin levels and an increase in venous thrombosis. *Blood* 1996; **88**: 3698–703.

118 Gehring NH, Frede U, Neu-Yilik G, *et al.* Increased efficiency of mRNA 3′ end formation: a new genetic mechanism contributing to hereditary thrombophilia. *Nat Genet* 2001; **28**: 389–92.

119 Cumming AM, Keeney S, Salden A, *et al.* The prothrombin gene G20210A variant: prevalence in a U.K. anticoagulant clinic population. *Br J Haematol* 1997; **98**: 353–5.

120 Rosendaal FR, Doggen CJ, Zivelin A, *et al.* Geographic distribution of the 20210 G to A prothrombin variant. *Thromb Haemost* 1998; **79**: 706–8.

121 Brown K, Luddington R, Williamson D, *et al.* Risk of venous thromboembolism associated with a G to A transition at position 20210 in the 3′-untranslated region of the prothrombin gene. *Br J Haematol* 1997; **98**: 907–9.

122 Hillarp A, Zoller B, Svensson PJ, Dahlback B. The 20210 A allele of the prothrombin gene is a common risk factor among Swedish outpatients with verified deep venous thrombosis. *Thromb Haemost* 1997; **78**: 990–2.

123 Emmerich J, Rosendaal FR, Cattaneo M, *et al.* Combined effect of factor V Leiden and prothrombin 20210A on the risk of venous thromboembolism – pooled analysis of 8 case-control studies including 2310 cases and 3204 controls. Study Group for Pooled-Analysis in Venous Thromboembolism. *Thromb Haemost* 2001; **86**: 809–16.

124 Samama MM, Rached RA, Horellou MH, *et al.* Pregnancy-associated venous thromboembolism (VTE) in combined heterozygous factor V Leiden (FVL) and prothrombin (FII) 20210 A mutation and in heterozygous FII single gene mutation alone. *Br J Haematol* 2003; **123**: 327–34.

125 Gerhardt A, Scharf RE, Zotz RB. Effect of hemostatic risk factors on the individual probability of thrombosis during pregnancy and the puerperium. *Thromb Haemost* 2003; **90**: 77–85.

126 Verhoef P, Kok FJ, Kluijtmans LA, *et al.* The 677C→T mutation in the methylenetetrahydrofolate reductase gene: associations with plasma total homocysteine levels and risk of coronary atherosclerotic disease. *Atherosclerosis* 1997; **132**: 105–13.

127 Ray JG, Shmorgun D, Chan WS. Common C677T polymorphism of the methylenetetrahydrofolate reductase gene and the risk of venous thromboembolism: meta-analysis of 31 studies. *Pathophysiol Haemost Thromb* 2002; **32**: 51–8.

128 Ogunyemi D, Ku W, Arkel Y. The association between inherited thrombophilia, antiphospholipid antibodies and lipoprotein A levels with obstetrical complications in pregnancy. *J Thromb Thrombolysis* 2002; **14**: 157–62.

129 Meglic L, Stegnar M, Milanez T, *et al.* Factor V Leiden, prothrombin 20210G→A, methylenetetrahydrofolate reductase 677C→T and plasminogen activator inhibitor 4G/5G polymorphism in women with pregnancy-related venous thromboembolism. *Eur J Obstet Gynecol Reprod Biol* 2003; **111**: 157–63.

130 Kraaijenhagen RA, in't Anker PS, Koopman MM, *et al.* High plasma concentration of factor VIIIc is a major risk factor for venous thromboembolism. *Thromb Haemost* 2000; **83**: 5–9.

131 Schambeck CM, Hinney K, Haubitz I, *et al.* Familial clustering of high factor VIII levels in patients with venous thromboembolism. *Arterioscler Thromb Vasc Biol* 2001; **21**: 289–92.

132 Hooper WC, El-Jamil M, Dilley A, *et al.* The relationship between the tissue plasminogen activator Alu I/D polymorphism and venous thromboembolism during pregnancy. *Thromb Res* 2001; **102**: 33–7.

133 Levine JS, Branch DW, Rauch J. The antiphospholipid syndrome. *N Engl J Med* 2002; **346**: 752–63.

134 Lockwood CJ, Romero R, Feinberg RF, *et al.* The prevalence and biologic significance of lupus anticoagulant and anticardiolipin antibodies in a general obstetric population. *Am J Obstet Gynecol* 1989; **161**: 369–73.

135 Perez MC, Wilson WA, Brown HL, Scopelitis E. Anticardiolipin antibodies in unselected pregnant women. Relationship to fetal outcome. *J Perinatol* 1991; **11**: 33–6.

136 Harris EN, Spinnato JA. Should anticardiolipin tests be performed in otherwise healthy pregnant women? *Am J Obstet Gynecol* 1991; **165**: 1272–7.

137 Crowther MA. Anticoagulant therapy for the thrombotic complications of the antiphospholipid antibody syndrome. *Thromb Res* 2004; **114**: 443–6.

138 Kearon C. Long-term management of patients after venous thromboembolism. *Circulation* 2004; **110**: 110–18.

139 de Swiet M, Floyd E, Letsky E. Low risk of recurrent thromboembolism in pregnancy. *Br J Hosp Med* 1987; **38**: 264.

140 Badaracco MA, Vessey MP. Recurrence of venous thromboembolic disease and use of oral contraceptives. *Br Med J* 1974; **1**: 215–17.

141   Howell R, Fidler J, Letsky E, de Swiet M. The risks of antenatal subcutaneous heparin prophylaxis: a controlled trial. *Br J Obstet Gynaecol* 1983; **90**: 1124–8.

142   Tengborn L, Bergqvist D, Matzsch T, *et al.* Recurrent thromboembolism in pregnancy and puerperium. Is there a need for thromboprophylaxis? *Am J Obstet Gynecol* 1989; **160**: 90–4.

143   Brill-Edwards P, Ginsberg JS, Gent M, *et al.* Safety of withholding heparin in pregnant women with a history of venous thromboembolism. Recurrence of Clot in This Pregnancy Study Group. *N Engl J Med* 2000; **343**: 1439–44.

144   Simioni P, Tormene D, Prandoni P, Girolami A. Pregnancy-related recurrent events in thrombophilic women with previous venous thromboembolism. *Thromb Haemost* 2001; **86**: 929.

145   Pabinger I, Grafenhofer H, Kyrle PA, *et al.* Temporary increase in the risk for recurrence during pregnancy in women with a history of venous thromboembolism. *Blood* 2002; **100**: 1060–2.

146   McLachlin J, Richards T, Paterson JC. An evaluation of clinical signs in the diagnosis of venous thrombosis. *Arch Surg* 1962; **85**: 738–44.

147   Bell WR, Simon TL, DeMets DL. The clinical features of submassive and massive pulmonary emboli. *Am J Med* 1977; **62**: 355–60.

148   Wells PS, Anderson DR, Bormanis J, *et al.* Value of assessment of pretest probability of deep-vein thrombosis in clinical management. *Lancet* 1997; **350**: 1795–8.

149   Wells PS, Anderson DR, Rodger M, *et al.* Excluding pulmonary embolism at the bedside without diagnostic imaging: management of patients with suspected pulmonary embolism presenting to the emergency department by using a simple clinical model and D-dimer. *Ann Intern Med* 2001; **135**: 98–107.

150   Wells PS, Anderson DR, Rodger M, *et al.* Evaluation of D-dimer in the diagnosis of suspected deep-vein thrombosis. *N Engl J Med* 2003; **349**: 1227–35.

151   Hull RD, Hirsh J, Carter CJ, *et al.* Diagnostic efficacy of impedance plethysmography for clinically suspected deep-vein thrombosis. A randomized trial. *Ann Intern Med* 1985; **102**: 21–8.

152   Kearon C. Diagnosis of pulmonary embolism. *CMAJ* 2003; **168**: 183–94.

153   McRae SJ, Ginsberg JS. The diagnostic evaluation of deep vein thrombosis. *Am Heart Hosp J* 2004; **2**: 205–10.

154   Ginsberg JS, Hirsh J, Rainbow AJ, Coates G. Risks to the fetus of radiological procedures used in the diagnosis of maternal venous thromboembolic disease. *Thromb Haemost* 1989; **61**(2): 189–96.

155   Kearon C. Excluding pulmonary embolism with helical (spiral) computed tomography: Evidence is catching up with enthusiasm. *CMAJ* 2003; **168**: 1430–1.

156   Winer-Muram HT, Boone JM, Brown HL, *et al.* Pulmonary embolism in pregnant patients: fetal radiation dose with helical CT. *Radiology* 2002; **224**: 487–92.

157   Kelly J, Rudd A, Lewis RR, Hunt BJ. Plasma D-dimers in the diagnosis of venous thromboembolism. *Arch Intern Med* 2002; **162**: 747–56.

158   Becker DM, Philbrick JT, Bachhuber TL, Humphries JE. D-dimer testing and acute venous thromboembolism. A shortcut to accurate diagnosis? *Arch Intern Med* 1996; **156**: 939–46.

159   Bremme K, Ostlund E, Almqvist I, *et al.* Enhanced thrombin generation and fibrinolytic activity in normal pregnancy and the puerperium. *Obstet Gynecol* 1992; **80**: 132–7.

160   Nolan TE, Smith RP, Devoe LD. Maternal plasma D-dimer levels in normal and complicated pregnancies. *Obstet Gynecol* 1993; **81**: 235–8.

161   Ballegeer V, Mombaerts P, Declerck PJ, *et al.* Fibrinolytic response to venous occlusion and fibrin fragment D-dimer levels in normal and complicated pregnancy. *Thromb Haemost* 1987; **58**: 1030–2.

162   Francalanci I, Comeglio P, Alessandrello Liotta A, *et al.* D-dimer plasma levels during normal pregnancy measured by specific ELISA. *Int J Clin Lab Res* 1997; **27**: 65–7.

163   Morse M. Establishing a normal range for D-dimer levels through pregnancy to aid in the diagnosis of pulmonary embolism and deep vein thrombosis. *J Thromb Haemost* 2004; **2**: 1202–4.

164   Wells PS, Hirsh J, Anderson DR, *et al.* Accuracy of clinical assessment of deep-vein thrombosis. *Lancet* 1995; **345**: 1326–30.

165   Chan WS, Ginsberg JS. Diagnosis of deep vein thrombosis and pulmonary embolism in pregnancy. *Thromb Res* 2002; **107**: 85–91.

166   Stein PD, Hull RD, Ghali WA, *et al.* Tracking the uptake of evidence: two decades of hospital practice trends for diagnosing deep vein thrombosis and pulmonary embolism. *Arch Intern Med* 2003; **163**: 1213–19.

167   Kearon C, Ginsberg JS, Hirsh J. The role of venous ultrasonography in the diagnosis of suspected deep venous thrombosis and pulmonary embolism. *Ann Intern Med* 1998; **129**: 1044–9.

168   Kearon C, Julian JA, Newman TE, Ginsberg JS. Noninvasive diagnosis of deep venous thrombosis. McMaster Diagnostic Imaging Practice Guidelines Initiative. *Ann Intern Med* 1998; **128**: 663–77.

169   Heijboer H, Buller HR, Lensing AW, *et al.* A comparison of real-time compression ultrasonography with impedance plethysmography for the diagnosis of deep-vein thrombosis in symptomatic outpatients. *N Engl J Med* 1993; **329**: 1365–9.

170   Lagerstedt CI, Olsson CG, Fagher BO, *et al.* Need for long-term anticoagulant treatment in symptomatic calf-vein thrombosis. *Lancet* 1985; **2**: 515–18.

171   Cogo A, Lensing AW, Koopman MM, *et al.* Compression ultrasonography for diagnostic management of patients with clinically suspected deep vein thrombosis: prospective cohort study. *BMJ* 1998; **316**: 17–20.

172   Birdwell BG, Raskob GE, Whitsett TL, *et al.* The clinical validity of normal compression ultrasonography in

outpatients suspected of having deep venous thrombosis. *Ann Intern Med* 1998; **128**: 1–7.

173 Chan WS, Chunilal SD, Lee AY, *et al.* Diagnosis of deep vein thrombosis during pregnancy: a pilot study evaluating the role of D-dimer and compression leg ultrasound during pregnancy [abstract]. *Blood* 2002; **100**: 275a.

174 Frede TE, Ruthberg BN. Sonographic demonstration of iliac venous thrombosis in the maternity patient. *J Ultrasound Med* 1988; **7**: 33–7.

175 Carpenter JP, Holland GA, Baum RA, *et al.* Magnetic resonance venography for the detection of deep venous thrombosis: comparison with contrast venography and duplex Doppler ultrasonography. *J Vasc Surg* 1993; **18**: 734–41.

176 Milne JA, Howie AD, Pack AI. Dyspnoea during normal pregnancy. *Br J Obstet Gynaecol* 1978; **85**: 260–3.

177 Kruip MJ, Slob MJ, Schijen JH, *et al.* Use of a clinical decision rule in combination with D-dimer concentration in diagnostic workup of patients with suspected pulmonary embolism: a prospective management study. *Arch Intern Med* 2002; **162**: 1631–5.

178 Hull RD, Raskob GE, Coates G, Panju AA. Clinical validity of a normal perfusion lung scan in patients with suspected pulmonary embolism. *Chest* 1990; **97**: 23–6.

179 Hull RD, Hirsh J, Carter CJ, *et al.* Diagnostic value of ventilation-perfusion lung scanning in patients with suspected pulmonary embolism. *Chest* 1985; **88**: 819–28.

180 The PIOPED Investigators. Value of the ventilation/perfusion scan in acute pulmonary embolism. Results of the prospective investigation of pulmonary embolism diagnosis (PIOPED). The PIOPED Investigators. *Jama* 1990; **263**: 2753–9.

181 Stein PD, Athanasoulis C, Alavi A, *et al.* Complications and validity of pulmonary angiography in acute pulmonary embolism. *Circulation* 1992; **85**: 462–8.

182 Hull RD, Raskob GE, Ginsberg JS, *et al.* A noninvasive strategy for the treatment of patients with suspected pulmonary embolism. *Arch Intern Med* 1994; **154**: 289–97.

183 Wells PS, Ginsberg JS, Anderson DR, *et al.* Use of a clinical model for safe management of patients with suspected pulmonary embolism. *Ann Intern Med* 1998; **129**: 997–1005.

184 Boiselle PM, Reddy SS, Villas PA, *et al.* Pulmonary embolus in pregnant patients: survey of ventilation–perfusion imaging policies and practices. *Radiology* 1998; **207**: 201–6.

185 Rathbun SW, Raskob GE, Whitsett TL. Sensitivity and specificity of helical computed tomography in the diagnosis of pulmonary embolism: a systematic review. *Ann Intern Med* 2000; **132**: 227–32.

186 Mullins MD, Becker DM, Hagspiel KD, Philbrick JT. The role of spiral volumetric computed tomography in the diagnosis of pulmonary embolism. *Arch Intern Med* 2000; **160**: 293–8.

187 Perrier A, Roy PM, Aujesky D, *et al.* Diagnosing pulmonary embolism in outpatients with clinical assessment, D-dimer measurement, venous ultrasound, and helical computed tomography: a multicenter management study. *Am J Med* 2004; **116**: 291–9.

188 van Strijen MJ, de Monye W, Schiereck J, *et al.* Single-detector helical computed tomography as the primary diagnostic test in suspected pulmonary embolism: a multicenter clinical management study of 510 patients. *Ann Intern Med* 2003; **138**: 307–14.

189 Musset D, Parent F, Meyer G, *et al.* Diagnostic strategy for patients with suspected pulmonary embolism: a prospective multicentre outcome study. *Lancet* 2002; **360**: 1914–20.

190 Schuster ME, Fishman JE, Copeland JF, *et al.* Pulmonary embolism in pregnant patients: a survey of practices and policies for CT pulmonary angiography. *AJR Am J Roentgenol* 2003; **181**: 1495–8.

191 Ginsberg JS, Bates SM. Management of venous thromboembolism during pregnancy. *J Thromb Haemost* 2003; **1**: 1435–42.

192 Chunilal SD, Eikelboom JW, Attia J, *et al.* Does this patient have pulmonary embolism? *JAMA* 2003; **290**: 2849–58.

193 Geerts WH, Pineo GF, Heit JA, *et al.* Prevention of venous thromboembolism: the Seventh ACCP Conference on Antithrombotic and Thrombolytic Therapy. *Chest* 2004; **126**: 338S–400S.

194 Hull RD, Raskob GE, Hirsh J, *et al.* Continuous intravenous heparin compared with intermittent subcutaneous heparin in the initial treatment of proximal-vein thrombosis. *N Engl J Med* 1986; **315**: 1109–14.

195 Barritt DW, Jordan SC. Anticoagulant drugs in the treatment of pulmonary embolism. A controlled trial. *Lancet* 1960; **1**: 1309–12.

196 Dempfle CE. Minor transplacental passage of fondaparinux *in vivo*. *N Engl J Med* 2004; **350**: 1914–15.

197 Flessa HC, Kapstrom AB, Glueck HI, Will JJ. Placental transport of heparin. *Am J Obstet Gynecol* 1965; **93**: 570–3.

198 Forestier F, Daffos F, Capella-Pavlovsky M. Low molecular weight heparin (PK 10169) does not cross the placenta during the second trimester of pregnancy study by direct fetal blood sampling under ultrasound. *Thromb Res* 1984; **34**: 557–60.

199 Forestier F, Daffos F, Rainaut M, Toulemonde F. Low molecular weight heparin (CY 216) does not cross the placenta during the third trimester of pregnancy. *Thromb Haemost* 1987; **57**: 234.

200 Ginsberg JS, Kowalchuk G, Hirsh J, *et al.* Heparin therapy during pregnancy. Risks to the fetus and mother. *Arch Intern Med* 1989; **149**: 2233–6.

201 Ginsberg JS, Hirsh J, Turner DC, *et al.* Risks to the fetus of anticoagulant therapy during pregnancy. *Thromb Haemost* 1989; **61**: 197–203.

202 Sanson BJ, Lensing AW, Prins MH, *et al.* Safety of low-molecular-weight heparin in pregnancy: a systematic review. *Thromb Haemost* 1999; **81**: 668–72.

203 Rodie VA, Thomson AJ, Stewart FM, *et al.* Low-molecular-weight heparin for the treatment of venous thromboembolism in pregnancy: a case series. *Br J Obstet Gynaecol* 2002; **109**: 1020–4.

204 Sorensen HT, Johnsen SP, Larsen H, *et al.* Birth outcomes in pregnant women treated with low-molecular-weight heparin. *Acta Obstet Gynecol Scand* 2000; **79**: 655–9.

205 Ulander VM, Stenqvist P, Kaaja R. Treatment of deep venous thrombosis with low-molecular-weight heparin during pregnancy. *Thromb Res* 2002; **106**: 13–7.

206 Smith MP, Norris LA, Steer PJ, *et al.* Tinzaparin sodium for thrombosis treatment and prevention during pregnancy. *Am J Obstet Gynecol* 2004; **190**: 495–501.

207 Rowan JA, McLintock C, Taylor RS, North RA. Prophylactic and therapeutic enoxaparin during pregnancy: indications, outcomes and monitoring. *Aust N Z J Obstet Gynaecol* 2003; **43**: 123–8.

208 Lepercq J, Conard J, Borel-Derlon A, *et al.* Venous thromboembolism during pregnancy: a retrospective study of enoxaparin safety in 624 pregnancies. *Br J Obstet Gynaecol* 2001; **108**: 1134–40.

209 Greer IA, Nelson-Piercy C. Low-molecular-weight heparins for thromboprophylaxis and treatment of venous thromboembolism in pregnancy: a systematic review of safety and efficacy. *Blood* 2005; **106**: 401–7.

210 Quick AJ. Experimentally induced changes in the prothrombin level of the blood: III. Prothrombin concentrations of newborn pups of a mother given Dicoumarol before parturition. *J Biol Chem* 1946; **164**: 371–6.

211 Hall JG, Pauli RM, Wilson KM. Maternal and fetal sequelae of anticoagulation during pregnancy. *Am J Med* 1980; **68**: 122–40.

212 Chan WS, Anand S, Ginsberg JS. Anticoagulation of pregnant women with mechanical heart valves: a systematic review of the literature. *Arch Intern Med* 2000; **160**: 191–6.

213 Hirsh J, Cade JF, Gallus AS. Fetal effects of coumadin administered during pregnancy. *Blood* 1970; **36**: 623–7.

214 Bates SM, Greer IA, Hirsh J, Ginsberg JS. Use of antithrombotic agents during pregnancy: the Seventh ACCP Conference on Antithrombotic and Thrombolytic Therapy. *Chest* 2004; **126**: 627S–644S.

215 Orme ML, Lewis PJ, de Swiet M, *et al.* May mothers given warfarin breast-feed their infants? *Br Med J* 1977; **i**: 1564–5.

216 McKenna R, Cole ER, Vasan U. Is warfarin sodium contraindicated in the lactating mother? *J Pediatr* 1983; **103**: 325–7.

217 Hull R, Delmore T, Carter C, *et al.* Adjusted subcutaneous heparin versus warfarin sodium in the long-term treatment of venous thrombosis. *N Engl J Med* 1982; **306**: 189–94.

218 Dolovich LR, Ginsberg JS, Douketis JD, *et al.* A meta-analysis comparing low-molecular-weight heparins with unfractionated heparin in the treatment of venous thromboembolism: examining some unanswered questions regarding location of treatment, product type, and dosing frequency. *Arch Intern Med* 2000; **160**: 181–8.

219 Shaughnessy SG, Hirsh J, Bhandari M, *et al.* A histomorphometric evaluation of heparin-induced bone loss after discontinuation of heparin treatment in rats. *Blood* 1999; **93**: 1231–6.

220 Douketis JD, Ginsberg JS, Burrows RF, *et al.* The effects of long-term heparin therapy during pregnancy on bone density. A prospective matched cohort study. *Thromb Haemost* 1996; **75**: 254–7.

221 Barbour LA, Kick SD, Steiner JF, *et al.* A prospective study of heparin-induced osteoporosis in pregnancy using bone densitometry. *Am J Obstet Gynecol* 1994; **170**: 862–9.

222 Dahlman TC. Osteoporotic fractures and the recurrence of thromboembolism during pregnancy and the puerperium in 184 women undergoing thromboprophylaxis with heparin. *Am J Obstet Gynecol* 1993; **168**: 1265–70.

223 Monreal M, Lafoz E, Olive A, *et al.* Comparison of subcutaneous unfractionated heparin with a low molecular weight heparin (Fragmin) in patients with venous thromboembolism and contraindications to coumarin. *Thromb Haemost* 1994; **71**: 7–11.

224 Pettila V, Kaaja R, Leinonen P, *et al.* Thromboprophylaxis with low-molecular-weight heparin (dalteparin) in pregnancy. *Thromb Res* 1999; **96**: 275–82.

225 Pettila V, Leinonen P, Markkola A, *et al.* Postpartum bone mineral density in women treated for thromboprophylaxis with unfractionated heparin or LMW heparin. *Thromb Haemost* 2002; **87**: 182–6.

226 Carlin AJ, Farquharson RG, Quenby SM, *et al.* Prospective observational study of bone mineral density during pregnancy: low-molecular-weight heparin versus control. *Hum Reprod* 2004; **19**: 1211–14.

227 Warkentin TE. Heparin-induced thrombocytopenia: pathogenesis and management. *Br J Haematol* 2003; **121**: 535–55.

228 Lindhoff-Last E, Nakov R, Misselwitz F, *et al.* Incidence and clinical relevance of heparin-induced antibodies in patients with deep vein thrombosis treated with unfractionated or low-molecular-weight heparin. *Br J Haematol* 2002; **118**: 1137–42.

229 Schindewolf M, Mosch G, Bauersachs RM, Lindhoff-Last E. Safe anticoagulation with danaparoid in pregnancy and lactation. *Thromb Haemost* 2004; **92**: 211.

230 Gould MK, Dembitzer AD, Doyle RL, *et al.* Low-molecular-weight heparins compared with unfractionated heparin for treatment of acute deep venous thrombosis. A meta-analysis of randomized, controlled trials. *Ann Intern Med* 1999; **130**: 800–9.

231 Lopaciuk S, Bielska-Falda H, Noszczyk W, *et al.* Low-molecular-weight heparin versus acenocoumarol in the secondary prophylaxis of deep vein thrombosis. *Thromb Haemost* 1999; **81**: 26–31.

232 Pini M, Aiello S, Manotti C, *et al.* Low-molecular-weight heparin versus warfarin in the prevention of recurrences after deep vein thrombosis. *Thromb Haemost* 1994; **72**: 191–7.

233 Ginsberg JS, Chan WS, Bates SM, Kaatz S. Anticoagulation of pregnant women with mechanical heart valves. *Arch Intern Med* 2003; **163**: 694–8.

234 Casele HL, Laifer SA, Woelkers DA, Venkataramanan R. Changes in the pharmacokinetics of the low-molecular-weight heparin enoxaparin sodium during pregnancy. *Am J Obstet Gynecol* 1999; **181**: 1113–17.

235 Shiach CR. Monitoring of low-molecular-weight heparin in pregnancy. *Hematology* 2003; **8**: 47–52.

236 Barbour LA, Oja JL, Schultz LK. A prospective trial that demonstrates that dalteparin requirements increase in pregnancy to maintain therapeutic levels of anti-coagulation. *Am J Obstet Gynecol* 2004; **191**: 1024–9.

237 Anand SS, Bates S, Ginsberg JS, *et al.* Recurrent venous thrombosis and heparin therapy: an evaluation of the importance of early activated partial thromboplastin times. *Arch Intern Med* 1999; **159**: 2029–32.

238 Hull RD, Raskob GE, Brant RF, *et al.* Relation between the time to achieve the lower limit of the APTT therapeutic range and recurrent venous thromboembolism during heparin treatment for deep vein thrombosis. *Arch Intern Med* 1997; **157**: 2562–8.

239 Chunilal SD, Young E, Johnston MA, *et al.* The APTT response of pregnant plasma to unfractionated heparin. *Thromb Haemost* 2002; **87**: 92–7.

240 Buller HR, Agnelli G, Hull RD, *et al.* Antithrombotic therapy for venous thromboembolic disease: the Seventh ACCP Conference on Antithrombotic and Thrombolytic Therapy. *Chest* 2004; **126**: 401S–428S.

241 Shaw RW, Bonnar J, Greer IA, *et al. Report of the RCOG Working Party on Prophylaxis against Thromboembolism in Gynecology and Obstetrics.* London: RCOG Press, 1995.

242 Kahn SR, Ginsberg JS. Relationship between deep venous thrombosis and the postthrombotic syndrome. *Arch Intern Med* 2004; **164**: 17–26.

243 Lindhagen A, Bergqvist A, Bergqvist D, Hallbook T. Late venous function in the leg after deep venous thrombosis occurring in relation to pregnancy. *Br J Obstet Gynaecol* 1986; **93**: 348–52.

244 Masuhr F, Mehraein S, Einhaupl K. Cerebral venous and sinus thrombosis. *J Neurol* 2004; **251**: 11–23.

245 Nagpal RD. Dural sinus and cerebral venous thrombosis. *Neurosurg Rev* 1983; **6**: 155–60.

246 Cantu C, Barinagarrementeria F. Cerebral venous thrombosis associated with pregnancy and puerperium. Review of 67 cases. *Stroke* 1993; **24**: 1880–4.

247 Weatherby SJ, Edwards NC, West R, Heafield MT. Good outcome in early pregnancy following direct thrombolysis for cerebral venous sinus thrombosis. *J Neurol* 2003; **250**: 1372–3.

248 Mehraein S, Ortwein H, Busch M, *et al.* Risk of recurrence of cerebral venous and sinus thrombosis during subsequent pregnancy and puerperium. *J Neurol Neurosurg Psychiatry* 2003; **74**: 814–16.

23

Venous thrombosis and ovarian stimulation

JACQUELINE CONARD, DELPHINE LEVY, ANNE GOMPEL

INTRODUCTION

Venous thrombosis occurs in about 1 per 1000 individuals per year in the general population and different environmental and biologic – acquired or congenital – conditions may increase the risk. Pregnancy is an important risk factor for venous thrombosis especially in the presence of additional risk factors such as bed rest, twin pregnancy, congenital thrombophilia, and antiphospholipid syndrome. More recently, severe, potentially life-threatening, thrombosis has been shown to be associated with the ovarian hyperstimulation syndrome (OHSS), a complication of ovulation induction or ovarian stimulation during *in vitro* fertilization (IVF) treatment.

OVULATION INDUCTION AND STIMULATION

Ovulation induction is a treatment for anovulatory or 'unexplained' infertility in the presence of normal sexual intercourse or insemination. A variety of regimens are used, including antiestrogens (such as clomiphene citrate, human menopausal gonadotrophin [hMG], and follicle-stimulating hormone [FSH]) to control follicular development and human chorionic gonadotropin (hCG) to trigger ovulation and for luteal support.[1] Pulsatile gonadotrophin-releasing hormone (GnRH) can also be administered to patients with hypothalamic amenorrhea. The aim is to recruit and achieve maturation of one or at most, two follicles. Antiestrogen therapy rarely results in OHSS, which is mainly observed in women with polycystic ovary syndrome. Treatments with hMG-FSH and hCG are usually incriminated in OHSS.

The main indication for ovulation induction is assisted reproductive technologies (ARTs) for IVF. Different protocols are used with combinations of GnRH analogs to downregulate the pituitary and exogenous gonadotrophins (FSH or hMG) to stimulate follicular development before. Oocytes are recovered 36 hours after hCG administration. Luteal support is achieved by administration of hCG or preferably progesterone (Box 23.1). The aim of this procedure is the recruitment and maturation of up to 15–20 follicles. After *in vitro* fecundation, one or two embryos are replaced and the others are frozen for subsequent transfer cycles. The protocols for ovulation induction increase serum

---

Box 23.1 ART protocol for IVF

- Menses
- Downregulation with GnRH analog
- Hyperstimulation with hMG or FSH
- hCG injection to trigger oocyte maturation (withheld when estradiol >12 675 pmol/L (3500 pg/mL) or more than 25 small- or intermediate-sized follicles)
- Oocyte retrieval 36 hours after hCG
- Embryo transfer (one to two embryos)
- Luteal support with progesterone
- Pregnancy

estrogen levels, but the increase in estrogen occurs more quickly and is of greater magnitude after IVF procedures.

OVARIAN HYPERSTIMULATION SYNDROME

Ovarian hyperstimulation syndrome is an iatrogenic, potentially life-threatening, complication of ovulation induction or ovarian stimulation during IVF.[2–9]

Clinical manifestations

The clinical manifestations of OHSS result from the sudden increase in vascular permeability at the ovarian level. This increased permeability in turn induces the development of a massive extravascular exudate predominantly located in the peritoneal cavity, leading to hypovolemia, oliguria or anuria, and electrolyte imbalance. The constitution of this third space results in a fall of the intravascular volume and hemoconcentration. The syndrome may be classified as mild, moderate, and severe[2,5,10,11] (Table 23.1). In mild cases, ovarian enlargement, abdominal distension, and weight gain are observed. In moderate cases, nausea and vomiting are present, and ovarian enlargement and abdominal distension are greater. Severe cases are associated with marked expansion of the third space (ascites, pleural effusion), electrolyte imbalance, hypotension, hypovolemia, oliguria, and high risk of thrombosis. The ovaries are greatly enlarged with multiple follicular cysts and corpora lutea. Women presenting with severe OHSS are at high risk of thrombosis and deaths have been reported, usually caused by cerebral thrombosis, renal failure, or cardiac tamponade.

Incidence

The incidence of OHSS may differ depending on the stimulation protocols used. In a large percentage of IVF cycles, women develop symptoms of mild hyperstimulation. The incidence of moderate to severe OHSS is reported at 1–10 percent of cycles, and the severe form in 0.25–2 percent of cycles.[5,7,10–13]

The syndrome occurs more frequently when polycystic ovaries are identified on ultrasound, in younger women due to greater ovarian responsiveness (often male factor couple infertility), and in women with high estradiol levels, number of follicles or number of oocytes retrieved.[5] It is also more common when ovarian stimulation protocols include gonadotrophins and long GnRH-agonist pituitary suppression (higher doses of gonadotrophins and younger patients). The occurrence is mainly dependent on hCG, either exogenous administration for the induction of ovulation, or endogenous increase, when pregnancy is established. Thus, OHSS is more common during pregnancy cycles, especially in the cases of multiple pregnancies. Consequently, it usually occurs after administration of hCG in high doses (5000–10 000 IU) and/or when pregnancy ensues (persistent endogenous hCG production). It is suspected that due to long half-life of hCG, it continues to stimulate the ovaries after ovulation.

Prevention

For prevention of OHSS during conventional ovulation induction treatments, hCG injection is withheld when serum estradiol levels are $\geq$4300 pmol/L (1200 pg/mL) or when more than two dominant follicles are seen on ultrasonography. During IVF, women are at risk of OHSS when estradiol levels are >12 675 pmol/L (3500 pg/mL) and when more than 25 small- or intermediate-sized follicles are present. Careful monitoring of women undergoing ovulation induction is mandatory. Avoiding or postponing (coasting) hCG administration when ovaries have been hyperstimulated can often prevent OHSS. Use of hCG for luteal support has been associated with an increased risk of OHSS, and hCG has been replaced by progesterone, considered to be safer.

Pathogenesis of ovarian hyperstimulation syndrome

The mechanism of OHSS is still unclear. Rapid angiogenesis in the ovary and an increase in capillary permeability,

Table 23.1 Grades of ovarian hyperstimulation syndrome

	Pathophysiology	Clinical signs	Ultrasound findings
Grade 1 Mild	Fluid accumulation	Weight gain Abdominal distension Discomfort	Enlarged ovaries >5 cm
Grade 2 Moderate	Further fluid accumulation	Nausea + vomiting Dyspnea	Further ovarian enlargement (8–12 cm) Ascites
Grade 3 Severe	Intravascular fluid loss ↓ cardiac output ↓ central venous pressure	Tense ascites Severe dyspnea Compromised circulation Thrombosis	Pleural and pericardial effusions Hepatorenal failure

together with rapid ovary enlargement are involved.[6] The causative role of estradiol was discussed initially since the severity of the syndrome correlates with plasma estradiol levels. The estrogen level is now considered as a marker of ovarian response, rather than the cause of OHSS.

Other factors have been involved in the pathophysiology of OHSS: activation of the ovarian prorenin–renin–angiotensin system;[5,14,15] inflammatory processes involving prostaglandins;[16] cytokines;[17–19] histamine; and vascular endothelial growth factor (VEGF).[20–22] The last, VEGF, seems to be the most important.[7] This factor originating from the ovarian follicle, is an important mediator of angiogenesis and stimulates capillary permeability. High levels have been found in the ascitic fluid in women with OHSS. Its serum level correlates with the severity of OHSS and depends on hCG administration, suggesting that OHSS following hCG administration may be mediated by VEGF.[7] The highest levels have been observed in women with polycystic ovaries, in whom the risk of OHSS is high.

However, if the OHSS is due to an increased level of VEGF secondary to an excessive degree of stimulation, it is difficult to explain why some women with large numbers of oocytes do not develop OHSS, and others with apparently average degree of stimulation develop OHSS. Attention has been focused on α_2-macroglobulin (α_2-M), a protein associated with remodeling processes of ovulation and with the maintenance of the corpus luteum, considered as a naturally occurring inhibitor of VEGF. A recent study examined whether there is a relation between serum VEGF levels, α_2-M levels and the development of OHSS in hyperstimulated women undergoing IVF (15 or more oocytes).[23] It showed no statistically significant difference in VEGF levels at the time of oocyte retrieval between hyperstimulated women who did or did not subsequently develop OHSS. In contrast, α_2-M levels were statistically higher in women who did not develop OHSS. Thus, α_2-M may act as a VEGF 'removing and inactivating' protein. It is suggested that α_2-M measurement at the time of oocyte retrieval may help to identify women for whom it is safe to proceed with embryo transfer from those for whom it is not, because of the risk of OHSS.

THROMBOSIS AND OVARIAN HYPERSTIMULATION SYNDROME

Venous and arterial thromboembolic manifestations were initially reported in 1964–65 during conventional ovulation induction in OHSS after hMG therapy[24,25] or after clomiphene acetate.[26] Since then, most of the reported cases were observed after ART.[27–29] Thrombosis has also been associated with administration of recombinant FSH.[18] The incidence of thrombosis has been estimated as 1/128 in severe OHSS. As OHSS is estimated to occur in 0.5–5 percent of the cycles, the risk for a thrombotic event during ART has been evaluated at 1 of 2650 to 1 of 6400 cycles[28] or 3 in 8000 cycles (0.04 percent).[29] Fifty-four cases of arterial

or venous thromboembolic events complicating OHSS were reported in a comprehensive review in 1997[28] and another literature review was published in 2003.[30]

Venous thromboses are more frequent (75 percent) than arterial ones.[28] Episodes of lower limb deep vein thrombosis and pulmonary embolism have been reported (possibly under-reported because they were considered as 'expected' in pregnancy), but unusual sites are also frequently involved. Indeed, 60 percent of cases have been observed in upper limb, neck and head veins.[28] Arterial thromboses are mostly intracerebral. Pulmonary embolism is infrequent. Few fatal or severe thrombotic events have been reported: death after thrombosis of the carotid or middle cerebral artery,[25,31] amputation of the lower limb following thrombosis of the femoral artery,[25] amputation of the forearm after thrombosis of the axillary artery recurring after thromboarterectomy,[32] coma, tetraplegia, and aphasia.[33]

Thrombosis occurs 6–70 days following hCG injection.[18,28,29,32,34–40] The mean observed delay between hCG and the thrombotic event is longer for venous compared with arterial thrombosis (38 days vs. 14 days, respectively). Thus, thromboembolic events usually occur some time after the peak estradiol concentration. Thrombosis is associated with pregnancy in 84 percent of the cases,[28] and especially twin or multiple pregnancies.

HEMOSTASIS CHANGES DURING *IN VITRO* FERTILIZATION AND OVARIAN HYPERSTIMULATION SYNDROME

Changes in coagulation and fibrinolysis observed during ovarian stimulation are similar to those observed during pregnancy.[41] Several circulating coagulation factors are increased (factor V, fibrinogen, von Willebrand factor), physiologic coagulation inhibition is impaired (decreased antithrombin and protein S levels), and fibrinolysis was first reported to decrease.[42–45] Coagulation activation markers, such as prothrombin fragment 1 + 2 and D-dimers are also increased.[45] Reevaluation of the fibrinolytic system found a decreased plasminogen inhibitor (PAI)-1 level, suggesting there is no impairment of fibrinolysis.[46] Activated protein C (APC) resistance has been measured with a clotting time (that is, activated partial thromboplastin time-[aPTT]) based assay during controlled stimulation (samples collected at estradiol minimum, days 5–8 before oocyte retrieval, estradiol maximum and at oocyte retrieval) and compared with normal cycle. No difference in APC resistance was found although there was a 10-fold increase in estradiol level.[47] In a more recent study, APC resistance was measured using a different test (thrombin generation initiated by tissue factor, extrinsic-tissue factor-based assay, instead of an intrinsic clotting assay) in 33 women due to undergo IVF.[48] Blood samples were obtained at baseline, after downregulation, hyperstimulation, and at luteal support. The APC resistance ratios increased slightly at downregulation, significantly during hyperstimulation and remained high during luteal support. Changes in coagulation inhibitors were moderate.

Coagulation changes are usually more pronounced in women with OHSS: higher levels of fibrinogen, von Willebrand factor, D-dimers, thrombin-antithrombin (TAT) complexes and fragment 1.2, low levels of prekallikrein and tissue factor pathway inhibitor.[42,49,50] *In vitro* fertilization is associated with rapid modifications of endogenous estradiol and progesterone levels. Correlation with estradiol levels have been found for parameters such as fibrinogen, D-dimers[50] and increased levels of estradiol (40-fold increase at hyperstimulation) correlated with APC resistance ratios ($P < 0.0005$).[48]

In women who become pregnant, the delay for normalization of prekallikrein is 3 weeks, whereas a rapid return to normal within 1 week after OHSS is observed in women with no pregnancy.[49] D-dimers and TAT complexes are also found to be higher in women with OHSS who have unsuccessful pregnancy outcomes.[50] Interestingly, in OHSS with pregnancy, increased coagulation activation is still present 3 weeks after OHSS[49] and protein S level is lower:[48,49] these findings might be useful in guiding clinicians about the appropriate duration of antithrombotic prophylaxis (if administered) after severe OHSS.

Procoagulant activities of blood monocytes mediated by tissue factor expression[51] and activation of the kinin system[52] have also been postulated as potential mediators of thrombosis in this syndrome. Elevated plasma von Willebrand factor, a marker of endothelial lesion, and low prekallikrein levels have been proposed as predictors of thrombotic complications in women with OHSS.[52,53]

MECHANISMS OF THROMBOSIS IN OVARIAN HYPERSTIMULATION SYNDROME

The pathogenesis of the reported thrombotic events is explained in part by the hypercoagulable state secondary to OHSS and by pregnancy, but it still remains obscure in the absence of OHSS. However, it is well known that venous thrombosis is frequently multifactorial.

Thrombosis is mostly associated with OHSS and hemoconcentration, the latter demonstrated by an increase in hematocrit. The resulting increase in blood viscosity together with hypercoagulability is likely a predisposing factor for thrombosis. It is difficult to determine which, if any of the measurable coagulation changes, contributes to promote thrombosis. Since OHSS-associated thrombosis is uncommon and comprehensive evaluation of the hemostatic and fibrinolytic pathways is not always available when it occurs, information about this is lacking. Hemostasis has been studied at different phases of IVF in women with severe OHSS but no thrombosis, and in isolated cases of women who experienced thrombosis related to IVF. Adding to the difficulty, protocols have changed over time: long and short protocols, with different drugs, at different doses. In some protocols, combined oral contraception,

a known risk factor of venous thrombosis, has been administered before starting the procedure and may induce a decrease in protein S levels for 4–6 weeks.[48,53]

Hyperestrogenism likely plays a role, contributing to a hypercoagulable state. Thrombosis frequently occurs after a lag time following OHSS, mainly in women who become pregnant. By itself, pregnancy increases the risk of thrombosis and might explain the occurrence of thrombosis in women with OHSS when they are pregnant. The few coagulation studies that have been done several weeks after the procedure when patients were pregnant showed that increased coagulation activation was still present 3 weeks after OHSS. Addition of changes related to OHSS to changes related to pregnancy increases the risk of thrombosis. However, in the general population of pregnant women, thrombosis is rarely observed at the very beginning of pregnancy and most changes in the coagulation and fibrinolytic systems increase as pregnancy progresses. In contrast, OHSS-associated thrombosis occurs almost exclusively during the first trimester of pregnancy. The vascular and inflammatory changes (liberation of cytokines) in OHSS may also particularly contribute to the hypercoagulable state in women with preexisting vascular risk factors such as congenital thrombophilia or antiphospholipid antibodies or systemic lupus erythematosus (SLE).[54,55]

Thrombophilia

As it is during pregnancy, congenital predisposition to venous thrombosis, namely thrombophilia, can be an important risk factor for OHSS-associated venous thrombosis.[56,57] Isolated cases of coagulation inhibitor deficiency or APC resistance have been reported in women with OHSS and thrombosis: antithrombin deficiency,[58] protein S deficiency,[29,59] APC resistance and factor V Leiden,[29,37,39,48,60,61] prothrombin (FII) G20210A,[29] combined factor V Leiden and factor II G20210A.[62] Screening for factor V Leiden and factor II G20210A has not been systematically performed in reported women with OHSS-associated thrombosis since these thrombophilias were described for the first time in 1994 and 1996, respectively. Concerning protein S interpretation, in some protocols, combined oral contraception is administered before starting the procedure and it must be taken into account when the assay is performed during the 6 weeks following discontinuation of this treatment.

Should screening for thrombophilia be performed in women who are candidates for IVF? Screening was performed in few series of women with severe OHSS, but contradictory results have been reported. In one study, thrombophilia was detected in 17 of the 20 patients who developed severe OHSS (8 decreased PS, 6 decreased AT, 7 MTHFR 677T, 5 antiphospholipid antibodies, 1 FV Leiden) and 11 of 41 controls (that is, women undergoing induction of ovulation without development of severe OHSS).[63] This high prevalence of thrombophilic abnormalities does not correspond to a permanent thrombophilia in all cases.

Abnormalities were observed during the acute phase of the severe OHSS in the patients or during the luteal phase of the treatment in the controls. Three women of this series developed thrombotic events: one had factor V Leiden and decreased protein S, one had antiphospholipid antibodies and decreased protein S and one had decreased antithrombin and MTHFR 677T. In another study, the prevalence of thrombophilias was not increased in 20 women who developed severe OHSS, compared with 40 women without severe OHSS and 100 healthy controls. The explanation for these discrepant results might be that in the latter study, tests were performed on samples obtained before the IVF treatment cycle so that changes related to OHSS were excluded. None of the women had thrombotic complications. The authors of this study concluded that systematic thrombophilia screening before IVF was neither justified nor cost effective.[64] An observational study included 305 consecutive women undergoing ovarian stimulation, who had thrombophilia screening.[65] Thrombotic events were observed in 4/747 cycles of ovarian stimulation (prevalence of 0.5 percent, 1.6 per 100 000 cycles/woman). Increased homocysteine level was the only change significantly associated with thrombosis.

More studies are needed, taking also into account the family history of venous thrombosis. A registry on thrombosis and thrombotic risk in women receiving ovarian stimulation for pregnancy, initiated by the International Society on Thrombosis and Haemostasis Subcommittee on Women's Health Issues, is available (konkleb@mail.med.upenn.edu). It might help in identifying risk factors of thrombosis and usefulness of thrombophilia screening. An association between thrombophilia and IVF failures was suggested in one study[66] but not confirmed by another.[67]

Antiphospholipid syndrome

Antiphospholipid syndrome is also a risk factor of thrombosis. In addition, estrogens play an important role in the pathogenesis of SLE and also increase the risk of thrombosis. Consequently, ovarian stimulation may exacerbate or induce SLE or favor thrombosis when anticardiolipin antibodies are present. No prospective study has been performed in women with SLE and no SLE was found in 535 women who underwent several cycles of controlled ovarian hyperstimulation.[68] A SLE flare was observed in two women with infertility who had subclinical SLE.[69] In another woman, who had elevated levels of anticardiolipin and antinuclear antibodies, ovulation induction was associated with inferior vena cava and left renal vein thrombosis during a febrile bacterial pneumonia.[70] Rechallenge of ovulation induction was associated with SLE flare and a death from probable pulmonary embolism.[71]

Head and neck vein thrombosis

Head and neck venous thrombi in OHSS are difficult to explain. Relative stasis of the legs and increase in intraabdominal pressure may decrease the venous return due to compression of the vena cava and iliac vessels and can explain the deep vein thrombosis events in the lower extremities. In contrast, thrombosis of the head and neck veins is unexpected. The recognized risk factors of these unusual thromboses are: congenital anatomic abnormality causing venous obstruction, unusual position or exercise, compression from tumor or indwelling central venous catheterization. One case of costoclavicular 'nipping' of the subclavian vein was reported;[59] no such cause was found in other women. Position of the head during sleep has been proposed as a local triggering factor.[72]

PREVENTION AND TREATMENT OF THROMBOSIS IN OVARIAN HYPERSTIMULATION SYNDROME

Prevention of severe OHSS is the primary measure to prevent thrombosis.[5,7] This includes pretreatment ultrasound scan for detection of polycystic ovaries requiring lowering of the dose of gonadotropin. In patients with overstimulated ovaries, dose of hCG to initiate oocyte ovulation is lowered and progesterone is preferred to hCG for luteal support. Recognized risk factors of OHSS are taken into account: serum estradiol more than 10 000 pmol/L (3000 pg/mL), 20 follicles or more of diameter of 12 mm or more. All of these measures are familiar to practitioners specialized in ovarian stimulation.

Thrombophilia screening should not be done in every woman before ovarian stimulation[64] but should be considered in women with a personal or family history of venous thrombosis, especially before the age of 50.[63] The screening includes prothrombin time, aPTT for the detection of lupus anticoagulant, anticardiolipin antibodies, antithrombin, protein C, and protein S assays, APC resistance or factor V Leiden mutation, factor II G20210A mutation, and homocysteine levels. Homozygous MTHFR 677T is not a major risk factor for venous thrombosis but may increase the risk of thrombosis when associated with other risk factors of thrombosis, and it has been associated with a fivefold increased risk for severe OHSS.[63] Thus, MTHFR screening may be added to the above mentioned tests. It must be remembered that hyperstimulated ovaries are also at high risk of hemorrhagic complications.

For prevention of thrombosis during OHSS, there are no precise specific guidelines. Graduated elastic compression stockings are recommended to prevent thrombosis in moderate and severe OHSS, especially when the hematocrit is high, because of the induced hemoconcentration and increased blood viscosity, and because of some degree of immobility of the patients. Prophylactic anticoagulant treatment depends on the presence of thrombophilia and history of thrombosis.

In severe OHSS, women are hospitalized and the prophylactic administration of unfractionated heparin by subcutaneous route (5000 U twice daily) is traditionally recommended during hospitalization, but the dose of heparin required is not well defined and internal jugular venous thrombosis has been reported despite prophylactic mini-dose heparin.[9,73] Information concerning the safety of administration of low-molecular-weight heparin (LMWH) is scarce at the beginning of pregnancy. However, LMWHs such as dalteparin, enoxaparin, or nadroparin at prophylactic dose (40 mg of enoxaparin or 5000 U dalteparin once daily) or higher doses for treatment were recently considered to be safe in two studies in pregnant women.[74,75] They are particularly suitable in this setting because it does not cross the placenta and, if compared to unfractionated heparin, appears to cause less osteoporosis with long-term use, and less heparin-induced thrombocytopenia. There is also the advantage of one injection a day for prophylaxis, instead of two injections when using unfractionated heparin. Use of LMWHs has been reported in women with OHSS at a daily dose of 5000 U dalteparin or 40 mg enoxaparin. This prophylaxis, when administered during the acute phase of OHSS only, seems insufficient to prevent thrombosis[29] and should probably be prolonged at least for 1 month when the woman is pregnant due to the significant hypercoagulation present during OHSS, that is maintained during the first month of pregnancy.

In women with factor V Leiden or factor II G20210A mutations, the question of prophylaxis in high risk situations is asked more and more frequently by clinicians. These genetic abnormalities predisposing to thrombosis are common in the Caucasian population (5–7 percent and 2–3 percent, respectively) and associated with a lower risk of thrombosis than other thrombophilias such as antithrombin, protein C, or protein S deficiencies: risk multiplied by 3–7 for the mutations, about 50 for the antithrombin deficiency.[76] In asymptomatic carriers of factor V or factor II heterozygous mutations (in the absence of IVF), clinical surveillance is usually recommended during pregnancy and prophylaxis is administered for 4–6 weeks in the postpartum period.[77] In women carrying these mutations and having no personal history of thrombosis, the risk of IVF-related thrombosis is probably moderate and prophylactic treatment may be appropriate after oocyte retrieval, or only when severe OHSS occurs. As above, the prophylaxis should probably be continued at least during the first month of pregnancy.

In women with personal history of deep vein thrombosis or pulmonary embolism, associated or not with thrombophilia, the risk of recurrent venous episode during OHSS is probably higher although it has not been evaluated. The feasibility of IVF may be questioned or discouraged in women at very high risk (such as antithrombin deficiency, previous massive embolism). In these women, when ovarian stimulation is decided, prophylactic treatment should be recommended from the start of the stimulation procedure with a temporary discontinuation of the treatment at the time of oocyte retrieval, or started after retrieval only. The appropriate dose of LMWH is unknown, but a slightly higher dose than one used for DVT prophylaxis seems reasonable. In these women at high risk of thrombosis, the

prophylaxis is justified throughout pregnancy and 6 weeks post partum, under strict clinical surveillance.

In SLE and antiphospholipid syndrome, independently or during IVF, subcutaneous unfractionated heparin (5000 IU subcutaneously every 12 hours) or LMWH (such as enoxaparin 40 mg every 24 hours) is started on day 1 of controlled ovarian stimulation and continued for several weeks.[77,78] Heparin is temporarily discontinued after the morning administration on the day prior to oocyte retrieval, and is reinitiated, in association with aspirin (75–100 mg/day), immediately after retrieval. The association of heparin and aspirin is also recommended to improve the pregnancy rate in the antiphospholipid syndrome.[79] For patients with prior antiphospholipid-related thrombotic events, heparin is proposed at therapeutic doses throughout any resultant pregnancy and 6 weeks postpartum. The use of graduated elastic compression elastic stockings is encouraged. Laboratory monitoring of prophylactic LMWH treatments is not presently required but platelet count is when the patient is receiving or has previously received unfractionated heparin.

CONCLUSIONS

Thrombosis is a rare but potentially fatal event during ovarian induction and IVF. Its pathophysiology and the reasons for thrombosis mainly occurring in the neck and head vessels remain mostly unknown. The prevention of thrombosis requires precise evaluation and more studies are needed to develop reliable guidelines.

KEY LEARNING POINTS

- Ovarian hyperstimulation is a risk factor for venous and arterial thrombosis.
- Thrombosis is rare, occurs mostly in the head and neck vessels.
- Reason for this unusual location of thrombosis is unknown.
- Thrombosis is more frequent after severe OHSS when women become pregnant.
- In women at risk of venous thrombosis (history of venous thrombosis and/or thrombophilia), the feasibility of IVF and need for anticoagulant prophylaxis must be considered.
- No clear guidelines are presently available for timing and dose of anticoagulant prophylaxis and such guidelines are required.

REFERENCES

1 Meirow D, Laufer N, Schenker JG. Ovulation induction and *in vitro* fertilization. *Gynecol Endocrinol* 1993; **6**: 211–24.

2   Schenker JG, Weinstein D: Ovarian hyperstimulation syndrome: A current survey. *Fertil Steril* 1978; **30**: 255–68.

3   Borenstein R, Elchalal U, Lunenfeld B, *et al.* Severe ovarian hyperstimulation syndrome: a reevaluated therapeutic approach. *Fertil Steril* 1989; **51**: 791–95.

4   Pride SM, James C St J, Ho Yuen B. The ovarian hyperstimulation syndrome. *Seminars Reproductive Endocrinol* 1990; **8**: 247–60.

5   Brinsden PR, Wada I, Tan SL, *et al.* Diagnosis, prevention and management of ovarian hyperstimulation syndrome. *Br J Obstet Gynaecol* 1995; **102**: 767–72.

6   Elchalal U, Schenker JG. The pathophysiology of ovarian hyperstimulation syndrome – view and ideas. *Hum Reprod* 1997; **12**: 1129–37.

7   Jacobs HS, Agrawal R. Complications of ovarian stimulation. *Baillieres Clin Obstet Gynaecol* 1998; **12**: 565–79.

8   Simon A, Revel A, Hurwitz A, Laufer N. The pathogenesis of ovarian hyperstimulation syndrome: a continuing enigma. *J Assist Reprod Genet* 1998; **15**: 202–9.

9   Whelan JG, Vlahos NF. The ovarian hyperstimulation syndrome. *Fertil Steril* 2000; **73**: 883–96.

10 Golan A, Ron-El R, Herman A, *et al.* Ovarian hyperstimulation syndrome: an update review. *Obstet Gynecol Surv* 1989; **44**: 430–40.

11 Navot D, Bergh PA, Laufer N. Ovarian hyperstimulation syndrome in novel reproductive technologies: prevention and treatment. *Fertil Steril* 1992; **58**: 249–61.

12 Forman RG, Frydman R, Egan D. Severe ovarian hyperstimulation syndrome using agonists of gonadotrophin releasing hormone for *in vitro* fertilization: a European series and a proposal for prevention. *Fertil Steril* 1990; **53**: 502–9.

13 MacDougall MJ, Tan SL, Balen A, Jacobs HS. A controlled study comparing patients with and without polycystic ovaries undergoing *in vitro* fertilization. *Hum Reprod* 1993; **8**: 233–7.

14 Navot D, Margalioth E, Laufer N, *et al.* Direct correlation between plasma rennin activity and severity of ovarian hyperstimulation syndrome. *Fertil Steril* 1987; **48**: 57–61.

15 Ong ACM, Eisen V, Rennie DP, *et al.* The pathogenesis of the ovarian hyperstimulation syndrome (OHS): a possible role for ovarian renin. *Clin Endocrinol* 1991; **34**: 43–9.

16 Schenker JG, Polishuk WZ. The role of prostaglandins in ovarian hyperstimulation syndrome. *Eur J Obstet Gynec Reprod Biol* 1976; **6/2**: 47–52.

17 Morris RS, Paulson RJ. Increased angiotensin-converting enzyme activity in a patient with severe ovarian hyperstimulation syndrome. *Fertil Steril* 1999; **71**: 562–3.

18 Loret de Mola JR, Kiwi R, *et al.* Subclavian deep vein thrombosis associated with the use of recombinant follicle-stimulating hormone (Gonal-F) complicating mild ovarian hyperstimulation syndrome. *Fertil Steril* 2000; **73**: 1253–5.

19 Abramov Y, Schenker JG, Lewin A, *et al.* Plasma inflammatory cytokines correlate to the ovarian hyperstimulation syndrome. *Hum Reprod* 1996; **11**: 1381–6.

20 McClure N, Leya J, Radwanska E, *et al.* Luteal phase support and severe ovarian hyperstimulation. *Hum Reprod* 1992; **7**: 758–64.

21 Krasnow JS, Berga SL, Gusik DS. Vascular permeability factor and vascular endothelial growth factor in ovarian hyperstimulation syndrome: a preliminary report. *Fertil Steril* 1996; **65**: 552–5.

22 Abramov Y, Barak V, Nisman B, Schenker JG. Vascular endothelial growth factor plasma levels correlate with the clinical picture in severe ovarian hyperstimulation syndrome. *Fertil Steril* 1997; 67: 261–5.

23 McElhinney B, Ardill J, Caldwell C, *et al.* Ovarian hyperstimulation syndrome and assisted reproductive technologies: why some and not others? *Hum Reprod* 2002, **17**: 1548–53.

24 Crooke AC, Butt WR, Carrington SP. Pregnancy in women with secondary amenorrhoea with human gonadotrophins. *Lancet* 1964; **1**: 184–8.

25 Mozes M, Bogokowsky H, Antebi E, *et al.* Thromboembolic phenomena after ovarian stimulation with human gonadotrophins. *Lancet* 1965; **2**: 1213–15.

26 Benshushan A, Shushan A, Paltiel O, *et al.* Ovulation induction with clomifene complicated by deep vein thrombosis. *Eur J Obstet Gynecol Reprod Biol* 1995; **62**: 261–2.

27 Benifla JL, Conard J, Naouri M, *et al.* Syndrome d'hyperstimulation ovarienne et thrombose. *J Gynecol Obstet Biol Reprod* 1994; **23**: 778–83.

28 Stewart JA, Hamilton PJ, Murdoch AP. Thromboembolic disease associated with ovarian stimulation and assisted conception techniques. *Hum Reprod* 1997; **12**: 2167–73.

29 Arya R, Shehata HA, Patel R, *et al.* Internal jugular vein thrombosis after assisted conception therapy. *Br J Haematol* 2001; **115**: 153–5.

30 Ou YC, Kao YL, Lai SL, *et al.* Thromboembolism after ovarian stimulation: successful management of a woman with superior sagittal sinus thrombosis after IVF and embryo transfer: case report. *Hum Reprod* 2003; **18**: 2375–81.

31 Cluroe AD, Synek BJ. A fatal case of ovarian hyperstimulation syndrome with cerebral infarction. *Pathology* 1995; **27**: 344–6.

32 Mancini A, Milardi D, Di Pietro ML, *et al.* A case of forearm amputation after ovarian stimulation for *in vitro* fertilization-embryo transfer. *Fertil Steril* 2001, 76: 198–200.

33 Humbert G, Delaunay P, Leroy J, *et al.* Accident vasculaire cerebral au cours d'un traitement par les gonadotrophines. *Nouv Presse Med* 1973; **2**: 28–30.

34 Stewart JA, Hamilton PJ, Murdoch AP. Upper limb thrombosis associated with assisted conception treatment. *Hum Reprod* 1997; **12**: 2174–5.

35 Moutos DM, Miller MM, Mahadevan MM. Bilateral internal jugular venous thrombosis complicating severe ovarian hyperstimulation syndrome after prophylactic albumin administration. *Fertil Steril* 1997; **68**: 174–6.

36 Aboulghar MA, Mansour RT, Serour GI, Amin YM. Moderate hyperstimulation syndrome complicated by deep cerebrovascular thrombosis. *Hum Reprod* 1998; **13**: 2088–91.

37 Todros T, Carmazzi CM, Bontempo S, *et al.* Spontaneous ovarian hyperstimulation syndrome an deep vein thrombosis in pregnancy. *Hum Reprod* 1999; **14**: 2245–8.

38 Tang OI, Ng E. HY, Cheng PW, Ho PC. Cortical vein thrombosis misinterpreted as intracranial haemorrhage in severe ovarian hyperstimulation syndrome. *Hum Reprod* 2000; **15**: 1913–16.

39 Ludwig M, Felberbaum RE, Diedrich K. Deep vein thrombosis during administration of HMG for ovarian stimulation. *Arch Gynecol Obstet* 2000; **263**: 139–41.

40 Belaen B, Geerinckx K, Vergauwe P, Thys J. Internal jugular vein thrombosis after ovarian stimulation. *Hum Reprod* 2001; **16**: 510–12.

41 Clark P, Brennand J, Conkie JA, *et al.* Activated protein C sensitivity, protein C, protein S and coagulation in normal pregnancy. *Thromb Haemost* 1998; **79**: 1166–70.

42 Phillips LL, Gladstone W, van der Wiele R. Studies of the coagulation and fibrinolytic systems in hyperstimulation syndrome after administration of human gonadotrophins. *J Reprod Med* 1975; **14**:138–43

43 Kim HC, Kemmann E, Shelden RM, Saidi P. Response of blood coagulation parameters to elevated endogenous 17β-estradiol levels induced by human menopausal gonadotropins. *Am J Obstet Gynecol* 1981; **140**: 807–10.

44 Aune B,Hoie KE, Oian P, Holst N, Osterud B. Does ovarian hyperstimulation for *in vitro* fertilization induce a hypercoagulable state? *Hum Reprod* 1991; **6**:925–7.

45 Biron C, Galtier-Dereure F, Rabesandratana H, *et al.* Hemostasis parameters during ovarian stimulation for *in vitro* fertilization: results of a prospective study. *Fertil Steril* 1997; **67**: 104–9.

46 Lox C, Cañez M, DeLeon F, *et al.* Hyperestrogenism induced by menotropins alone or in conjunction with luprolide acetate in *in vitro* fertilization cycles: the impact of hemostasis. *Fertil Steril* 1995; **63**: 566–70.

47 Wramsby ML, Bàkarewa MI, Blomlbäck M, Bremme AK. Response to activated protein C during normal menstrual cycle and ovarian stimulation. *Human Reprod* 2000; **15**: 795–7.

48 Curvers J, Nap AW, Thomassen MC, *et al.* Effect of *in vitro* fertilization treatment and subsequent pregnancy on the protein C pathway. *Br J Haematol* 2001; **115**: 400–7.

49 Kodama H, Fukuda J, Karube H, *et al.* Status of the coagulation and fibrinolytic systems in ovarian hyperstimulation syndrome. *Fertil Steril* 1996; **66**: 417–24.

50 Rogolino A, Coccia ME, Fedi S, *et al.* Hypercoagulability, high tissue factor and low tissue factor pathway inhibitors levels in severe ovarian hyperstimulation syndrome: possible association with clinical outcome. *Blood Coagul Fibrinolysis* 2003; **14**: 277–82.

51 Balasch J, Reverter JC, Fabregues F, *et al.* Increased induced monocyte tissue factor expression by plasma from patients with severe ovarian hyperstimulation syndrome. *Fertil Steril* 1996; **66**: 608–13.

52 Kodama H, Takeda S, Fukuda J, *et al.* Activation of plasma kinin system correlates with severe coagulation disorders in patients with ovarian hyperstimulation syndrome. *Hum Reprod* 1997; **12**: 891–895.

53 Todorow S, Schricker ST, Siebzehnruebl ER, *et al.* Von Willebrand factor: an endothelial marker to monitor *in-vitro* fertilization patients with ovarian hyperstimulation syndrome. *Hum Reprod* 1993; **8**: 2039–46.

54 Ellis MH, Ben Nun I, Rathaus V, *et al.* Internal jugular vein thrombosis in patients with ovarian hyperstimulation syndrome. *Fertil Steril* 1988; **69**: 140–2.

55 Birdsall MA, Lockwood GM, Ledger WL, *et al.* Antiphospholipid antibodies in women having *in-vitro* fertilization. *Hum Reprod* 1996; **11**: 1185–9.

56 Conard J, Horellou MH, Van Dreden P, *et al.* Thrombosis and pregnancy in congenital deficiencies in AT III, protein C or protein S: study of 78 women. *Thromb Haemost* 1990; **63**: 319–20.

57 Simioni P, Sanson BJ, Prandoni P, *et al.* Incidence of venous thromboembolism in families with inherited thrombophilia. *Thromb Haemost* 1998; **81**: 198–202.

58 Kligman I, Noyes N, Benadiva CA, *et al.* Massive deep vein thrombosis in a patient with antithrombin III deficiency undergoing ovarian stimulation for *in vitro* fertilization. *Fertil Steril* 1995; **63**: 673–6.

59 Boulieu D, Ninet J, Pinede L, *et al.* Thrombose veineuse précoce de siège inhabituel, en début de grossesse après stimulation ovarienne. *Contracept Fertil Sex* 1989; **17**: 725–7.

60 Horstkamp B, Lubke MK, Kentenich H *et al.* Internal jugular vein thrombosis caused by resistance to activated protein C as a complication of ovarian hyperstimulation after *in-vitro* fertilization. *Hum Reprod* 1996; **11**: 280–2.

61 Brechmann J, Unterberg C. Superior vena cava thrombosis after *in vitro* fertilization. *Dtsch Med Wochenschr* 2000; **125**: 1429–32.

62 McGowan BM, Kay LA, Perry DJ. Deep vein thrombosis followed by internal jugular vein thrombosis as a complication of *in vitro* fertilization in a woman heterozygous for the prothrombin 3′ UTR and factor V Leiden mutations. *Am J Hematol* 2003; **73**: 276–8.

63 Dulitzky M, Cohen SB, Inbal A, *et al.* Increase prevalence of thrombophilia among women with severe ovarian hyperstimulation syndrome. *Fertil Steril* 2002; **77**: 463–7.

64 Fabregues F, Tassies D, Reverter JC, *et al.* Prevalence of thrombophilia in women with severe ovarian hyperstimulation syndrome and cost-effectiveness of screening. *Fertil Steril* 2004; **81**: 989–95.

65 Grandone E, Colaizzo D, Vergura P, *et al.* Age and homocysteine plasma levels are risk factors for thrombotic complications after ovarian stimulation. *Hum Reprod* 2002; **19**: 1796–9.

66 Grandone E, Colaizzo D, Lo Bue A, *et al.* Inherited thrombophilia and *in vitro* fertilization implantation failure. *Fertil Steril* 2001; **76**: 201–2.

67 Martinelli I, Taioli E, Ragni G, *et al.* Embryo implantation after assisted reproductive procedures and maternal thrombophilia. *Haematologica* 2003; **88**: 789–93.

68 Bruce IN, Laskin CA. Sex hormones in systemic lupus erythematosus: a controversy for modern times. *J Rheumatol* 1997; **24**: 1461–3.

69 Ben-Chetrit A, Ben-Chetrit E. Systemic lupus erythematosus induced by ovulation induction treatment;. *Arthritis Rheum* 1994; **37**: 1614–17.

70 Le Thi Huong D, Wechsler B, Piette JC, *et al.* Risks of ovulation-induction therapy in systemic lupus erythematosus. *Br J Rheumatol* 1996; **35**: 1184–6.

71 Casoli P, Tumiati B, La Sala G. Fatal exacerbation of systemic lupus erythematosus after induction of ovulation. *J Rheumatol* 1997; **24**: 1639–40.

72   Weber RR, Shackelford HL, Bernhart WR. Position-induced internal jugular vein thrombosis. *W V Med J* 1988; **84:** 509–11.

73   Hignett M, Spence J, Claman P. Internal jugular vein thrombosis: a late complication of ovarian hyperstimulation syndrome despite minidose heparin prophylaxis. *Hum Reprod* 1995; **10**: 3121–3.

74   Sanson BJ, Lensing AWA, Prins MH, *et al.* Safety of low-molecular-weight heparin in pregnancy: a systematic review. *Thromb Haemost* 1999; **8**1: 668–72.

75   Lepercq J, Conard J, Borel-Derlon A, *et al.* Venous thromboembolism during pregnancy: a retrospective study of enoxaparin safety in 624 pregnancies. *Br J Obstet Gynaecol* 2001; **108**: 1134–40.

76   Rosendaal FR. Risk factors for venous thrombotic disease. *Thromb Haemost* 1999; **82**: 610–19.

77   Bates SM, Greer IA, Hirsh J, Ginsberg JS. Use of antithrombotic agents during pregnancy: the Seventh ACCP conference on antithrombotic and thrombolytic therapy. *Chest* 2004; **126**; 637S–644S.

78   Wechsler B, Huong DT, Vauthier-Brouzes D, *et al.* Can we advise ovulation induction in patients with SLE? *Scand J Rheumatol* 1998; **107**(Suppl): 53–9.

79   Scherl G, Feinman M, Zouves C, *et al.* High fecundity rates following *in-vitro* fertilization and embryo transfer in antiphospholipid antibody positive women treated with heparin and asprin. *Hum Reprod* 1994; **9**: 2278–83.

24

Thrombophilia and pregnancy complications

SCOTT M NELSON, IAN A GREER

INTRODUCTION

There is increasing recognition that thrombophilias may contribute to abnormal placentation and placental damage. Early in pregnancy this may manifest as miscarriage, which may be recurrent. In later pregnancy, thrombophilias have been associated with stillbirth, preeclampsia, placental abruption, and intrauterine growth restriction (IUGR). These complications are the leading causes of maternal and fetal adverse pregnancy outcome, with a significant psychosocial impact and economic burden secondary to preterm delivery. The aim of this chapter is to review the contribution of thrombophilia to adverse perinatal outcomes and address the role of potential therapeutic interventions.

HAEMOSTATIC CHANGES OF PREGNANCY

Normal pregnancy may be regarded as an acquired thrombophilic state[1,2] due to increased concentrations of coagulation factors, a reduction in endogenous anticoagulants, and suppressed fibrinolytic activity.[3] Although these changes help maintain placental function during pregnancy and meet delivery's haemostatic challenge, they may also, if exaggerated, predispose to thrombosis and placental vascular complications. These changes are considered in detail in Chapter 21. In brief the concentrations of factors V, VII, VIII, IX, X, XII, and von Willebrand factor increase significantly in pregnancy, accompanied by a pronounced increase

in fibrinogen levels which increase up to twofold from non-pregnant levels.[3] Protein C and antithrombin levels remain within the normal nonpregnant range[4,5] but Protein S (which exists in plasma in two forms: the functionally active free protein S and protein S complexes with C4B-binding protein, which is inactive) falls substantially from early in pregnancy in association with an increase in the C4B-binding protein.[6,7] Activated protein C (APC) resistance is not only associated with factor V Leiden, but is also acquired in association with antiphospholipid antibodies,[8] cancer,[9] and the hormonal changes of pregnancy.[10] At term, 45 percent of pregnant women have an APC sensitivity ratio below the 95th centile for the normal range for nonpregnant women of similar age.[11] Furthermore, the acquired APC resistance of pregnancy correlates directly with thrombin generation in terms of thrombin–antithrombin complexes and indirectly with birthweight.[12] This indicates the potential involvement of alterations in the coagulation system impacting on perinatal outcome. In general the reduction in APC ratio is directly related to its value in the nonpregnant state, being most pronounced in women with the highest APC ratio. Although a reduced response to APC is found in women with antiphospholipid antibodies, the APC ratio has not been found to correlate with antiphospholipid antibodies levels.[13] Indeed, whereas both IgG anticardiolipin and lupus anticoagulant do not change across gestation, they increase significantly post partum.[13] In contrast, autoantibodies to other phospholipid antigens are not increased after delivery.[14] Plasma fibrinolytic activity is reduced during pregnancy, remains low during labor and delivery, but returns to normal shortly after delivery.[3] This is mainly due to increases in plasminogen activator inhibitor (PAI)-1 and PAI-2. The latter is produced by trophoblast and therefore concentrations vary with birthweight, and quantity and quality of placental tissue. Thrombin-activatable fibrinolysis inhibitor (TAFI) is not altered in pregnancy.[15]

HEREDITARY THROMBOPHILIA

Thrombophilic risk factors are common and are found in 15–25 percent of Caucasian populations. Many of the heritable thrombophilias exert their effects by disruption of the endogenous anticoagulant systems, and the antithrombin and protein C/protein S systems.[16] Heritable thrombophilias include deficiencies of the endogenous anticoagulants, antithrombin, and protein C and protein S; genetic mutations in procoagulant factors such as factor V Leiden (*FVL*) and prothrombin G20210A, and the thermolabile (C677T) variant of the methylene tetrahydrofolate reductase (*MTHFR*) gene. Other relatively common thrombophilias with a combination of both heritable and acquired components include elevated factor VIIIc concentrations, hyperhomocysteinemia and acquired APC resistance. The main acquired thrombophilias are anticardiolipin antibodies and lupus anticoagulant. In recent years there has been a rapid increase in the understanding of the contribution of these thrombophilic conditions to venous thromboembolism (VTE), with at least 50 percent of cases of VTE in pregnancy being associated with a known thrombophilia,[17] with attention now being turned to their role in pregnancy complications.

The relative prevalence of these thrombophilias is variable (Table 24.1) with data derived from both asymptomatic populations and women presenting with VTE.[16,17] Qualitative or quantitative deficiencies in antithrombin, protein C and protein S are uncommon (see Table 24.1), with a combined prevalence of <10/1000.[18] Collectively they will present in <10 percent of cases with VTE. In contrast, 2–7 percent of people in Western European

Table 24.1 Prevalence rates for thrombophilia in a European population

Thrombophilic defect	Prevalence (%)
Factor V Leiden heterozygous	2–7
Prothrombin G20210A heterozygous	2
Antithrombin deficiency	0.25–0.55
Protein C deficiency	0.20–0.33
Protein S deficiency	0.03–0.13
MTHFR C677T homozygous	10
Antiphospholipid antibodies	1–5

populations are heterozygous for FVL,[18] however, it is uncommon in other populations, such as Taiwan Chinese, where only 0.2 percent are heterozygous for FVL.[19] Factor V Leiden will usually be identified in 20–40 percent of women with a pregnancy-associated VTE.[20] Activated protein C resistance can also result from problems other than FVL, including antiphospholipid syndrome and other genetic defects in the factor V molecule such as factor V Cambridge or the HR2 haplotype. Although factor V Cambridge is uncommon, the HR2 haplotype is relatively common and has been reported to carry an excess risk of VTE in high-risk patients.[21] Activated protein C resistance is commonly acquired in pregnancy, with 40 percent of pregnant women affected,[6] possibly due to gestational increases in factor V and factor VIII. Such acquired changes are important, as in the nonpregnant state both high levels of factor VIII and APC resistance are associated with an increased risk of VTE independent of the FVL status. Obviously this widely prevalent acquired thrombophilia may interact with an inherited thrombophilia to enhance risk further, and such risk may apply not only to VTE but also adverse pregnancy outcomes. Prothrombin G20210A is present in 2 percent of the Western European population[22] and in approximately 6 percent of patients with VTE, including gestational VTE,[23] and in almost 20 percent of those with a strong family history of VTE.[22] Again this thrombophilia is uncommon in the Taiwan Chinese, where only around 0.2 percent are heterozygous for prothrombin G20210A.[19]

Homozygosity for *MTHFR* C677T is associated with hyperhomocysteinemia. This genotype is not directly related to thrombosis but predisposes to arterial and venous thrombosis where there is concomitant B vitamin deficiency[24] by provoking hyperhomocysteinemia. About 10 percent of individuals in Western European populations are homozygous for this genetic variant. However, such homozygotes do not appear to be at increased risk of pregnancy-related VTE.[24,25] The reasons for this are unclear but may be attributable to the pregnancy-related physiologic reductions in homocysteine levels and/or the effects of folic acid supplementation in pregnancy.[26]

ACQUIRED THROMBOPHILIA

Although pregnancy itself is a physiologic thrombophilic state, many other causes of acquired thrombophilia are found in pregnancy, including antiphospholipid syndrome (APS), ulcerative colitis, diabetes mellitus, Cushing syndrome, preeclampsia, nephrotic syndrome, malignancy, myeloproliferative disorders, liver disease, and ovarian hyperstimulation. The majority of these act through changes in the endogenous coagulation system. However, antiphospholipid antibodies, which have a clear role in adverse pregnancy outcome, represent a heterogeneous collection of autoantibodies united by their reactivity with negatively charged phospholipids components of cell membranes. Although antiphospholipid is an accepted term in respect of

---

Box 24.1 International consensus statement on preliminary criteria for the classification of the APS[27]

Antiphospholipid antibody syndrome is present if at least one of the clinical criteria and one of the laboratory criteria that follow are met:*

Clinical criteria

1 Vascular thrombosis:[†]

One or more clinical episodes[†] of arterial, venous, or small vessel thrombosis,[§] in any tissue or organ. Thrombosis must be confirmed by objective validated criteria (that is, unequivocal findings of appropriate imaging studies or histopathologic examination). For histopathologic confirmation, thrombosis should be present without significant evidence of inflammation in the vessel wall

2 Pregnancy morbidity

(a) One or more unexplained deaths of a morphologically normal fetus at or beyond the tenth week of gestation, with normal fetal morphology documented by ultrasound or by direct examination of the fetus, or

(b) One or more premature births of a morphologically normal neonate before the 34th week of gestation because of: (i) eclampsia or severe preeclampsia defined according to standard definitions,[28] or (ii) recognized features of placental insufficiency,[¶] or

(c) Three or more unexplained consecutive spontaneous abortions before the tenth week of gestation, with maternal anatomic or hormonal abnormalities and paternal and maternal chromosomal causes excluded

In studies of populations of patients who have more than one type of pregnancy morbidity, investigators are strongly encouraged to stratify groups of subjects according to a, b, or c above

Laboratory criteria

1 Lupus anticoagulant (LA) present in plasma, on two or more occasions at least 12 weeks apart, detected according to the guidelines of the International Society on Thrombosis and Haemostasis (Scientific Subcommittee on LAs/phospholipid-dependent antibodies)[29,30]

2 Anticardiolipin (aCL) antibody of IgG and/or IgM isotype in serum or plasma, present in medium or high titer (that is, >40 GPL or MPL, or >the 99th percentile), on two or more occasions, at least 12 weeks apart, measured by a standardized enzyme-linked immunosorbent assay (ELISA)[31–33]

3 Anti-β_2 glycoprotein-I antibody of IgG and/or IgM isotype in serum or plasma (in titer >the 99th percentile), present on two or more occasions, at least 12 weeks apart, measured by a standardized ELISA, according to recommended procedures[34]

*Classification of APS should be avoided if less than 12 weeks or more than 5 years separate the positive aPL test and the clinical manifestation

[†]Coexisting inherited or acquired factors for thrombosis are not reasons for excluding patients from APS trials. However, two subgroups of APS patients should be recognized, according to: (a) the presence, and (b) the absence of additional risk factors for thrombosis. Indicative (but not exhaustive) such cases include: age (>55 in men, and >65 in women), and the presence of any of the established risk factors for cardiovascular disease. (Hypertension, diabetes mellitus, elevated low-density lipoprotein [LDL] or low high-density lipoprotein [HDL]-cholesterol, cigarette smoking, family history of premature cardiovascular disease, body mass index [†]30 kg/m², microalbuminuria, estimated glomerular filtration rate <60 mL/min), inherited thrombophilias, oral contraceptives, nephrotic syndrome, malignancy, immobilization, and surgery. Thus, patients who fulfill criteria should be stratified according to contributing causes of thrombosis.

[†]A thrombotic episode in the past could be considered as a clinical criterion, provided that thrombosis is proved by appropriate diagnostic means and that no alternative diagnosis or cause of thrombosis is found.

[§]Superficial venous thrombosis is not included in the clinical criteria

[¶]Generally accepted features of placental insufficiency include: (i) abnormal or nonreassuring fetal surveillance test(s), for example, a nonreactive nonstress test, suggestive of fetal hypoxemia, (ii) abnormal Doppler flow velocimetry waveform analysis suggestive of fetal hypoxemia, for example, absent end-diastolic flow in the umbilical artery, (iii) oligohydramnios, for example, an amniotic fluid index of 5 cm or less, or (iv) a postnatal birth weight less than the 10th percentile for the gestational age.

---

the clinical syndrome, it is a misnomer in that the autoantibodies of clinical relevance are directed against phospholipid-binding proteins, or conformation epitopes involving the binding proteins, and not against the phospholipid antigens *per se*. Thus, many antiphospholipid antibodies require β_2-glycoprotein-I (β_2-GP-1), a phospholipid-binding plasma protein with weak anticoagulant activity, for binding to acidic phospholipids such as phosphatidylserine and cardiolipin. An international consensus statement on preliminary criteria for the classification of APS states that a patient with APS must meet at least one of the two clinical criteria (vascular thrombosis or complications of pregnancy, as defined in

Box 24.1) and at least one of two laboratory criteria. Antiphospholipid syndrome is considered in more depth in Chapter 8.

The prevalence of antiphospholipid autoantibodies (LA and aCL) in the general obstetric population has been reported as approximately 2 percent,[35] which is comparable with those found in healthy young control subjects where the prevalence is 1–5 percent.[36] The range in prevalence reflects inter-laboratory differences in cut-off levels used, variation in assay methods for detection of antibodies and population profiles.[37] The prevalence in selected populations with fetal loss is higher.

HEMOSTASIS AND MECHANISM FOR ADVERSE PREGNANCY OUTCOME

Successful pregnancy is dependent upon trophoblast invasion into the uterine vasculature and on the development and maintenance of an adequate uteroplacental circulation in the mother. The architecture and function of the placenta require certain hemostatic features and give rise to potential target sites for pathologic coagulation including maternal uteroplacental circulation, the basal plate, the intervillous space, the villous surface, and the fetoplacental vasculature. Disruption by thrombosis at any of these sites may lead to impaired blood flow and consequently the perinatal complications of miscarriage, IUGR, preeclampsia with fetal compromise, and stillbirth.

Hemostatic mechanisms within the placenta may be disturbed by either maternal or fetal signals, as although maternal blood flows in placental intervillous spaces, the cells in contact are embryonic trophoblast cells. Therefore, systemic blood components such as coagulation factors, protein C or protein S are of maternal origin, whereas cellular regulatory components such as the initiator of blood coagulation tissue factor (TF), or the anticoagulant proteins – thrombomodulin, the endothelial protein C receptor and annexin V – are of fetal origin and operate at the interface. Some components may be derived from both maternal and embryonic origin such as tissue factor pathway inhibitor (TFPI), locally secreted by endothelial cells and trophoblasts fibrinolytic system: tissue plasminogen activator (tPA) and urokinase (uPA), which can be secreted from vessel cells following stimuli of cytokines or growth factors. Balance of these prothrombotic and anticoagulant factors is essential for normal placental development.

The main activator of coagulation, TF, is a glycoprotein produced by monocytes and endothelial cells, fibroblasts, macrophages, and placental trophoblasts. It has been localized to trophoblasts lining intervilli spaces and the presence of large amounts of ready-to-use TF seems to be essential for the maintenance of hemostasis in the placenta and uterus.[2] Lack of functional TF causes lethal defects in mice before e11.5, which is associated with abnormalities of vasculature in the yolk sac. Disruption of the TF pathway inhibitor gene has consequences almost identical to those of the elimination of the TF gene. This can be studied in a transgenic mouse which expresses low amounts of human TF (L-TF) and no murine TF. L-TF mice have a 14–18 percent incidence of fatal postpartum hemorrhage, suggesting that TF plays a role in uterine hemostasis.[38] L-TF mated with L-TF had a 42 percent incidence of fatal mid-gestational hemorrhage. Placentas of low TF embryos were abnormal and contained numerous maternal blood pools in the labyrinth.[38]

Thrombomodulin, a membrane receptor participating in the activation of protein C, was initially isolated and characterized in crude extracts of human placenta.[39] Thrombomodulin is located on the endothelium of placental vessels and also on the apical membranes of syncytiotrophoblasts, with a 2.3-fold increase of thrombomodulin by term compared with first-trimester placentas.[40] This high level of thrombomodulin expression was associated with a significantly increased ability to activate protein C. Thrombomodulin protein expression and biologic activity were also found in syncytial membranes prepared from placentas.[40] Increased plasma and urinary thrombomodulin levels were reported in preeclamptic pregnancies, suggesting a potential involvement of placental thrombomodulin in this complication.[40] Increased thrombomodulin resulting from placental vascular damage was considered to be a marker for placental abruption.[41] Studies of thrombomodulin knockout mice have demonstrated that thrombomodulin-null mice succumb to complete early mid-gestation (e8.5) growth arrest, followed by the rapid resorption and lethal consumptive coagulopathy of all mutant embryos within 24 hours. The growth arrest and abortion of thrombomodulin-null mice is caused by a failure of placental trophoblast function, because the development of thrombomodulin-null mice proceeds normally as long as thrombomodulin expression is selectively maintained only in this particular type of cell.[42] Maternal anti-coagulation therapy with either warfarin or low-molecular-weight heparin (LMWH) delays resorption of $TM^{-/-}$ embryos but does not overcome the observed growth defect. This is attributable to incomplete inhibition of coagulation factor function as selective reduction of embryonic tissue factor to <1 percent of normal levels completely rescues thrombomodulin knockout-mice, in contrast to maternal reduction which did not.[43]

Protein C which inactivates factors Va and VIIIa, and controls fibrin degradation by attenuating the activity of PAI-1, is also essential for development. Total genetic deficiency of protein C results in death in the early neonatal period secondary to disseminated intravascular coagulation and widespread microvascular thrombosis.[44] Maternal protein C expression is also required to sustain pregnancies beyond the early embryonic period, as demonstrated by transgenic mouse studies.[45] Thus, a lack of APC either due to a thrombomodulin deficiency or low maternal protein C levels, facilitates TF to cause unfettered coagulation disrupting development. The downstream events of this include the generation of thrombin, conversion of the thrombin substrate fibrinogen into fibrin, and subsequent generation of fibrin split products, resulting in the death of trophoblast. In support of this is the frequently reported association between fibrin depositions and trophoblast apoptosis in pathologic human pregnancy.[46,47] In human and mouse trophoblasts, the tissue and urokinase-type plasminogen activators are abundantly expressed,[48–50] with both distinct fast-acting inhibitors of plasminogen activator, PAI-1 and PAI-2, present in normal human placenta tissue. However, mainly endothelial cells synthesize PAI-1, the physiologic inhibitor of both urokinase and tPA. Overexpression of PAI-1 may compromise normal fibrin clearance mechanisms and promote pathologic fibrin deposition, when the clotting cascade is activated. The presence of PAI-1 and the expression of mRNA have been studied in normal and pathologic pregnancies.[51,52] Plasma and placental PAI-1 levels are significantly elevated in pregnant women with severe preeclampsia, with localization of increased mRNA and protein expression to placental villous syncytiotrophoblasts from women with preeclampsia compared to normal pregnancies.[53] Hypertensive pregnancies have also been shown to have higher placental PAI-2 and fibrinoid material.[54] The overexpression of PAI could effect the rapid degradation of fibrin at the trophoblast surface. Thrombomodulin, in addition to inhibiting coagulation, also inhibits fibrin degradation by enhancing the activation of plasma carboxypeptidase U and TAFI.[55,56] Thrombomodulin thus prevents placental injury not only by suppressing the formation of thrombin and fibrin, but also by limiting the generation of fibrin split products.

Collectively these results demonstrate that close regulation of the hemostatic systems is required at the fetomaternal interface, with trophoblast not only potentially predisposing the placental vascular bed to organ-specific thrombosis, but also closely regulating hemostasis.[57] It can therefore modify the potential response to inherited and acquired thrombophilia of the mother, with abnormalities in this interaction presenting with various clinical scenarios including miscarriage, IUGR, preeclampsia, abruption, and stillbirth.

THROMBOPHILIA AND ADVERSE PREGNANCY OUTCOME

Miscarriage is common affecting 25 percent of conceptions; greater attention therefore focuses on women with recurrent pregnancy loss. Recurrent fetal loss is a frequent problem, with three or more successive losses affecting 1–2 percent of women of reproductive age and two or more successive losses affecting around 5 percent. A small number of such pregnancy losses are due to identifiable anatomic, chromosomal, endocrinological, or immunological problems in the mother or fetus. However, in the majority of cases of recurrent fetal losses, at least in the past, no cause has been identified. Recent data show that prothrombotic

changes, secondary to both acquired and inherited thrombophilias are associated with a substantial proportion of these fetal losses (Table 24.2). The most compelling evidence is derived from studies in women with antiphospholipid antibodies, which show that anticardiolipin antibodies (odds ratio [OR] 3.40, 95 percent confidence interval [CI] 1.33 to 8.68) and lupus anticoagulants (OR 2.97, 95 percent CI 1.03 to 8.56) are associated not only with increased thrombin generation but also with increased risk of early fetal loss. Furthermore prevention of fetal loss in these women is achievable by antithrombotic therapy, in particular heparin and low-dose aspirin.[59] There is therefore growing interest in whether other forms of inherited and acquired thrombophilias also predispose women to adverse pregnancy outcome and whether this can be ameliorated by antithrombotic interventions.

Hereditary thrombophilia is a relatively common finding in women with early fetal loss. A recent systematic review by Robertson et al. examined 25 studies with 7167 women and the association between thrombophilia and inherited early pregnancy loss, and showed a positive association overall (Table 24.2).[58] In particular significant associations were observed in carriers of homozygous FVL (OR 2.71, 95 percent CI 1.32 to 5.58), heterozygous FVL (OR 1.68, 95 percent CI 1.09 to 2.58) and prothrombin heterozygosity (OR 2.49, 95 percent CI 1.24 to 5.00). On examining the risk of recurrent first trimester loss FVL (OR 1.91, 95 percent CI 1.01 to 3.61), prothrombin heterozygosity (OR 2.70, 95 percent CI 1.37 to 5.34) still showed an association with recurrent loss, as did the acquired thrombophilias of anticardiolipin antibodies (OR 5.05, 95 percent CI 1.82 to 14.01) and hyperhomocysteinemia (OR 4.21, 95 percent CI 1.28 to 13.87). Indeed this association with fetal loss extended in to the second trimester and was stronger for both FVL (OR 4.12, 95 percent CI 1.93 to 8.81) and prothrombin heterozygosity (OR 8.60, 95 percent CI 2.18 to 33.95). This systematic review partially addresses some of the inconsistencies between the previously reported case control and cohort studies, which may reflect problems

Table 24.2   Risk of early loss in woman with thrombophilia

Thrombophilic defect	Thrombophilia n/N	No thrombophilia n/N	OR (95% CI)
Factor V Leiden homozygous	37/76	484/1010	2.71 (1.32 to 5.58)
Factor V Leiden heterozygous	172/243	1632/2689	1.68 (1.09 to 2.58)
Prothrombin heterozygous	53/75	657/1356	2.49 (1.24 to 5.00)
MTHFR homozygous	53/75	534/907	1.40 (0.77 to 2.55)
Antithrombin deficiency	2/8	54/196	0.88 (0.17 to 4.48)
Protein C deficiency	2/3	34/73	2.29 (0.20 to 26.43)
Protein S deficiency	3/4	33/72	3.55 (0.35 to 35.72)
Anticardiolipin antibodies	127/149	869/1956	3.40 (1.33 to 8.68)
Lupus anticoagulants	59/107	581/1728	2.97 (1.03 to 9.76)
Acquired activated protein C resistance	102/113	63/199	4.04 (1.67 to 9.76)
Hyperhomocysteinemia	33/37	128/235	6.25 (1.37 to 28.42)

Data derived from Robertson et al.[58]
n, number of events; N, number of women studies in each category.

with small sample size, and clearly supports an association with both acquired and inherited thrombophilia and early, recurrent, and late fetal loss.

In addition to recurrent fetal loss there is now evidence linking thrombophilia to an unexplained first pregnancy loss. In a prospective cohort study of 2480 pregnant women, 106 women had APC resistance which was not attributable to FVL.[60] This cohort was characterized by an increased risk of second trimester fetal loss, although no increase in preeclampsia, small for gestational age babies, first trimester fetal loss, or abnormal blood loss was observed. The 'NOHA first' study also describes a large carefully designed case–control study nested in a cohort of nearly 32 700 women of whom 18 percent had pregnancy loss with first gestation.[61] The analysis compared 3496 pairs of women with an unexplained pregnancy loss with normal pregnancy controls and examined the incidence of FVL and factor II G20210A in these groups. The findings of the multivariate analysis clearly demonstrated an overall association between unexplained first pregnancy loss between 10 and 39 weeks gestation and the two thrombophilic risk factors FVL (OR 3.46, 95 percent CI 2.53 to 4.72) and factor II G20210A (OR 2.60, 95 percent CI 1.86 to 3.64), although no association was observed in losses prior to 10 weeks. As unexplained first pregnancy loss occurred in about 10.9 percent of gestations, these findings have substantial clinical impact and suggest that all women who have a first unexplained pregnancy loss after 10 weeks of gestation should be screened for thrombophilia.

The widespread vascular damage of preeclampsia associated with endothelial dysfunction, enhanced coagulation, and fibrin deposition suggests a role for thrombophilia as a potentially modifiable risk factor. Intrauterine growth restriction is also associated with thrombosis and placental infarction on the maternal side, again implicating the hemostatic system. Thus, not only could women with thrombophilia be predisposed to failure to establish an adequate placenta and therefore experience fetal loss, but potentially also late pregnancy complications. Indeed in women with antiphospholipid antibodies there is evidence of an increase in thrombin generation[62,63] and thrombotic placental infarction.[64] The

risk of later pregnancy complications in this group of women is even increased despite treatment with low-dose aspirin and heparin.[59,65] For example, gestational hypertension complicates 17 percent of such ongoing pregnancies, antepartum hemorrhage 7 percent, preterm delivery 24 percent, and 15 percent of the neonates are small for gestational age.[66,67]

Since the original association of preeclampsia with antiphospholipid syndrome in 1989[68] and inherited thrombophilia in 1995,[69] a number of case–control and cohort studies have examined the association with thrombophilia. Some of these have supported the association whereas others have refuted it. Robertson et al. examined 25 studies with 11 183 women detailing the risk of thrombophilia and preeclampsia (Table 24.3).[58] The risk of preeclampsia was significantly associated with heterozygous FVL (OR 2.19, 95 percent CI 1.46 to 3.27), heterozygous prothrombin (OR 2.54, 95 percent CI 1.52 to 4.23), MTHFR homozygosity (OR 1.37, 95 percent CI 1.07 to 1.76), aCL antibodies (OR 2.73, 95 percent CI 1.65 to 4.51), and hyperhomocysteinemia (OR 3.49, 95 percent CI 1.21–10.11). Preeclampsia was the only outcome for which a significant association with homozygosity for MTHFR C677T was found. Overall the increase in risk of preeclampsia with thrombophilia is modest. Thrombophilia is not considered an etiological factor for preeclampsia but rather may contribute to the severity of preeclampsia because of an exaggerated effect on the hemostatic system in women with thrombophilia.[70,71]

The association of thrombophilia with IUGR is more controversial. A number of case–control studies have demonstrated an association, whereas other studies have refuted this occurrence. An association has been demonstrated in women with severe IUGR, but not in milder cases. Martinelli et al. studied 63 women with history of IUGR, defined as birthweight under the 10th percentile, and 93 parous women with uneventful pregnancies.[72] Among women with IUGR, 13 percent had FVL compared with 2.2 percent controls (OR 6.9, 95 percent CI 1.4 to 33.5), and 12 percent had prothrombin mutation compared with 2.2 percent in controls (OR 5.9, 95 percent CI 1.2 to 29.4). In a regression analysis model these thrombophilias were independently associated with IUGR. A

Table 24.3   Risk of preeclampsia in woman with thrombophilia

Thrombophilic defect	Thrombophilia n/N	No thrombophilia n/N	OR (95% CI)
Factor V Leiden homozygous	4/5	608/1143	1.87 (0.44 to 7.88)
Factor V Leiden heterozygous	161/249	1790/3673	2.19 (1.46 to 3.27)
Prothrombin heterozygous	42/71	937/2028	2.54 (1.52 to 4.23)
MTHFR homozygous	221/481	1234/3205	1.37 (1.07 to 1.76)
Antithrombin deficiency	1/1	57/131	3.89 (0.16 to 97.19)
Protein C deficiency	3/3	60/104	5.15 (0.26 to 102.22)
Protein S deficiency	14/20	158/402	2.83 (0.76 to 10.57)
Anticardiolipin antibodies	130/217	803/2428	2.73 (1.65 to 4.51)
Lupus anticoagulants	63/89	426/981	1.45 (0.70 to 4.61)
Hyperhomocysteinemia	37/41	257/364	3.49 (1.21 to 10.11)

Data derived from Robertson et al.[57]
n, number of events; N, number of women studies in each category.

later report from the same group tested these mutations in neonates weighing less than 2500 g.[73] Neonates delivered by mothers with FVL or prothrombin mutations accounted for 30 percent of newborns weighing less than 1000 g, 18.7 percent ranging from 1001 g to 2499 g, and only 9.5 percent weighing 2500 g or more. Overall, 27.6 percent of neonates of mothers with the mutations weighed less than 2500 g compared with 13.9 percent in neonates of mothers without mutations (OR 2.4, 95 percent CI 1.5 to 3.7). Infante-Rivard *et al.* did not find an association between thrombophilic mutations and IUGR less than 10th percentile.[74] In this study the prevalence of thrombophilia in mothers of 493 newborns with IUGR and 472 controls did not differ significantly. However, a third of the studied population was not white and the degree of IUGR was mild, with mean birth weight of 2393 ± 606 g and 83 percent of newborns delivered at 36–40 weeks' gestation. In contrast, in the study by Kupferminc *et al.* the mean birth weight was 1387 ± 616 g and mean gestational week was 33 ± 4.0.[75] Similarly, Martinelli *et al.* reported a mean gestational week at delivery of 35 ± 3 and a mean birthweight of 1584 ± 586 g.[72] These differences suggest that the studies are dealing with noncomparable fetal and neonatal populations with different clinical relevance. An overview of these IUGR data[58] is shown in Table 24.4, detailing women from five studies (n = 195) including the study by Yusada *et al.*,[76] which examined the risk of IUGR in the presence of antiphospholipid antibodies. These studies suggest a general trend of increased IUGR risk in women with

thrombophilia, and in combination with previous subgroup analysis, there is a suggestion that this effect would be greatest in women with severe IUGR.[77]

Placental abruption is a devastating clinical condition. Although only occurring in 0.5 percent of gestations, it carries a high fetal mortality and significant maternal risk. Risk factors for placental abruption include preeclampsia, prior abruption, sudden uterine decompression, chemical teratogens, external trauma, and uterine malformations.[79] A potential association with thrombophilia is suggested by a number of studies. Wiener-Megnagi *et al.* studied 27 women who had abruption and 29 control subjects matched for age, parity, and ethnic origin.[78] In the group of patients making up the cases, 63 percent had an APC ratio of 2.5 or less, compared with 17 percent of control subjects with an OR of 8.16 (*P* = 0.001). Of 15 patients, 8 were found to have FVL, compared with one heterozygote in the control group (3.4 percent). In another study thrombophilia was found in 70 percent of 20 women with placental abruption,[79] and the odds ratio for factor II 20210G > A mutation was 8.9 (95 percent CI 1.8 to 43.6), whereas the odds ratio for FVL was 4.9 (95 percent CI, 1.0 to 17.4). The finding of an increased incidence of venous thrombosis in first-degree relatives of women with placental abruption also suggests a higher prevalence of thrombophilia. An overview of these data on abruption is shown in Table 24.5,[58] with the strongest association being seen in women who are heterozygous for prothrombin OR 7.71 (95 percent CI 3.01 to 19.76).

Table 24.4   Risk of intrauterine growth restriction in woman with thrombophilia

Thrombophilic defect	Thrombophilia n/N	No thrombophilia n/N	OR (95% CI)
Factor V Leiden homozygous	1/1	60/153	4.64 (0.19 to 115.68)
Factor V Leiden heterozygous	25/49	512/1147	2.68 (0.59 to 12.13)
Prothrombin heterozygous	25/44	583/1375	2.92 (0.62 to 13.70)
MTHFR homozygous	62/121	460/961	1.24 (0.84 to 1.82)
Anticardiolipin antibodies	7/60	15/800	6.91 (2.70 to 17.68)

Data derived from Robertson *et al.*[57]
n, number of events; N, number of women studies in each category.

Table 24.5   Risk of abruption in woman with thrombophilia

Thrombophilic defect	Thrombophilia n/N	No thrombophilia n/N	OR (95% CI)
Factor V Leiden homozygous	3/3	24/53	8.43 (0.41 to 171.20)
Factor V Leiden heterozygous	13/28	64/332	4.70 (1.13 to 19.59)
Prothrombin heterozygous	10/20	44/400	7.71 (3.01 to 19.76)
MTHFR homozygous	3/14	40/183	1.47 (0.40 to 5.35)
Antithrombin deficiency	1/2	26/54	1.08 (0.06 to 18.12)
Protein C deficiency	1/1	22/66	5.93 (0.23 to 151.58)
Protein S deficiency	4/8	19/59	2.11 (0.47 to 9.34)
Anticardiolipin antibodies	6/12	44/111	1.42 (0.42 to 4.77)
Acquired activated protein C resistance	5/13	18/54	1.25 (0.36 to 4.37)
Hyperhomocysteinemia	32/42	96/195	2.40 (0.36 to 15.89)

Data derived from Robertson *et al.*[57]
n, number of events; N, number of women studies in each category.

ANTITHROMBOTIC THERAPY

Given the evidence for thrombophilia in the etiology of some adverse pregnancy outcomes, clinicians are increasingly using antithrombotic therapy in women at risk of such complications, despite limited evidence of benefit. Thromboprophylaxis in pregnancy centers on the use of unfractionated heparin (UFH) or LMWH due to the fetal hazards of coumarins[80] (see Chapter 11). Coumarin embryopathy is characterized by midface hypoplasia, stippled chondral calcification, scoliosis, short proximal limbs and short phalanges, and affects 5 percent of fetuses exposed to the drug between 6 and 9 weeks gestation. In addition coumarin use has been associated with an increase in delayed neurodevelopment independent of the increased risk of hemorrhage in the mother and fetus.[81] Neither UFH[82] nor LMWH[83,84] cross the placenta, as determined by measuring anti-Xa activity in fetal blood, and thus there is no evidence of teratogenesis or risk of fetal hemorrhage. Although for many years UFH was the standard anticoagulant used during and outwith pregnancy, LMWH has now replaced UFH for the acute treatment of VTE in the nonpregnant population. In Europe and Australasia LMWH is now the preferred choice for prevention and treatment of VTE in pregnancy.[85] The advantages of LMWH over UFH include an enhanced ratio of anti-Xa (anti-thrombotic) to anti-IIa (anticoagulant), resulting in a reduced risk of bleeding, stable and predictable pharmacokinetics with increased bioavailability and half-life, allowing less frequent fixed or weight-based dosing without the need for monitoring, subcutaneous administration, less activation of platelets, with less binding to platelet factor 4 substantially reducing the risk of heparin-induced thrombocytopenia (HIT).[86] A major concern with the widespread use of UFH in pregnancy has been the 2 percent risk of symptomatic heparin-induced osteoporotic fracture in pregnancy.[86] LMWHs are associated with a substantially lower risk of this devastating complication.[76]

Until recently the data on the efficacy of LMWH in pregnancy as evidenced by incidence of recurrent or new VTE, and the safety of LMWHs, measured by the incidence of severe bleeding, allergic skin reaction, HIT and osteoporosis was limited to individual studies and a systematic review several years ago when data were much more limited.[87] To try to provide accurate quantification of risk for use of LMWH in pregnancy Greer and Nelson-Piercy performed a systematic review of 64 studies encompassing 2777 pregnancies that reported outcomes but excluding women receiving LMWH for mechanical heart valves.[88] In 174 patients the indication for LMWH was treatment of acute VTE, with 2 women (1.15 percent) experiencing recurrent VTE. This compares favorably with recurrence rates of 5–8 percent reported in trials carried out in nonpregnant patients treated with LMWH or UFH followed by coumarin therapy who were followed up for 3 or 6 months. In 2603 pregnancies LMWH was used for either thromboprophylaxis (n = 1348), prevention of adverse pregnancy

outcome (n = 535) or unspecified prophylaxis (n = 720). In the 2603 women receiving thromboprophylactic doses 0.54 percent of women experienced a DVT, 0.19 percent a pulmonary embolus and 0.12 percent an unspecified VTE. Thus the risk of VTE in pregnancy despite LMWH thromboprophylaxis was 0.84 percent. These data demonstrate that LMWHs provide effective thromboprophylaxis in pregnancy, and although not directly comparable, the risk of VTE was 2.4 percent in a cohort of women with a single previous VTE subsequently managed during pregnancy without any specific thromboprophylaxis.[89] In addition to these venous thrombotic events, 0.54 percent of women experienced an arterial thrombosis while on prophylaxis with LMWH, however, all of these events were transient ischemic attacks in women on LMWH because of antiphospholipid syndrome. With respect to bleeding complications, significant antepartum hemorrhage occurred in 0.42 percent, postpartum hemorrhage in 0.92 percent and a wound hematoma in 0.65 percent. It is reassuring therefore to observe that use of LMWH was not associated with an increased risk of bleeding peripartum. Further, the incidence of these bleeding episodes combined was 1.99 percent, which compares favorably with the rate of massive hemorrhage (defined as blood loss >1500 mL) of 0.7 percent as determined in a prospective study of patients who were not receiving LMWH.[90]

Greer and Nelson-Piercy[88] also reported that allergic skin reactions were observed in 1.84 percent of patients and were more common with the use of dalteparin and nadroparin than with enoxaparin. A low platelet count, defined as $<100 \times 10^9/L$ was only observed in 0.08 percent of women, and there were no cases of thrombosis associated with HIT.[76] This is consistent with previous reports in other patient groups of a substantially lower incidence of HIT with LMWH use compared to UFH. However, as nurture gestational thrombocytopenia can complicate up to 7 percent of pregnancies, and thrombocytopenia also occurs with preeclampsia[91] this may represent underreporting of thrombocytopenia or bias towards not attributing it to LMWH use. Nonetheless the low rate of HIT in this study is reassuring. It is also consistent with the recent recommendation of the American College of Chest Physicians (ACCP) that there is no need to monitor platelet counts in pregnant patients treated exclusively with LMWH,[92] as it is the use of UFH which often sensitizes women to heparin and the occurrence of HIT on subsequent LMWH exposure. Only one clinically evident osteoporotic complication was reported in this systematic review, and this was a single well-documented case of postpartum osteoporotic vertebral fracture in a woman who had received a high dose (15 000 IU daily) of dalteparin for a total of 36 weeks. However, there has been a report of three osteoporotic fractures secondary to tinzaparin use in pregnancy in a single center.[93] At present it is unclear whether this was related to specific patients factors or was tinzaparin specific or was a dose-related effect. It therefore appears that LMWH is safe in pregnancy and effective for thromboprophylaxis. On this basis, LMWH is now being extended as therapy for placental vascular conditions where excessive thrombosis is implicated in the pathogenesis.

THERAPEUTIC INTERVENTIONS FOR ACQUIRED AND INHERITED THROMBOPHILIA

The use of antithrombotic therapy, in particular aspirin and heparin, has been particularly studied in fetal loss related to antiphospholipid syndrome,[59] and addressed in a Cochrane review. A total of 849 participants were enrolled in 13 trials,[59] which were heterogeneous with regard to the trial design and the interventions studied. Three trials compared aspirin with placebo or standard care (n = 135).[94-96] Six explored the efficacy of heparin combined with aspirin; two of these used low-molecular-weight heparin (LWMH) combined with aspirin (n = 140) and compared this to aspirin alone[97] or intravenous immunoglobulin (IVIG).[98] The others used unfractionated heparin combined with aspirin; two compared the combination to aspirin alone (n = 140);[99,100] one compared low-dose with high-dose heparin both combined with aspirin (n = 50);[101] and one compared the combination with prednisone and aspirin (n = 45).[102] Two trials compared heparin with placebo or aspirin (n = 241).[103,104] Three trials used IVIG; in one study all participants received aspirin and heparin with the addition of either IVIG or placebo (n = 16).[105] Another study included above compared IVIG to LMWH and aspirin (n = 42).[98] The third study compared IVIG to prednisone and aspirin (n = 82).[106]

Of the interventions examined, only UFH combined with aspirin was shown to reduce the incidence of pregnancy loss (relative risk [RR] 0.46, 95 percent CI 0.29 to 0.71) when compared with aspirin alone.[59] Low-molecular-weight heparin combined with aspirin had no statistically significant effect when compared to aspirin alone (RR 0.78, 95 percent CI 0.39 to 1.57) or intravenous immunoglobulin (IVIG) (RR 0.37, 95 percent CI 0.12 to 1.16); however, the point estimates are in the direction of benefit, although the confidence intervals are wide. No head-to-head study comparing LMWH and unfractionated heparin were included and, therefore, the relative effects of UFH versus LMWH are essentially unknown in this situation. However, if the effect is mediated through the antithrombotic effects of LMWH then the superior properties of LMWH compared to UFH in heparin would be expected to be of value. One recent study reported that the combination of LMWH and aspirin is as effective as UFH and aspirin in women with recurrent pregnancy loss, with 21 of 25 patients on LMWH delivering a viable fetus compared to 20 out of 25 in the UFH group.[107] Comparing all studies, the treatment advantage of UFH was maintained with the composite adverse pregnancy outcomes of 'pregnancy loss or intrauterine growth restriction (IUGR)' (RR 0.57, 95 percent CI 0.39 to 0.83) and 'pregnancy loss or premature delivery' (RR 0.65, 95 percent CI 0.47 to 0.91). The LMWH studies did not

provide IUGR data but they did include premature delivery data. The risk of 'pregnancy loss or premature delivery' when LMWH combined with aspirin was compared to aspirin or IVIG was similar to the UFH studies, although they do not reach statistical significance (RR 0.70, 95 percent CI 0.39 to 1.29 and RR 0.49, 95 percent CI 0.18 to 1.34, respectively). High-dose UFH did not differ from low-dose UFH in its effects. Thrombocytopenia was either not reported or did not occur, except in one study where it was described as mild in two women receiving LMWH.[98] Intriguingly the use of aspirin alone showed no effect over placebo. Therefore, although inconclusive there is the suggestion that it is the heparin which is having the beneficial effect in these combination regimens.

When the LMWH and UFH studies are pooled there is a 35 percent reduction in pregnancy loss or premature delivery (RR 0.65, 95 percent CI 0.49 to 0.86).[59] The rationale for this pooling within the Cochrane dataset is unclear as the two types of heparin have quite different biologic characteristics, despite recent evidence of equal efficacy.[107] However, on the basis of this pooling of data it is now recommended that all women with recurrent miscarriage should be screened for antiphospholipid syndrome and affected women treated with low-dose aspirin and LMWH, such as enoxaparin or dalteparin.

Antithrombotic therapy in women with inherited thrombophilia and recurrent pregnancy loss has been examined in small and predominantly uncontrolled trials or observational studies. Administration of LMWH (enoxaparin 20 mg/day), to women with primary early recurrent fetal loss and impaired fibrinolytic capacity, resulted in normalization of fibrinolysis. Sixteen of 20 conceived and a live birth occurred in 13 (81 percent).[108] A systematic review of LMWH use reported pregnancy outcomes in 2215 pregnancies treated with LMWH.[88] Successful outcome was defined as a live birth and excluded neonatal deaths. The studies were subdivided as: treatment with LMWH in 370 pregnancies with a history of recurrent pregnancy loss, of these 85.4 percent had successful outcomes, and in 1845 pregnancies where LMWH was given for thromboprophylaxis or the treatment of VTE, 96.6 percent had a successful outcome. A further study showed that LMWH use in 61 pregnancies in 50 women with a history of thrombophilia and recurrent fetal loss resulted in 46 live births (75 percent) compared with a success rate of only 20 percent in these 50 women in prior gestations without antithrombotic therapy.[109] Carp et al. reported that antenatal treatment with enoxaparin in women with hereditary thrombophilia is associated with live birth in 26 (70.2 percent) of 37 compared with 21 (43.8 percent) in untreated patients,[110] but this was a cohort study rather than a controlled trial. These preliminary results were encouraging and further evidence has been generated by the LIVE-ENOX trial examining two dose regimen of enoxaparin, 40 mg or 80 mg/day in women with recurrent pregnancy loss.[111,112] Of the 166 women completing the study, 135 gestations resulted in live births: 70 (84.3 percent) in the 40 mg/day group and 65 (78.3 percent) in the 80 mg/day group. There was no significant difference in pregnancy outcome between the 40 mg/day and 80 mg/day enoxaparin groups. The live birth rate with enoxaparin prophylaxis was 78.0 percent for women with APC resistance and FVL, 84.4 percent for *MTHFR* gene C677T homozygotes and hyperhomocysteinemia, 76.9 percent for antiphospholipid syndrome and 81.3 percent for other types of thrombophilia. Differences in live birth rate between types of thrombophilia were not statistically significant ($P = 0.484$). There has been considerable debate about this trial.[113] As Lindqvist and Merlo[114] rightly point out the study has many limitations, particularly the absence of an untreated control group, the heterogeneous entry criteria and the risk of regression toward the mean, with the use of a historic comparison group. However, at present, given that we have no effective treatment for recurrent pregnancy loss other than possibly LMWH, which carries minimal risk in pregnancy, clinicians, and patients will continue to use and request such therapy until data from randomized controlled trials are available,[113] so emphasizing the pressing need for adequately controlled randomized trials in this area.

To further complicate the debate over antithrombotic treatment for pregnancy loss, a recent study by Gris *et al.* demonstrated that treatment with 40 mg enoxaparin daily in women with a thrombophilia (FVL, prothrombin G20210A or protein S deficiency) and one previous pregnancy loss after 10 weeks gestation, resulted in a significantly better live birth rate (86 percent) compared with low-dose aspirin alone (29 percent).[115] As there was no untreated group and as the pregnancy success rate is relatively high after one miscarriage, it is difficult to assess the implications of these results.

When the data from the studies described above are combined, there is significant circumstantial evidence that LMWH may improve the pregnancy outcome in women with thrombophilia and pregnancy loss. Therefore, until results from randomized controlled trials are available we would suggest that clinicians consider the use of prophylaxis with LMWH, such as 40 mg enoxaparin daily, throughout gestation, in women with thrombophilia and a pregnancy loss after 10 weeks in their first pregnancy or who have experienced recurrent pregnancy loss.

SCREENING FOR INHERITED THROMBOPHILIA IN PREGNANCY

The association of thrombophilias with VTE in pregnancy and adverse perinatal outcome, and the realization that treatment with anticoagulants may prevent some adverse events,[100] has prompted calls for widespread screening of the antenatal population. We have previously demonstrated that universal screening for FVL in pregnancy is not cost-effective in terms of the cost for management of VTE complications.[116] Similarly even use of selective screening based on a personal or family (in a first-degree relative)

history of VTE was not cost-effective for pregnancy management. However, this study did not address any of the maternal or neonatal costs associated with perinatal complications, instead concentrating on diagnosis and VTE treatment costs. Of the 967 women in the cohort 30 had FVL and of these 6 (20 percent) had a vascular complication which was defined as miscarriage, stillbirth, VTE, IUGR, or preeclampsia. Only 1 of the 87 women identified within the overall cohort with a vascular complication had a VTE, therefore the majority of vascular events were not related to VTE but rather to obstetric complications. Preeclampsia and IUGR are the leading causes of iatrogenic prematurity and the care of both the mother and the premature infants is associated with significant costs.

In a subsequent study some of these issues regarding maternal costs were addressed using a hypothetical population of 10,000 women and population-based prevalence figures for adverse pregnancy events and the following thrombophilias: FVL; prothrombin G20210A; antithrombin, protein C, and protein S deficiencies; lupus anticoagulants and anticardiolipin antibodies. The cost-effectiveness of universal prepregnancy screening was calculated[117] with the assumption that the intervention would have a 50 percent reduction in adverse vascular events, consistent with their previous study.[115] In this model, universal screening, with enhanced antenatal care, and management of complications cost £5 384 320, in contrast with £525 815 if screening was not undertaken. Based on a reduction of adverse events from 2921 to 2861 this was associated with an incremental cost-effectiveness ratio of £81 436.05. Based on these values, universal screening for thrombophilia is not cost-effective. Unfortunately, this study did not take into account neonatal costs, and the economic consequences of preterm delivery are also huge. For example babies born before 28 weeks are associated with average inpatient health service costs of £22 000 (1998 costs) in the first 10 years of life alone and require further substantial investment in outpatient and educational/other support services.[118] Consideration of these neonatal costs and taking into account the reduction in psychological morbidity may have altered the overall conclusion in favor of universal screening. This is obviously dependent on the assumption that aspirin and LMWH are an effective intervention for all of these vascular complications.

CONCLUSION

There is clear evidence that certain inherited and acquired thrombophilias are associated with adverse pregnancy outcome, however, the exact pathogenic mechanism by which this damage to the uteroplacental unit occurs and why some women with thrombophilias express vascular complications but others do not remains elusive. Similarly the mechanism by which antithrombotic therapy alters the interaction between the maternal and fetal compartments is not clear and requires further study. The combination of aspirin and LMWH is an effective therapy for recurrent pregnancy loss in antiphospholipid syndrome, and extension of such therapy to women with heritable thrombophilia and late or recurrent fetal loss should be considered pending the results of randomized controlled trials. The uteroplacental complications of preeclampsia, IUGR and abruption require further study, as these conditions are associated with significant vascular damage, which may be amenable to antithrombotic therapy even in the absence of a documented thrombophilia.

KEY LEARNING POINTS

- Pregnancy is an acquired prothrombotic state due to the physiologic changes of the hemostatic system.
- Inherited or acquired thrombophilic states will synergistically interact with these physiologic changes.
- Thrombophilic changes are associated with adverse perinatal outcome by disruption of trophoblast development.
- The antithrombotic therapy of LMWH and aspirin improves perinatal outcome in the acquired thrombophilic state of antiphospholipid syndrome.
- The antithrombotic therapy of LMWH and aspirin may also improve perinatal outcome in women with inherited thrombophilia.

REFERENCES

1   Brenner B. Haemostatic changes in pregnancy. *Thromb Res* 2004; **114**: 409–14.

2   Lanir N, Aharon A, Brenner B. Haemostatic mechanisms in human placenta. *Best Pract Res Clin Haematol* 2003; **16**: 183–95.

3   Stirling Y, Woolf L, North WR, *et al.* Haemostasis in normal pregnancy. *Thromb Haemost* 1984; **52**: 176–82.

4   Bremme K, Ostlund E, Almqvist I, *et al.* Enhanced thrombin generation and fibrinolytic activity in normal pregnancy and the puerperium. *Obstet Gynecol* 1992; **80**: 132–7.

5   Kjellberg U, Andersson NE, Rosen S, *et al.* APC resistance and other haemostatic variables during pregnancy and puerperium. *Thromb Haemost* 1999; **81**: 527–31.

6   Clark P, Brennand J, Conkie JA, *et al.* Activated protein C sensitivity, protein C, protein S and coagulation in normal pregnancy. *Thromb Haemost* 1998; **79**: 1166–70.

7   Faught W, Garner P, Jones G, Ivey B. Changes in protein C and protein S levels in normal pregnancy. *Am J Obstet Gynecol* 1995; **172**(1 Pt 1): 147–50.

8   Bokarewa MI, Bremme K, Falk G, *et al.* Studies on phospholipid antibodies, APC-resistance and associated mutation in the coagulation factor V gene. *Thromb Res* 1995; **78**: 193–200.

9   Haim N, Lanir N, Hoffman R, *et al.* Acquired activated protein C resistance is common in cancer patients and is associated with venous thromboembolism. *Am J Med* 2001; **110**: 91–6.

10 Clark P, Sattar N, Walker ID, Greer IA. The Glasgow Outcome, APCR and Lipid (GOAL) Pregnancy Study: significance of pregnancy-associated activated protein C resistance. *Thromb Haemost* 2001; **85**: 30–5.

11 Mathonnet F, de Mazancourt P, Bastenaire B, *et al.* Activated protein C sensitivity ratio in pregnant women at delivery. *Br J Haematol* 1996; **92**: 244–6.

12 Clark P, Walker ID, Greer I. Acquired activated protein-C resistance in pregnancy and association with increased thrombin generation and fetal weight. *Lancet* 1999; **353**: 292–3.

13 Bokarewa MI, Wramsby M, Bremme K. Reactivity against phospholipids during pregnancy. *Hum Reprod* 1998; **13**: 2633–5.

14 el Roeiy A, Myers SA, Gleicher N. The prevalence of autoantibodies and lupus anticoagulant in healthy pregnant women. *Obstet Gynecol* 1990; **75**(3 Pt 1): 390–6.

15 Chetaille P, Alessi MC, Kouassi D, *et al.* Plasma TAFI antigen variations in healthy subjects. *Thromb Haemost* 2000; **83**: 902–5.

16 Greer IA. Prevention of venous thromboembolism in pregnancy. *Best Pract Res Clin Haematol* 2003; **16**: 261–78.

17 Greer IA. Inherited thrombophilia and venous thromboembolism. *Best Pract Res Clin Obstet Gynaecol* 2003; **17**: 413–25.

18 Walker ID. Congenital thrombophilia. *Baillieres Clin Obstet Gynaecol* 1997; **11**: 431–45.

19 Zheng H, Tzeng CC, Butt C, *et al.* An extremely low prevalence of Factor V Leiden, FIIG20210A and FXIIIV34L in Taiwan Chinese population. *Thromb Haemost* 2002; **87**: 1081–2.

20 Zoller B, Holm J, Dahlback B. Resistance to activated protein C due to a factor V gene mutation: the most common inherited risk factor of thrombosis. *Trends Cardiovasc Med* 1996; **6**: 45–53.

21 Margaglione M, Bossone A, Coalizzo D, *et al.* FV HR2 haplotype as additional inherited risk factor for deep vein thrombosis in individuals with a high-risk profile. *Thromb Haemost* 2002; **87**: 32–6.

22 Poort SR, Rosendaal FR, Reitsma PH, Bertina RM. A common genetic variation in the 3'-untranslated region of the prothrombin gene is associated with elevated plasma prothrombin levels and an increase in venous thrombosis. *Blood* 1996; **88**: 3698–703.

23 McColl MD, Walker ID, Greer IA. A mutation in the prothrombin gene contributing to venous thrombosis during pregnancy. *Br J Obstet Gynaecol* 1998; **105**: 923–5.

24 McColl MD, Ellison J, Reid F, *et al.* Prothrombin 20210 G→A, MTHFR C677T mutations in women with venous

thromboembolism associated with pregnancy. *Br J Obstet Gynaecol* 2000; **107**: 565–9.

25 Gerhardt A, Scharf RE, Beckmann MW, *et al.* Prothrombin and factor V mutations in women with a history of thrombosis during pregnancy and the puerperium. *N Engl J Med* 2000; **342**: 374–80.

26 Ellison J, Clark P, Walker ID, Greer IA. Effect of supplementation with folic acid throughout pregnancy on plasma homocysteine concentration. *Thromb Res* 2004; **114**: 25–7.

27 Miyakis S, Lockshin MD, Atsumi T, *et al.* International consensus statement on an update of the classification criteria for definite antiphospholipid syndrome (APS). *J Thromb Haemost* 2006; **4**: 295–306.

28 ACOG practice bulletin. Diagnosis and management of preeclampsia and eclampsia. Number 33, January 2002. American College of Obstetricians and Gynecologists. *Int J Gynaecol Obstet* 2002; **77**: 67–75.

29 Wisloff F, Jacobsen EM, Liestol S. Laboratory diagnosis of the antiphospholipid syndrome. *Thromb Res* 2002; **108**: 263–71.

★ 30 Brandt JT, Triplett DA, Alving B, Scharrer I. Criteria for the diagnosis of lupus anticoagulants: an update. On behalf of the Subcommittee on Lupus Anticoagulant/ Antiphospholipid Antibody of the Scientific and Standardisation Committee of the ISTH. *Thromb Haemost* 1995; **74**: 1185–90.

31 Tincani A, Allegri F, Sanmarco M, *et al.* Anticardiolipin antibody assay: a methodological analysis for a better consensus in routine determinations – a cooperative project of the European Antiphospholipid Forum. *Thromb Haemost* 2001; **86**: 575–83.

32 Harris EN, Pierangeli SS. Revisiting the anticardiolipin test and its standardization. *Lupus* 2002; **11**: 269–75.

★ 33 Wong RC, Gillis D, Adelstein S, *et al.* Consensus guidelines on anti-cardiolipin antibody testing and reporting. *Pathology* 2004; **36**: 63–8.

34 Reber G, Tincani A, Sanmarco M, *et al.* Proposals for the measurement of anti-beta2-glycoprotein I antibodies. Standardization group of the European Forum on Antiphospholipid Antibodies. *J Thromb Haemost* 2004; **2**: 1860–2.

35 Lockwood CJ, Romero R, Feinberg RF, *et al.* The prevalence and biologic significance of lupus anticoagulant and anticardiolipin antibodies in a general obstetric population. *Am J Obstet Gynecol* 1989; **161**: 369–73.

36 Petri M. Epidemiology of the antiphospholipid antibody syndrome. *J Autoimmun* 2000; **15**: 145–51.

37 Robert JM, Macara LM, Chalmers EA, Smith GC. Inter-assay variation in antiphospholipid antibody testing. *Br J Obstet Gynaecol* 2002; **109**: 348–9.

● 38 Erlich J, Parry GCN, Fearns C, *et al.* Tissue factor is required for uterine hemostasis and maintenance of the placental labyrinth during gestation. *Proc Natl Acad Sci U S A* 1999; **96**: 8138–43.

39 Salem HH, Maruyama I, Ishii H, Majerus PW. Isolation and characterization of thrombomodulin from human placenta. *J Biol Chem* 1984; **259**: 12246–51.

40 Fazel A, Vincenot A, Malassine A, *et al.* Increase in expression and activity of thrombomodulin in term human syncytiotrophoblast microvilli. *Placenta* 1998; **19**: 261–8.

41 Magriples U, Chan DW, Bruzek D, *et al.* Thrombomodulin: a new marker for placental abruption. *Thromb Haemost* 1999; **81**: 32–4.

● 42 Isermann B, Hendrickson SB, Hutley K, *et al.* Tissue-restricted expression of thrombomodulin in the placenta rescues thrombomodulin-deficient mice from early lethality and reveals a secondary developmental block. *Development* 2001; **128**: 827–38.

43 Isermann B, Sood R, Pawlinski R, *et al.* The thrombomodulin-protein C system is essential for the maintenance of pregnancy. *Nat Med* 2003; **9**: 331–7.

● 44 Jalbert LR, Rosen ED, Moons L, *et al.* Inactivation of the gene for anticoagulant protein C causes lethal perinatal consumptive coagulopathy in mice. *J Clin Invest* 1998; **102**: 1481–8.

● 45 Lay AJ, Liang Z, Rosen ED, Castellino FJ. Mice with a severe deficiency in protein C display prothrombotic and proinflammatory phenotypes and compromised maternal reproductive capabilities. *J Clin Invest* 2005; **115**: 1552–61.

46 Ratts VS, Tao X-J, Webster CB, *et al.* Expression of BCL-2, BAX and BAK in the trophoblast layer of the term human placenta: a unique model of apoptosis within a syncytium. *Placenta* 2000; **21**: 361–6.

47 Toki T, Horiuchi A, Ichikawa N, *et al.* Inverse relationship between apoptosis and Bcl-2 expression in syncytiotrophoblast and fibrin-type fibrinoid in early gestation. *Mol Hum Reprod* 1999; **5**: 246–51.

48 Teesalu T, Blasi F, Talarico D. Expression and function of the urokinase type plasminogen activator during mouse hemochorial placental development. *Dev Dyn* 1998; **213**: 27–38.

49 Strickland S, Richards WG. Invasion of the trophoblasts. *Cell* 1992; **71**: 355–7.

50 Hu ZY, Liu YX, Liu K, *et al.* Expression of tissue type and urokinase type plasminogen activators as well as plasminogen activator inhibitor type-1 and type-2 in human and rhesus monkey placenta. *J Anat* 1999; **194** (Pt 2): 183–95.

51 Estelles A, Gilabert J, Grancha S, *et al.* Abnormal expression of type 1 plasminogen activator inhibitor and tissue factor in severe preeclampsia. *Thromb Haemost* 1998; **79**: 500–8.

52 Kruithof EK, Tran-Thang C, Gudinchet A, *et al.* Fibrinolysis in pregnancy: a study of plasminogen activator inhibitors. *Blood* 1987; **69**: 460–6.

53 Estelles A, Gilabert J, Keeton M, *et al.* Altered expression of plasminogen activator inhibitor type 1 in placentas from pregnant women with preeclampsia and/or

intrauterine fetal growth retardation. *Blood* 1994; **84**: 143–50.

54 He S, Bremme K, Blomback M. Increased blood flow resistance in placental circulation and levels of plasminogen activator inhibitors types 1 and 2 in severe preeclampsia. *Blood Coagul Fibrinolysis* 1995; **6**: 703–8.

55 Wang W, Nagashima M, Schneider M, *et al*. Elements of the primary structure of thrombomodulin required for efficient thrombin-activable fibrinolysis inhibitor activation. *J Biol Chem* 2000; **275**: 22942–7.

56 Nesheim M, Wang W, Boffa M, *et al*. Thrombin, thrombomodulin and TAFI in the molecular link between coagulation and fibrinolysis. *Thromb Haemost* 1997; **78**: 386–91.

57 Sood R, Kalloway S, Mast AE, *et al*. Feto-maternal cross-talk in the placental vascular bed: control of coagulation by trophoblast cells. *Blood* 2006; **107**: 3173–80.

58 Robertson L, Wu O, Langhorne P, *et al*. Thrombophilia in pregnancy: a systematic review. *Br J Haematol* 2006; **132**: 171–96.

59 Empson M, Lassere M, Craig J, Scott J. Prevention of recurrent miscarriage for women with antiphospholipid antibody or lupus anticoagulant. *Cochrane Database Syst Rev* 2005; CD002859.

60 Lindqvist PG, Svensson P, Dahlback B. Activated protein C resistance – in the absence of factor V Leiden – and pregnancy. *J Thromb Haemost* 2006; **4**: 361–6.

61 Lissalde-Lavigne G, Fabbro-Peray P, *et al*. Factor V Leiden and prothrombin G20210A polymorphisms as risk factors for miscarriage during a first intended pregnancy: the matched case–control 'NOHA first' study. *J Thromb Haemost* 2005; **3**: 2178–84.

62 Rand JH, Wu XX, Giesen P. A possible solution to the paradox of the 'lupus anticoagulant': antiphospholipid antibodies accelerate thrombin generation by inhibiting annexin-V. *Thromb Haemost* 1999; **82**: 1376–7.

63 Vincent T, Rai R, Regan L, Cohen H. Increased thrombin generation in women with recurrent miscarriage. *Lancet* 1998; **352**: 116.

64 Van Horn JT, Craven C, Ward K, *et al*. Histologic features of placentas and abortion specimens from women with antiphospholipid and antiphospholipid-like syndromes. *Placenta* 2004; **25**: 642–8.

65 Lassere M, Empson M. Treatment of antiphospholipid syndrome in pregnancy – a systematic review of randomized therapeutic trials. *Thromb Res* 2004; **114**(5–6): 419–26.

66 Stone S, Khamashta MA, Poston L. Placentation, antiphospholipid syndrome and pregnancy outcome. *Lupus* 2001; **10**: 67–74.

67 Shehata HA, Nelson-Piercy C, Khamashta MA. Management of pregnancy in antiphospholipid syndrome. *Rheum Dis Clin North Am* 2001; **27**: 643–59.

68 Branch DW, Andres R, Digre KB, *et al*. The association of antiphospholipid antibodies with severe preeclampsia. *Obstet Gynecol* 1989; **73**: 541–5.

69 Dekker GA, de Vries JI, Doelitzsch PM, *et al*. Underlying disorders associated with severe early-onset preeclampsia. *Am J Obstet Gynecol* 1995; **173**: 1042–8.

70 Mello G, Parretti E, Marozio L, *et al*. Thrombophilia is significantly associated with severe preeclampsia: results of a large-scale, case-controlled study. *Hypertension* 2005; **46**: 1270–4.

71 Kupferminc MJ, Fait G, Many A, *et al*. Severe preeclampsia and high frequency of genetic thrombophilic mutations. *Obstet Gynecol* 2000; **96**: 45–9.

72 Martinelli P, Grandone E, Colaizzo D, *et al*. Familial thrombophilia and the occurrence of fetal growth restriction. *Haematologica* 2001; **86**: 428–31.

73 Grandone E, Margaglione M, Colaizzo D, *et al*. Lower birth-weight in neonates of mothers carrying factor V G1691A and factor II A(20210) mutations. *Haematologica* 2002; **87**: 177–81.

74 Infante-Rivard C, Rivard GE, Yotov WV, *et al*. Absence of association of thrombophilia polymorphisms with intrauterine growth restriction. *N Engl J Med* 2002; **347**: 19–25.

75 Kupferminc MJ, Eldor A, Steinman N, *et al*. Increased frequency of genetic thrombophilia in women with complications of pregnancy. *N Engl J Med* 1999; **340**: 9–13.

76 Yasuda M, Takakuwa K, Tokunaga A, Tanaka K. Prospective studies of the association between anticardiolipin antibody and outcome of pregnancy. *Obstet Gynecol* 1995; **86**(4 Pt 1): 555–9.

77 Younis JS, Samueloff A. Gestational vascular complications. *Best Pract Res Clin Haematol* 2003; **16**: 135–51.

78 Wiener-Megnagi Z, Ben Shlomo I, Goldberg Y, Shalev E. Resistance to activated protein C and the Leiden mutation: high prevalence in patients with abruptio placentae. *Am J Obstet Gynecol* 1998; **179**(6 Pt 1): 1565–7.

79 Prochazka M, Happach C, Marsal K, *et al*. Factor V Leiden in pregnancies complicated by placental abruption. *Br J Obstet Gynaecol* 2003; **110**: 462–6.

80 Bates SM, Ginsberg JS. Anticoagulants in pregnancy: fetal effects. *Baillieres Clin Obstet Gynaecol* 1997; **11**: 479–88.

81 Wesseling J, Van Driel D, Heymans HSA, *et al*. Coumarins during pregnancy: long-term effects on growth and development of school-age children. *Thromb Haemost* 2001; **85**: 609–13.

82 Flessa HC, Kapstrom AB, Glueck HI, Will JJ. Placental transport of heparin. *Am J Obstet Gynecol* 1965; **93**: 570–3.

83 Forestier F, Daffos F, Capella-Pavlovsky M. Low molecular weight heparin (PK 10169) does not cross the placenta during the second trimester of pregnancy: study by direct fetal blood sampling under ultrasound. *Thromb Res* 1984; **34**: 557–60.

84 Forestier F, Daffos F, Rainaut M, Toulemonde F. Low molecular weight heparin (CY 216) does not cross the

placenta during the third trimester of pregnancy. *Thromb Haemost* 1987; **57**: 234.

85 Greer IA. Prevention and management of venous thromboembolism in pregnancy. *Clin Chest Med* 2003; **24**: 123–37.

86 Nelson-Piercy C. Hazards of heparin: allergy, heparin-induced thrombocytopenia and osteoporosis. *Baillieres Clin Obstet Gynaecol* 1997; **11**: 489–509.

87 Sanson BJ, Lensing AW, Prins MH, *et al*. Safety of low-molecular-weight heparin in pregnancy: a systematic review. *Thromb Haemost* 1999; **81**: 668–72.

88 Greer IA, Nelson-Piercy C. Low-molecular-weight heparins for thromboprophylaxis and treatment of venous thromboembolism in pregnancy: a systematic review of safety and efficacy. *Blood* 2005; **106**: 401–7.

89 Brill-Edwards P, Ginsberg JS, Gent M, *et al*. Safety of withholding heparin in pregnant women with a history of venous thromboembolism. Recurrence of clot in this Pregnancy Study Group. *N Engl J Med* 2000; **343**: 1439–44.

90 Waterstone M, Bewley S, Wolfe C. Incidence and predictors of severe obstetric morbidity: case-control study. *BMJ* 2001; **322**: 1089–93.

91 Burrows RF, Kelton JG. Thrombocytopenia at delivery: a prospective survey of 6715 deliveries. *Am J Obstet Gynecol* 1990; **162**: 731–4.

92 Warkentin TE, Greinacher A. Heparin-induced thrombocytopenia: recognition, treatment, and prevention: the Seventh ACCP Conference on Antithrombotic and Thrombolytic Therapy. *Chest* 2004; **126**(3 Suppl): 311S–337S.

93 Byrd L, Johnston TA, Shiach C, Hay CRM. Osteoporotic fracture and low molecular weight heparin. *J Obstet Gynaecol* 2004; **24**(Suppl 1): S11.

94 Cowchock S, Reece EA. Do low-risk pregnant women with antiphospholipid antibodies need to be treated? Organizing Group of the Antiphospholipid Antibody Treatment Trial. *Am J Obstet Gynecol* 1997; **176**: 1099–100.

95 Pattison NS, Chamley LW, Birdsall M, *et al*. Does aspirin have a role in improving pregnancy outcome for women with the antiphospholipid syndrome? A randomized controlled trial. *Am J Obstet Gynecol* 2000; **183**: 1008–12.

96 Tulppala M, Marttunen M, Soderstrom-Anttila V, *et al*. Low-dose aspirin in prevention of miscarriage in women with unexplained or autoimmune related recurrent miscarriage: effect on prostacyclin and thromboxane A2 production. *Hum Reprod* 1997; **12**: 1567–72.

97 Farquharson RG, Quenby S, Greaves M. Antiphospholipid syndrome in pregnancy: a randomized, controlled trial of treatment. *Obstet Gynecol* 2002; **100**: 408–13.

98 Triolo G, Ferrante A, Ciccia F, Accardo-Palumbo A, *et al*. Randomized study of subcutaneous low molecular weight heparin plus aspirin versus intravenous immunoglobulin in the treatment of recurrent fetal loss associated with

antiphospholipid antibodies. *Arthritis Rheum* 2003; **48**: 728–31.

99 Kutteh WH. Antiphospholipid antibody-associated recurrent pregnancy loss: treatment with heparin and low-dose aspirin is superior to low-dose aspirin alone. *Am J Obstet Gynecol* 1996; **174**: 1584–9.

100 Rai R, Cohen H, Dave M, Regan L. Randomised controlled trial of aspirin and aspirin plus heparin in pregnant women with recurrent miscarriage associated with phospholipid antibodies (or antiphospholipid antibodies). *BMJ* 1997; **314**: 253–7.

101 Kutteh WH, Ermel LD. A clinical trial for the treatment of antiphospholipid antibody-associated recurrent pregnancy loss with lower dose heparin and aspirin. *Am J Reprod Immunol* 1996; **35**: 402–7.

102 Cowchock FS, Reece EA, Balaban D, *et al*. Repeated fetal losses associated with antiphospholipid antibodies: a collaborative randomized trial comparing prednisone with low-dose heparin treatment. *Am J Obstet Gynecol* 1992; **166**: 1318–23.

103 Laskin CA, Bombardier C, Hannah ME, *et al*. Prednisone and aspirin in women with autoantibodies and unexplained recurrent fetal loss. *N Engl J Med* 1997; **337**: 148–53.

104 Silver RK, MacGregor SN, Sholl JS, *et al*. Comparative trial of prednisone plus aspirin versus aspirin alone in the treatment of anticardiolipin antibody-positive obstetric patients. *Am J Obstet Gynecol* 1993; **169**: 1411–17.

105 Branch DW, Peaceman AM, Druzin M, *et al*. A multicenter, placebo-controlled pilot study of intravenous immune globulin treatment of antiphospholipid syndrome during pregnancy. The Pregnancy Loss Study Group. *Am J Obstet Gynecol* 2000; **182**(1 Pt 1): 122–7.

106 Vaquero E, Lazzarin N, Valensise H, *et al*. Pregnancy outcome in recurrent spontaneous abortion associated with antiphospholipid antibodies: a comparative study of intravenous immunoglobulin versus prednisone plus low-dose aspirin. *Am J Reprod Immunol* 2001; **45**: 174–9.

107 Noble LS, Kutteh WH, Lashey N, *et al*. Antiphospholipid antibodies associated with recurrent pregnancy loss: prospective, multicenter, controlled pilot study comparing treatment with low-molecular-weight heparin versus unfractionated heparin. *Fertil Steril* 2005; **83**: 684–90.

108 Gris JC, Quere I, Monpeyroux F, *et al*. Case-control study of the frequency of thrombophilic disorders in couples with late foetal loss and no thrombotic antecedent – the Nimes Obstetricians and Haematologists Study 5 (NOHA5). *Thromb Haemost* 1999; **81**: 891–9.

109 Brenner B, Hoffman R, Blumenfeld Z, *et al*. Gestational outcome in thrombophilic women with recurrent pregnancy loss treated by enoxaparin. *Thromb Haemost* 2000; **83**: 693–7.

110 Carp H, Dolitzky M, Inbal A. Thromboprophylaxis improves the live birth rate in women with consecutive

recurrent miscarriages and hereditary thrombophilia. *J Thromb Haemost* 2003; **1**: 433–8.

● 111   Brenner B, Bar J, Ellis M, *et al.* Effects of enoxaparin on late pregnancy complications and neonatal outcome in women with recurrent pregnancy loss and thrombophilia: results from the Live-Enox study. *Fertil Steril* 2005; **84**: 770–3.

● 112   Brenner B, Hoffman R, Carp H, *et al.* Efficacy and safety of two doses of enoxaparin in women with thrombophilia and recurrent pregnancy loss: the LIVE-ENOX study. *J Thromb Haemost* 2005; **3**: 227–9.

113   Walker ID, Kujovich JL, Greer IA, *et al.* The use of LMWH in pregnancies at risk: new evidence or perception? *J Thromb Haemost* 2005; **3**: 778–93.

114   Lindqvist PG, Merlo J. Low-molecular-weight heparin for repeated pregnancy loss: is it based on solid evidence? *J Thromb Haemost* 2005; **3**: 221–3.

● 115   Gris JC, Mercier E, Quere I, *et al.* Low-molecular-weight heparin versus low-dose aspirin in women with one fetal loss and a constitutional thrombophilic disorder. *Blood* 2004; **103**: 3695–9.

● 116   Clark P, Twaddle S, Walker ID, *et al.* Cost-effectiveness of screening for the factor V Leiden mutation in pregnant women. *Lancet* 2002; **359**: 1919–20.

117   Wu O, Robertson L, Twaddle S, *et al.* Screening for thrombophilia in high-risk situations: a meta-analysis and cost-effectiveness analysis. *Br J Haematol* 2005; **131**: 80–90.

118   Petrou S. The economic consequences of preterm birth during the first 10 years of life. *Br J Obstet Gynaecol* 2005; **112**(Suppl 1): 10–15.

25

Heart disease in pregnancy

SARAH GERMAIN, CATHERINE NELSON-PIERCY

IMPORTANCE OF CARDIAC DISEASE IN PREGNANCY

Cardiac disease in pregnancy is relatively rare in the United Kingdom, United States, and other developed countries, although still common in developing countries. Disease patterns are changing in the former, with a decline in rheumatic heart disease, but an increase in congenital and ischemic heart disease. Women with congenital heart disease are now surviving into adulthood, after corrective surgery as children, with the potential for childbearing, but often more complicated pregnancies. Increasing maternal age, as well as rising rates of cigarette smoking, obesity, and diabetes among women, means ischemic heart disease is encountered more frequently.

Although uncommon, cardiac disease is the leading cause of maternal death in the United Kingdom according to the latest *Confidential Enquiry into Maternal and Child Health* report (2000–02).[1] The report warns that heart disease is still potentially dangerous in pregnancy. The most common causes of the 44 deaths in this group in the report were cardiomyopathy, thoracic aortic aneurysm dissection and myocardial infarction. Women with pulmonary vascular disease are a particularly high-risk group, with a mortality of around 30 percent in Eisenmenger's syndrome and 30–50 percent in pulmonary hypertension (primary and secondary).

PHYSIOLOGIC CHANGES IN PREGNANCY

Hemostatic changes

Pregnancy is a hypercoagulable state, with an increase in procoagulant factors such as fibrinogen and factor VIII, a decrease in the endogenous anticoagulant protein S,[2] suppressed fibrinolysis and venous stasis, resulting in an increased risk of thromboembolism.[3] In addition estrogens interfere with collagen deposition within the media of muscular arteries, and circulating elastase can break up elastic lamellae and weaken the aortic media.[3] This weakening of vessel walls may predispose to dissection, even in women without an underlying connective tissue disorder.

Hemodynamic changes

The hemodynamic changes of pregnancy are as profound as those associated with training and exercise.[4] Most occur in the first and second trimesters, with relatively less in the third trimester. Maternal heart rate is increased from as early as 2–5 weeks of pregnancy, and continues to rise until late third trimester.[4,5] At term, values are 20 percent above those in the nonpregnant state (10–20 beats/min).[6] Circulating blood volume increases from 6 weeks, reaching a plateau by early third trimester, with levels increased 40–50 percent on nonpregnancy.[7] Levels are even higher in multiple pregnancies. The relatively larger increase in plasma volume over red blood cell mass results in a physiologic anemia.[8] Cardiac output rises by 30–50 percent,[6] due to a combination of increased heart rate and increased stroke volume.[9,10] This begins early in the first trimester, reaches a maximum by mid second trimester,[11] and then may start to fall again.[5,12] Pregnancy therefore results in a hyperdynamic circulation. Myocardial contractility and thickness are increased,[4] due to the volume load of pregnancy and vasodilatation, with mild left ventricular hypertrophy.[12]

Maternal blood pressure (BP) decreases until about 20 weeks of pregnancy, and then gradually increases again, reaching pre-pregnancy levels by term.[12] The decrease in diastolic BP is more marked than that of systolic BP. Systemic and pulmonary vascular resistance are also reduced.[6] These decreases in BP and resistance are due to a combination of endogenous gestational hormones, circulating prostaglandins, and a low resistance vascular bed in the placenta.[10,11] Decreased systemic vascular resistance results in a reduction in left ventricular (LV) afterload and therefore increased LV systolic function. This peaks at about 20 weeks and then plateaus until term.

During labor and delivery each contraction results in an extra 300–500 mL of blood returning back into the systemic circulation. Cardiac output is also increased due to the sympathetic response caused by pain and anxiety, with associated rise in heart rate and BP.[10,11] Conversely, if a pregnant woman is placed in the supine position, venocaval compression can occur due to obstruction by the gravid uterus, resulting in reduced cardiac preload/venous return and cardiac output by up to 25 percent, and therefore a risk of hypotension. Blood pressure also increases during labor.[12] Immediately after delivery the venocaval compression is relieved and autotransfusion from the emptied and contracted uterus can lead to a further increase in cardiac output of 60–80 percent.[10,11] There is then a dramatic decrease in cardiac output and volume loading.[4] Most of the hemodynamic changes of pregnancy resolve by 2–6 weeks post partum.[11,12] Some occur early, with systemic vascular resistance back to prelabor levels by 1 hour, whereas changes such as the ventricular hypertrophy take longer to resolve.[4]

SYMPTOMS AND SIGNS OF CARDIAC DISEASE

Symptoms

One of the difficulties in assessing women with possible heart disease is that many of the symptoms and signs of normal pregnancy can mimic those associated with cardiovascular pathology. Symptoms include dyspnea, orthopnea (due to pressure on the diaphragm by the gravid uterus), syncope (supine hypotensive syndrome due to venocaval compression), palpitations (due to rise in heart rate and increased awareness), and lightheadedness.

Signs

Signs include a loud first heart sound, presence of a third heart sound (in up to 84 percent), a benign ejection systolic murmur or continuous murmur, features of a hyperdynamic circulation (including a bounding and often collapsing pulse), a forceful and sometimes displaced apex beat, distended jugular veins (with prominent a and v waves and brisk x and y descents), and lower limb edema (due to venous obstruction by the gravid uterus and decreased colloid osmotic pressure).[13]

Heart murmurs are common in pregnancy, especially as gestation progresses, due to the increased cardiac output.[6] The benign ejection systolic murmur of pregnancy can occur in up to 96 percent of women. It is mid-systolic, soft (1/6 or 2/6), and found at the lower left sternal edge (pulmonary area). Continuous murmurs include a cervical venous hum and a 'mammary soufflé', the latter being due to increased mammary blood flow.[6] Any other murmurs should be investigated. The murmurs of mitral and aortic stenosis are accentuated in pregnancy due to the increased blood volume and cardiac output. Conversely the murmurs of aortic and mitral regurgitation are attenuated because of lowered systemic vascular resistance.

INVESTIGATIONS IN PREGNANCY

Chest radiograph

If clinically indicated a chest radiograph should be taken in pregnancy, as there is minimal risk of radiation exposure to the fetus with abdominal shielding.[14] Features on the chest radiograph that can be found in normal pregnancy are straightening of the left upper heart border (due to prominence of the pulmonary conus), increased cardiothoracic ratio and horizontal position (secondary to raised diaphragm), and increased pulmonary vascular markings (because of rise in cardiac output and pulmonary blood volume).[13] In the early postpartum period, small bilateral pleural effusions can be noted, but these resolve spontaneously within 1–2 weeks.

Electrocardiogram

Electrocardiogram (ECG) changes include left axis deviation, small Q wave and inverted T wave in lead III, inferior/lateral ST depression, and T wave inversion.[10] These are due to changes in heart position with diaphragmatic elevation. There may also be atrial and ventricular ectopics, which are usually benign.[9]

Echocardiogram

Transthoracic echocardiography poses no risk to mother or fetus. In pregnancy there is a slight increase in systolic and diastolic LV dimensions, a moderate increase in the size of the other chambers, progressive dilatation of pulmonary, mitral, and tricuspid valve annuli with functional regurgitation, and small pericardial effusions (in up to 44 percent by third trimester).[6]

EFFECT OF PREGNANCY ON HEART DISEASE

Physiologic changes in pregnancy can lead to cardiovascular symptoms and signs, such as palpitations, extrasystoles and ejection systolic murmur, but these are rarely pathologic. Clinically significant heart disease during pregnancy has a prevalence of approximately 1 percent,[6] but for these women there is an increased risk of adverse maternal, fetal, and neonatal outcomes. Pregnancy can pose particular problems for a number of reasons. The heart has less reserve than the respiratory system and may not be able to adequately increase cardiac output as required.

The American College of Obstetricians and Gynecologists have divided cardiac disease into that associated with minimal, moderate, and major risk of maternal complications or death (see Table 25.1). Other conditions included by some in the high-risk group are severe aortic stenosis (with or without symptoms), mitral stenosis with New York Heart Association (NYHA) III or IV, and mitral or aortic regurgitation with NYHA III or IV.[11] Women with pulmonary hypertension are a particularly high-risk group, with a very high rate of maternal mortality (30–40 percent) and adverse neonatal events.[15] Important factors affecting the outcome/safety in pregnancy include the presence and severity of pulmonary hypertension, presence of cyanosis, hemodynamic significance of the lesion, NYHA functional class, LV function, and degree of left heart obstruction (mitral or aortic valve areas or aortic valve gradient).[9] Maternal complications include arrhythmias, cardiac decompensation and heart failure, thromboembolism, cerebrovascular accident (CVA), and death. Risks to the fetus/neonate include intrauterine growth restriction (IUGR), premature delivery, respiratory distress syndrome, intraventricular hemorrhage, and death.

In a recent Canadian study[16] adverse maternal cardiac events occurred in 13 percent of completed pregnancies. Women were at high risk if they had decreased LV function (ejection fraction <40 percent), left heart obstruction (aortic valve area <1.5 cm^2 or mitral valve area <2.0 cm^2), a previous cardiovascular event (heart failure, transient ischemic attack [TIA], or CVA), or were NYHA class II or higher. The risk of complications was 4 percent if there were none of these risk factors, 27 percent if one, and 62 percent if two or more. The three women who died in their series had two or more risk factors. Predictors of neonatal complications were similar: NYHA class II or higher, left heart obstruction, use of anticoagulation during pregnancy, smoking during pregnancy, multiple pregnancy, and maternal age less than 20 or more than 35 years. Fetal mortality was 4 percent in the presence of one or more risk factor, compared to 2 percent if there were none.

Table 25.1 Maternal risk associated with cardiac disease in pregnancy*

Maternal risk of complications or death	Conditions
Minimal (<1%)	Atrial septal defect
	Ventricular septal defect
	Patent ductus arteriosus
	Pulmonic/tricuspid disease
	Corrected Fallot's tetralogy
	Bioprosthetic valve
	Mitral stenosis (NYHA I and II)
	Marfan syndrome with normal aorta
Moderate (5–15%)	Mitral stenosis with atrial fibrillation
	Artificial valve
	Mitral stenosis (NYHA III and IV)
	Aortic stenosis
	Aortic coarctation (uncomplicated)
	Uncorrected Fallot tetralogy
	Previous myocardial infarction
Major (>15%)	Pulmonary hypertension
	Eisenmenger syndrome
	Aortic coarctation (complicated)
	Marfan syndrome with aortic involvement
	Peripartum cardiomyopathy

*Adapted from Ramsey et al.[10]
NYHA, New York Heart Association.

EFFECT OF HEART DISEASE ON PREGNANCY

Pregnant women with cardiac disease require a multidisciplinary approach, with involvement of cardiologists/physicians with expertise in pregnancy, obstetricians with expertise in high-risk pregnancy, fetal medicine, pediatricians, and obstetric anesthetists. Regular antenatal visits and monitoring should be carried out to try to preempt or respond quickly to any problems. Ideally women should have a cardiovascular assessment pre-pregnancy, and then at least during each trimester and in the event of any change in symptoms. A careful plan for issues around labor and delivery should be agreed, documented and circulated widely and prominently, including provision for out-of-hours or emergency complications or delivery.

If the mother has congenital heart disease then there is an increased risk of congenital heart disease in the baby, and these women should be offered a detailed fetal cardiac anomaly scan. The background risk of a fetal cardiac anomaly in the general population is 0.4–0.6 percent, and this is increased about 10-fold if a first-degree relative is affected.[11] There is a higher recurrence rate in left heart obstructive lesions, and in autosomal dominant conditions such as

Marfan syndrome. Women with cardiac conditions have particular associated maternal and fetal risks, for example the risk of premature delivery, are discussed below. They should be counseled carefully regarding these and prepared as much as possible for likely outcomes.

Women at very high risk of cardiac complications during pregnancy, including a significant risk of maternal mortality, such as those with Eisenmenger syndrome, and severe pulmonary hypertension, should be carefully counseled and advised to avoid pregnancy. If they present during pregnancy then difficult decisions will need to be made, and must involve discussion between the patient and various specialists, whether to advise continuation with the pregnancy or not. It is important that women who decide against medical advice to continue with a pregnancy are reassured that they will be fully supported by their medical caregivers.

ETIOLOGY

The etiology of heart disease can be divided into congenital or acquired causes. Congenital cardiac lesions include common conditions such as ventricular and atrial septal defects, patent ductus arteriosus, and valve lesions (for example, bicuspid aortic valve). There are also much rarer conditions, often involving multiple cardiac defects, such as Fallot tetralogy, transposition of the great arteries, and a single ventricle. Underlying syndromes can also predispose to cardiac disease, for example Marfan. Acquired causes include ischemic heart disease, rheumatic heart disease, cardiomyopathies, and aortic dissection or aneurysm.

GENERAL MANAGEMENT

Some general principles of management can be applied to all cardiac conditions that are encountered in pregnancy. A multidisciplinary approach is crucial, with the involvement of all interested parties, including the pregnant woman and her partner. Ideally the planning should begin before pregnancy, or at least early on in gestation, before major problems have developed. Good communication between all the parties involved is of prime importance, with clear documentation of decisions made, in both the woman's notes and on the delivery suite. Strategies should be in place in case out-of-hours and/or emergency delivery are required.

Advice to any particular woman will depend on a number of factors including her underlying cardiac lesion and functional status. Appropriate investigations should be carried out to assess the nature and severity of the lesion, thus enabling a degree of risk stratification. Surgery or other procedures may be recommended prior to embarking on pregnancy. As well as current status, maternal life expectancy and therefore ability to care for the child, is also an important factor to be considered.

SPECIFIC CONDITIONS

Valvular heart disease

MITRAL STENOSIS

Background

Mitral stenosis is the most common cardiac lesion associated with rheumatic heart disease.[9] It is usually asymptomatic prior to pregnancy, as it has a natural history of 10–20 years on average before symptoms develop. Women can therefore present for the first time with symptoms in pregnancy, with decompensation secondary to the adaptive physiologic changes of tachycardia, increased blood volume and cardiac output, and the presence of arrhythmias, resulting in raised left atrial pressure.[6] Women are particularly vulnerable in the late second and third trimesters, labor and delivery, and early postpartum period when these hemodynamic changes are most marked. The commonest complication is pulmonary edema due to the increased left atrial pressure.[9] Arrhythmias are also common, in particular atrial fibrillation,[11] which can itself precipitate failure because of the increased heart rate and loss of atrial systole.

Women are at higher risk if they have severe stenosis ($<1.5\,cm^2$), moderate or severe symptoms, are diagnosed late in pregnancy, or have had cardiac event(s) before pregnancy (including abnormal functional class).[6] But it is important to remember that a woman's condition may deteriorate and she may become symptomatic in pregnancy even if she is undiagnosed or NYHA I/II before pregnancy. Maternal mortality is reported as being up to 5 percent overall, but is less than 1 percent if minimal symptoms.[17] Fetal mortality increases with deteriorating maternal functional capacity, with a rate of 30 percent if NYHA class IV.[18]

A recent study from South Africa[19] showed a 51 percent maternal complication rate, mostly in the third trimester or early postpartum, with the most common being pulmonary edema. Risk of cardiac events was predicted by late antenatal presentation, first presentation in pregnancy, and moderate or severe symptoms before pregnancy.

Management

If stenosis is mild or moderate then features of volume overload/pulmonary edema can be treated with diuretics and oxygen, and lifestyle measures such as limiting salt intake and reducing physical activity.[3] β-Blockers also improve symptoms, by decreasing heart rate, increasing diastolic filling time, and therefore reducing the risk of pulmonary edema.[20] Arrhythmias such as atrial fibrillation should be treated as normal (see below). Diuretics are safe to use in pregnancy,[21] but there is some caution over β-blockers because of reports of IUGR associated with the use of atenolol in the first half of pregnancy.[22] Despite this there is extensive experience of β-blockers in pregnancy and they are generally considered safe to use.[20,21] As with any drug in pregnancy, a risk–benefit assessment needs to be made for the particular pregnant woman. Other issues that need to be considered are anticoagulation (see later), because of the increased risk of intracardiac thrombus and systemic embolus with mitral stenosis, an enlarged left atrium, and atrial fibrillation, and continued penicillin prophylaxis if there is a history of acute rheumatic fever and carditis.[3] Penicillins are safe to use in pregnancy.[23]

If the mitral stenosis is severe (NYHA class III or IV, or valve area $<1.0\,\text{cm}^2$) then pregnancy should be delayed until valvotomy (balloon, open, or closed) or valve replacement has been carried out, as women are then able to tolerate pregnancy with fewer complications.[3] If they present for the first time in pregnancy with severe disease then balloon mitral valvuloplasty can be carried out, usually during the second trimester, allowing a normal vaginal delivery and good fetal outcome.[3,24] Radiation exposure should be reduced by uterus shielding and limited fluoroscopy, or alternatively the procedure performed under transesophageal echocardiography guidance. Balloon mitral valvuloplasty can also be carried out during pregnancy if medical treatment fails, although in both cases the valve needs to be noncalcified with minimal regurgitation.[24]

The complication rate for valvotomy in pregnancy is lowest for the percutaneous balloon procedure, with a 1 percent risk of major complications.[9] The risks are much higher for the surgical repair, with the closed procedure having mortality of 5–15 percent for the fetus and 3 percent for the mother, and the figures for the open operation are even higher at 15–33 percent for the fetus and 5 percent for the mother.[9]

Vaginal delivery should be the aim, unless there are obstetric indications for cesarean section, with an epidural to optimize pain control and allow assisted delivery to avoid pushing during the second stage.[6] Pulmonary artery catheters can be used before and during delivery to facilitate management if there is severe disease, especially as the left atrial pressure and pulmonary wedge pressure can increase by a further 8–10 mm Hg during labor.[6] The supine/lithotomy positions should be avoided where possible during labor and delivery, and careful monitoring of fluid balance carried out to avoid overload.

MITRAL VALVE PROLAPSE

Mitral valve prolapse is one of the more common cardiac problems in pregnancy,[10] and is usually asymptomatic and well tolerated. The hemodynamic changes in pregnancy often mean that the associated late systolic murmur and midsystolic click become less obvious.[10] Complications such as thromboembolism and endocarditis are rare, and antibiotic prophylaxis is not required unless there is associated mitral regurgitation or the mitral valve is thickened.[10]

MITRAL REGURGITATION

Background

Mitral regurgitation occurs less frequently than mitral stenosis. If there is no significant LV dysfunction then pregnancy can be well tolerated as the decreased peripheral vascular resistance leads to reduction in afterload and therefore decreases the degree of regurgitation.[6]

Management

If a woman is symptomatic then mitral valve surgery before pregnancy is recommended,[6] but this will not improve any LV dysfunction which is already present, and may still leave her at increased risk during pregnancy. If a woman develops heart failure during pregnancy then she should be treated with diuretics and digoxin. Surgery can usually be avoided unless she has acute severe deterioration in status or there are ruptured chordae tendineae. If surgery is needed then it is best to aim for repair rather than replacement, especially as this will avoid the need for anticoagulation.[3]

AORTIC STENOSIS

Background

Aortic stenosis encountered in pregnancy is usually due to a congenital bicuspid valve,[3] but can be caused by rheumatic heart disease.[10] It is encountered less commonly than other valvular lesions, since patients are usually older and male. In comparison with mitral stenosis, clinical symptoms can present late in the course of the disease.[10] Complications occur mainly with severe aortic stenosis, because of the decreased capacity to increase cardiac output appropriately. Abnormally raised LV systolic and filling pressures can precipitate or exacerbate heart failure or ischemia.[11] As the ventricle is noncompliant and hypertrophied it is sensitive to falls in preload, and therefore venous return needs to be maintained and hypotension avoided, to prevent myocardial, cerebral, or uteroplacental ischemia. There is also an association between a bicuspid aortic valve and cystic medial necrosis, which may predispose these women to spontaneous aortic dissection (see later section), usually in the third trimester.[3]

Management

If women are seen before pregnancy with an outflow gradient peak of more than 50 mm Hg they should be advised to delay conception until surgical correction.[3] If there is only mild or moderate obstruction and LV function is normal, then these women can usually be managed conservatively during pregnancy. If symptoms develop before the end of the first trimester, then women are at high risk of decompensation,[6] and some physicians would recommend terminating the pregnancy, although even therapeutic abortion carries significant maternal mortality.[10] Aortic valve replacement and palliative aortic balloon valvuloplasty have been performed during pregnancy, but there is some associated maternal and fetal risk.[6] In a review of a number of small studies, with a total of 106 pregnancies in 65 patients, the maternal mortality was 11 percent and perinatal mortality 4 percent.[25] Most of these deaths occurred in the earlier studies, and in the 25 pregnancies managed more recently, there was deterioration of maternal function in 20 percent, but no maternal mortality.[11]

AORTIC REGURGITATION

Background

Aortic regurgitation is usually due to either a dilated aortic annulus (for example in Marfan), a bicuspid aortic valve, or previous endocarditis.[6] As with mitral regurgitation, the decrease in systemic vascular resistance associated with pregnancy results in a reduction in the degree of regurgitation.[10] Women with abnormal functional capacity or LV dysfunction are likely to be at high risk of maternal and/or fetal complications, although there are little outcome data available.[6]

Management

If treatment is required, then symptoms can usually be managed medically, with diuretics and vasodilators, such as hydralazine and nifedipine.[6] Angiotensin-converting enzyme inhibitors are contraindicated in pregnancy because of reported associations with oligohydramnios, renal tubular dysplasia, neonatal renal failure, and hyocalvaria.[21] Surgical repair or replacement is usually only required if there are severe symptoms (NYHA class III or IV).[3] All of these women should have their volume status and BP carefully monitored during labor and delivery.

PULMONARY STENOSIS

Pulmonary stenosis is usually well tolerated in pregnancy, if the degree of stenosis is mild or has previously been corrected with valvuloplasty or surgery.[10] Patients may be asymptomatic, even with severe pulmonary stenosis, but right heart failure or arrhythmias can be precipitated by pregnancy because of the increased hemodynamic load.[10] Therefore, correction pre-pregnancy should be considered if possible, although balloon valvuloplasty during pregnancy is feasible.[3]

PROSTHETIC HEART VALVES

General issues

The main issues to be considered in women with prosthetic heart valves regarding pregnancy are the need for anticoagulation, and the risks of valve failure and infective endocarditis. Mechanical valves usually have better long-term valve survival, but in young women appear to be associated with greater morbidity and decreased maternal survival, and also carry the need for anticoagulation.[26] Maternal mortality with mechanical valves is 1–4 percent, usually due to complications of thrombosis.[6] Women with metal valve replacements require antibiotic prophylaxis regardless of the mode of delivery.[27] This is discussed in more detail in the section on infective endocarditis.

Anticoagulation

- Risks

Anticoagulation is a controversial issue during pregnancy, because of the need to balance maternal versus fetal interests. Women with bioprosthetic or homograft valves do not require anticoagulation unless atrial fibrillation or intracardiac thrombus are also present.[6] Those with mechanical prosthetic valves need lifelong anticoagulation, and this must continue throughout pregnancy,[28] especially as it is a procoagulant state.[11] There are no large clinical trials to give clear guidance on which regimen is best from the maternal or fetal points of view. The risk of prosthetic valve thrombosis depends on a number of factors including valve type, location, number of valves, presence of atrial fibrillation, left atrial size, previous thrombosis, and adequacy of anticoagulation. The risk is decreased with the newer bileaflet valves (for example, CarboMedics) compared with the first generation ball and cage valves (Starr Edwards) and single tilting disk valves (Bjork-Shiley), and is also less with aortic valve compared to mitral valve replacements.[9]

Warfarin crosses the placenta and is known to have teratogenic effects.[29] If used between 6 weeks' and 12 weeks' gestation there is an associated embryopathy, including stippled epiphyses and nasal hypoplasia.[30,31] Even if it is not used until the second and third trimesters there is still an increased risk of central nervous system defects, miscarriage, and stillbirth.[29] Central nervous system abnormalities include impaired brain growth due to fetal intracranial hemorrhage and scarring, dorsal midline dysplasia with agenesis of corpus callosum, Dandy–Walker malformation, midline cerebellar atrophy, and ventral midline dysplasia characterized by optic atrophy. There is also an increased risk of fetal cerebral hemorrhage during delivery especially if forceps assistance is required.[3] These complications may be dose related, as two studies have shown the adverse effects occurred more commonly if a dose of more than 5 mg/day was used.[32,33] One review[28] demonstrated an embryopathy risk of 6.4 percent (95 percent confidence interval [CI] 4.6 percent to 8.9 percent) if used throughout pregnancy, but this increased risk was eliminated if heparin was substituted between 6 weeks' and 12 weeks' gestation.

Heparin, both unfractionated heparin (UFH) and low-molecular-weight heparin (LMWH), is safe from a fetal point of view, as it does not cross the placenta.[29] The main problem with using heparin instead of warfarin during pregnancy is that even at full doses it has been associated with an increased risk of valve thrombosis, embolic events, and even death.[34,35] Although it has been suggested that this may just be due to inadequate dosing, the true incidence of treatment failure is unknown. Other complications associated with UFH include osteoporosis and thrombocytopenia.[29] Compared with UFH, LMWH has a longer half-life and increased bioavailability. This means it has a more predictable anticoagulant effect, with less need for monitoring and fewer side effects, and allows outpatient use.[29] There has been recent concern over a statement from Aventis Pharmaceuticals regarding treatment failures and potential teratogenicity of the LMWH enoxaparin, but numbers were small with poor quality data.[36] There is therefore an urgent need for better studies in this area to aid clinical decision making.

A review by Chan et al.[34] of 976 women with mechanical heart valves using anticoagulation during pregnancy demonstrated a 2.5 percent risk of major bleeding, usually at the time of delivery. Warfarin carried the lowest maternal risk, with 3.9 percent thromboembolism and 1.8 percent death rates, but it had the highest rate of fetal loss at 30 percent and embryopathy at 6 percent. If warfarin was used between 6 weeks' and 12 weeks' gestation then there was twice the fetal loss rate compared to UFH during the same period, but using heparin during the first trimester more than doubled the risk of maternal thromboembolism and death (9.2 percent and 4.2 percent). The highest maternal risks (25 percent thromboembolism and 7 percent death) were associated with UFH. In this study a large proportion of the women had older style mechanical valves, which carry an increased thrombotic risk. Another study by Meschengieser et al.[35] showed a risk of embolic episodes of 4.9 percent with heparin compared with 0.3 percent with warfarin. More recent reports where dose-adjusted regimens of LMWH have been used are much more encouraging.[37]

- Management

The three main strategies that can therefore be adopted for anticoagulation during pregnancy are: (i) using warfarin throughout; (ii) using high-dose heparin throughout (UFH or LMWH); and (iii) using high-dose UFH/LMWH from 6 weeks' to 12 weeks' gestation, and then swapping to warfarin for the rest of the pregnancy. Aspirin may be added if there is a particularly high risk of thrombosis,[28] although this increases the risk of bleeding. With regimens (i) and (iii), women need to be converted from warfarin to heparin around 36 weeks, to allow time for reversal of its anticoagulant effects prior to delivery, because of the risks of both fetal intracerebral hemorrhage (due to immaturity of fetal liver) and maternal peripartum hemorrhage.[29] Around the time of delivery women on subcutaneous UFH or LMWH may be switched over to intravenous heparin, which can then be stopped once labor is established. After delivery, anticoagulation can be restarted once hemostasis is achieved, initially with heparin, and then warfarin restarted 2–3 days post partum. Both heparin and warfarin are safe to use while breastfeeding.[3]

If warfarin is used the target international normalized ratio (INR) range should be 2.5–3.5 (American College of Chest Physicians). With UFH, the activated partial thromboplastin time (aPTT) should be maintained between 2.0 and 2.5 (17 500–20 000 U every 12 hours).[29,38] A dose of 100 anti-Xa U/kg twice daily of LMWH should be given. When LMWH is used outside pregnancy there is usually no need for monitoring, but when managing women with metal heart valves in pregnancy it has been recommended that anti-Xa levels should be measured 4–6 hours post injection, and a peak level of greater than 1–1.2 U/mL maintained.[29,38] If significant bleeding occurs or urgent delivery is required, then warfarin can be reversed with fresh frozen plasma and vitamin K, and heparin with protamine sulfate. Vitamin K should be avoided if possible as it makes a woman very difficult to re-anticoagulate afterward.

The first regimen is the safest for the mother, but as discussed above carries with it the increased risk of fetal complications, whereas the second regime will be best from a fetal perspective, but is associated with a higher rate of valve thrombosis and maternal death. Therefore, women need to be counseled carefully regarding the risks associated with each option, and be as fully involved in the decision making as possible.

Valve failure

There is a concern that pregnancy may cause accelerated structural deterioration of tissue valves, leading to premature valve failure, and need for reoperation, but recent studies seem to show that this is not the case. In a study of 232 cases of prosthetic heart valves,[26] mechanical valves had a higher risk of thromboembolism and 10-year mortality compared with bioprosthetic valves, but a lower rate of valve loss. Pregnancy did not increase the rate of failure of either type of valve replacement.

INFECTIVE ENDOCARDITIS

Background

The incidence of infective endocarditis in pregnancy is reported to be 0.006 percent.[39] It is therefore a rare complication of pregnancy, but a potentially fatal one, with 10–30 percent maternal mortality. Endocarditis was the cause of 10 percent of cardiac-related maternal deaths between 1985 and 1996, mostly due to heart failure or an embolic event.[13] Fetal mortality is also high. A recent review[40] showed 22.1 percent maternal and 14.7 percent fetal mortality. Infection may be acquired at the time of delivery, but may also occur antenatally.

Infective endocarditis is a difficult diagnosis to make in pregnancy, since new murmurs and changes in existing murmurs can be a normal feature. Predisposing factors include congenital heart disease, and intravenous drug abuse. Rheumatic heart disease is now much less common in the developed world as an underlying cause.

Prophylaxis

According to recent guidelines, antibiotic prophylaxis is recommended in individuals who have a higher risk for developing endocarditis than the general population and is particularly important for individuals in whom endocardial infection is associated with high morbidity and mortality

Table 25.2   Endocarditis risk associated with various cardiac conditions and recommendations for antibiotic prophylaxis*

Risk category	Conditions	Prophylaxis recommended
High	Prosthetic valves (metal, bioprosthetic and homografts)	Yes
	Previous bacterial endocarditis	
	Complex cyanotic congenital heart disease (Fallot, transposition of great arteries)	
	Surgically corrected systemic-pulmonary shunts/conduits	
Moderate	Other congenital cardiac malformations	Probably
	Acquired valvular disease	
	Hypertrophic cardiomyopathy	
	Mitral valve prolapse with mitral regurgitation or thickened valve leaflets	
Low	Isolated secundum atrial septal defect	No
	Surgically repaired atrial or ventricular septal defect, patent ductus arteriorus	
	Mitral valve prolapse without regurgitation	
	Physiologic heart murmurs	
	Cardiac pacemakers	

* Adapted from Nelson-Piercy.[9]

(Table 25.2).[27] There is not universal consensus over recommendations for antibiotic prophylaxis during pregnancy, labor, and delivery. Some clinicians would state that prophylaxis is not required unless there is evidence of clinically overt infection, although most would use it in high-risk patients.[3] Many would also include moderate-risk women, considering the benefits far outweigh the risks, since antibiotics are relatively cheap, and endocarditis is potentially fatal. Early studies suggested that there was a low incidence of bacteremia associated with uncomplicated vaginal delivery (1–5 percent), but later studies have shown that bacteremia is actually more common than might be expected, suggesting that vaginal delivery should still be covered with antibiotics.[41]

The recommended antibiotic regimen is 2 g amoxicillin plus 1.5 mg/kg gentamicin intravenously at the onset of labor/rupture of membranes/prior to cesarean section, and then 500 mg amoxicillin orally 6 hours later (intramuscularly or intravenously if unable to take orally).[42] If the woman is allergic to penicillin, then 1 g vancomycin or 400 mg teicoplanin intravenously can be used instead of amoxicillin.

Treatment of endocarditis

If a pregnant woman develops symptoms of infective endocarditis then delivery should be considered, regardless of gestation, because of the associated high fetal and maternal mortality.[40]

Other congenital heart disease

With advances in medical and surgical treatments, larger numbers of women with congenital heart disease are now surviving into the reproductive age group. Even if the lesions have been surgically corrected, they may still have residual defects. Women with pulmonary hypertension, cyanosis, or severe LV outflow obstruction are at particularly high risk of cardiac complications during pregnancy. There is an increased risk of congenital heart disease in the offspring, especially with outflow tract obstruction.[11]

LEFT-TO-RIGHT SHUNTS

Left-to-right shunts include atrial (ASD) and ventricular (VSD) septal defects, and patent ductus arteriosus (PDA). In the absence of pulmonary hypertension, pregnancy and delivery are usually well tolerated.[11] With left to right shunts, the right (in ASD or VSD) or left (in PDA) ventricle is volume overloaded, but the increase in cardiac output in pregnancy, that could cause difficulties, is countered by the decrease in peripheral vascular resistance.

If there is a large shunt, or preexisting raised pulmonary artery pressure, then pulmonary hypertension can develop or worsen, and arrhythmias and ventricular dysfunction can occur.[10] If systemic vasodilatation and/or increased pulmonary resistance cause transient right-to-left shunting, then there is a risk of paradoxical embolization.[11]

COARCTATION OF THE AORTA

If coarctation of the aorta is not corrected then maternal mortality in pregnancy can be up to 3 percent.[11] In one early study 8 of 14 deaths were due to aortic rupture, the high-risk period being the third trimester and peripartum.[43] However, a more recent study, of 87 pregnancies, had no maternal deaths and only one early neonatal death.[44] Risks are higher if there are associated cardiac defects, aortopathy, or longstanding hypertension;[10] IUGR, and premature labor and delivery are more common. Hypertension is difficult to control in these women, since treating upper body hypertension may lead to excessive hypotension below the level of the coarctation with fetal compromise. Following coarctation repair the risk of dissection and rupture is reduced but not completely eliminated.[11]

CYANOTIC HEART DISEASE

General

In pregnant women with cyanotic heart disease the reduced systemic vascular resistance and rise in cardiac output exacerbate the degree of right-to-left shunting, leading to worsening of maternal hypoxemia and cyanosis.[11] Polycythemia, secondary to the hypoxia, results in an increased risk of thromboembolism, including paradoxical embolism. The fetus tolerates cyanosis poorly, and there is a high incidence of fetal loss, IUGR, stillbirth, and premature delivery. Prognosis is particularly poor if maternal arterial oxygen saturation is less than 80 percent, hematocrit exceeds 60–65 percent or hemoglobin is greater than 200 g/L, or if she has recurrent syncope.[10]

A report[45] of 96 pregnancies in 44 women, with a variety of cyanotic congenital heart defects, showed 32 percent maternal cardiac events (including 1 death), 37 percent prematurity, and 43 percent live birth rate. If the maternal arterial oxygen saturation was <85 percent then the live birth rate was only 12 percent.

Tetralogy of Fallot

Tetralogy of Fallot is the most common form of cyanotic congenital heart disease, comprising of a large VSD, overriding aorta, right ventricular (RV) outflow obstruction (pulmonary stenosis), and RV hypertrophy. If the defects are corrected surgically then the 20-year survival is more than 75 percent.[10] If not, then less than 5 percent survive beyond 25 years.

Women with Fallot that has been successfully corrected are usually low risk during pregnancy.[11] They may still encounter problems, if they have residua or sequelae, for example: arrhythmias, a residual shunt, RV or LV dysfunction (caused by previous volume overload), RV outflow tract obstruction, pulmonary regurgitation, or pulmonary hypertension (caused by effects of a previous, palliative, modified Blalock–Taussig shunt between the subclavian and pulmonary arteries).[11] The size of the VSD and degree of pulmonary stenosis will be important determinants of risk.

Single ventricle, tricuspid atresia, and Fontan circulation

In people with tricuspid atresia and double inlet ventricle there is only one effective ventricle, usually the left, leading to mixing of the systemic and pulmonary venous returns. The degree of cyanosis will depend on the amount of pulmonary blood flow. It is not possible to completely correct the defect surgically, since there is only one effectively functioning ventricle. The Fontan operation aims to 'physiologically correct' the defect, by connecting the right atrium directly to the pulmonary artery and closing the ASD, so the LV pumps exclusively oxygenated blood from the lungs. The functional outcome is not perfect, as people still have a limited ability to increase their cardiac output, but it does relieve the cyanosis and removes the effects of long-term volume overload on the single ventricle.

In a series of 33 pregnancies in 21 women after successful Fontan operations,[46] 45 percent went to term with no maternal mortality. Two of the women had cardiac complications (atrial flutter in one woman, and ventricular dysfunction, aortic regurgitation and atrioventricular valve regurgitation in the other) and the first trimester miscarriage rate was high at 39 percent. The 10-year survival post-Fontan operation in the nonpregnant population is only 60–80 percent,[11] and so women should be counseled regarding this before conception, since there are implications not just for pregnancy itself but also for raising the child.

Transposition of the great arteries

Transposition of the great arteries was traditionally repaired by the Mustard or Senning procedure, which involved placing an atrial 'baffle' to divert blood, with the anatomic right ventricle having to support the systemic circulation. Complications in adult life following this repair include sinus node dysfunction, atrial arrhythmias, and dysfunction of the systemic (right) ventricle.[11] Connolly et al.[47] looked at 60 pregnancies in 22 of these women and showed relatively good outcomes: 83 percent had live births, 12 percent required cesarean section, 1 had a premature delivery at 29 weeks' gestation, and 2 had maternal complications (1 had congestive heart failure with atrioventricular valve regurgitation and the other was a woman with multiple problems including preeclampsia, congestive heart failure, endocarditis and myocardial infarction). Another study[48] examined 45 pregnancies in 19 women, with 60 percent live births, 27 percent miscarriages, and 13 percent termination of pregnancy. Five of the women (26 percent) developed cardiovascular complications: heart failure (3), worsening cyanosis (1), and CVA (1), with no maternal deaths. One of the live offspring had congenital heart disease.

The current repair of choice is the arterial switch, which returns the left ventricle to being the systemic ventricle.[11] Few of these women have as yet reached reproductive age, so there are no data about how they tolerate pregnancy and delivery.

Pulmonary hypertension and Eisenmenger syndrome

• General

Pulmonary hypertension can be primary, or secondary to Eisenmenger or lung disease. It is a serious problem, as vascular resistance is fixed and pulmonary blood flow cannot be increased, leading to refractory hypoxemia.[9] In a review of 125 pregnancies[49] in women with either Eisenmenger, primary hypertension or secondary pulmonary hypertension, all groups did poorly. Maternal mortality was 36 percent, 30 percent, and 56 percent, respectively, and overall neonatal mortality was 13 percent. Women are at particularly high risk if systolic pulmonary artery pressure is greater than 75 percent of systolic pressure.

● Eisenmenger syndrome

Eisenmenger syndrome occurs when pulmonary hypertension and pulmonary vascular obstructive disease develop secondary to an uncorrected left-to-right shunt, such as a VSD or ASD.[50] Left-to-right shunting results in chronically increased pulmonary artery pressure and flow, and this eventually leads to irreversibly raised pulmonary vascular resistance and hypertension and shunt reversal. Once pulmonary hypertension develops the underlying defect is inoperable and heart-lung transplant is the only effective surgical treatment.

Pregnancy poses a major risk in these patients, as the concomitant vasodilatation and reduced peripheral vascular resistance results in increased right-to-left shunting, worsening maternal cyanosis, and adversely affects the fetus.[11] There is progressive failure in maintaining pulmonary blood flow, arterial oxygen saturation, and cardiac output. Patients have a particularly poor prognosis if they have syncope, severe hypoxemia (arterial oxygen saturation <85 percent), and/or increased right heart filling pressure, as they are associated with advanced pulmonary vascular disease, severely impaired right ventricular function, decreased cardiac output, and inadequate oxygenation.[13]

For women with Eisenmenger syndrome the maternal mortality is 30–40 percent,[15] and has remained virtually unchanged over the past 50 years. Perinatal mortality has decreased though, from 28 percent to 8 percent, but only 15 percent of infants are born at term.[15] Complications tend to occur around term and in the first week postpartum.[9] Most maternal deaths are attributable to thromboembolism, hypovolemia or preeclampsia, with refractory hypoxemia at the end.[9] Spontaneous abortion and preterm labor are common, with perinatal mortality mainly due to prematurity.[11]

● Primary pulmonary hypertension

Primary pulmonary hypertension is a rare condition of unknown etiology, that carries a substantial risk of morbidity and mortality, especially in pregnancy.[10] It affects women more than men, and the peak incidence in the third and fourth decades of life coincides with the reproductive years. The mean survival after onset of symptoms is only 2–3 years, with most dying from intractable right ventricular failure or sudden death due to atrial tachyarrhythmias.[10]

Women may become symptomatic during pregnancy for the first time, due to the physiologic increases in blood volume, peripheral vasodilatation, and hypertension. The hypercoagulable state in pregnancy can also lead to pulmonary emboli or thrombi, which worsen the pulmonary hypertension. The diagnosis is often missed initially, as symptoms such as fatigue, dyspnea, and dizziness, are attributed to pregnancy itself. Maternal mortality is 30–50 percent,[10,49] with the greatest risk around delivery and the first week postpartum. If women tolerate pregnancy with a successful outcome, then they have a better long-term prognosis.

● Management

Preconceptual counseling should stress the extreme risk of undertaking pregnancy with pulmonary hypertension regardless of the cause.[9] If the woman presents when she is already pregnant, then most clinicians would offer termination of the pregnancy and effective contraception or sterilization. There is still a 7 percent maternal mortality associated with elective termination of the pregnancy, so it is best to avoid pregnancy if at all possible.[9]

If the woman wishes to continue with the pregnancy then she should be hospitalized for bedrest from at least mid-gestation. Supplemental oxygen can be given to decrease pulmonary vascular resistance and shunt flow, and thromboprophylaxis is given antenatally until 6 weeks post partum.[51] There are a number of case reports where inhaled nitric oxide, a potent selective pulmonary vasodilator, has been used during the peripartum period to decrease pulmonary hypertension and improve oxygenation.[52] Intravenous epoprostenol (prostacyclin) has also been used for a similar purpose.[53] Other, less selective, vasodilators should not be used, as these will cause a concomitant lowering of systemic pressure and exacerbate hypoxemia.[9] Delivery needs to be in a unit with intensive care facilities for both mother and baby. There is no good evidence regarding vaginal delivery versus cesarean section, or regional versus general anesthetic. Hypotension should be avoided and both mother and fetus monitored carefully. The particularly high-risk period is during delivery and the first week post partum,[9] and these women should stay in hospital for at least 2 weeks' post delivery. Often women still die despite all the above optimal management and in the United Kingdom, the number of women dying from pulmonary hypertension in pregnancy has remained constant for the past 40 years.[1]

Aortic dissection

Inherited collagen abnormalities, such as Marfan and Ehlers–Danlos, and congenital abnormalities, such as aortic coarctation and bicuspid aortic valve, are associated with a risk of aortic dissection.[13] The risk during pregnancy for women with these conditions is even higher, particularly during the third trimester or around the time of delivery. This is probably due to the associated hemodynamic and hemostatic changes,[11] including vascular wall structural changes and increased blood volume and cardiac output resulting in increased hemodynamic shear stress, and hormonal factors causing similar changes to cystic medial necrosis. In addition pregnancy itself seems to increase the risk of dissection of the aorta and its branches. Dissection has been one of the leading cardiac causes of maternal death over the past 10 years.[1]

Symptoms include acute severe chest, abdominal, or back pain. Chest radiograph may show a widened mediastinum but can be normal. Recommended investigations if dissection is suspected include transesophageal echo, magnetic resonance imaging, computed tomography (with contrast), and aortogram.

MARFAN SYNDROME

Background

Marfan syndrome is an autosomal dominant condition. Eighty percent have cardiac involvement (mainly mitral valve prolapse and mitral regurgitation).[54] The main cardiovascular complications of concern during pregnancy are spontaneous aortic dissection and/or rupture. Dissection can occur at any point along the aorta, but most commonly originates in the ascending portion. Dissection occurs most often in the third trimester or the early postpartum period.[54]

The high-risk group are those with enlargement of the aortic root greater than 4–4.5 cm and/or progressive dilatation.[9] Those with normal cardiac findings should be able to have a safe pregnancy and uncomplicated vaginal delivery, although dissection can still occur even with a normal aortic root measurement,[55] especially if there is a family history of aortic dissection or sudden death. The risk of dissection or rupture during pregnancy with an aortic root of less than 4 cm is about 1 percent. In the series by Lipscomb et al.,[55] 4 of 36 women with Marfan had an aortic dissection, even though none had significant cardiovascular abnormalities limiting function before pregnancy. Although a previous series[56] looking at 45 pregnancies in 21 patients showed no significant aortic root changes or increase in obstetric complications in women with a normal aortic root before pregnancy, 3 of 9 women with roots more than 4 cm did have a dissection or rapid dilatation. If the root is greater than 4 cm, the risk of dissection during pregnancy is about 10 percent.

Management

If a woman with Marfan is contemplating pregnancy, she requires a screening echocardiogram to assess the aortic root dimension. If it is greater than 4.5 cm then elective repair would be advised before conception.[3,9] If an aortic root over 4.5 cm is not picked up until the woman is already pregnant, and especially if there is progressive dilatation over time, then some clinicians would advise the pregnancy should be terminated, to allow prompt repair.[3]

Recommendations for managing these women during pregnancy include 4–8 weekly echocardiograms to detect any progressive aortic root dilatation, and the use of prophylactic β-blockers, to reduce risk of aortic dilatation, dissection and regurgitation (especially if hypertensive or aortic root dilatation is already present).[9] If aortic root measurements are less than 4.5 cm, and stable, then a vaginal delivery should be aimed for. Adequate analgesia is needed to avoid wide blood pressure surges during labor or delivery, and measures used to shorten the second stage. If the aortic root is enlarged to greater than 4.5 cm, or dilating during pregnancy, then elective cesarean section with regional anesthesia should be recommended.[55]

Ischemic heart disease

BACKGROUND

The incidence of ischemic heart disease (IHD) in pregnancy is <1/10 000 pregnancies,[10] but is becoming more common with increasing maternal age. Further risk factors include smoking, diabetes, obesity, hypertension and hypercholesterolemia, and multiparous women are also at increased risk.[9] Ischemic heart disease most commonly presents in the third trimester, peripartum, or early postpartum period.

Compared to IHD in the general nonpregnant population, the etiology is more likely to be nonatherosclerotic, for example coronary artery thrombosis or dissection.[9] One study[57] showed the breakdown of causes to be: atherosclerosis 43 percent, coronary thrombosis without atherosclerosis 21 percent, coronary dissection 16 percent, aneurysm 4 percent, spasm 1 percent, and normal coronary arteries 29 percent. Atherosclerosis tends to occur in women with known risk factors, and presents earlier, that is, third trimester rather than peri/postpartum, whereas postpartum the cause is more likely to be coronary artery dissection, usually involving the left anterior descending artery. Other causes that should be considered are coronary arteritis, coronary artery embolism (from prosthetic valves, infective endocarditis or mitral stenosis), congenital coronary anomalies, cocaine misuse, and use of ergot derivatives (such as ergotamine and bromocriptine) or vasoactive drugs to control uterine bleeding because of the risk of vasospasm. The resultant myocardial ischemia most commonly involves the anterior heart wall.[57]

The maternal death rate for myocardial infarction (MI) in pregnancy can be up to 50 percent, and usually occurs at the time of infarction or within 2 weeks, often in relation to labor and delivery. Roth and Elkayam[57] examined 125 cases and found 21 percent maternal mortality and 13 percent fetal mortality. Hankins showed 35 percent maternal mortality, with 20 percent occurring at the time of MI.[58] Two-thirds of the women had their event in the third trimester, when the mortality was greatest (45 percent), especially if they delivered within 2 weeks of the MI (50 percent). This was often associated with congestive cardiac failure or arrhythmias. If the woman survived then she had an increased risk of spontaneous abortion or unexplained stillbirth.

MANAGEMENT

As for the nonpregnant individual, initial diagnosis is made by a combination of history, ECG features, cardiac enzymes or biomarkers, and echocardiogram findings. The troponins are now the cardiac biomarkers most commonly used. They are very cardiac specific, and studies have shown that levels are not affected by labor (even if prolonged)[59] or by cesarean section,[60] although they appear to increase but remain within the normal range in preeclampsia.[61] The traditional cardiac enzyme creatinine kinase lacks cardiac specificity, as it is also present in the uterus, and therefore levels will be affected by labor.[10] Echocardiogram can be used to look for abnormal wall motion associated with myocardial ischemia, to evaluate LV ejection fraction, and to exclude structural abnormalities. Coronary angiogram can also be performed to allow direct assessment of the coronary arteries.

Initial treatment should generally be as for nonpregnant individuals, including oxygen, aspirin, nitrates, heparin and β-blockers. Intravenous and intracoronary thrombolysis, percutaneous transluminal coronary angioplasty, and coronary artery bypass surgery have all been performed successfully in pregnancy.[62–64] Experience with thrombolysis is limited, with a significant risk of maternal hemorrhage and fetal loss, especially if given at the time of delivery, and some would consider pregnancy to be a relative contraindication to thrombolysis.[21] For any particular individual therefore, a careful risk–benefit assessment needs to be made, taking into consideration a range of factors including gestation and timing of delivery. Since maternal mortality is significantly higher if women deliver within 2 weeks of an MI, then delivery should be delayed beyond this period if possible.[10]

If a woman with a previous history of IHD becomes pregnant, then she should continue secondary prevention agents, including aspirin and β-blocker, but lipid-lowering drugs should be stopped[9] as there is concern over risk of fetal abnormality with first trimester use and limited safety data in later pregnancy. There are only limited data for women with a previous MI regarding their outcome in future pregnancies, although the usual prognostic factors, including LV function and active myocardial ischemia, should be considered.

Cardiomyopathies

PERIPARTUM

Background

The definition of peripartum cardiomyopathy (PPCM) is development of cardiac failure in the last month of pregnancy or within 5 months of delivery, in the absence of both an identifiable cause and of recognizable heart disease prior to the last month of pregnancy (for example, dilated cardiomyopathy), and with evidence of LV dysfunction on echocardiogram (LV ejection fraction <45 percent, LV end diastolic pressure >2.7 cm/m^2 or fractional shortening <30 percent).[9,65] It has an incidence of 1 in 3000–15000 live births in the United Kingdom and United States,[66] but is higher in certain countries such as Haiti, where the rate is 1:350–400.[67]

The etiology of PPCM is unknown, although there are a number of theories. The most widely accepted is that it is an immune process.[68] Features of myocarditis are often found on endomyocardial biopsy, although the figure ranges from 9 percent to 100 percent in different studies.[66,69,70] Autoantibodies have been identified against a range of cardiac antigens, including actin, myosin, smooth muscle, adenine nucleotide translocator or branched chain

α-keto acid dehydrogenase.[65] One suggestion is that these are cross-reacting antibodies, which have developed as an immune response to fetal antigens in the maternal circulation. Viral infection may also play a role, especially as viral replication in known to be increased in pregnancy.[66] Other theories regarding the etiology of peripartum cardiomyopathy include exaggeration of the hemodynamic response to pregnancy; selenium deficiency rendering the heart more susceptible to injury from viral infection, hypotension or hypocalcemia (selenium levels are decreased in pregnancy due to interaction with prolactin);[71,72] prolonged tocolysis (in a rabbit model β-agonists such as ritodrine and terbutaline lead to impaired cardiac function);[73,74] relaxin causing relaxation of cardiac skeleton; and various genetic factors.

Risk factors for PPCM include multiple pregnancy, multiparity, increasing maternal age, preeclampsia and gestational hypertension, African descent, prolonged tocolysis, and a positive family history.[75] PPCM can present with cardiac failure, arrhythmias, or venous or arterial thromboembolic events (pulmonary embolus, CVA, or atrial or ventricular emboli). In comparison with dilated cardiomyopathy[76] there is no difference in presenting clinical features, although there is a higher incidence of myocarditis on biopsy, and women tend to have a bipolar prognosis, with either a dramatic improvement within 6 weeks, or rapid deterioration and death.

A number of series have been published looking at both maternal and fetal outcome with PPCM. Overall, full recovery occurs in 7–52 percent, with maternal mortality ranging from 6 percent to 60 percent, and 7–14 percent require transplantation. Perinatal mortality and morbidity are increased, as are premature delivery rates. Felker et al.[77] showed 43 percent recovered, 7 percent died, and 7 percent received transplants. In the series by Witlin et al.[78] 7 percent recovered, while of those with persistent cardiomyopathy 19 percent died, 12 percent required transplantation and 69 percent were stable on treatment. In an older study by Demarkis et al.[79] 52 percent had resolution of LV function by 6 months of whom none died, whereas of the 48 percent with persistent LV dysfunction at this point, 85 percent died with an average survival of 4.7 years. Prognostic factors for survival included higher LV ejection fraction and smaller LV end-diastolic diameter, whereas those with symptoms at 2 weeks postpartum, black women, multiparous women, and those older than 30 years had a poorer prognosis.

Outcome after cardiac transplantation for PPCM is generally good. Aziz et al.[80] presented three women, with myocarditis negative biopsies, all of whom underwent successful transplantation. Keogh et al.[81] demonstrated a 30 percent higher early rejection rate and need for cytotoxic treatment than patients receiving transplants for dilated cardiomyopathy, although survival at 2 years was still 88 percent. In the series by Rickenbacher et al.[82] patients with PPCM had a similar outcome to dilated cardiomyopathy, with 75 percent survival at 1 year and 60 percent at 5 years.

The outcome of subsequent pregnancies in women with previous PPCM is largely dependent on the assessment of

LV function at 6 months post presentation. Elkayam et al.[83] looked at 60 pregnancies in 44 women. In a subsequent pregnancy, those with normal LV function at 6 months had no maternal deaths, 21 percent developed symptoms, 11 percent had a premature delivery, and 4 percent had an abortion. The outcome was much worse in those with impaired LV function at 6 months, with 19 percent maternal deaths, 44 percent becoming symptomatic, 37 percent requiring premature delivery, and 25 percent having an abortion. Similarly, Witlin et al.[78] showed that one woman whose LV dysfunction resolved by 6 months remained asymptomatic in two further pregnancies, whereas of five women with persistent cardiomyopathy, four decompensated (with one death) and one remained stable. In the series by Sutton et al.[84] the four women with normal LV function at 6 months remained asymptomatic with stable LV function with future pregnancies, although Ceci et al.[85] reported that a woman with resolved LV dysfunction had recurrent PPCM in a subsequent pregnancy.

Management

Initial investigations should include ECG, chest radiograph, and echocardiogram. The ECG features are normal sinus rhythm or sinus tachycardia, atrial arrhythmias, LV hypertrophy, Q waves, ST changes, and T wave inversion.[66] Chest radiograph may show cardiomegaly,[66] and echocardiogram demonstrates LV dysfunction and excludes other causes.[65] Some clinicians would also advocate carrying out endomyocardial biopsy, especially if women do not respond to standard treatment.[80]

The principles for initial treatment are treatment of heart failure and anticoagulation.[66] Preload can be decreased by the use of diuretics and oral nitrates, and afterload reduced by hydralazine, nitrates, or amlodipine antenatally, and with angiotensin-converting enzyme inhibitors or angiotensin receptor antagonists postnatally. Inotropes, such as digoxin, dobutamine, and dopamine, will increase myocardial contractility. β-Blockers will reduce sympathetic nervous system activation. Anticoagulation is important because of the risk of thromboembolism, and the various options, involving heparin and/or warfarin, are discussed in an earlier section. If women fail to respond to 2 weeks of standard medical treatment, and endomyocardial biopsy is positive for myocarditis, then immunosuppression should be considered.[65] Intravenous immunoglobulins have been demonstrated to increase LV ejection fraction,[86] whereas a newer drug, pentoxifylline, inhibits production of the proinflammatory cytokine tumor necrosis factor α and has been shown to improve cardiac function.[87] In severe cases of PPCM the last resort is cardiac transplantation, if a suitable donor can be found in time.[82] Intraarterial balloon pumps or left ventricular assist devices have been used as bridges to transplantation (or recovery) in these situations.[81,88,89]

Women who have had PPCM require echocardiography assessment after 6 months to measure LV function and determine likely prognosis. If they have normal LV function at rest and on exercise then 6–12 months of treatment is recommended, after which they can stop medication.[90] If LV function is normal at rest but reduced on exercise, then the advice is a 'long period' of treatment with an angiotensin-converting enzyme inhibitor and/or β-blocker.[90] In those women whose LV function is still impaired at rest, lifelong treatment is recommended.[90] Dobutamine stress echocardiography is useful to identify reduced contractile reserve even with normal/recovered LV function.[11]

One of the most difficult management issues is how to advise these women regarding future pregnancies. Even if LV function appears to have recovered at six months, subsequent pregnancies can still cause marked deterioration in function. This may be due to persistent subclinical myocardial dysfunction that is unmasked by the hemodynamic changes of pregnancies, or may be reactivation of the underlying idiopathic pathological process responsible for the initial cardiomyopathy. The studies described above show that there are few deaths in this group with recovered LV function, even if it declines again in a future pregnancy. Patients should be fully counseled regarding the potential consequences if they chose to undertake another pregnancy.

HYPERTROPHIC CARDIOMYOPATHY

Background

Most cases of hypertrophic cardiomyopathy are familial and autosomal dominant.[9] Women can be asymptomatic, with the diagnosis being made through family screening. Symptoms include syncope, presyncope, and 'angina-like' chest pain. The risks for these women during pregnancy are similar to those with aortic stenosis. The LV outflow tract obstruction prevents augmentation of cardiac output, and therefore they cannot respond adequately to hemodynamic stresses such as hypotension or hypovolemia.[9] Elevated LV systolic and filling pressures can also precipitate heart failure and/or ischemia. Pregnancy is usually well tolerated, as long as hypotension and hypovolemia are avoided.[9]

Management

β-Blockers should be continued in pregnancy, or can be started if women develop symptoms.[91] Hypovolemia should be corrected rapidly and adequately if it develops. The BP should be carefully monitored if the woman has epidural analgesia or anesthesia, because the associated vasodilatation and hypotension can cause an increase in the degree of LV outflow tract obstruction.[9]

Arrhythmias

BACKGROUND

Palpitations and an increased heart rate are common features of normal pregnancy, but development of a serious arrhythmia is uncommon in a structurally normal heart.[21] Structural abnormalities should be excluded if a new arrhythmia occurs. Pregnancy can also exacerbate the frequency or severity of previously known arrhythmias. Only 10 percent of those with symptoms of dizziness, syncope, or palpitations actually have an underlying arrhythmia.[92] Bradycardia is unusual among women of childbearing age: postpartum sinus bradycardia can persist for several days, although it does not usually require treatment.[21]

MANAGEMENT

Atrial and ventricular ectopics

Atrial and ventricular premature complexes are common and do not usually correlate with symptoms.[9]

Sinus tachycardia

Women with a sinus tachycardia should be investigated for possible occult blood loss, infection, heart failure, thyrotoxicosis, and pulmonary embolus, where appropriate. If these are excluded no treatment is required.[9]

Supraventricular tachycardia

Supraventricular tachycardia is the most common arrhythmia in pregnancy,[93] although it rarely presents for the first time in pregnancy[94] – 22 percent of women with a previous supraventricular tachycardia have an exacerbation in pregnancy.[94] Fifty percent will not respond to vagal maneuvers, and therefore drug treatment is required in the acute situation.[93] Adenosine, propranolol, or verapamil can be used, although adenosine is probably the best in pregnancy, since there is no placental transfer and fewer side effects than verapamil.[93,95,96] For prophylaxis sotalol, propranolol, or flecainide can be safely used.[21]

Atrial fibrillation and flutter, ventricular tachycardia, and fibrillation

These arrhythmias are usually associated with structural cardiac abnormalities, and need to be treated promptly. Management is usually as for the nonpregnant individual. Pacing (temporary and permanent), cardioversion, and implantable defibrillators are all safe in pregnancy.[97,98] Natale et al. studied 44 pregnancies in women with implantable defibrillators and all had good maternal and fetal outcomes.[99]

Antiarrhythmic drugs

A general principle during pregnancy is to try to avoid drugs unless symptoms are severe or life-threatening. In particular if possible prescribing during the first trimester should be avoided, and the oldest most established drugs should be used where possible.[100] Table 25.3 summarizes current advice regarding the different classes of antiarrhythmics.

Cardiac transplantation

BACKGROUND

Pregnancy in women with heart transplants is becoming more frequent as more women in this group consider childbearing, since the first report of a successful pregnancy and

Table 25.3 Use of antiarrhythmic drugs in pregnancy[19,25]

Class	Drugs
IA	**Quinidine** has the most experience during pregnancy **Procainamide** can also be used for wide complex tachycardia **Disopyramide** should be avoided because it can induce uterine contractions
IB	**Lidocaine** is not teratogenic and is safe in pregnancy
IC	**Flecainide** is often used for fetal tachycardias, and is also safe to use for maternal arrhythmias
II	**β-Blockers** such as **propranolol**, **atenolol**, **labetalol** and **metoprolol** have been used extensively in pregnancy. There is a risk of fetal bradycardia, and also concern that atenolol is associated with low birthweight infants
III	**Amiodarone** is associated with fetal bradycardia and hypothyroidism,[101] and increased prematurity, and should be avoided where possible **Sotalol** is a potassium channel blocker as well as a β-blocker and can be used in pregnancy
IV	**Verapamil** has been used to treat both maternal and fetal tachyarrhythmias, but care should be taken with intravenous use because of the risk of profound maternal hypotension. The concomitant use of verapamil and β-blockers should be avoided **Diltiazem** is usually avoided as skeletal abnormalities have been reported in animal studies
Other	**Adenosine** is safe to use in pregnancy There is wide experience with **digoxin**, although digoxin toxicity should be avoided as it can cause fetal death

normal vaginal delivery in a cardiac transplant recipient by Lowenstein *et al.* in 1988.[102]

Hemodynamic considerations in the transplanted heart include sensory denervation, loss of vagal stimulus, and hypersensitivity to circulating catecholamines.[10,103] Sensory denervation can lead to asymptomatic myocardial ischemia and/or early graft rejection. Vagal denervation can result in a baseline tachycardia. The development of arrhythmias may indicate catecholamine supersensitivity or excess, and possible rejection or ischemia. Transplant recipients usually have a reduced cardiac output and ventricular compliance, with high central venous pressures, and during exertion ventricular diastolic pressures increase dramatically. The hemodynamic changes of pregnancy, namely increased blood volume, cardiac output and heart rate, may result in cardiac overload in these patients.

There are increased risks for both the mother and fetus, although many are able to have a successful delivery of a healthy infant. One study of 32 pregnancies in heart[29] or heart-lung[3] transplant patients showed 44 percent developed hypertension and 22 percent preeclampsia, 22 percent required treatment for rejection, 13 percent developed an infection during pregnancy, 41 percent delivered prematurely, and 33 percent required delivery by cesarean section.[104] Maternal complications are mainly related to the immunosuppressant drugs used, which need to be continued to avoid chronic rejection, and to the effects of the hemodynamic changes of pregnancy on the transplanted heart.[105] They include an increased risk of hypertension and preeclampsia, cardiac failure, gestational diabetes, infection, premature rupture of membranes, and adrenal insufficiency, as well as higher rates of anemia, cholestatic jaundice, and postnatal depression.[103] The fetus is at increased risk of spontaneous abortion due to infection, adrenal insufficiency, IUGR and low birthweight, and prematurity.[103] Dashe *et al.* showed a 38 percent preterm delivery rate with 24 percent small for gestational age.[106] The immunosuppressant drugs also have potential teratogenic effects, although extrapolation from studies of pregnancies in women with renal and liver transplants would suggest that ciclosporin, tacrolimus, prednisolone, and azathioprine are all safe and one review of 30 cases found no congenital anomalies or fetal/neonatal death.[107]

Branch *et al.*[108] looked at 47 pregnancies in 35 heart transplant recipients, and compared women undergoing their first pregnancy with those who had at least one previous pregnancy after transplantation. The live birth rate was 75–83 percent, which is similar to that for other organ transplant patients. There was a high incidence of low birthweight and prematurity (40 percent for primiparous women and 50 percent for multiparous women compared with 11 percent for nontransplant population). Subsequent pregnancies did not significantly increase the incidence of complications for mother or baby, or increase the risk of graft failure. There was a slight increase in the mean rejection rate per year after pregnancy in the multiparous group. There were eight maternal deaths during the follow-up period: three due to voluntary cessation of immunosuppression (one related to postnatal depression); two due to allograft vasculopathy (1.7 and 5.6 years postpartum); and one due to each of acute rejection (3.5 years post-partum), sudden death (2.8 years postpartum), and *Cryptosporidium* meningitis (1.9 years postpartum). A large study by Johnson *et al.* looking at why females are at increased risk of rejection after heart transplantation compared with males, found previous pregnancy a significant risk factor $(P < 0.0001)$[109] although there does not appear to be an increased risk of rejection during pregnancy itself or the immediate postpartum period.

MANAGEMENT

Ideally, women who have had a heart transplant should be counseled prior to becoming pregnant. Issues to be considered include risk of both fetal and maternal complications during pregnancy, review of medication for potential adverse fetal effects, and maternal long-term prognosis. An important issue when considering embarking on pregnancy and child rearing, is the risk of maternal death unrelated to pregnancy. Cardiac transplant patients have a high early mortality, with 15–20 percent dying within 1 year of the operation.[110] Thereafter there is a fairly constant mortality of 4 percent per year, with only 50 percent alive after 10 years and 15 percent after 20 years.[110]

It is generally advised to wait for 1–2 years after transplantation before attempting to conceive.[10,111] The majority of acute rejection occurs within the first 6–12 months, and this period will allow time to ensure the function of the graft is adequate and stable, and to stabilize the immunosuppressive regimen. Favorable outcomes have been achieved, even when women have become pregnant less than 1 year post transplantation. During pregnancy regular surveillance for rejection should not be interrupted,[10] and immunosuppressive drugs need to be continued and regular monitoring of drug levels is essential. The benefits of immunosuppression outweigh any associated fetal risks. During labor and delivery, the baseline tachycardia due to vagal denervation may require treatment with β-blockers.[10] Prior to regional anesthesia, adequate hydration is important to improve preload. Cesarean section should only be carried out for obstetric reasons, although there is a higher overall risk of requiring cesarean section in this group.[10]

It is important to counsel women post partum regarding appropriate contraception.[112] Barrier methods can be used, but intrauterine devices may not be suitable if there is an increased risk of infection.[103] Caution should be taken with the combined oral contraceptive pill, since immunosuppressants often give these women arterial hypertension, although this is less of a problem with the newer low-dose estrogen pills.[103]

Cardiopulmonary bypass

Cardiac disease in pregnancy can usually be managed medically, however, occasionally surgical intervention is required, usually necessitating cardiopulmonary bypass. Operating on a pregnant woman brings with it particular problems, as there are now two patients to be considered, and the best interests of the mother and fetus may not coincide.[113] The maternal mortality associated with cardiac surgery has fallen over the past 40–50 years, since cardiopulmonary bypass was first used during pregnancy in 1959 for a pulmonary valvotomy and ASD closure.[114] The risk to the mother is now similar to that for nonpregnant women, but fetal mortality remains high. Reviews of published case series over the past 20–30 years quote morbidity and mortality rates for the mother of 7.5–24 percent and 0–6 percent, respectively, and corresponding figures for the fetus of 9–10 percent and 12.5–30 percent.[113–115]

The fetus appears to be at greater risk with maternal cardiac surgery than with other types of operation during pregnancy. The highest mortality rates were associated with aortic-arterial dissection repair and pulmonary embolectomy.[113] This is probably related to maternal clinical status at time of operation and to length of time on bypass. A careful balance needs to be obtained between maintaining adequate placental perfusion while providing appropriate conditions for cardiac surgery to be performed. Potential insults to the mother and fetus during cardiopulmonary bypass are hypothermia, hemodilution, inhibition of coagulation, and nonpulsatile blood flow.[115] Pomini et al.[115] showed that hypothermia during bypass was one of the major determinants of poor fetal outcome, with 24 percent mortality, while there were no fetal deaths if normothermic conditions were used. In contrast, the maternal mortality was not affected by temperature. Hypothermia appears to increase uterine contractions, decrease placental oxygen exchange, and impair fetal myocardial conduction. This needs to be balanced however, by the need for maternal myocardial protection during surgery. Experimental work on lamb fetuses[116] has suggested that intermittent/pulsatile rather than continuous blood flow results in increased placental blood flow, and prevents a rise in placental vascular resistance, possibly through nitric oxide release.[117] Low flow rates also appear to cause hypoxia and hypercapnia.

From the maternal point of view it is better to operate in early pregnancy, as hemodynamic changes increase as gestation progresses, and women are at higher risk if surgery is performed immediately after delivery.[113] The best outcome from the fetal point of view is obtained if one waits until viability is reached, then deliver by cesarean section and carry out the cardiac surgery immediately afterward at the same operation.[113]

Parry and Westaby considered the different physiological responses to cardiopulmonary bypass of the mother, the fetus, and the fetoplacental unit.[114] Cardiopulmonary bypass results in maternal uterine contractions, especially during rewarming after hypothermia. This leads to placental hypoperfusion and insufficiency, and secondary fetal hypoxia. It is thought to be due to dilution of the stabilizing effects of progesterone, and can be minimized by administering progesterone, β_2-agonists, or intravenous alcohol. The fetal response to cardiopulmonary bypass is bradycardia, probably due to the placental hypoperfusion caused by uterine contractions. This is improved by increasing the perfusion rate. The fetoplacental unit initially develops a progressive respiratory acidosis when the fetus is first removed from bypass. This is due to increased prostaglandin synthesis causing a rise in placental vascular resistance. Later there is a metabolic acidosis, probably caused by catecholamines released as part of the fetal stress response. Indomethacin and steroids have been used experimentally to block both prostaglandin synthesis and the fetal stress response.

The main recommendations regarding cardiac surgery involving cardiopulmonary bypass in pregnancy are therefore:[113–115]

- Use medical interventions (such as balloon valvuloplasty) wherever possible, thus avoiding the need for surgery altogether.
- Keep time on bypass to a minimum.
- Use high flow (>5 L/min), high pressure (>70–75 mm Hg), normothermic conditions for bypass, avoid hypothermia, and consider pulsatile rather than continuous flow.
- Monitor fetal heart rate and uterine activity using cardiotocography, and adjust the flow rate and pharmacologic interventions accordingly.
- Be careful using drugs such as halothane that have tocolytic properties.
- If fetus is viable, then deliver by cesarean section immediately before carrying out the cardiac surgery.
- If surgery is carried out prior to delivery, then facilities must be available to carry out cesarean section if required.

Cardiopulmonary arrest

Cardiopulmonary arrest is a rare complication of pregnancy, with an incidence of 1:30 000 late pregnancies, but if it does occur then the chance of maternal survival is poor.[118] Important causes to consider in the pregnant woman are hemorrhage, placental abruption, pulmonary embolism, amniotic fluid embolism, eclampsia, and drug toxicity.[119] This is in contrast to cardiac arrest in the nonpregnant individual, where a primary cardiac cause, such as a myocardial infarction, is much more common.[119] Table 25.4 summarizes some of the physiologic changes of pregnancy, the difficulties they can cause when attempting resuscitation, and some of the adaptations that can be made to overcome these.

During pregnancy there are two people to resuscitate, but emphasis must be on effective life support for the mother, as this is the best way to optimize fetal outcome. The principles for basic and advanced life support are essentially the same as those for nonpregnant individuals,[119] taking into account the adaptations outlined in the table opposite. Attempts should be made to quickly identify the underlying cause of

Table 25.4   Resuscitation in pregnancy*

	Physiologic changes of pregnancy	Difficulties in resuscitation	Adaptations
Airway	Anatomic changes, e.g. obesity of neck Laryngeal edema	Maintaining clear airway Intubation	Incline laterally for suction, inserting airways, etc. Head tilt/jaw thrust to obtain clear airway quickly Suction to aspirate vomit
Breathing	Increased ventilation Increased oxygen demand Reduced chest compliance Reduced functional residual capacity Incompetent gastroesophageal sphincter, increased intragastric pressure and risk of regurgitation	Greater oxygen requirement Increased risk of pulmonary aspiration More difficult to see rise and fall of chest	Cricoid pressure until intubated with cuffed tube Higher inflation pressures for effective ventilation
Circulation	Rib flaring Raised diaphragm Breast hypertrophy General obesity Venocaval compression by gravid uterus impeding venous return and cardiac output	External chest compression difficult, e.g. determining hand position for compressions Supine position needs to be avoided Applying apical pad for debrillation	Left lateral position (Cardiff wedge, pillows, 'human wedge' using assistant's knees[120]) Manual displacement of uterus to left Raise patient's legs Possibly move hand position further up sternum (no specific guidelines available though) Care in placing defibrillation pads and using paddles, including moving dependent breast out of the way Better to use adhesive electrodes rather than paddles

*Adapted from Morris and Stacey.[118]

the arrest, and appropriate treatment(s) initiated. If an occult internal hemorrhage has occurred, then hypovolemic arrest can ensue, due to the large maternal blood volume. Blood needs to be cross-matched urgently and intravenous fluid replacement commenced, with early surgical intervention if required. If magnesium has been used to treat or prevent eclampsia, and high magnesium levels are suspected, then consider giving calcium chloride.

Outside pregnancy, anoxia develops within 3–4 minutes of cardiopulmonary arrest, but in pregnant women it can occur even more quickly.[118] The fetus can tolerate hypoxia for longer. If basic and/or advanced life support are not successful within 5 minutes then cesarean section should be performed.[116,121,122] There will probably not be time to obtain a formal theater pack, and a simple scalpel alone may need to be used, depending on the geographic location of the arrest. Timing and speed are critical in determining the optimal outcome for both mother and fetus. Resuscitation should be continued while the delivery is being carried out, and once the abdominal cavity has been entered then transabdominal open cardiac massage can be used. Delivery of the fetus is an important part of

the resuscitation attempt, since it allows complete relief of the venocaval compression, improves thoracic compliance and aids ventilation.

Since an obstetric arrest is such a rare occurrence in any particular unit, the resuscitation and emergency cesarean section drills need to be practiced using dummies, to allow all personnel who may be involved in the actual event to keep their skills up to date.[118] Successful resuscitation attempts require a multidisciplinary approach, and this is particularly true when the arrest occurs in a pregnant woman.

KEY LEARNING POINTS

- Although cardiac disease in pregnancy is still relatively rare, congenital and ischemic heart disease are being faced more frequently, as life expectancy and maternal age and comorbidities are increasing.
- The physiologic adaptation to pregnancy includes marked hemostatic and hemodynamic changes.

- Cardiovascular symptoms and signs in pregnancy can be due to these physiologic changes, without indicating underlying pathology, but severe and new symptoms need to be investigated further.
- In the 1 percent of pregnant women with cardiac disease, pregnancy can cause worsening of function and decompensation, because of reduced cardiac reserve and inability to increase cardiac output adequately. Those with pulmonary hypertension are at particularly high risk.
- Maternal complications of heart disease in pregnancy include arrhythmias, cardiac failure, and thromboembolism. Fetal complications include IUGR, congenital heart disease, premature delivery, and intrauterine death.
- Management should be multidisciplinary, and start with pre-pregnancy assessment and counseling regarding individual risk and likely prognosis.
- Specific management will depend on the particular cardiac condition, but may include pharmacologic agents such as antiarrhythmics, anticoagulants, diuretics, and antibiotic prophylaxis; invasive procedures such as valvuloplasty; or rarely surgical interventions such as valve replacement. Prescribing should take into account any drug effects on the fetus.
- In general, vaginal delivery should be the aim, unless there are obstetric indications for cesarean section. Exceptions include Marfan syndrome with aortic root dilatation.

REFERENCES

1 Royal College of Obstetrics Gynaecology. *Why Mothers Die 2000–2. Confidential Enquiry into Maternal Deaths.* London: RCOG Press, 2004.

2 Oruc S, Saruc M, Koyuncu FM, Ozdemir E. Changes in the plasma activities of protein C and protein S during pregnancy. *Aust N Z J Obstet Gynaecol* 2000; **40**: 448–50.

★ 3 ACC/AHA guidelines for the management of patients with valvular heart disease. A report of the American College of Cardiology/American Heart Association. Task Force on Practice Guidelines (Committee on Management of Patients with Valvular Heart Disease). *J Am Coll Cardiol* 1998; **32**: 1486–588.

4 Hunter S, Robson SC. Adaptation of the maternal heart in pregnancy. *Br Heart J* 1992; **68**: 540–3.

5 van Oppen AC, van der Tweel I, Alsbach GP, *et al.* A longitudinal study of maternal hemodynamics during normal pregnancy. *Obstet Gynecol* 1996; **88**: 40–6.

6 Reimold SC, Rutherford JD. Valvular heart disease in pregnancy. *N Engl J Med* 2003; **349**: 52–9.

7 Thornburg KL, Jacobson SL, Giraud GD, Morton MJ. Hemodynamic changes in pregnancy. *Semin Perinatol* 2000; **24**: 11–4.

8 Whittaker PG, Macphail S, Lind T. Serial hematologic changes and pregnancy outcome. *Obstet Gynecol* 1996; **88**: 33–9.

9 Nelson-Piercy C. Heart disease in pregnancy. *Acta Anaesth Belg* 2002; **53**: 321–6.

10 Ramsey PS, Ramin KD, Ramin SM. Cardiac disease in pregnancy. *Am J Perinatol* 2001; **18**: 245–65.

11 Siu SC, Colman JM. Heart disease and pregnancy. *Heart* 2001; **85**: 710–15.

12 Duvekot JJ, Peeters LL. Maternal cardiovascular hemodynamic adaptation to pregnancy. *Obstet Gynecol Surv* 1994; **49**: S1–14.

13 Tan JY-L. Cardiovascular disease in pregnancy. *Curr Obstet Gynaecol* 2004; **14**:155–65.

14 Damilakis J, Perisinakis K, Prassopoulos P, *et al.* Conceptus radiation dose and risk from chest screen-film radiography. *Eur Radiol* 2003; **13**: 406–12.

15 Yentis SM, Steer PJ, Plaat F. Eisenmenger's syndrome in pregnancy: maternal and fetal mortality in the 1990s. *Br J Obstet Gynaecol* 1998; **105**: 921–2.

16 Siu SC, Sermer M, Colman JM, *et al.* Cardiac Disease in Pregnancy (CARPREG) Investigators. Prospective multicenter study of pregnancy outcomes in women with heart disease. *Circulation* 2001; **104**: 515–21.

17 Clark S. Cardiac disease in pregnancy. *Crit Care Clin* 1991; **7**: 777–97.

18 Brady K, Duff P. Rheumatic heart disease in pregnancy. *Clin Obstet Gynecol* 1989; **32**: 21–40.

19 Desai DK, Adanlawo M, Naidoo DP, *et al.* Mitral stenosis in pregnancy: a four-year experience at King Edward VIII Hospital, Durban, South Africa. *Br J Obstet Gynaecol* 2000; **107**: 953–8.

20 al Kasab SM, Sabag T, al Zaibag M, *et al.* Beta-adrenergic receptor blockade in the management of pregnant women with mitral stenosis. *Am J Obstet Gynecol* 1990; **163**: 37–40.

21 James PR. Cardiovascular disease. *Best Prac Res Clin Obstet Gynecol* 2001; **15**: 903–11.

22 Shehata HA, Nelson-Piercy C. Drugs to avoid. *Best Prac Res Clin Obstet Gynecol* 2001; **15**: 971–86.

23 Rubin P. Drug treatment during pregnancy. *BMJ* 1998; **317**: 1503–6.

24 Loya YS, Desai DM, Sharma S. Mitral and pulmonary balloon valvotomy in pregnant patients. *Indian Heart J* 1993; **45**: 57–9.

25 Lao T, Sermer M, MaGee L, *et al.* Congenital aortic stenosis and pregnancy – a reappraisal. *Am J Obstet Gynecol* 1993; **169**: 540–55.

26 North RA, Sadler L, Stewart AW, *et al.* Long-term survival and valve-related complications in young women with cardiac valve replacements. *Circulation* 1999; **99**: 2669–76.

27 Dajani AS, Taubert KA, Wilson W. Prevention of bacterial endocarditis. Recommendations by the American Heart Association. *JAMA* 1997; **277**: 1794–801.

28 Chan WS. What is the optimal management of pregnant women with valvular heart disease in pregnancy? *Haemostasis* 1999; **29**: 105–6.

29   Gibson PS, Rosene-Montella K. Anticoagulants. *Best Pract Res Clin Obstet Gynecol* 2001; **15**: 847–61.

30   Hall JG, Pauli RM, Wilson KM. Maternal and fetal sequelae of anticoagulation during pregnancy. *Am J Med* 1980; **68**: 122–40.

31   Stevenson RE, Burton OM, Ferlauto GJ, Taylor HA. Hazards of oral anticoagulation during pregnancy. *JAMA* 1980; **243**: 1549–51.

32   Cotrufo M, De Feo M, De Santo LS, *et al.* Risk of warfarin during pregnancy with mechanical valve prostheses. *Obstet Gynecol* 2002; **99**: 35–40.

33   Vitale N, De Feo M, De Santo LS, *et al.* Dose-dependent fetal complications of warfarin in pregnant women with mechanical heart valves. *J Am Coll Cardiol* 1999; **33**: 1637–41.

34   Chan WS, Anand S, Ginsberg JS. Anticoagulation of pregnant women with mechanical heart valves: a systematic review of the literature. *Arch Intern Med* 2000; **160**: 191–6.

35   Meschengieser SS, Fondevila CG, Santarelli MT, Lazzari MA. Anticoagulation in pregnant women with mechanical heart valve prostheses. *Heart* 1999; **82**: 23–6.

36   Oran B, Lee-Parritz A, Ansell J. Low-molecular-weight heparin for the prophylaxis of thromboembolism in women with prosthetic mechanical heart valves during pregnancy. *Thromb Haemostat* 2004; **92**: 747–51.

37   Ginsberg JS, Chan WS, Bates SM, Kaatz S. Anticoagulation of pregnant women with mechanical heart valves. *Arch Intern Med* 2003; **163**: 694–8.

38   Ginsberg JS. Use of antithrombotic agents during pregnancy. *Chest* 2001; **119**: 122S–131S.

39   Montoya ME, Karnath BM, Ahmad M. Endocarditis during pregnancy. *South Med J* 2003; **96**: 1156–7.

40   Campuzano K, Roque H, Bolnick A, *et al.* Bacterial endocarditis complicating pregnancy: case report and systematic review of the literature. *Arch Gynecol Obstet* 2003; **268**: 251–5.

41   Sugrue D, Blake S, Troy P, MacDonald D. Antibiotic prophylaxis against infective endocarditis after normal delivery: is it necessary? *Br Heart J* 1980; **44**: 499–502.

42   Task Force Members. Guidelines on prevention, diagnosis and treatment of infective endocarditis. The Task Force on Infective Endocarditis of the European Society of Cardiology. *Eur Heart J* 2004; **25**: 267–76.

43   Deal K, Wooley CF. Coarctation of the aorta and pregnancy. *Ann Intern Med* 1973; **78**: 706–10.

44   Connolly H, Ammash N, Warnes C. Pregnancy in women with coarctation of the aorta. *J Am Coll Cardiol* 1996; **27**: 43A.

45   Presbitero P, Somerville J, Stone S, *et al.* Pregnancy in cyanotic congenital heart disease. Outcome of mother and fetus. *Circulation* 1994; **89**: 2673–6.

46   Canobbio MM, Mair DD, van der Velde M, Koos BJ. Pregnancy outcomes after the Fontan repair. *J Am Coll Cardiol* 1996; **28**: 763–7.

47   Connolly HM, Grogan M, Warnes CA. Pregnancy among women with congenitally corrected transposition of great arteries. *J Am Coll Cardiol* 1999; **33**: 1692–5.

48   Therrien J, Barnes I, Somerville J. Outcome of pregnancy in patients with congenitally corrected transposition of the great arteries. *Am J Cardiol* 1999; **84**: 820–4.

49   Weiss BM, Zemp L, Seifert B, Hess OM. Outcome of pulmonary vascular disease in pregnancy: a systematic overview from 1978 through 1996. *J Am Coll Cardiol* 1998; **31**: 1650–7.

50   Lieber S, Dewilde P, Huyghens L, *et al.* Eisenmenger's syndrome and pregnancy. *Acta Cardiol* 1985; **40**: 421–4.

51   Avila WS, Grinberg M, Snitcowsky R, *et al.* Maternal and fetal outcome in pregnant women with Eisenmenger's syndrome. *Eur Heart J* 1995; **16**: 460–4.

52   Goodwin TM, Gherman RB, Hameed A, Elkayam U. Favorable response of Eisenmenger syndrome to inhaled nitric oxide during pregnancy. *Am J Obstet Gynecol* 1999; **180**: 64–7.

53   Barst RJ, Rubin LJ, Long WA, *et al.* A comparison of continuous intravenous epoprostenol (Prostacyclin) with conventional therapy for primary pulmonary hypertension. *N Engl J Med* 1996; **334**: 296–301.

54   Task Force on the Management of Cardiovascular Diseases During Pregnancy of the European Society of Cardiology. Expert consensus document on management of cardiovascular diseases during pregnancy. *Eur Heart J* 2003; **24**: 761–81.

55   Lipscomb KJ, Smith JC, Clarke B, *et al.* Outcome of pregnancy in women with Marfan's syndrome. *Br J Obstet Gynaecol* 1997; **104**: 201–6.

56   Rossiter JP, Repke JT, Morales AJ, *et al.* A prospective longitudinal evaluation of pregnancy in the Marfan syndrome. *Am J Obstet Gynecol* 1995; **173**: 1599–606.

57   Roth A, Elkayam U. Acute myocardial infarction associated with pregnancy. *Ann Intern Med* 1996; **125**: 751–62.

58   Hankins GD, Wendel GD Jr, Leveno KJ, Stoneham J. Myocardial infarction during pregnancy: a review. *Obstet Gynecol* 1985; **65**: 139–46.

59   Shivvers SA, Wians FH Jr, Keffer JH, Ramin SM. Maternal cardiac troponin I levels during normal labor and delivery. *Am J Obstet Gynecol* 1999; **180**: 122.

60   Koscica KL, Bebbington M, Bernstein PS. Are maternal serum troponin I levels affected by vaginal or cesarean delivery? *Am J Perinatol* 2004; **21**: 31–4.

61   Fleming SM, O'Gorman T, Finn J, *et al.* Cardiac troponin I in pre-eclampsia and gestational hypertension. *Br J Obstet Gynaecol* 2000; **107**: 1417–20.

62   Schumacher B, Belfort MA, Card RJ. Successful treatment of acute myocardial infarction during pregnancy with tissue plasminogen activator. *Am J Obstet Gynecol* 1997; **176**: 716–19.

63   Sullebarger JT, Fontanet HL, Matar FA, Singh SS. Percutaneous coronary intervention for myocardial infarction during pregnancy: a new trend? *J Invasive Cardiol* 2003; **15**: 725–8.

64 Silberman S, Fink D, Berko RS, *et al.* Coronary artery bypass surgery during pregnancy. *Eur J Cardiothorac Surg* 1996; **10**: 925–6.

♦ 65 Pearson GD, Veille JC, Rahimtoola S, *et al.* Peripartum cardiomyopathy. National Heart, Lung, and Blood Institute and Office of Rare Diseases (National Institutes of Health) Workshop Recommendations and Review. *JAMA* 2000; **283**: 1183–8.

66 Brown CS, Bertolet BD. Peripartum cardiomyopathy: a comprehensive review. *Am J Obstet Gynecol* 1998; **178**: 409–14.

67 Fett JD. Peripartum cardiomyopathy. Insights from Haiti regarding a disease of unknown etiology. *Minn Med* 2002; **85**: 46–8.

68 Ansari AA, Fett JD, Carraway RE, *et al.* Autoimmune mechanisms as the basis for human peripartum cardiomyopathy. *Clin Rev Allergy Immunol* 2002; **23**: 301–24.

69 Midei MG, DeMent SH, Feldman AM, *et al.* Peripartum myocarditis and cardiomyopathy. *Circulation* 1990; **81**: 922–8.

70 Rizeq MN, Rickenbacher PR, Fowler MB, Billingham ME. Incidence of myocarditis in peripartum cardiomyopathy. *Am J Cardiol* 1994; **74**: 474–7.

71 Fett JD, Ansari AA, Sundstrom JB, Combs GF. Peripartum cardiomyopathy: a selenium disconnection and auto-immune connection. *Int J Cardiol* 2002; **86**: 311–16.

72 Kothari SS. Aetiopathogenesis of peripartum cardiomyopathy: prolactin-selenium interaction? *Int J Cardiol* 1997; **60**: 111–14.

73 Lampert MB, Hibbard J, Weinert L, *et al.* Peripartum heart failure associated with prolonged tocolytic therapy. *Am J Obstet Gynecol* 1993; **168**: 493–5.

74 Russo LR, Besinger RE, Tomich PG, Thomas JX Jr. Effect of chronic tocolytic therapy on maternal ventricular function in pregnant rabbits. *Am J Obstet Gynecol* 1996; **175**: 847–52.

75 Mehta NJ, Mehta RN, Khan IA. Peripartum cardiomyopathy: clinical and therapeutic aspects. *Angiology* 2001; **52**: 759–62.

76 O'Connell JB, Costanzo-Nordin MR, Subramanian R, *et al.* Peripartum cardiomyopathy: clinical, hemodynamic, histologic and prognostic characteristics. *J Am Coll Cardiol* 1986; **8**: 52–6.

77 Felker GM, Thompson RE, Hare JM, *et al.* Myocarditis and long-term survival in peripartum cardiomyopathy. *Am Heart J* 2000; **140**: 785–91.

78 Witlin AG, Mabie WC, Sibai BM. Peripartum cardiomyopathy: an ominous diagnosis. *Am J Obstet Gynecol* 1997; **176**: 182–8.

79 Demarkis JG, Rahimtoola SH, Sutton GC, *et al.* Natural course of peripartum cardiomyopathy. *Circulation* 1971; **44**: 1053–61.

80 Aziz TM, Burgess MI, Acladious NN, *et al.* Heart transplantation for peripartum cardiomyopathy: a report of three cases and a literature review. *Cardiovasc Surg* 1999; **7**: 565–7.

81 Keogh A, Macdonald P, Spratt P, *et al.* Outcome in peripartum cardiomyopathy after heart transplantation. *J Heart Lung Transplant* 1994; **13**: 202–7.

82 Rickenbacher PR, Rizeq MN, Hunt SA, *et al.* Long-term outcome after heart transplantation for peripartum cardiomyopathy. *Am Heart J* 1994; **127**: 1318–23.

● 83 Elkayam U, Tummala PP, Rao K, *et al.* Maternal and fetal outcomes of subsequent pregnancies in women with peripartum cardiomyopathy. *N Engl J Med* 2001; **344**: 1567–71.

84 Sutton MSJ, Cole P, Plappert M, *et al.* Effects of subsequent pregnancy on left ventricular function in peripartum cardiomyopathy. *Am Heart J* 1991; **121**: 1776–8.

85 Ceci O, Berardesca C, Caradonna F, *et al.* Recurrent peripartum cardiomyopathy. *Eur J Obstet Gynecol Reprod Biol* 1998; **76**: 29–30.

86 Bozhurt B, Villaneuva FS, Holubkov R, *et al.* Intravenous immune globulin in the therapy of peripartum cardio-myopathy. *J Am Coll Cardiol* 1999; **34**: 177–80.

87 Sliwa K, Skudicky D, Candy G, *et al.* The addition of pentoxifylline to conventional therapy improves outcome in patients with peripartum cardiomyopathy. *Eur J Heart Fail* 2002; **4**: 305–9.

88 Tandler R, Schmid C, Weyand M, Scheld HH. Novacor LVAD bridge to transplantation in peripartum cardiomyopathy. *Eur J Cardiothorac Surg* 1997; **11**: 394–6.

89 Lewis R, Mabie WC, Burlew B, Sibai BM. Biventricular assist device as a bridge to cardiac transplantation in the treatment of peripartum cardiomyopathy. *South Med J* 1997; **90**: 955–8.

90 Ardehali H, Kasper EK, Baughman KL. Peripartum cardiomyopathy. *Minerva Cardioangiol* 2003; **51**: 41–8.

91 Oakley GD, McGarry K, Limb DG, Oakley CM. Management of pregnancy in patients with hypertrophic cardiomyopathy. *Br Med J* 1979; **1**: 1749–50.

92 Shotan A, Ostrzega E, Mehra A, *et al.* Incidence of arrhythmias in normal pregnancy and relation to palpitations, dizziness, and syncope. *Am J Cardiol* 1997; **79**: 1061–4.

93 Mason BA, Ricci-Goodman J, Koos BJ. Adenosine in the treatment of maternal paroxysmal supraventricular tachycardia. *Obstet Gynecol* 1992; **80**: 478–80.

94 Lee SH, Chen SA, Wu TJ, *et al.* Effects of pregnancy on first onset and symptoms of paroxysmal supraventricular tachycardia. *Am J Cardiol* 1995; **76**: 675–8.

95 Joglar JA, Page RL. Treatment of cardiac arrhythmias during pregnancy: safety considerations. *Drug Saf* 1999; **20**: 85–94.

96 Robins K, Lyons G. Supraventricular tachycardia in pregnancy. *Br J Anaesth* 2004; **92**: 140–3.

97 Page RL. Treatment of arrhythmias during pregnancy. *Am Heart J* 1995; **130**: 871–6.

98 Jaffe R, Gruber A, Fejgin M, *et al.* Pregnancy with an artificial pacemaker. *Obstet Gynecol Surv* 1987; **42**: 137–9.

99   Natale A, Davidson T, Geiger MJ, Newby K. Implantable cardioverter-defibrillators and pregnancy: a safe combination? *Circulation* 1997; **96**: 2808–12.

100 Joglar JA, Page RL. Antiarrhythmic drugs in pregnancy. *Curr Opin Cardiol* 2001; **16**: 40–5.

101 Magee LA, Downar E, Sermer M, *et al.* Pregnancy outcome after gestational exposure to amiodarone in Canada. *Am J Obstet Gynecol* 1995; **172**: 1307–11.

102 Lowenstein BR, Vain NW, Perrone SV, *et al.* Successful pregnancy and vaginal delivery after heart transplantation. *Am J Obstet Gynecol* 1988; **158**: 589–90.

103 Bordignon S, Aramayo AM, Nunes e Silva D, *et al.* Pregnancy after cardiac transplantation. Report of one case and review. *Arq Bras Cardiol* 2000; **75**: 519–22.

104 Wagoner LE, Taylor DO, Olsen SL, *et al.* Immuno-suppressive therapy, management, and outcome of heart transplant recipients during pregnancy. *J Heart Lung Transplant* 1993; **12**: 993–9.

105 Delforge C, Kartheuser R, De Plaen JF, *et al.* Pregnancy after cardiac transplantation. *Transplant Proc* 1997; **29**: 2481–3.

106 Dashe JS, Ramin KD, Ramin SM. Pregnancy following cardiac transplantation. *Prim Care Update Ob Gyns* 1998; **5**: 257–62.

107 Scott JR, Wagoner LE, Olsen SL, *et al.* Pregnancy in heart transplant recipients: management and outcome. *Obstet Gynecol* 1993; **82**: 324–7.

108 Branch KR, Wagoner LE, McGrory CH, *et al.* Risks of subsequent pregnancies on mother and newborn in female heart transplant recipients. *J Heart Lung Transplant* 1998; **17**: 698–702.

109 Johnson MR, Naftel DC, Hobbs RE, *et al.* The incremental risk of female sex in heart transplantation: a multiinstiutional study of peripartum cardiomyopathy and pregnancy. Cardiac Transplant Research Database Group. *J Heart Lung Transplant* 1997; **16**: 801–12.

110 Anyanwu A, Treasure T. Prognosis after heart transplantation. *BMJ* 2003; **326**: 509–10.

111 Armenti VT, Radomski JS, Moritz MJ, *et al.* Report for the National Transplantation Pregnancy Registry (NTPR): outcomes of pregnancy after transplantation. *Clin Transpl* 2000: 123–34.

112 Spina V, Aleandri V, Salvi M. Contraception after heart transplantation. *Minerva Ginecol* 1998; **50**: 539–43.

113 Weiss BM, von Segesser LK, Alon E, *et al.* Outcome of cardiovascular surgery and pregnancy: a systematic review of the period 1984–96. *Am J Obstet Gynecol* 1998; **179**: 1643–53.

114 Parry AJ, Westaby S. Cardiopulmonary bypass during pregnancy. *Ann Thorac Surg* 1996; **61**: 1865–9.

115 Pomini F, Mercogliano D, Cavalletti C, *et al.* Cardiopulmonary bypass in pregnancy. *Ann Thorac Surg* 1996; **61**: 259–68.

116 Champsaur G, Parisot P, Martinot S, *et al.* Pulsatility improves hemodynamics during fetal bypass. Experimental comparative study of pulsatile versus steady flow. *Circulation* 1994; **90**: II47–50.

117 Vedrinne C, Tronc F, Martinot S, *et al.* Effects of various flow types on maternal hemodynamics during fetal bypass: is there nitric oxide release during pulsatile perfusion? *J Thorac Cardiovasc Surg* 1998; **116**: 432–9.

118 Morris S, Stacey M. Resuscitation in pregnancy. *BMJ* 2003; **327**: 1277–9.

119 *Advanced Life Support Course. Provider Manual*, 4th ed. Resuscitation Council (UK) and ERC, 2000.

120 Goodwin AP, Pearce AJ. The human wedge: a manoeuvre to relieve aortocaval compression in resuscitation during late pregnancy. *Anaesthesia* 1992; **47**: 433–4.

121 Whitten M, Irvine LM. Postmortem and perimortem cesarean section: what are the indications? *J R Soc Med* 2000; **93**: 6–9.

122 Page-Rodriguez A, Gonzalez-Sanchez JA. Perimortem cesarean section of twin pregnancy: case report and review of the literature. *Acad Emerg Med* 1999; **6**: 1072–4.

26

Preeclampsia, hypertension, and intrauterine growth restriction

LOUISE BYRD, LOUISE KENNY, PHILIP BAKER

DEFINITION

Arterial pressure is distributed continuously in the population at large and the dividing line between normotension and hypertension is arbitrary. This is also true for pregnant women, in whom an arbitrary threshold is adopted. In clinical practice the threshold of abnormality is set low to identify at-risk cases, but this results in many women being identified with hypertension and/or proteinuria who are not at increased risk of adverse experiences. For the purposes of classification, hypertension in pregnancy is defined as a diastolic blood pressure of >110 mm Hg on any one occasion OR >90 mm Hg on two or more consecutive occasions, 4 hours apart. Proteinuria in pregnancy is defined as a total protein excretion >300 mg per 24 hours OR two clean-catch mid-stream or catheter specimens of urine collected 4 hours apart with 2+ on reagent strip (adapted from Davey and MacGillivray[1]). Although diastolic hypertension is used in categorizing the disorder, this does not indicate that systolic hypertension is unimportant and severe systolic hypertension is associated with significant risk to the mother.

Blood pressure should be measured with the patient in the sitting position with a cuff appropriate for the size of the patient's arm. The standard bladder used in sphygmomanometer cuffs (23 × 12 cm) 'under-cuffs' about a quarter of the antenatal population resulting in overdiagnosis of hypertension. 'Over-cuffing' underestimates measurements, but usually by less than 5 mm Hg, and is preferable in cases of doubt. Keeping the rate of deflation during measurement to 2–3 mm/s will prevent overdiagnosing diastolic hypertension. Phases I and V of the Korotkoff sounds identify the systolic and diastolic limits, respectively, correlating more accurately with outcome than phase IV.[2] Digit preference, the practice of rounding the final digit of the blood pressure to 0, occurs in more than 80 percent of antenatal measurements and should be avoided.

Women who are hypertensive and pregnant should be subdivided into those with chronic hypertension and those with pregnancy-induced or gestational hypertension (PIH). Women with PIH are further subdivided: the majority have non-proteinuric PIH, a condition associated with minimal maternal or perinatal mortality/morbidity, whereas a minority have proteinuric PIH, which is associated with major pregnancy complication (preeclampsia).[3]

The term 'pregnancy-induced hypertension' usually implies hypertension caused by, but unrelated to, other pathology associated with the pregnancy, a diagnosis that is difficult to make until after the pregnancy has ended. Hypertension and proteinuria define preeclampsia, but they are not fundamental to the etiology and are more indicative of 'end-organ damage'. If any organ system known to be potentially affected by preeclampsia is involved (liver, kidney, blood, and placenta) the possibility of the disease must be suspected. Hypertension and proteinuria alone cannot always be relied upon to define the disease, but for pragmatic reasons these signs remain hallmarks for definition.

Based on the recommendation of Davey and Mac-Gillivray,[1] the International Society for the Study of Hypertension in Pregnancy (ISSHP) uses the term 'gestational hypertension' to cover all women with PIH whether proteinuric or not, as long as previously they had been neither

Box 26.1 The ISSHP classification (modified and abbreviated)

(A) Gestational hypertension and/or proteinuria developing during pregnancy, labor or the puerperium in a previously normotensive nonproteinuric woman
- Gestational hypertension (without proteinuria)
- Gestational proteinuria (without hypertension)
- Gestational proteinuric hypertension (preeclampsia)

(B) Chronic hypertension (before the twentieth week of pregnancy) and chronic renal disease (proteinuria before the twentieth week of pregnancy)
- Chronic hypertension (without proteinuria)
- Chronic renal disease (proteinuria with or without hypertension)
- Chronic hypertension with superimposed preeclampsia (new onset proteinuria)

(C) Unclassified hypertension and/or proteinuria

(D) Eclampsia

hypertensive nor proteinuric (Box 26.1). It is imperative that every effort is made to accurately classify women with hypertension in pregnancy as having chronic hypertension, nonproteinuric PIH, or preeclampsia. The etiology and management of the three conditions are quite different.

PREECLAMPSIA

Pathophysiology

Although the etiology of preeclampsia is still unclear, it is now widely believed that a cascade of events leads to the clinical syndrome. This cascade is considered to be initiated by a genetic predisposition, which, in turn, leads to a faulty interplay between the invading extravillous trophoblast cells (of fetal origin) and the immunologically active decidual cells (of maternal origin).

The development of the human hemochorial placenta and the maintenance of a successful pregnancy are dependent on the proliferation, migration, and invasion of trophoblast into the maternal decidua and myometrium in early pregnancy. The process of trophoblast invasion leads to the transformation of the spiral arteries supplying the intervillous space. These small, narrow-caliber arteries are gradually converted into large sinusoidal vessels, as the endothelium and the internal elastic lamina are replaced by trophoblast. These changes transform the vascular supply to a low-pressure, high-flow system, allowing an adequate blood flow to the placenta and fetus.

In preeclampsia two lesions occur in the spiral arteries. First, only the most superficial decidual portion of the spiral artery is invaded by the trophoblast; there is a lack of remodeling, and the maternal spiral arteries do not undergo the physiologic vasodilation that normally occurs between 8 and 18 weeks of gestation.[4] The diminished dilatation, associated increased resistance within the uteroplacental circulation, and impaired intervillous blood flow, probably result in an inadequately perfused placenta. At this stage there is no clinical disease. The second, and probably subsequent lesion within the spiral arteries, is acute atherosis, with aggregates of fibrin, platelets, and lipid-laden macrophages partially or completely blocking these arteries.[5] Consequent placental hypoperfusion, with subsequent ischemia, has then been postulated as causing the secretion of a factor or factors into the maternal circulation, which then causes activation of the vascular endothelium.[6] An increase in lipid peroxidation, both locally, within the placenta, and systemically, suggests that oxidative stress (an imbalance between free radical synthesis and antioxidant defence) may be involved in the endothelial cell changes. Endothelial cell activation is a key mediator in the maternal syndrome of preeclampsia. The ubiquitous nature of the vascular endothelium accounts for the widespread clinical manifestations of the disease (see later).

The mechanisms governing trophoblast invasion in both normal and compromised pregnancies are controversial and as yet not completely elucidated. A plethora of factors have been implicated including the enzymology of extracellular matrix degradation, trophoblast differentiation, and transcriptional regulation, human leukocyte antigen G, and transforming growth factors. In the past decade tremendous progress has been made in unraveling the cellular and molecular mechanisms leading to these events. With the advent of increased availability of novel gene knockout and transgenic mice, it is expected that knowledge in this area will continue to increase exponentially.

Incidence

The incidence of preeclampsia varies, depending both on the definition used and the population studied. In some recent prospective studies, the incidence has been as low as 2.2 percent, even in a primigravid population in which the condition is known to have the highest incidence.[7] The incidence of nonproteinuric PIH is approximately three times greater.

Mortality and morbidity

Even in developed countries, women still die from preeclampsia and eclampsia.[8] In the United Kingdom fewer than 10 women die each year, nonetheless eclampsia has an associated mortality of 2 percent.[9] Worldwide however, hypertensive disease accounts for approximately 100 000 maternal deaths per year. Because of concern for the potential consequences of preeclampsia and the difficulty in identifying those women who will progress to such complications, many women require intensive surveillance. Up to a quarter of antenatal admissions are as a direct result of monitoring and managing women with hypertension. Perinatal mortality is also increased with preeclampsia.

Early-onset preeclampsia is associated with intrauterine growth restriction (IUGR – see later). Placental involvement also explains the association with placental abruption. As delivery is the only cure, the hypertensive diseases of pregnancy have become the commonest cause of iatrogenic prematurity. They account for 15 percent of all premature births, but up to a quarter of very-low-birthweight babies.

There is strong evidence linking size at birth to health in adulthood, that is, that there are fetal origins of adult disease.[10] Thus, the small babies that result from pregnancies affected by preeclampsia have an increased risk of health problems in adult life, including an increased risk of developing hypertension, heart disease and diabetes. Additional and significant learning disabilities and low IQ has also been noted in this group.

Management

SCREENING FOR PREECLAMPSIA

History

More than a third of preeclampsia occurs in women with risk factors; a careful history will identify many of these risks. A family history in a first-degree relative increases the risk of preeclampsia four to eightfold.[11] In addition a woman has double the risk of preeclampsia if pregnant by a partner who had previously fathered a pregnancy affected by preeclampsia. An immunological element to the disease process is evidenced by the effect of exposure to the paternal foreign antigen, either via the fetus or the partner. This explains why preeclampsia occurs more commonly in first pregnancies (15 times the risk in parous women[12]), and why both miscarriages and terminations of pregnancy provide some reduction in this risk. A longer interval between pregnancies, which may be associated with a change in partner, seems to increase the risk, whereas nonbarrier methods of contraception and increased duration of sexual cohabitation reduce the risk.[13] Teenage mothers and pregnancies conceived by donor insemination have an increased risk of preeclampsia.

Underlying medical disorders, particularly with renal or vascular disturbance such as chronic hypertension, increase the risk of preeclampsia;[14] emphasizing the importance of the maternal susceptibility in the disease process. All forms of glucose intolerance including gestational diabetes are associated with an increased risk. This may be related to obesity, which is an independent risk factor.[15] Women with antiphospholipid syndrome[16] and multiple pregnancies are at increased risk.[12] Molar pregnancies have also been associated with preeclampsia presenting in early pregnancy,[17] as have pregnancies complicated by hydrops fetalis[18] or chromosomal anomalies.[19] Women with a history of preeclampsia, particularly those requiring delivery before 37 weeks, have about a 20 percent chance of disease recurrence.

Biophysical tests

The detection of raised blood pressure in early gestation, even within the normal blood pressure range, is a weak indicator of the subsequent risk of preeclampsia. The use of ambulatory automated monitoring removes many of the errors of standard sphygmomanometry but these ambulatory devices may under-read in preeclampsia. Isometric exercise testing and the roll over test have been investigated. However problems with reproducibility and poor predictive values are such that these have not been introduced into clinical practice. The angiotensin II sensitivity test, which assesses the blood pressure response to infusion of the vasoconstrictor angiotensin II, is invasive, time-consuming and costly. Although promising in initial small studies, it has shown poor predictive values in larger studies.[20]

Doppler analysis of the uterine artery waveform shows promise as a screening technique, with reasonable sensitivity and specificity. It is relatively quick, noninvasive, and inexpensive. In pregnancies at increased risk of preeclampsia, a high resistance blood flow pattern in the uterine arteries is found in mid-pregnancy, indicated by an increased pulsatility index with a diastolic notch. The later this test is performed, the better the predictive values. At 20 weeks' gestation, in a low-risk population, approximately 1 in 5 women with an abnormal waveform will develop preeclampsia;[21] the predictive value is considerably greater at 24 weeks.

At present screening tests allow women to be targeted for increased surveillance and prophylactic therapies. The importance of such tests will escalate if an adequate treatment to prevent preeclampsia is established.

Biochemical tests

Although various blood tests may identify at-risk women, none qualifies as an effective predictive test.[22] The detection of raised second trimester human chorionic gonadotrophin and maternal serum α-fetoprotein values, for example, has been associated with a twofold increase in preeclampsia, probably reflecting the disease process that occurs at the uteroplacental interface, but both lack sensitivity and specificity. Many markers of endothelial activation have been shown to be increased in preeclampsia. Some markers will rise before the clinical manifestations of the disease, but as there is invariably overlap between the women who are subsequently normal, and those who do develop preeclampsia, this limits their clinical usefulness. Similar rises have been seen in the placental protein, inhibin A.[23] Urinary excretion of calcium, microalbuminuria and prostacyclin metabolites, as well as urinary kallikrein:creatinine ratio, have also been investigated. Further work may eventually establish a combination of tests which could be clinically useful.[24]

THE ROLE OF PROPHYLAXIS

A variety of agents have been studied for prophylaxis of preeclampsia. Aspirin, calcium, and fish oils have gained the most attention in this regard, although other substances such as magnesium, zinc, and even rhubarb have been investigated. Low-dose aspirin, a cyclooxygenase enzyme inhibitor, reverses the imbalance that occurs in preeclampsia between the vasoconstrictor thromboxane A_2 and the vasodilator prostacyclin by inhibiting platelet thromboxane production. A Cochrane review of 42 randomized trials demonstrated a 15 percent relative risk reduction in the risk of preeclampsia associated with the use of aspirin or other antiplatelet agents.[25] In addition, these trials demonstrated an 8 percent reduction in the risk of preterm delivery and a 14 percent reduction in the risk of death to the baby, while confirming the safety of the drug(s). The dose, timing, and populations to be targeted still need to be established.

In the 10 trials (6864 women) that investigated the role of calcium, there was a moderate reduction in the incidence of preeclampsia. However, if women had an adequate calcium intake prior to the study, this effect was not sustained. The role of calcium supplementation in developed countries is uncertain, and is the subject of an ongoing World Health Organization trial. Fish oils containing n-3 fatty acids are thought to modify platelet thromboxane A_2 production. Trials to date have not, however, shown any reduction in preeclampsia. The potential role of oxidative stress in the etiology of the maternal syndrome of preeclampsia (see earlier), has resulted in the study of the antioxidants vitamins C and E. In a high-risk population (selected on the basis of abnormal uterine artery Doppler waveform analysis), vitamins C and E supplementation (1000 mg of vitamin C and 400 IU of vitamin E), was given from the second trimester. A reduction in the likelihood of developing preeclampsia, by at least 50 percent, was demonstrated.[26] These finding have been investigated further in large multicenter trials. The first of these, reported by Poston et al.,[27] was the Vitamins in Pregnancy (VIP) trial which examined the effects of these vitamins in a multicenter, randomized, placebo-controlled trial with a cohort of 2410 women with risk factors for preeclampsia. Of 2404 women treated, 2395 were included in the analysis. Antioxidant vitamin therapy did not reduce the risk of preeclampsia (15 percent [n = 181] vs. 16 percent [n = 187], relative risk [RR] 0.97, 95 percent confidence interval [CI] 0.80 to 1.17). There was no reduction in the risk of severe preeclampsia, gestational hypertension, preterm delivery due to preeclampsia, development of HELLP syndrome (hemolysis, elevated liver enzyme levels and a low platelet count), eclampsia, or severe proteinuria. Antioxidants were associated with an increased use of magnesium sulfate (4 percent [n = 47] vs. 2 percent [n = 26], RR 1.81, 95 percent CI 1.13 to 2.91) and intravenous antihypertensive therapy (3 percent [n = 31] vs. 1 percent [n = 16], RR 1.94, 95 percent CI 1.07 to 3.53). With respect to fetal and neonatal outcomes treatment with antioxidants was associated with an increased risk of low birthweight (28 percent [n = 387] vs. 24 percent [n = 335], RR 1.15, 95 percent CI 1.02 to 1.30), stillbirth (1 percent [n = 19] vs. 0.5 percent [n = 7], RR 2.70,

95 percent CI 1.02 to 7.14) and fetal acidosis as determined by arterial cord pH < 7 (3 percent [n = 20/675] vs. 1 percent [n = 9/657], RR 2.18, 95 percent CI 1.00 to 4.76). The authors therefore concluded that high-dose antioxidant vitamin supplementation is not beneficial in the prevention of preeclampsia and may indeed be detrimental to the fetoplacental unit. Rumbold et al.[28] subsequently reported a randomized trial of 1000 mg of vitamin C and 400 IU vitamin E daily compared with placebo given through pregnancy in 1877 nulliparous women. Again no benefit was found with regard to risk of preeclampsia, but there was no increased risk of adverse outcomes for the fetus. Thus the potential of such antioxidant therapy seen in early trials has not been confirmed in larger randomized trials in different populations.

MATERNAL AND FETAL ASSESSMENT

The first task is to confirm the diagnosis of preeclampsia (see above) to ensure that iatrogenic morbidity does not ensue. Care in assessing blood pressure will prevent misdiagnosis (see earlier). Errors in the interpretation of proteinuria are also common with dipstick urine analysis. Twenty-four-hour collections of urine are traditionally performed but newer automated devices that can be used by the bedside and relate proteinuria to serum creatinine, may be preferable. Every effort should be made to identify women at risk of life-threatening complications. This is a multisystem disorder. Other organ involvement must be considered (see later). For pragmatic reasons, other signs, such as epigastric pain, have not been introduced to define the disease, but are equally important.

MANAGEMENT REMOTE FROM TERM

Early-onset preeclampsia is frequently associated with placental insufficiency which can result in IUGR, abruption of the placenta and even fetal death. Fetal wellbeing must be carefully considered in all cases. A symphyseal fundal height should be carefully measured in all women who present with preeclampsia, in addition to an enquiry as to fetal movements. Ultrasound assessment is important to confirm fetal growth, assess the amniotic fluid volume and obtain umbilical artery Doppler waveforms. Suspected fetal compromise is a frequent indication for delivery in preeclampsia. Involvement of other organ systems in the affected women must be sought:

- Platelets are consumed due to the endothelial activation. A platelet count of more than $50 \times 10^9/L$ is likely to support normal hemostasis, but a falling platelet count, particularly to less than $100 \times 10^9/L$ may indicate a need to deliver.
- Hypovolemia results in an increased hematocrit, with an apparent rise in the hemoglobin concentration. Preeclampsia can cause disseminated intravascular coagulation, and clotting disorders must be assessed in severe cases or where there is thrombocytopenia.

- Uric acid, a measure of renal tubular function, is used to assess the disease severity, although severe disease can still occur with a normal uric acid level. Very high levels of uric acid are associated with acute fatty liver of pregnancy. Raised urea and creatinine are associated with late renal involvement but are not useful as an early indicator of disease severity, although serial measurements may identify renal disease progression.
- Liver dysfunction can occur. Aspartate aminotransferase (AST) and other transaminases indicate hepatocellular damage. (It should be remembered that the normal range for transaminases is approximately 20 percent lower than the nonpregnant range.) Elevated levels may again indicate a need to deliver because of concern for developing maternal compromise. Preeclampsia can have serious hepatic complications including subcapsular hematoma, liver rupture, and hepatic infarction. If proteinuria excretion is high (usually >3 g/24 hours), circulating albumen levels may fall, increasing the risk of pulmonary edema. The mother may become nephrotic with associated increased risk of venous thrombosis. A raised AST can be associated with either hemolysis or liver involvement; lactate dehydrogenase levels are also elevated in the presence of hemolysis. A severe variant of preeclampsia is known as HELLP syndrome. Hemolysis, elevated liver enzymes and low platelets are the hallmarks of this disorder.

Corticosteroids should be given to enhance fetal lung maturity and are safe in preeclampsia. Steroid therapy may assist in the recovery of HELLP syndrome and have been used in the postpartum period. It is not unusual to see a slight improvement in biochemical parameters associated with corticosteroid use. The hypertension of preeclampsia can cause direct arterial injury including cerebral hemorrhage, which may be fatal. To prevent such injury severe hypertension should be avoided. Blood pressures greater than or equal to 170/110 mm Hg (mean arterial pressure [MAP] of greater than or equal to 140 mm Hg) require urgent therapy[29] (see below). The rationale for treating moderate hypertension, that is blood pressure greater than 140/90 mm Hg but less than 170/110 mm Hg, is less clear. Treatment at this level may, by reducing placental blood flow, compromise fetal growth, without affording any maternal benefit.[29]

Where antihypertensives are considered then the relative safety of methyldopa makes it a popular choice. Oral administration can achieve an adequate therapeutic response within 12 hours, provided a sufficient dose (500–750 mg) is given. However a faster-acting alternative, popular in British obstetric practice, is labetalol. This drug is well tolerated, with good short-term fetal/neonatal safety. In practice, the choice of agent probably matters less than the clinician's familiarity with it.

In women with established preeclampsia, delivery should be considered once fetal lung maturity has been achieved (likely at about 32 weeks' gestation). This is particularly important if there is evidence of maternal multiorgan involvement and/or fetal compromise. However, asymptomatic women with preeclampsia, presenting between 26 and 32 weeks, can often be managed conservatively in an attempt to achieve improved perinatal survival, without substantial risk to the mother. This does however require close inpatient supervision, in a unit with adequate numbers of appropriately skilled staff. Trials have confirmed the advantages of a cautiously expectant approach.[30] Indications for delivery include an inability to control hypertension, deteriorating liver or renal function, progressive fall in platelets or neurologic complications. A nonreactive cardiotocography with decelerations or a fetal condition that is clearly deteriorating may, depending on gestation, also warrant delivery.

LABOR WARD MANAGEMENT OF PREECLAMPSIA

A set protocol, familiar to all staff, should be followed when a women has severe preeclampsia. The two main reasons why women die, as reported by the *Confidential Enquiries into Maternal Death*, are cerebral hemorrhage and adult or acute respiratory distress syndrome,[8] consequent on severe hypertension and excess fluid intake. Control of blood pressure and fluid balance is therefore crucial.

Intrapartum blood pressure control

Blood pressure should be measured frequently (every 15 minutes). To facilitate this, and to show trends in blood pressure, automated sphygmomanometers may be used. However as these devices under-read the blood pressure in preeclampsia, absolute blood pressure measurements should be confirmed with a mercury sphygmomanometer. As intracerebral hemorrhage is an important cause of death,[8] MAPs should be used to guide management, and most protocols recommend the instigation of antihypertensive therapy at MAP of >125 mm Hg. Regimens do vary, although there is an increasing trend towards regional protocols. As hypertension arises secondary to vasospasm antihypertensive drugs act by relaxing vascular smooth muscle. A smooth and sustained reduction in pressure is preferable to sudden, short-term changes.

Hydralazine, a potent vasodilator, has long been favored. By directly inhibiting the contractility of smooth muscle it reduces systemic vascular resistance, resulting in an increase in cardiac output, with an additional increase in cerebral blood flow (the latter accounting for the headache frequently observed during its use). A surge in noradrenaline correlates with the tachycardia that ensues, and may also explain the anxiety, restlessness and hyperreflexia seen in as many as 50 percent of patients.[31] Norepinephrine may also cause vasoconstriction within the uteroplacental circulation, thereby predisposing to 'fetal distress'.[32] Metaanalysis has recently concluded that this should no longer be the drug of first choice.[33] A popular alternative is labetalol, a potent α- and β-adrenoceptor antagonist. This lowers the blood pressure rapidly but without associated tachycardia, and appears to have no effect on placental blood flow. It is administered orally (200 mg) or intravenously as a bolus of 20 mg, followed at 10 minutes intervals by 40, 80, and 80 mg boluses, up to a cumulative dose of 220 mg. Once the MAP is <125 mm Hg, an infusion of 40 mg/h is commenced, doubling (if necessary) at 30-minute intervals, until a satisfactory response or a dose of 160 mg/h is attained. Colloid should be infused prior to treatment if the baby is undelivered, to protect the uteroplacental circulation, prevent hypotension, and fetal distress.

If one agent is ineffective, or if side effects occur, another agent can be used. Other alternatives include sodium nitroprusside and nifedipine. Care must be taken with the former as fetal toxicity is possible, although normal fetal survival has been reported.[34] Nifedipine, a calcium-channel blocker, should no longer be used sublingually as it has been shown to cause precipitate drops in blood pressure with consequent detrimental effects on placental, and hence fetal, blood flow. Slow-release tablets are an alternative. There is a theoretical risk of potentiation if used with magnesium sulfate,[35] and its antitocolytic effect may predispose to postpartum hemorrhage.[36]

Fluid management

As women with preeclampsia can have a reduced intravascular volume, leaky capillary membranes and low albumen levels, they are prone to pulmonary edema. Renal failure is a rare complication of preeclampsia that usually follows acute blood loss, when there has been inadequate transfusion, or as a result of profound hypotension. Oliguria, without a rising serum urea or creatinine, is a manifestation of severe preeclampsia and not of incipient renal failure. Administration of intravenous fluid in response to oliguria must be performed with caution. Most protocols limit fluid intake (in the form of intravenous crystalloid) to approximately 1 mL/kg per hour. A Foley catheter should be inserted and strict fluid balance recorded.

In well-perfused women with no signs of blood loss and/or hemolysis and a creatinine level of less than 100 mmol/L, oliguria (<400 mL/24 hour) requires no treatment *per se*. Such reduced urinary output will be transient and will usually correct itself. Repetitive fluid challenges should be avoided. Occasionally central venous pressure (CVP) monitoring is useful. If the CVP is high (>8 mm Hg) with persistent oliguria, a dopamine infusion can be considered (1 μg/kg per minute). A rising creatinine (greater than 100 mmol/L) with oliguria (with or without increasing serum potassium levels) is more likely to represent structural deficit within the kidneys and is not therefore going to be corrected with fluids. Instead such infusions will only overflow into the lungs, causing respiratory compromise. These women may require hemodialysis or hemofiltration, and the advice of a renal physician should be sought. The administration of diuretics will improve urine output temporarily, while further decreasing the circulating volume and exacerbating any electrolyte imbalance. Furosemide should therefore be used with caution, and only be given if there are signs of pulmonary edema. In particularly difficult cases, pulmonary artery catheterization should be considered.

ANTICONVULSANT THERAPY

A patient who requires anticonvulsant therapy also requires urgent delivery. This can only happen once the patient is stabilized, which requires protection and maintenance of a patent airway, administration of anticonvulsants, and control of any associated hypertension. Magnesium sulfate is now established as the anticonvulsant of first choice to control an eclampsia.[37] It is likely to act by reversing the vasospasm within the cerebral circulation. In addition to reducing the incidence of further seizures, benefits of magnesium sulfate over both diazepam and phenytoin, include a significantly lower need for maternal ventilation, less pneumonia, and fewer intensive care admissions. Magnesium sulfate acts as a membrane stabilizer, a vasodilator, and it reduces intracerebral ischemia. It is usually given as a 2 g intravenous loading dose and a maintenance infusion at 1–2 g/h. A maximum of 8 g can be administered. In cases of oliguria, care must be taken as magnesium sulfate is renally excreted. Early signs of toxicity are detected by absence of patella reflexes, ultimately respiratory arrest and muscle paralysis or cardiac arrest will occur. The antidote is 10 mL of 10 percent calcium gluconate given intravenously. Although effective in most cases, there is evidence that about 10 percent of women have a further seizure after starting magnesium sulfate.[38] Nevertheless, an eclamptic seizure is usually self-limiting and prolonged seizures warrant a brain scan to exclude other pathology, particularly an intracerebral bleed.

Even with severe preeclampsia, eclampsia is rare (<1 percent). The Magpie trial evaluated magnesium sulfate versus placebo in women with preeclampsia, and demonstrated a clear benefit of *prophylactic* therapy. Magnesium sulfate halved the risk of eclampsia and probably reduced the risk of maternal death. There did not appear to be any substantive harmful short-term effects on either mother or baby.[39] The difficulty, however, is not how, but who to treat. About 40 percent of all cases are either completely or partially unheralded; many have only moderate hypertension before having a seizure, and others unexpectedly convulse at home without prior documentation of disease.

ANESTHESIA

A general anesthetic can be particularly dangerous in women with preeclampsia as endotracheal intubation can cause severe hypertension. Neuraxial anesthesia is therefore the preferred method of analgesia for labor and anesthesia for operative deliveries but a coagulopathy must be excluded. A platelet count of greater than 80×10^9/L is adequate for hemostasis and most obstetric anesthetists will insert a regional block under these circumstances. Care must be taken to avoid arterial hypotension, in view of the vasoconstriction and reduced intravascular volume. This is particularly so following postpartum hemorrhage, when central invasive monitoring may need to be considered.

Delivery

Ultimately treatment necessitates delivery. The mode of delivery is determined amongst other things by the speed in which it must be expedited, the ability of the fetus to withstand labor, and the chances of successful induction. Where possible a vaginal delivery is the preferred option. It is worth considering that:

- Oxytocin has an antidiuretic effect. If given in large volumes it can result in hyponatremia, pulmonary edema, and convulsions. In addition oxytocin causes a peripheral vasodilation, with reflex tachycardia. In women with severe preeclampsia, the resultant increase in cardiac output can stress a possibly compromised heart, resulting in heart failure.
- Ergometrine may provoke an increase in blood pressure. Women with severe preeclampsia are particularly susceptible; the increase produced can result in a headache, eclampsia, or even death.
- A reduced intravascular space in preeclampsia means that blood loss is less well tolerated.

Postpartum care

A third of cases of eclampsia occur post partum, and intensive monitoring must therefore be maintained for 48 hours following delivery. Although eclampsia has been reported beyond this time it is unlikely to be associated with serious morbidity. Blood pressure is frequently at its highest 3–4 days after delivery. Antihypertensive therapy may therefore need to be continued following delivery and even after discharge home. In the absence of fetal considerations the most effective therapy can be used and drugs such as methyldopa discontinued.

All women who have had severe preeclampsia should be reviewed at a hospital postnatal clinic 6–12 weeks after delivery. Blood pressure should be measured and urinalysis performed. Tests of renal and liver function should also be undertaken; residual disease may merit referral to a physician. Underlying predispositions to preeclampsia (particularly in multiparas), such as inherited thrombophilias or antiphospholipid syndrome should be excluded. The postnatal visit also provides an excellent opportunity to discuss complications of the pregnancy, and the planned management of any future pregnancy.

CHRONIC HYPERTENSION

Chronic hypertension is detected either by an antecedent medical history or by a raised blood pressure in the first half of pregnancy. The physiologic decline in the blood pressure in early pregnancy is exaggerated in women with chronic hypertension so that they may be normotensive. Conversely in later pregnancy the physiologic increase of blood pressure in pregnancy is exaggerated.[40] A woman with chronic hypertension may be normotensive initially, developing hypertension only in the third trimester, thus presenting as PIH. Not uncommonly the presentation is of mild hypertension in the second half of pregnancy without any antecedent readings.

Chronic hypertension in pregnancy is a major predisposing factor for preeclampsia. The risk is about five times higher than in normotensive women. Preeclampsia superimposed on chronic hypertension tends to be recurrent. The signs of preeclampsia in this group of women are the same as in other women except that the blood pressure levels start from a higher baseline. When proteinuria develops this is inevitably associated with IUGR. The easiest diagnostic guide is maternal plasma urate levels. Values below 0.30 mmol/L would not support a diagnosis of preeclampsia. Women with chronic hypertension, who do not develop preeclampsia, can usually expect a normal, uncomplicated perinatal outcome.[41] There is some evidence for a modest increase in the incidence of IUGR in women with chronic hypertension.[42] Opinion is divided as to whether there is an increased risk of placental abruption within this group.

Although there is no direct evidence that any of the commonly used antihypertensive drugs (with the exception of angiotensin-converting enzyme inhibiters) are teratogenic there may be more subtle effects on fetal growth and development. Therefore any women with mild to moderate hypertension should discontinue treatment prior to conception. Because of the physiologic fall in blood pressure by the 12th week of pregnancy many women in this group may only require medication in the late trimester if at all. In women with higher blood pressure the value of treatment is debated. Outside pregnancy treatment is instigated to prevent long-term complications. In pregnancy the concern is the short term. There is no evidence that treating chronic hypertension reduces the risk of superimposed preeclampsia,[43] nor is there any evidence to support a particular fetal benefit. Indeed long-term use of antihypertensives themselves has been associated with modest fetal growth restriction. This may be due to a specific drug effect or consequent on a reduction in placental perfusion following a lowering of arterial pressure.

INTRAUTERINE GROWTH RESTRICTION

One of the most challenging areas currently facing obstetricians is the detection and management of pregnancies where the growth of the fetus is poor. There is little doubt that these fetuses experience not only increased rates of perinatal morbidity and mortality, but also higher levels of morbidity extending into adult life.

As many as 40 percent of so-called unexplained stillbirths are small for gestation (SGA). About 30 percent of cases of sudden infant death syndrome are SGA at birth and the overall mortality of babies with IUGR is as much as eightfold greater than appropriately grown babies. These babies are also at high risk of perinatal hypoxia and acidemia, operative delivery, and neonatal encephalopathy. Paradoxically, these babies have a slightly reduced incidence of respiratory distress syndrome presumably because of the intrauterine stress resulting in increased surfactant production.

It is possible that babies with IUGR are at increased risk of early cognitive/neurologic impairment and cerebral palsy, compared with those who are normal weight at birth. Long-term data in adults have also suggested that there are similar significant differences in academic achievement and professional attainment among these two groups, with better performances in those adults who had a normal birthweight. Finally it would also appear that the uterine environment to which the fetus is exposed can lead to 'programming' which then has consequences for adult health, the so-called 'Barker Hypothesis'. Being SGA is associated with an increased risk of hypertension, glucose intolerance and atheromatous vascular disease in later life.[44]

In defining SGA the WHO suggests that the cut-off should be made at the 10th centile, thus labeling 10 percent of all infants as SGA. Chard et al. argue that the majority of SGA babies are in fact 'healthy but small'.[45] They suggest that the diagnosis of IUGR should be reserved for those infants who fail to reach their genetic growth potential. A better definition would perhaps be 'fetuses whose growth velocity slows down or stops completely'. Pivotal to this definition is the determination of each fetus's growth potential. It is this group of fetuses with IUGR that are most at risk of the sequelae associated with poor growth.

The determinants of fetal size are multifactorial. Maternal size is of greater importance than paternal build. Additional factors include ethnicity and socioeconomic status. Fetal sex is also relevant, with male fetuses being on average some 200 g heavier than their female counterparts at term. The etiology of SGA can be divided into maternal factors (including diet, smoking, renal disease), fetal factors (genetic constitution, structural abnormality, infection), and placental factors (mosaicism). The use of ratios which attempt to correct for these confounding variables may correlate better with perinatal outcome.[46] Pregnancy-specific complications are also associated with IUGR. Preeclampsia is perhaps the best known (see earlier), and the focus of this chapter. Maternal disease severity and fetal involvement however do not always correlate; some babies of women who have eclampsia at term have normal birthweight.[47] It must be noted that not all babies with IUGR will be SGA, and not all infants who are SGA will have IUGR (only some 15 percent), which can also afflict larger infants. It does not, however, seem to affect pregnancy outcomes unless the fetus has an abdominal circumference under the 5th centile.[48] It is therefore logical to concentrate on this group.

In clinical practice once IUGR is diagnosed in SGA babies management options are limited to close surveillance and timely delivery, balancing the risks of continuing with the pregnancy against the risks of prematurity. This is based on the assumption that timely delivery will improve the outcome. However, a randomized controlled trial of timed delivery to the compromised fetus there was insufficient evidence to favor either immediate or delayed delivery as there was no difference in overall mortality and/or morbidity in either group. On this basis decisions will continue to be made case by case. Biometric tests are designed to predict size and if performed longitudinally, growth; biophysical tests, on the other hand, assess fetal wellbeing. Methods employed include abdominal palpation, symphyseal fundal height, ultrasound biometry and estimated fetal weight, cardiotocography, biophysical profiles, and Doppler flow velocimetry.

About a third of growth-restricted fetuses can be detected clinically, either by palpation or by measuring the symphyseal fundal height (SFH).[49] Serial assessment of the SFH, plotted on customized charts (adjusted for variables such as maternal height, weight, parity, and ethnic group), results in increased antenatal detection of SGA babies and fewer hospital investigations for fetal growth.[50] Such measurements need to be supplemented by ultrasound biometry. Whereas a single assessment of the abdominal circumference and/or an estimated fetal weight by ultrasound, especially when plotted on a customized chart, is the most accurate means of predicting SGA,[51] serial measurements (performed at least 2 weeks apart) are superior in the prediction of IUGR.[52]

The use of amniotic fluid volume in the evaluation of fetal wellbeing is well established. Phelan et al. introduced the concept of the amniotic fluid index (AFI),[53] as an alternative to the vertical diameter of the deepest pool. This is a semiquantitative technique, in which the pregnant woman has her uterus divided into four quadrants, by two imaginary lines, vertically along the linea nigra and horizontally across the umbilicus. The vertical diameter of the largest pocket in each segment is determined and the sum of each quadrant is the AFI. Oligohydramnios is defined as less than 5 cm, and polyhydramnios as greater than 25 cm. Normal values have been constructed for each gestation.[54] A reduced AFI is associated with increased perinatal mortality.

There is compelling evidence from a systemic review that umbilical artery Doppler waveform, when used to monitor high risk fetuses, results in reduced perinatal morbidity and mortality.[55] A study comparing cardiotocography, biophysical profiles, and Doppler found that only the latter had value in predicting poor perinatal outcome in SGA fetuses.[56] Biophysical profiles may be useful when Doppler becomes abnormal, as they have a good negative predictive value in high-risk populations.[57] Umbilical artery Doppler waveform demonstrates that, in normal pregnancy, there is forward flow from the fetus to the placenta throughout the cardiac cycle. However in the placentae of fetuses with IUGR there is increased vascular resistance, which leads to reduced flow in the diastolic component of the fetal cardiac cycle (end diastolic flow), in the umbilical artery. Progressive degrees of placental pathology leads, in turn, to absent and then reversed end diastolic flow. The degree of abnormality in the umbilical artery Doppler waveform correlates well with the risk of fetal hypoxia. In high-risk pregnancies with absent end diastolic flow, 80 percent of fetuses will be hypoxic and 46 percent acidemic, with the relative risk of perinatal mortality being 1.0 where end diastolic flow is present, 4.0 with absent end diastolic flow and 10.6 with reversed end diastolic flow.[58]

It is apparent that the interval between the loss of end diastolic flow and fetal demise may vary from days to weeks and that the onset of cardiotocographic abnormalities is very late in the process – at which stage, fetal damage may well be irreversible. Thus, particularly at the extremes of viability, much interest has been paid to methods of fetal surveillance that would allow pregnancy to be prolonged in cases of IUGR with absent end diastolic flow. In these fetuses, so-called brain sparing can be detected by changes in Doppler waveform indices of the middle cerebral artery (MCA), which represent increased flow. Long-term follow-up of fetuses demonstrating increased MCA flow indicate that it is a benign adaptive mechanism. Although this increase in cerebral blood flow occurs sequentially after reduced growth velocity and loss of umbilical artery end diastolic flow, reversal of this adaptation is sudden and is associated with a poor prognosis. Thus serial assessment of the MCA waveform does not give suitable forewarning of deterioration for it to be clinically helpful.

Many other arterial waveforms have been assessed, in an attempt to more accurately predict early decompensation in IUGR with absent end diastolic flow , all to no avail. However examination of the fetal venous systems has indicated an increased pulsatility in the umbilical veins and vena cava, with reversed flow during atrial contraction in the ductus venous (reversed 'a' wave) in fetuses with absent end diastolic flow. These all seem to give adequate warning of fetal decompensation, with the latter being particularly promising in clinical practice.[59] If a diagnosis of IUGR is made after 34 weeks' gestation, then delivery is indicated. Under 34 weeks' gestation, steroids should be administered prior to delivery if possible. Between 28 and 34 weeks' gestation, the presence of reversed end diastolic flow should prompt delivery. The management of absent end diastolic flow under 34 weeks' gestation and indeed reversed end diastolic flow under 28 weeks' gestation is more controversial. Optimal surveillance strategies have not been established.[49]

It is recommended that pregnancies complicated by IUGR and absent end diastolic flow in the umbilical artery should be managed by clinicians with a special interest in fetal medicine, in units capable of providing intensive neonatal care. Growth-restricted fetuses are at high risk of intrapartum hypoxia and acidemia. At gestations under 37 weeks, delivery by cesarean section is usually the best option. For those in whom labor is induced continuous electronic fetal monitoring, with early recourse to fetal scalp sampling, is recommended. Prostaglandins and oxytocin must be used with great care, because of the risk of uterine hypertonicity and fetal compromise.

IMPLICATIONS FOR MATERNAL HEALTH

Epidemiologic studies have recently demonstrated a relationship between a pregnancy complicated by preeclampsia and an increased risk of maternal coronary heart disease in later life. A study of 374 Icelandic women with a past history of pregnancy-induced hypertension indicated the death rate, from coronary heart disease, was significantly higher (1.47, 95 percent CI 1.05 to 2.02) than expected from analysis of population data, during corresponding periods. The relative risk of dying from coronary heart disease was further increased among women who had had eclampsia (RR 2.61, 95 percent CI 1.11 to 6.12) or preeclampsia (RR 1.90, 95 percent CI 1.02 to 3.52) compared with those with hypertension alone.[59] Overall the reported increased relative risk of death from ischemic heart disease in these women is 1.7 which translates to an absolute risk of about an additional four deaths per 10 000 women years.[60] This figure would be increased with additional risk factors such as age, smoking and body mass index.

The pathophysiologies of both ischemic heart disease and preeclampsia have been independently and comprehensively investigated. Data would suggest common pathways, including impaired insulin sensitivity, dyslipidemia, and coagulation disturbance. The specific vascular lesion of preeclampsia, that is, the acute atherosis in the intima of the spiral arterioles of the placental bed, is similar to that seen in arteriosclerosis.

Like coronary heart disease, preeclampsia is probably not associated with a single causative factor, but instead an accumulation of factors, both maternal (adiposity, insulin resistance and phenotype) and fetal (placentation), that work together to produce a 'vascular stress' such that the threshold for disease risk is exceeded. The inflammatory and metabolic response to pregnancy is exaggerated, and the usual buffering mechanisms are no longer adequate. In such an individual this threshold for clinical cardiovascular disease is breached; first during pregnancy and again in later life, when other acquired cardiovascular risk factors, such as age, are encountered. In this way, adverse pregnancy outcome may reveal women at increased risk of metabolic and vascular diseases in later life. This link between pregnancy complications and risk of vascular disease provides an important opportunity for identifying those individuals at risk. This is vital if lifestyle changes, such that would modify this disease risk, could then be instigated.

Intervention for women with a past history or preeclampsia could be focused on the perimenopausal years, a time when risk of vascular disease increases rapidly, or even earlier. Screening in these women would take the form of routine coronary heart disease assessment, which would include measurement of blood pressure, fasting lipids (total cholesterol, triglyceride and high-density lipoprotein cholesterol) and glucose concentrations. Derivation of coronary heart disease risk, using widely available risk factor charts based on equations derived from the Framingham heart study, could then be undertaken. Guidelines for the primary prevention of coronary heart disease[60] recommend that the use of cholesterol-lowering drugs, antihypertensive agents, and aspirin should be based on the individual's projected 'cardiac risk', and not on measurements of individual parameters alone. For cholesterol-lowering treatment, individuals should have a projected risk of sustaining a coronary heart disease event in a 10-year period of ⩾30 percent, but a risk of only ⩾15 percent for initiating antihypertensive or aspirin treatment.[61]

To help ensure that appropriate women are screened and given relevant health education, the family physician needs to be informed and involved. Interventions could start at the routine 6-week postpartum review when these women could be made aware of their potentially increased risk for coronary heart disease and counseled appropriately regarding lifestyle modification, such as diet and exercise.

There is the potential for modification of risk factors in advance of a subsequent pregnancy or in early pregnancy. Increased physical activity in women who are sedentary may result in a better pregnancy outcome for both mother and child. Work to date has indicated that increasing exercise during pregnancy may both increase birthweight,[62] and reduce the risk of gestational diabetes.[63] Clearly, such data are encouraging, and would suggest that complications are not simply genetically determined, but that lifestyle factors play a major role.

The majority of the above findings come from observational studies, with a relatively small number of cases or endpoints. There is, however, an urgent need to explore vascular and metabolic risk factors and their association to adverse pregnancy outcome, with larger cohorts and longer periods of follow-up, adequate control groups, and proper attention to confounding factors such as smoking. Such knowledge has great potential to impact not only on women's health but also on the health of future generations.

KEY LEARNING POINTS

- Preeclampsia is a multisystem disorder involving the placenta, liver, kidneys, blood, cardiovascular and neurological systems; hypertension and proteinuria are diagnostic signs.
- Both maternal and fetal morbidity and mortality are more likely to occur with early-onset disease.
- In spite of many tests being investigated, preeclampsia cannot be accurately predicted.
- Cerebral hemorrhage and adult respiratory distress are common causes of death in preeclampsia, therefore acute management focuses on controlling blood pressure and restricting fluid intake.

- Early-onset preeclampsia is frequently associated with placental insufficiency, which can result in IUGR, abruption of the placenta and even fetal death. Fetal wellbeing must be carefully considered in all cases. Suspected fetal compromise is a frequent indication for delivery in preeclampsia.
- Preeclamptic hypertension can cause direct arterial injury, which can, in turn, predispose to possibly fatal cerebral hemorrhage. To prevent this injury severe hypertension should be avoided. Blood pressures greater than 170/110 mm Hg (MAP of greater than or equal to 140 mm Hg) require urgent therapy.
- In practice the choice of antihypertensive agent probably matters less than the clinician's familiarity with it.
- Magnesium sulfate is now established as the anticonvulsant of first choice to control an eclamptic fit.
- Epidemiologic studies have recently demonstrated a relation between a pregnancy complicated by preeclampsia and an increased risk of maternal coronary heart disease in later life.
- This link between pregnancy complications and risk of vascular disease provides an important opportunity for identifying those individuals at risk.
- Interventions could start at the routine 6-week postpartum review when these women could be made aware of their potentially increased risk for coronary heart disease and counseled appropriately regarding lifestyle modification, such as diet and exercise.

REFERENCES

1   Davey DA, MacGillivray I. The classification and definition of the hypertensive disorders of pregnancy. *Am J Obstet Gynecol* 1988; **1**: 892–8.
2   Shennan A, Gupta M, Halligan A, *et al.* Lack of reproducibility in pregnancy of Korotkoff Phase IV as measured by mercury sphygmomanometry. *Lancet* 1996; **347**: 139–42.
3   Hayman R, Baker PN. *Hypertension in Pregnancy: Definition, Diagnosis and Investigation. 1997 a CME Self-assessment Test.* London: RCOG Press.
4   Robertson WB, Brosens I, Dixon HG. The pathological response of the vessels of the placental bed to hypertensive pregnancy. *J Pathol Bacteriol* 1967; **93**: 581–92.
5   Robertson WB, Brosens I, Dixon HG. Uteroplacental vascular pathology. *Eur J Obstet Gynaecol Reprod Biol* 1975; **5**: 47–65.
6   Roberts JM, Taylor RN, Musci TJ, *et al.* Pre-eclampsia: an endothelial cell disorder. *Am J Obstet Gynecol* 1989; **161**: 1200–4.
7   Higgins JR, Walshe JJ, Halligan A, *et al.* Can 24-hour ambulatory blood pressure measurement predict the

development of hypertension in primigravidae? *Br J Obstet Gynaecol* 1997; **104**: 356–62.

8   Department of Health. *Why Mothers Die. Report on Confidential Enquiries into Maternal Deaths in the United Kingdom 1997–1999*. London: The Stationery Office, 2001.

9   Douglas KA, Redman CWG. Eclampsia in the United Kingdom. *BMJ* 1994; **309**: 1395–400.

10 Barker DJP, Bull AR, Osmond C. Fetal and placental size and risk of hypertension in adult life. *BMJ* 1990; **301**: 259–61.

11 Cincotta RB, Brennecke SP. Family history of pre-eclampsia as a predictor for pre-eclampsia in primigravidas. *Int J Gynecol Obstet* 1998; **60**: 23–7.

12 MacGilliary I. Some observations on the incidence of pre-eclampsia. *J Obstet Gynaecol Br Commonwealth* 1959; **65**: 536–9.

13 Robillard PY, Husley TC. Association of pregnancy-induced-hypertension, pre-eclampsia, and eclampsia with duration of sexual cohabitation before conception. *Lancet* 1988; **159**: 1452–5.

14 Butler NR, Bonham DG. *Perinatal Mortality*. Edinburgh: Churchill Livingstone, 1963: 87–100.

15 Ros HS, Cnattingius S, Lipworth L. Comparison of risk factors for pre-eclampsia and gestational hypertension in a population-based cohort study. *Am J Epidemiol* 1998; **47**: 1062–70.

16 Branch DW, Andres R, Digre KB, *et al*. The association of antiphospholipid antibodies with severe pre-eclampsia. *Obstet Gynecol* 1989; **73**: 541–5.

17 Chun D, Braga C, Chow C, Lok L. Clinical observation on some aspects of hydatidiform moles. *J Obstet Gynaecol Br Commonwealth* 1964; **71**: 180–4.

18 Jeffcoate TNA, Scott JS. Some observations on the placental factor in pregnancy toxaemia. *Am J Obstet Gynecol* 1959; **77**: 475–89.

19 Rijhsinghani A, Yankowitz J, Strauss RA, *et al*. Risk of pre-eclampsia in second trimester triploid pregnancies. *Obstet Gynecol* 1997; **90**: 884–8.

20 Kyle PM, Buckley D, Kissaine J, *et al*. The angiotensin sensitivity test and low dose aspirin are ineffective methods to predict and prevent hypertensive disorders in nulliparous pregnancy. *Am J Obstet Gynecol* 1995; **173**: 865–72.

21 Mires GJ, Williams FL, Leslie J, Howie PW. Assessment of uterine arterial notching as a screening test for adverse pregnancy outcome. *Am J Obstet Gynecol* 1998; **179**: 1317–23.

22 Stamilio DM, Sehdev HM, Morgan MA, *et al*. Can antenatal clinical and biochemical markers predict the development of severe pre-eclampsia? *Am J Obstet Gynecol* 2000; **182**: 589–94.

23 Cuckle H, Sehmi I, Jones R. Maternal serum inhibin A can predict pre-eclampsia. *Br J Obstet Gynaecol* 1998; **105**: 1101–3.

24 Chappell LC, Seed PT, Briley A, *et al*. A longitudinal study of biochemical variables in women at risk of preeclampsia. *Am J Obstet Gynecol* 2002; **187**: 127–36.

♦ 25 Duley L, Henderson-Smart D, Knight M, King J. Anti-platelet drugs for prevention of pre-eclampsia and its consequences: systematic review. *BMJ* 2001; **322**: 329–33.

26 Chappell LC, Seed PT, Briley AL, *et al*. Prevention of pre-eclampsia by antioxidants: a randomized trial of vitamins C and E in women at increased risk of pre-eclampsia. *Lancet* 1999; **354**: 810–16.

27 Poston L, Briley AL, Seed PT, *et al*. Vitamins in Pre-eclampsia (VIP) Trial Consortium. Vitamin C and vitamin E in pregnant women at risk for pre-eclampsia (VIP trial): randomised placebo-controlled trial. *Lancet* 2006; **367**: 1119–20.

28 Rumbold AR, Crowther CA, Haslam RR, *et al*. ACTS Study Group. Vitamins C and E and the risks of preeclampsia and perinatal complications. *N Engl J Med* 2006; **354**: 1841–3.

29 Von Dadelszen P, Ornstein MP, Bull SB, *et al*. Fall in mean arterial pressure and fetal growth restriction in pregnancy hypertension: a meta-analysis. *Lancet* 2000; **355**: 87–92.

30 Sabai BM, Mercer BM, Schiff E, Friedman SA. Aggressive versus expectant management of severe pre-eclampsia at 28–32 weeks gestation: a randomised control trial. *Am J Obstet Gynecol* 1994; **171**: 818–22.

31 Assali NS, Kaplan S, Oighenstein S, Suyemoto R. Hemodynamic effects of l-hyralaziinophthalazine in human pregnancy; results of intravenous administration. *J Clin Invest* 1953; **32**: 922–30.

32 Vink GJ, Moodley J. The effect of low dose dihydrallazine on the fetus in the emergency treatment of hypertension in pregnancy. *S Afr Med J* 1982; **62**: 475–7.

33 Magee LA, Ornstein MP, von Dadelszen P. Fortnightly review: management of hypertension in pregnancy. *BMJ* 1999; **318**: 1332–6.

34 Goodlin RC. Safety of sodium nitroprusside. *Obstet Gynecol* 1983; **62**: 270.

35 Iseri LT, French JH. Magnesium: nature's physiological calcium blocker. *Am Heart J* 1984; **108**: 188–94.

36 Ulmsten U. Treatment of normotensive and hypertensive with preterm labour using oral nifedipine, a calcium antagonist. *Arch Gynecol* 1984; **246**: 69–72.

● 37 Which anticonvulsant for women with eclampsia? Evidence from the Collaborative Eclampsia Trial. *Lancet* 1995; **345**: 1455–63.

38 Sawhney H, Sawhney IM, Mandal R, *et al*. Efficacy of magnesium sulphate and phenytoin in the management of eclampsia. *J Obstet Gynecol Res* 1999; **25**: 333–8.

● 39 The Magpie collaborative group. Do women with pre-eclampsia, and their babies, benefit from magnesium sulphate? The magpie trial: a randomised placebo-controlled trial. *Lancet* 2002; **359**: 1877–90.

40 Chesley EM, Agamanolis DP, Banker BQ, Victor M. Hypertensive encephalopathy: a clinicopathologic study of 20 cases. *Neurology* 1978; **28**: 928–39.

41 Chamberlain G, Philipp E, Howlett B, Masters K. *British Births 1970. Vol 2: Obstetric Care*. London: Heinemann Medical Books, 1978.

42 Haelterman E, Breart G, Paris LJ, *et al.* Effect of uncomplicated chronic hypertension on the risk of small-for-gestational age birth. *Am J Epidemiol* 1997; **1**: 689–95.

43 Sibai BM, Mabie BC, Shamsa F, *et al.* A comparison of no medication versus methyldopa or labetalol in chronic hypertension during pregnancy. *Am J Obstet Gynecol* 1990; **1**: 960–6.

44 Barker DJ. The long-term outcome of retarded fetal growth. *Clin Obstet Gynecol* 1997; **40**: 853–63.

45 Chard T, Yoong A, Macintosh M. The myth of fetal growth retardation at term. *Br J Obstet Gynaecol* 1993; **100**: 1076–81.

46 Wilcox MA, Johnson IR, Maynard PV, *et al.* The individualised birthweight ratio: a more logical outcome measure of pregnancy than birthweight alone. *Br J Obstet Gynaecol* 1993; **100**: 342–47.

47 Bobrow CS, Soothill PW. Fetal growth velocity: a cautionary tale. *Lancet* 1999; **3**: 1460.

48 The Grit study Group. A randomized trial of timed delivery for compromised preterm fetus: short term outcomes and Bayesian interpretation. *Br J Obstet Gynaecol* 2003; **110**: 27–32.

49 Coomarasamy A, Fisk NM, Gee H, Robson SC. *The Investigation and Management of the Small-for-gestational-age Fetus.* RCOG Guidelines No 31. London: RCOG, 2002.

50 Gardosi JO, Mongelli JM, Mul T. Intrauterine growth retardation. *Baillieres Clin Obstet Gynecol* 1995; **9**: 445–63.

51 Chang TC, Robson SC, Boys RJ, Spencer JA. Prediction of the small for gestational age infant: which ultrasonic measurement is best? *Obstet Gynecol* 1992; **80**: 1030–8.

52 Chang TC, Robson SC, Spencer JA, Gallivan S. Identification of fetal growth retardation: comparison of Doppler waveform indices and serial ultrasound measurements of abdominal circumference and fetal weight. *Obstet Gynecol* 1993; **82**: 230–6.

53 Phelan JP, Ahn MO, Smith CV, *et al.* Amniotic fluid index measurements during pregnancy. *J Reprod Med* 1987; **32**: 601.

54 Bastide A, Manning F, Morrison I, *et al.* Ultrasound evaluation of amniotic fluid: outcome of pregnancies with severe oligohydramnios. *Am J Obstet Gynecol* 1986; **154**: 895–900.

55 Alfirevic Z, Neilson JP. Doppler ultrasonography in high risk pregnancies: systemic review with meta-analysis. *Am J Obstet Gynecol* 1995; **172**: 1379–87.

56 Soothill PW, Ajayi RA, Campbell S, Nicolides KH. Prediction of morbidity in small and normally grown fetuses by fetal heart rate variability, biophysical score and umbilical artery Doppler studies. *Br J Obstet Gynaecol* 1993; **100**: 742–5.

57 Dayal AK, Manning FA, Bereck DJ, *et al.* Fetal death after normal biophysical score: an eighteen-year experience. *Am J Obstet Gynecol* 1999; **181**: 1231–6.

58 Karsdorp VH, van Vugt JM, van Geijn HP, *et al.* Clinical significance of absent or reversed end diastolic velocity waveforms in umbilical artery. *Lancet* 1994; **344**: 1664–68.

59 Hecher K, Hackeloer BJ. Cardiotocogram compared to Doppler investigation of the fetal circulation in the premature growth-retarded fetus: longitudinal observations. *Ultrasound Obstet Gynecol* 1997; **9**: 152–61.

60 Sattar N, Greer IA. Pregnancy complications and maternal cardiovascular risk: opportunities for intervention and screening? *BMJ* 2002; **325**: 157–60.

61 Joint British recommendations on prevention of coronary heart disease in clinical practice. British Cardiac Society, British Hyperlipidaemia Association, British Hypertension Society, endorsed by the British Diabetic Association. *Heart* 1998; **80**(Suppl 2): S1–29.

62 Clapp JF, Little KD. The interaction between regular exercise and selected aspects of women's health. *Am J Obstet Gynecol* 1995; **173**: 2–9.

63 Carpenter MW. The role of exercise in pregnant women with diabetes mellitus. *Clin Obstet Gynecol* 2000; **43**: 56–64.

27

Thrombocytopenia in pregnancy

KATHRYN E WEBERT, JOHN G KELTON

INTRODUCTION

Thrombocytopenia is defined as a reduction in the number of circulating platelets to less than the laboratory's normal value, which is typically less than 150×10^9/L. It is important to note that the normal range for an individual's platelet count has been determined in healthy, but not pregnant individuals. Therefore, this value may not necessarily reflect the normal range in pregnant women.

NORMAL PLATELET COUNT IN AN UNCOMPLICATED PREGNANCY

In general, the platelet count of a healthy woman with an uncomplicated pregnancy falls by about 10 percent during the pregnancy with the greatest decrease occurring in the third trimester.[1] Approximately 8 percent of women will experience a severe decrease in their platelet count leading to moderate thrombocytopenia. Therefore, it is possible that mild thrombocytopenia is a physiologic variant that requires neither intervention nor specific therapy.[2,3]

EVALUATION OF A PREGNANT WOMAN WITH THROMBOCYTOPENIA

History and physical examination

When evaluating a pregnant woman with thrombocytopenia the physician should consider three questions:

- What is the etiology of the thrombocytopenia?
- What is the risk to the mother?
- What is the risk to the fetus?

It is important to elicit the duration of the hemostatic impairment. Questions about a history of bleeding and spontaneous or easy bruising help to establish chronicity. The woman should be asked about drug use including prescription drugs, over-the-counter medications, herbal remedies, and illicit drugs. For example, it is important to determine if she has recently ingested an antiplatelet agent, such as aspirin or alcohol, which interferes with platelet function and can trigger bleeding or bruising. She should also be questioned about systemic symptoms, such as joint symptoms, rash, fevers, and night sweats as these symptoms are suggestive of secondary thrombocytopenia, which include systemic lupus erythematosus (SLE), human immunodeficiency virus (HIV) infection, and lymphoproliferative disorders (Box 27.1), and also about risk factors for HIV. In addition, she should be asked about any family members with a history of thrombocytopenia or bleeding disorders as this would be suggestive of inherited causes of thrombocytopenia, such as von Willebrand disease, type IIb or congenital thrombocytopenia. Finally, an obstetrical history should be obtained with specific attention paid to thrombocytopenia, complications in previous pregnancies, and any history of pregnancy loss. A history of pregnancy loss may be associated with the presence of an antiphospholipid antibody.

The physical examination should focus on evidence of hemostatic impairment and signs of an underlying cause of thrombocytopenia. Many patients with thrombocytopenia are asymptomatic. Only at very low platelet counts are petechiae observed. Petechiae are tiny, red dots found on dependent parts of the body and at sites of trauma. They represent minute collections of red cells that have leaked from blood vessels. Petechiae are specific for thrombocytopenia. Large bruises or purpura are often observed on the limbs and trunk and have a lower specificity. The risk of bleeding increases progressively from asymptomatic patients, to patients with petechiae and purpura, to

---

Box 27.1 Secondary causes of thrombocytopenia (adapted from Webert and Kelton[4])

Infections
- Human immunodeficiency virus
- Varicella zoster virus
- Epstein–Barr virus

Collagen vascular disease
- SLE
- Rheumatoid arthritis
- Progressive systemic sclerosis
- Sjögren's syndrome

Lymphoproliferative disorders
- Chronic lymphocytic leukemia
- Hodgkin disease
- Non-Hodgkin lymphoma

Other
- Antiphospholipid antibody syndrome
- Autoimmune thyroid dysfunction
- Sarcoidosis
- Post-bone marrow transplantation
- Inflammatory bowel disease
- Autoimmune hemolytic anemia (Evan's syndrome)
- Bullous pemphigoid
- Myasthenia gravis

---

patients who have mucous membrane bleeding, which is typically manifested by blood blisters in the mouth. Blood blisters usually occur on the bite margins of the oral mucosa and tongue. They indicate that the patient is at significant risk for bleeding and that treatment is urgently required. Physical exam should focus on the examination of the joints, lymph nodes, spleen, and liver since abnormalities in these areas may indicate a secondary cause of thrombocytopenia. The pregnant woman's blood pressure should be measured to rule out a hypertensive disorder of pregnancy.

Laboratory evaluation

One of the most important first steps is to review the peripheral blood film, looking for pseudothrombocytopenia. Pseudothrombocytopenia is a laboratory artifact that causes spontaneous platelet agglutination and results in platelets clumps seen in the peripheral blood film. Automated determination of the platelet count will be inaccurate, as the machine will not recognize the larger platelet aggregates as platelets. Pseudothrombocytopenia commonly occurs because of agglutination of the patient's platelets in ethylenediaminetetraacetic acid (EDTA). This disorder occurs in approximately 0.1 percent of blood samples and is typically caused by an EDTA-dependent autoantibody that agglutinates platelets at low calcium concentrations. This can be avoided by using an anticoagulant other than EDTA to collect the blood sample. This condition is of no clinical significance and does not appear to be more common in pregnancy. Another cause of pseudothrombocytopenia is platelet satellitism. In this condition, platelets form rosettes around neutrophils or monocytes. Other less common causes of pseudothrombocytopenia include agglutination of platelet by monoclonal paraproteins or platelet-reactive cold agglutinins. Hemoglobin and white blood cell count should be evaluated. Cytopenias involving other cell lines are suggestive of disorders of the bone marrow such as myeloproliferative or myelodysplastic syndromes.

The platelet count helps to determine the woman's bleeding risk. People with mild thrombocytopenia (platelet count $<150 \times 10^9$/L but $>50 \times 10^9$/L) have a low risk of bleeding. Those with severe thrombocytopenia (platelet count $<20 \times 10^9$/L) have a higher risk of bleeding and can experience spontaneous bleeding. The peripheral blood film may lead to the diagnosis of the condition causing the thrombocytopenia. Fragmented red cells or schistocytes are observed in thrombotic thrombocytopenic purpura (TTP), hemolytic uremic syndrome (HUS), disseminated intravascular coagulation (DIC), and hypertensive disorders of pregnancy, such as preeclampsia. Leukoerythroblastic changes in the peripheral film, such as teardrop-shaped red blood cells, nucleated red blood cells, and immature white cells, suggest infiltration of the bone marrow. The presence of abnormal circulating cells, such as lymphoblasts or myeloblasts, suggests a malignant process. Typical changes on the peripheral blood film such as megaloblastic red blood cells and hypersegmented neutrophils suggest the diagnosis of vitamin B_{12} or folate deficiency. The finding of atypical lymphocytes raises the possibility of a viral infection. Finally, the finding of giant platelets on the peripheral blood film suggests the diagnosis of certain congenital thrombocytopenias.

Examination of the bone marrow should be considered if the etiology of the thrombocytopenia is uncertain after the initial evaluation. In addition, a bone marrow examination should be performed when abnormalities are seen on the peripheral blood film or when multiple blood cell lineages are affected. The finding of normal or increased numbers of megakaryocytes in the marrow is supportive of a diagnosis of peripheral destruction or sequestration of the platelets. Other laboratory tests that may be indicated include: urinalysis (to check for proteinuria); creatinine; liver function tests and liver transaminases; other coagulation parameters, such as fibrinogen, international normalized ratio (INR) and prothrombin time (PT); anti-nuclear antibody (ANA); rheumatoid factor (RF); anticardiolipin antibodies; antiphospholipid antibodies; thyroid-stimulating hormone (TSH); and testing for HIV infection.

ETIOLOGY OF THROMBOCYTOPENIA IN PREGNANCY

Thrombocytopenia is common in pregnancy. In fact, a prospective study of approximately 15 000 mother and newborn pairs demonstrated that thrombocytopenia occurs in 7 percent of women.[5] The most common causes of thrombocytopenia were incidental thrombocytopenia of pregnancy (74 percent), thrombocytopenia complicating hypertensive disorders of pregnancy (21 percent), and thrombocytopenia associated with immunologic disorders such as idiopathic thrombocytopenic purpura (ITP) and SLE (4 percent). Other less common causes of thrombocytopenia include thrombotic thrombocytopenic purpura and hemolytic uremic syndrome (TTP-HUS), DIC, acute fatty liver of pregnancy, antiphospholipid antibody syndrome, thrombocytopenia secondary to medications, and HIV infection.

The etiology of thrombocytopenia is classified by pathogenic mechanism. These mechanisms include decreased production of platelets, increased destruction of platelets, and decreased numbers of circulating platelets (because of increased sequestration of platelets in the spleen or dilutional causes) (Table 27.1). Thrombocytopenia in pregnancy can also be caused by mechanisms such as acute fatty liver of pregnancy, and others may be due to underlying maternal medical conditions, either previously diagnosed or undiagnosed (Box 27.2). The timing of when the thrombocytopenia occurs in pregnancy may provide a clue as to its etiology (Table 27.2). A summary of the clinical findings of various causes of thrombocytopenia is provided in Table 27.3.

INCIDENTAL THROMBOCYTOPENIA OF PREGNANCY

Introduction/clinical presentation

Incidental thrombocytopenia of pregnancy, sometimes designated as gestational thrombocytopenia, is the most common cause of thrombocytopenia in pregnancy and has been estimated to occur in approximately 60–70 women per 1000 live births.[5] Affected women are otherwise well and healthy.[2,5] The thrombocytopenia is typically detected in the late second or third trimester.[7] Most women with gestational thrombocytopenia have platelet counts between 100×10^9/L and 150×10^9/L.[2]

Incidental thrombocytopenia of pregnancy is a diagnosis of exclusion. A woman is diagnosed with incidental thrombocytopenia of pregnancy if she has mild thrombocytopenia (platelet count $>70 \times 10^9$/L but $<150 \times 10^9$/L) and no other cause of thrombocytopenia (such as hypertension). A woman with mild thrombocytopenia should have a review of her blood film to rule out other abnormalities and a physical exam to exclude other causes of thrombocytopenia such as hypertension or hypersplenism.

Occasionally, people with incidental thrombocytopenia of pregnancy have a platelet count less than 70×10^9/L. Similarly, patients with mild ITP can have a platelet count greater than 70×10^9/L. Therefore, there may be instances in which it is difficult to distinguish between the two disorders. As the obstetrical management of women with mild thrombocytopenia is similar, the differentiation is less important. However, since ITP can result in a decreased neonatal platelet count (see subsequent section), neonatal platelet count should be monitored.

Pathophysiology

The pathophysiology of incidental thrombocytopenia of pregnancy is unknown. It is possible that this condition is simply representative of a shift in the normal distribution of the maternal platelet count that occurs with pregnancy. The distribution of platelet counts of pregnant women with incidental thrombocytopenia is illustrated in Figure 27.1. Consequently, we believe that this condition represents a normal physiologic variant of pregnancy.

Treatment

No treatment is required for incidental thrombocytopenia of pregnancy. Obstetrical care should not be modified and may include epidural anesthetic and vaginal delivery as indicated. The maternal platelet count typically returns to normal within 6 weeks of delivery, but the thrombocytopenia may recur in subsequent pregnancies. In a large prospective case series, the fetal platelet count was normal with no risk to the fetus demonstrated.[5] If the infant is thrombocytopenic, an alternative diagnosis, such as neonatal alloimmune thrombocytopenia, should be considered.

Table 27.1   Etiology of thrombocytopenia by pathophysiologic mechanism (adapted from Webert and Kelton[6])

Pathophysiologic mechanism	Relative frequency
Decreased platelet production	
Acquired	
Marrow infiltration: metastatic cancer, hematologic malignancies (leukemia, lymphoma, myeloma), myelofibrosis, storage disorders, granulomatous disorders (sarcoidosis)	+++
Marrow aplasia: aplastic anemia, post-chemotherapy, post-radiation therapy	+++
Amegakaryocytic thrombocytopenia	++
Ineffective thrombopoiesis: myelodysplasia, secondary to toxins (alcohol), folate and vitamin B_{12} deficiency, paroxysmal nocturnal hemoglobinuria	+
Congenital	
Wiskott–Aldrich syndrome and variants	+
Bernard Soulier syndrome	+
May–Hegglin anomaly	+
Alport syndrome and variants	+
Other	+
Increased platelet destruction	
Immune mechanisms	
Autoimmune	
Idiopathic thrombocytopenic purpura	+++++
Evan syndrome	++
Secondary to other disorders	
Lymphoproliferative disorders, systemic lupus erythematosus, human immunodeficiency virus infection, thyroid dysfunction, hypogammaglobulinemia, antiphospholipid antibody syndrome	+++
Alloimmune	
Neonatal alloimmune thrombocytopenia	++
Posttransfusion purpura	+
Refractoriness to platelet transfusions	+++
Immune complex mediated	++
Drug-induced	++
Non-immune mechanisms	
Disseminated intravascular coagulation	+++
Thrombotic thrombocytopenic purpura, hemolytic uremic syndrome	++
Sepsis	++++
Malignant hypertension	++
Hypertensive disorders of pregnancy	+++
Hypersplenism	+++
Abnormal vascular surfaces	++
von Willebrand disease, type IIB	+
Decreased numbers of circulating platelets (sequestration)	
Splenomegaly	++++
Extracorporeal circulation	++
Dilutional disorders	++
Hypothermia	++

THROMBOCYTOPENIA ASSOCIATED WITH HYPERTENSIVE DISORDERS OF PREGNANCY

Clinical presentation/introduction

Hypertension in pregnancy is common, occurring in approximately 20 percent of all women. It is the second most common cause of thrombocytopenia in pregnancy.[2] It has been demonstrated to occur with an incidence of 13–15 per 1000 live births or in approximately 1–2 percent of all pregnancies.[2] There are four main hypertensive disorders in pregnancy: chronic hypertension; gestational hypertension; preeclampsia/eclampsia; and preeclampsia

Box 27.2 Causes of thrombocytopenia during pregnancy

Common causes
- Incidental thrombocytopenia of pregnancy*
- Hypertensive disorders of pregnancy (preeclampsia)*
- Primary autoimmune thrombocytopenia:
  - ITP
- Secondary autoimmune thrombocytopenia:
  - SLE
  - Antiphospholipid antibody syndrome
  - Related to medication/drugs
  - HIV infection
  - Other
- Hemolysis, elevated liver enzymes, low platelets (HELLP) syndrome*

Rare causes
- DIC
- TTP-HUS
- Folate deficiency
- Viral infection
- Hematologic malignancies
- Hypersplenism
- Congenital causes of decreased platelet production (for example, Bernard Soulier syndrome)

*Cause unique to pregnancy.

occurring in a woman with chronic hypertension (discussed in Chapter 26). The platelet count in women with preeclampsia or eclampsia may be decreased whereas it tends to be normal in women with chronic or gestational hypertension. Therefore, only preeclampsia and eclampsia will be discussed further.

Preeclampsia and eclampsia

Preeclampsia is defined as hypertension and proteinuria occurring after 20 weeks' gestation in a woman with no history of hypertension. Preeclampsia is associated with clinical manifestations that may include hypertension, proteinuria, edema, central nervous system symptoms (for example, headache, blurred vision, or scotoma), pulmonary edema, microangiopathic hemolytic anemia, and thrombocytopenia. When the woman also has seizures not attributable to another cause, she is said to have eclampsia. Preeclampsia is common and is estimated to occur in 3–14 percent of all pregnancies.[8,9] Eclampsia has been estimated to occur in 0.05–0.10 percent of pregnancies.[9] The incidence of both conditions tends to be lower in developed countries compared with underdeveloped countries.[9]

Thrombocytopenia occurs in about 33 percent of women with preeclampsia.[10] The thrombocytopenia is typically mild to moderate in severity, with counts generally in the range

Table 27.2 Etiology of thrombocytopenia based on gestational age

First trimester (1–12 weeks)	Second trimester (13–27 weeks)	Third trimester (28+ weeks)
ITP	ITP	Hypertensive disorders of pregnancy
Thrombocytopenia secondary to a preexisting condition or a condition not related to pregnancy	Gestational thrombocytopenia	TTP-hemolytic uremic syndrome
		Acute fatty liver of pregnancy
		Disseminated intravascular coagulation

ITP, idiopathic thrombocytopenic purpura; TTP, thrombotic thrombocytopenic purpura.

Table 27.3 Clinical findings of various causes of thrombocytopenia in pregnancy

	TTP-HUS	Preeclampsia	Eclampsia	HELLP	DIC
Thrombocytopenia	++	+	+	+	+
Hemolytic anemia	++	+	+	+	+
Abnormal coagulation parameters (i.e. INR, PTT)	−	−	−	−	+
Renal insufficiency	+	−	−	−	+/−
Proteinuria	−	+	+	+	−
Neurologic abnormalities (focal)	++	+/−	+/−	+/−	−
Neurologic abnormalities (mental status changes)	++	−	−	−	−
Seizures	+	−	++	−	−
Hypertension	−	++	++	+	−
Fever	+	−	−	−	+/−
Liver enzyme abnormalities	−	+/−	+	+	−
Gastrointestinal symptoms	+	+	+	+	+/−
Edema	−	+	+	+	−

++, severe; +, mild-moderate; +/−, not consistently present; −, not present.
DIC, disseminated intravascular coagulation; TTP-HUS, thrombotic thrombocytopenic purpura/hemolytic uremic syndrome.

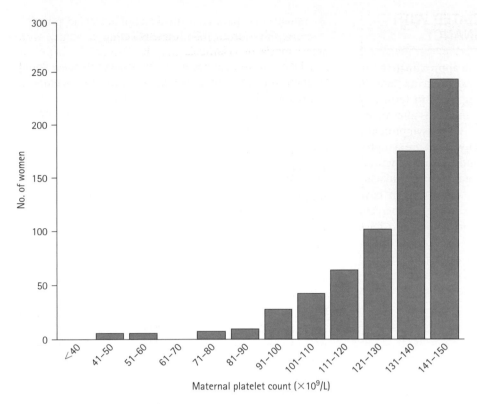

Figure 27.1 Frequency histogram of the platelet counts of pregnant women with incidental thrombocytopenia of pregnancy managed at a single institution during a 6-year period. Data from Burrows RF, Kelton JE. Platelets and pregnancy. (Redrawn from Lee RV, Barrow WM, Cotton DB, et al. (eds) *Correct obstetric medicines* vol. 2, St. Louis, MO, Mosby, 1993; pp. 83–106, Copyright 1993, with permission from Elsevier.)

of 50×10^9/L to 100×10^9/L. The thrombocytopenia may precede the finding of hypertension.[11]

HELLP syndrome

The HELLP syndrome (*h*emolysis, *e*levated *l*iver enzyme levels and *l*ow *p*latelet count) occurs in approximately 4–20 percent of women with preeclampsia[9] or approximately 0.3 percent of all pregnancies and is part of the spectrum of hypertensive disorders. The clinical manifestations of the HELLP syndrome include abdominal pain, proteinuria, hypertension, jaundice, nausea, and vomiting. Laboratory findings include elevated hepatic transaminases, elevated lactate dehydrogenase, anemia, and thrombocytopenia.

Pathophysiology

The pathophysiology of preeclampsia and eclampsia is not well understood but is characterized by vascular endothelial damage and dysfunction in the placenta, kidneys and brain.[9] The thrombocytopenia is thought to be due to platelet consumption[12] yet the mechanism of the platelet consumption remains unknown but does not appear to be due to the activation of the coagulation cascade.[11] Researchers have demonstrated that approximately 45 percent of thrombocytopenic preeclamptic patients have elevated levels of platelet-associated IgG, which suggests that immune mechanisms contribute to the thrombocytopenia.[11]

In addition to the thrombocytopenia, many patients with preeclampsia also have evidence of impaired platelet function, as measured by *in vitro* and *in vivo* tests of platelet function.[11] Also, studies have demonstrated that, in addition to the decreased platelet count, the circulating platelets have increased markers of activation, such as P-selectin, CD63, and platelet endothelial cell adhesion molecule (PECAM-1) using sensitive assays for coagulation.[13]

Treatment

The treatment of hypertensive disorders of pregnancy is discussed in Chapter 26. The thrombocytopenia generally responds to lowering of the blood pressure. It has been suggested that platelet transfusions should be given for a maternal platelet count less than 20×10^9/L prior to vaginal delivery and for a maternal platelet count less than 50×10^9/L prior to a caesarean section delivery.[9] However, our approach is to only give platelet transfusions if there is evidence of bleeding after delivery.

Fetal/maternal outcome

The maternal platelet count typically returns to normal within days of delivery; however, the occasional woman will have persistent thrombocytopenia for weeks.[14] The fetus generally has a normal platelet count unless there is another underlying disorder causing the fetal thrombocytopenia.

THROMBOCYTOPENIA ASSOCIATED WITH ACUTE FATTY LIVER OF PREGNANCY

Acute fatty liver of pregnancy occurs in approximately 1 in 7000–16 000 deliveries.[15–18] It typically occurs late in pregnancy with most cases occurring close to term and some women developing symptoms and signs after delivery. Although some women present with asymptomatic elevation of liver transaminases, other women are symptomatic with signs and symptoms including nausea, vomiting, abdominal pain, decreased mental status, headache, jaundice, and bleeding. In addition, some women have associated diabetes insipidus. Approximately 50 percent of women with acute fatty liver of pregnancy also have preeclampsia.

The typical laboratory findings of acute fatty liver of pregnancy are increased liver transaminases with progression to fulminant liver failure. Thrombocytopenia occurs in only a minority of patients.

Pathophysiology

Acute fatty liver of pregnancy is characterized by microvesicular fatty infiltrates of hepatocytes with no associated inflammation or necrosis.[19] The associated thrombocytopenia is usually attributed to concomitant DIC.

Treatment

Acute fatty liver of pregnancy typically resolves after delivery. Women should be provided with supportive care as required. Thrombocytopenia, if present, resolves as the DIC and acute fatty liver of pregnancy resolves. Platelet transfusions may be considered in pregnant women with severe thrombocytopenia and bleeding. The fetal platelet counts are generally normal unless there is another underlying process.

PRIMARY AUTOIMMUNE THROMBOCYTOPENIA: IDIOPATHIC THROMBOCYTOPENIC PURPURA

Introduction/clinical presentation

One of the most common autoimmune disorders that physicians manage is ITP, a disorder of both children and adults. Adults with ITP can present in one of three ways:

- many patients will be asymptomatic and have thrombocytopenia that is discovered incidentally
- patients will give a history of easy bruising that may have occurred for many years and, frequently, worsened with the ingestion of a substance that interferes with platelet function, such as aspirin or alcohol

- patients may have an acute onset of petechiae, purpura, and mucous membrane bleeding.

ITP occurs in young women and frequently these young women will become pregnant. In fact, ITP occurs in approximately 1–2 per 1000 live births[3] and accounts for about 3 percent of all women who are thrombocytopenic at the time of delivery.[5]

Pathophysiology

Idiopathic thrombocytopenic purpura is an autoimmune disorder caused by immunoglobulins directed against platelet antigens. In most patients with ITP, there is evidence of immunoglobulin G (IgG) antibodies with specificity for platelet antigens carried on platelet glycoprotein IIb/IIIa and/or glycoprotein Ib/IX. Platelets that are coated with the IgG autoantibodies are cleared by Fcγ receptors on the surface of reticuloendothelial cells, predominantly in the spleen and liver. Maternal IgG is actively transported across the placenta; therefore, the fetus may be at risk of developing thrombocytopenia *in utero* and at the time of delivery secondary to maternal antibodies. Rarely, the neonatal thrombocytopenia can be severe (discussed subsequently), and there have been reports of babies of mothers with ITP having severe hemorrhagic complications.[20–24]

Diagnosis

The diagnosis of ITP should be suspected in an otherwise healthy pregnant woman who presents with isolated thrombocytopenia. Many women presenting with mild or moderate thrombocytopenia during pregnancy will have a known history of ITP. Others may be diagnosed with ITP for the first time during pregnancy because of thrombocytopenia discovered on routine blood testing. Rarely, women will be diagnosed with ITP because of the onset of hemostatic impairment manifested by bruising, petechiae, and bleeding. As mentioned previously, there are various causes of thrombocytopenia in pregnancy which should be considered, including incidental thrombocytopenia of pregnancy. It may not be possible to differentiate mild ITP from incidental thrombocytopenia of pregnancy.

The diagnosis of ITP is one of exclusion. Primary immune thrombocytopenia is suggested by the absence of symptoms suggesting other secondary forms of immune thrombocytopenia, such as SLE, antiphospholipid antibody syndrome, lymphoproliferative disorders, and viral illness. The patient's medication use should be reviewed to rule out thrombocytopenia secondary to drugs. Blood pressure should be evaluated to rule out a hypertensive disorder of pregnancy.

The diagnosis of ITP during pregnancy does not require special laboratory testing.[25] With the exception of the thrombocytopenia, the complete blood count should be normal. Examination of the peripheral blood film should not reveal any red blood cell fragments, which would be suggestive of a microangiopathic hemolytic anemia (for example, TTP-HUS, DIC). Liver enzymes should be checked and patients with risk factors for HIV should be tested.[25] There is currently no diagnostic test which is specific for the diagnosis of ITP. Various assays have been developed to detect platelet-associated IgG (PAIgG); however, because the results are not sufficiently specific or sensitive, the routine use of these tests is not justified in suspected ITP.[25,26]

Treatment

Women with ITP should not be discouraged from becoming pregnant if their platelet counts are greater than 50×10^9/L. Women with platelet counts less than 20×10^9/L after splenectomy and other treatments can successfully deliver healthy babies, but will require careful monitoring during pregnancy.[24] However, all women with ITP, regardless of their platelet count, should be counseled before pregnancy that they will require monitoring and possible intervention during pregnancy. Furthermore, all pregnancies with ITP carry a potential risk to both the mother and the fetus.

The management of a pregnant woman with ITP requires collaboration between the obstetrician, hematologist, anesthetist, and neonatologist. As the maternal platelet count tends to fall during pregnancy, the maternal platelet count should be checked at least once a month during the first and second trimester of pregnancy, once every 2 weeks in the third trimester, and more frequently closer to term.[3,27]

TREATMENT OF NONPREGNANT ADULTS

For adults with ITP who are not pregnant, it is recommended that the following patients receive treatment: patients with a platelet count less than $20-30 \times 10^9$/L; and patients with a platelet count less than 50×10^9/L and signs and symptoms of bleeding or risk factors for bleeding.[25] The main therapeutic options for ITP include corticosteroids, intravenous immunoglobulins (IVIg), anti-Rh immunoglobulin (anti-D), and splenectomy. In cases of ITP refractory to the main therapies, other treatments for the nonpregnant patient include danazol, vinca alkaloids, cyclophosphamide, plasma exchange, and combination chemotherapy. Initial therapy generally includes high-dose corticosteroids (for example, prednisone at a dose of 1–2 mg/kg per day). Because corticosteroid therapy may take several days to weeks to increase the platelet count, if the patient is symptomatic with a platelet count less than 30×10^9/L, IVIg should also be given. The dose of IVIg usually used is 1 g/kg per day for 1 day. Some physicians prefer anti-D instead of IVIg. The main advantage of this treatment regimen is its shorter infusion time.[28] Potential disadvantages are the risk of alloimmune hemolysis associated with the therapy and the fact that the woman must be

Rh(D)-positive to benefit from the therapy. The dose of anti-D administered is usually 50–70 μg/kg.

TREATMENT DURING PREGNANCY

There are few studies comparing the management of ITP in pregnant women compared with that in nonpregnant patients.[25] A pregnant woman with ITP likely requires treatment if her platelet count is less than 30×10^9/L in the first and second trimesters or less than 50×10^9/L in the third trimester or if she is having bleeding symptoms.[25]

We generally recommended that pregnant women who require treatment receive IVIg as first line therapy.[3] Corticosteroids, while favored by many physicians because they are effective and inexpensive, may be associated with an increased risk of hypertensive disorders of pregnancy and can exacerbate gestational diabetes and bone loss.[27] Therefore, corticosteroids are not recommended as initial treatment for pregnant women.[3,25] The experience with anti-D to treat ITP in pregnancy is limited, although a small pilot study involving eight women concluded that the treatment was effective and appeared to be safe for both mother and fetus.[28] Splenectomy should be avoided if possible, and delayed until the second trimester when the risk of miscarriage is decreased.[25] Because of the size of the uterus, splenectomy is technically more difficult in the third trimester of pregnancy. Treatment with potentially teratogenic medications, such as danazol, vinca alkaloids, and cyclophosphamide should be avoided.

Maternal outcome

In the past 15 years, there has been a shift in thinking about ITP in pregnancy. It is now generally agreed that most pregnant women with ITP can successfully carry a child without morbidity or mortality. Early case reports suggested that ITP in pregnancy carried high morbidity for mothers and babies. It was often suggested that mothers with ITP avoid pregnancy or deliver by caesarean section, to avoid the potentially detrimental effects of a vaginal delivery on a thrombocytopenic baby.[20,29–31] However, recent studies have suggested more optimistic maternal and fetal outcomes in a pregnancy complicated by ITP.[24] Maternal complications are uncommon and are usually bleeding secondary to surgical incisions and lacerations of the birth canal.[7]

MODE OF DELIVERY

It is safe to manage these mothers with routine vaginal delivery unless caesarean delivery is required for obstetrical indications. At the time of delivery, it may be reasonable to increase the platelet count to allow for epidural anesthesia as many anesthetists will not perform an epidural unless the platelet count is greater than 80×10^9/L.[32] As the fetus may be thrombocytopenic (see below), it is considered best to avoid the use of fetal scalp electrodes, fetal blood sampling, ventouse deliveries, and rotational forceps as these procedures may expose the baby to hemorrhagic risk.[26]

Fetal outcome

About 10 percent of the babies born to these mothers will be thrombocytopenic with the platelet nadir occurring several days after delivery. Very severe thrombocytopenia is uncommon and should suggest an alternative diagnosis, such as alloimmune neonatal thrombocytopenia. For example, an analysis of prospective and retrospective studies of the past 10 years, which included 1243 infants born in 1235 pregnancies complicated by ITP, indicated that severe neonatal thrombocytopenia (neonatal platelet count $<20 \times 10^9$/L) occurred in only 4 percent of neonates and that moderate neonatal thrombocytopenia (neonatal platelet count $<50 \times 10^9$/L) occurred in only 9 percent of neonates.[3] A retrospective analysis of obstetrical patients with ITP over an 11-year period conducted at our institution indicated that 4.6 percent of babies had severe thrombocytopenia and 9 percent of babies had moderate thrombocytopenia.[24]

IMPACT OF MATERNAL INTERVENTIONS ON PLATELET COUNT

There is no evidence that maternal therapeutic interventions during pregnancy will predictably result in an increase in the fetal platelet count.[33,34]

PREDICTORS OF NEONATAL THROMBOCYTOPENIA

In general, neonatal thrombocytopenia cannot be reliably predicted by any maternal factor or serological test. Furthermore, a maternal response to a therapeutic intervention does not necessarily predict a fetal response. The most reliable predictor of fetal thrombocytopenia is the history of delivery of a previously affected infant.[24,35,36] There is also a suggestion that babies of mothers who have undergone splenectomy may have thrombocytopenia more frequently than those of nonsplenectomized mothers, although this finding has not been consistent in all studies.[36–38]

INVASIVE TECHNIQUES FOR DETERMINING THE FETAL PLATELET COUNT

The fetal platelet count may be determined before delivery by various mechanisms including percutaneous umbilical blood sampling (PUBS) and by fetal scalp sampling. The former involves the ultrasound-guided removal of fetal blood from the umbilical vein. This procedure is technically difficult and has been associated with fetal bleeding and death.[39–42] In a review of 195 pregnancies complicated by ITP in which PUBS was used, the procedure-related complication rate was 5 percent.[42] As the risk of potentially

lethal bleeding in babies born to mothers with ITP is less than 1 percent, the procedure of PUBS is considered to carry too great a risk to be used routinely in pregnancies complicated by ITP.[3,25]

Fetal scalp sampling involves the collection of fetal blood via a scalp incision prior to delivery. This procedure requires that the fetal head be engaged in the pelvis, the cervical membranes are ruptured and the maternal cervix is dilated.[43] This procedure has been demonstrated frequently to give fetal scalp platelet counts that differ by as much as 35 percent from the true fetal platelet count.[3] Therefore, we have discontinued fetal scalp sampling at our institution as we do not feel it is reliable enough to guide management.

SECONDARY AUTOIMMUNE THROMBOCYTOPENIA

Immune thrombocytopenia can occur in association with a variety of systemic disorders. These disorders tend to involve immune dysregulation and include infections, collagen vascular diseases, lymphoproliferative disorders, and other autoimmune diseases (see Box 27.1, p. 375). The thrombocytopenia generally improves with treatment of the underlying condition but may also require therapies as described for ITP.

THROMBOCYTOPENIA ASSOCIATED WITH SYSTEMIC LUPUS ERYTHEMATOSUS

Thrombocytopenia can occur in up to 25 percent of patients with SLE. The thrombocytopenia is usually caused by autoantibodies. Some patients will have concomitant platelet dysfunction characterized by increased bleeding and bruising. A subset of patients with SLE or SLE-like disorders have antiphospholipid antibodies (see below). The treatment of the thrombocytopenia is similar to that for ITP, although the response to splenectomy may be slightly lower.[44]

Antiphospholipid antibody syndrome

Antiphospholipid antibodies can be classified as either lupus anticoagulants or anticardiolipin antibodies. Lupus anticoagulants are antibodies which interfere with phospholipid-dependent coagulation reactions, commonly detected by an unexplained elevation of the patient's prothrombin time. These antibodies are immunoglobulins with specificity for negatively charged phospholipids. They tend to be heterogeneous in their epitope specificity with most binding protein complexes including β_2-glycoprotein I. Another class of antibodies, the anticardiolipin antibodies, is detected by an enzyme-linked immunosorbent assay (ELISA) using cardiolipin as the antigen. Cardiolipin is the same antigen that is detected in the Venereal Disease Research Laboratory (VDRL) test for syphilis, which explains why these patients will also have a false-positive VDRL test. The two classes of antibodies are distinct, but have overlapping specificities. Most anticardiolipin antibodies actually recognize an epitope on β_2-glycoprotein I. The term 'antiphospholipid antibodies' is applied to both sets of antibodies (see Chapter 8).

Antiphospholipid antibodies can occur in isolation, termed primary antiphospholipid antibody syndrome, or may be associated with other disorders, such as systemic lupus erythematosus, infection, malignancy, or medications. Antiphospholipid antibodies are associated with both venous and arterial thrombosis. The antiphospholipid antibody syndrome includes any combination of arterial and venous thrombosis and unexplained recurrent fetal losses in the presence of antiphospholipid antibodies. In addition, many of these patients will also have thrombocytopenia and a vascular rash termed livedo reticularis. Thrombocytopenia is common occurring in approximately 25–50 percent of patients with antiphospholipid antibodies.[45] Patients can have other hematologic abnormalities including platelet dysfunction, autoimmune hemolytic anemia, and leukopenia.

CRITERIA FOR DIAGNOSIS OF ANTIPHOSPHOLIPID ANTIBODY SYNDROME

The preliminary classification criteria for the diagnosis of antiphospholipid antibody syndrome were formulated during a workshop in 1998 (Box 27.3).[46] The clinical criteria for diagnosis include vascular thrombosis (both arterial and venous) and pregnancy morbidity. The laboratory criteria include the presence of high-titer anticardiolipin antibody or lupus anticoagulant.

PATHOPHYSIOLOGY

The mechanisms by which antiphospholipid antibodies cause pregnancy loss, thrombosis, and thrombocytopenia are not known. It is possible that antiphospholipid antibodies cause an imbalance between the anticoagulation and the procoagulation systems by interfering with normal proteins which are involved in the regulation of coagulation.[48] Proteins which have been demonstrated to be targets of antiphospholipid antibodies include β_2-glycoprotein I, prostacyclin, prothrombin, factor XII, protein C, protein S, annexin V, tissue plasminogen activator, and tissue factor.[49–53] Antiphospholipid antibodies may also cause activation of endothelial cells.[53–55]

Fetal loss in antiphospholipid antibody syndrome is likely due to abnormal placental function due to thrombosis during the development of the maternoplacental circulation[53] or due to abnormalities of early trophoblast invasion.[56] Cases of fetal loss have been associated with the pathologic findings of narrowing of the spiral arterioles, intimal thickening, acute atherosis, fibrinoid necrosis, thrombosis, and infarction.[53]

Box 27.3 Criteria for the classification of the antiphospholipid antibody syndrome Adapted from: Wilson et al.[46]

Clinical criteria

1 Vascular thrombosis
   (a) One or more clinical episodes or arterial, venous, or small vessel thrombosis in any tissue or organ AND
   (b) Thrombosis must be confirmed by imaging or Doppler studies or histopathology, with the exception of superficial venous thrombosis AND
   (c) For histopathologic confirmation, thrombosis should be present without significant evidence of inflammation in the vessel wall

2 Pregnancy morbidity
   (a) One or more unexplained deaths of a morphologically normal fetus (documented by ultrasound or by direct examination of the fetus) at or beyond the tenth week of gestation OR
   (b) One or more premature births of a morphologically normal neonate at or before the 34th week of gestation because of severe preeclampsia or eclampsia, or severe placental insufficiency OR
   (c) Three or more unexplained consecutive spontaneous abortions before the tenth week of gestation with maternal anatomic or hormonal and paternal and maternal chromosomal causes excluded.

Laboratory criteria

1 Anticardiolipin antibody of IgG and/or IgM isotype in blood, present in medium or high titer, on at least two occasions at least 6 weeks apart, measured by standard ELISA for β_2-glycoprotein I-dependent anticardiolipin antibodies OR

2 Lupus anticoagulant present in plasma, on at least two occasions at least 6 weeks apart, detected according to the guidelines of the International Society of Thrombosis and Hemostasis (Scientific Subcommittee on Lupus Anticoagulants/Phospholipid-dependent Antibodies),[47] in the following steps:
   (a) Prolonged phospholipid-dependent coagulation demonstrated on a screening test (e.g. activated partial thromboplastin time, kaolin clotting time, dilute Russell's viper venom time, dilute prothrombin time, Textarin time).
   (b) Failure to correct the prolonged coagulation time of the screening test by mixing with normal platelet-poor plasma.
   (c) Shortening or correction of the prolonged coagulation time on the screening rest by the addition of excess phospholipid.
   (d) Exclusion of other coagulopathies (e.g. factor VIII inhibitor, heparin)

Definite antiphospholipid antibody syndrome is considered to be present if at least one of the clinical criteria and one of the laboratory criteria are met.

TREATMENT

During pregnancy, patients with antiphospholipid antibody syndrome may be at risk for thrombocytopenia, fetal loss, and thrombosis.

Women with antiphospholipid antibodies only

There is controversy as to how pregnant women with persistently positive antiphospholipid antibodies but no history of complications should be treated. It is generally agreed that the routine screening of women without history of complications for antiphospholipid antibodies should not be performed as there is no indication for pharmacologic therapy in these women.[57] This is supported by the results of a randomized clinical study in which the pregnancy outcomes in women with antiphospholipid antibodies considered to be at low risk for pregnancy complications who were treated with standard care were similar to women who were treated with low dose aspirin.[58] Some experts would treat these patients with low dose aspirin (80–100 mg/day),[59,60] whereas most would simply follow the pregnancy closely and prescribe no medication.[61]

Women with thrombocytopenia

Because the thrombocytopenia is usually mild, treatment aimed at raising the platelet count is rarely necessary.

Women with a history of arterial or venous thrombotic events

Women with previous arterial or venous thrombosis require prophylaxis with heparin during pregnancy and in the postpartum period. In general, it is recommended that therapeutic doses of low-molecular-weight heparin be used during the pregnancy and intravenous unfractionated heparin be used for emergency situations and at the time of delivery.[48,61] However, the heparin dose for each patient should be individualized with consideration given to the number and severity of previous events, the associated risk factors for the thrombotic events, and her risk of bleeding.[57] Low-molecular-weight heparin is preferred over unfractionated heparin because it causes less heparin-induced thrombocytopenia and heparin-induced osteoporosis. Warfarin may be used in the postpartum period with the target INR being 2.0–3.0.[62] Oral anticoagulants should not be used during pregnancy as they are teratogenic. Although there is no evidence for its use, some physicians also recommend the administration of low-dose aspirin.[61]

Women with a history of pregnancy losses

Women with previous pregnancy losses (both early and late) are generally treated with low-dose heparin (that is, prophylactic dose low-molecular-weight heparin) alone or in combination with low-dose aspirin in an attempt to increase the live birth rate.[48,61] Clinical trials have demonstrated that the combination of heparin plus low-dose aspirin to be superior to aspirin alone or no therapy in women with a history of recurrent pregnancy loss with antiphospholipid antibodies.[63–66] The optimal duration of heparin therapy remains an unanswered question. High-dose IVIg therapy has also been suggested to be effective in some women with antiphospholipid antibodies and a history of pregnancy losses and/or thrombotic events.[67,68] However, these results have not been confirmed by all studies[69] and a metaanalysis failed to demonstrate that IVIg were effective in women with recurrent spontaneous miscarriage.[70] Therefore, it is currently recommended that IVIg is only used to treat women who cannot receive heparin and low-dose aspirin or those who have failed treatment with heparin and low-dose aspirin.[71] Corticosteroids do not improve the live birth rate and increase the risk of preterm delivery, gestational hypertension, and gestational diabetes.[72]

FETAL/MATERNAL OUTCOME

Studies have demonstrated that women with antiphospholipid antibodies have lower live birth rates when compared with women without antiphospholipid antibodies (62–84 percent vs. 90–98 percent).[57,73–76] If the woman has a history of an unsuccessful pregnancy, the chance of the next pregnancy being successful without treatment is approximately 25 percent.[59] However, women with antiphospholipid antibodies with a history of obstetric complications who are treated with heparin and aspirin have been demonstrated to have improvement of their low birth rate to approximately 80 percent.[64] Preeclampsia is more common in women with antiphospholipid antibody syndrome with one study demonstrating preeclampsia to occur in 51 percent of these women and severe preeclampsia to occur in 27 percent of these women.[77] Babies born to women with antiphospholipid antibody syndrome have an increased rate of fetal distress (approximately 50 percent) and fetal growth impairment (approximately 33 percent).[77]

THROMBOCYTOPENIA ASSOCIATED WITH HUMAN IMMUNODEFICIENCY VIRUS INFECTION

Thrombocytopenia is common and occurs in approximately 20 percent of patients with symptomatic HIV infection and 10 percent of symptomatic seropositive patients.[78] Thrombocytopenia may be the presenting manifestation of HIV infection and the risk of HIV should be assessed in any patient with ITP. Patients have immune-mediated destruction of their platelets, similar to ITP. Other mechanisms that may contribute to the thrombocytopenia include a defect in platelet production due to direct infection of megakaryocytes and the suppressive effects of medications. Patients with severe thrombocytopenia should be treated similarly to patients with ITP. Most patients respond to steroid therapy; however, only 10–20 percent will have a sustained response.[79] A transient improvement in the platelet count is induced by IVIg, but patients will require repeated treatments.[80] Splenectomy will induce improvement in most patients and there is no evidence that it increases the rate of progression to acquired immunodeficiency syndrome.[81] Treatment with antiretroviral medications also has a beneficial effect on the thrombocytopenia.[81,82]

THROMBOCYTOPENIA ASSOCIATED WITH LYMPHOPROLIFERATIVE DISORDERS

Immune thrombocytopenia commonly complicated chronic lymphocytic leukemia (CLL). This should be differentiated from thrombocytopenia of underproduction of platelets, which is seen in the spent stage of CLL. Immune thrombocytopenia is seen in 1–2 percent of patients with Hodgkin disease and can predate or post-date the diagnosis of the illness.[83] When it occurs after the illness, it does not necessarily indicate a relapse of the disease. In some patients, the thrombocytopenia will resolve with the treatment of the underlying malignancy. In others, the thrombocytopenia requires specific treatment. These patients should be treated similarly to patients with ITP.

DRUG-INDUCED THROMBOCYTOPENIA

Many drugs can cause thrombocytopenia and the mechanism is usually due to autoantibodies. The medications most commonly implicated include heparin, quinidine, sulfonamides, and gold; however, virtually every medication has been associated with thrombocytopenia.

Patients with drug induced thrombocytopenia typically have moderate to severe thrombocytopenia. Thrombocytopenia is usually seen within 1–2 weeks after beginning a medication, but it may occur in patients who have been taking the medication for several years. The platelet destruction is usually IgG mediated. The thrombocytopenia usually resolves within days of stopping the causative drug. In cases of severe thrombocytopenia, the patient may be treated with reticuloendothelial cell blockage using either IVIg or intravenous Rh(D) immune globulin. Treatment with corticosteroids is less effective. In cases of life-threatening hemorrhage, platelet transfusions may be required. Patients should not take the drug causing the thrombocytopenia again as it will likely cause thrombocytopenia with subsequent exposure.

HEPARIN-INDUCED THROMBOCYTOPENIA

Heparin-induced thrombocytopenia (HIT) usually develops between 5 and 8 days after initiation of heparin therapy; however, if the patient has been exposed to heparin within the past 3 months, it may occur earlier. Patients with HIT frequently develop thrombotic complications, especially deep venous thrombosis, skin lesions, and uncommon thrombotic events such as adrenal gland thrombosis and hemorrhage. The condition is caused by an IgG antibody which recognizes a complex of heparin and platelet factor-4 (PF-4). The PF-4/heparin/IgG complexes bind to platelet Fc receptors causing platelet activation and microparticle formation resulting in activation of coagulation.

The frequency of HIT varies among clinical settings. The risk of thrombocytopenia appears to be related to the type, dose, and duration of heparin administration. For example, unfractionated heparin is more immunogenic than low-molecular-weight heparin. Furthermore, different patient populations have different risks of forming HIT-IgG. For example, the risk of HIT-IgG is higher in orthopedic patients than in medical patients. Although cases have occurred, HIT has been demonstrated to be rare in pregnancy.[84] Fausett and colleagues performed a retrospective cohort study comparing the incidence of HIT in pregnant and nonpregnant women. Among the 244 heparin-treated pregnant women there were no cases of HIT compared to 10 cases (4 percent) in the control group. It has been hypothesized that the lower incidence of HIT might have been due to the fact that the pregnant women were healthier and younger than the control group or that pregnancy may be associated with an altered immune response at the level of the heparin/PF-4 complexes.[84]

Diagnosis

The diagnosis of HIT should be considered in all patients receiving heparin therapy who develop thrombocytopenia or the clinical manifestations discussed previously. Serologic tests can be used to confirm the diagnosis of HIT. Enzyme immunoassays measure the binding of platelet antibodies to a complex of heparin and PF-4. The gold standard tests are biological assays, such as the serotonin release assay.[85,86]

Treatment

Treatment of HIT involves discontinuation of heparin and the patient should be treated with an agent that inhibits thrombin generation, such as lepirudin, bivalirudin, argatroban, or a nonheparin glycosaminoglycan with predominant anti-factor Xa activity, such as danaparoid.[87] Fondaparinux, a novel anticoagulant with anti-factor Xa and factor IXa activity may also be effective for the treatment of HIT; however, its efficacy and optimal dosing have not yet been established.[87] Warfarin should not be used to treat acute HIT because it can trigger warfarin-induced limb gangrene. All medications suggested for the treatment of HIT (lepirudin, bivalirudin, argatroban, danaparoid, and fondaparinux) are classified as belonging to category B which means that they have been demonstrated to cause no fetal damage in high-dose animal studies; however, human data are limited.[87] The direct thrombin inhibitors have been demonstrated to cross the placenta in low doses.[88] In contrast, danaparoid and fondaparinux do not appear to cross the placenta[89] and, therefore, may be the medications of choice for the treatment of HIT in pregnancy.[87]

THROMBOTIC THROMBOCYTOPENIC PURPURA AND HEMOLYTIC UREMIC SYNDROME

Clinical presentation

Thrombotic thrombocytopenic purpura and HUS are syndromes which present with abnormalities in various systems. Historically, the syndrome of TTP was thought to be a pentad consisting of microangiopathic hemolytic anemia, thrombocytopenia, acute renal insufficiency, fluctuating neurologic abnormalities, and fever. The syndrome of HUS was diagnosed if the neurologic symptoms and fever were not present and if the renal insufficiency was prominent. Although it may be argued that the two conditions represent distinct syndromes, the clinical features of TTP and HUS are similar and it is often difficult to distinguish between the two, so the conditions are often practically described as TTP-HUS. A notable exception to this is postdiarrheal HUS which often occurs in children and is usually caused by bacteria such as *Escherichia coli* O157:H7.

Combined TTP-HUS is an uncommon disorder and has been estimated to occur with an incidence of 3.7 cases per 1 000 000 individuals,[90] but this appears to be increasing.[91] It is more common in young women. Although it tends to have an acute onset with no initiating factors, TTP-HUS has been noted to occur in association with several conditions including pregnancy.[92,93] In fact, women who are either pregnant or postpartum have been demonstrated to account for 10–25 percent of patients with TTP-HUS.[94]

Associations with other disorders have been noted and include *E. coli* O157:H7 infection,[95] bone marrow transplantation,[96] HIV infection[97–99] and the use of certain medications including ciclosporin, cisplatin, and mitomycin.[96,100] In pregnancy, TTP-HUS most commonly presents close to term or post partum.[101] The most common presenting symptoms include gastrointestinal abnormalities and hypertension.[102] The disorder is commonly confused with others that occur late in pregnancy, including preeclampsia, eclampsia, and the HELLP syndrome.[102] In fact, it has been noted that, in many women, these conditions may only be distinguished by the course of the illness following delivery as TTP-HUS would not be expected to improve without specific therapy.[101]

Pathophysiology

Patients with familial (congenital) HUS have reduced levels of the ADAMTS-13 protease which is directed against von Willebrand factor.[103] The decreased protease levels are due to a congenital deficiency of the protease (either congenital or acquired). The decreased levels of ADAMTS-13 result in increased levels of unusually large von Willebrand factor multimers, which could cause increased platelet aggregation and platelet thrombi. However, decreased levels of ADAMTS-13 protease are not found in all cases of sporadic TTP-HUS and it is likely that multiple factors contribute to the pathogenesis of TTP-HUS. For example, in some patients, deficiency of the ADAMTS-13 protease alone may be enough to cause the syndrome. In others, other risk factors, such as pregnancy, obesity, or the factor V Leiden mutation, may be required to be present.[102]

Treatment

Adults with TTP-HUS should be treated with plasma exchange.[91,104] If plasma exchange is not immediately available, the patient should be treated with infusions of fresh frozen plasma until they are able to undergo plasma exchange. Other therapies which have been suggested for poorly responsive or resistant TTP-HUS include antiplatelet agents, corticosteroids, vincristine, IVIg infusion, and splenectomy.[105–108]

Often, in pregnancy, it may not be possible to definitely diagnose TTP-HUS. The differential diagnosis of these women can include preeclampsia, eclampsia, and HELLP in addition to TTP-HUS. In such instances, it has been suggested that the decision to begin plasma exchange treatment should be based on the opinion that spontaneous recovery following delivery is unlikely, and that progressive multiorgan failure and death are possible.[101] It is unclear what recommendations should be made with respect to women with a history of TTP-HUS and future pregnancies. There are reports in the literature of women who have had pregnancies complicated by TTP-HUS who have had subsequent pregnancies which were uncomplicated.[109] However, there are also examples of women who have had recurrent TTP-HUS apparently precipitated by pregnancy.[110]

Fetal/maternal outcome

Prior to the availability of treatment with plasma exchange, over 80 percent of patients with TTP died.[111] Currently, if plasma exchange is used appropriately, over 80 percent of patients survive the syndrome.[104,112] Case series reviewing TTP-HUS occurring in pregnancy have demonstrated the condition to be associated with high maternal mortality and long-term morbidity such as chronic renal disease and residual neurologic deficit. In addition, when the syndrome occurred early in the pregnancy, preterm delivery and intrauterine death were frequent complications.[113] Fetal death is often secondary to placental infarction due to thrombosis. Fetal survival may be improved by initiation of prompt and effective maternal therapy. There have been no reports of transmission of maternal TTP to the baby.

DISSEMINATED INTRAVASCULAR COAGULATION

Disseminated intravascular coagulation is a coagulopathic disorder which results from the activation of both the clotting and fibrinolytic systems resulting in an excess of thrombin and plasmin and both hemorrhagic and thrombotic manifestations. It results from the general stimulation of coagulation activity by release of procoagulant substances into the blood.[114] It is not a primary condition, but is the result of a wide array of diverse conditions which cause tissue factor release, cell necrosis or damage, or introduction of foreign substances into the circulation. The common causes of DIC are listed in Box 27.4. Pregnancy-related causes include placental abruption, amniotic fluid embolism, septic abortion and intrauterine infection, retained dead fetus, hydatidiform mole, placenta accrete, preeclampsia and eclampsia, acute fatty liver of pregnancy, and prolonged shock.[114] Placental abruption is the most common cause of obstetrical DIC.

Box 27.4 Causes of disseminated intravascular coagulation (DIC)

- Infections
  - Gram-negative septicemia
  - Meningococcemia
  - Rocky Mountain spotted fever
  - Viral infections
- Malignant neoplasms
- Acute leukemia (especially acute promyelocytic leukemia)
- Liver disease
- Obstetric complications*
  - Placental abruption
  - Preeclampsia and eclampsia
  - HELLP syndrome
  - Amniotic fluid embolism
  - Retained dead fetus
  - Intrauterine sepsis
  - Hydatidiform mole
  - Placenta accrete
  - Large fetomaternal bleed
  - Acute fatty liver of pregnancy
- Connective tissue diseases
- Massive trauma
- Head injury
- Extensive burns
- Heat stroke
- Shock
- Massive transfusion
- Abdominal aortic aneurysm
- Giant hemangioma (Kasabach–Merritt syndrome)
- Snake bites
- Spider bites

*Cause unique to pregnancy.

Clinical presentation

There is a large spectrum of manifestations of DIC, ranging from patients who are asymptomatic with laboratory abnormalities to patients with symptoms of both hemorrhagic and thrombotic complications. The laboratory features of DIC include thrombocytopenia, prolongation of the INR and PTT, decreased levels of plasma fibrinogen and coagulation factors V and VIII, and elevated levels of fibrin degradation products. Examination of the peripheral blood film may reveal evidence of microangiopathic hemolytic anemia such as schistocytes and increased reticulocytes.

Pathophysiology

Disseminated intravascular coagulation occurs when there is activation of the coagulation system with excess production of thrombin. Because of the activation of coagulation, there is intravascular fibrin deposition which results in thrombosis of small vessels and resultant organ dysfunction. The deposition of fibrin may also result in microangiopathic hemolytic anemia. There is consumption of clotting factors and platelets which may result in bleeding. Finally, the deposited fibrin results in increased fibrinolysis and production of fibrin degradation products which may further interfere with coagulation and cause impairment of myometrial function.

The factors which cause the massive activation of the clotting cascade include the release of tissue factor into the circulation, injury to endothelial cells resulting in the exposure of tissue factor, and/or enhanced expression of tissue factor by monocytes in response to endotoxin and cytokines.[115] In pregnancy, triggers of the process of DIC include endothelial damage, the release of placental tissue, amniotic fluid, incompatible red cells, or bacterial products into the maternal circulation.[114]

Treatment

The treatment of DIC should be directed at prompt diagnosis and treatment of the underlying disease process. The presence of DIC is an indication for immediate evacuation of the uterus, if retained dead fetus or placenta is suspected.[115] The patient should be supported with transfusions of blood products, including platelets, plasma, cryoprecipitate, coagulation factors, and red cells as required. Rarely, systemic anticoagulation with heparin may be indicated; however, its effectiveness remains unproved.

POSTTRANSFUSION PURPURA

In cases of posttransfusion purpura, the patient, usually a woman, develops severe thrombocytopenia 5–12 days after receiving a transfusion of a blood product containing platelets. The thrombocytopenia is often severe (platelet count $<10 \times 10^9$/L). Posttransfusion purpura occurs when a woman produces an alloantibody to a specific platelet antigen that she lacks, usually PL^{A1}. The syndrome most commonly occurs in multiparous women because previous pregnancies lead to their sensitization. Patients who have previously been transfused are also at risk.

Diagnosis

The diagnosis of posttransfusion purpura is made by the identification of a platelet-specific antibody in a patient with acute onset of thrombocytopenia 5–12 days after receiving a transfusion of a blood product. Although it is most commonly seen after transfusion of packed red blood cells, all blood products, including plasma, can cause the reaction.

Treatment

Posttransfusion purpura is self-limiting with recovery occurring within 1–3 weeks. However, because the condition can result in severe bleeding, treatment with plasmapheresis or IVIg should be considered. Platelet transfusions should be avoided except in cases of life-threatening hemorrhage.

NEONATAL ALLOIMMUNE THROMBOCYTOPENIA

Neonatal alloimmune thrombocytopenia results in fetal, not maternal thrombocytopenia, but is discussed here for completeness. It is caused by maternal alloimmunization to antigens found on the fetal platelets. It is uncommon and is estimated to effect approximately 1 in 1000–1 in 5000 live births.[116–118]

Neonatal alloimmune thrombocytopenia is mediated by alloantibodies in maternal plasma directed against fetal platelet glycoproteins inherited from the father. The maternal immune system produces IgG antibodies which cross the placenta and bind to fetal platelet antigens, resulting in increased destruction and clearance of fetal platelets. The most common alloantibody to cause this disorder is targeted against a platelet glycoprotein termed PL^{A1} (HPA-1a) located on platelet glycoprotein IIIa.

Unlike hemolytic disease of the newborn, most cases of neonatal alloimmune thrombocytopenia occur in the mother's first pregnancy. Subsequent pregnancies are generally affected with similar or increased severity. This disorder causes severe and often life-threatening fetal thrombocytopenia that can occur *in utero*. Treatment of neonatal alloimmune thrombocytopenia includes maternal intravenous immunoglobulin infusions, maternal steroids, and fetal platelet transfusions.

KEY LEARNING POINTS

- When evaluating a pregnant woman with thrombocytopenia, three questions should be considered: (i) What is the etiology of the thrombocytopenia? (ii) What is the risk to the mother? and (iii) What is the risk to the fetus.
- Thrombocytopenia in pregnancy is common and occurs in approximately 7 percent of all pregnancies.
- The most common cause of thrombocytopenia in pregnancy is incidental thrombocytopenia of pregnancy. Other causes of thrombocytopenia in pregnancy include thrombocytopenia complicating hypertensive disorders of pregnancy, and thrombocytopenia associated with immunological disorders (such as idiopathic thrombocytopenic purpura).
- The management of incidental thrombocytopenia of pregnancy is observation and it does not require modification of obstetrical care.
- All women with ITP, regardless of their platelet count, should be counseled before pregnancy that they will require monitoring and possible intervention during pregnancy. All pregnancies with ITP carry a potential risk to the mother and the fetus.
- In women with antiphospholipid antibody syndrome, heparin alone or in combination with aspirin is indicated to prevent the recurrence of obstetric complications and thrombosis.

ACKNOWLEDGMENTS

K Webert is supported by a Novo Nordisk/Canadian Blood Services Research Fellowship in Hemostasis. J Kelton is a Canada Research Chairholder.

The authors would like to thank A Santos for his help with the figures.

REFERENCES

1 Verdy E, Bessous V, Dreyfus M, *et al.* Longitudinal analysis of platelet count and volume in normal pregnancy. *Thromb Haemost* 1997; **77**: 806–7.

2 Burrows RF, Kelton JG. Incidentally detected thrombocytopenia in healthy mothers and their infants. *N Engl J Med* 1988; **319**: 142–5.

3 Gill KK, Kelton JG. Management of idiopathic thrombocytopenic purpura in pregnancy. *Semin Hematol* 2000; **37**: 275–89.

4 Webert KE, Kelton JG. Disorders of platelet number and function. In: Warrell DA, Cox TM, Firth JD, Benz EJ, eds.

Oxford Textbook of Medicine, 4th ed. Oxford: Oxford University Press, 2003: 748–57.

5   Burrows RF, Kelton JG. Fetal thrombocytopenia and its relation to maternal thrombocytopenia. *N Engl J Med* 1993; **329**: 1463–6.

6   Webert KE, Kelton JG. Immune-mediated thrombocytopenia. In: Gresele P, Page C, Fuuster V, Vermylen J, eds. *Platelets in Thrombotic and Non-thrombotic Disorders*. Cambridge: Cambridge University Press, 2002: 542–55.

7   Kam PCA, Thompson SA, Liew ACS. Thrombocytopenia in the parturient. *Anaesthesia* 2004; **59**: 255–64.

8   Lindheimer MD. Hypertension in pregnancy. *Hypertension* 1993; **22**: 127–37.

9   Mushambi MC, Halligan AW, Williamson K. Recent developments in the pathophysiology and management of pre-eclampsia. *Br J Anaesth* 1996; **76**: 133–48.

10 Kelton JG. Heparin-induced thrombocytopenia: an overview. *Blood Rev* 2002; **16**: 77–80.

11 Burrows RF, Hunter DJ, Andrew M, Kelton JG. A prospective study investigating mechanism of thrombocytopenia in preeclampsia. *Obstet Gynecol* 1987; **70**: 334–8.

12 Gibson B, Hunter D, Neame PB, Kelton JG. Thrombocytopenia in preeclampsia and eclampsia. *Semin Thromb Hemost* 1982; **8**: 234–47.

13 Harlow FH, Brown MA, Brighton TA, *et al.* Platelet activation in the hypertensive disorders of pregnancy. *Am J Obstet Gynecol* 2002; **187**: 688–95.

14 Shehata N, Burrows R, Kelton JG. Gestational thrombocytopenia. *Clin Obstet Gynecol* 1999; **42**: 327–34.

15 Pockros PJ, Peters RL, Reynolds TB. Idiopathic fatty liver of pregnancy: findings in ten cases. *Medicine (Baltimore)* 1984; **63**: 1–11.

16 Reyes H, Sandoval L, Wainstein A, *et al.* Acute fatty liver of pregnancy: a clinical study of 12 episodes in 11 patients. *Gut* 1994; **35**: 101–16.

17 Usta IM, Barton JR, Amon EA, *et al.* Acute fatty liver of pregnancy: an experience in the diagnosis and management of fourteen cases. *Am J Obstet Gynecol* 1994; **171**: 1342–7.

18 Castro MA, Fassett MJ, Reynolds TB, *et al.* Reversible peripartum liver failure: a new perspective on the diagnosis, treatment, and cause of acute fatty liver of pregnancy, based on 28 consecutive cases. *Am J Obstet Gynecol* 1999; **181**: 389–95.

19 Bacq Y, Riely CA. Acute fatty liver of pregnancy: the hepatologist's view. *Gastroenterologist* 1993; **1**: 257–64.

20 Hwa HL, Chen RJ, Chen YC, *et al.* Maternal and fetal outcome of pregnant women with idiopathic thrombocytopenic purpura: a retrospective analysis of 25 pregnancies. *J Formos Med Assoc* 1993; **92**: 957–61.

21 Sharon R, Tatarsky I. Low fetal morbidity in pregnancy associated with acute and chronic idiopathic thrombocytopenic purpura. *Am J Hematol* 1994; **46**: 87–90.

22 Tampakoudis P, Bili H, Lazaridis E, *et al.* Prenatal diagnosis of intracranial hemorrhage secondary to maternal idiopathic thrombocytopenic purpura: a case report. *Am J Perinatol* 1995; **12**: 268–70.

23 Iyori H, Fujisawa K, Akatsuka J. Thrombocytopenia in neonates born to women with autoimmune thrombocytopenic purpura. *Pediatr Hematol Oncol* 1997; **14**: 367–73.

24 Webert KE, Mittal R, Sigouin C, *et al.* A retrospective 11-year analysis of obstetric patients with idiopathic thrombocytopenic purpura. *Blood* 2003; **102**: 4306–11.

25 George JN, Woolf SH, Raskob GE, *et al.* Idiopathic thrombocytopenic purpura: a practice guideline developed by explicit methods for the American Society of Hematology. *Blood* 1996; **88**: 3–40.

26 British Committee for Standards in Haematology General Haematology Task Force. Guidelines for the investigation and management of idiopathic thrombocytopenic purpura in adults, children and in pregnancy. *Br J Haematol* 2003; **120**: 574–96.

27 Cines DB, Blanchette VS. Immune thrombocytopenic purpura. *N Engl J Med* 2002; **346**: 995–1008.

28 Michel M, Novoa MV, Bussel JB. Intravenous anti-D as a treatment for immune thrombocytopenic purpura (ITP) during pregnancy. *Br J Haematol* 2003; **123**: 142–6.

29 Territo M, Finklestein J, Oh W, *et al.* Management of autoimmune thrombocytopenia in pregnancy and in the neonate. *Obstet Gynecol* 1973; **41**: 579–84.

30 Murray JM, Harris RE. The management of the pregnant patient with idiopathic thrombocytopenic purpura. *Am J Obstet Gynecol.* 1976; **126**: 449–51.

31 Kryc JJ, Corrigan JJ, Jr. Idiopathic thrombocytopenic purpura during pregnancy: a pediatric viewpoint. *Am J Pediatr Hematol Oncol* 1983; **5**: 21–5.

32 Letsky EA, Greaves M. Guidelines on the investigation and management of thrombocytopenia in pregnancy and neonatal alloimmune thrombocytopenia. Maternal and Neonatal Haemostasis. Working Party of the Haemostasis and Thrombosis Task Force of the British Society for Haematology. *Br J Haematol* 1996; **95**: 21–6.

33 Silver RM, Branch DW, Scott JR. Maternal thrombocytopenia in pregnancy: time for a reassessment. *Am J Obstet Gynecol* 1995; **173**: 479–82.

34 Bessho T, Ida A, Minagawa K, Koyama K. Effects of maternally administered immunoglobulin on platelet counts of neonates born to mothers with autoimmune thrombocytopenia: re-evaluation. *Clin Exp Obstet Gynecol* 1997; **24**: 53–7.

35 Christiaens GC, Nieuwenhuis HK, Bussel JB. Comparison of platelet counts in first and second newborns of mothers with immune thrombocytopenic purpura. *Obstet Gynecol* 1997; **90**: 546–52.

36 Yamada H, Kato EH, Kishida T, *et al.* Risk factors of neonatal thrombocytopenia in pregnancy complicated by idiopathic thrombocytopenic purpura. *Ann Hematol* 1998; **76**: 211–14.

37 Yamada, H, Kato EH, Kobashi G, *et al.* Passive immune thrombocytopenia in neonates of mothers with idiopathic thrombocytopenic purpura: incidence and risk factors. *Semin Thromb Hemost* 1999; **25**: 491–6.

38 Fujimura K, Harada Y, Fujimoto T, *et al.* Nationwide study of idiopathic thrombocytopenic purpura in pregnant women and the clinical influence on neonates. *Int J Hematol* 2002; **75**: 426–33.

39 Moise KJ, Jr, Carpenter RJ, Jr, Cotton DB, *et al.* Percutaneous umbilical cord blood sampling in the evaluation of fetal platelet counts in pregnant patients with autoimmune thrombocytopenic purpura. *Obstet Gynecol* 1988; **72**: 346–50.

40 Duchatel F, Oury JF, Mennesson B, Muray JM. Complications of diagnostic ultrasound-guided percutaneous umbilical blood sampling: analysis of a series of 341 cases and review of the literature. *Eur J Obstet Gynecol Reprod Biol* 1993; **52**: 95–104.

41 Garmel SH, Craigo SD, Morin LM, *et al.* The role of percutaneous umbilical blood sampling in the management of immune thrombocytopenic purpura. *Prenat Diagn* 1995; **15**: 439–45.

42 Payne SD, Resnik R, Moore TR, *et al.* Maternal characteristics and risk of severe neonatal thrombocytopenia and intracranial hemorrhages in pregnancies complicated by autoimmune thrombocytopenia. *Am J Obstet Gynecol* 1997; **177**: 149–55.

43 McCrae KR, Samuels P, Schreiber AD. Pregnancy-associated thrombocytopenia: pathogenesis and management. *Blood* 1992; **80**: 2697–714.

44 Hall S, McCormick JL, Jr, Greipp PR, *et al.* Splenectomy does not cure the thrombocytopenia of systemic lupus erythematosus. *Ann Intern Med* 1985; **102**: 325–8.

★ 45 Crowther MA, Burrows RF, Ginsberg J, Kelton JG. Thrombocytopenia in pregnancy: diagnosis, pathogenesis and management. *Blood Rev* 1996; **10**: 8–16.

46 Wilson WE, Gharavi AE, Koike T, *et al.* International consensus statement on preliminary classification criteria for definite antiphospholipid syndrome: report of an international workshop. *Arthritis Rheum* 1999; **42**: 1309–11.

47 Brandt JT, Triplett DA, Alving B, Scharrer I. Criteria fro the diagnosis of lupus anticoagulants: an update. *Thromb Haemost* 1995; **74**: 1185–90.

48 Galli M, Barbui T. Antiphospholipid syndrome: definition and treatment. *Semin Thromb Hemost* 2003; **29**: 195–203.

49 Oosting JD, Derksen RHWM, Bobbink IWG, *et al.* Antiphospholipid antibodies directed against a combination of phospholipids with prothrombin, protein C or protein S – an explanation for their pathogenic mechanisms. *Blood* 1993; **81**: 2618–25.

50 Matsuda J, Saitoh N, Gohchi K, *et al.* Anti-annexin V antibody in systemic lupus erythematosus patients with lupus anticoagulant and/or anticardiolipin antibody. *Am J Hematol* 1994; **47**: 56–8.

51 Cugno M. Dominguez M, Cabibbe M, *et al.* Antibodies to tissue-type plasminogen activator in plasma from patients with primary antiphospholipid syndrome. *Br J Haematol* 2000; **108**: 871–5.

52 Jones DW, Mackie IJ, Gallimore MJ, Winter M. Antibodies to factor XII and recurrent fetal loss in patients with the antiphospholipid syndrome. *Br J Haematol* 2001; **113**: 550–2.

◆ 53 Branch DW, Khamashta MA. Antiphospholipid syndrome: obstetric diagnosis, management, and controversies. *Obstet Gynecol* 2003; **101**: 1333–44.

54 Simantov R, LaSala JM, Lo SK, *et al.* Activation of cultured vascular endothelial cells by antiphospholipid antibodies. *J Clin Invest* 1995; **96**: 2211–19.

55 Del Papa N, Guidali L, Sala A, *et al.* Endothelial cells as target for antiphospholipid antibodies. Human polyclonal and monoclonal anti-beta 2-glycoprotein I antibodies react *in vitro* with endothelial cells through adherent beta 2-glycoprotein I and induce endothelial activation. *Arthritis Rheum* 1997; **40**: 551–61.

56 Regan L, Rai R. Thrombophilia and pregnancy loss. *J Reprod Immunol* 2002; **55**: 163–80.

◆ 57 Derkson RHWM, Khamashta MA, Branch DW. Management of the obstetric antiphospholipid syndrome. *Arthritis Rheum* 2004; **50**: 1028–39.

58 Cowchuck S, Reece EA, and the Organizing Group of the Antiphospholipid Antibody Treatment Trial. Do low-risk pregnant women with antiphospholipid antibodies need to be treated? *Am J Obstet Gynecol* 1997; **176**: 1099–100.

59 Roubey RAS. Treatment of the antiphospholipid syndrome. *Curr Opin Rheumatol* 2002; **14**: 238–42.

★ 60 Alarcón-Segovia D, Boffa MC, Branch W, *et al.* Prophylaxis of the antiphospholipid syndrome: a consensus report. *Lupus* 2003; **12**: 499–503.

61 Tincani A, Branch W, Levy RA, *et al.* Treatment of pregnant patients with antiphospholipid syndrome. *Lupus* 2003; **12**: 524–9.

● 62 Crowther MA, Ginsberg JS, Julian J *et al.* A comparison of two intensities of warfarin for the prevention of recurrent thrombosis in patients with the antiphospholipid antibody syndrome. *N Engl J Med* 2003; **349**: 1133–8.

● 63 Kutteh WH. Antiphospholipid antibody-associated recurrent pregnancy loss: treatment with heparin and low-dose aspirin is superior to low-dose aspirin alone. *Am J Obstet Gynecol* 1996; **174**: 1584–9.

● 64 Rai R, Cohen H, Dave M, Regan L. Randomised controlled trial of aspirin and aspirin plus heparin in pregnant women with recurrent miscarriage associated with phospholipid antibodies (or antiphospholipid antibodies). *BMJ* 1997; **314**: 253–7.

65 Backos M, Rai R, Baxter N, Chilcott IT, *et al.* Pregnancy complications in women with recurrent miscarriage associated with antiphospholipid antibodies treated with low dose aspirin and heparin. *Br J Obstet Gynaecol* 1999; **106**: 102–7.

66 Empson M, Lassere M, Craig JC, Scott JR. Recurrent pregnancy loss with antiphospholipid antibody: a

systematic review of therapeutic trials. *Obstet Gynecol* 2002; **99**: 135–44.

67   Clark AL, Branch DW, Silver RM, *et al.* Pregnancy complicated by the antiphospholipid syndrome: outcomes with intravenous immunoglobulin therapy. *Obstet Gynecol* 1999; **93**: 437–41.

68   Branch DW, Peaceman AM, Druzin M, *et al.* A multicenter, placebo-controlled pilot study of intravenous immune globulin treatment of antiphospholipid syndrome during pregnancy. The Pregnancy Loss Study Group. *Am J Obstet Gynecol* 2000; **182**: 122–7.

69   Triolo G, Ferrante A, Ciccia F, *et al.* Randomized study of subcutaneous low-molecular-weight heparin plus aspirin versus intravenous immunoglobulin in the treatment of recurrent fetal loss associated with antiphospholipid antibodies. *Arthritis Rheum* 2003; **48**: 728–31.

70   Daya D, Gunby J, Clark DA. Intravenous immunoglobulin therapy for recurrent spontaneous abortion: a meta-analysis. *Am J Reprod Immunol* 1998; **39**: 69–76.

71   Galli M, Barbui T. Antiphospholipid antibodies and pregnancy. *Best Pract Res Clin Haematol* 2003; **16**: 211–25.

72   Laskin CA, Bombardier C, Hannah ME, *et al.* Prednisone and aspirin in women with autoantibodies and unexplained recurrent fetal loss. *N Engl J Med* 1997; **337**: 148–53.

73   Lockwood CJ, Romero R, Feinburg RF, *et al.* The prevalence and biologic significance of lupus anticoagulant and anticardiolipin antibodies in a general obstetric population. *Am J Obstet Gynecol* 1989; **161**: 369–73.

74   Pattison NS, Chamley LW, McKay EJ, *et al.* Antiphospholipid antibodies in pregnancy: prevalence and clinical associations. *Br J Obstet Gynaecol* 1993; **100**: 909–13.

75   Lynch A, Marlar R, Murphy J, *et al.* Antiphospholipid antibodies in predicting adverse pregnancy outcome: a prospective study. *Ann Intern Med* 1994; **120**: 470–5.

76   Yasuda M, Takakuwa K, Tokunaga A, Tanaka K. Prospective studies of the association between anticardiolipin antibody and outcome of pregnancy. *Obstet Gynecol* 1995; **86**: 555–9.

77   Branch DW, Silver RM, Blackwell JL, *et al.* Outcome of treated pregnancies in women with antiphospholipid syndrome: an update of the UTAH experience. *Obstet Gynecol* 1992; **80**: 614–20.

78   Sloand EM, Klein HG, Banks SM, *et al.* Epidemiology of thrombocytopenia in HIV infection. *Eur J Haematol* 1992; **48**: 168–72.

79   Walsh C, Krigel R, Lennette E, Karpatkin S. Thrombocytopenia in homosexual patients. Prognosis, response to therapy, and prevalence of antibody to the retrovirus associated with the acquired immuno-deficiency syndrome. *Ann Intern Med* 1985; **103**: 542–5.

80   Gillis S, Eldor A. Immune thrombocytopenic purpura in adults: clinical aspects. *Baillieres Clin Haematol* 1998; **11**: 361–72.

81   Coyle TE. Hematologic complications of human immunodeficiency virus infection and the acquired immunodeficiency syndrome. *Med Clin North Am* 1997; **81**: 449–70.

82   Marroni M, Gresele P, Vezza R, *et al.* Thrombocytopenia in HIV infected patients. Prevalence and clinical spectrum. *Recenti Prog Med* 1995; **86**: 103–6.

83   Rudders RA, Aisenberg AC, Schiller AL. Hodgkin's disease presenting as 'idiopathic' thrombocytopenic purpura. *Cancer* 1972; **30**: 220–30.

84   Fausett MB, Vogtlander M, Lee RM, *et al.* Heparin-induced thrombocytopenia is rare in pregnancy. *Am J Obstet Gynecol* 2001; **185**: 148–52.

85   Kelton JG, Hunter DJS, Neame PB. A platelet function defect in pre-eclampsia. *Obstet Gynecol* 1985; **65**: 107–9.

86   Warkentin TE, Heddle NM. Laboratory diagnosis of immune heparin-induced thrombocytopenia. *Curr Hematol Rep* 2003; **2**: 148–57.

87   Warkentin TE, Aird WC, Rand JH. Platelet-endothelial interactions: sepsis, HIT, and antiphospholipid syndrome. *Hematology (Am Soc Hematol Educ Program)* 2003: 497–519.

88   Markwardt F, Fink G, Kaiser B, *et al.* Pharmacological survey of recombinant hirudin. *Pharmazie* 1988; **43**: 202–7.

89   Lagrange F, Vergnes C, Brun JL, *et al.* Absence of placental transfer of pentasaccharide (Fondaparinux, Arixtra) in the dually perfused human cotyledon *in vitro*. *Thromb Haemost* 2002; **87**: 831–5.

90   Torok TJ, Holman RC, Chorba TL. Increasing mortality from thrombotic thrombocytopenic purpura in the United States – analysis of national mortality data. 1968–1991. *Am J Hematol* 1995; **50**: 84–90.

91   Rock GA. Management of thrombotic thrombocytopenic purpura. *Br J Haematol* 2000; **109**: 496–507.

92   Caggiano V, Fernando LP, Schneider JM, *et al.* Thrombotic thrombocytopenic purpura: report of fourteen cases – occurrence during pregnancy and response to plasma exchange. *J Clin Apheresis* 1983; **1**: 71–85.

93   George JN. The association of pregnancy with thrombotic thrombocytopenic purpura-hemolytic uremic syndrome. *Curr Opin Hematol* 2003; **10**: 339–44.

94   Proia A, Paesano R, Torcia F, *et al.* Thrombotic thrombocytopenic purpura and pregnancy: a case report and a review of the literature. *Ann Hematol* 2002; **81**: 210–14.

95   Chart H, Smith HR, Scotland SM, *et al.* Serological identification of *Escherichia coli* O157:H7 infection in haemolytic uraemic syndrome. *Lancet* 1991; **337**: 138–40.

96   Atkinson K, Biggs JC, Hayes J, *et al.* Cyclosporin A associated nephrotoxicity in the first 100 days after allogeneic bone marrow transplantation: three distinct syndromes. *Br J Haematol* 1983; **54**: 59–67.

97   Jokela J, Flynn T, Henry K. Thrombotic thrombocytopenic purpura in a human immunodeficiency virus (HIV)-seropositive homosexual man. *Am J Hematol* 1987; **25**: 341–434.

98 Meisenberg BR, Robinson WL, Mosley CA, *et al.* Thrombotic thrombocytopenic purpura in human immunodeficiency (HIV)-seropositive males. *Am J Hematol* 1988; **27**: 212–15.

99 Leaf AN, Laubenstein LJ, Raphael B, *et al.* Thrombotic thrombocytopenic purpura associated with human immunodeficiency virus type 1 (HIV-1) infection. *Ann Intern Med* 1988; **109**: 194–7.

100 Murgo AJ. Thrombotic microangiopathy in the cancer patient including those induced by chemotherapeutic agents. *Semin Hematol* 1987; **24**: 161–77.

★ 101 McMinn JR, George JN. Evaluation of women with clinically suspected thrombotic thrombocytopenic purpura-hemolytic uremic syndrome during pregnancy. *J Clin Apheresis* 2001; **16**: 202–9.

102 George JN, Vesely SK, Terrell DR. The Oklahoma Thrombotic Thrombocytopenic Purpura-Hemolytic Uremic Syndrome (TTP-HUS) Registry: a community perspective of patients with clinically diagnosed TTP-HUS. *Semin Hematol* 2004; **41**: 60–7.

103 Levy GG, Nicholos WC, Lian EC, *et al.* Mutations in a member of the ADAMTS gene family cause thrombotic thrombocytopenic purpura. *Nature* 2001; **413**: 475–6.

◆ 104 Rock GA, Shumak KH, Buskard NA, *et al.* Comparison of plasma exchange with plasma infusion in the treatment of thrombotic thrombocytopenic purpura. Canadian Apheresis Study Group. *N Engl J Med* 1991; **325**: 393–7.

105 Schreeder MT, Prchal JT. Successful treatment of thrombotic thrombocytopenia purpura by vincristine. *Am J Hematol* 1983; **14**: 75–8.

106 Wong P, Itoh K, Yoshida S. Treatment of thrombotic thrombocytopenic purpura with intravenous gamma globulin [letter]. *N Engl J Med* 1986; **314**: 385–6.

107 O'Connor NT, Bruce-Jones P, Hill LF. Vincristine therapy for thrombotic thrombocytopenic purpura. *Am J Hematol* 1992; **39**: 234–6.

◆ 108 Crowther MA, Heddle N, Hayward CP, *et al.* Splenectomy done during hematologic remission to prevent relapse in patients with thrombotic thrombocytopenic purpura. *Ann Intern Med* 1996; **125**: 294–6.

109 Doan JT, Vesely SK, Holloway NM, George JN. The potential risks with future pregnancies after thrombotic thrombocytopenic purpura-hemolytic uremic syndrome. *Blood* 2000; **96**: 629a.

110 Natelson EA, White D. Recurrent thrombotic thrombocytopenic purpura in early pregnancy: effect of uterine evacuation. *Obstet Gynecol* 1985; **66**(Suppl 3): 54S–56S.

111 Amorosi EL, Ultmann JE. Thrombotic thrombocytopenic purpura: report of 16 cases and review of the literature. *Medicine* 1966; **45**: 139–59.

◆ 112 Vesely SK, George JN, Lammle B, *et al.* ADAMTS13 activity in thrombotic thrombocytopenic purpura-hemolytic uremic syndrome: relation to presenting features and clinical outcomes in a prospective cohort of 142 patients. *Blood* 2003; **102**: 60–8.

113 Egerman RS, Witlin AG, Friedman SA, Sibai BM. Thrombotic thrombocytopenic purpura and hemolytic uremic syndrome in pregnancy: review of 11 cases. *Am J Obstet Gynecol* 1996; **175**: 950–6.

114 Letsky EA. Disseminated intravascular coagulation. *Best Pract Res Clin Obstet Gynaecol* 2001; **15**: 623–44.

115 Leung LLK. Pathogenesis and etiology of disseminated intravascular coagulation. In: *UpToDate*, Rose BD (ed.) *UpToDate*, Watham, MA, 2004.

116 Burrows RF, Kelton JG. Platelets and pregnancy. In: Lee RV, Barron WM, Cotton DB, *et al.*, eds. *Current Obstetric Medicine*, Vol 2. St Louis, MO: Mosby, 1993: 83–106.

◆ 117 Bussel JB, Zabusky MR, Berkowitz RL, McFarland JG. Fetal alloimmune thrombocytopenia. *N Engl J Med* 1997; **337**: 22–6.

118 Levy JA, Murphy LD. Thrombocytopenia in pregnancy. *J Am Board Fam Pract* 2002; **15**: 290–7.

28

Gestational diabetes

SARAH E CAPES, HERTZEL C GERSTEIN

INTRODUCTION

Gestational diabetes mellitus (GDM), defined as glucose intolerance recognized for the first time during pregnancy and normally resolving after pregnancy, may result in pregnancy complications such as fetal macrosomia, shoulder dystocia, and operative delivery. It is increasingly recognized that a diagnosis of GDM is also associated with long-term health risks for the mother and child, which include increased risk of type 2 diabetes and other vascular risk factors later in life. The link between GDM and vascular disease is best understood by considering that the metabolic changes that are required to support a growing fetus lead to increasing demands on the maternal metabolic and cardiovascular systems. The increased demand can unmask underlying malfunction in these systems, such that pregnancy can be considered a metabolic 'stress test' for the mother.[1] Thus a diagnosis of GDM might be considered a 'failed' stress test that is a marker of susceptibility to disease later in life. This chapter will provide an overview of clinical aspects of GDM, with a primary focus on its long-term implications for vascular health in affected women.

PATHOPHYSIOLOGY

Gestational diabetes mellitus is characterized by profound insulin resistance combined with an inability to secrete sufficient insulin in response to a glucose challenge. Using euglycemic clamp techniques, women with GDM have been shown to have lower insulin sensitivity throughout pregnancy compared with weight-matched pregnant women without GDM. This reduction in insulin sensitivity has also been demonstrated in the pregravid period in women destined to develop GDM; indeed, the difference in insulin sensitivity between women with and without GDM is greatest before the pregnancy and in early gestation, but persists into late gestation.[2] It develops when the pancreas is unable to respond by secreting sufficient insulin to maintain normal glucose levels, usually becoming manifest in the second half of pregnancy. The pathophysiology of GDM may differ between lean and obese women with GDM, favoring a prominent defect in the ability to secrete insulin in response to a glucose challenge in lean women with GDM, versus more prominent insulin resistance in obese women with GDM.[2]

As well as its effects on glucose metabolism, insulin resistance may result in other metabolic disturbances, including impaired suppression of maternal free fatty acids and abnormal protein synthesis and degradation. The resulting excesses in nutrient availability to the fetus may contribute to fetal macrosomia, a well-recognized complication of GDM.

SCREENING AND DIAGNOSIS

Screening for GDM is a controversial topic.[3] Debate continues regarding the impact of GDM on pregnancy outcomes, the effectiveness of treatment in improving outcomes, and the possible negative effects of screening (which include an increase in obstetrical intervention for women with a diagnosis of GDM). Indeed, professional organizations across North America have remarkably different views on whether or how women should be screened for GDM, with recommendations ranging from universal screening[4] to selective screening (that is, recommending no glucose testing for women at low risk)[5] to no screening.[6] Furthermore, diagnostic criteria for a diagnosis of GDM remain controversial, since cut-points to distinguish pregnancies at high risk of adverse outcomes from those at low risk have not been clearly defined. Despite these controversies, there is value in establishing a diagnosis of GDM, both to improve pregnancy outcomes in high-risk women, and to identify women at high risk of long-term complications (discussed later in the chapter). This section will provide an overview of current approaches to screening and diagnosis of GDM. The controversies surrounding screening and diagnosis of GDM have been reviewed in detail elsewhere.[6,7]

Risk factors for gestational diabetes mellitus

The Nurses' Health Study is a prospective cohort study of 14 613 American women who reported a singleton pregnancy between 1990 and 1994. It identified the following risk factors for a self-reported diagnosis of GDM: increasing maternal age, family history of diabetes mellitus, nonwhite ethnicity, higher body mass index (BMI), weight gain in early adulthood, and cigarette smoking. Pregravid vigorous exercise was associated with a nonsignificant decrease in risk.[8] In another prospective cohort study, 909 normotensive and nondiabetic women were questioned about physical activity early in gestation. It found that any physical activity in the year before pregnancy and during pregnancy reduced the risk of developing GDM by more than 50 percent versus inactivity (relative risk [RR] 0.31, 95 percent confidence interval [CI] 0.12 to 0.79).[9]

Screening for gestational diabetes mellitus

Several approaches are currently in use worldwide to screen women for GDM. In North America, a two-step approach is most often used. In the two-step approach, patients are screened for GDM with a glucose challenge test, in which 50 g of glucose is given by mouth. Blood glucose is drawn 1 hour later, and those with a glucose level above the cutoff (either 7.2 mmol/L [130 mg/dL] or 7.8 mmol/L [140 mg/dL]) go on to have an oral glucose tolerance test. Depending on the cutoff used, the glucose challenge test identifies between 80 percent and 90 percent of women with GDM.[7] However, false positive results are common. Indeed, the 50 g glucose challenge test is positive in up to 25 percent of pregnant women, and one researcher found that fewer than 1 in 5 women with a positive glucose challenge met criteria for a diagnosis of GDM by the oral glucose tolerance test.[10] The World Health Organization (WHO) approach, commonly used outside North America, consists of a single step, 75 g oral glucose tolerance test to both screen and diagnose GDM. By convention, screening is usually conducted between 24 weeks' and 28 weeks' gestation, although there is no clinical trial evidence to support that this is the best time to screen. Women with strong risk factors for GDM probably should be screened earlier and if negative, should be rescreened during subsequent trimesters. No methodologically sound randomized controlled trials have been done to evaluate the effectiveness of a policy of screening for GDM (either universal screening or selective screening of women with risk factors) versus routine care without screening for GDM. Furthermore, there is no consensus as to whether the one-step WHO approach is more or less predictive of adverse pregnancy outcomes than a two-step approach. Nevertheless, the one-step WHO approach identifies at least twice as many women with GDM than the two-step approach.[7]

Diagnosis of gestational diabetes mellitus

The diagnosis of GDM requires a single oral glucose tolerance test. This differs from the diagnostic test for nonpregnant individuals, for which two abnormal tests on two different days are generally required. In North America, both the 100 g, 3-hour and the 75 g, 2-hour test are used (Table 28.1). There is no universal agreement regarding glucose levels that best identify pregnancies at high risk of adverse outcomes. Results from the international Hyperglycemia and Adverse Pregnancy Outcome (HAPO) Study should help to clarify this issue.[11]

OVERVIEW OF MANAGEMENT

Women who are newly diagnosed with GDM should be instructed to follow an appropriate diet. For women who are close to ideal weight at the start of the pregnancy, a diet consisting of 30 kcal/kg of present weight (40 percent carbohydrates, 20 percent protein, 40 percent fat), and consisting of three meals and three snacks, should be prescribed. Physical activity as appropriate for pregnancy should be encouraged. Women should monitor their capillary glucose before breakfast and 1 or 2 hours after meals. About 85 percent of women can achieve adequate glycemic control with diet alone. If glycemic targets are not met within 2 weeks, insulin therapy should be initiated. Current guidelines from the Canadian Diabetes Association recommend a target fasting glucose of less than 5.3 mmol/L (95 mg/dL) and 2-hour postprandial glucose of less than 6.7 mmol/L (121 mg/dL).[4] The American Diabetes Association recommends that insulin be initiated when medical nutrition therapy is unable to maintain glucose levels at or below a fasting value of 5.8 mmol/L (105 mg/dL) or a 1-hour postprandial value of 8.6 mmol/L (155 mg/dL) or a 2-hour postprandial value of 7.2 mmol/L (130 mg/dL).[5] Although some research has found oral hypoglycemic agents to be effective

Table 28.1   Diagnosis of gestational diabetes mellitus (GDM)

	Diagnostic test – oral glucose tolerance test							
	American Diabetes Association (100 g)*		Canadian Diabetes Association (75 g)*		National Diabetes Data Group (100 g)*		World Health Organization (75 g)†	
Glucose level	(mmol/L)	(mg/dL)	(mmol/L)	(mg/dL)	(mmol/L)	(mg/dL)	(mmol/L)	(mg/dL)
Fasting	5.3	95	5.3	95	5.8	105	7.0	126
1-hour	10	180	10.6	191	10.6	190	–	–
2-hour	8.6	155	8.9	160	9.2	165	7.8	140
3-hour	7.8	140	–	–	8.1	145	–	–

* Two or more glucose levels must meet or exceed these levels for a diagnosis of GDM.

† One or more glucose level must meet or exceed these levels for a diagnosis of GDM.

in treating GDM,[12] further study is needed to establish their safety. Oral hypoglycemic agents are not approved for use in pregnancy in either Canada or the United States.

The evidence that treating mild GDM improves pregnancy outcomes is weak. A recent Cochrane systematic review of dietary interventions for mild hyperglycemia in pregnancy was able to identify only 4 randomized controlled trials (enrolling a total of 612 women) that compared primary dietary therapy for GDM versus no treatment. These studies did not show any difference in high birthweight or C-section rate between treated and untreated groups. The review concluded that the current published evidence is insufficient to evaluate diet therapy for GDM.[13] Similarly, there are few randomized controlled trials comparing intensive insulin therapy for severe hyperglycemia in GDM, versus less intensive treatment. One trial that randomized insulin-requiring GDM women to postprandial versus preprandial glucose monitoring showed that the postprandial monitoring group achieved significantly better glycemic control (glycosylated hemoglobin 6.5 percent vs. 8.1 percent, $P = 0.006$). This group also had a significantly lower risk of large-for-gestational age infant (12 percent vs. 42 percent, $P = 0.01$), a lower risk of neonatal hypoglycemia (3 percent vs. 21 percent, $P = 0.05$), and a lower rate of delivery by cesarean section because of cephalopelvic disproportion (12 percent vs. 36 percent, $P = 0.04$).[14] This study provides some evidence that intensive insulin therapy can improve pregnancy outcomes for women with GDM and severe hyperglycemia.

Some investigators have evaluated the use of ultrasound measures to guide treatment of GDM, allowing therapy to be targeted to those women at highest risk of pregnancy complications. For example, one study evaluated a policy of withholding insulin for women with GDM and fasting glucose <5.5 mmol/L, if the fetal abdominal circumference was less than the 70th percentile. This policy led to a 38 percent reduction in insulin use with no increase in neonatal morbidity. The study concluded that the combination of fasting glucose and ultrasound determination of fetal abdominal circumference can be used to identify pregnancies at low risk of macrosomia, from whom insulin therapy can be safely withheld.[15]

The effect of treating GDM or impaired glucose tolerance (IGT) in pregnancy was the subject of a recent Cochrane group systematic review. The review identified only three methodologically sound randomized controlled trials that enrolled a total of 223 women. All three trials involved women with IGT, since none of the trials involving women with GDM met the authors' criteria for inclusion. The review found that treating IGT in pregnancy lowered the risk of neonatal hypoglycemia (RR 0.25, 95 percent CI 0.07 to 0.86) but did not have a significant impact on other outcomes such as abdominal operative delivery rates, reduction in birthweight greater than the 90th percentile, or admission to special care baby units.[16] However, a recent randomized trial in gestational diabetes compared dietary advice, blood glucose monitoring, and insulin therapy as needed with routine care. This trial has provided critical evidence that identifying and treating gestational diabetes can substantially reduce the risk of adverse perinatal outcomes (composite primary outcome of perinatal death, shoulder dystocia, bone fracture, and nerve palsy of 1 percent vs. 4 percent; adjusted relative risk, 0.33, 95 percent CI 0.14 to 0.75) without increasing the rate of cesarean delivery.[17]

In conclusion, there is some evidence that insulin therapy to lower glucose in GDM can improve clinical pregnancy outcomes, at least in patients with more severe hyperglycemia. There is insufficient evidence to evaluate dietary therapy for women with mild GDM. Well-designed clinical trials, with enrolment of high-risk women and an intervention producing adequate separation in glycemic control between treatment and control groups, as well as clinically relevant outcome measures, are required.

IMPLICATIONS OF GESTATIONAL DIABETES MELLITUS FOR FUTURE VASCULAR HEALTH

Implications for vascular health for the mother

Gestational diabetes mellitus has been linked to increased long-term risk of traditional vascular risk factors such as

Box 28.1 Vascular risk factors associated with gestational diabetes mellitus

- Type 2 diabetes
- Obesity

For the mother
- Dyslipidemia
  - Increased total cholesterol, LDL and triglycerides
  - Increased small dense LDL
- Higher systolic and diastolic blood pressure
- Increased BMI
- Hypercoagulability
- Increased inflammation
- Microalbuminuria
- Metabolic syndrome

For the child
- Early-onset type 2 diabetes mellitus

type 2 diabetes mellitus, hypertension, and dyslipidemia. Furthermore, changes in nontraditional vascular risk factors, such as hypercoagulability and inflammation, have also been noted in women with previous GDM (Box 28.1). To date, however, there have been no prospective studies of the incidence of cardiovascular events in women with a past history of GDM. Evidence supporting the relation of GDM to vascular risk factors is reviewed below.

TYPE 2 DIABETES

What is the risk of developing type 2 diabetes mellitus after GDM?

Estimates of the rate at which women with previous GDM develop type 2 diabetes vary greatly. A published systematic review of the literature found crude rates of conversion from GDM to type 2 diabetes mellitus ranging from 2.6 percent to 70 percent over follow-up periods ranging from 6 weeks to 28 years post partum in 28 cohort studies.[18] Much of the variability among studies could be attributed to important differences in factors such as completeness of follow-up, duration of follow-up after the index GDM pregnancy, diagnostic criteria used to diagnose diabetes, and selection of the study cohort. Indeed, most of the published studies examining this issue do not meet key criteria required for a valid prognostic study, namely:[19]

- the enrollment of an inception cohort identified at a uniformly early point in the disease in question (that is, gestational diabetes)
- at least 80 percent complete follow-up of the cohort
- objective criteria for the outcome of interest (that is, diabetes in the nonpregnant state).

Studies that do not meet these criteria may overestimate the rate of conversion from GDM to type 2 diabetes. For example, one common methodologic problem that was found in these studies was the performance of postpartum glucose tolerance testing only in women with past GDM who presented for follow-up based on clinical grounds, rather than in an unselected, prospectively followed cohort of women with GDM.[20-22] In one study, only 18 percent of all women with GDM presented for postpartum glucose tolerance testing[23] and in another study, those women who presented for follow-up were more than twice as likely to have required insulin during the pregnancy than women who did not attend for postpartum glucose tolerance testing.[24] Thus these studies would tend to identify a high-risk subset of women with gestational diabetes who would tend to have higher rates of type 2 diabetes postpartum. Other studies were not methodologically sound because of less than 80 percent follow-up of women with GDM[25-27] or failure to define criteria for a diagnosis of diabetes in the postpartum period.[28]

A literature review for cohort studies meeting the above three key methodologic criteria identified only three studies suitable for inclusion[29-31] (Table 28.2). Over mean follow-up ranging from 3.9 to 6 years after the GDM pregnancy, the incidence of type 2 diabetes ranged from 7 percent (in mostly white American women) to 30 percent (in Zuni Indian women). Predictors of higher risk of conversion from GDM to type 2 diabetes included higher fasting glucose at the time of diagnosis of GDM;[29] higher maternal BMI before pregnancy[29,30] and at diagnosis of GDM;[30] preterm delivery;[29] abnormal glucose tolerance in the first 2 months post partum;[29] longer time since the index GDM pregnancy[30] and more weight gain during that time;[30] use of insulin in pregnancy;[30] and diabetes in a first-degree relative.[30] Interestingly, one of the three studies found that more than 20 percent of Danish women with a previous diagnosis of GDM who developed diabetes post partum actually had type 1 diabetes; these women were leaner and younger than those who developed type 2 diabetes.

Does GDM cause type 2 diabetes mellitus?

Another interesting question is whether the metabolic stress of pregnancy itself might have long-lasting diabetogenic effects on the mother. In theory, the state of insulin resistance that is induced by pregnancy and that increases demand on pancreatic β-cells may stress a susceptible β-cell, increasing the probability of developing type 2 diabetes later on. This question has been explored in large epidemiologic studies in the general population, in which parity has been associated with slightly increased risk of diabetes mellitus and IGT in some studies[32] but not others.[33,34] However, at least one study has suggested that an additional pregnancy in women with previous GDM may increase the risk of developing type 2 diabetes mellitus. In a prospective study of 666 Latino women with GDM, who did not have diabetes at their first postpartum visit and who were followed for a mean of 22 months after the index pregnancy, the risk of type 2 diabetes mellitus was threefold higher in women who had an additional pregnancy

Table 28.2   Incidence of type 2 diabetes (DM) in women with gestational diabetes mellitus (GDM)

Author(s)	Study population	Outcome criteria	Follow–up	Results
Damm et al.[29]	298 Danish women with diet-controlled GDM identified prospectively and 57 controls with normal OGTT in pregnancy	DM diagnosed by WHO criteria with 75 g OGTT	81% of eligible GDM women had follow-up OGTT; median follow-up 6 years post partum	At follow-up, 3.7% of GDM women were on insulin, 13.7% had diabetes based on OGTT or a fasting capillary glucose >7.8 mmol/L, and 17% had IGT Overall, 34% of GDM women had abnormal glucose tolerance compared with 5.3% of controls (RR 6.54, 1.98 to 21.55). Median interval between pregnancy and diagnosis of DM was 48 months
Coustan et al.[30]	350 American women (91% white) with GDM identified retro-spectively via chart review	DM diagnosed by a 75 g OGTT	100% of subjects who consented to be studied had the OGTT at mean 30–47 months postpartum	Prevalence of DM at follow-up was 7%, and 4% had IGT
Benjamin et al.[31]	51 Zuni women with GDM and normal controls identified prospectively	Clinical diagnosis of DM or random glucose >11 or positive 75 g OGTT	92% of eligible GDM women had glucose tolerance status determined at mean 4.8 years post partum	Incidence of DM at follow-up was 30% in women with past GDM versus 6% of controls; 94% of GDM women had normal glucose tolerance in the early postpartum period

OGTT, oral glucose tolerance test.

compared to those who did not. Specifically, the annual incidence of type 2 diabetes mellitus was 30.9 percent vs. 11.9 percent (adjusted relative risk 3.34 [95 percent CI 1.8 to 6.19]). Weight gain after the index pregnancy further increased the risk (with every 4.5 kg [10 lb] gain almost doubling the incidence of type 2 DM) even after adjusting for the effect of an additional pregnancy and other confounders.[35]

LIPID ABNORMALITIES

Normal pregnancy is characterized by an increase in lipid levels, with an increasingly proatherogenic lipid profile as pregnancy progresses. A longitudinal study of 17 pregnant women and 12 nonpregnant control women showed that lipid levels were no different between the two groups during the first trimester. However, total cholesterol and low-density lipoprotein (LDL) levels increased progressively in the pregnant women, peaked in the third trimester, and returned to baseline postpartum. Triglyceride levels also increased more than 200 percent in the pregnant women. Furthermore, an increase in small dense LDL (LDL3) cholesterol was noted in the pregnant women. These small dense LDL are retained in arterial intima, are more easily oxidized, and once oxidized they are taken up into macrophages where they form foam cells and atherosclerotic plaques.[36] Several investigators have hypothesized that the proatherogenic lipid changes seen in normal pregnancy might increase the

woman's risk of subsequent cardiovascular disease. This hypothesis is supported by data from the Framingham and National Health and Nutrition Examination Survey (NHANES) studies,[37] which both showed a positive correlation between cardiovascular events and increasing number of pregnancies. At least one study has shown that the proatherogenic changes in lipid profile seen in pregnancy are exaggerated in the diabetic pregnancy. Indeed, a small cohort study comparing lipid profiles in normal pregnant women versus pregnant women with GDM found that the pregnancy-related increase in lipid levels occurred earlier in women with GDM, and the LDL and triglyceride peaks were higher in the GDM women.[38] This implies that women with GDM are exposed to higher lipid levels for a longer period of time during their pregnancies than women without GDM.

In addition to having an atherogenic lipid profile intrapartum, women with past GDM are likely to have such a profile several years after the index pregnancy. For example, a prospective cohort study enrolled 56 women with past GDM and 48 control mothers, 5–6 years after the index pregnancy. The two groups were similar in age, weight, BMI, and parity (although the women with past GDM were significantly more likely to have a first-degree relative with diabetes). Total cholesterol, triglycerides and LDL-cholesterol levels were significantly higher in women with past GDM compared with controls. Systolic blood pressure was also significantly higher in women with past GDM (122 mm Hg vs. 117 mm Hg, $P = 0.01$).[39]

There are several possible explanations for these differences. First, increased insulin resistance and/or insulin deficiency is likely to be associated with both the development of GDM and, later in life, dyslipidemia and elevated blood pressure. Second, women with GDM might have an inherited dyslipidemia. Third, lifestyle differences between the two groups might contribute to the differences in lipid profile and blood pressure. Regardless, it is clear that a history of GDM is a marker for dyslipidemia after the pregnancy. In summary, women with GDM have been shown to have exaggerated pregnancy-related rises in lipid levels compared to women with normal pregnancies, and women with past GDM are also more likely to have dyslipidemia years after the index pregnancy.

HYPERTENSION

Several large cohort studies have shown a clear positive association between glucose intolerance in pregnancy and hypertensive disorders in pregnancy.[40] Long-term studies also suggest that women with GDM are at increased risk of hypertension later in life. For example, a case–control study compared blood pressure in 20 Swedish women with a past history of GDM 2–4 years earlier, versus 20 control women matched for age, who had had at least one pregnancy and had no history of GDM. The mean age of women in this study was 36 years. All women with past GDM had normal glucose levels and HbA$_{1c}$ post partum. The investigators found that women with a history of GDM had significantly higher systolic and diastolic blood pressure (although all the women were normotensive). Those with past GDM also had higher BMI (mean BMI 24.6 kg/m^2) up to 4 years after the index pregnancy and were more likely to have family history of cardiovascular disease.[41] Similarly, a prospective study that followed 106 women with previous GDM and 101 control women for up to 11 years postpartum reported a trend towards higher systolic blood pressure in those women with past GDM compared with controls ($P = 0.06$).[42]

OTHER CARDIOVASCULAR RISK FACTORS

Normal pregnancy is characterized by changes in several factors that have been associated with cardiovascular risk in nonpregnant populations. For example, increases in coagulation factors, acquired resistance to the endogenous anticoagulant activated protein C and a reduction in protein S (its cofactor), and impaired fibrinolysis through increases in plasminogen activator inhibitor (PAI)-1 and PAI-2 have been noted during pregnancy.[43] Furthermore, normal pregnancy is characterized by a substantial inflammatory response: granulocytes and monocytes show a significantly higher expression of CD11b and CD64 in pregnant women compared with nonpregnant women, and increases in intracellular reactive oxygen species in granulocytes, monocytes and lymphocytes have been noted in pregnant women (although to a lesser degree than seen in preeclamptic patients and septic patients).[44]

The increases in some of these nontraditional cardiovascular risk factors may be exaggerated in pregnancies complicated by GDM. For example, greater subclinical inflammation (as indicated by higher white blood cell counts in early pregnancy) has been linked to increased risk of GDM in a prospective cohort study of 2753 women.[45] Cytokines (such as interleukin-6 and tumor necrosis factor α) released during inflammation induce insulin resistance and also increase secretion of cortisol and growth hormone. These inflammatory changes, which may be more marked in women with GDM, are associated with the future development of cardiovascular disease, diabetes mellitus, and death in nonpregnant populations.[46] Similarly, the hypercoagulability of pregnancy may be exaggerated in GDM.[47]

An increase in some nontraditional CV risk factors also has been noted several years after the index pregnancy in women with previous GDM. For example, a case–control study was done to compare the prevalence of microalbuminuria in 72 women with a history of GDM 5–6 years previously, compared with 35 control women without a history of GDM who were matched for age, parity, and time since last pregnancy. None of the women with previous GDM had been diagnosed with diabetes since the pregnancy. Median urine albumin excretion rate was significantly higher in the women with past GDM compared with controls (15.6 mg/24 h vs. 6.4 mg/24 h, p < .0001) and 30.5 percent of women with past GDM had microalbuminuria (>21 mg/24 h).[48] In the nonpregnant population, microalbuminuria has been clearly linked to increased risk of cardiovascular events.[49] Another study showed that the prevalence of metabolic syndrome was 4.4 times higher in women with a past history of GDM compared with control women without GDM; indeed, by 11 years after delivery, 27.2 percent of women with GDM and 8.2 percent of controls had developed insulin resistance syndrome (defined using criteria recommended by the Expert Panel on Detection, Evaluation and Treatment of High Blood Cholesterol in Adults[50]). The risk was highest in women who were both obese before the pregnancy and developed GDM.[42]

In summary, there is some evidence that metabolic, coagulation, and inflammatory risk factors for cardiovascular disease are greater during pregnancies complicated by GDM compared with normal pregnancies. Furthermore, adverse cardiovascular risk factor profiles may be present years after the index pregnancy in women with previous GDM.

VASCULAR DISEASE

There is ample evidence that GDM is associated with an increase in traditional and nontraditional cardiovascular risk factors during the pregnancy, as well as years after the index pregnancy. However, there is little research into whether these adverse risk factor profiles translate into increased risk of cardiovascular events in later life. One case–control study compared macrovascular and microvascular function between 20 Swedish women with past GDM 2–4 years previously versus 20 age-matched control women with no history of GDM. The mean age of women in the study was 36 years, and all women were normotensive and normoglycemic at the time of study. The investigators found that women with past GDM had increased wall stiffness in the common carotid artery, and diminished vasodilation in the skin microvessels of hand and foot in response to acetylcholine (indicating endothelial dysfunction).[41] To date, no study has compared the incidence of cardiac events in women with and without a past history of GDM.

Implications for future vascular health for the fetus

Maternal hyperglycemia during pregnancy may also have long-term effects on the fetus. There is increasing evidence that the diabetic environment *in utero* may program the fetus for childhood obesity and diabetes susceptibility. For example, in Pima Indians, a population with a high prevalence of type 2 diabetes, babies born to mothers with diabetes during pregnancy are at increased risk of childhood obesity and diabetes compared with babies who were not exposed to a diabetic environment *in utero*.[51] A study of 58 sibling pairs from 19 Pima Indian families, in which at least one sibling was born before and one after the mother was diagnosed with diabetes, found that the risk of diabetes was almost fourfold higher in siblings born after the mother was diagnosed (odds ratio 3.7, $P = 0.02$) and the mean BMI was 2.6 kg/m^2 higher at age 13 in offspring of diabetic versus nondiabetic pregnancies ($P = 0.003$).[52]

Similarly, in the Framingham Offspring Study of 2527 individuals followed for 20 years (mean age 54), those people with a family history of maternal diabetes were more likely to develop abnormal glucose tolerance than those with a family history of paternal diabetes (odds ratio 1.6, 95 percent CI 1.1 to 2.4); furthermore, individuals with a family history of maternal diabetes with onset before age 50 were about three times more likely to develop diabetes than those whose mothers developed diabetes after age 50.[53] In another study of 14 881 American children aged 9–14 years, children whose mothers had GDM were 40 percent more likely to be overweight in adolescence compared with children of mothers with no GDM history (odds ratio 1.4, 95 percent CI 1.1 to 2.0). The increased risk of adolescent overweight was attenuated somewhat by adjustment for maternal BMI and birthweight.[54]

Further support for the diabetogenic effect of the hyperglycemic environment *in utero* comes from a study showing that offspring of women with type 1 diabetes (an autoimmune disease which does not confer genetic risk of type 2 diabetes to offspring) had higher body mass index (BMI), greater insulin resistance, and a projected threefold increased risk of type 2 diabetes at age 5–15 compared with controls.[55] Impaired glucose tolerance is seen in both macrosomic and nonmacrosomic offspring of diabetic mothers.[56]

The effect of diabetes treatment on these long-term outcomes for the child is unknown. In the Pima Indian population, historical improvements in the management of diabetes in pregnancy since the 1960s have not greatly reduced the burden of diabetes experienced by children born to diabetic mothers.[57]

Summary: implications of gestational diabetes mellitus for future vascular health

It is clear that a diagnosis of GDM has important health implications for both the mother and the fetus. For the mother, GDM is associated with exaggerated metabolic responses to pregnancy, including abnormal elevations in lipid levels and inflammatory markers. After the pregnancy, women with GDM are at increased risk of type 2 diabetes, dyslipidemia, hypertension, and microalbuminuria, all factors that increase their risk of cardiovascular disease. Although the magnitude of any increased risk of cardiovascular events in women with past GDM is not known, the evidence suggests that a diagnosis of GDM should be considered a marker for future vascular disease. For the fetus, observational studies suggest that exposure to hyperglycemia *in utero* may be associated with increased risk of childhood obesity and early-onset of type 2 diabetes. However, more research is needed to determine whether or not intervention to treat hyperglycemia in pregnancy can improve health outcomes for the child.

LONG-TERM FOLLOW-UP OF WOMEN WITH PAST GESTATIONAL DIABETES MELLITUS

Women with a history of GDM should be considered at high risk of cardiovascular disease. Fortunately, since GDM generally is diagnosed at least 20 years before the onset of clinical CVD in women, there is ample opportunity to intervene and potentially to lower the risk. Long-term follow-up of these women should include regular screening for diabetes, hypertension, dyslipidemia and vascular disease. Both the Canadian and American Diabetes Associations recommend that an oral glucose tolerance should be done at least 6 weeks' post partum to rule out persistent diabetes, and should be followed by periodic screening for diabetes.[4,5] Healthy lifestyle measures, including weight loss and regular exercise, have been shown to lower the risk of type 2 diabetes by more than half in individuals at high risk[58] and should be encouraged for all women with GDM. Specific recommendations regarding weight loss and exercise should be individualized for each patient. Pharmacologic treatment with agents such as metformin[58] and acarbose[59] also has been shown to lower the risk of type 2 diabetes in individuals with prediabetic states and also should be considered in high-risk women with past GDM.

KEY LEARNING POINTS

- Gestational diabetes is a disease characterized by profound insulin resistance combined with an inability to secrete sufficient insulin in response to a glucose challenge.
- Risk factors for gestational diabetes include increasing maternal age, family history of diabetes mellitus, nonwhite ethnicity, higher BMI, weight gain in early adulthood, and cigarette smoking. Physical activity before and during pregnancy is protective.
- Several different approaches for screening and diagnosis of gestational diabetes are used worldwide. There is no universal agreement on how to best identify pregnancies at high risk of adverse outcomes.
- Insulin can improve clinical pregnancy outcomes, at least in patients with severe hyperglycemia. There is insufficient evidence to evaluate dietary therapy for women with mild GDM.
- Women with a history of gestational diabetes are at risk of diabetes, hypertension, and vascular disease in later life.
- The hyperglycemic environment *in utero* may increase the risk of obesity and early onset type 2 diabetes in the offspring of women with gestational diabetes.
- Weight loss, exercise, and treatment with metformin or acarbose may lower the risk of type 2 diabetes in women with past gestational diabetes.
- Women with past gestational diabetes should be screened regularly for diabetes, hypertension, dyslipidemia, and vascular disease.

REFERENCES

◆ 1   Williams D. Pregnancy: a stress test for life. *Curr Opin Obstet Gynecol* 2003; **15**: 465–71.

2   Catalano PM, Kirwan JP, Haugel-de Mouzon S, King J. Gestational diabetes and insulin resistance: role in short- and long-term implications for mother and fetus. *J Nutr* 2003; **133**: 1674S–1683S.

3   Stephenson MJ. Screening for gestational diabetes mellitus: a critical review. *J Fam Pract* 1993; **37**: 277–83.

★ 4   Canadian Diabetes Association Clinical Practice Guidelines Expert Committee. Canadian Diabetes Association 2003 clinical practice guidelines for the prevention and management of diabetes in Canada. *Can J Diabetes* 2003; **27**(Suppl 2): S99–S105.

★ 5   American Diabetes Association. Clinical Practice Recommendations 2004. *Diabetes Care* 2004; **27**(Suppl 1): S88–S90.

6   Berger H, Crane J, Farine D, *et al.* Screening for gestational diabetes mellitus. *J Obstet Gynaecol Can* 2002; **24**: 894–912.

◆ 7   Brody SC, Harris R, Lohr K. Screening for gestational diabetes mellitus: a summary of the evidence for the US Preventive Services Task Force. *Obstet Gynecol* 2003; **101**: 380–92.

● 8   Solomon CG, Willett WC, Carey VJ, *et al.* A prospective study of pregravid determinants of gestational diabetes mellitus. *JAMA* 1997; **278**: 1078–83.

9   Dempsey JC, Sorensen TK, Williams MA, *et al.* Prospective study of gestational diabetes mellitus risk in relation to maternal recreational physical activity before and during pregnancy. *Am J Epidemiol* 2004; **159**: 663–70.

10   Sermer M, Naylor CD, Gare DJ, *et al.* Impact of time since last meal on the gestational glucose challenge test. The Toronto Tri-Hospital Gestational Diabetes Project. *Am J Obstet Gynecol* 1994; **171**: 607–16.

11   HAPO Study Cooperative Research Group. The Hyperglycemia and Adverse Pregnancy Outcome (HAPO) Study. *Int J Gynaecol Obstet* 2002; **78**: 69–77.

12   Langer L, Conway DL, Berkus MD, *et al.* A comparison of glyburide and insulin in women with gestational diabetes mellitus. *N Engl J Med* 2000; **343**: 1134–8.

◆ 13   Walkinshaw SA. Dietary regulation for 'gestational diabetes'. *Cochrane Database Syst Rev* 1996; **2**: CD000070. DOI: 10.1002/14651858.CD000070.pub2.

● 14   de Veciana M, Major CA, Morgan MA, *et al.* Postprandial versus preprandial blood glucose monitoring in women with gestational diabetes mellitus requiring insulin therapy. *N Engl J Med* 1995; **333**: 1237–41.

15   Kjos SL, Schaefer-Graf U, Sardesi S, *et al.* A randomized controlled trial using glycemic plus fetal ultrasound parameters versus glycemic parameters to determine insulin therapy in gestational diabetes with fasting hyperglycemia. *Diabetes Care* 2001; **24**: 1904–10.

◆ 16   Tuffnell DJ, West J, Walkinshaw SA. Treatments for gestational diabetes and impaired glucose tolerance in pregnancy. *Cochrane Database Syst Rev* 2003; **1**: CD003395. DOI:10.1002/14651858.CD003395.

● 17   Crowther CA, Hiller JE, Moss JR, *et al.* Effect of treatment of gestational diabetes mellitus on pregnancy outcomes. *N Engl J Med* 2005; **352**: 2477–86.

◆ 18   Kim C, Newton KM, Knopp RH. Gestational diabetes and the incidence of type 2 diabetes. *Diabetes Care* 2002; **25**: 1862–7.

19   Laupacis A, Wells G, Richardson WS, Tugwell P. Users' guides to the medical literature. V. How to use an article about prognosis. Evidence-Based Medicine Working Group. *JAMA* 1994; **272**: 234–7.

20   Ko G, Chan J, Tsang L, *et al.* Glucose intolerance and other cardiovascular risk factors in Chinese women with a history of gestational diabetes mellitus. *Aust N Z J Obstet Gynaecol* 1999; **39**: 478–83.

21   Lam KS, Li DF, Lauder IJ, *et al.* Prediction of persistent carbohydrate intolerance in patients with gestational diabetes. *Diabetes Res Clin Pract* 1991; **12**: 181–6.

22   Farrell J, Forrest JM, Storey GNB, *et al.* Gestational diabetes – infant malformations and subsequent

maternal glucose tolerance. *Aust N Z J Obstet Gynecol* 1986; **26**: 11–16.

23 Conway DL, Langer O. Effects of new criteria for type 2 diabetes on the rate of postpartum glucose intolerance in women with gestational diabetes. *Am J Obstet Gynecol* 1999; **181**: 610–14.

24 Catalano PM, Vargo KM, Bernstein IM, Amini SB. Incidence and risk factors associated with abnormal postpartum glucose tolerance in women with gestational diabetes. *Am J Obstet Gynecol* 1991; **165**: 914–19.

25 Buchanan T, Xiang A, Kjos S, *et al*. Antepartum predictors of the development of type 2 diabetes in Latino women 11–26 months after pregnancies complicated by gestational diabetes. *Diabetes* 1999; **48**: 2430–6.

26 Metzger BE, Cho NH, Roston SM, Radvany R. Prepregnancy weight and antepartum insulin secretion predict glucose tolerance five years after gestational diabetes mellitus. *Diabetes Care* 1993; **16**: 1598–605.

27 Pettitt DJ, Knowler WC, Baird HR, Bennett PH. Gestational diabetes: infant and maternal complications of pregnancy in relation to third-trimester glucose tolerance in Pima Indians. *Diabetes Care* 1980; **3**: 458–64.

28 Mohammed N, Dooley J. Gestational diabetes and subsequent development of NIDDM in aboriginal women of northwestern Ontario. *Int J Circumpolar Health* 1998; **57**(Suppl 1): 355–8.

29 Damm P, Kohl C, Bertelsen A, Molsted-Pedersen L. Predictive factors for the development of diabetes in women with previous gestational diabetes. *Am J Obstet Gynecol* 1992; **167**: 607–16.

30 Coustan DR, Carpenter MW, O'Sullivan PS, Carr SR. Gestational diabetes: predictors of subsequent disordered glucose metabolism. *Am J Obstet Gynecol* 1993; **168**: 1139–45.

31 Benjamin E, Winters D, Mayfield J, Gohdes D. Diabetes in pregnancy in Zuni Indian women. *Diabetes Care* 1993; **16**: 1231–5.

32 Kritz-Silverstein D, Barrett-Connor E, Wingard DL. The effect of parity on the later development of non-insulin-dependent diabetes mellitus or impaired glucose tolerance. *N Engl J Med* 1989; **321**: 1214–19.

33 Boyko EJ, Alderman BW, Keane EM, Baron AE. Effects of childbearing on glucose tolerance and NIDDM prevalence. *Diabetes Care* 1990; **13**: 848–54.

34 Manson JE, Rimm EB, Colditz GA, *et al*. Parity and incidence of non-insulin-dependent diabetes mellitus. *Am J Med* 1992; **93**: 13–18.

35 Peters RK, Kjos SL, Xiang A, Buchanan TA. Long-term diabetogenic effect of single pregnancy in women with previous gestational diabetes mellitus. *Lancet* 1996; **347**: 227–30.

36 Toescu S, Nuttall SL, Martin U, *et al*. Oxidative stress and normal pregnancy. *Clin Endocrinol* 2002; **57**: 609–13.

37 Ness RB, Harris T, Cobb J, *et al*. Number of pregnancies and the subsequent risk of cardiovascular disease. *N Engl J Med* 1993; **328**: 1528–33.

38 Toescu V, Nuttall SL, Kendall MJ, *et al*. Women with gestational diabetes should be targeted to reduce cardiovascular risk [letter]. *BMJ* 2002; **325**: 966.

39 Meyers-Seifer CH, Vohr BR. Lipid levels in former gestational diabetic mothers. *Diabetes Care* 1996; **19**: 1351–6.

40 Joffe GM, Esterlitz JR, Levine RJ, *et al*. for the Calcium for Preeclampsia Prevention (CPEP) Study Group. *Am J Obstet Gynecol* 1998; **179**: 1032–7.

41 Hu J, Norman M, Wallensteen M, Gennser G. Increased large arterial stiffness and impaired acetylcholine-induced skin vasodilatation in women with previous gestational diabetes mellitus. *Br J Obstet Gynaecol* 1998; **105**: 1279–87.

42 Verma A, Boney CM, Tucker R, Vohr BR. Insulin resistance syndrome in women with prior history of gestational diabetes mellitus. *J Clin Endocrinol Metab* 2002; **87**: 3227–35.

43 Greer IA. Thrombosis in pregnancy: maternal and fetal issues. *Lancet* 1999; **353**: 1258–65.

44 Sacks GP, Studena K, Sargent IL, Redman CWG. Normal pregnancy and preeclampsia both produce inflammatory changes in peripheral blood leukocytes akin to those of sepsis. *Am J Obstet Gynecol* 1998; **179**: 80–6.

45 Wolf M, Sauk J, Shah A, Smirnakis KV, *et al*. Inflammation and glucose intolerance – a prospective study of gestational diabetes mellitus. *Diabetes Care* 2004; **27**: 21–7.

46 Blake GJ, Ridker PM. Inflammatory bio-markers and cardiovascular risk prediction. J Int Med 2002; **252**: 283–94.

47 Bellart J, Gilabert R, Fontcuberta J, *et al*. Coagulation and fibrinolysis parameters in normal pregnancy and gestational diabetes. *Am J Perinatol* 1998; **15**: 479–86.

48 Friedman S, Rabinerson D, Bar J, *et al*. Microalbuminuria following gestational diabetes. Acta *Obstet Gynecol Scand* 1995; **74**: 356–60.

49 Gerstein HC, Mann JF, Yi Q, *et al*. HOPE Study Investigators. Albuminuria and risk of cardiovascular events, death, and heart failure in diabetic and nondiabetic individuals. *JAMA* 2001; **286**: 421–6.

50 Executive Summary of the Third Report of the National Cholesterol Education Program (NCEP) Expert Panel on Detection, Evaluation, and Treatment of High Blood Cholesterol in Adults (Adult Treatment Panel III). *JAMA* 2001; **285**: 2486–97.

51 Pettitt DJ, Aleck KA, Baird HR, *et al*. Congenital susceptibility to NIDDM. Role of intrauterine environment. *Diabetes* 1988; **37**: 622–8.

52 Dabelea D, Hanson RL, Lindsay RS, *et al*. Intrauterine exposure to diabetes conveys risks for type 2 diabetes and obesity: a study of discordant sibships. *Diabetes* 2000; **49**: 2208–11.

53 Meigs JB, Cupples LA, Wilson PW. Parental transmission of type 2 diabetes: the Framingham Offspring Study. *Diabetes* 2000; **49**: 2201–7.

54 Gillman MW, Rifas-Shiman S, Berkey CS, *et al.* Maternal gestational diabetes, birth weight, and adolescent obesity. *Pediatrics* 2003; **111**: e221–6.

55 Weiss PA, Scholz HS, Haas J, Tamussino KF, Seissler J, Borkenstein MH. Long-term follow-up of infants of mothers with type 1 diabetes: evidence for hereditary and nonhereditary transmission of diabetes and precursors. *Diabetes Care* 2000; **23**: 905–11.

56 Silverman BL, Metzger BE, Cho NH, Loeb CA. Impaired glucose tolerance in adolescent offspring of diabetic mothers. Relationship to fetal hyperinsulinism. *Diabetes Care* 1995; **18**: 611–17.

57 Lindsay RS, Hanson RL, Bennett PH, Knowler WC. Secular trends in birth weight, BMI, and diabetes in the offspring of diabetic mothers. *Diabetes Care* 2000; **23**: 1249–54.

● 58 Knowler WC, Barrett-Connor E, Fowler SE, *et al.* for the Diabetes Prevention Program Research Group. Reduction in the incidence of type 2 diabetes with lifestyle intervention or metformin. *N Engl J Med* 2002; **346**: 393–403.

● 59 Chiasson JL, Josse RG, Gomis R, Hanefeld M, *et al.* STOP-NIDDM Trail Research Group. Acarbose for prevention of type 2 diabetes mellitus: the STOP-NIDDM randomised trial. *Lancet* 2002; **359**: 2072–7.

29

Pregnancy and programming

NAVEED SATTAR, IAN A GREER

INTRODUCTION

Considerable data link low birthweight due to intrauterine growth restriction (IUGR) to increased risk of vascular disease in the offspring's later adult life. This is considered to be the result, in part, of programming through fetal nutrition.[1] These data support the hypothesis that pregnancy outcome in terms of birthweight is linked to the individual's subsequent health. In contrast, much less attention has focused on the relation between adverse pregnancy outcomes, such as preeclampsia, gestational diabetes, preterm delivery, and IUGR, and the mother's subsequent health. Interesting data have accumulated linking the maternal vascular, metabolic, and inflammatory complications of pregnancy to an increased risk of vascular disease in later life. This chapter reviews the emerging evidence to support this fascinating concept, addresses potential mechanisms, and discusses potential clinical implications.

A key factor underlying cardiovascular disease and, in particular coronary heart disease (CHD) is the metabolic syndrome. The metabolic syndrome is a spectrum of metabolic abnormalities associated with insulin resistance, which is manifest as relative hyperglycemia, hyperlipidemia, and coagulation disturbance. The normal physiologic response to pregnancy represents a transient excursion into a metabolic syndrome, where several components are acquired: a relative degree of insulin resistance, significant hyperlipidemia, and an increase in coagulation factors.[2,3] Normal pregnancy also involves upregulation of the inflammatory cascade, including an increased white cell count.[4] In the nonpregnant population, such upregulation is a recent addition to the cardiovascular risk arena, as markers of inflammation such as C-reactive protein, interleukin-6, serum amyloid A and white cell count have been found to independently predict cardiovascular events and diabetes[5,6] although the causality of such markers is currently debated. All these metabolic changes of pregnancy are likely to be driven by hormonal changes, either directly or indirectly via regulation of early fat acquisition and its rapid mobilization in the second half of pregnancy.[7] Such metabolic responses could be considered as 'stress' tests on maternal carbohydrate and lipid pathways, and vascular function. In this way, adverse pregnancy outcome may 'unmask' women at increased risk of metabolic and vascular diseases in later life (Fig. 29.1).[8]

COMPLICATIONS OF PREGNANCY

Gestational diabetes

Perhaps the best-studied example of this phenomenon is glucose metabolism in pregnancy. If the mother fails to compensate adequately for the increase in gestational insulin resistance by enhancing pancreatic insulin secretion, she will experience glycemic dysregulation (manifest as an abnormal glucose tolerance test), and she will have a 30 percent risk of developing type 2 diabetes in later life.[9] In fact, it appears that pregnancy itself may accelerate the development of type 2 diabetes in susceptible women.[10] Consistent with an increased diabetes risk, women with a history of gestational diabetes demonstrate subtle yet significant differences in lipid levels, blood pressure, inflammatory markers and adiponectin, and microvascular and large vessel function subsequent to pregnancy, relative to

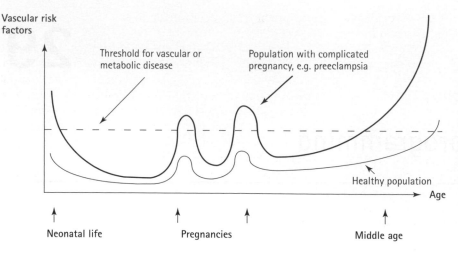

Figure 29.1 Vascular risk factors expressed in middle age, but not clearly identifiable in early adulthood, are identifiable during 'excursions' into the 'metabolic syndrome of pregnancy'. Expression of risk factors is increased in pregnancies complicated by, for example, preeclampsia or gestational diabetes, with associated increase in risk in later life. (Modified from Sattar and Greer.[8])

control women, even if they remain glucose tolerant.[11–13] Based on our current knowledge of risk factors, all these observations predict an increased risk for CHD in women with previous gestational diabetes. Although the latter has as yet not been directly proved, recent evidence demonstrates a reduction in the progression of carotid atherosclerosis with an insulin sensitizing agent (glitazones) in women with history of gestational diabetes.[14]

Hypertensive complications

Preeclampsia, which complicates 2–4 percent of pregnancies, remains one of the commonest causes of maternal and fetal morbidity and mortality. However, early and more recent data addressing the long-term consequences for the mother are conflicting. The early work of Leon Chesley and others[15,16] suggested that women with pregnancies complicated by pregnancy-induced hypertension and eclampsia did not develop later chronic hypertension, but others[17] have found an increase in risk of hypertension, especially where the hypertensive problem arises before 30 weeks' gestation. There does appear to be agreement, however, that mothers who experience uncomplicated pregnancies have a lower incidence of subsequent hypertension, compared with the general female population of similar age and race.[15] Recent studies demonstrate that women with a history of preeclampsia have higher circulating levels of fasting insulin, lipid and, coagulation factors post partum, relative to controls with matched body mass index.[18,19] They also appear to exhibit a specific defect in endothelium-dependent vascular function, relative to women with a history of a healthy pregnancy, independent of maternal obesity, blood pressure, and metabolic disturbances associated with insulin resistance or dyslipidemia.[20] Finally, we recently demonstrated elevated intercellular adhesion molecule (ICAM)-1 levels in such women.[21]

This pattern of metabolic and vascular changes in women with a history of preeclampsia is near identical to the abnormalities seen in this condition at diagnosis, namely exaggerated lipid and insulin levels, disturbed hemostatic parameters and endothelial dysfunction.[8] It is not surprising, therefore, that the specific vascular lesion of preeclampsia – acute atherosis with lipid-laden foam cells in the placental bed – is similar to that observed in atherosclerosis. Thus, the genotypes and phenotypes underlying vascular disease may also underlie preeclampsia.

The above changes in risk markers in women with a history of preeclampsia predict that they may be at an increased CHD risk. Jonsdottir and colleagues[22] examined causes of death in 374 women with a history of hypertensive complications, and noted that their death rate from CHD complications was significantly higher (1.47, 95 percent confidence interval [CI] 1.05 to 2.02) than expected from analysis of population data from public health and census reports during corresponding periods. Moreover, they noted that the relative risk of dying from CHD was significantly higher among women who had had eclampsia (relative risk [RR] 2.61, 95 percent CI 1.11 to 6.12) or preeclampsia (RR 1.90, 95 percent CI 1.02 to 3.52), compared with those with hypertension alone.[22] A prospective cohort study, using the Royal College of General Practitioners oral contraceptive study data, also reported that a history of preeclampsia increased the risk of cardiovascular conditions in later life. For total ischemic heart disease the relative risk was 1.7 (1.3 to 2.2). Furthermore, they found that the increased risk could not be explained by underlying chronic hypertension.[23] Similarly, a retrospective cohort study from Scotland, using hospital discharge data[24] reported an association between preeclampsia and subsequent ischemic heart disease in the mother (hazard ratio 2.0, 95 percent CI 1.5 to 2.5). Finally, Irgens and colleagues[25] were able to confirm a higher CHD mortality in women with preeclampsia, and in addition noted an exceptionally high relative risk of death from cardiovascular causes among women with preeclampsia and a preterm delivery – hazard ratio of 8.12 (95 percent CI 4.31 to 15.33) compared with women without preeclampsia reaching term. Prospective evaluation of women in pregnancy with long-term follow-up is now required to elaborate the mechanisms underlying this association.

Low–birthweight babies

Intriguingly, recent retrospective studies[26,27] have noted a 7–11-fold increase in risk of death from cardiovascular causes in women who delivered a baby less than 2500 g relative to women with babies greater than or equal to 3500 g. These findings appeared not to be confounded by socio-economic status, and the magnitudes of association were too great to be explained by maternal smoking. The observations suggest a link between maternal risk factors for CHD and fetal programming. Again, the maternal genotypes and phenotypes associated with increased risk of CHD may also underlie IUGR and fetal programming. In turn, this will lead to a continual cycling of risk factors through generations.

Preliminary data from our group (Kanagalingam *et al.*, unpublished data, 2006) suggests that women with a history of IUGR pregnancy demonstrate greater plasma cholesterol to high-density lipoprotein (HDL)-cholesterol ratio, triglyceride, ICAM-1, C-reactive protein (CRP) and interleukin (IL)-6 despite similar body mass index. Some, but not all of these changes could be related to a higher rate of smoking (>60 percent continued to smoke) among mothers with a history of IUGR pregnancy. Hence, smoking is a major preventable risk factor for IUGR pregnancy and also subsequent CHD risk.

Preterm delivery

Women with a history of preterm delivery (<37 weeks) had around a twofold increased risk for CHD in observational studies.[24,27] Although reliable data on maternal smoking – a major potential confounder – were not available in these studies, maternal smoking appeared not to be a confounder in this relation; such women were not at increased risk of smoking-related cancers. Preterm labor is recognized to be an inflammatory phenomenon,[28] with a leukocyte infiltrate in the cervical and uterine tissues, even in the absence of infection. One could speculate, therefore, that the association between preterm labor and CHD might relate to upregulation of chronic inflammatory pathways. Women with a 'proinflammatory' phenotype may develop greater upregulation of the chronic inflammatory pathways, beyond that seen in normal pregnancy, leading to preterm labor. This would help explain why these same women will be at increased risk of CHD in later life, as inflammation is an independent predictor, albeit modestly so, of CHD in men and women.[29] Again, confirmation of this important observation is needed in future, ideally prospective studies, along with an exploration of the inflammatory mechanisms common to both clinical problems.

Spontaneous pregnancy loss

As well as complications arising in the latter half of pregnancy, Smith and colleagues recently demonstrated a specific association between spontaneous abortion and maternal risk of ischemic heart disease.[30] They speculated that the association might occur via acquired and inherited thrombophilias, since these not only predict spontaneous pregnancy loss but have also been associated with CHD. In addition, polycystic ovarian syndrome or diabetes may also explain their findings, but such data were not available to the researchers.

Placental syndromes

More recently, Ray and colleagues[31] determined CHD risk in women with a history of placental syndromes. Maternal placental syndromes, including the hypertensive disorders of pregnancy and abruption or infarction of the placenta, probably originate from diseased placental vessels. They argued that since such syndromes arise most often in women who have metabolic risk factors for cardiovascular disease, including obesity, pre-pregnancy hypertension, diabetes mellitus, and dyslipidemia, a higher CHD risk should be apparent in such women in later life. Their results confirmed their hypothesis: the adjusted hazard ratio for CHD was 2.0 (95 percent CI 1.7 to 2.2) for women who had had a maternal placental syndrome compared with in women who had not. Of further interest, this risk was higher in the combined presence of a maternal placental syndrome and poor fetal growth (3.1, 2.2 to 4.5) or a maternal placental syndrome and intrauterine fetal death (4.4, 2.4 to 7.9), relative to neither. Table 29.1 summarizes links between pregnancy complications and subsequent metabolic and vascular disease risk.

POTENTIAL MECHANISMS LINKING PREGNANCY COMPLICATIONS TO CORONARY HEART DISEASE IN LATER LIFE

Although it is possible that the occurrence of the pregnancy complication 're-sets' mothers metabolism in an adverse direction and, thus, 'directly' increases future risk for metabolic and vascular diseases, it is far more likely that 'occult' cardiovascular risk factors exist prior to pregnancy in such women. Such 'occult' factors are exacerbated by the metabolic stress of pregnancy, and contribute to the occurrence of complications. Aging also exacerbates the same factors, and contributes to the elevated CHD risk in later life, in the same group of women.

The nature of these 'occult' risk factors is not entirely clear. One readily identifiable risk factor predictive of several pregnancy complications is obesity. Obesity is strongly linked to elevated risk for preeclampsia; the incidence of preeclampsia rises by about 0.5 percent for every 1 unit elevation in early or pre-pregnancy body mass index.[32]

Table 29.1 Association of adverse pregnancy outcomes with diabetes or coronary heart disease risk factor status and vascular morbidity/mortality

Pregnancy outcome	Incidence in pregnancy (%)	Risk factors shown to be perturbed after pregnancy	Association with risk of diabetes, CHD mortality or morbidity (Hazard ratios [95% CI])
Gestational diabetes	1.9–5*	Lipids[11] Blood pressure[11] Large vessel function[12,13]	↑ risk of type 2 diabetes, especially if recurrence of gestational diabetes in a subsequent pregnancy. No data on CHD risk
Preeclampsia	2–4	Small vessel lipids[18] Clotting[18] Fasting insulin[19] Large vessel function[20] ICAM-1[21]	1.9 (1.0 to 3.5) vs. PIH alone[22] 1.7 (1.3 to 2.2) vs. no preeclampsia[23] 2.0 (1.5 to 2.5) vs. no preeclampsia[24] 8.12 (4.31 to 15.33) if PET plus preterm delivery[25]
Low birthweight (<2500 g)	5	Chol:HDL-c ratio ICAM-1 CRP/IL-6 Smoking rate (unpublished data)	11.3 (3.5 to 36.1) vs. ≥3500 g[24] 7.1 (2.6 to 18.7) vs. ≥3500 g[26]
Preterm delivery (<37 weeks)	5–6	Not studied	1.8 (1.3 to 2.5) vs. term delivery[24] 2.1 (1.2 to 3.5) vs. term delivery[27]
Spontaneous pregnancy loss	–	Not studied	1.53 (1.13 to 2.06)[30]
Placental syndrome (PIH/PET; abruption; placental infarction)	7	Not studied	2.0 (0.7 to 2.2) vs. no placental syndrome 3.1 (2.2 to 4.5) if combined with poor fetal growth[31]

*Dependent on population studied, ethnic group and diagnostic criteria.
CHD, coronary heart disease; CRP, C-reactive protein; HDL, high-density lipoprotein; ICAM, intercellular adhesion molecule; IL, interleukin; PET, preeclampsia; PIH, pregnancy-induced hypertension.

Unsurprisingly, obesity also increases the risk of gestational hypertension and diabetes. Perhaps less well appreciated is the link between obesity and risk for spontaneous pregnancy loss. In terms of mechanisms, our group has recently demonstrated significant perturbations in all conventional risk factors, in insulin, CRP, and leptin concentrations, and in endothelial-dependent blood flow in obese pregnant women in the third trimester, relative to a lean group.[33] Of interest, using statistical methods, Bodnar et al. suggested that approximately a third of the total effect of body mass index on preeclampsia risk is mediated through inflammation and triglyceride levels.[34] However, an important recent prospective study suggested that the elevated CHD risk in women with a history of preeclampsia could not be accounted for simply by greater maternal obesity.[35] Whether the same is true for other pregnancy complications, linked to obesity, remains to be tested.

In contrast, very lean women are at elevated risk of having a very low-birthweight baby. Other factors, such as greater prevalence of smoking and poor maternal nutrition, might, in part, explain the association of this pathogenesis with subsequent CHD risk in the mother. Our preliminary observation of a sustained higher rate of smoking in women with IUGR pregnancies would certainly support this. Clearly, future studies are required to identify the nature of the 'occult' CHD risk factors predictive of pregnancy complications. Such knowledge would be critical to enable future preventative studies.

CLINICAL IMPLICATIONS

Screening for diabetes?

A major problem in the prevention of vascular disease has been the difficulties in identifying individuals at risk at an early enough stage to benefit from interventions such as lifestyle modification. For example, by the time type 2 diabetes is diagnosed, around 30–50 percent of patients will have evidence of vascular disease. Clearly, women with a history of gestational diabetes are candidates for screening for diabetes. This should take the form of fasting plasma glucose measurement, between 6 weeks and 6 months post partum, with subsequent assessments guided by initial results. A diagnosis of diabetes is now made if plasma glucose is ≥7 mmol/L on two occasions. If a result between 6.1 mmol/L and 6.9 mmol/L is recorded on two occasions, then an oral glucose tolerance test is advised. All women should be counseled about their elevated risk of developing type 2 diabetes in the future, and the benefits of lifestyle modification. This is important, as improved diet and physical activity has recently been proved to prevent the onset of type 2 diabetes in individuals at high risk.[36,37] Even if initial plasma glucose concentrations are normal, regular checks are warranted, particularly with the recurrence of gestational diabetes in a second pregnancy, to allow early identification and treatment of asymptomatic diabetes.

Need to quantify subsequent CHD risk?

Similarly, if other adverse pregnancy outcomes (preeclampsia, IUGR and preterm labor) are confirmed as indicators of increased vascular risk in mothers, these women may benefit from screening and primary prevention strategies. Such intervention could be focused on the perimenopausal years, a time when risk of vascular disease increases rapidly, or even earlier. This may be particularly relevant in mothers with low-birthweight babies (<2500 g), in whom relative risks for CHD appear increased severalfold (see Table 29.1). In addition, as hazard ratios for complications appear additive, a woman with multiple pregnancy complications, for example, preeclampsia combined with preterm delivery (<37 weeks) and a baby in the bottom quintile of birth weight, is at severalfold increased risk of CHD.[24] It is notable that the *absolute* risk of CHD in women in their forties is very low, thus, only factors which increase risk severalfold should be targeted.

Screening in these women should take the form of routine cardiovascular assessment – including measurement of blood pressure, fasting lipids (total cholesterol, triglyceride and HDL-cholesterol) and glucose concentrations – and the derivation of CVD risk using widely available risk factor charts. In the United Kingdom, currently practice is to consider treatment with cholesterol-lowering agents once risk for any cardiovascular event exceeds 20 percent over the next 10 years.[38] To help ensure that appropriate women are screened and given relevant health education, adverse pregnancy outcomes could be used in general practitioner/family physician computer databases for targeted health screening programs. Indeed, such interventions could start at the routine 6 weeks' postpartum review when these women could be made aware of their potentially increased risk for CHD.

Opportunity to modify risk pre–pregnancy?

The second implication of an association between maternal CHD risk and adverse pregnancy outcome is the potential for modification of risk factors in advance of a subsequent pregnancy or in early pregnancy. For example, increased physical activity in women who are sedentary may result in a better pregnancy outcome for both mother and child. Indeed, there are preliminary data to support this hypothesis; increasing exercise during pregnancy may increase birthweight[39] and reduce the risk of gestational diabetes[40]

and preeclampsia.[41] Clearly, such data would suggest that complications are not simply genetically determined, but that lifestyle factors play a major role. At present this remains largely speculative, and further research is needed to address this important question. Of interest, however, a recent trial[42] randomizing nonsmoking white women with singleton pregnancies (N = 290), and with no previous pregnancy-related complications, to either continue their usual diet or to adopt a diet that promoted fish, low-fat meats and dairy products, oils, whole grains, fruits, vegetables, and legumes from gestational week 17 to 20 to birth, demonstrated a substantially reduced risk of preterm delivery (RR 0.10, 95 percent CI 0.01 to 0.77). Clearly, these data need replication in larger studies.

Of major concern is the rise in incidence of obesity worldwide, a phenomenon that includes women of the reproductive age. We recently demonstrated a near doubling in the prevalence of obesity over the past decade in mothers (average age ~28 years) booking for antenatal care in our hospital; presently around 1 in 5 such women are frankly obese (body mass index > 30 kg/m^2).[43] It is clear that obesity in mothers is strongly linked to gestational diabetes, preeclampsia, spontaneous miscarriage, increased caesarean section rates and significant increased fetal morbidity. In the United States, where obesity rates are generally even higher, the American College of Obstetricians and Gynecologists has recently issued guidance on the impact of obesity on pregnancy.[44] In the United Kingdom, recent guidelines on exercise in pregnancy from the Royal College of Obstetricians have supported continued exercise in pregnancy and concluded that in most cases, exercise is safe for both the mother and fetus during pregnancy and will contribute to a number of health benefits such as reduced risk of gestational diabetes.[45]

Future large prospective studies should determine whether simple activities such as walking for 30 min/day can help reduce risk of a number of pregnancy complications such as preeclampsia and gestational diabetes, particularly in those at risk (e.g. BMI >25 kg/m^2). Such studies should also assess for potential benefits to the offspring in longer-term follow-up studies.

FETAL PROGRAMMING

A detailed discussion of fetal programming is beyond the scope of this chapter and the reader is referred to comprehensive reviews on the topic.[46–50] However, a number of general observations can be made. First, a number of epidemiologic studies worldwide have demonstrated a relation between poor early growth and an increased susceptibility to insulin resistance, visceral obesity, type 2 diabetes, and other features of the metabolic syndrome in adulthood. Such relations appear to be stronger than that linking low birthweight to adult CHD risk. The mechanisms for such observations remain complex but include programming of neuroendocrine pathways, appetite control, blood pressure, lipid axis or genetic factors.[46–50] With respect to the latter, it is now clear that since insulin is a growth factor *in utero*, genes coding for insulin resistance could link low birthweight to subsequent risk for diabetes in adulthood.[51]

Second, other observations suggest a synergistic effect of low birthweight and adult obesity for the risk for type 2 diabetes.[52] In other words, obesity seems more harmful to metabolic pathways in adults who were born at low birthweight. Part of the mechanism for this association may relate to an increased propensity for intraabdominal fat accumulation in offspring of low birthweight,[50] perhaps as a protective mechanism against future starvation or infection, but further studies are required to confirm this.

Third, an increased risk of diabetes is not confined to adults born at low birthweight but also extends to those at the other end of the spectrum of birthweight. Clearly, part of the mechanism for the latter association relates to large babies born to mothers with gestational diabetes. Recent data from India[53] suggest that maternal diabetes is associated with adiposity and higher glucose and insulin concentrations in female offspring at 5 years. In that study, the absence of similar associations in offspring of diabetic fathers suggests a programming effect in the diabetic intrauterine environment.

Finally, recent data worryingly links maternal obesity (independent of maternal gestational diabetes) with fetal-neonatal obesity, with obvious implications for future metabolic disease in the offspring. As a result, some researchers have argued[54] that the worldwide epidemic of adolescent obesity may be contributed to by maternal obesity, which leads to an abnormal metabolic milieu *in utero* during gestation. In other words, maternal obesity may beget obesity in offspring so leading to the propagation of a vicious cycle. There is intense interest in the latter question such that major research bodies (for example, National Institutes of Health) have issued calls for further direct research into this important area.

CONCLUSION

In conclusion, it is now clear that many complications of pregnancy signal an increased relative risk for vascular disease in mothers, and babies born at the extremes of the birth spectrum are also at elevated risk. Thus, there is an urgent need to explore vascular and metabolic risk factors and their association to adverse pregnancy outcomes, since such knowledge has great potential to impact not only on women's health but also the health of future generations. We cannot influence genotype, but there is the possibility of altering phenotype. Therefore, improving the maternal risk factor status and metabolic profiles prior to, or early in, pregnancy – for example by stopping smoking, increasing physical activity in sedentary women, improved diet, and weight loss in obese women – could benefit fetal development and reduce vascular risk of future generations.

KEY LEARNING POINTS

- Women with a history of adverse pregnancy outcome appear to be at increased risk of metabolic and vascular diseases in later life.
- Pregnancy complications and coronary heart disease may have common disease mechanisms.
- Offspring born at extremes of the birthweight spectrum are at higher risk of metabolic diseases in later life reflecting both genetic factors and influence of intrauterine environment.
- Women with a history of gestational diabetes should be screened for type 2 diabetes and be given counseling and appropriate lifestyle advice.
- Women who have had a very low birthweight baby or combined complications seem to be at severalfold increased risk of mortality from cardiovascular causes and should be screened for vascular risk factors in their late thirties.
- The possibility that maternal vascular risk factors, potentially 'modifiable' before pregnancy, correlate with increased risk of preterm delivery and low birthweight, and thus fetal programming, requires further investigation.
- Future studies to determine effects of maternal physical activity and improved diet on risk of pregnancy complications and fetal outcome are urgently required.

REFERENCES

1 Godfrey KM, Barker DJ. Fetal nutrition and adult disease. *Am J Clin Nutr* 2000; **71**: 1344S–52S.

2 Greer IA. Thrombosis in pregnancy: maternal and fetal issues. *Lancet* 1999; **10**: 1258–65.

3 Martin U, Davies C, Hayavi S, *et al*. Is normal pregnancy atherogenic? *Clin Sci* 1999; **96**: 421–5.

4 Sacks GP, Studena K, Sargent IL, Redman CWG. Normal pregnancy and pre-eclampsia both produce inflammatory changes in peripheral blood leukocytes akin to those of sepsis. *Am J Obstet Gynecol* 1998; **179**: 80–6.

5 Haffner S. Do interventions to reduce coronary heart disease reduce the incidence of type 2 diabetes? A possible role for inflammatory factors. *Circulation* 2001; **103**: 346–7.

6 Lowe GD. Circulating inflammatory markers and risks of cardiovascular and non-cardiovascular disease. *J Thromb Haemos* 2005; **3**: 1618–27.

7 Sattar N, Gaw A, Packard CJ, Greer IA. Potential pathogenic roles of aberrant lipoprotein and fatty acid metabolism in pre-eclampsia. *Br J Obstet Gynaecol* 1996; **103**: 614–20.

8 Sattar N, Greer IA. Pregnancy complications and maternal cardiovascular risk: opportunities for intervention and screening? *BMJ* 2002; **325**: 157–60.

9 Kaufmann RC, Schleyhahn FT, Huffman DG, Amankwah KS. Gestational diabetes diagnostic criteria: long-term

maternal follow-up. *Am J Obstet Gynecol* 1995; **172**: 621–5.

10 Peters RK, Kjos SL, Xiang A, Buchanan TA. Long-term diabetogenic effect of single pregnancy in women with previous gestational diabetes mellitus. *Lancet* 1996; **347**: 227–30.

11 Meyers-Seifer CH, Vohr BR. Lipid levels in former gestational diabetic women. *Diabetologia* 1996; **19**: 1351–6.

12 Hu J, Norman M, Wallensteen M, Gennser G. Increased larger arterial stiffness and impaired acetylcholine-induced skin vasodilatation in women with previous gestational diabetes. *Br J Obstet Gynaecol* 1998; **105**: 1279–87.

13 Heitritter SM, Solomon CG, Mitchell GF, *et al.* Subclinical inflammation and vascular dysfunction in women with previous gestational diabetes mellitus. *J Clin Endocrinol Metab* 2005; **90**: 3983–8.

14 Xiang AH, Peters RK, Kjos SL, *et al.* Effect of thiazolidinedione treatment on progression of subclinical atherosclerosis in premenopausal women at high risk for type 2 diabetes. *J Clin Endocrinol Metab* 2005; **90**: 1986–91.

15 Chesley LC, Annitto JE, Cosgrove RA. The remote prognosis of eclamptic women: sixth periodic report. *Am J Obstet Gynecol* 1976; **124**: 446–59.

16 Fisher KA, Luger A, Spargo BH, Lindheimer MD. Hypertension in pregnancy: clinical-pathological correlations and remote prognosis. *Medicine* 1981; **60**: 267.

17 Sibai B, A Ae-N, Gonzalez-Ruiz A. Severe pre-eclampsia-eclampsia in young primigravid women: subsequent pregnancy outcome and remote prognosis. *Am J Obstet Gynecol* 1986; **155**: 1011–16.

18 He S, Silveira A, Hamsten A, *et al.* Haemostatic, endothelial and lipoprotein parameters and blood pressure levels in women with a history of pre-eclampsia. *Thromb Haemost* 1999; **81**: 538–42.

19 Laivuori H, Tikkanen MJ, Ylikorkala O. Hyperinsulinaemia 17 years after pre-eclamptic first pregnancy. *J Clin Endocrinol Metab* 1996; **81**: 2908–11.

20 Chambers JC, Fusi L, Malik IS, *et al.* Association of maternal endothelial dysfunction with preeclampsia. *JAMA* 2001; **285**: 1607–12.

21 Sattar N, Ramsay J, Crawford L, *et al.* Classic and novel risk factor parameters in women with a history of preeclampsia. *Hypertension* 2003; **42**: 39–42.

22 Jonsdottir LS, Arngrimsson R, Geirsson RT, *et al.* Death rates from ischaemic heart disease in women with a history of hypertension in pregnancy. *Acta Obstet Gynecol Scand* 1995; **74**: 772–6.

23 Hannaford P, Ferry S, Hirsch S. Cardiovascular sequelae of toxaemia of pregnancy. *Heart* 1997; **77**: 154–8.

24 Smith GCS, Pell JP, Walsh D. Pregnancy complications and maternal risk of ischaemic heart disease: a retrospective cohort study of 129 290 births. *Lancet* 2001; **357**: 2002–6.

25 Irgens HU, Reisaeter L, Irgens LM, Lie RT. Long term mortality of mothers and fathers after pre-eclampsia: population based cohort study. *BMJ* 2001; **24**: 1213–17.

26 Davey-Smith G, Harding S, Rosato M. Relation between infants' birth weight and mothers' mortality: prospective observational study. *BMJ* 2000; **320**: 839–40.

27 Davey-Smith G, Whitley E, Gissler M, Hemminki E. Birth dimensions of offspring, premature birth, and the mortality of mother. *Lancet* 2000; **356**: 2066–7.

28 Thomson AJ, Telfer JF, Young A, *et al.* Leukocytes infiltrate the myometrium during human parturition: further evidence that labour is an inflammatory process. *Hum Reprod* 1999; **14**: 229–36.

29 Danesh J, Wheeler JG, Hirschfield GM, *et al.* C-reactive protein and other circulating markers of inflammation in the prediction of coronary heart disease. *N Engl J Med* 2004; **350**: 1387–97.

30 Smith GC, Pell JP, Walsh D. Spontaneous loss of early pregnancy and risk of ischaemic heart disease in later life: retrospective cohort study. *BMJ* 2003; **326**: 423–4.

31 Ray JG, Vermeulen MJ, Schull MJ, Redelmeier DA. Cardiovascular health after maternal placental syndromes (CHAMPS): population-based retrospective cohort study. *Lancet* 2005; **19**: 1797–803.

32 O'Brien TE, Ray JG, Chan WS. Maternal body mass index and the risk of preeclampsia: a systematic overview. *Epidemiology* 2003; **14**: 368–74.

33 Ramsay JE, Ferrell WR, Crawford L, *et al.* Maternal obesity and dysregulation of metabolic, vascular and inflammatory pathways: relevance for pregnancy complications? *J Clin Endocinol Metab* 2002; **87**: 4231–7.

34 Bodnar LM, Ness RB, Harger GF, Roberts JM. Inflammation and triglycerides partially mediate the effect of prepregnancy body mass index on the risk of preeclampsia. *Am J Epidemiol* 2005; **15**: 1198–206.

35 Wilson BJ, Watson MS, Prescott GJ, *et al.* Hypertensive diseases of pregnancy and risk of hypertension and stroke in later life: results from cohort study. *BMJ* 2003; **326**: 845.

36 Tuomilehto J, Lindstrom J, Eriksson JG, *et al.* Finnish Diabetes Prevention Study Group. Prevention of type 2 diabetes mellitus by changes in lifestyle among subjects with impaired glucose tolerance. *N Engl J Med* 2001; **344**: 1343–50.

37 Hu FB, Manson JE, Stampfer MJ, *et al.* Diet, lifestyle, and the risk of type 2 diabetes mellitus in women. *N Engl J Med* 2001; **345**: 790–7.

38 British Cardiac Society; British Hypertension Society; Diabetes UK, *et al.* JBS 2: Joint British Societies' guidelines on prevention of cardiovascular disease in clinical practice. *Heart* 2005; **91**(Suppl 5): v1–52.

39 Clapp JF 3rd, Kim H, Burciu B, Lopez B. Beginning regular exercise in early pregnancy: effect on fetoplacental growth. *Am J Obstet Gynecol* 2000; **183**: 1484–8.

40 Dornhorst A, Michela R. Risk and prevention of type 2 diabetes in women with gestational diabetes. *Diabetes Care* 1998; **21**(Suppl 2): 43B–9B.

41   Sorensen TK, Williams MA, Lee IM, *et al*. Recreational physical activity during pregnancy and risk of preeclampsia. *Hypertension* 2003; **41**: 1273–80.

42   Khoury J, Henriksen T, Christophersen B, Tonstad S. Effect of a cholesterol-lowering diet on maternal, cord, and neonatal lipids and pregnancy outcome: a randomized clinical trial. *Am J Obstet Gynecol* 2005; **193**: 1292–301.

43   Kanagalingam MG, Forouhi NG, Greer IA, Sattar N. Changes in booking body mass index over a decade: retrospective analysis from a Glasgow Maternity Hospital. *Br J Obstet Gynaecol* 2005; **112**: 1431–3.

44   American College of Obstetricians and Gynecologists. ACOG Committee Opinion number 315, September 2005. Obesity in pregnancy. *Obstet Gynecol* 2005; **106**: 671–5.

45   Royal College of Obstetricians. Exercise in pregnancy, January 2006. Available at: www.rcog.org.uk/resources/Public/pdf/exercise_pregnancy_rcog_statement4.pdf (accessed June 2006).

46   Alexander BT. Fetal programming of hypertension. *Am J Physiol Regul Integr Comp Physiol* 2006; **290**: R1–10.

47   Martin-Gronert MS, Ozanne SE. Programming of appetite and type 2 diabetes. *Early Hum Dev* 2005; **81**: 981–8.

48   Stocker CJ, Arch JR, Cawthorne MA. Fetal origins of insulin resistance and obesity. *Proc Nutr Soc* 2005; **64**: 143–51.

49   Phillips DI. Fetal programming of the neuroendocrine response to stress: links between low birth weight and the metabolic syndrome. *Endocr Res* 2004; **30**: 819–26.

50   Remacle C, Bieswal F, Reusens B. Programming of obesity and cardiovascular disease. *Int J Obes Relat Metab Disord* 2004; **28**(Suppl 3): S46–53.

51   Hattersley AT, Tooke JE. The fetal insulin hypothesis: an alternative explanation of the association of low birthweight with diabetes and vascular disease. *Lancet* 1999; **22**: 1789–92.

52   Hales CN, Barker DJ, Clark PM, *et al*. Fetal and infant growth and impaired glucose tolerance at age 64. *BMJ* 1991; **26**: 1019–22.

53   Krishnaveni GV, Hill JC, Leary SD, Fall CH. Anthropometry, glucose tolerance, and insulin concentrations in Indian children: relationships to maternal glucose and insulin concentrations during pregnancy. *Diabetes Care* 2005; **28**: 2919–25.

54   Catalano PM. Obesity and pregnancy – the propagation of a viscous cycle? *J Clin Endocrinol Metab* 2003; **88**: 3505–6.

HORMONAL THERAPY IN WOMEN

PART 3

HORMONAL THERAPY IN WOMEN

30

Oral contraceptive use and venous thromboembolism: epidemiology, mechanisms, and patient management

FRANCESCO DENTALI, JAMES D DOUKETIS

INTRODUCTION

The oral contraceptive (OC) is one of the most widely used drugs worldwide. It is estimated that 100 million women use a typical OC consisting of an estrogen and a progestin component, which is available in an oral and, more recently, transdermal preparations.[1] Approximately 13 million women use a progestin-only contraceptive, which has comparable contraceptive efficacy as the combined estrogen-progestin formulations, and is available in an oral, intramuscular, intrauterine, and subdermal formulations.[2]

The first OC was approved for use as a contraceptive in United States in 1959, and contained 150 μg of mestranol and 10 mg of norethynodrel. Two years later, the first thromboembolic side effect was reported, when a nurse developed pulmonary embolism shortly after starting an OC.[3] Since then, the estrogen content of OC has been reduced with the purpose of minimizing the adverse effects and the progestin has also changed over the time but this change was related more to the chemical composition rather than the dose. In 1967, a case–control study showed that OC users had a threefold increased risk of venous thromboembolism (VTE) in comparison with nonusers.[4] Since then, 41 additional case–control studies,[5–45] 3 prospective cohort studies,[46–48] and 1 randomized controlled trial[49] have confirmed that the risk of VTE in OC users is twofold to fourfold higher than in nonusers. However, the estimated absolute risk for developing VTE remains low, increasing from 1 per 10 000 person years, to 3–4 per 10 000 person years during the time when the OC is used.

In the past two decades, several inherited or acquired abnormalities in the coagulation system have been discovered which are associated with a hypercoagulable state. Factor V Leiden and the prothrombin gene mutation G20210A are common in the general population, particular in Caucasians. Several studies have shown that the absolute risk of VTE in women who use OCs and have a prothrombotic blood disorder is higher than expected from the addition of these risks, thereby suggesting a possible enhancement in their individual effect on thrombosis risk. Despite considerable advances in our understanding of the association between the OC and the risk for VTE and its interplay with prothrombotic blood abnormalities on this risk, several questions remain unclear or unanswered. Furthermore, there are few studies that address the practical clinical management of women who are assessed regarding the risks of VTE with contraceptive use. The objectives of this chapter are to address unresolved issues regarding the association between the OC and VTE, and to provide clinicians with suggested management guidelines of patients who are at risk for VTE in whom contraceptive therapy is being considered.

WHAT IS THE RISK FOR VENOUS THROMBOEMBOLISM WITH DIFFERENT TYPES OF CONTRACEPTIVE?

Oral contraceptives can be administered as a monophasic, which is taken every day for at least 21 days each cycle, or a biphasic or triphasic preparations, in which the dose of both compounds varies over the administration cycle. Preparations that contain only progestin can be administered in several ways: as an intramuscular depot injection, every three months; as an oral preparation, which requires that the pill is taken at the same time daily for optimal efficacy; intrauterine preparations that are impregnated into an intrauterine device; and subdermal implants, which provide long-term contraception over a 4–5-year period.

As stated above, the first OC contained 150 μg of mestranol and 10 mg of norethynodrel. Since then, the estrogen content of OC (usually consisting of ethinylestradiol) has been reduced, mainly to minimize prothrombotic adverse effects, first to 50 μg and then to 30–35 μg, and some preparations contain only 15–20 μg of ethinylestradiol. The progestin has also changed over the time but this change involves the chemical composition rather than the dose. Progestins (and their respective OC) are classified as first, second, or third generation. Norethisterone, norethynodrel, lynestrenol, and ethynodiol acetate are contained in first-generation OCs. Norgestrel, levonorgestrel, and norgestrione are contained in second-generation OCs. Desogestrogel, gestodene, and norgestimate are contained in third-generation OCs. Oral contraceptives containing cyproterone acetate and drospirenone are not yet categorized.

Most studies have shown that the risk of VTE is approximately twice as high in users of OC containing higher estrogen doses in comparison to users of OCs containing lower estrogen doses. Thus, Gerstman et al. have demonstrated that risk of VTE is higher in users of OC containing more than 50 μg compared with VTE risk in users of OC containing less than 50 μg.[20] Bloemenkamp et al. have shown that the risk of VTE is greater in users of OCs containing 50 μg as opposed to less than 35 μg of ethinylestradiol.[13] Although the risk for VTE is increased in users of an OC containing low doses of estrogen (30–35 μg of ethinylestradiol), there is little evidence regarding the risk for VTE in users of an OC containing very low doses of estrogen (15–20 μg of ethinylestradiol). However, it is reasonable to assume some increase in risk in such preparations, although the absolute risk is not known.

In terms of the effect of the progestin component of the OC on VTE risk, three studies in mid-1990s showed that third-generation OCs, containing desogestrel or gestodene, was associated with a higher risk for VTE compared with

second-generation OCs.[22,37,39] Since then, additional studies found a greater VTE risk in users of third-generation OCs than in users of second-generation OCs, although the difference was not always statistically significant.[8,13,23,34,38,40,41,43–45] Thus, two cohort studies found that the incidence of VTE among new users of third- and second-generation OCs was 9.0/10 000 person years and 2–4/10 000 person years, respectively, yielding a relative risk of 3.5 (95 percent confidence interval [CI] 1.4 to 8.8).[37,38] Furthermore, two recent meta-analyses have concluded that there is a small but statistically significant greater risk for VTE with third-generation than second-generation OCs.[50,51]

In support of these clinical observations, multiple biochemical studies compared OCs with a different progestin component showed that third-generation preparations have more pronounced effects on procoagulant, anticoagulant, and fibrinolytic pathways than second-generation preparations.[52–55] Furthermore, use of third-generation OCs may lead to a greater tendency toward developing acquired resistance to activated protein C, and a greater decrease in protein S levels than second-generation OC preparations.[52] The risk for VTE associated with OCs containing the newer progestin, cyproterone, is less well defined. However, one study found a threefold to fourfold higher risk of VTE among cyproterone users in comparison with women who used levonorgestrel.[56] Currently, there are no data available on the thrombotic risk of drospirenone, a progestin analog of spironolactone.

Most epidemiologic studies have reported VTE risk in users of monophasic OCs. Monophasic combination OCs provide a constant daily dose of estrogen and progestin, whereas biphasic or triphasic OCs provide varying doses of both components given through a 21-day cycle. Two cohort studies have suggested that that the risk of VTE associated with multiphasic levonorgestrel OCs is similar to that of monophasic levonorgestrel OCs.[7,37] However, the paucity of studies addressing this issue precludes definitive conclusions. A progestin-only contraceptive is considered by gynecologic authorities as a safer alternative contraceptive for high-risk women, despite the fact there are only limited observational data on thrombotic risk.[2,33,34,40,57–60] Data from the World Health Organization Collaborative Study showed a small, nonsignificant increase in risk for VTE in association with oral and injectable progestin-only contraceptives.[2] Vasilakis et al. found a modest, nonsignificant, positive association between venous thromboembolism and exposure to progestins alone used for contraception, whereas they found a substantial association with the higher dose progestins used for other therapeutic indications.[58] Two studies have confirmed this association, showing a fivefold to sixfold increased risk of VTE when higher doses of progestin were used for therapeutic indications such as menstrual disorders.[58,60] Furthermore, in these three studies women with history of VTE or other known risk factors were excluded. Overall, there was no clear evidence of increased risk of VTE when progestin-only preparations were used for contraception. On the other hand, use of higher doses of progestins may be associated with an increased risk of VTE.[58,60] Finally, there are no studies that assessed the risk of VTE in users of transdermal OCs or combination contraceptive vaginal ring.

WHAT IS THE EFFECT OF THE DURATION OF ORAL CONTRACEPTIVE USE ON THE RISK FOR VENOUS THROMBOEMBOLISM?

Several studies have investigated the effect of the duration of OC use on the risk for VTE.[8,15,21,34,61–64] Earlier studies assessing the duration of OC use described that the association between OC use and VTE was unrelated to duration of use.[17,24,35] Conversely, more recent studies demonstrate that the risk is highest during the first 6 months to 1 year of OC use, particularly among first-time users.[8,15,21,34,61–64] This later finding suggests the existence of a subgroup of women who are at risk for VTE soon after starting the OC. The increased risk of VTE is apparent within the initial 6 months after the start of the OC, appears to diminish thereafter but does not disappear during the subsequent years of use.[15] The risk associated with reexposure after a period of no use is similar to, and not higher than, that associated with first-time use.[65]

It has been suggested that women who developed VTE soon after the start of the OC may have a preexisting tendency for VTE and that OC may act as a catalyst for the development of clinically overt thromboembolism in women with an inherited or acquired prothrombotic blood abnormality.[66] In one study, in women who developed VTE during early use of OC, thrombophilia was more often present than among those who develop VTE during prolonged use.[15] On the other hand, in women who develop VTE after long-term OC use, the effect of OC on the pathogenesis of VTE is less clear. In those patients, OC may act as a contributory factor that, coupled with other clinical factors such as comorbid disease, may result in the development of VTE. Otherwise, OC may be an innocent bystander, with the development of VTE being due to other nonhormonal factors.

WHAT IS THE MECHANISM FOR THE ASSOCIATION BETWEEN ORAL CONTRACEPTIVE USE AND VENOUS THROMBOEMBOLISM?

In 1971 von Kaulla *et al.* reported an increased level of thrombin generation and decreased levels of antithrombin in women taking OCs.[67] However, until recently, it was uncertain whether the use of low-dose OCs disturbed the hemostatic balance in favor of a prothrombotic state. Potential prothrombotic effects included increases in the levels of coagulation factors VII and VIII, and decreases in the levels of the endogenous anticoagulants antithrombin

III and protein S.[68–71] Overall, these prothrombotic changes were considered counterbalanced, at least partially, by such antithrombotic effects as increases in the levels of other anticoagulant proteins and increased fibrinolysis. Furthermore, the changes in levels of coagulation factors during OC use were such that they typically remained within the normal range.[68–71] Recent studies on the effects of second-generation and third-generation OC on the procoagulant, anticoagulant, and fibrinolytic pathways, in contrast, indicate that OCs have a net prothrombotic effect.[52–54] Quantitatively, the prothrombotic effects appear to be greater with third-generation OCs, which also appear to be associated with a greater risk for VTE compared with second-generation OCs.[52]

Effects of the oral contraceptive on thrombin generation and fibrinolysis

Recent studies have confirmed that the levels of prothrombin, factor VII, factor VIII, factor X, fibrinogen, and prothrombin fragment 1 + 2 are increased and the levels of factor V are decreased during the use of oral contraceptives.[72] The increase in prothrombin and factor VII and the decrease in factor V were significantly more pronounced with third-generation OCs than with second-generation OCs.[72] Moderately increased levels of prothrombin and factor VIII are associated with an increased risk of VTE.[73,74] Furthermore, a decrease in factor V may contribute to the prothrombotic side effects of OCs, since factor V may exhibit anticoagulant activity from its ability to act as a cofactor in the inactivation of activated factor VIII that is mediated by activated protein C.[75,76]

The measurements of the plasma levels of the individual proteins involved in fibrinolysis suggest that OC use enhances fibrinolytic activity.[68–71,77] However, a functional clot lysis test that simultaneously measured the activity of the fibrinolytic system and the ability of thrombin-activatable fibrinolysis inhibitor (TAFI) to inhibit fibrinolysis indicated that the increased fibrinolytic activity during the use of OCs is counterbalanced by an increased activity of the TAFI system.[77] This may be due to the finding that TAFI levels and thrombin generation are elevated during OC use, and this effect appears more pronounced with third- than second-generation OCs.[77]

Effects of the oral contraceptive on activated protein C resistance

Since 1993, APC resistance is a recognized risk factor for VTE.[78] About 1 year later, several groups reported that APC resistance is caused by a point mutation in the factor V gene (R506Q) resulting in the replacement of an arginine residue at a predominant cleavage site for APC.[79,80] Since the mutation was first discovered in Leiden, the mutated molecule is often called factor V Leiden. As a consequence of this mutation, the downregulation of factor V activation in carriers of the factor V Leiden mutation is impaired, resulting in enhanced thrombin formation in individuals with the mutation, a phenomenon which explains the increased risk for VTE in carriers of the factor V Leiden mutation.[81]

An acquired form of APC resistance associated with OC use may occur in the absence of the factor V Leiden mutation.[52,82–85] A cross-sectional study, in which APC resistance was determined in plasma from 60 women not using OC and from 125 women using either a second- or third-generation OC, indicated that independent of the kind of OC used, plasma from women using OC was considerably more resistant to APC than plasma from non-OC users.[52] Furthermore, it was found that the APC resistance of plasma is significantly higher with third-generation OC use than with second-generation OC use, and appears similar to the APC resistance of heterozygous carriers of the factor V Leiden mutation who are nonusers of the OC.[52] Since resistance to activated protein C, even in the absence of factor V Leiden, is an independent risk factor for VTE, these observations support the theory that acquired resistance to activated protein C contributes to the increased risk for VTE in OC users. The molecular basis of acquired resistance to activated protein C during OC use is unknown. Decreased levels of plasma protein S, the cofactor of activated protein C, explain only partly the resistance to activated protein C found with OC use.[54]

WHAT IS THE EFFECT OF PROTHROMBOTIC BLOOD ABNORMALITIES ON THE RISK FOR VENOUS THROMBOEMBOLISM IN WOMEN USING ORAL CONTRACEPTIVES?

In terms of inherited prothrombotic blood abnormalities, the factor V Leiden mutation is the most common, occurring in 2–5 percent of Caucasians.[86,87] This blood abnormality is characterized by an impaired anticoagulant response to activated protein C due to a point mutation in the factor V gene, which results in a single amino acid change that destroys a cleavage site for activated protein C.[88] The abnormal factor V Leiden protein is inactivated at a 10-fold slower rate than normal, and persists longer in the circulation, resulting in increased thrombin generation and a prothrombotic state.[88] The prothrombin gene G20210A mutation occurs in 1–2 percent of Caucasians, and is thought to exert its prothrombotic effect through enhanced activation of prothrombin.[89] Elevated plasma levels of factor VIII are also common in the general population, although their effect on the risk for VTE is not clear. Inherited deficiencies of endogenous anticoagulants protein C, protein S, and antithrombin III are uncommon, with a combined prevalence of 1–2 percent in the general population.[90,91] Other inherited blood abnormalities, such as the thermolabile variant of methylene tetrahydrofolate reductase C677T, the 4G/5G variant of plasminogen activator inhibitor-1, and the factor XIII G100T variant, are not associated with an increased risk for VTE.[92,93] Acquired prothrombotic blood abnormalities include hyperhomocysteinemia, usually due to vitamin B6 or folate deficiency, and the antiphospholipid antibody syndrome, which occurs in the presence of a lupus anticoagulant or elevated anticardiolipin antibodies.[94,95]

In OC users, the presence of a prothrombotic blood abnormality may further increase the risk for VTE. The first indication for a potential synergistic effect between an inherited prothrombotic blood abnormality and the OC was derived from the Leiden Thrombophilia Study, a population-based case–control study that compared 155 consecutive premenopausal women with a first episode of venous thrombosis with a population of 169 population controls.[7] This study found that heterozygous carriers of the factor V Leiden mutation who used an OC had approximately 35-fold higher risk for VTE compared to nonusers of the OC without this mutation (odds ratio [OR] = 34.7, 95 percent CI 7.8 to 154). In a further analysis that involved this database, it was estimated that use of a third-generation OC increased the thrombotic risk of 50-fold in heterozygous carriers of the factor V Leiden mutation.[37] The results of this study suggested a multiplicative interaction between OC use and the factor V mutation on the risk for VTE.[7] This study also provided data about the risk for VTE in OC users with elevated factor VIII levels, as the risk for VTE in such individuals was 10-fold higher compared with the risk in nonusers of the OC without elevated factor VIII (OR 10.3, 95 percent CI 3.7 to 28.9).[96] Other population-based case–control studies confirmed the increased risk of a first episode of VTE among carriers of the factor V Leiden mutation who use the OC.[14,43] In a case–control study, Andersen et al.[41] found that the risk for VTE among OC users with either a deficiency of antithrombin, protein C or protein S, or the factor V Leiden mutation was considerably higher than nonusers of the OC without these abnormalities (OR 63.3, 95 percent CI 6.2 to 648.4 and OR 52.5, 95 percent CI: 3.7–738, respectively).[43] Finally, Martinelli et al. showed that use of the OC in heterozygous carriers of the factor V Leiden or prothrombin 20210A mutations was associated with a 16- and 20-fold increased risk for VTE, respectively, compared with nonusers of the OC without these mutations.[14] There are no studies, to our knowledge, regarding the risk of OC use in women with hyperhomocysteinemia.

CLINICAL MANAGEMENT SCENARIOS

Should screening for thrombophilia be done in women who are starting the oral contraceptive?

The increased risk of VTE in women with thrombophilia who use the OC means that screening for prothrombotic blood abnormalities might be considered, with the aim of preventing OC-associated VTE. However, it has been argued that screening of all women who intend to use or already use the OC would not be a realistic task to prevent fatal VTE.[97] For instance, Vandenbroucke *et al.* calculated the estimated annual incidence of VTE in factor V Leiden carriers who use the pill is 28.5 per 10 000 woman years.[97] Assuming a case-fatality rate of 2 percent, they estimated an annual death rate of 5.7 per 100 000, thereby inferring that 400 000 women would have to be screened to prevent one VTE-related death. Thus, universal genetic screening does not seem to be justified although the actual risks and benefits of genetic screening remain to be investigated. On the other hand, selective screening in women with prior VTE or family history of VTE in first-degree relatives (parents, siblings) before starting the OC is reasonable. We acknowledge, however, that a positive personal or family history of VTE may not identify all women with a prothrombotic tendency who may be more susceptible to develop OC-associated VTE. Consequently, decisions regarding the use of the OC in such patents should be based on best available estimates of the risks, health benefits of the OC and, perhaps most importantly, patient preferences.

Should an oral contraceptive be considered for women with an asymptomatic prothrombotic blood abnormality?

In women with asymptomatic thrombophilia who do not have a prior history of VTE, counseling should be provided on the risk of OC-associated VTE and on alternative forms of contraception with the aim that the patient will partake in the clinical decision-making process. This open discussion is warranted because the risk of OC-associated VTE will vary depending on the prothrombotic blood abnormality. Thus, in heterozygous carriers of the factor V Leiden or prothrombin G20210A mutations, the risk for VTE, although greatly increased relative to OC users who do not take the OC, should be weighed against potential health benefits of the OC. This can be better achieved if the absolute risk of VTE with OC use is considered, which is 28–50 cases per 10 000 woman years of OC use.[97] This may be considered acceptable for some women and unacceptably high for others. This risk should be weighed against the health and social consequences of unplanned pregnancy if the OC is not used. In healthy women, VTE is more frequent during pregnancy than during OC use, with an estimated incidence of 1 case per 1000 deliveries and a 1–2 percent case-fatality rate.[98,99]

In women with a deficiency of antithrombin III or protein C, it is prudent to avoid OCs because of the reported absolute risk for VTE with OC use of 400 per 10 000 patient-years of OC use.[100] The OC-related VTE risk in carriers of protein S deficiency is uncertain but is likely increased. Another management option for contraception in women with asymptomatic thrombophilia is a progestin-only contraceptive. These preparations are thought to be associated with a lower risk for VTE compared to combined estrogen-progestin OCs, presumably because the estrogen component of the OC is considered to harbor the prothrombotic effects.[101] However, there are no studies that have addressed the safety of progestin-only contraceptives in women with asymptomatic thrombophilia or in whom a history of VTE is unknown.

What is the management of women using oral contraceptives who develop venous thromboembolism?

Women who develop VTE while using an OC should discontinue the OC, at least temporarily. Indirect evidence suggests that VTE that occurs during the use of OC is less likely to recur when the OC is stopped, as stopping the OC may have the effect of removing an ongoing prothrombotic stimulus.[21,22] Anticoagulant therapy should be started as in women who develop VTE without associated OC use. Oral anticoagulants, administered to achieve an international normalized ratio (INR) of 2.0–3.0, should be initiated together with therapeutic dose of unfractionated or low-molecular-weight heparin. Heparin should be discontinued after 4–6 days of therapy when INR is >2.0 for 2 consecutive days. The optimal duration of anticoagulant therapy is less clear. In patients who develop VTE during exposure to a transient risk factor, such as surgery, 3 months of treatment is considered sufficient, whereas in patients who develop VTE during exposure to a permanent risk factor, such as advanced cancer or paralysis, long-term or indefinite treatment is recommended.[102] The duration of treatment in patients with unprovoked VTE is controversial, although at least 6 months of treatment is recommended.[102] Some experts recommended that patients who develop VTE while using OC should be treated for 3 months, as such OC is considered a transient and reversible risk factor.[103] This approach appears reasonable in women who develop VTE within months of starting OC, whereas in women who develop VTE after they have used OC for several years, the argument that OC is a transient reversible risk factor is less compelling. In such women, the OC may be only an innocent bystander, and not the factor that provoked the thrombotic event. Consequently, anticoagulant therapy for 3 months may be insufficient. Overall, the duration of anticoagulant therapy should be individualized because for some women 3 months of therapy may be reasonable, whereas for others a therapy of 6 months or longer should be considered.

What is the management of women using oral contraceptives who require elective surgery?

To date, in OC users who require elective surgery, there is no compelling evidence that OC needs to be temporarily discontinued before and after surgery. Some experts suggest that there is the potential that perioperative use of OC will further increase the risk for DVT beyond that conferred by the surgical procedure and postoperative immobility.[48,101] A prospective cohort study found a nonstatistically significant doubling of the risk of postoperative VTE in women who used OC during the month of surgery compared with those who stopped their OC use more than 1 month before surgery.[48] However, the absolute incidence of VTE in young women remains low and OC is a relatively weak risk factor for VTE compared with the risk associated with surgery and any possible additive effect of OC is unlikely to be important in terms of the overall VTE risk.

However, appropriate methods of thromboprophylaxis should be considered in such patients, particularly if there is anticipated postoperative immobility or in patients who are undergoing high-risk procedures such as major orthopedic surgery.

CONCLUSIONS AND PRIORITIES FOR FUTURE RESEARCH

Associations between exposure and disease observed in observational studies do not constitute proof of causality. In addition, although the magnitude of an association between risk and disease is usually expressed as relative risk or odds ratio, the importance of any given association for the individual patient is best determined by the absolute risk. However, data from several studies have clearly demonstrated an increased risk of venous thrombosis in women taking OCs, although the absolute risk is low. Several modifications of hemostasis have been observed, but the clinical significance of the effects of OC on markers of thrombin generation, fibrinolysis, and activated protein C resistance remains unclear.

Women with a history of VTE with or without thrombophilia should avoid OCs as a prior history is the strongest risk factor for recurrence. Women with asymptomatic thrombophilia and no history of VTE should be counseled on the risks of thrombosis and encouraged to consider alternative forms of contraception although the risk varies in this group. However, use of alternative, nonhormonal contraception may lead to more unplanned pregnancies and their attendant VTE risk. In healthy women and in carriers of the factor V Leiden or prothrombinG20210A mutations, VTE seems to be more frequent during pregnancy than during OC. Given their higher thrombotic risk third-generation OCs should be avoided and second generation or progestin unopposed ones should be preferred. However, due to the low absolute risk of VTE associated with the use of third generation ones for the individual patient, current evidence does not support a recommendation that women already using third-generation OC should stop taking them. Moreover, some women may benefit from the further minimization of androgenic activity provided by these products.

Progestin-only contraceptives are considered to be a safer option than combination OC especially in women with a known inherited hypercoagulable state or a previous history of VTE. However, these two types of OC have never been directly compared and the safety of using progestin-only contraceptives in those settings remains largely unknown. Finally, the VTE risk associated with the use of norethindrone and norgestimate, which are among the most commonly used progestins in the United States, and with transdermal and vaginal ring contraceptives is essentially unknown.

KEY LEARNING POINTS

- The risk of VTE is approximately twice as high in users of OC containing higher estrogen doses in comparison to users of OCs containing lower estrogen doses.
- Third-generation OCs, containing desogestrel or gestodene, are associated with a higher risk for VTE compared with second-generation OCs.
- Overall, there is no clear evidence of increased risk of VTE when progestin-only preparations are used for contraception, but use of higher doses of progestins may be associated with an increased risk of VTE.
- Levels of prothrombin, factor VII, factor VIII, factor X, fibrinogen, and prothrombin fragment 1 + 2 are increased and the levels of factor V are decreased during the use of oral contraceptives.
- In OC users, the presence of a prothrombotic blood abnormality may further increase the risk for VTE.
- Selective screening in women with prior VTE or family history of VTE in first-degree relatives (parents, siblings) before starting the OC is a reasonable decision.
- In women with asymptomatic thrombophilia who do not have a prior history of VTE, counseling should be provided on the risk of OC-associated VTE and on alternative forms of contraception because the risk of OC-associated VTE will vary depending on the prothrombotic blood abnormality.
- Women who develop VTE while using an OC should discontinue the OC, at least temporarily. There is indirect evidence suggesting VTE that occurs during the use of OC is less likely to recur when the OC is stopped, as stopping the OC may have the effect of removing an ongoing prothrombotic stimulus.

REFERENCES

1 United Nations Population Division, Department of Economic and Social Affairs. *World Contraceptive Use 2001.* New York, NY: United Nations, 2002.

2 World Health Organization Collaborative Study of Cardiovascular Disease and Steroid Hormone Contraception. Cardiovascular disease and use of oral and injectable progestogen-only contraceptives and combined injectable contraceptives: results of an international, multicenter, case-control study. *Contraception* 1998; **57**: 315–24.

3 Jordan WM. Pulmonary embolism. *Lancet* 1961; **ii**: 1146–7.

4   [Not authors listed] Oral contraception and thrombo-
     embolic disease. *J R Coll Gen Pract* 1967; **13**: 267–79.

5   Valla D, Le MG, Poynard T, *et al*. Risk of hepatic vein
     thrombosis in relation to recent use of oral
     contraceptives: a case-control study. *Gastroenterology*
     1986; **90**: 807–11.

6   Thorogood M, Mann J, Murphy M, Vessey M. Risk
     factors for fatal venous thromboembolism in young
     women: a case-control study. *Int J Epidemiol* 1992; **21**:
     48–52.

● 7   Vandenbroucke JP, Koster T, Briet E, *et al*. Increased risk
     of venous thrombosis in oral-contraceptive users who are
     carriers of factor V Leiden mutation. *Lancet* 1994; **344**:
     1453–7.

● 8   Spitzer WO, Lewis MA, Heinemann LAJ, *et al*. on behalf
     of Transnational Research Group on Oral Contraceptives
     and the Health of Young Women. Third generation oral
     contraceptives and risk of venous thromboembolic
     disorders: an international case-control study. *BMJ* 1996;
     312: 83–8.

● 9   Grodstein F, Stampfer MJ, Goldhaber SZ, *et al*.
     Prospective study of exogenous hormones and risk of
     pulmonary embolism in women. *Lancet* 1996; **348**:
     983–7.

10 Realini JP, Encarnacion CE, Chintapalli KN, Rees CR. Oral
     contraceptives and venous thromboembolism: a case-
     control study designed to minimize detection bias. *J Am
     Board Fam Pract* 1997; **10**: 315–21.

11 Martinelli I, Sacchi E, Landi G, *et al*. High risk of cerebral-
     vein thrombosis in carriers of a prothrombin-gene
     mutation and in users of oral contraceptives. *N Engl J
     Med.* 1998; **338**: 1793–7.

12 de Bruijn SFTM, Stam J, Koopman MMW, Vandenbroucke JP.
     For the Cerebral Venous Sinus Thrombosis Study Group.
     Case-control study of risk of cerebral sinus thrombosis in
     oral contraceptive users and in carriers of hereditary
     prothrombotic conditions. *BMJ* 1998; **316**: 589–92.

13 Bloemenkamp KWM, Rosendaal FR, Buller HR, *et al*.
     Risk of venous thrombosis with use of current low-dose
     oral contraceptives is not explained by diagnostic
     suspicion and referral bias. *Arch Intern Med* 1999; **159**:
     65–70.

14 Martinelli I, Taioli E, Bucciarelli P, *et al*. Interaction
     between the G20210A mutation of the prothrombin gene
     and oral contraceptive use in deep vein thrombosis.
     Arterioscler Thromb Vasc Biol 1999; **19**: 700–3.

15 Bloemenkamp KWM, Rosendaal FR, Helmerhorst FM,
     Vandenbroucke JP. Higher risk of venous thrombosis
     during early use of oral contraceptives in women with
     inherited clotting defects. *Arch Intern Med* 2000; **160**:
     49–52.

16 Parkin L, Skegg DCG, Wilson M, *et al*. Oral contraceptives
     and fatal pulmonary embolism. *Lancet* 2000; **355**:
     2133–4.

17 Helmrich SP, Rosenberg L, Kaufman DW, *et al*. Venous
     thromboembolism in relation to oral contraceptive use.
     Obstet Gynecol 1987; **69**: 91–5.

18 Gerstman BB, Piper JM, Freiman JP, *et al*. Oral
     contraceptive oestrogen and progestin potencies and the
     incidence of deep venous thromboembolism. *Int J
     Epidemiol* 1990; **19**: 931–6.

19 Hirvonen E, Idanpaan-Heikkila J. Cardiovascular death
     among women under 40 years of age using low-estrogen
     oral contraceptives and intrauterine devices in Finland
     from 1975 to 1984. *Am J Obstet Gynecol* 1990; **163**:
     281–4.

20 Gerstman BB, Piper JM, Tomita DK, *et al*. Oral
     contraceptive estrogen dose and the risk of deep venous
     thromboembolic disease. *Am J Epidemiol* 1991; **133**:
     32–7.

21 Poulter NR, Chang CL, Farley TMM, *et al*.; for the World
     Health Organization Collaborative Study of
     Cardiovascular Disease and Steroid Hormone
     Contraception Investigators. Venous thromboembolic
     disease and combined oral contraceptives: results of an
     international multicentre case-control study. *Lancet*
     1995; **346**: 1575–82.

22 Jick H, Jick SS, Gurewich V, *et al*. Risk of idiopathic
     cardiovascular death and nonfatal venous
     thromboembolism in women using oral contraceptives
     with differing progestagen components. *Lancet* 1995;
     346: 1589–93.

23 Heinemann LAJ, Lewis MA, Assmann A, Thiel C. Case-
     control studies on venous thromboembolism: bias due
     to design? A methodological study on venous
     thromboembolism and steroid hormone use.
     Contraception 2002; **65**: 207–14.

24 Sartwell PE, Masi AT, Arthes FG, *et al*. Thromboembolism
     and oral contraceptives: an epidemiologic case-control
     study. *Am J Epidemiol* 1969; **90**: 365–80.

25 Greene GR, Sartwell PE. Oral contraceptive use in patients
     with thromboembolism following surgery, trauma, or
     infection. *Am J Public Health* 1972; **62**: 680–5.

26 Anonymous. Oral contraceptives and venous
     thromboembolic disease, surgically confirmed gallbladder
     disease, and breast tumours: report from the Boston
     Collaborative Drug Surveillance Programme. *Lancet* 1973;
     1: 1399–404.

27 Grounds M. Anovulants: thrombosis and other associated
     changes. *Med J Aust* 1974; **2**: 440–6.

28 Stolley PD, Tonascia JA, Tockman MS, *et al*. Thrombosis
     with low-estrogen oral contraceptives. *Am J Epidemiol*
     1975; **102**: 197–208.

29 Maguire MG, Tonascia JA, Sartwell PE, *et al*. Increased
     risk of thrombosis due to oral contraceptives: a further
     report. *Am J Epidemiol* 1979; **110**: 188–95.

30 Petitti DB, Wingerd J, Pellegrin F, Ramcharan S. Oral
     contraceptives, smoking, and other factors in relation to
     risk of venous thromboembolic disease. *Am J Epidemiol*
     1978; **108**: 480–5.

31 Petitti DB, Wingerd J, Pellegrin F, Ramcharan S. Risk of
     vascular disease in women: smoking, oral contraceptives,
     noncontraceptive estrogens, and other factors. *JAMA*
     1979; **242**: 1150–4.

32 Porter JB, Hunter JR, Jick H, Stergachis A. Oral contraceptives and nonfatal vascular disease. *Obstet Gynecol* 1985; **66**: 1–4.

33 Farmer RDT, Lawrenson RA, Thompson CR, *et al.* Population-based study of risk of venous thromboembolism associated with various oral contraceptives. *Lancet* 1997; **349**: 83–8.

34 Lidegaard Ø, Edstrom B, Kreiner S. Oral contraceptives and venous thromboembolism: a five-year national case-control study. *Contraception* 2002; **65**: 187–96.

35 Vessey MP, Doll R. Investigation of relation between use of oral contraceptives and thromboembolic disease. *Br Med J* 1968; **2**: 199–205.

36 Vessey MP, Doll R. Postoperative thromboembolism and the use of oral contraceptives. *Br Med J* 1970; **3**: 123–6.

37 Bloemenkamp KWM, Rosendaal FR, Helmerhorst FM, *et al.* Enhancement by factor V Leiden mutation of risk of deep-vein thrombosis associated with oral contraceptives containing a third-generation progestagen. *Lancet* 1995; **346**: 1593–6.

38 Jick H, Kaye JA, Vasilakis-Scaramozza C, Jick SS. Risk of venous thromboembolism among users of third-generation oral contraceptives compared with users of oral contraceptives with levonorgestrel before and after 1995: cohort and case-control analysis. *BMJ* 2000; **321**: 1190–5.

39 Farley TMM, Meirik O, Chang CL, *et al.*, for the World Health Organization Collaborative Study of Cardiovascular Disease and Steroid Hormone Contraception Investigators. Effect of different progestagens in low oestrogen oral contraceptives on venous thromboembolic disease. *Lancet* 1995; **346**: 1582–8.

40 Lidegaard Ø, Edström B, Kreiner S. Oral contraceptives and venous thromboembolism: a case-control study. *Contraception* 1998; **57**: 291–301.

41 Andersen BS, Olsen J, Nielsen GL, *et al.* Third generation oral contraceptives and heritable thrombophilia as risk factors of non-fatal venous thromboembolism. *Thromb Haemost* 1998; **79**: 23–31.

42 Farmer RDT, Todd J-C, Lewis MA, *et al.* The risks of venous thromboembolic disease among German women using oral contraceptives: a database study. *Contraception* 1998; **57**: 67–70.

43 Herings RMC, Urquhart J, Leufkens HGM. Venous thromboembolism among new users of different oral contraceptives. *Lancet* 1999; **354**: 127–8 [published correction appears in *Lancet* 1999; **354**: 1478].

44 Burnhill MS. The use of a large-scale surveillance system in Planned Parenthood Federation of America Clinics to monitor cardiovascular events in users of combination oral contraceptives. *Int J Fertil Womens Med* 1999; **44**: 19–30.

45 Farmer RD, Lawrenson RA, Todd J-C, *et al.* A comparison of the risks of venous thromboembolic disease in association with different combined oral contraceptives. *Br J Clin Pharmacol* 2000; **49**: 580–90.

46 [No authors listed]. Oral contraceptives, venous thrombosis, and varicose veins: Royal College of General Practitioners' Oral Contraception Study. *J R Coll Gen Pract* 1978; **28**: 393–9.

47 Porter JB, Hunter JR, Danielson DA, *et al.* Oral contraceptives and nonfatal vascular disease: recent experience. *Obstet Gynecol* 1982; **59**: 299–302.

48 Vessey M, Mant D, Smith A, Yeates D. Oral contraceptives and venous thromboembolism: findings in a large prospective study. *Br Med J (Clin Res Ed)* 1986; **292**: 526.

49 Fuertes-de la Haba A, Curet JO, Pelegrina I, Bangdiwala I. Thrombophlebitis among oral and nonoral contraceptive users. *Obstet Gynecol* 1971; **38**: 259–63.

50 Koster T, Small R-A, Rosendaal FR, Helmerhorst FM. Oral contraceptives and venous thromboembolism: a quantitative discussion of the uncertainties. *J Intern Med* 1995; **238**: 31–7.

51 Kemmeren JM, Algra A, Grobbee DE. Third generation oral contraceptives and risk of venous thrombosis: meta-analysis. *BMJ* 2001; **323**: 131–4.

52 Rosing J, Tans G, Nicolaes GA, *et al.* Oral contraceptives and venous thrombosis: different sensitivities to activated protein C in women using second and third-generation oral contraceptives. *Br J Haematol* 1997; **97**: 233–8.

53 Rosing J, Middeldorp S, Curvers J, *et al.* Low-dose oral contraceptives and acquired resistance to activated protein C: a randomised cross-over study. *Lancet* 1999; **354**: 2036–40.

54 Tans G, Curvers J, Middeldorp S, *et al.* A randomized cross-over study on the effects of levonorgestrel- and desogestrel-containing oral contraceptives on the anticoagulant pathways. *Thromb Haemost* 2000; **84**: 15–21.

55 Mackie IJ, Piegsa K, Furs SA, *et al.* Protein S levels are lower in women receiving desogestrel-containing combined oral contraceptives (COCs) than in women receiving levonorgestrel-containing COCs at steady state and on cross-over. *Br J Haematol* 2001; **113**: 898–904.

56 Vasilakis-Scaramozza C, Jick H. Risk of venous thromboembolism with cyproterone or levonorgestrel contraceptives. *Lancet* 2001; **358**: 1427–9.

57 Lewis MA, Heinemann LAJ, MacRae KD, *et al.*, with the Transnational Research Group on Oral Contraceptives and the Health of Young Women. The increased risk of venous thromboembolism and the use of third generation progestagens: role of bias in observational research. *Contraception* 1996; **54**: 5–13.

58 Vasilakis C, Jick H, Melero-Montes MM. Risk of idiopathic venous thromboembolism in users of progestagens alone. *Lancet* 1999; **354**: 1610–11.

59 Heinemann LA, Assmann A, DoMinh T, Garbe E. Oral progestogen-only contraceptives and cardiovascular risk: results from the Transnational Study on Oral Contraceptives and the Health of Young Women. *Eur J Contracept Reprod Health Care* 1999; **4**: 67–73.

60 Poulter NR, Chang CL, Farley TMM, Meirik O. Risk of cardiovascular diseases associated with oral progestagen

preparations with therapeutic indications [letter]. *Lancet* 1999; **354**: 1610.

61   Bottinger LE, Westerholm B. Oral contraceptives and thromboembolic disease. *Acta Med Scand* 1971; **190**: 455–63.

62   Suissa S, Blais L, Spitzer WO, *et al.* First-time use of newer oral contraceptives and the risk of venous thromboembolism. *Contraception* 1997; **56**: 141–6.

63   Farley TMM, Meirik O, Marmot MG, *et al.* Oral contraceptives and risk of venous thromboembolism: impact of duration of use. *Contraception* 1998; **57**: 61–5.

64   Poulter NR, Farley TMM, Chang CL, *et al.* Safety of combined oral contraceptive pills. *Lancet* 1996; **347**: 547.

65   Suissa S, Spitzer WO, Rainville B, *et al.* Recurrent use of newer oral contraceptives and the risk of venous thromboembolism. *Hum Reprod* 2000; **15**: 817–21.

66   MacGillavry MR, Prins MH. Oral contraceptives and inherited thrombophilia: a gene-environment interaction with a risk of venous thrombosis? *Semin Thromb Hemost* 2003; **29**: 219–26.

67   Von Kaulla E, Droegemueller W, Aoki N, Von Kaulla KN. Antithrombin 3 depression and thrombin generation acceleration in women taking oral contraceptives. *Am J Obstet Gynecol* 1971; **109**: 868–73.

68   Bonnar J. Coagulation effects of oral contraception. *Am J Obstet Gynecol* 1987; **157**: 1042–8.

69   Stubblefield PG. Cardiovascular effects of oral contraceptives: a review. *Int J Fertil* 1989; **34**(Suppl): 40–9.

70   Kluft C, Lansink M. Effect of oral contraceptives on haemostasis variables. *Thromb Haemost* 1997; **78**: 315–26.

71   Winkler UH. Blood coagulation and oral contraceptives: a critical review. *Contraception* 1998; **57**: 203–9.

72   Middeldorp S, Meijers JCM, van den Ende AE, *et al.* Effects on coagulation of levonorgestrel- and desogestrel-containing low dose oral contraceptives: a cross-over study. *Thromb Haemost* 2000; **84**: 4–8.

73   Koster T, Blann AD, Briët E, Vandenbroucke JP, Rosendaal FR. Role of clotting factor VIII in effect of von Willebrand factor on occurrence of deep-vein thrombosis. *Lancet* 1995; **345**: 152–5.

74   Kraaijenhagen RA, Anker PS, Koopman MM, *et al.* High plasma concentration of factor VIIIc is a major risk factor for venous thromboembolism. *Thromb Haemost* 2000; **83**: 5–9.

75   Shen L, Dahlbäck B. Factor V and protein S as synergistic cofactors to activated protein C in degradation of factor VIIIa. *J Biol Chem* 1994; **269**: 18735–8.

76   Váradi K, Rosing J, Tans G, *et al.* Factor V enhances the cofactor function of protein S in the APC-mediated inactivation of factor VIII: influence of the factor VR506Q mutation. *Thromb Haemost* 1996; **76**: 208–14.

77   Meijers JCM, Middeldorp S, Tekelenburg W, *et al.* Increased fibrinolytic activity during use of oral contraceptives is counteracted by an enhanced factor XI-independent downregulation of fibrinolysis: a randomized cross-over study of two low-dose oral contraceptives. *Thromb Haemost* 2000; **84**: 9–14.

78   Dahlbäck B, Carlsson M, Svensson PJ. Familial thrombophilia due to a previously unrecognised mechanism characterized by poor anticoagulant response to activated protein C: prediction of a cofactor to activated protein C. *Proc Natl Acad Sci U S A* 1993; **90**: 1004–8.

79   Bertina RM, Koeleman BPC, Koster T, *et al.* Mutation in blood coagulation factor V associated with resistance to activated protein C. *Nature* 1994; **369**: 64–7.

80   Zoller B, Dahlback B. Linkage between inherited resistance to activated protein C and factor V gene mutation in venous thrombosis. *Lancet* 1994; **343**: 1536–8.

81   Rosing J, Tans G. Effects of oral contraceptives on hemostasis and thrombosis. *Am J Obstet Gynecol* 1999; **180**(6 Pt 2): S375–82.

82   Østerud B, Robertsen R, Åsvang GB, Thijssen F. Resistance to activated protein C is reduced in women using oral contraceptives. *Blood Coagul Fibrinolysis* 1994; **5**: 853–4.

83   Olivieri O, Friso S, Manzato F, *et al.* Resistance to activated protein C in healthy women taking oral contraceptives. *Br J Haematol* 1995; **91**: 465–70.

84   Henkens CMA, Bom VJJ, Seinen AJ, van der Meer J. Sensitivity to activated protein C: influence of oral contraceptives and sex. *Thromb Haemost* 1995; **73**: 402–4.

85   Lowe GDO, Rumley A, Woodward M, *et al.* Activated protein C resistance and the FV:R506Q mutation in a random population sample – associations with cardiovascular risk factors and coagulation variables. *Thromb Haemost* 1999; **81**: 918–24.

86   Rees DC, Cox M, Clegg JB. World distribution of factor V Leiden. *Lancet* 1995; **346**: 1133–4.

87   Ridker PM, Miletich JP, Hennekens CH, Buring JE. Ethnic distribution of factor V Leiden in 4047 men and women: implications for venous thromboembolism screening. *JAMA* 1997; **277**: 1305–7.

88   Crowther MA, Kelton JG. Congenital thrombophilic states associated with venous thrombosis: a qualitative overview and proposed classification system. *Ann Intern Med* 2003; **138**: 128–34.

89   Rosendaal FR, Doggen CJ, Zivelin A, *et al.* Geographic distribution of the 20210 G to A prothrombin variant. *Thromb Haemost* 1998; **79**: 706–8.

90   Tait RC, Walker ID, Perry DJ, *et al.* Prevalence of antithrombin deficiency in the healthy population. *Br J Haematol* 1994; **87**:106–12.

91   Tait RC, Walker ID, Reitsma PH, *et al.* Prevalence of protein C deficiency in the healthy population. *Thromb Haemost* 1995; **73**: 87–93.

92   den Heijer M. Hyperhomocysteinaemia as a risk factor for venous thrombosis: an update of the current evidence. *Clin Chem Lab Med* 2003; **11**: 1404–7.

93   Kearon C, Crowther M, Hirsh J. Management of patients with hereditary hypercoagulable disorders. *Annu Rev Med* 2000; **51**: 169–85.

94   Selhub J, D'Angelo A. Hyperhomocysteinemia and thrombosis: acquired conditions. *Thromb Haemost* 1997; **78**: 527–31.

95   Levine JS, Branch DW, Rauch J. The antiphospholipid syndrome. *N Engl J Med* 2000; **346**: 752–63.

96   Bloemenkamp KWM, Helmerhorst FM, Rosendaal FRR, Vandenbroucke JP. Venous thrombosis, oral contraceptives and high factor VIII levels. *Thromb Haemost* 1999; **82**: 1024–7.

97   Vandenbroucke JP, van der Meer FJM, Helmerhorst FM, RosendaalFR. Factor V Leiden: should we screen oral contraceptive users and pregnant women? *BMJ* 1996; **313**: 1127–30.

98   McColl MD, Ramsay JE, Tait RC, *et al.* Risk factors for pregnancy associated venous thromboembolism. *Thromb Haemost* 1997; **78**: 1183–8.

99   Lindqvist, P, Dahlback B, Marsal, K. Thrombotic risk during pregnancy: a population study. *Obstet Gynecol* 1999; **94**: 595–9.

100 Pabinger I, Schneider B, and the GTH Study Group on Natural Inhibitors. Thrombotic risk of women with hereditary antithrombin III-, protein C- and protein S-deficiency taking oral contraceptive medication. *Thromb Haemost* 1994; **7**: 548–52.

101 Gomes MP, Deitcher SR. Risk of venous thromboembolic disease associated with hormonal contraceptives and hormone replacement therapy: a clinical review. *Arch Intern Med* 2004; **164**: 1965–76.

102 Schulman S. Unresolved issues in anticoagulant therapy. *J Thromb Haemost* 2003; **1**:1464–70.

103 Buller HR, Agnelli G, Hull RD, *et al.* Antithrombotic therapy for venous thromboembolic disease: The Seventh ACCP Conference on Antithrombotic and Thrombolytic Therapy. *Chest* 2004; **126**: 401S–428S.

31

The oral contraceptive pill, mechanisms of vascular risk, and practical prescribing strategies for women with thrombotic problems

KITTY W M BLOEMENKAMP, FRANS M HELMERHORST

INTRODUCTION

Oral contraceptives have been available since the 1960s and are now used by more than 100 million women throughout the world.[1] The effects of oral contraceptives continue to be of immense interest, because these are the most frequently and very often long-term used drugs by healthy women in the developed world.

In one classification system of oral contraceptives the progestogens are classified as first, second, third and fourth generation. The first generation includes: ethynodiol acetate, lynestrenol, norethisterone (acetate), and norethynodrel. The second generation includes: norgestrel, levonorgestrel, and norgestrione. The third generation includes: desogestrel, gestodene, and norgestimate. The fourth generation includes: chlormadinone and cyproterone acetate (both C21 derivatives). A miscellaneous group includes mainly C21 steroids, such as dydrogesterone, medrogestone, medroxyprogesterone acetate, and the natural progesterone. In currently available oral contraceptives ethinyl estradiol in the amount of 20 μg, 30 μg, 35 μg, or 50 μg is combined in several ways with the different progestogens, either mono, bi or triphasic, and in various dosages.[2–5]

Besides having beneficial effects – the highly effective protection against pregnancy – oral contraceptives like all medicines also show adverse effects. Even a small increase in risk will affect a large number of users, who are often young and healthy. Ever since oral contraceptives have been marketed, reports have appeared on links between oral contraceptive use and cardiovascular disease, including both venous and arterial thrombosis.[6–8] Oral contraceptives influence the hemostatic, carbohydrate, lipid, and endothelium systems, mechanisms regulating blood pressure and probably as yet unknown systems, as a result of which there is an increased risk of cardiovascular disease.[9–16] In venous as well in arterial thrombosis the final event leading to the disease will be clot formation – nevertheless the risk factors are different (Boxes 31.1 and 31.2).

Cardiovascular side effects can be distinguished in venous thrombosis (deep vein thrombosis, pulmonary embolism, ischemic stroke) and arterial thrombosis (acute myocardial infarction, ischemic stroke, hemorrhagic stroke, and peripheral arterial occlusive disease).

VENOUS THROMBOSIS

Venous thrombosis is a common disease with an overall annual incidence of 1–3 in 1000 persons.[17] The most frequent forms are deep vein thrombosis of the legs and pulmonary embolism. Less frequent are thrombosis of the retinal veins, mesenteric veins, cerebral sinus veins, arm veins, and the portal vein (Budd–Chiari syndrome).[18] The pathogenesis of venous thrombosis is complex and not totally understood. Virchow's triad is still helpful for global understanding: changes of the vessel wall, slowing of the

Box 31.1 Risk factors for venous thrombosis

Acquired
- Surgery
- Malignancies
- Trauma
- Immobilization
- Pregnancy, puerperium
- Use of oral contraceptives
- Use of hormone replacement therapy
- Ovulation induction
- *In vitro* fertilization
- Age
- Previous thrombosis
- Antiphospholipid syndrome

Inherited
- Antithrombin deficiency
- Protein C deficiency
- Protein S deficiency
- APC resistance/factor V Leiden
- Prothrombin (20210 A) mutation
- Dysfibrinogenemia

Mixed/unknown
- Hyperhomocysteinemia
- High factor VIII levels
- APC resistance in absence of FVL
- High levels of factor IX
- High levels of factor XI
- High levels of thrombin-activatable fibrinolysis inhibitor (TAFI)

Box 31.2 Risk factors for arterial thrombosis

Acquired
- Pregnancy, puerperium
- Use of oral contraceptives
- Use of hormone replacement therapy
- Ovulation induction?
- *In vitro* fertilization?
- Age
- Smoking
- Hypertension
- Hypercholesterolemia
- Diabetes mellitus
- Lack of exercise
- Antiphospholipid syndrome

Inherited
- APC resistance/factor V Leiden?
- Prothrombin (20210 A) mutation?

Mixed/unknown
- Hyperhomocysteinemia
- High factor VIII levels?
- High levels of factor IX?

bloodstream, and alterations in composition of the blood cells.[19] During the past decades it has become clear that the causes of venous thrombosis include hereditary and acquired factors (Box 31.1), although there is still a group of patients in which venous thrombosis occurs in the absence of obvious predisposing factors, the so-called idiopathic cases.[20–22]

Venous thrombosis is a multicausal disease, in which several risk factors (acquired or genetic) need to be present simultaneously. The risk of thrombosis rises sharply with the number of risk factors. Since age is a strong risk factor for thrombosis, the number of risk factors required for thrombosis decreases with age.[22] The incidence of venous thrombosis in young women in the fertile age is low and depends on predisposing factors such as pregnancy, oral contraceptive use, hormone replacement therapy, use of hormones during *in vitro* fertilization, and ovulation induction, carrier ship of a coagulation defect or combinations of risk factors.[6,8]

Epidemiologic studies (cohort and case–control studies) showed that oral contraceptive use was a clear risk factor for venous thrombosis and studies with healthy volunteers

(randomized and cross-sectional studies) showed that oral contraceptives alter various hemostatic variables, inducing a slight tilt towards a prothrombotic state.[23] To reduce the cardiovascular risk during oral contraceptive use, the estrogen type was changed from mestranol into ethinyl estradiol and the estrogen content was lowered from 100 μg to 50 μg ethinyl estradiol and subsequently less. The decrease from 100 μg to 50 μg seemed effective in decreasing the risk of arterial and venous disease. Nevertheless, the lowering of the estrogen content to less than 50 μg ethinyl estradiol and at the same time, the efforts to produce newer types of progestogens with the purpose of reduction of the risk of thrombotic disease did not lead to the expected further decrease in the incidence of venous thrombosis.[6,8,23,24]

In 1995 several studies showed that the newer 'third-generation' oral contraceptives, which contained desogestrel or gestodene as progestogens, had higher risks of venous thrombosis than the older 'second-generation' oral contraceptives, which contained mainly levonorgestrel.[25–28] Subsequent studies had variable results.[29–37] The original studies were heavily criticized, and it was hypothesized that the observed higher risk for oral contraceptives containing desogestrel or gestodene was completely explained by bias and confounding.

From several papers and a recent metaanalyses it can be concluded that low-dose oral contraceptives with a third-generation progestogen confer a higher risk (by a factor 1.5–1.8) of venous thrombosis than the previous generation of oral contraceptives.[24,38] These differences in risk appear to be real and cannot be accounted for by methodologic problems in the studies or the analyses.[23] The higher risk associated with oral contraception with a third-generation progestogen compared with previous generations was also present in women without factor V Leiden and without a positive family history, that is, preferential prescription because of family history could not explain the findings.[27] For the venous thrombosis risk of preparations containing the newer progestogen cyproterone acetate there are some epidemiologic data, suggesting a threefold to fourfold increased risk of thrombosis.[39] Conflicting results have been published about the thrombotic safety of oral contraceptives containing drospirenone. In contrast with the results of a study conducted by the manufacturer of the drospirenone-containing pill, findings of a laboratory study and the Dutch Pharmacovigilance Centre suggest an increased risk of thrombosis in users of the drospirenone-pill.[40–43] Therefore we have to await the results of larger ongoing observational studies to assess the risk.

Susceptibility to prothrombotic states

Reduced sensitivity to the anticoagulant action of activated protein C (APC resistance) was described by Dahlbäck et al. in 1993.[44] Factor V Leiden mutation (substitution of adenine for guanine at nucleotide 1691)[45] leads to resistance to APC and is commonly found among patients with venous thrombosis; up to 20 percent of patients with deep vein thrombosis are carriers.[46] The risk of venous thrombosis in factor V Leiden carriers is fourfold to eightfold increased in heterozygotes and 50-fold to 100-fold increased in homozygotes.[47] The prevalence of factor V Leiden in populations varies and is estimated between 3 percent and 5 percent in Caucasians.[48,49]

In 1994 an interaction between the newly discovered inherited coagulation disorder[45] and oral contraceptive use was described[50] (Fig. 31.1). In noncarriers who use oral contraceptives, the risk of venous thrombosis was increased fourfold, in carrier nonusers the risk was increased eightfold, and in users of oral contraceptives who also carried the factor V Leiden mutation the risk rose by 30–50-fold.[50] This susceptibility has been confirmed in other studies[31,51] and is even higher in the few women who are homozygous for factor V Leiden.[47] The risk of carriers using a desogestrel (third generation)-containing oral contraceptive as compared with noncarrier nonusers was found to be increased by almost 50-fold.[27]

The prevalence of other inherited coagulation defects, such as deficiencies of protein C, protein S, or antithrombin, which are risk factors of venous thrombosis, is much lower than that of factor V Leiden; their prevalence is estimated at less than 1 percent.[52–54] Although the evidence is derived from small observational studies and case reports these inherited coagulation defects also appear to synergistically lead to an excess risk of venous thrombosis among oral contraceptive users.[54–56] A mutation in the prothrombin gene (the substitution of adenine for guanine at nucleotide 20210) has been recently discovered[57] and seems to be a moderate risk factor for thrombosis, and has a prevalence of 2–4 percent among Caucasians.[57,58] Martinelli et al.[59] showed also an increased risk of venous thrombosis in prothrombin mutation carriers who used oral contraceptives.

Recent observational studies showed that the risk for venous thrombosis is highest during initial oral contraceptive use. This suggests a subgroup of women who are at immediate risk of thrombosis when exposed to oral contraceptives. In a case–control study[60] it was found that among women with thrombophilia (protein C, protein S, or antithrombin deficiency; factor V Leiden or prothrombin 20210 A mutation), the risk to develop deep vein thrombosis during the first 6 months of oral contraceptive use (as compared with prolonged use) was increased 19-fold (95 percent confidence interval [CI] 1.9 to 175.7). It was concluded that women with inherited clotting defects who use oral contraceptives develop venous thrombosis not only more often, but also sooner, which confirms an old clinical impression.[61] Therefore venous thrombosis in the first year of oral contraceptive use may indicate the presence of an inherited clotting defect.[60]

Elevated plasma levels of factor VIII are a risk factor for venous thrombosis and mediate the effects of non-O blood group and increase level of von Willebrand factor.[62,63]

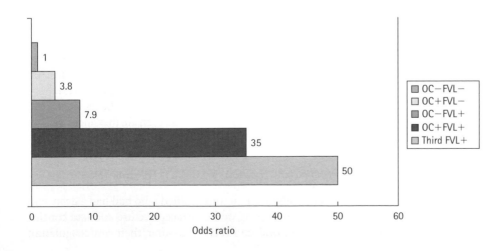

	OC−FVL−
	OC+FVL−
	OC−FVL+
	OC+FVL+
	Third FVL+

Figure 31.1 Interaction factor V Leiden and oral contraceptive use and the risk of venous thrombosis. (Source: Bloemenkamp et al.[27] and Vandenbroucke et al.[50])

These findings are in accordance with data reported in the 1960s, describing that the risk was higher in people with blood group A as compared with people with blood group O, or more generally 'non-O' versus O,[64–67] especially during the use of oral contraceptives or during pregnancy or puerperium.[64,68–71] We found that oral contraceptive use yielded an odds ratio of 3.8 (95 percent CI 2.4 to 6.0) and high factor VIII levels ($\geq$150 IU/dL), and an odds ratio of 4.0 (95 percent CI 2.0 to 8.0) relative to low factor VIII levels (<100 IU/dL). The joint effect of oral contraceptive use and high factor VIII resulted in an odds ratio of 10.3 (95 percent CI 3.7 to 28.9), which points to additive effects of the two risk factors.[72] A recent study pointed toward a synergistic effect.[73]

A case report in which one of a monozygotic twin pair developed deep vein thrombosis after they had started using oral contraceptives on the same day and were on the same holiday trip (both sisters were heterozygotic carriers of factor V Leiden mutation),[74] shows us that gene–environment interaction is complex and still not fully understood.

Biologic mechanism

PROCOAGULANT EFFECTS

A recent randomized crossover study[11] compared the effect on procoagulation between an oral contraceptive containing 150 μg levonorgestrel (a so-called second-generation oral contraceptive) and an oral contraceptive containing 150 μg desogestrel (a so-called third-generation oral contraceptive). The plasma concentrations of factors II, VII, X, and fibrinogen all increased during use of both oral contraceptives (factor VII and factor II more during use of the desogestrel containing oral contraceptive). The plasma concentrations of factor VII increased, and of factor V decreased, changes which were more prominent during the use of the desogestrel-containing oral contraceptive. Prothrombin fragment 1 + 2, a marker of clotting activation, increased, whereas concentrations of other activation markers such as thrombin–antithrombin complexes and soluble fibrin remained unchanged. Several studies also found above described changes in procoagulation.[1,2,75,76] Kemmeren et al. compared the effect of combined oral contraceptives containing desogestrel or levonorgestrel with the effect of progestogen-only oral contraceptives containing desogestrel or levonorgestrel on the coagulation system in the absence or presence of factor V Leiden. Desogestrel-containing oral contraceptives had a more pronounced effect on the coagulation system than levonorgestrel containing oral contraceptives, which may be explained by a less effective compensation of the thrombotic effect of ethinyl estradiol by desogestrel relative to levonorgestrel.[13]

ANTICOAGULANT EFFECTS

Recently, several studies reported that oral contraceptives induce an increased resistance to APC in women who did not carry factor V Leiden.[12,76–80] Resistance to APC, independent of the presence of factor V Leiden, is a risk factor for venous thrombosis. One problem when comparing these studies is that different assays to measure APC resistance were used (intrinsic vs. extrinsic pathway, 'in house' vs. 'commercial'). Although all tests show that oral contraceptive use increases resistance to the anticoagulant action of activated protein C, the tests seem to differ in their sensitivity to sex steroids. One assay (prothrombin time-based), developed by Rosing, shows high sensitivity for use of oral contraceptives, of all types, and even distinguishes between different 'generations' of oral contraceptives in accordance with the epidemiologic findings. Women who used third-generation-containing oral contraceptives were less sensitive to APC than women using second-generation-containing oral contraceptives and had APC sensitivity test results that did not differ from heterozygous female carriers of factor V Leiden who did not use oral contraceptives.[14,80,81] As resistance to APC, even in absence of factor V Leiden, is a risk factor for venous thrombosis,[82,83,84] these observations support the theory that acquired resistance to APC contributes to the increased risk of thrombosis in oral contraceptive users. The molecular basis of acquired resistance to APC during the use of oral contraceptives is unknown. Furthermore was it recently confirmed that the thrombin generation-based APC-resistance test discriminates well between oral contraceptives with a high risk of thrombosis (desogestrel and gestodene, cyproterone acetate) and oral contraceptives with a lower thrombotic risk (levonorgestrel).[85,86] In the study of van Vliet et al., cyproterone acetate and drospirenone-containing oral contraceptive users were less sensitive to APC than levonorgestrel-containing oral contraceptive users, which predicts an increased risk of thrombosis.[85] Oral contraceptives increase plasma levels of protein C and decrease plasma levels of protein S: the effect of oral contraceptives on plasma levels of antithrombin is reported inconsistently.[2,3,11,13,14,75]

FIBRINOLYTIC EFFECTS

Oral contraceptive use induces changes in variables in the fibrinolytic system, for example, increase in plasminogen, tissue plasminogen activator (tPA) activity, plasmin–α_2-antiplasmin complexes and D-dimer, decrease of levels of plasminogen activator inhibitor (PAI)-1 antigen, PAI-1 activity, and tPA antigen. All these changes suggest an increased fibrinolytic activity,[9,75] which may be a response to an induced prothrombotic state. These changes have not been shown to be different between levonorgestrel and desogestrel containing oral contraceptives.[15,16] The levels of TAFI increased on levonorgestrel, and even further increased on desogestrel.[15]

HEMOSTATIC SYSTEM IN FORMER THROMBOSIS PATIENTS

In one study women were studied who had had a deep vein thrombosis during oral contraceptive use and had continued using oral contraceptives after their anticoagulation treatment had been stopped. It was found that in former thrombosis patients several of the effects of oral contraceptives were more pronounced than in the healthy women: specifically on factor VII, antithrombin, normalized APC-sensitivity ratios (n-APC-sr), and protein C.[87]

CONCLUSIONS REGARDING THE HEMOSTATIC EFFECT

When investigating the effect of oral contraceptive use on hemostatic variables, we find that procoagulation is stimulated, anticoagulation is inhibited and fibrinolysis is stimulated. How to interpret these findings remains difficult. The concept that the increase in procoagulation is clinically counterbalanced by an increase in fibrinolysis[88] seems illogical, since we do not know what the impact is of the changes in the different haemostatic systems, that is, what the net result will be. Moreover, to date no effect of variation in the fibrinolytic system on the risk of thrombosis has been demonstrated, that is, fibrinolysis appears to play at most a minor role here. Furthermore the levels of coagulation variables remained mostly within the normal range during oral contraceptive use.[9–16] To estimate the net effect, we have to go back to epidemiologic studies which investigate clinical endpoints, instead of intermediate endpoints (plasma levels of hemostatic variables). However, hemostatic studies have improved our understanding. Current low-dose oral contraceptives stimulate procoagulation, inhibit anticoagulation, and stimulate fibrinolysis, and even anti-fibrinolysis might be increased.[10–16] And there is now evidence that even small functional differences in hemostatic variables can be considered as risk factors for venous thrombosis, such as elevated levels of factor II, factor VIII, and fibrinogen[57,72,89] and decreased levels of n-APC-sr.[82] Overall, oral contraceptive use seems to influence all parts of the hemostatic system toward a prothrombotic state. Possibly, it is the combination of the alterations of these several hemostatic variables that leads to an increased risk of venous thrombosis. Oral contraceptives induce changes in procoagulant, anticoagulant, and fibrinolytic parameters resulting in a net prothrombotic effect.[23] This prothrombotic effect can be measured globally by a thrombin generation-based APC resistance test.[10] The test outcome predicts the risk of venous thrombosis, supporting the epidemiologic observations: users of oral contraceptives containing gestodene, desogestrel, and cyproterone acetate were found more resistant to the anticoagulant action of APC by this test than users of oral contraceptives containing levonorgestrel.[10,85,86]

Prescription

HEALTHY FIRST-TIME USERS

Oral contraceptive use increases the risk of venous thrombosis three to five times. Third-generation-containing oral contraceptives have a 1.5-fold increased risk of venous thrombosis compared with second-generation (levonorgestrel)-containing oral contraceptives. This taken into account with no other beneficial effects (efficacy, subjective side effects, cycle control) of third-generation oral contraceptives compared with second-generation oral contraceptives;[90] second-generation oral contraceptives should generally be the first choice to prescribe, especially in first-time users. Cyproterone acetate containing oral contraceptives seem to have a venous thrombosis risk in the range of the third-generation oral contraceptives. Van Vliet *et al.* advise that even in the absence of sound clinical outcome data do not prescribe drospirenone-containing combined oral contraceptives as a first choice for women starting oral contraceptives.[85] Before switching from one oral contraceptive to another, a women should be counseled about the benefits and risks of the different preparations.

AFTER VENOUS THROMBOSIS

It is unknown what the chances are to develop a recurrent venous thrombosis once a women developed venous thrombosis during oral contraceptive use and either continues or discontinues using oral contraceptives. In an older study[91] 42 women who developed venous thrombosis during oral contraceptive use were compared with 42 women who developed venous thrombosis without oral contraceptives. The risk of recurrent venous thrombosis related to pregnancy was identical. The risk of recurrence, not associated with pregnancy was fourfold increased in the group of women who had their first thrombosis without oral contraceptives in comparison to the group who had their first thrombosis with oral contraceptives. The results were not influenced by oral contraceptive use during the follow-up period.

The risk of recurrent venous thrombosis is greatly increased among patients who have had more than one thromboembolic episode and among patients who have cancer, the lupus anticoagulant, or a hereditary deficiency of an inhibitor of coagulation. Patients with these risk factors receive long-term secondary thromboprophylaxis and were therefore not included in a recent study on the risk of recurrent venous thrombosis. In this study 175 women were enrolled who developed a first venous thromboembolism during oral contraceptive use.[92] In this study these women were advised to refrain from further oral contraceptive use. The cumulative probability of recurrence at 5 years was 5.9 percent (95 percent CI 0.6 to 11.1) among these women and 4.3 percent (95 percent CI 0 to 10.1; $P = 0.8$) among the 60 women in the same age groups in whom the first event was idiopathic. Among women who were taking oral contraceptives, the relative risk of recurrence was 0.8 (95 percent CI 0.1 to 4.0; $P = 0.8$) and remained unchanged after adjustment for age and other possibly confounding factors.

The choice to discontinue or not to start oral contraceptive use after a women has developed venous thrombosis is not completely evidence based. Nevertheless logical reasoning along the lines that venous thrombosis is a multicausal disease would imply that the fewer risk factors that exist, the smaller the risk of recurrence. This agrees with the recommendations of the World Health Organization

(WHO) to discontinue or not to start using oral contraceptives if a woman has a personal history of venous thrombosis.[93]

USE OF ORAL CONTRACEPTIVES IN SYMPTOMATIC CARRIERS OF CLOTTING DEFECTS (HETEROZYGOUS, HOMOZYGOUS, AND COMBINED DEFECTS)

Among women with thrombogenic mutations, oral contraceptive users have a 2–20-fold higher risk of thrombosis than of nonusers.[27,50,60] Therefore the use of oral contraceptives is contraindicated in known carriers of clotting defects (heterozygous, homozygous, and combined defects),[93] especially since nowadays reliable alternative methods of contraception are available. Routine screening is not appropriate because of the rarity of the conditions and the high costs of screening.[94]

PRESCRIBING ORAL CONTRACEPTIVES IN WOMEN WITH A FAMILY HISTORY OF VENOUS THROMBOSIS IN A FIRST-DEGREE FAMILY MEMBER

If a woman has a positive family history of venous thrombosis, this could point toward carriership of a clotting defect. Most of the inherited clotting defects have an autosomal dominant inheritance pattern. There are no consistent data regarding the thrombotic risk in users of oral contraceptives with an inherited clotting defect and personal history of venous thrombosis. Selective screening on the basis of clinical judgment, and family and personal history, instead of universal screening, may be useful before oral contraceptives are prescribed. This in the view of adequate counseling of women in their contraception choice and pregnancy. Nonetheless, the actual risks and benefits of such practice remain to be examined.

CURRENT VENOUS THROMBOSIS

During current venous thrombosis oral contraceptives are contraindicated, unless a woman is fully anticoagulated.[93]

ARTERIAL THROMBOSIS

Epidemiology: a historical perspective

In the WHO technical report *Cardiovascular Disease and Steroid Hormone Contraception*[8] there is an excellent overview on the association between arterial disease, acute myocardial infarction (AMI), and oral contraceptives. The history began classically with a case report.[95] In the earliest epidemiologic studies of the 1960s an association was not found, whereas in the subsequent three decades a relative risk (RR) between 0.9 and 5 was observed in six case–control[96–101] and three cohort studies.[102–104] Several types of bias have been addressed, but considered to be minimal.

The relative risk was alike for developed and developing countries. Duration and past using of oral contraceptives had no relation with the disease.[8] A similar and consistent relation between the pill and AMI was observed in oral contraceptive users with a threefold increased risk of other arterial diseases as ischemic stroke[8,105] and peripheral artery disease with a fourfold increased risk.[106]

Reduction in the estrogen dose of combined oral contraceptives did not influence the risk of arterial thrombosis in contrast to venous thrombosis.[8,106–108] The type of progestogens in the combined oral contraceptive pill modulates the risk of venous thrombosis: third-generation progestogens (desogestrel and gestodene)[109] increased the risk twofold relative to levonorgestrel, a second-generation progestogen.[23] Third-generation pills have been developed for their favorable effect on the lipid profile,[110] suggesting that they would confer a lower risk of arterial thrombosis than oral contraceptives containing a second-generation progestogen. Small[100–111] and two large studies[108,112] showed contradictory results. The MICA study from the UK[112] demonstrated a twofold increased risk for oral contraceptives containing a third-generation progestogen relative to second-generation progestogens, whereas the Risk of Arterial Thrombosis In relation to Oral Contraceptives (RATIO) study from the Netherlands[108] reported the opposite. Although both studies were large, neither could exclude the absence of a difference. As there were no obvious biases in either study that could explain this difference, it is most likely that the difference in risk of myocardial infarction between oral contraceptives with a third- or a second-generation progestogen, if any, is small. In the RATIO study, there was no difference between oral contraceptives with a second- or a third-generation progestogen with regard to the risk of ischemic stroke, or the risk of peripheral artery disease.[106,107]

Risk factors

The three main risk factors (Box 31.2) of arterial disease – smoking, hypertension, and diabetes – appeared to make the difference: 'Women who do not smoke, who have their blood pressure checked, and who do not have hypertension or diabetes, are at no increased risk of AMI.' The data suggest that treated hypertension is still a risk factor. Treated diabetes, hypercholesterolemia, and family history of heart disease were not sufficiently addressed in the early studies.[8] In the RATIO study,[108] the overall risk of myocardial infarction for oral contraceptive users was increased twofold. However, it was much higher for women who also smoked (14-fold), had hypertension (6-fold), had hypercholesterolemia (25-fold), had diabetes (17-fold) or were obese (5-fold). For ischemic stroke, with an overall twofold increased risk, these interactive effects with conventional risk factors were also seen, although they were less striking: women who also had hypertension had an eightfold increased risk, those who also smoked a fourfold increased risk, and those with hypercholesterolemia an 11-fold increased risk. Almost all young women with peripheral artery disease are smokers, and the combination of smoking and oral contraceptive use led to a 36-fold increased risk in the RATIO study. Similarly, very high relative risks were found for the combination of oral contraceptive use with hypercholesterolemia (50-fold increased risk) and with diabetes (40-fold increased risk).[113]

Coagulation

Coagulation abnormalities play a minor role in arterial disease in contrast with venous thrombosis. Oral contraceptives users with factor V Leiden or prothrombin 20210A mutation have a similar risk of AMI as women without these mutations. Although in the RATIO study an increased risk of myocardial infarction was observed for women with elevated levels of factor VIII or IX (twofold to threefold increased risk for levels exceeding the 90th percentile of the distribution in the population), this risk was not enhanced more than expected by oral contraceptive use.[113]

Effect on lipid metabolism

The estrogen, ethinyl estradiol, increases triglycerides, high-density lipoprotein (HDL)-cholesterol, and its major apolipoprotein, whereas low density lipoprotein (LDL)-cholesterol is decreased. Progestogens have opposite effects on these parameters and both type and dose of the progestogen are important for the final effect on lipid metabolism.[110] After short-term use of third generation oral contraceptives a better HDL-cholesterol profile has been reported than for second-generation oral contraceptives in young healthy women and a favorable effect on the risk of myocardial infarction based on this increase in HDL-cholesterol was subsequently postulated.[114,115] In their RATIO trial, investigating 218 patients and 769 healthy control women, Tanis et al. concluded that the duration of low-dose oral contraceptive use did not influence the risk of myocardial infarction. Third-generation oral contraceptive users had a higher HDL-cholesterol, but mean differences in HDL-cholesterol levels between second- and third-generation oral contraceptives attenuated with increasing age.[116]

Effect on blood pressure

The slightly elevated, sometimes decreased blood pressure observed during oral contraceptive use is clinically irrelevant. Known is that women with hypertension have an increased risk of arterial disease. Scientifically sound data with arterial disease as a clinically relevant outcome among women using oral contraceptives and with (adequately treated) hypertension is not available.[8,93]

Prescription

FOR HEALTHY FIRST-TIME USERS

Although the incidence of AMI is quite low in women of reproductive age, it is advisable to check potential users and potential AMI women for their blood pressure and/or diabetes. In the highly recommendable WHO publication *Medical Eligibility Criteria for Contraceptive Use*[93] we can see the overall advice about smoking, although no smoking at all is the basic line.

For women age is indeed a risk factor of cardiovascular events, however in combination with smoking, WHO recommends the following:[93]

- <15 cigarettes/day. This is a situation where the theoretical or proved risks usually outweigh the advantages of using the method, in this case the combined oral contraceptives.
- >15 cigarettes/day. This is a situation, which represents an unacceptable health risk if the combined oral contraceptive method is used. Unpublished WHO data from 1997 found no increase in relative risk of AMI among current progestogen-only pill users relative to nonusers.[8]
- High blood pressure. WHO says: 'For all categories of hypertension, classifications are based on the assumption that no other risk factors for cardiovascular disease exist. When multiple risk factors do exist, risk of cardiovascular disease may increase substantially. A single reading of blood pressure level is not sufficient to classify a woman as hypertensive.' Three categories are mentioned by WHO:
  - History of hypertension, where blood pressure CANNOT be evaluated (including hypertension in pregnancy). Since women who did not have a blood pressure check before oral contraceptive use had an increased risk of acute myocardial infarction and stroke, an evaluation of cause and level of hypertension is recommended, as soon as feasible. It is a situation where the theoretical or proved risks usually outweigh the advantages of using the method, in this case the combined oral contraceptives.
  - Adequately controlled hypertension. There are no data that may support the hypothesis that oral contraceptive users with adequately controlled and monitored hypertension are at reduced risk of acute myocardial infarction and stroke compared with untreated hypertensive oral contraceptive users. WHO decided that in this situation the theoretical or proved risks of oral contraceptive use usually outweigh the advantages.
  - Elevated blood pressure levels (properly taken measurements), systolic 140–159 mm Hg or diastolic 90–99 mm Hg. Among women with hypertension, oral contraceptive users were at increased risk of stroke, acute myocardial infarction, and peripheral

arterial disease compared with nonusers. It is a situation where the theoretical or proved risks usually outweigh the advantages of using the method, in this case the combined oral contraceptives.

- Systolic >160 mm Hg or diastolic >100 mm Hg: a condition which represents an unacceptable health risk if the contraceptive method is used.
- Vascular disease: a condition which represents an unacceptable health risk if the contraceptive method is used.
- History of high blood pressure during pregnancy (where current blood pressure is measurable and normal). Women who had a history of high blood pressure in pregnancy, who also used oral contraceptives, had an increased risk of myocardial infarction, compared with oral contraceptive users who did not have a history of high blood pressure during pregnancy. The absolute risks of AMI in this population remained small. A condition where the advantages of using the method generally outweigh the theoretical or proved risks.
- Diabetes mellitus. History of gestational disease, a condition for which there is no restriction for the use of the contraceptive method.
- Nonvascular disease
  - Noninsulin dependent, a condition where the advantages of using the method generally outweigh the theoretical or proved risks.
  - Insulin-dependent, a condition where the advantages of using the method generally outweigh the theoretical or proved risks.
- Nephropathy/retinopathy/neuropathy. The category should be assessed according to the severity of the condition. Then the prescriber can choose between a condition where the advantages of using the method generally outweigh the theoretical or proved risks, or a condition where the theoretical or proved risks usually outweigh the advantages of using the method.
- Other vascular disease or diabetes of >20 years' duration. The category should be assessed according to the severity of the condition. Then the prescriber can choose between a condition where the advantages of using the method generally outweigh the theoretical or proved risks, or a condition where the theoretical or proved risks usually outweigh the advantages of using the method.
- Known hyperlipidemias. Routine screening is not appropriate because of the rarity of the conditions and the high cost of screening. Although some types of hyperlipidemias are risk factors for vascular disease, the category should be assessed according to the type, its severity, and the presence of other cardiovascular risk factors. Then the prescriber can choose between a condition where the advantages of using the method generally outweigh the theoretical or proved risks, or a condition where the theoretical or proved risks usually outweigh the advantages of using the method.
- Multiple risk factors for arterial disease. When a woman has multiple major risk factors, any of which

alone would substantially increase the risk of cardiovascular disease, use of oral contraceptives may increase her risk to an unacceptable level.

FOR WOMEN WITH A HISTORY OF A CARDIOVASCULAR EVENT

Current and history of ischemic heart disease or stroke: a condition which represents an unacceptable health risk if the contraceptive method is used.

FOR WOMEN WITH VALVULAR HEART DISEASE

Uncomplicated, a condition where the advantages of using the method generally outweigh the theoretical or proved risks. Complicated (pulmonary hypertension, risk of atrial fibrillation, history of subacute bacterial endocarditis) condition which represents an unacceptable health risk if the contraceptive method is used.

FOR WOMEN WITH MIGRAINE

Among women with migraine, women who also had aura have a higher risk of stroke than those without aura. Among women with migraine, those who use oral contraceptives have been shown to have a twofold to fourfold increased risk of stroke compared with women who did not use oral contraceptives.

Without aura

- Age <35 years. Initiation of use: a condition for which there is no restriction for the use of the contraceptive method. Continuation of use: a condition where the advantages of using the method generally outweigh the theoretical or proved risks.
- Age >35 Initiation of use: a condition where the advantages of using the method generally outweigh the theoretical or proven risks. Continuation of use: a condition where the theoretical or proved risks usually outweigh the advantages of using the method.

With aura, at any age

A condition which represents an unacceptable health risk if the contraceptive method is used.

CONCLUSIONS

Oral contraceptives users have a twofold to fivefold increased risk of cardiovascular disease. Women taking third-generation oral contraceptives have an almost twofold increased risk of venous thrombosis when compared with second-generation oral contraceptives. Women who do not smoke, who have their blood pressure checked, and who do not have hypertension or diabetes, are at no increased risk of AMI. The difference in risk of myocardial infarction when comparing third-generation with second-generation oral contraceptives, if any, is small. This taken into account with no other beneficial effects (efficacy, subjective side effects, cycle control) of third-generation oral contraceptives compared with second-generation oral contraceptives, second-generation oral contraceptives should generally be the first choice to prescribe, especially in first-time users.

Further epidemiologically sound research is needed on the influence of progestogen-only methods, oral contraceptives containing newer progestogens, and new contraceptive methods with different delivery systems (vaginal ring, transdermal patches, implants, intrauterine devices and combined injectables) on the risk of cardiovascular disease.

KEY LEARNING POINTS

- Oral contraceptives induce changes in procoagulant, anticoagulant and fibrinolytic parameters resulting in a net prothrombotic effect. Oral contraceptives users have a twofold to fivefold increased risk of cardiovascular disease.
- Women taking third-generation oral contraceptives have an almost twofold increased risk of venous thrombosis compared with those taking older-generation oral contraceptives. Therefore second-generation oral contraceptives should generally be the first choice to prescribe, especially in first-time users.
- The choice to discontinue or not to start oral contraceptive use after a women developed venous thrombosis is not completely evidence based. Nevertheless the recommendation is to discontinue or not to start using oral contraceptives if a woman has a personal history of venous thrombosis
- Among women with thrombogenic mutations, oral contraceptive users have a 2–20-fold higher risk of thrombosis than of nonusers. Therefore the use of oral contraceptives is contraindicated in known carriers of clotting defects (heterozygous, homozygous, and combined defects), especially, as nowadays reliable alternative methods of contraception are available.
- Women who do not smoke, who have their blood pressure checked, and who do not have hypertension or diabetes, are at no increased risk of AMI.
- The difference in risk of myocardial infarction when comparing third-generation with second-generation oral contraceptives, if any, is small. This taken into account with no other beneficial effects (efficacy, subjective side effects, cycle control) of third-generation oral contraceptives compared with second-generation oral contraceptives; second-generation oral contraceptives should generally be the first choice to prescribe, especially in first-time users.
- Further epidemiologically sound research is needed on the influence of progestogen only methods, oral contraceptives containing newer progestogens and

new contraceptive methods with different delivery systems (vaginal ring, transdermal patches, implants, intrauterine devices and combined injectables) on the risk of cardiovascular disease.

REFERENCES

1 United Nations Department for Economic and Social Information and Policy Analysis Population Division. *Levels and Trends of Contraceptive Use as Assessed in 1994.* New York: United Nations, 1996.

2 Robinson GE. Lowdose combined oral contraceptives. *Br J Obstet Gynaecol* 1994; **101**: 1036–42.

3 Fotherby K, Caldwell ADS. New progestogens in oral contraception. *Contraception* 1994; **49**: 132.

4 Diczfalusy E. *The Contraceptive Revolution: an Era of Scientific and Social Development.* Carnforth, UK: Parthenon Publishing, 1997.

5 Oral contraception. In: Speroff L, Fritz MA, Glass RH, Kase NG, eds. *Clinical Gynecologic Endocrinology and Infertility*, 7th ed. Baltimore: Lipincott, Williams and Wilkins, 2005.

6 Bloemenkamp KWM, Helmerhorst FM, Rosendaal FR, Vandenbroucke JP. Thrombophilias and gynaecology. *Best Pract Res Clin Obstet Gynaecol* 2003; **17**: 509–28.

7 Hannaford P. The collection and interpretation of epidemiological data about the cardiovascular risks associated with the use of steroid contraceptives. *Contraception* 1998; **57**: 137–42.

8 *Cardiovascular Disease and Steroid Hormone Contraception.* Report of a WHO scientific group. Geneva: World Health Organization, 1998 (WHO Technical Report Series, No. 877).

9 Winkler UH. Effects on hemostatic variables of desogestrel and gestodene-containing oral contraceptives in comparison with levonorgestrel-containing oral contraceptives: a review. *Am J Obstet Gynecol* 1998; **179**: S51–61.

10 Rosing J, Middeldorp S, Curvers J, *et al.* Low-dose oral contraceptives and acquired resistance to activated protein C: a randomized cross-over study. *Lancet* 1999; **354**: 2036–40.

11 Middeldorp S, Meijers JCM, van den Ende AE, *et al.* Effects on coagulation of levonorgestrel and desogestrel containing low dose oral contraceptives: a cross-over study. *Thromb Haemost* 2000; **84**: 4–8.

12 Kemmeren JM, Algra A, Meijers JC, *et al.* Effect of second- and third-generation oral contraceptives on the protein C system in the absence or presence of the factor V Leiden mutation: a randomized trial. *Blood* 2004; **103**: 927–33.

13 Kemmeren JM, Algra A, Meijers JC, *et al.* Effects of second and third generation oral contraceptives and their respective progestagens on the coagulation system in the absence or presence of the factor V Leiden mutation. *Thromb Haemost.* 2002; **87**: 199–205.

14 Tans G, Curvers J, Middeldorp S, *et al.* A randomized cross-over study on the effects of levonorgestrel- and desogestrel-containing oral contraceptives on the anticoagulant pathways. *Thromb Haemost.* 2000; **84**: 15–21.

15 Meijers JCM, Middeldorp S, Tekelenburg W, *et al.* Increased fibrinolytic activity during use of oral contraceptives is counteracted by an enhanced factor XI-independent downregulation of fibrinolysis; a randomized cross-over study of two low-dose oral contraceptives. *Thromb Haemost* 2000; **84**: 9–14.

16 Kemmeren JM, Algra A, Meijers JC, *et al.* Effect of second- and third-generation oral contraceptives on fibrinolysis in the absence or presence of the factor V Leiden mutation. *Blood Coagul Fibrinolysis* 2002; **13**: 373–81.

17 Kierkegaard A. Incidence of acute deep vein thrombosis in two districts. A phlebographic study. *Acta Chir Scand* 1980; **146**: 267–9.

18 Colman RW, Hirsch J, Marder VJ, Salzman EW. *Hemostasis and Thrombosis. Basic Principles and Clinical Practice*, 3rd edn. Philadelphia: JB Lippincott Company, 1994: 1283–4.

19 Virchow R. Thrombose und embolie. Gefässen entzündung und septische infektion. In: Virchow R, ed. *Gesammelte abhandlungen zur wissenschaftlichen Medicin.* Frankfurt: Meidinger, Sohn un Co, 1856: 219–732.

20 Lane DA, Mannucci PM, Bauer KA, *et al.* Inherited thrombophilia: part 1. *Thromb Haemost* 1996; **76**: 651–2.

21 Lane DA, Mannucci PM, Bauer KA, *et al.* Inherited thrombophilia: part 2. *Thromb Haemost* 1996; **76**: 824–34.

22 Rosendaal FR. Venous thrombosis: a multi-causal disease. *Lancet* 1999; **353**: 1167–73.

23 Vandenbroucke JP, Rosing J, Bloemenkamp KWM, *et al.* Oral contraceptives and the risk of venous thrombosis. *N Engl J Med* 2001; **344**: 1527–35.

24 Kemmeren JM, Algra A, Grobbee DE. Third generation oral contraceptives and risk of venous thrombosis: meta-analysis. *BMJ* 2001; **323**: 131–4.

25 World Health Organization Collaborative Study of Cardiovascular Disease and Steroid Hormone Contraception. Effect of different progestagens in low oestrogen oral contraceptives on venous thromboembolic disease. *Lancet* 1995; **346**: 1582–8.

26 Jick H, Jick SS, Gurewich V, *et al.* Risk of idiopathic cardiovascular death and non-fatal venous thromboembolism in women using oral contraceptives with differing progestagen components. *Lancet* 1995; **346**: 1589–93.

27 Bloemenkamp KWM, Rosendaal FR, Helmerhorst FM, *et al.* Enhancement by factor V Leiden mutation of risk of deep-vein thrombosis associated with oral contraceptives containing a third-generation progestagen. *Lancet* 1995; **346**: 1593–6.

28 Spitzer WO, Lewis MA, Heinemann LAJ, *et al.* on behalf of Transnational Research Group on Oral Contraceptives and the Health of Young women. Third generation oral contraceptives and risk of venous thromboembolic disorders: an international case-control study. *BMJ* 1996; **312**: 83–8.

29 Farmer RDT, Lawrenson RA, Thompson CR, *et al.* Population-based study of risk of venous thromboembolism associated with various oral contraceptives. *Lancet* 1997; **349**: 83–8.

30 Suissa S, Blais L, Spitzer WO, *et al.* First-time use of newer oral contraceptives and the risk of venous thromboembolism. *Contraception* 1997; **56**: 141–6.

31 Andersen BS, Olsen J, Nielsen GL, *et al.* Third-generation oral contraceptives and heritable thrombophilia as risk factors of non-fatal venous thromboembolism. *Thromb Haemost* 1998; **79**: 23–31.

32 Lidegaard Ø, Edström B, Kreiner S. Oral contraceptives and venous thromboembolism. A case-control study. *Contraception* 1998; **57**: 291–301.

33 Lewis MA, MacRae KD, Kühl-Habich D, *et al.* The differential risk of oral contraceptives: the impact of full exposure history. *Hum Reprod* 1999; **14**: 1493–9.

34 Herings RMC, Urquhart J, Leufkens HGM. Non-causal explanations for the increased risk of venous thromboembolism among users of third-generation oral contraceptives. *Pharmacoepidemiol Drug Saf* 1996; **5**: S1–S119.

35 Herings RMC, Urquhart J, Leufkens HGM. Venous thromboembolism among new users of different oral contraceptives. *Lancet* 1999; **354**: 127–8.

36 Mellemkjaer L, Sørensen HT, Dreyer L, *et al.* Admission for and mortality from primary venous thromboembolism in women of fertile age in Denmark, 1977–95. *BMJ* 1999; **319**: 820–1.

37 Bloemenkamp KWM, Rosendaal FR, Büller HR, *et al.* Risk of venous thrombosis with use of current low-dose oral contraceptives is not explained by diagnostic suspicion and referral bias. *Arch Intern Med* 1999; **159**: 65–70.

38 Hennessy S, Berlin JA, Kinman JL, *et al.* Risk of venous thromboembolism from oral contraceptives containing gestodene and desogestrel versus levonorgestrel: a meta-analysis and formal sensitivity analysis. *Contraception* 2001; **64**: 125–33.

39 Vasilakis-Scaramozza C, Jick H. Risk of venous thromboembolism with cyproterone or levonorgestrel contraceptives. *Lancet* 2001; **358**: 1427–9.

40 Heuser P, Tonga K, Hopkins R, *et al.* Specific oral contraceptive use and venous thromboembolism resulting in hospital admission. *N Z Med J* 2004; **117**: U1176.

41 Seaman HE, de Vries CS, Farmer RD. Venous thromboembolism associated with cyproterone acetate in combination with ethinyloestradiol (Dianette): observational studies using the UK General Practice Research Database. *Pharmacoepidemiol Drug Saf* 2004; **13**: 427–36.

42 Van Grootheest K, Vrieling T. Thromboembolism associated with the new contraceptive Yasmin. *BMJ* 2003; **326**: 257.

43 Heinemann LA, Dinger J. Safety of a new oral contraceptive containing drospirenone. *Drug Saf* 2004; **27**: 1001–18.

44 Dahlbäck B, Carlsson M, Svensson PJ. Familial thrombophilia due to previously unrecognized mechanism characterized by poor anticoagulant response to activated protein C: prediction of a cofactor to activated protein C. *Proc Natl Acad Sci U S A* 1993; **90**: 1004–8.

45 Bertina RM, Koeleman RPC, Koster T, *et al*. Mutation in blood coagulation factor V associated with resistance to activated protein C. *Nature* 1994; **369**: 64–7.

46 Koster T, Rosendaal FR, Ronde H de, *et al*. Venous thrombosis due to poor anticoagulant response to activated protein C: Leiden Thrombophilia Study. *Lancet* 1993; **342**: 1503–6.

47 Rosendaal FR, Koster T, Vandenbroucke JP, Reitsma PH. High risk of thrombosis in patients homozygous for factor V Leiden (activated protein C resistance). *Blood* 1995; **85**: 1504–8.

48 Rees DC, Cox M, Clegg JB. World distribution of factor V Leiden. *Lancet* 1995; **346**: 1133–4.

49 Ridker PM, Miletich JP, Hennekens CH, Buring JE. Ethnic distribution of factor V Leiden in 4047 men and women: implications for venous thromboembolism screening. *JAMA* 1997; **277**: 1305–7.

50 Vandenbroucke JP, Koster T, Briet E, *et al*. Increased risk of venous thrombosis in oral contraceptive users who are carriers of factor V Leiden mutation. *Lancet* 1994; **344**: 1453–7.

51 Hellgren M, Svenson PJ, Dahlback B. Resistance to activated protein C as a basis for venous thromboembolism associated with pregnancy and oral contraceptives. *Am J Obstet Gynecol* 1995; **173**: 210–13.

52 Heijboer H, Brandjes DPM, Büller HR, *et al*. Deficiencies of coagulation-inhibiting and fibrinolytic proteins in outpatients with deep-vein thrombosis. *N Engl J Med* 1990; **323**: 1512–16.

53 Koster T, Rosendaal FR, Briët E, *et al*. Protein C deficiency in a controlled series of unselected outpatients: an infrequent but clear risk factor for venous thrombosis (Leiden Thrombophilia Study). *Blood* 1995; **85**: 2756–61.

54 Simioni P, Sanson BJ, Prandoni, *et al*. Incidence of venous thromboembolism in families with inherited thrombophilia. *Thromb Haemost* 1999; **81**: 198–202.

55 Pabinger I, Schneider B. Thrombotic risk of women with hereditary antithrombin III, protein C and protein S deficiency taking oral contraceptive medication. The GTH Study Group on Natural Inhibitors. *Thromb Haemost* 1994; **71**: 548–52.

56 Girolami A, Simioni P, Girolami B, Zanardi S. The role of drugs, paticularly oral contraceptives, in triggering thrombosis in congenital defects of coagulation inhibitors: a study of six patients. *Blood Coagul Fibrinolysis* 1991; **2**: 673–8.

57 Poort SR, Rosendaal FR, Reitsma PH, Bertina RM. A common genetic variation in the 3′ untranslated region of the prothrombin gene is associated with elevated plasma prothrombin levels and an increase in venous thrombosis. *Blood* 1996; **88**: 3698–703.

58 Rosendaal FR, Doggen CJ, Zivelin A, *et al*. Geographic distribution of the 20210 G to A prothrombin variant. *Thromb Haemost* 1998; **79**: 706–8.

59 Martinelli I, Taioli E, Bucciarelli P, *et al*. Interaction between the G20210A mutation of the prothrombin gene and oral contraceptive use in deep vein thrombosis. *Arterioscler Thromb Vasc Biol* 1999; **19**: 700–3.

60 Bloemenkamp KWM, Rosendaal FR, Helmerhorst FM, Vandenbroucke JP. Higher risk of venous thrombosis during early use of oral contraceptives in women with inherited clotting defects. *Arch Intern Med* 2000; **160**: 49–52.

61 Vessey MP, Doll R. Investigation of relation between use of oral contraceptives and thromboembolic disease. *BMJ* 1968; **2**: 199–205.

62 Koster T, Blann AD, Briet E, *et al*. Role of clotting factor VIII in effect of von Willebrand factor on occurrence of deep-vein thrombosis. *Lancet* 1995; **345**: 152–5.

63 Kamphuisen PW, Houwing-Duistermaat JJ, van Houwelingen HC, *et al*. Familial clustering of factor VIII and von Willebrand factor levels. *Thromb Haemost* 1998; **79**: 323–7.

64 Jick H, Slone D, Westerholm B, *et al*. Venous thromboembolic disease and ABO blood type. A cooperative study. *Lancet* 1969; **1**: 539–42.

65 Talbot S, Wakley EJ, Ryrie D, Langman MJ. ABO blood groups and venous thromboembolic disease. *Lancet* 1970; **1**: 1257–9.

66 Bates M. Venous thromboembolic disease and ABO blood type. *Lancet* 1971; **1**: 239.

67 Talbot S, Wakley EJ, Langman MJ. A19 A29 B, and O blood groups, Lewis blood groups, and serum triglyceride and cholesterol concentrations in patients with venous thromboembolic disease. *Lancet* 1972; **1**: 1152–4.

68 Hill H, Loudon NB, Pitcher CS, Pocock VM. Venous thromboembolic disease and ABO blood type. *Lancet* 1969; I: 623.

69 Mourant AE, Kopec AC, Domaniewska-Sobczak K. Blood groups and blood clotting. *Lancet* 1971; **1**: 223–7.

70 Westerholm B, Wiechel B, Eklund G. Oral contraceptives, venous thromboembolic disease, and ABO blood type. *Lancet* 1971; **Sept 18**: 664.

71 Allan TM. ABO blood groups and venous thromboembolism. *Lancet* 1971; ii: 1209–10.

72 Bloemenkamp KWM, Helmerhorst FM, Rosendaal FR, Vandenbroucke JP. Venous thrombosis, oral contraceptives and high factor VIII levels. *Thromb Haemost* 1999; **82**: 1024–7.

73 Legnani C, Cini M, Cosmi B, *et al*. Risk of deep vein thrombosis: interaction between oral contraceptives and high factor VIII levels. *Haematologica* 2004; **89**: 1347–51.

74 Bloemenkamp KWM. Oral contraceptives, venous thrombosis and the role of coagulation defects. Academic Thesis, Chapter 10. Venous thrombosis in a monozygotic twin who used oral contraceptives, Leiden, the Netherlands, 1999: 151–5; ISBN 90-9013299-6,

75 Kluft C, Lansink M. Effect of oral contraceptives on haemostasis variables. *Thromb Haemost* 1997; **78**: 315–26.

76 Henkens CMA, Bom VJJ, Seinen AJ, Meer van der J. Sensitivity to activated protein C; Influence of oral contraceptives and sex. *Thromb Haemost* 1995; **73**: 402–4.

77 Østerud B, Robertsen R, Svang GB, Thijssen F. Resistance to activated protein C is reduced in women using oral contraceptives. *Blood Coagul Fibrinolysis* 1994; **5**: 853–4.

78 Olivieri O, Friso S, Manzato F, *et al*. Resistance to activated protein C in healthy women taking oral contraceptives. *Br J Haematol* 1995; **91**: 465–70.

79 Bokarewa MI, Falk G, StenLinder M, *et al*. Thrombotic risk factors and oral contraception. *J Lab Clin Med* 1995; **126**: 294–8.

80 Rosing J, Tans G, Nicolaes GAF, *et al*. Oral contraceptives and venous thrombosis; different sensitivities to activated protein C in women using second and third-generation oral contraceptives. *Br J Haematol* 1997; **97**: 233–8.

81 Kluft C, de Maat MPM, Heinemann LAJ, *et al*. Importance of levonorgestrel dose in oral contraceptives for effects on coagulation. *Lancet* 1999; **354**: 832–3.

82 De Visser MCH, Rosendaal FR, Bertina RM. A reduced sensitivity for activated protein C in the absence of factor V Leiden increases the risk of venous thrombosis. *Blood* 1999; **93**: 1271–6.

83 Rodegheiro F, Tosetto A. Activated protein C resistance and factor V Leiden mutation are independent risk factors for venous thromboembolism. *Ann Intern Med* 1999; **130**: 643–50.

84 Tans G, van Hylckama Vlieg A, Thomassen MC, *et al*. Activated protein C resistance determined with a thrombin generation-based test predicts for venous thrombosis in men and women. *Br J Haematol* 2003; **122**: 465–70.

85 van Vliet HA, Winkel TA, Noort I, *et al*. Prothrombotic changes in users of combined oral contraceptives containing drospirenone and cyproterone acetate. *J Thromb Haemost* 2004; **2**: 2060–2.

86 Alhenc-Gelas M, Plu-Bureau G, Guillonneau S, *et al*. Impact of progestagens on activated protein C (APC) resistance among users of oral contraceptives. *J Thromb Haemost* 2004; **2**: 1594–600.

87 Bloemenkamp KWM, Rosendaal FR, Helmerhorst FM, *et al*. Hemostatic effects of oral contraceptives in women who developed deep-vein thrombosis while using oral contraceptives. *Thromb Haemost* 1998; **80**: 382–7.

88 Consensus Development Meeting. Metabolic aspects of oral contraceptives of relevance for cardiovascular diseases. *Am J Obstet Gynecol* 1990; **162**: 1335–7.

89 Koster T, Rosendaal FR, Reitsma PH, *et al*. Factor VII and fibrinogen levels as risk factors for venous thrombosis. A case-control study of plasma levels and DNA polymorphisms, Leiden Thrombophilia Study. *Thromb Haemost* 1994; **71**: 719–22.

90 Maitra N, Kulier R, Bloemenkamp KW, Helmerhorst FM, Gulmezoglu AM. Progestogens in combined oral contraceptives for contraception. *Cochrane Database Syst Rev* 2004: CD004861.

91 Badaracco MA, Vessey MP. Recurrence of venous thromboembolic disease and use of oral contraceptives. *Br Med J* 1974; **1**: 215–17.

92 Kyrle PA, Minar E, Bialonczyk C, *et al*. The risk of recurrent venous thromboembolism in men and women. *N Engl J Med* 2004; **350**: 2558–63.

93 World Health Organization. *Improving Access to Quality Care in Family Planning. Medical Eligibility Criteria for Contraceptive Use*, 3rd edition WHO 2004. Available at: www.who.int/reproductive-health/ publications/mec/mec.pdf

94 Vandenbroucke JP, van der Meer FJ, Helmerhorst FM, Rosendaal FR. Factor V Leiden: should we screen oral contraceptive users and pregnant women? *BMJ* 1996; **313**: 1127–30.

95 Boyce J, Fawcett JW, Noall EWP. Coronary thrombosis and Conovid. *Lancet* 1963; **i**: 111.

96 Rosenberg L, Hennekens CH, Rosner B, *et al*. Oral contraceptive use in relation to nonfatal myocardial infarction. *Am J Epidemiol* 1980; **111**: 59–66.

97 Thorogood M, Mann J, Murphy M, Vessey M. Is oral contraceptive use still associated with an increased risk of fatal myocardial infarction? Report of a case–control study. *Br J Obstet Gynaecol* 1991; **98**: 1245–53.

98 D'Avanzo B, La Vecchia C, Negri E, *et al*. Oral contraceptive use and risk of myocardial infarction: an Italian case–control study. *J Epidemiol Community Health* 1994; **48**: 324–5.

99 Sidney S, Petitti DB, Quesenberry CP Jr, *et al*. Myocardial infarction in users of low-dose oral contraceptives. *Obstet Gynecol* 1996; **88**: 939–44.

100 World Health Organization. Acute myocardial infarction and combined oral contraceptives: results of an international multicentre case–control study. WHO Collaborative Study of Cardiovascular Disease and Steroid Hormone Contraception. *Lancet* 1997; **349**: 1202–9.

101 Lewis MA, Heinemann LA, Spitzer WO, *et al*. The use of oral contraceptives and the occurrence of acute myocardial infarction in young women. Results from the Transnational Study on Oral Contraceptives and the Health of Young Women. *Contraception* 1997; **56**: 129–40.

102 Mant D, Villard-Mackintosh L, Vessey MP, Yeates D. Myocardial infarction and angina pectoris in young women. *J Epidemiol Community Health* 1987; **41**: 215–19.

103 Stampfer MJ, Willett WC, Colditz GA, *et al*. A prospective study of past use of oral contraceptive agents and risk of

cardiovascular diseases. *N Engl J Med* 1988; **319**: 1313–17.

104 Croft P, Hannaford P. Risk factors for acute myocardial infarction in women. *BMJ* 1989; **298**: 674.

105 World Health Organization. Ischaemic stroke and combined oral contraceptives: results of an international, multicentre, case–control study. WHO Collaborative Study of Cardiovascular Disease and Steroid Hormone Contraception. *Lancet* 1996; **348**: 498–505.

106 van den Bosch MAAJ, Kemmeren JM, Tanis BC, *et al.* The RATIO study: oral contraceptives and the risk of peripheral arterial disease in young women. *J Thromb Haemost* 2003; **1**: 439–44.

107 Kemmeren JM, Tanis BC, van den Bosch MA, *et al.* Risk of Arterial Thrombosis in Relation to Oral Contraceptives (RATIO) study: oral contraceptives and the risk of ischemic stroke. *Stroke* 2002; **33**: 1202–8.

108 Tanis BC, van den Bosch MA, Kemmeren JM, *et al.* Oral contraceptives and the risk of myocardial infarction. *N Engl J Med* 2001; **345**: 1787–93.

109 Henzl MR, Edwards JA. Pharmacology of progestins. 17-alpha-hydroxyprogesterone derivatives and progestins of the first and second generation. In: Sitruk-Ware R, Mishell DR, eds. *Progestins and Antiprogestins in Clinical Practice*. New York: Marcel Dekker, 2000: 101–32.

110 Godsland IF, Crook D, Simpson R, *et al.* The effects of different formulations of oral contraceptive agents on lipid and carbohydrate metabolism. *N Engl J Med* 1990; **323**: 1375–81.

111 Jick H, Jick S, Myers MW, Vasilakis C. Risk of acute myocardial infarction and low-dose combined oral contraceptives. *Lancet* 1996; **347**: 627–8.

112 Dunn N, Thorogood M, Faragher B, *et al.* Oral contraceptives and myocardial infarction: results of the MICA case–control study. *BMJ* 1999; **318**: 1579–84.

113 Rosendaal FR, van Hylckama Vlieg A, Tanis BC, Helmerhorst FM. Estrogens, progestogens and thrombosis. *J Thrombosis Haemost* 2003; **1**: 1371–80.

114 Kloosterboer HJ, Rekers H. Effects of three combined oral contraceptive preparations containing desogestrel plus ethinyl estradiol on lipid metabolism in comparison with two levonorgestrel preparations. *Am J Obstet Gynecol* 1990; **163**: 370–3.

115 Marz W, Jung-Hoffmann C, Heidt F, *et al.* Changes in lipid metabolism during 12 months of treatment with two oral contraceptives containing 30 micrograms ethinylestradiol and 75 micrograms gestodene or 150 micrograms desogestrel. *Contraception* 1990; **41**: 245–58.

116 Tanis BC. Lipid levels after long term use of second and third generation oral contraceptives. Thesis, B C Tanis. Arterial thrombosis in young women: role of oral contraceptives and coagulation factors. Thesis Leiden 2003. ISBN: 90–9017251–3.

32

Postmenopausal hormone replacement therapy and cardiovascular disease

EMMANUEL OGER, GENEVIÈVE PLU-BUREAU, PIERRE-YVES SCARABIN

INTRODUCTION

Cardiovascular disease has become the leading cause of death for women in developing countries. Coronary heart disease (CHD) and stroke kill twice as many women as all cancers combined. Moreover, women are more likely to die from cardiovascular disease than men.[1] Despite this growing epidemic, the incidence of CHD remains substantially lower in women than in men of the same age. These sex-related differences in CHD have not been adequately explained in terms of lifestyle or traditional risk factors, and it is generally believed that women are protected by female sex hormones.

Epidemiologic evidence suggests that women's protection against CHD is mediated through estrogen. Arterial disease is uncommon in premenopausal women and bilateral oophorectomy increases the risk of CHD.[2,3] In addition, early menopause is associated with an increased risk of CHD, suggesting that longer exposure to endogenous estrogen may be cardioprotective.[4,5] However, there is no clear evidence for rebound acceleration in CHD risk around the age of 50 years among women and there is no closing of the gap between the sexes with advancing age.[6] Thus, whether the menopause itself plays a role in the development of CHD remains unclear, and the rise in CHD rates after the age of 50 years may be related to the aging process rather than to the decline in endogenous estrogen levels.

More convincing evidence for a protective effect of estrogen on CHD arose from observational studies of hormone therapy (HT) among postmenopausal women. By the mid-1990s, a decreased risk of CHD was the main expected benefit of HT in postmenopausal women and conjugated equine estrogen (CEE) was one of the most frequently prescribed medication in the United States. However, large prevention trials in the United States failed to confirm the protective effect of HT on CHD.[7,8] In addition, there was clear evidence that oral estrogen would increase the risk of venous thromboembolism (VTE).[9] Thus, the cardiovascular effects of estrogen are far more complex than initially assumed and depend on the HT regimen as well as clinical outcomes.

This chapter reviews the literature about the cardiovascular risk among women using HT by clinical outcome (CHD, stroke or VTE) and study design (observational study or randomized trial). Current data on selective estrogen receptor modulators (SERMs) are also included.

HORMONE REPLACEMENT AND RISK FOR CORONARY HEART DISEASE

Evidence from observational studies

CASE–CONTROL STUDIES

Table 32.1 summarizes the findings from six hospital-based case–control studies.[10–15] All these studies assessed the risk of a first nonfatal myocardial infarction (MI) using the World Health Organization (WHO) criteria. Cases

Table 32.1 Case–control studies comparing the risk of a first nonfatal myocardial infarction between users of hormone therapy and nonusers

Authors	Country	Mean age years (range)	No. of cases	Odds ratio (95% CI) Crude	Odds ratio (95% CI) Adjusted
Rosenberg et al., 1976[10]	USA, Canada, NZ, UK, Israel	(40–75)	336		0.85 (0.38 to 1.91)
Jick et al., 1978[11]	USA	(39–45)	14	4.25 (0.94 to 19.3)	
Rosenberg et al., 1980[12]	USA	45 (30–50)	99	0.77 (0.42 to 1.40)	
Szklo et al., 1984[13]	USA	(35–64)	39		0.61 (0.20 to 1.88)
La Vecchia et al., 1987[14]	Italy	<55	168		2.95 (0.80 to 10.8)
Rosenberg et al., 1993[15]	USA	(45–69)	477		0.90 (0.70 to 1.20)

Oral estrogens were mostly conjugated equine estrogens.

were identified through discharge diagnostic indices. Clear definition of menopausal status was not provided and this is of concern because some studies enrolled women aged 45 years or under.

A major difficulty with case–control studies is the proper selection of controls. Hospital-based studies used hospitalized patients as controls, except one study which enrolled women listed in the telephone directory and who had published telephone numbers.[15] Exclusion of all diseases potentially related to estrogen use should be considered. All but one study[11] used such exclusion criteria. Information on exposure to estrogen was collected through face-to-face interview[10,12–14] or by telephone.[11,15] Current use of estrogen encompassed a wide range of definitions, that is, use within the months before hospitalization.[10,12] However, some studies did not even provide any definition and in such instance ever use was a more suitable definition than current use.[11,13,14] Type and dose of estrogens were not specified in two studies.[13,14] In the others, the most common type of estrogen used was CEE given mostly alone and the majority of users had taken CEE for more than 1 year. The adjusted risk estimate was mostly available. For two studies[11,12] odds ratios were calculated from raw data. No study reported a significant association of HT with a first nonfatal MI. However, these small-sample-sized studies had a limited statistical power. Two case–control studies showed a nonsignificant increase in CHD risk.

COHORT STUDIES

The oldest study reported a retrospective analysis of a hospital-based cohort of hypoestrogenic women followed up at least 5 years in one US clinical center.[16] However, events occurring in the first 5 years were not taken into account. Only the crude relative risk was calculated from raw data (relative risk 0.33, 95 percent confidence interval [CI] 0.18 to 0.58). Another study with major methodologic flaws was performed among postmenopausal healthy women from a single private practice. Women were offered CEE and were followed up for a minimum of 3 years.[17] Eighty-one long-term users were compared with the remaining

76 women who declined estrogen. Five controls experienced an MI compared with 1 treated woman (age-adjusted relative risk 0.34, 95 percent CI 0.09 to 1.34). Both studies were excluded from the quantitative assessment.

All other cohort studies have been community based, including the landmark Framingham Study[18] and the Nurses' Health Study[19,20] (Table 32.2). The Lipid Research Clinics Prevalence Study[21] enrolled subjects either randomly selected from a community-based target or because of elevated lipid levels. The other cohort studies used a nested case–control design. The diagnosis of acute MI was based on well-defined criteria. Cases were identified through a medical review of records on a biennial basis[18] or discharge diagnostic indices of hospitals known to serve the study population,[22–26] computerized search,[27–32] or self report by mailed questionnaire.[19,20] Death certificates, medical records, or vital statistics were used to ascertain CHD deaths.[20–22,28,33–38] Clear definition of menopausal status was not provided except in a few studies[18,20,24,30,31,39] and this is of concern because some of these studies enrolled women aged 45 or even under.[20,21,28,33] Most studies did not state that they excluded women with diseases potentially related to estrogen.

Information on exposure was collected through pharmacy computerized files, by face-to-face interview or by mailed self-questionnaire. Current use of estrogen was defined as use at the time of hospitalization or death for cases.[40] In some studies any definition was not provided[30,37,41] or information was collected only at baseline without any updating during the follow-up period and in such instance ever use was more suitable than current use. One study updated information biennially.[19,20] Type and dose of estrogens were not specified in most studies. In the others, the most common type of estrogen used was CEE. With regard to the route of estrogen administration, a cohort study conducted in United Kingdom suggested that oral and transdermal therapies have a similar cardioprotective effect.[32]

Some studies investigated the association between CHD and estrogen use according to the dose and duration of use. In the Nurses' Health Study[19,20] hormone use during each 2-year period was established from a woman's report at the

Table 32.2 Cohort studies comparing the risk of coronary heart disease between users of hormone therapy and nonusers

Authors	Country	Mean age, years (range)	No. of cases	Risk ratio (95% CI) Crude	Risk ratio (95% CI) Adjusted
Nonfatal MI as endpoint					
Wilson *et al.*, 1985[18]	USA	(50–83)	51		1.87 (0.89 to 3.95)
Stampfer *et al.*, 1985[19]	USA	(30–55)	65		0.34 (0.14 to 0.82)
Henderson *et al.*, 1988[22]	USA	73	178		0.72 (0.53 to 0.97)
Hernandez *et al.*, 1990[27]	USA	(50–64)	120	0.70 (0.39 to 1.28)	
Sourander *et al.*, 1998[28]	Finland	(40–69)	362		1.05 (0.76 to 1.46)
Lokkegaard *et al.*, 2003[39]	Denmark	>45	20		0.97 (0.57 to 1.65)
Ferrara *et al.*, 2003[40]	USA	>50	854		0.88 (0.72 to 1.07)
Pfeffer *et al.*, 1978[23]	USA	70 (44–100)	185	0.62 (0.33 to 1.16)	0.68 (0.32 to 1.42)
Croft *et al.*, 1989[41]	UK	70 (44–100)	NA		0.80 (0.30 to 1.80)
Mann *et al.*, 1994[29]	UK	(45–64)	1521	0.82 (0.66 to 1.01)	0.83 (0.66 to 1.03)
Sidney *et al.*, 1997[24]	USA	(45–74)	438	0.75 (0.54 to 1.02)	0.96 (0.66 to 1.40)
Heckbert *et al.*, 1997[31]	USA	(30–79)	850	0.63 (0.50 to 0.78)	0.70 (0.55 to 0.89)
Varas-Lorenzo *et al.*, 2000[32]	UK	(50–74)	1013	0.72 (0.59 to 0.88)	0.72 (0.59 to 0.89)
Pasty *et al.*, 2001[26]	USA	67 (30–79)	232	0.89 (0.65 to 1.23)	
Chilvers *et al.*, 2003[25]	UK	(35–65)	559	0.78 (0.62 to 0.97)	0.74 (0.55 to 0.99)
Fatal CHD as end point					
Bush *et al.*, 1987[21]	USA	(40–69)	24	0.25 (0.06 to 1.07)	
Petitti *et al.*, 1987[33]	USA	(18–54)	11		0.30 (0.10 to 1.30)
Criqui *et al.*, 1988[34]	USA	(50–79)	87	0.75 (0.45 to 1.24)	0.99 (0.59 to 1.67)
Henderson *et al.*, 1988[22]			149		0.59 (0.42 to 0.82)
Folsom *et al.*, 1995[35]	USA	(55–69)	290		0.82 (0.47 to 1.43)
Cauley *et al.*, 1997[36]	USA	>65	152		0.49 (0.26 to 0.93)
Sourander *et al.*, 1998[28]			84		0.19 (0.05 to 0.77)
Grodstein *et al.*, 2000[20]	USA	(30–55)	921	0.52 (0.46 to 0.61)	0.61 (0.52 to 0.71)
Ferrara *et al.*, 2003[40]			256		0.88 (0.60 to 1.30)
Ross *et al.*, 1981[37]	USA	73 (?–80)	133		0.57 (0.33 to 0.99)
Adam *et al.*, 1981[38]	UK	(50–59)	76	0.75 (0.14 to 3.95)	
Beard *et al.*, 1989[30]	USA	(40–59)	86	0.66 (0.36 to 1.23)	0.55 (0.24 to 1.30)
Chilvers *et al.*, 2003[25]	UK	(35–65)	41	0.41 (0.27 to 0.61)	

Oral estrogens were mostly conjugated equine estrogens.
CHD, coronary heart disease; MI, myocardial infarction.

start of the period and thus misclassification cannot be ruled out. The reduced risk of CHD in current users of CEE was smaller among women taking higher doses ($\geq$1.25 mg) than among women taking 0.625 mg or 0.3 mg. The same pattern of CHD risk was observed among diabetic women.[40]

META-ANALYSIS OF STUDIES

Table 32.3 shows the overall relative risk estimate according to both study designs and the endpoint. Data from case–control studies showed an almost null effect, but was rather imprecise. Results from cohort studies display a significant decreased risk for CHD. A stronger association was found for CHD death than for nonfatal MI and it is noteworthy that confidence intervals do not overlap. No heterogeneity between the studies was detected. To sum up, observational studies suggested that HT might reduce CHD. All these studies had methodologic limitations and an overall overestimation of the estrogen benefit was likely.

Results of randomized controlled trials

The first large trial designed to investigate the cardioprotective effect of estrogen was conducted in men with a history of CHD.[47] Begun in the 1960s, the Coronary Drug Project was a double-blind, placebo-controlled secondary prevention trial. Intervention was either CEE at a daily dose of 2.5 mg or 5.0 mg or placebo. The estrogen arms were stopped early because of excess clotting and cardiovascular disease. The first large trials of HT among postmenopausal women were planned in the United States about 25 years later. All the randomized trials of HT set up to assess cardiovascular disease are summarized in Table 32.4 and Figure 32.1.

Table 32.3 Metaanalysis of the association between hormone therapy and coronary heart disease among postmenopausal women according to the study design

Study design	No. of studies	No. of cases	Endpoint	Homogeneity*	Risk ratio (95% CI)
Case–control	6	1133	Nonfatal MI	>0.10	0.92 (0.74–1.16)
Cohort	15	6448	Nonfatal MI	>0.10	0.81 (0.74–0.88)
	13	2310	Fatal CHD	>0.10	0.61 (0.55–0.68)

*P value.

CHD, coronary heart disease; MI, myocardial infarction.

Table 32.4 Randomized trials of hormone therapy set up to assess cardiovascular disease

Study	Country	Clinical background Mean age, years (range)	Number*	Duration of follow-up	Active treatment (daily)	Primary endpoint	Main findings
Heart and Estrogen/ Progestin Study[7]	USA	Previous CHD 67 years (44–79)	2763	4.1 years	0.625 mg CEE +2.5 mg MPA	CHD death nonfatal MI	No difference in CHD risk
Estrogen in Venous Thromboembolism Trial[42]	Norway	Previous VTE	140	1.3 years	2 mg E2 + 1 mg NETA	VTE recurrence	Stopped early. Increased risk of VTE recurrence
Women's Estrogen for Stroke Trial[43]	USA	Previous stroke 71 yrs (>44)	664	2.8 years	1 mg 17β-E2	Stroke recurrence	Increased risk of fatal stroke
Women's Health Initiative[8,44]	USA	(i) Healthy women with intact uterus 63 years (50–79)	16 608	5.2 years	0.625 mg CEE +2.5 mg MPA	CHD death nonfatal MI	Stopped early. Increased risk of breast cancer. Risks exceeding benefits
		(ii) Healthy women without uterus 64 years (50–79)	10 739	7 years	0.625 mg CEE	CHD death nonfatal MI	Stopped early Increased risk of stroke
Estrogen in the Prevention of Reinfarction Trial[45]	UK	Previous MI 62 years (50–69)	1017	2 years	2 mg E2 valerate	CHD death nonfatal MI	No difference in CHD risk
Papworth HT Atherosclerosis study[46]	UK	Angiographically proved CHD 67 years	255	31 months	80 µg 17β-E2 ± 120 µg NETA patch		Nonsignificant increase in CHD risk

*Approximately equal numbers in placebo and active treatment group.

CEE, MPA, E2, and NETA denote conjugated equine estrogens, medroxyprogesterone acetate, estradiol, and norethisterone acetate, respectively.

CHD, coronary heart disease; MI, myocardial infarction; VTE, venous thromboembolism.

HERS

The Heart and Estrogen/progestin Replacement Study (HERS) was the first clinical trial designed to investigate whether estrogen plus progestin therapy reduced CHD risk in postmenopausal women with previous CHD.[7] Begun in 1993, HERS was a multicenter, randomized, double-blind, placebo-controlled trial that enrolled 2763 postmenopausal women (mean age 66.7 years) with an intact uterus.

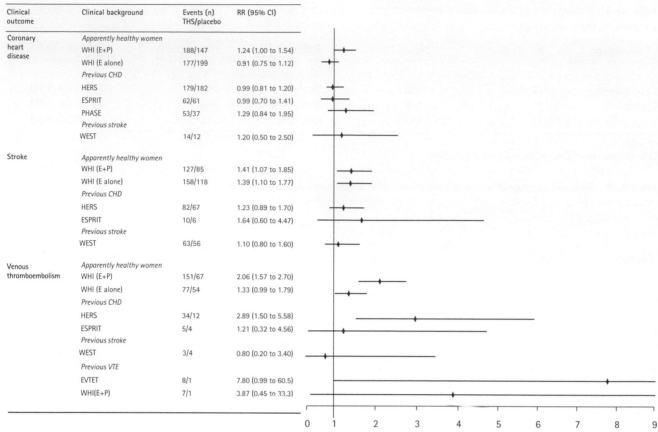

Clinical outcome	Clinical background	Events (n) THS/placebo	RR (95% CI)
Coronary heart disease	*Apparently healthy women*		
	WHI (E+P)	188/147	1.24 (1.00 to 1.54)
	WHI (E alone)	177/199	0.91 (0.75 to 1.12)
	Previous CHD		
	HERS	179/182	0.99 (0.81 to 1.20)
	ESPRIT	62/61	0.99 (0.70 to 1.41)
	PHASE	53/37	1.29 (0.84 to 1.95)
	Previous stroke		
	WEST	14/12	1.20 (0.50 to 2.50)
Stroke	*Apparently healthy women*		
	WHI (E+P)	127/85	1.41 (1.07 to 1.85)
	WHI (E alone)	158/118	1.39 (1.10 to 1.77)
	Previous CHD		
	HERS	82/67	1.23 (0.89 to 1.70)
	ESPRIT	10/6	1.64 (0.60 to 4.47)
	Previous stroke		
	WEST	63/56	1.10 (0.80 to 1.60)
Venous thromboembolism	*Apparently healthy women*		
	WHI (E+P)	151/67	2.06 (1.57 to 2.70)
	WHI (E alone)	77/54	1.33 (0.99 to 1.79)
	Previous CHD		
	HERS	34/12	2.89 (1.50 to 5.58)
	ESPRIT	5/4	1.21 (0.32 to 4.56)
	Previous stroke		
	WEST	3/4	0.80 (0.20 to 3.40)
	Previous VTE		
	EVTET	8/1	7.80 (0.99 to 60.5)
	WHI(E+P)	7/1	3.87 (0.45 to 33.3)

Figure 32.1 Randomized trials of hormone therapy set up to assess cardiovascular disease.

Intervention was 0.625 mg CEE plus 2.5 mg medroxyprogesterone acetate (MPA) or placebo. The primary outcome was the occurrence of nonfatal MI or CHD death. During an average follow-up of 4.1 years, 179 women in the HT group and 182 women in the placebo group experienced a nonfatal MI or fatal CHD event (relative risk 0.99, 95 percent CI 0.81–1.22), despite a 11 percent lower low-density lipoprotein (LDL)-cholesterol and 10 percent higher high-density lipoprotein (HDL)-cholesterol level in the HT group.[48] Within the overall null effect, there was a significant time trend, with more CHD events in the HT group than in the placebo group in year 1 and fewer in years 4 and 5.

WEST

The Women's Estrogen for Stroke Trial (WEST) study was designed in 1993 as a randomized, placebo-controlled trial of HT for the secondary prevention of cerebrovascular disease.[43] However, secondary outcomes included nonfatal MI. This trial was conducted in 664 postmenopausal women (mean age, 71 years) who had recently had an ischemic stroke or transient ischemic attack. Women were randomly assigned to receive either 1 mg of 17β-estradiol per day or placebo. During a mean follow-up period of 2.8 years, there were 14 MI among the women in the estradiol group, and 12 among those in the placebo group (relative risk 1.2, 95 percent CI 0.5 to 2.5).

WHI

The Women's Health Initiative (WHI) study focused on strategies which could potentially reduce the incidence of CHD, breast and colorectal cancer, and fractures in postmenopausal women. Between 1993 and 1998, the WHI enrolled 161 809 postmenopausal women in the age range of 50–79 years into a set of clinical trials (trials of low-fat dietary pattern, calcium, and vitamin D supplementation, and two trials of postmenopausal HT) and an observational study at 40 clinical centers in the United States.

The estrogen plus progestin component of the WHI was a randomized controlled primary prevention trial in which 16 608 postmenopausal women with an intact uterus were randomly assigned to receive CEE (0.625 mg/day) plus MPA (2.5 mg/day) or placebo. The primary outcome was CHD, with breast cancer as the primary adverse outcome. A global index included the two primary outcomes plus stroke, pulmonary embolism, endometrial cancer, colorectal cancer, hip fracture, and death due to other causes. On May 31, 2002, after a mean of 5.2 years of follow-up (planned duration 8.5 years), the data and safety monitoring board recommended stopping the trial of estrogen plus progestin versus placebo because the statistic test for breast cancer exceeded the stopping boundary for this adverse effect and the overall risks exceeded the benefits.[8] Combined HT was associated with a hazard ratio for CHD of 1.24 (nominal 95 percent CI 1.00 to 1.54) with 188 events in the HT group and 147 events in the placebo group.[49] Absolute rates of CHD were 39 cases per 10 000 person years and 33 cases per 10 000 person years for HT and placebo, respectively. Absolute excess risk attributable to estrogen plus progestin was not large (less than 10 events per 10 000 person years). An elevated risk of CHD appeared to emerge soon after randomization and there was evidence for a decreasing risk of CHD with time. Higher baseline levels of LDL-cholesterol were associated with an excess risk of CHD. The hazard ratio for the global index was 1.15 (95 percent CI 1.03 to 1.28).

Despite the early termination of the WHI estrogen plus progestin trial, the WHI estrogen-alone was continued for assessing the health risks and benefits. A total of 10 739 postmenopausal women, aged 50–79 years, with prior hysterectomy, were randomly assigned to receive either 0.625 mg/day of CEE or placebo.[44] The primary outcome was CHD incidence (nonfatal MI and CHD death). Invasive breast cancer incidence was the primary safety outcome. A global index of risks and benefits was also used for summarizing overall effects. On February 2, 2004, despite the fact that no predefined stopping boundaries had been crossed, the National Institutes of Health (NIH) decided to stop the intervention phase of the trial because the risk of stroke was increased and there was no reason to expect future favorable effects of CEE on CHD risk. After an average follow-up of 6.8 years, estrogen alone was associated with a hazard ratio for CHD of 0.91 (nominal 95 percent CI 0.75 to 1.12) with 177 events in the HT group and 199 events in the placebo group. There was a significant trend of slightly elevated hazard ratios in the early follow-up period that diminished over time. Subgroup analysis showed a nonsignificant trend to lower CHD risk in younger women. Results for the global index were 1.01 (95 percent CI 0.91 to 1.12) and the estimated excess risk for all events in the global index was a nonsignificant 2 events per 10 000 person years.

ESPRIT

The EStrogen in the Prevention of ReInfarction Trial (ESPRIT) study was set up in United Kingdom to assess the effect of unopposed estradiol valerate on CHD risk in postmenopausal women who had survived their first MI.[45] The study was a randomized, blinded, placebo-controlled, secondary prevention trial among 1017 women aged 50–69 years. Women received either estradiol valerate (2 mg/day) or placebo for 2 years. Primary outcomes were reinfarction or cardiac death, and all-cause mortality. The frequency of re-infarction or cardiac death did not differ between treatment groups at 24 months (relative risk 0.99, 95 percent CI 0.70 to 1.41), and there was no significant difference in all-cause mortality (relative risk 0.79, 95 percent CI 0.50 to 1.27).

PHASE

The Papworth HT Atherosclerosis (PHASE) study was a randomized controlled trial of transdermal estrogen among 255 postmenopausal women with angiographically proved CHD.[46] Women (mean age 66 years) were randomly assigned to a 17β-estradiol patch (80 μg/day) or no treatment. Women without a uterus received estrogen alone whereas women with an intact uterus received estradiol alone for 14 days, followed by patches delivering 17β-estradiol (80 μg/day) plus norethisterone (120 μg/day) for 14 days. The primary endpoints were cardiac mortality, nonfatal MI or hospitalization with unstable angina. After an average of 31 months, the CHD event rate was 15.4 per 100 patient years for the HT group compared with 12.6 per 100 patient years for the control group (relative risk 1.29, 95 percent CI 0.84 to 1.95).

Divergent findings from observational studies and clinical trials

The majority of observational studies showed a clear decrease in CHD risk among postmenopausal women using HT. However, randomized trials failed to confirm a cardioprotective effect of HT. These divergent findings may be related to differences between study designs, studied populations, and hormone regimens.

In observational studies, women who use HT are often healthier than nonusers and confounding bias may occur when there is a failure to fully control for health related factors. Education level and socioeconomic status may have an important impact on the HT-related cardiovascular risk. Some observational studies that adjusted for socioeconomic status showed no cardioprotective effect of HT.[50] However, other studies, including the Nurses' Health Study, have adequately controlled for socioeconomic status and still found a decreased risk of CHD among HT users.[20] Protective effect of HT in observational studies may be also due in part to compliance bias. In fact, women who adhere to HT (or placebo in trials) tend to adhere to other protective types of behavior and have a substantially lower rate of mortality.[51] Thus, compliance bias may explain why HT-related cardioprotective effect is more pronounced for CHD death than for nonfatal MI.

Another problem related to cohort studies is that information about treatment is collected at a certain interval in cohort studies. This design would not capture information on women who both initiated hormone use and have a MI within this interval. Such women would be considered to be nonusers of hormones which would explain an overestimated cardioprotection associated with hormone use.

Women in the trials were older than women included in observational studies and differential effect of HT on CHD risk by age could be relevant to the divergent findings between observational studies and trials. In the Nurses' Health Study, the age range at inclusion was 33–55 years in comparison with an average age close to 65 years in the WHI. In the WHI estrogen-alone, subgroup analysis showed a clear but nonsignificant trend to lower CHD risk in younger women. Nevertheless, the WHI opposed-estrogen trial and

HERS reported no significant difference in risk of CHD between women who were aged 50–60 years at baseline and the older women. Differences in body-mass index could be also relevant to the discrepancy between observational data and trials. The mean body mass index was close to 30 in the WHI and it was about 25 in the Nurses' Health Study. Women in observational studies tend to be thinner and have lower levels of endogenous estrogen. Beneficial effect of HT may depend largely upon endogenous hormonal status.

The timing of initiation of estrogen may be an important factor influencing the effects of HT on CHD. In most observational studies, HT use began within 2 years after menopause. In both HERS and WHI, women were post-menopausal for at least 10 years at the time of inclusion. It is quite possible that HT may be beneficial in younger women with minimal atherosclerotic lesions, but may not delay progression of complicated plaques in older women. Thus, the Estrogen Replacement and Atherosclerosis trial[52] found no effect of HT on the progression of coronary artery atherosclerosis among women with history of CHD. By contrast, the Estrogen in the Prevention of Atherosclerosis trial showed that estrogen alone could decrease the progression of subclinical carotid atherosclerosis among younger women without CHD.[53] Experimental data from animal models lend support to these clinical findings. Administration of estrogen can prevent the development of atherosclerosis when given to monkeys immediately after oophorectomy, whereas no reduction in atherosclerosis plaque is found when HT is initiated after several years.[54]

Differences in hormone regimens could explain in part the discrepancy between observational studies and trials. CEE was commonly used in both trials and observational studies. However, few observational studies have suggested a cardioprotective effect of CEE combined with MPA.

In addition, most of combined HT users took MPA on a cyclical basis. By contrast, a continuous combined regimen was used in WHI and HERS. It is quite possible that MPA may attenuate favorable effects of estrogen. The decrease in CHD risk among HT users in WHI estrogen-alone trial, although nonsignificant, is consistent with this hypothesis.

HORMONE REPLACEMENT AND RISK FOR STROKE

The impact of HT on stroke has been evaluated through observational and randomized trials. Clinical outcomes of interest were all stroke, ischemic, or hemorrhagic stroke (fatal or nonfatal).

Evidence from observational studies

CASE–CONTROL STUDIES

Table 32.5 summarizes the findings from six case–control studies. All these studies were conducted in Anglo-Saxon countries. A difficulty related to studies of stroke is the definition of clinical event. The more recent studies used strict criteria for this definition. The classification of event as an ischemic stroke required the rapid onset of a neurologic deficit that persisted at least 24 hours with no apparent cause other than that of vascular origin, or evidence of infarction on brain imaging procedures, at surgery or at autopsy. Stroke was defined as hemorrhagic if there was some evidence of blood in the subarachnoidal space or ventricles or dense intraparenchymal blood on brain imaging procedures, blood at surgery, angiography or autopsy.

Table 32.5 Case–control studies comparing the risk of stroke between users of hormone therapy and nonusers.

Authors	Country	Mean age, years (range)	No. of cases	Endpoint	Odds ratio (95% CI) Crude	Odds ratio (95% CI) Adjusted
Pfeffer and Van Dens 1976[55]	USA	(40–100)	174	Nonfatal stroke		0.97 (0.65 to 1.44)
			96	Ischemic		1.13 (0.71 to 1.77)
Pfeffer et al., 1978[23]			19	Hemorrhagic		0.86 (0.00 to 9.10[23])
Rosenberg et al., 1980[56]	USA	(>45)	198	Ischemic	1.16 (0.75 to 1.77)	
Thompson et al., 1989[57]	UK	(45–69)	244	Stroke F + NF	1.20 (0.81 to 1.76)	
Petitti et al., 1998[58]	USA	(45–74)	349	Ischemic F + NF		1.03 (0.65 to 1.65)
			83	Hemorrhagic F + NF		0.33 (0.12 to 0.96)
Thrift et al., 1996[59]	Australia	(15–75+)	105	Stroke F + NF	0.41	0.36 (0.14 to 0.95)
Lemaitre et al., 2002[60]	USA	(30–79)	726	Ischemic E + P	0.61 (0.45 to 0.83)	0.97 (0.69 to 1.37)
			726	Ischemic E	0.74 (0.58 to 0.95)	0.94 (0.72 to 1.23)
			213	Hemorrhagic E + P	0.72 (0.43 to 1.20)	0.74 (0.43 to 1.28)
			213	Hemorrhagic E	1.12 (0.77 to 1.63)	1.06 (0.71 to 1.56)

E, estrogen only; E + P, estrogen + progestin treatment; F, fatal; NF, nonfatal.

Earlier studies used only clinical criteria. Some studies validated events through medical database or deaths registry. Mostly all these studies assessed the risk of first stroke. Some studies analyzed nonfatal events[55,56] whereas the others analyzed fatal and nonfatal strokes together.[57–60]

Cases were identified through discharge diagnosis code. Clear definition of menopausal status was not provided in all studies and this is of concern because some studies enrolled very young women aged 45 years or even under.[59,60] Information on exposure to estrogen was differently collected through face-to-face interview, by telephone, or computerized pharmacy database.[60] The type of estrogen use was not similar in all studies. The majority of the studies analyzed unopposed conjugated equine estrogen, but some studies analyzed all forms of oral estrogen with no molecular distinction. Some recent studies assessed the risks of stroke according to unopposed or opposed estrogen.[58,60] Risk estimates for ischemic and hemorrhagic stroke were available in all but two case–controls studies.[56,59] Adjusted risk estimates were mostly available. For two studies,[56,57] only crude odds ratios were available.

Only two case–control studies showed a significant decreased risk for stroke. The study conducted by Thrift et al. in Australia analyzed 105 women with no clear definition of menopausal status.[59] Only 11 women in the case group were exposed to estrogen and 29 women in the control group. The odds ratio for stroke was based on all events without distinction between ischemic and hemorrhagic stroke. Fatal and nonfatal strokes were mixed. The corresponding odds ratio was 0.36 (95 percent CI 0.14 to 0.95). In a larger case–control study conducted by Petitti et al.[58] a decreased risk of hemorrhagic stroke was observed in current hormone users as compared with never users (odds ratio 0.33, 95 percent CI 0.12 to 0.96).[58] In this study, postmenopausal hormone use was not associated with any change in the risk of ischemic stroke. Estimated risks for a first fatal or nonfatal stroke ranged from 0.61 to 1.20 in the other studies and none of those estimates were significant. No difference was detected between unopposed or opposed regimens.

COHORT STUDIES

Fifteen studies were found and five were excluded. Methodologic limitations are described earlier in the chapter for one study.[16] Three other studies had no internal controls.[61–63] The fifth study enrolled women with a previous MI.[64] Table 32.6 summarizes the findings from the remaining 10 selected cohort studies[18,20,21,28,33,35,65–75] and overall risk estimate is based on those latter data.

Risk of first nonfatal or fatal stroke was assessed. The distinction between ischemic or hemorrhagic stroke was available in only four cohort studies for ischemic events and two cohort studies for hemorrhagic stroke. Diagnosis of stroke was based on well-defined criteria in the more recent studies. Cases were identified through a medical review of records on a biennial basis, through discharge diagnostic indices of hospitals known to serve the study population,

computerized search from register, or self report by mailed questionnaire. Death certificates, medical records or vital statistics were used to ascertain stroke deaths. The definition of menopausal status or estrogen exposure had the similar limitations than in case–control studies.

In some studies information on exposure was collected only at baseline without any updating during the follow-up period. Only oral estrogen use was evaluated with or without progestin. No study evaluated transdermal estrogen.

METAANALYSIS OF STUDIES

Table 32.7 shows the overall relative risk estimate according to the study design. With regard to cohort studies, tests for heterogeneity were highly significant and, therefore, random-effect models were used to estimate the risk for stroke associated with HT use. Overall these studies suggested that HT increased the risk of ischemic stroke and had no effect on hemorrhagic stroke. All these observational studies had methodologic limitations.

Results of randomized controlled trials

HERS

Stroke incidence and stroke death were used as secondary cardiovascular outcomes in HERS.[76] A total of 149 strokes occurred over a mean of 4.1 years. As expected, most (85 percent) of the strokes were ischemic; 8 percent were hemorrhagic and 8 percent could not be classified. Combined HT was associated with a nonsignificant increase in the risk of stroke (relative risk 1.23, 95 percent CI 0.89 to 1.70). The effect of HT on the risk of stroke was somewhat more pronounced for fatal strokes (relative risk 1.61, 95 percent CI 0.73 to 3.55) than for nonfatal strokes (relative risk 1.18, 95 percent CI 0.83 to 1.66). There was no clear difference in the risk for ischemic and hemorrhagic strokes.

WEST

The primary endpoint of WEST was death from any cause or nonfatal stroke.[43] After an average of 2.8 years, there were 63 strokes (12 fatal strokes and 51 nonfatal strokes) among the women in the estradiol group, and 56 (4 fatal strokes and 52 nonfatal strokes) among those in the placebo group (risk ratio 1.1, 95 percent CI 0.8 to 1.6). Estrogen did not reduce the risk of death alone (relative risk 1.2, 95 percent CI 0.8 to 1.8) or the risk of nonfatal stroke (relative risk 1.0, 95 percent CI 0.7 to 1.4). Hormone therapy was associated with an increased risk of fatal stroke (relative risk 2.9, 95 percent CI 0.9 to 9.0).

ESPRIT

This secondary prevention trial of postmenopausal women who had survived a first MI included stroke as a secondary

Table 32.6   Cohort studies comparing the risk of stroke between users of hormone therapy and nonusers.

Authors	Country	Mean age, years (range)	No. of cases	Endpoint	Risk ratio (95% CI)	
					Crude	Adjusted
Petitti et al., 1979,[65] 1987[33]	USA	(18–54)	?	Stroke	0.9 (0.4 to 1.8)	0.6 (0.2 to 2.2)
			9	Stroke F		
Wilson et al., 1985[18]	USA	(50–83)	45	All stroke		2.27 (1.21 to 4.23)
			21	Ischemic		2.60 (1.26 to 5.38)
Pedersen et al., 1997[67]	Denmark	>44	144	Stroke F + NF		1.26 (0.82 to 1.92)
Lokkegaard et al., 2003[66]			89	Stroke NF		1.54 (1.07 to 2.46)
			38	Stroke F		0.75 (0.28 to 1.99)
			99	Total Ischemic		1.63 (0.98 to 2.70)
			77	Ischemic NF		1.75 (1.02 to 3.01)
			80	Hemorrhagic		0.74 (0.41 to 1.32)
Bush et al., 1987[21]	USA Canada	(40–69)	8	Stroke F	0.40 (0.01 to 3.07)	
Paganini-Hill et al., 1988[68]	USA	73 median	63	Ischemic F 1988		0.53 (0.31 to 0.91)
Henderson et al., 1991[69]						
Paganini-Hill et al., 1995[70]				Ischemic F 1991		0.63
Boysen et al., 1988[71]	Denmark	(45–74)	238	Stroke	0.41 (0.27 to 0.62)	
Lindenstrom et al., 1993[72]						
Stampfer et al., 1991[73]	USA	(30–55)	550	All stroke		1.13 (0.94 to 1.35)
Grodstein et al., 1996,[74] 2000[20]			574	Ischemic		1.26 (1.00 to 1.61)
			224	Hemorrhagic		0.93 (0.64 to 1.34)
Finucane et al., 1993[75]	USA	55–74	250	Stroke F + NF		0.69 (0.47 to 1.00)
				Stroke F		0.37 (0.14 to 0.92)
Folsom et al., 1995[35]	USA	55–69	90	Stroke F		0.95 (0.37 to 2.43)
Sourander et al., 1998[28]	Finland	>56	111	Stroke F + NF		0.86 (0.42 to 1.75)
				Stroke F		0.16 (0.02 to 1.18)

F, fatal; NF, nonfatal.

Table 32.7   Metaanalysis of the association between hormone therapy and stroke among postmenopausal women according to the study design

Study design	No. of studies	Homogeneity*	Risk ratio (95% CI)[†]	Risk ratio (95% CI)[‡]
Case–control				
All stroke	6	>0.10	0.97 (0.84 to 1.11)	1.18 (1.01 to 1.38)
Ischemic	4	>0.10	0.99 (0.85 to 1.16)	1.16 (0.93 to 1.45)
Hemorrhagic	3	>0.10	0.85 (0.62 to 1.15)	0.66 (0.30 to 1.47)
Cohort				
All stroke	10	0.001	0.92 (0.79 to 1.06)	0.88 (0.63 to 1.23)
Ischemic	4	0.04	1.31 (1.08 to 1.59)	1.30 (0.83 to 2.06)
Hemorrhagic	2	>0.10	0.87 (0.64 to 1.20)	0.76 (0.44 to 1.32)

*P value;
[†]Fixed-effect model;
[‡]Random-effect model.

outcome event.[45] Stroke arose more frequently in women receiving oral estradiol than women taking placebo. However, the risk ratio for stroke (relative risk 1.64, 95 percent CI 0.60 to 1.47) was not significant.

WHI

The WHI trial included stroke as a secondary outcome. In the estrogen plus progestin component of the WHI, the stroke rates were higher in women receiving HT (relative risk 1.41, nominal 95 percent CI 1.07 to 1.85), with most of the elevation occurring in nonfatal elevation.[8] Prior history of stroke did not confer additional risk. No significant interaction with baseline characteristics was found for the effect of estrogen plus progestin on stroke. There was no significant trend with time.

In the estrogen-alone WHI trial,[44] stroke diagnostic was supported by imaging studies in most cases (90 percent had computed tomography/magnetic resonance imaging studies available). The risk of stroke was increased for women receiving HT (relative risk 1.39, nominal 95 percent CI 1.10 to 1.77), with an elevation more pronounced for nonfatal events. Subgroups analysis and test for trend with time led to negative findings.

Consistent findings from observational studies and clinical trials

Although the risk ratios for stroke are somewhat lower in observational studies than in randomized trials, there is a good consistency between both approaches with respect to the impact of HT on this clinical outcome. Large cohort studies such as the Nurses' Health Study investigated the association between HT use and major cardiovascular outcomes, including CHD and stroke. However, it remains unclear why divergent findings between observational studies and trials were observed only for CHD. Study designs were similar and confounding factors were taken into account in the same way. CHD may be more subject to confounding than other outcomes and the reasons for such discrepancy require further investigations.

HORMONE REPLACEMENT AND RISK FOR VENOUS THROMBOEMBOLISM

Despite evidence that oral estrogen activates blood coagulation in postmenopausal women and might induce thrombosis, HT has long been believed to have little effect on the risk of VTE. Recent data showed that VTE was an important adverse outcome of HT.

Evidence from observational studies

EARLY OBSERVATIONAL STUDIES 1974–1992

By the mid-1990s, case–control studies had failed to provide evidence for an association between HT and VTE.[16,65,77–79] However, these studies had some methodologic limitations, including lack of well-defined diagnostic criteria for VTE, selection bias, inadequate control of confounding variable and lack of statistical power.

RECENT OBSERVATIONAL STUDIES 1996–2003

Since October 1996, nine studies have overcome the limitations of the early studies and consistently reported a twofold to threefold increased risk of VTE. Four case–control studies used information collected through health databases in the United States,[80,81] United Kingdom,[82] and Italy.[83] The four other case–control studies obtained data from interviews of hospitalized women.[84–87] Grodstein et al. reported data from the landmark Nurses' Health Cohort Study.[88] In all studies, the clinical endpoint was a well-documented first episode of idiopathic VTE, either deep venous thrombosis (DVT) or pulmonary embolism (PE), except for the Nurses' Health Study which was restricted to the risk of PE.[88] It is worth noticing that Hoibraaten et al.[86] and Smith et al.[81] included women with a secondary VTE. A subgroup analysis restricted to women with an idiopathic VTE was displayed and we used this estimate in the quantitative assessment.

Matched controls were selected among women hospitalized for a disease thought to be unrelated to HT use or among women randomly chosen from the source cohort. Controls were selected from among hospitalized women. Definition of current use of HT used different time windows from 1,[84] 3,[87] 6[80,82] and up to 24 months.[88] Prevalence of current estrogen replacement therapy use among controls varied largely from 2.3 percent in Italy, 12–25 percent in the United Kingdom, 25–37 percent in the United States to 32 percent in France.

Potentially confounding variables were taken into account by matching and adjustment. Recall bias was avoided in cohort studies or in studies using information from healthcare databases. In the other case–control studies, participants were interviewed by trained research assistant using pictures of available HT packages. Referral bias was best avoided in studies which examined the risk for PE, a more severe condition than DVT.

RISK FOR VENOUS THROMBOEMBOLISM RELATED TO ORAL ESTROGEN

In most of the studies of oral estrogen, CEE was used. Table 32.8 shows crude and adjusted risk ratios for VTE among current oral estrogen replacement therapy users compared to never users. It is worth emphasizing that none of the studies found an increased VTE risk among past HT users. Data from observational studies were homogeneous and consistently showed a severalfold increased risk for VTE in current users of CEE. This pooled estimate was close to the relative risk observed in the cohort study (Table 32.9).

Use of esterified estrogens was not associated with an increased risk for VTE in one case–control study.[81] Scarabin et al. reported that 17β-estradiol users had a twofold increased risk of VTE.[87] No significant difference in VTE risk was found between users of unopposed oral estrogen and combined estrogen-progestin regimen except in one study comparing estrogen plus progestin to estrogen alone (odds ratio 1.60, 95 percent CI 1.13 to 2.26).[81]

Information on the duration of estrogen replacement therapy was available in six studies. Daly et al.,[85] Perez et al.,[82] and Hoibraaten et al.[86] reported data on the risk for

Table 32.8 Crude and adjusted risk ratios for venous thromboembolism associated with hormone therapy among postmenopausal women

Study design Authors	Route of estrogen administration	No. of exposed cases	Risk ratio (95% CI)	
			Crude	Adjusted
Case–control studies				
Boston CDSP, 1974[78]	Oral	4	2.3 (0.4 to 8.3)	1.9 (0.4 to 7.8)
Pettiti *et al.*, 1979[65]	Oral	NA	0.7 (0.2 to 2.5)*	
Devor *et al.*, 1992[79]	Oral	6	0.8 (0.3 to 2.4)	
Daly *et al.*, 1996[85]	Oral	37	3.6 (1.8 to 7.2)	4.6 (2.1 to 10)
	Transdermal	5	2.2 (0.7 to 7.5)	2.0 (0.5 to 7.6)
Daly *et al.*, 1996[84]	Oral	4	NA	2.2 (0.6 to 7.9)
Jick *et al.*, 1996[80]	Oral	21	3.6 (1.6 to 7.8)	
Perez Gutthann *et al.*, 1997[82]	Oral	20	1.1 (0.7 to 1.7)	2.1 (1.3 to 3.6)
	Transdermal	7	1.0 (0.5 to 2.2)	2.1 (0.9 to 4.6)
Hoibraaten *et al.*, 1999[86]	Oral†‡	42	1.5 (0.8 to 2.7)	NA
	Transdermal	2	0.6 (0.0 to 3.1)	NA
Scarabin *et al.*, 2003[87]	Oral†	32	3.7 (1.9 to 7.1)	3.9 (2.0 to 7.6)
	Transdermal	30	1.0 (0.5 to 1.7)	1.0 (0.5 to 1.7)
Smith *et al.*, 2004[81]	Oral†	NA	1.7 (1.2 to 2.4)	
Cohort study				
Grodstein *et al.*, 1996[88]	Oral	22	1.7 (0.9 to 3.0)	2.1 (1.2 to 3.8)

CDSP, Collaborative Drug Surveillance Program.
*90% CI.
Oral estrogen was CEE in all but five studies †:17β-estradiol, §§: estradiol valerate.
The more adjusted risk ratios are shown.
‡Idiopathic venous thromboembolism only.

Table 32.9 Overall measures of association between venous thromboembolism and hormone therapy among postmenopausal women

Route of administration Study design	No. of studies	Homogeneity			Risk ratio (95% CI)
		χ^2	df	*P* value	
Oral ERT					
Case–control	7	11.2	6	>0.05	2.2 (1.8 to 2.7)
Cohort	1				2.1 (1.2 to 3.8)
Transdermal ERT					
Case–control	4	1.9	3	>0.10	1.1 (0.7 to 1.9)

ERT, estrogen replacement therapy.

VTE according to the duration of estrogen replacement therapy, but these data encompassed oral and transdermal estrogen replacement therapy. No clear association between VTE risk and the duration of current oral estrogen use was observed. The risk for VTE was however higher during the first year of use than in the subsequent years with adjusted odds ratios ranging from 3.0 to 8.1 (pooled estimate 4.8, 95 percent CI 3.1 to 7.3).

As far as the estrogen dose was concerned, Jick *et al.* found a higher risk of VTE among women who used CEE at 1.25 mg or more per day compared with lower dosage, that is, 0.325 mg/day (odds ratio 6.9, 95 percent CI 1.5 to 33 and odds ratio 2.1, 95 percent CI 0.4 to 11, respectively).[80] A dose-dependent association was also reported by Smith *et al.*[81] No association of estrogen dose and duration of HRT use with VTE risk was found in the prospective cohort study conducted by Grodstein *et al.*[88] nor in three case–control studies.[82,84,85,87]

RISK FOR VENOUS THROMBOEMBOLISM RELATED TO THE TRANSDERMAL ESTROGEN

Two case–control studies[82,85] reported no clear difference between the oral and transdermal routes of estrogen administration, but these results were based on only five and seven cases who used transdermal estrogen. In these studies, crude and adjusted odds ratios for VTE among women using transdermal estrogen compared with nonusers did not significantly differ from 1. In the study by Hoibraaten *et al.*, only 2 cases out of 176 and 7 controls out of 352 were exposed to transdermal estrogen.[86] Another study assessed the risk for VTE in postmenopausal women predominantly using transdermal estrogen, but odds ratios were based on only six women who used HT and results according to the route of estrogen administration were not shown.[83] More recently, the EStrogen and THromboEmbolism Risk (ESTHER) study,[87] a hospital-based multicenter case–control study of HT in French women, reported data based on 30 cases using transdermal estrogen. In contrast with oral estrogen, no significant association of transdermal estrogen with VTE was found (odds ratio 0.9, 95 percent CI 0.5 to 1.6). Overall, estimation based on these four case–control studies yielded a VTE risk close to 1 (odds ratio 1.1, 95 percent CI 0.7 to 1.9) (see Table 32.9).

Evidence from randomized clinical trials

EVTET

The Estrogen in Venous Thromboembolism Trial (EVTET), a randomized double-blind trial, compared 2 mg estradiol plus 1 mg norethisterone acetate to placebo in postmenopausal women with previously verified VTE.[42] The study stopped prematurely after a mean follow-up of 1 year and 4 months. Eight women in the estrogen replacement therapy group and one woman in the placebo group developed VTE. The rate of VTE recurrence was 8.5 per 100 patient years (95 percent CI 2.6 to 14.4) in the HT group and 1.1 per 100 patient years (95 percent CI 0 to 3.2) in the placebo group.

HERS

VTE was used as a secondary outcome in HERS.[7] More women in the hormone group experienced VTE (relative risk 2.89, 95 percent CI 1.50 to 5.58). The risk remained elevated over the 4 years of follow-up with no clear time trend.

WEST

Women were monitored for VTE events.[43] Diagnosis required an objective test. Only 7 women (1 percent) experienced VTE during an average follow-up of 2.8 years. The estimated risk ratio for VTE related to oral 17β-estradiol was 0.8 (95 percent CI 0.2 to 3.4).

ESPRIT

In this secondary prevention trial after a first MI, 9 women (0.9 percent) reported VTE during the 2-year study period.[48]

VTE was not significantly associated with estradiol valerate use (relative risk 1.2, 95 percent CI 0.3 to 4.5).

WHI

Findings for VTE by evaluating centrally adjudicated cases occurring during an average follow-up of 5.6 years in the estrogen plus progestin component of the WHI were recently reported.[89] Nonprocedure-related VTE rate was higher in women receiving HT (adjusted hazard ratio 2.54, 95 percent CI 1.81 to 3.56). Among women who had a prior history of VTE the estimated risk of recurrence related to HT was higher (hazard ratio 3.87, 95 percent CI 0.45 to 33). Older age, obesity, and factor V Leiden mutation added to the risk associated with HT use. There was a significant trend in the hazard ratio over time showing diminishing risk with increasing time.

In the estrogen-alone WHI trial,[44] the risk of VTE was slightly increased in women receiving HT (relative risk 1.33, nominal 95 percent CI 0.99 to 1.79). In a per-protocol analysis censuring nonadherent participants, a greater risk for pulmonary embolism was observed (relative risk 1.99). No significant trend over time was detected.

Synthesis of evidence from observational studies and randomized trials

This quantitative review found consistent data from observational studies and randomized trials showing that current use of oral estrogen is associated with a twofold increased risk for VTE. Observational studies reported highest risk in the first year. Data from the WHI trial supported this finding but data from the HERS trial did not. Risk was somewhat higher in trials that included women with cardiovascular disease who in addition were older than healthy postmenopausal women enrolled in primary prevention trials or observational studies. Women aged 50–59 had an estimated annual incidence of first VTE of 0.8 per thousand.[89] Absolute risk excess related to current use of oral estrogen remained low (1.1–1.8 per 1000 women years). Conversely, recurrence rate was higher and absolute risk excess was substantial, yielding to 14–51 women treated with oral estrogen for 1 year to cause 1 additional event.

With regard to transdermal estrogen, data are scant. Pooled estimates from observational data yielded no association between transdermal estrogen and VTE. These findings suggest that transdermal estrogen replacement therapy might be safer than oral estrogen with respect to VTE, but no definite and valid conclusion can be drawn. Definitive support for the safety of the transdermal route of estrogen administration regarding VTE should be a placebo-controlled randomized trial.

Biologic plausibility of findings

Biologic evidence lends support to the elevated VTE risk among users of oral estrogen and to the difference between routes of estrogen administration. Randomized trials have recently shown that oral estrogen increased plasma levels of markers for *in vivo* thrombin activation (prothrombin fragment 1 + 2) and lowered antithrombin activity in postmenopausal women, whereas transdermal estrogen had little or no effect on coagulation and fibrinolysis.[90–95] In addition, oral estrogen significantly decreases total protein S plasma level.[91,96]

Activated protein C (APC) resistance has emerged as a risk factor for venous thrombosis.[97,98] Although this phenotype is mostly related to a mutation in the factor V gene (R506Q or Leiden mutation),[99] APC resistance detected in the absence of any thrombogenic mutation is also an independent risk factor for VTE.[100] An acquired resistance to activated protein C has been found in users of oral estrogen replacement therapy (ERT),[101] but two randomized trials recently showed that these results did not apply to users of transdermal ERT.[95,102] Changes in prothrombin fragment 1 + 2 plasma level were positively and significantly correlated with changes in endogenous thrombin potential (ETP)-based APCsr in factor V Leiden non-carriers allocated to oral ERT. These biologic data show that oral estrogen induces an APC resistance and activates blood coagulation, but these deleterious effects on coagulation did not apply to transdermal estrogen. These results emphasize the potential importance of the route of estrogen administration in prescribing HT.

A major difference between oral and transdermal estrogen administration is the hepatic first-pass effect. Oral estrogen administration leads to high hormone concentrations in the liver and promotes hepatic protein synthesis. In addition, oral estrogen replacement therapy results in a ratio of estrone to estradiol close to 5, whereas transdermal estrogen replacement therapy leads to a more physiologic ratio close to 1.

SELECTIVE ESTROGEN RECEPTOR MODULATORS AND CARDIOVASCULAR RISK

Selective estrogen receptor modulators (SERMs), including both tamoxifen and raloxifene, are molecules that bind with high affinity to estrogen receptors and may exhibit either estrogen-agonistic or estrogen-antagonistic effects, according to the target. Tamoxifen is use as an adjuvant treatment of breast cancer which reduces recurrence and mortality in women with hormone-dependant breast cancer. This treatment has been proposed to primary prevention of breast cancer in women at high risk. Four trials have now reported on the use of tamoxifen as prophylaxis to prevent breast cancer. Relevant information is also available on side effects, in particular cardiovascular disease. All the tamoxifen prevention trails compared 20 mg tamoxifen daily for at least 5 years with placebo.

Tamoxifen had been shown to alter lipid and lipoprotein metabolism, which could reduce the risk of coronary artery disease. It seemed appropriate to evaluate the effect on these endpoints. But with agonist estrogenic effect of tamoxifen on coagulation factors, an increased risk of venous thromboembolism is expected. The National Surgical Adjuvant Breast and Bowel Project P-1 Study (NSABP)[103] was set up to explore these issues. The other trials[104–106] are smaller. Table 32.10 summarizes the results of these trials. Venous thromboembolism events were increased in all studies. An updated metaanalysis of all

Table 32.10   Cardiovascular events associated with tamoxifen in four primary breast cancer prevention studies

| Authors | Country | Endpoints | Number* | No. of Events | | Risk ratio (95% CI) |
				Tamoxifen	Placebo	
Fisher *et al.*, 1998[103]	USA	Fatal MI	13 175	7	8	0.88 (0.27 to 2.77)
		Nonfatal MI		24	20	1.20 (0.64 to 2.30)
		Stroke		38	24	1.59 (0.93 to 2.77)
		Pulmonary embolism		18	6	3.01 (1.15 to 9.27)
		Deep venous thrombosis		35	22	1.60 (0.91 to 2.86)
Powles *et al.*, 1998[105]	UK	Pulmonary embolism	2471	3	2	NA
		Deep venous thrombosis		4	2	NA
Veronesi *et al.*, 1998[104]	Italy	Pulmonary embolism	3837	1	1	NA
		Deep venous thrombosis		6	3	NA
		Stroke		9	5	NA
Cuzick *et al.*, 2002[106]	UK	Pulmonary embolism	7044	13	10	
		Deep venous thrombosis		24	5	
		All VTE events		43	17	2.5 (1.5 to 4.4)
		Stroke		13	11	NA
		MI		5	5	NA

*Approximately equal numbers in placebo and active treatment group.
MI, myocardial infarction; NA, not available; VTE, venous thromboembolic events.

available data was published in 2003[107] and reported an increased risk of VTE (relative risk 1.9, 95 percent CI 1.4 to 2.6). No significant increase in MI rate was observed in the NSABP trial. Thirty-one MIs occurred in tamoxifen group (6681 women) versus 28 in placebo group (6707 women). There was a nonsignificant increase risk of stroke with 24 events in placebo group versus 38 in tamoxifen group (relative risk 1.59, 95 percent CI 0.93 to 2.77).

Another trial is in progress with other anti-estrogenic agents for minimizing the cardiovascular side effects. The results of the direct comparison with raloxifene in the Study of Tamoxifen And Raloxifene (STAR) trial are awaited with great interest. Raloxifene was evaluated in one large randomized trial, the Multiple Outcomes Raloxifene Evaluation (MORE) study.[108] This trial enrolled 7705 women who were at least 2 years postmenopausal and had osteoporosis, defined as low bone mineral density or radiographically apparent vertebral fracture. There was a long list of exclusion criteria and 14 674 women were screened but not randomized. Women were randomly allocated to receive daily either placebo (n = 2576) or 60 mg (n = 2557) or 120 mg of raloxifene (n = 2572). All women received daily supplements of calcium and cholecalciferol. Participants were followed up to 36 months. The primary endpoints were incident vertebral fractures and bone mineral density. All categories of adverse events were reported including cardiovascular events, VTE, and mortality. Cardiovascular events, including coronary events and cerebrovascular events were centrally and blindly adjudicated. Criteria used to define VTE were not provided. A secondary analysis was conducted. Overall, raloxifene did not affect the risk of cardiovascular events. However in the subgroup of 1035 women with an unfavorable risk profile at baseline, raloxifene significantly lowered the risk of subsequent cardiovascular events compared with placebo (relative risk 0.60, 95 percent CI 0.38 to 0.95). After 36 months, 57 women reported VTE, 8 in the placebo group (0.3 percent), 25 (1.0 percent) in 60 mg raloxifene group and 24 (0.1 percent) in the 120 mg raloxifene group. The relative risk for VTE related to raloxifene compared with placebo was 3.1 (95 percent CI 1.5 to 6.2).

The Raloxifene Use for The Heart (RUTH) trial enrolled 10 101 postmenopausal women between June 1998 and August 2000 in 26 countries.[109] Half of the women had documented CHD and the remainder had multiple risk factors, including lower extremity arterial disease, smoking, hypertension, hyperlipidemia, diabetes mellitus, or age above 70 years. The mean age of women was 68 years and they were an average of 19 years postmenopausal. The primary endpoint is any coronary event, including coronary death, nonfatal MI or acute coronary syndrome.

RECOMMENDATIONS AND FUTURE RESEARCH DIRECTIONS

Hormone therapy offers well-established clinical benefit for menopausal symptoms. Treatment of menopausal symptoms remains the primary indication for HT but hormone regimen should not be initiated or continued for the purpose of preventing cardiovascular disease. A healthy lifestyle and a good medical care are the basis for preventing cardiovascular disease. Such therapies, including statins, angiotensin-converting enzyme inhibitors, and β-blockers, have been proved in clinical trials to reduce CHD risk in postmenopausal women.

Current data have limited ability to investigate the wide variety of hormone treatments available, especially the transdermal route of estrogen administration and progesterone. In addition, it is quite possible that HT may be beneficial among women aged 45–55 before the development of cardiovascular disease. Therefore, the effects of HT in younger women as well as the timing of initiation of HT require further studies.

Clinical research has to continue into genetic factors influencing the response to HT, different estrogen and progestogen formulations, different modes of delivery, lower dose options and alternative regimens (SERMs such as raloxifene and tamoxifen, phytoestrogens). This research will assist patients and clinicians in making treatment decisions on the basis of an individual's benefits and risks.

KEY LEARNING POINTS

- Epidemiologic evidence for a cardioprotective effect of estrogen in women is limited.
- Decreased risk of coronary heart disease has been for a long time the main expected benefit of HT among postmenopausal women, but randomized trials failed to confirm the cardioprotective effect of estrogen.
- Treatment of menopausal symptoms remains the primary indication for HT.
- Hormone therapy may increase the risk for both coronary heart disease and stroke and should not be used for the prevention of cardiovascular disease. Other means have been proved in clinical trials to reduce CHD risk in postmenopausal women.
- Oral estrogen increases the risk of VTE, but there is some evidence that transdermal estrogen is safer.
- Current data have limited ability to investigate the wide variety of hormone regimens available, especially the transdermal route of estrogen administration and progesterone. The effects of HT in younger women who have just reached menopause require further investigation.

ACKNOWLEDGMENT

We thank Sophie Guillonneau for her technical assistance.

REFERENCES

1   [No authors listed]. The greatest threat to women's health. *Lancet* 2003; **362**: 1165.

2   Gordon T, Kannel WB, Hjortland MC, McNamara PM. Menopause and coronary heart disease. The Framingham Study. *Ann Intern Med* 1978; **89**: 157–61.

3   Colditz GA, Willett WC, Stampfer MJ, *et al*. Menopause and the risk of coronary heart disease in women. *N Engl J Med* 1987; **316**: 1105–10.

4   van der Schouw YT, van der GY, Steyerberg EW, *et al*. Age at menopause as a risk factor for cardiovascular mortality. *Lancet* 1996; **347**: 714–18.

5   Hu FB, Grodstein F, Hennekens CH, *et al*. Age at natural menopause and risk of cardiovascular disease. *Arch Intern Med* 1999; **159**: 1061–6.

6   Tunstall-Pedoe H. Myth and paradox of coronary risk and the menopause. *Lancet* 1998; **351**: 1425–7.

7   Hulley S, Grady D, Bush T, *et al*. Randomized trial of estrogen plus progestin for secondary prevention of coronary heart disease in postmenopausal women. Heart and Estrogen/progestin Replacement Study (HERS) Research Group. *JAMA* 1998; **280**: 605–13.

8   Rossouw JE, Anderson GL, Prentice RL, *et al*. Risks and benefits of estrogen plus progestin in healthy postmenopausal women: principal results From the Women's Health Initiative randomized controlled trial. *JAMA* 2002; **288**: 321–33.

9   Oger E, Scarabin PY. Assessment of the risk for venous thromboembolism among users of hormone replacement therapy. *Drugs Aging* 1999; **14**: 55–61.

10 Rosenberg L, Armstrong B, Jick H. Myocardial infarction and estrogen therapy in post-menopausal women. *N Engl J Med* 1976; **294**: 1256–9.

11 Jick H, Dinan B, Rothman KJ. Noncontraceptive estrogens and nonfatal myocardial infarction. *JAMA* 1978; **239**: 1407–9.

12 Rosenberg L, Slone D, Shapiro S, *et al*. Noncontraceptive estrogens and myocardial infarction in young women. *JAMA* 1980; **244**: 339–42.

13 Szklo M, Tonascia J, Gordis L, Bloom I. Estrogen use and myocardial infarction risk: a case-control study. *Prev Med* 1984; **13**: 510–16.

14 La Vecchia C, Franceschi S, Decarli A, *et al*. Risk factors for myocardial infarction in young women. *Am J Epidemiol* 1987; **125**: 832–43.

15 Rosenberg L, Palmer JR, Shapiro S. A case–control study of myocardial infarction in relation to use of estrogen supplements. *Am J Epidemiol* 1993; **137**: 54–63.

16 Hammond CB, Jelovsek FR, Lee KL, *et al*. Effects of long-term estrogen replacement therapy. I. Metabolic effects. *Am J Obstet Gynecol* 1979; **133**: 525–36.

17 Lafferty FW, Fiske ME. Postmenopausal estrogen replacement: a long-term cohort study. *Am J Med* 1994; **97**: 66–77.

18 Wilson PW, Garrison RJ, Castelli WP. Postmenopausal estrogen use, cigarette smoking, and cardiovascular morbidity in women over 50. The Framingham Study. *N Engl J Med* 1985; **313**: 1038–43.

19 Stampfer MJ, Willett WC, Colditz GA, *et al*. A prospective study of postmenopausal estrogen therapy and coronary heart disease. *N Engl J Med* 1985; **313**: 1044–9.

20 Grodstein F, Manson JE, Colditz GA, *et al*. A prospective, observational study of postmenopausal hormone therapy and primary prevention of cardiovascular disease. *Ann Intern Med* 2000; **133**: 933–41.

21 Bush TL, Barrett-Connor E, Cowan LD, *et al*. Cardiovascular mortality and noncontraceptive use of estrogen in women: results from the Lipid Research Clinics Program Follow-up Study. *Circulation* 1987; **75**: 1102–9.

22 Henderson BE, Paganini-Hill A, Ross RK. Estrogen replacement therapy and protection from acute myocardial infarction. *Am J Obstet Gynecol* 1988; **159**: 312–17.

23 Pfeffer RI, Whipple GH, Kurosaki TT, Chapman JM. Coronary risk and estrogen use in postmenopausal women. *Am J Epidemiol* 1978; **107**: 479–97.

24 Sidney S, Petitti DB, Quesenberry CP, Jr. Myocardial infarction and the use of estrogen and estrogen-progestogen in postmenopausal women. *Ann Intern Med* 1997; **127**: 501–8.

25 Chilvers CE, Knibb RC, Armstrong SJ, *et al*. Post menopausal hormone replacement therapy and risk of acute myocardial infarction – a case–control study of women in the East Midlands, UK. *Eur Heart J* 2003; **24**: 2197–205.

26 Psaty BM, Smith NL, Lemaitre RN, *et al*. Hormone replacement therapy, prothrombotic mutations, and the risk of incident nonfatal myocardial infarction in postmenopausal women. *JAMA* 2001; **285**: 906–13.

27 Hernandez AM, Walker AM, Jick H. Use of replacement estrogens and the risk of myocardial infarction. *Epidemiology* 1990; **1**: 128–33.

28 Sourander L, Rajala T, Raiha I, *et al*. Cardiovascular and cancer morbidity and mortality and sudden cardiac death in postmenopausal women on oestrogen replacement therapy (ERT). *Lancet* 1998; **352**: 1965–9.

29 Mann RD, Lis Y, Chukwujindu J, Chanter DO. A study of the association between hormone replacement therapy, smoking and the occurrence of myocardial infarction in women. *J Clin Epidemiol* 1994; **47**: 307–12.

30 Beard CM, Kottke TE, Annegers JF, Ballard DJ. The Rochester Coronary Heart Disease Project: effect of cigarette smoking, hypertension, diabetes, and steroidal estrogen use on coronary heart disease among 40- to 59-year-old women, 1960 through 1982. *Mayo Clin Proc* 1989; **64**: 1471–80.

31 Heckbert SR, Weiss NS, Koepsell TD, *et al*. Duration of estrogen replacement therapy in relation to the risk of incident myocardial infarction in postmenopausal women. *Arch Intern Med* 1997; **157**: 1330–6.

32 Varas-Lorenzo C, Garcia-Rodriguez LA, Perez-Gutthann S, Duque-Oliart A. Hormone replacement therapy and

incidence of acute myocardial infarction. A population-based nested case–control study. *Circulation* 2000; **101**: 2572–8.

33   Petitti DB, Perlman JA, Sidney S. Noncontraceptive estrogens and mortality: long-term follow-up of women in the Walnut Creek Study. *Obstet Gynecol* 1987; **70**: 289–93.

34   Criqui MH, Suarez L, Barrett-Connor E, McPhillips J, *et al.* Postmenopausal estrogen use and mortality. Results from a prospective study in a defined, homogeneous community. *Am J Epidemiol* 1988; **128**: 606–14.

35   Folsom AR, Mink PJ, Sellers TA, *et al.* Hormonal replacement therapy and morbidity and mortality in a prospective study of postmenopausal women. *Am J Public Health* 1995; **85**: 1128–32.

36   Cauley JA, Seeley DG, Browner WS, *et al.* Estrogen replacement therapy and mortality among older women. The study of osteoporotic fractures. *Arch Intern Med* 1997; **157**: 2181–7.

37   Ross RK, Paganini-Hill A, Mack TM, *et al.* Menopausal oestrogen therapy and protection from death from ischaemic heart disease. *Lancet* 1981; **1**: 858–60.

38   Adam S, Williams V, Vessey MP. Cardiovascular disease and hormone replacement treatment: a pilot case–control study. *Br Med J (Clin Res Ed)* 1981; **282**: 1277–8.

39   Lokkegaard E, Pedersen AT, Heitmann BL, *et al.* Relation between hormone replacement therapy and ischaemic heart disease in women: prospective observational study. *BMJ* 2003; **326**: 426.

40   Ferrara A, Quesenberry CP, Karter AJ, *et al.* Current use of unopposed estrogen and estrogen plus progestin and the risk of acute myocardial infarction among women with diabetes: the Northern California Kaiser Permanente Diabetes Registry, 1995–1998. *Circulation* 2003; **107**: 43–8.

41   Croft P, Hannaford PC. Risk factors for acute myocardial infarction in women: evidence from the Royal College of General Practitioners' oral contraception study. *BMJ* 1989; **298**: 165–8.

42   Hoibraaten E, Qvigstad E, Arnesen H, *et al.* Increased risk of recurrent venous thromboembolism during hormone replacement therapy – results of the randomized, double-blind, placebo-controlled estrogen in venous thromboembolism trial (EVTET). *Thromb Haemost* 2000; **84**: 961–7.

43   Viscoli CM, Brass LM, Kernan WN, *et al.* A clinical trial of estrogen-replacement therapy after ischemic stroke. *N Engl J Med* 2001; **345**: 1243–9.

44   Anderson GL, Limacher M, Assaf AR, *et al.* Effects of conjugated equine estrogen in postmenopausal women with hysterectomy: the Women's Health Initiative randomized controlled trial. *JAMA* 2004; **291**: 1701–12.

45   Cherry N, Gilmour K, Hannaford P, *et al.* Oestrogen therapy for prevention of reinfarction in postmenopausal women: a randomised placebo controlled trial. *Lancet* 2002; **360**: 2001–8.

46   Clarke SC, Kelleher J, Lloyd-Jones H, *et al.* A study of hormone replacement therapy in postmenopausal women with ischaemic heart disease: the Papworth HRT atherosclerosis study. *Br J Obstet Gynaecol* 2002; **109**: 1056–62.

47   The Coronary Drug Project. Findings leading to discontinuation of the 2.5-mg day estrogen group. The coronary Drug Project Research Group. *JAMA* 1973; **226**: 652–7.

48   Hulley S, Furberg C, Barrett-Connor E, *et al.* Noncardiovascular disease outcomes during 6.8 years of hormone therapy: Heart and Estrogen/progestin Replacement Study follow-up (HERS II). *JAMA* 2002; **288**: 58–66.

49   Manson JE, Hsia J, Johnson KC, *et al.* Estrogen plus progestin and the risk of coronary heart disease. *N Engl J Med* 2003; **349**: 523–34.

50   Humphrey LL, Chan BK, Sox HC. Postmenopausal hormone replacement therapy and the primary prevention of cardiovascular disease. *Ann Intern Med* 2002; **137**: 273–84.

51   Petitti DB. Coronary heart disease and estrogen replacement therapy. Can compliance bias explain the results of observational studies? *Ann Epidemiol* 1994; **4**: 115–8.

52   Herrington DM, Reboussin DM, Brosnihan KB, *et al.* Effects of estrogen replacement on the progression of coronary-artery atherosclerosis. *N Engl J Med* 2000; **343**: 522–9.

53   Hodis HN, Mack WJ, Lobo RA, *et al.* Estrogen in the prevention of atherosclerosis. A randomized, double-blind, placebo-controlled trial. *Ann Intern Med* 2001; **135**: 939–53.

54   Mikkola TS, Clarkson TB. Estrogen replacement therapy, atherosclerosis, and vascular function. *Cardiovasc Res* 2002; **53**: 605–19.

55   Pfeffer RI, Van Den NS. Estrogen use and stroke risk in postmenopausal women. *Am J Epidemiol* 1976; **103**: 445–56.

56   Rosenberg SH, Fausone V, Clark R. The role of estrogens as a risk factor for stroke in postmenopausal women. *West J Med* 1980; **133**: 292–6.

57   Thompson SG, Meade TW, Greenberg G. The use of hormonal replacement therapy and the risk of stroke and myocardial infarction in women. *J Epidemiol Community Health* 1989; **43**: 173–8.

58   Petitti DB, Sidney S, Quesenberry CP, Jr., Bernstein A. Ischemic stroke and use of estrogen and estrogen/progestogen as hormone replacement therapy. *Stroke* 1998; **29**: 23–8.

59   Thrift AG, McNeil JJ, Forbes A, Donnan GA. Risk factors for cerebral hemorrhage in the era of well-controlled hypertension. Melbourne Risk Factor Study (MERFS) Group. *Stroke* 1996; **27**: 2020–5.

60   Lemaitre RN, Heckbert SR, Psaty BM, *et al.* Hormone replacement therapy and associated risk of stroke in postmenopausal women. *Arch Intern Med* 2002; **162**: 1954–60.

61 Hunt K, Vessey M, McPherson K. Mortality in a cohort of long-term users of hormone replacement therapy: an updated analysis. *Br J Obstet Gynaecol* 1990; **97**: 1080–6.

62 Falkeborn M, Persson I, Terent A, *et al.* Hormone replacement therapy and the risk of stroke. Follow-up of a population-based cohort in Sweden. *Arch Intern Med* 1993; **153**: 1201–9.

63 Schairer C, Adami HO, Hoover R, Persson I. Cause-specific mortality in women receiving hormone replacement therapy. *Epidemiology* 1997; **8**: 59–65.

64 Angeja BG, Shlipak MG, Go AS, *et al.* Hormone therapy and the risk of stroke after acute myocardial infarction in postmenopausal women. *J Am Coll Cardiol* 2001; **38**: 1297–301.

65 Petitti DB, Wingerd J, Pellegrin F, Ramcharan S. Risk of vascular disease in women. Smoking, oral contraceptives, noncontraceptive estrogens, and other factors. *JAMA* 1979; **242**: 1150–4.

66 Lokkegaard E, Jovanovic Z, Heitmann BL, *et al.* Increased risk of stroke in hypertensive women using hormone therapy: analyses based on the Danish Nurse Study. *Arch Neurol* 2003; **60**: 1379–84.

67 Pedersen AT, Lidegaard O, Kreiner S, Ottesen B. Hormone replacement therapy and risk of non-fatal stroke. *Lancet* 1997; **350**: 1277–83.

68 Paganini-Hill A, Ross RK, Henderson BE. Postmenopausal oestrogen treatment and stroke: a prospective study. *BMJ* 1988; **297**: 519–22.

69 Henderson BE, Paganini-Hill A, Ross RK. Decreased mortality in users of estrogen replacement therapy. *Arch Intern Med* 1991; **151**: 75–8.

70 Paganini-Hill A. Estrogen replacement therapy and stroke. *Prog Cardiovasc Dis* 1995; **38**: 223–42.

71 Boysen G, Nyboe J, Appleyard M, *et al.* Stroke incidence and risk factors for stroke in Copenhagen, Denmark. *Stroke* 1988; **19**: 1345–53.

72 Lindenstrom E, Boysen G, Nyboe J. Lifestyle factors and risk of cerebrovascular disease in women. The Copenhagen City Heart Study. *Stroke* 1993; **24**: 1468–72.

73 Stampfer MJ, Colditz GA, Willett WC, *et al.* Postmenopausal estrogen therapy and cardiovascular disease. Ten-year follow-up from the nurses' health study. *N Engl J Med* 1991; **325**: 756–62.

74 Grodstein F, Stampfer MJ, Manson JE, *et al.* Post-menopausal estrogen and progestin use and the risk of cardiovascular disease. *N Engl J Med* 1996; **335**: 453–61.

75 Finucane FF, Madans JH, Bush TL, *et al.* Decreased risk of stroke among postmenopausal hormone users. Results from a national cohort. *Arch Intern Med* 1993; **153**: 73–9.

76 Simon JA, Hsia J, Cauley JA, *et al.* Postmenopausal hormone therapy and risk of stroke: The Heart and Estrogen-progestin Replacement Study (HERS). *Circulation* 2001; **103**: 638–42.

77 Quinn DA, Thompson BT, Terrin ML, *et al.* A prospective investigation of pulmonary embolism in women and men. *JAMA* 1992; **268**: 1689–96.

78 [No authors listed]. Surgically confirmed gallbladder disease, venous thromboembolism, and breast tumors in relation to postmenopausal estrogen therapy. A report from the Boston Collaborative Drug Surveillance Program, Boston University Medical Center. *N Engl J Med* 1974; **290**: 15–9.

79 Devor M, Barrett-Connor E, Renvall M, *et al.* Estrogen replacement therapy and the risk of venous thrombosis. *Am J Med* 1992; **92**: 275–82.

80 Jick H, Derby LE, Myers MW, *et al.* Risk of hospital admission for idiopathic venous thromboembolism among users of postmenopausal oestrogens. *Lancet* 1996; **348**: 981–3.

81 Smith NL, Heckbert SR, Lemaitre RN, *et al.* Esterified estrogens and conjugated equine estrogens and the risk of venous thrombosis. *JAMA* 2004; **292**: 1581–7.

82 Perez GS, Garcia Rodriguez LA, Castellsague J, Duque OA. Hormone replacement therapy and risk of venous thromboembolism: population-based case–control study. *BMJ* 1997; **314**: 796–800.

83 Varas-Lorenzo C, Garcia-Rodriguez LA, Cattaruzzi C, *et al.* Hormone replacement therapy and the risk of hospital-ization for venous thromboembolism: a population-based study in southern Europe. *Am J Epidemiol* 1998; **147**: 387–90.

84 Daly E, Vessey MP, Painter R, Hawkins MM. Case-control study of venous thromboembolism risk in users of hormone replacement therapy. *Lancet* 1996; **348**: 1027.

85 Daly E, Vessey MP, Hawkins MM, *et al.* Risk of venous thromboembolism in users of hormone replacement therapy. *Lancet* 1996; **348**: 977–80.

86 Hoibraaten E, Abdelnoor M, Sandset PM. Hormone replacement therapy with estradiol and risk of venous thromboembolism – a population-based case-control study. *Thromb Haemost* 1999; **82**: 1218–21.

87 Scarabin PY, Oger E, Plu-Bureau. Differential association of oral and transdermal oestrogen-replacement therapy with venous thromboembolism risk. *Lancet* 2003; **362**: 428–32.

88 Grodstein F, Stampfer MJ, Goldhaber SZ, *et al.* Prospective study of exogenous hormones and risk of pulmonary embolism in women. *Lancet* 1996; **348**: 983–7.

89 Cushman M, Kuller LH, Prentice R, *et al.* Estrogen plus progestin and risk of venous thrombosis. *JAMA* 2004; **292**: 1573–80.

90 Conard J, Samama M, Basdevant A, *et al.* Differential AT III-response to oral and parenteral administration of 17 beta-estradiol. *Thromb Haemost* 1983; **49**: 252.

91 Hoibraaten E, Os I, Seljeflot I, Andersen TO, *et al.* The effects of hormone replacement therapy on hemostatic variables in women with angiographically verified coronary artery disease: results from the estrogen in women with atherosclerosis study. *Thromb Res* 2000; **98**: 19–27.

92 Teede HJ, McGrath BP, Smolich JJ, *et al.* Postmenopausal hormone replacement therapy increases coagulation

activity and fibrinolysis. *Arterioscler Thromb Vasc Biol* 2000; **20**: 1404–9.

93 Vehkavaara S, Silveira A, Hakala-Ala-Pietila T, *et al.* Effects of oral and transdermal estrogen replacement therapy on markers of coagulation, fibrinolysis, inflammation and serum lipids and lipoproteins in postmenopausal women. *Thromb Haemost* 2001; **85**: 619–25.

94 Scarabin PY, Alhenc-Gelas M, Plu-Bureau, *et al.* Effects of oral and transdermal estrogen/progesterone regimens on blood coagulation and fibrinolysis in postmenopausal women. A randomized controlled trial. *Arterioscler Thromb Vasc Biol* 1997; **17**: 3071–8.

95 Oger E, Alhenc-Gelas M, Lacut K, *et al.* Differential effects of oral and transdermal estrogen/progesterone regimens on sensitivity to activated protein C among postmenopausal women: a randomized trial. *Arterioscler Thromb Vasc Biol* 2003; **23**: 1671–6.

96 Marque V, Alhenc-Gelas M, Plu-Bureau, *et al.* The effects of transdermal and oral estrogen/progesterone regimens on free and total protein S in postmenopausal women. *Thromb Haemost* 2001; **86**: 713–4.

97 Dahlback B. Resistance to activated protein C caused by the factor VR506Q mutation is a common risk factor for venous thrombosis. *Thromb Haemost* 1997; **78**: 483–8.

98 Rodeghiero F, Tosetto A. Activated protein C resistance and factor V Leiden mutation are independent risk factors for venous thromboembolism. *Ann Intern Med* 1999; **130**: 643–50.

99 Bertina RM, Koeleman BP, Koster T, *et al.* Mutation in blood coagulation factor V associated with resistance to activated protein C. *Nature* 1994; **369**: 64–7.

100 de Visser MC, Rosendaal FR, Bertina RM. A reduced sensitivity for activated protein C in the absence of factor V Leiden increases the risk of venous thrombosis. *Blood* 1999; **93**: 1271–6.

101 Hoibraaten E, Mowinckel MC, de Ronde H, *et al.* Hormone replacement therapy and acquired resistance to activated protein C: results of a randomized, double-blind, placebo-controlled trial. *Br J Haematol* 2001; **115**: 415–20.

102 Post MS, Christella M, Thomassen LG, *et al.* Effect of oral and transdermal estrogen replacement therapy on hemostatic variables associated with venous thrombosis: a randomized, placebo-controlled study in postmenopausal women. *Arterioscler Thromb Vasc Biol* 2003; **23**: 1116–21.

103 Fisher B, Costantino JP, Wickerham DL, *et al.* Tamoxifen for prevention of breast cancer: report of the National Surgical Adjuvant Breast and Bowel Project P-1 Study. *J Natl Cancer Inst* 1998; **90**: 1371–88.

104 Veronesi U, Maisonneuve P, Costa A, *et al.* Prevention of breast cancer with tamoxifen: preliminary findings from the Italian randomised trial among hysterectomised women. Italian Tamoxifen Prevention Study. *Lancet* 1998; **352**: 93–7.

105 Powles T, Eeles R, Ashley S, *et al.* Interim analysis of the incidence of breast cancer in the Royal Marsden Hospital tamoxifen randomised chemoprevention trial. *Lancet* 1998; **352**: 98–101.

106 Cuzick J, Forbes J, Edwards R, *et al.* First results from the International Breast Cancer Intervention Study (IBIS-I): a randomised prevention trial. *Lancet* 2002; **360**: 817–24.

107 Cuzick J, Powles T, Veronesi U, *et al.* Overview of the main outcomes in breast-cancer prevention trials. *Lancet* 2003; **361**: 296–300.

108 Barrett-Connor E, Grady D, Sashegyi A, *et al.* Raloxifene and cardiovascular events in osteoporotic postmenopausal women: four-year results from the MORE (Multiple Outcomes of Raloxifene Evaluation) randomized trial. *JAMA* 2002; **287**: 847–57.

109 Wenger NK, Barrett-Connor E, Collins P, *et al.* Baseline characteristics of participants in the Raloxifene Use for The Heart (RUTH) trial. *Am J Cardiol* 2002; **90**: 1204–10.

33

Hormone replacement therapy and venous thromboembolism: risks, mechanisms, and patient management

JAMES D DOUKETIS

INTRODUCTION

The past decade has witnessed remarkable changes in our understanding of the risks and benefits of hormone replacement therapy (HRT), which is defined as an estrogen formulation with or without a progestin and is usually administered in an oral or transdermal (patch) form. Observational studies performed in the 1990s suggested that users of HRT had a two to three times greater risk of developing venous thromboembolism (VTE), which includes deep vein thrombosis and pulmonary embolism, than nonusers of HRT.[1–7] These findings were subsequently confirmed in randomized placebo-controlled trials, the most important of which were the Hormone Replacement Therapy Study (HERS) and the Women's Health Initiative (WHI) study.[8,9]

Based on the findings from these trials, HRT is no longer recommended for the primary or secondary prevention of cardiovascular disease or osteoporosis by gynecologic groups and other experts.[10–13] However, HRT remains an effective treatment for women with menopausal symptoms, such as vasomotor flushing and mood instability, and is recommended for short-term (<2 year) use in such patients.[14] The scope of this clinical problem is considerable, as 25 percent of women will have menopausal symptoms for 1 year or longer and in 5 percent of such women these symptoms can be debilitating.[15] Although there are nonhormonal treatments available for menopausal symptoms, such as clonidine or venlafaxine (an antidepressant), these agents require further investigation in clinical trials to assess efficacy compared with HRT. Consequently, it is likely that HRT will continue, at least for the foreseeable future, as an important and widely used treatment for menopausal women, although for short-time use.

Clinical management issues relating to HRT use and VTE risk are frequently encountered in clinical practice for three reasons. First, VTE is a common vascular disease, the most common vascular disease in premenopausal women and the third most common vascular disease in postmenopausal women, after coronary artery disease and stroke. Second, an increasing number of women are being identified with risk factors for VTE, either inherited (for example, factor V Leiden mutation) or acquired (for example, obesity). Third, pharmacologic treatment of menopausal symptoms with

HRT may be required in a considerable proportion of women who reach the menopause.

Against this background, there are three objectives of this chapter: (i) to assess the risk for VTE with HRT, according to the type and duration of treatment; (ii) to assess possible mechanisms of HRT-related VTE, including the effect of inherited and acquired thrombophilia on the risk for VTE; and (iii) to provide practical management approaches for frequently encountered clinical scenarios relating to HRT use and VTE risk.

WHAT IS THE RISK FOR VENOUS THROMBOEMBOLISM WITH DIFFERENT TYPES OF HORMONE REPLACEMENT THERAPY?

Estrogen–progestin hormone replacement therapy

Combined estrogen-progestin HRT is recommended for women with an intact uterus because unopposed or estrogen-only HRT is associated with an increased risk for endometrial cancer.[16] In the 1990s, several observational studies, summarized in Table 33.1, provided evidence that women who used estrogen-progestin HRT had a twofold to threefold higher risk of developing VTE than nonusers of estrogen-progestin HRT.[1–7]

The findings from these observational studies were corroborated in three randomized, placebo-controlled trials, also summarized in Table 33.1, that involved women without prior history of VTE.[8,9,18] The first trial, HERS, investigated oral conjugated equine estrogen (CEE), 0.625 mg daily, combined with oral medroxyprogesterone acetate (MPA), 2.5 mg daily in 2763 women with coronary artery disease (mean age 67 years) to assess the potential cardioprotective effect of HRT.[8] Apart from the principal finding that HRT does not decrease the risk for nonfatal myocardial

infarction and cardiovascular death, HRT users had a twofold increased risk for developing VTE (hazard ratio [HR] 2.08, 95 percent confidence interval [CI] 1.28 to 3.40). The risk was comparable for the development of deep vein thrombosis (HR 1.98, 95 percent CI 1.14 to 3.45) and for pulmonary embolism (HR 2.86, 95 percent CI 1.13 to 7.26). In terms of the absolute risk for VTE when assessed over the mean follow-up period of 6.8 years, the risk for VTE in users and nonusers of HRT was 5.9 events/1000 patient years, and 2.8 events/1000 patient years, respectively. The risk of VTE in the placebo group is somewhat higher than the 1–2 events/1000 patient years observed in studies that assessed the risk for VTE in the general population,[19] and may reflect differences in populations studied. There is emerging evidence suggesting that atherosclerotic vascular disease, which includes coronary artery disease, may predispose patients (such as those in HERS) to VTE by common mechanisms, possibly related to lipid abnormalities.[20] Estrogen-only and transdermal HRT preparations were not studied in HERS.

The second trial, the Estrogen Replacement and Atherosclerosis (ERA) study investigated the effects of estrogen-progestin HRT (0.625 mg CEE + 2.5 mg MPA), estrogen-only HRT (0.625 mg CEE), or placebo on the progression of coronary atherosclerosis in 309 postmenopausal women with coronary artery disease (mean age 66 years).[18] After a mean follow-up of 3.2 years, VTE occurred in 2 women (2 percent) who received estrogen-progestin HRT, 5 women (5 percent) who received estrogen-only HRT, and 1 woman (1 percent) who received placebo, and the difference across groups was not statistically significant ($P = 0.16$).

The third trial is the WHI,[9] a landmark study that involved approximately 16 000 postmenopausal women between the ages of 50 and 79 (mean age 64 years), and assessed CEE, 0.625 mg daily, and MPA, 2.5 mg daily. This study was principally designed to assess whether HRT would decease the risk for cardiovascular disease and what effect it had on breast cancer risk. Apart from the principal findings

Table 33.1 HRT and risk for VTE

| Authors/study | Study design | Risk of VTE according to type of HRT (risk ratio; 95% confidence interval) | | | |
		Oral E-only	Oral E+P	Transdermal E-only	Transdermal E+P
Daly et al.[1]	Case–control, matched, hospital based	3.2 (1.4 to 7.4)	5.3 (1.9 to 14.6)	2.0 (0.5 to 7.6)	
Jick et al.[2]	Case–control, matched, population based	4.1 (1.8 to 9.3)	2.4 (0.8 to 7.3)	NA	
Pérez Guttham et al.[3]	Nested case–control, population based	1.9 (1.0 to 3.8)	2.2 (1.4 to 3.5)	2.1 (0.9 to 4.6)	
Varas Lorenzo et al.[4]	Nested case–control, population based	1.4 (0.4 to 4.6)	5.0 (1.5 to 16.7)	2.3 (1.0 to 5.3)	
Grodstein et al.[5]	Prospective cohort, registered nurses	2.1 (1.2 to 3.8)		NA	
Høibraaten et al.[6]	Case–control, matched, hospital based	1.2 (0.8 to 1.9)		NA	
Douketis et al.[7]	Case–control, women with suspected VTE	1.2 (0.6 to 2.6)	2.7 (1.4 to 5.1)	NA	
Scarabin et al.[17]	Case–control, matched, hospital based	1.3 (0.1 to 18.8)	3.5 (1.9 to 6.8)	0.8 (0.3 to 2.5)	1.0 (0.3 to 3.3)
HERS[8]	Randomized controlled trial	NA	2.7 (1.4 to 5.0)	NA	
WHI[9]	Randomized controlled trial	1.3 (0.99 to 1.8)	2.1 (1.3 to 3.6)	NA	

E-only, estrogen-only HRT; E+P, combined estrogen-progestin HRT; HRT, hormone replacement therapy; NA, not available; VTE, venous thromboembolism.

of this study, that estrogen-progestin HRT increased the risk for cardiovascular events and breast cancer, HRT was associated with a twofold increased risk for VTE (HR 2.11, 95 percent CI 1.58 to 2.82). As in the HERS study, the risk was comparable for deep vein thrombosis (HR 2.07, 95 percent CI 1.49 to 2.87) and pulmonary embolism (HR 2.13, 95 percent CI 1.39 to 3.25).

Taken together, there are remarkably consistent findings regarding the association between HRT and VTE across different study designs (case–control, cohort, randomized trials) and patient populations.

Estrogen-only hormone replacement therapy

Estrogen-only HRT is typically used in women who have had a hysterectomy and, consequently, will not have as widespread use as estrogen-progestin HRT. Observational studies that investigated estrogen-only HRT found variable results, with findings summarized in Table 33.1. In three case–control studies,[3,4,6] estrogen-only HRT was not associated with a statistically significant increased risk for VTE, whereas three other studies reported a twofold to fourfold increased risk for VTE.[1,2,5] The HERS and ERA studies did not assess estrogen-only HRT. In the WHI study, there was a trend toward an increased risk for VTE with estrogen-only HRT although the risk did not attain statistical significance (HR 1.33, 95 percent CI 0.99 to 1.79).[21]

Overall, the strength of the association between estrogen-only HRT and VTE appears to be less than with estrogen-progestin HRT, although an estrogen-only HRT is still likely to be associated with an increased risk for VTE.

Transdermal hormone replacement therapy

Transdermal HRT is administered by a patch and can consist of combined estrogen-progestin or estrogen-only preparations. Transdermal HRT is widely used in Europe, whereas its use in North America is infrequent.[17] Transdermal HRT bypasses first pass hepatic metabolism that occurs with oral HRT, and it has been postulated that this pharmacokinetic property may account for the biochemical and clinical differences between oral and transdermal HRT.[22,23] As outlined below, transdermal HRT may be less likely to induce a prothrombotic state compared with oral HRT.

In terms of clinical studies that investigated the effects of transdermal HRT on the risk for VTE, there are fewer studies compared with oral HRT. An approximately twofold increased risk for VTE was found in two case–control studies that investigated transdermal HRT, with hazard ratios of 2.0 (95 percent CI 0.5 to 7.6), 2.1 (95 percent CI 0.9 to 4.6), and 2.3 (95 percent CI 1.0 to 5.3).[3,4] However, these studies were small, and fivefold to sevenfold increased risk for VTE with transdermal HRT could not be excluded. In another, larger, case–control study, which involved 536 patients, there was an increased risk for VTE

in users of oral HRT (HR 3.5, 95 percent CI 1.8 to 6.8), but no increased risk for VTE in users of transdermal HRT (HR 0.9, 95 percent CI 0.5 to 1.6).[17]

In summary, estrogen-progestin HRT is associated with about a twofold to threefold increased risk for VTE, estrogen-only HRT appears to be associated with a lower risk for VTE, whereas transdermal HRT may not be associated with an increased risk for VTE.

WHAT IS THE EFFECT OF THE DURATION OF HORMONE REPLACEMENT THERAPY ON THE RISK FOR VENOUS THROMBOEMBOLISM?

Determining the effect of the duration of HRT on the risk for VTE is clinically relevant because if the risk is dependent of the duration of exposure, this may help ascertain whether an episode of VTE is causally linked to VTE. For example, if the risk of VTE is limited to the initial 6–12 month period after starting HRT, episodes that are remote from this period of risk may not be causally linked to HRT. The clinical implication would be that such an episode of VTE may be considered unprovoked (or idiopathic), warranting consideration for long-term (>6 months) anticoagulation. On the other hand, an episode of VTE occurring soon after the start of HRT may be considered secondary to the HRT so that after withdrawing HRT, short-term (≤3 months) anticoagulant therapy may be sufficient.

Several studies have investigated the effect of the duration of HRT on the risk for VTE.[1–9] As outlined in Table 33.2, the pattern that appears to emerge is one of a heightened risk during the first year after the start of treatment that diminishes but does not disappear during the subsequent 4–5 years. This clustering of events soon after the start of HRT followed by a lessened but persistent risk over the long-term suggests two possible mechanisms for HRT-associated VTE. The first mechanism, analogous to a multiple hit pathogenesis, involves women who have a preexisting tendency for VTE and who on exposure to HRT develop clinically overt thromboembolism. Thus, HRT may act as a catalyst for the development of VTE in women with an inherited or acquired prothrombotic blood abnormality. This mechanism has been suggested for women who developed VTE soon after the start of the oral contraceptive. In one study, women who developed VTE within 1 year of starting an oral contraceptive were more likely to have inherited thrombophilia (that is, deficiencies of protein C or protein S) compared with women who developed VTE after a longer period of exposure to an oral contraceptive.[17] On the other hand, in women who develop VTE after long-term HRT use, the effect of HRT on the pathogenesis of VTE may be less prominent. In such women, one may speculate that HRT may have more subtle biochemical effects that, coupled with other clinical factors such as comorbid disease, may result in the development of VTE. Alternatively, HRT may be an innocent bystander, with the development of VTE being due to other nonhormonal factors. Finally, HRT may interact with, as of

Table 33.2   Effect of duration of oral HRT on risk for VTE

Authors/study	Risk of VTE according to duration of HRT*					
	1–6 months	1–12 months	12–24 months	24–36 months	36–48 months	> or ≥60 months
Daly et al.[1]	NA	6.7 (2.1 to 21.3)	4.4 (1.6 to 11.9)	1.9 (0.5 to 7.8)		2.1 (0.8 to 6.1)
Jick et al.[2]	NA	6.7 (1.5 to 30.8)	NA	NA	NA	4.4 (1.6 to 12.2)
Pérez Guttham et al.[3]	4.6 (2.5 to 8.4)	NA	1.1 (0.6 to 2.1)	1.1 (0.6 to 2.1)	1.1 (0.6 to 2.1)	1.1 (0.6 to 2.1)
Varas-Lorenzo et al.[4]		2.9 (1.2 to 6.9)	0.0 (0 to 4.1)	0.0 (0 to 4.1)	0.0 (0 to 4.1)	0.0 (0 to 4.1)
Grodstein et al.[5]	2.6 (1.2 to 5.2)	2.6 (1.2 to 5.2)	2.6 (1.2 to 5.2)	2.6 (1.2 to 5.2)	2.6 (1.2 to 5.2)	1.9 (0.9 to 4.0)
Høibraaten et al.[6]	NA	3.54 (1.5 to 8.2)	0.66 (0.4 to 1.1)	0.66 (0.4 to 1.1)	0.66 (0.4 to 1.1)	0.66 (0.4 to 1.1)
Douketis et al.[7]					NA	NA
Scarabin et al.[17]	NA	10.1 (1.1 to 92)	5.7 (1.4 to 23)	5.0 (1.4 to 18)	5.0 (1.4 to 18)	2.0 (0.8 to 4.7)
HERS[8]	NA	3.3	4.1	2.4	1.5	1.5
WHI[9]	NA	3.6	2.3	1.7	1.8	2.5

*Time periods approximate.
HRT, hormone replacement therapy; NA, not available; VTE, venous thromboembolism.

yet, undetermined inherited or acquired prothrombotic blood abnormalities or other genetic polymorphisms in the development of VTE.

WHAT IS THE MECHANISM FOR THE ASSOCIATION BETWEEN HORMONE REPLACEMENT THERAPY AND VENOUS THROMBOEMBOLISM?

The mechanism of HRT-associated VTE is not known. Proposed mechanisms include a procoagulant state related to HRT-associated increased thrombin generation, impaired fibrinolysis, or acquired activated protein C (APC) resistance.[24–26]

Effects of hormone replacement therapy on thrombin generation and fibrinolysis

Most studies that investigated the effects of HRT on the coagulation system have limited clinical relevance because nonspecific parameters of coagulation were assessed, such as fibrinogen, coagulation factor VII, and plasminogen, which are not reliable predictors of an increased risk for VTE. Measuring the effects of HRT on markers of thrombin generation (that is, fibrinopeptide A [FPA], prothrombin fragment 1+2 [F1+2], and thrombin-antithrombin [TAT] complex, and markers of fibrinolysis (that is, plasminogen, tissue plasminogen activator inhibitor [PAI]-1) may provide a more reliable assessment of the risk for VTE. Studies that have assessed the effects of HRT on F1+2, FPA, and TAT have yielded mixed results with no clear tendency toward a prothrombotic diathesis.[27–37] On the other hand, there appears to be a more consistent effect of HRT to decrease PAI-1 activity, thereby enhancing fibrinolytic activity.[27–37]

Effects of hormone replacement therapy on activated protein C resistance

Activated protein C resistance is an established risk factor for VTE and, in most patients, this prothrombotic abnormality is related to the presence of R506Q mutation in factor V Leiden. An acquired form of APC resistance can occur in the absence of the factor V Leiden mutation and may be associated with an increased risk for VTE. Acquired resistance to APC has been described with oral contraceptive use and, therefore, it has been postulated whether a similar effect can occur in users of HRT. In a randomized trial in 140 women (mean age 56 years) with previous VTE who received estrogen-progestin HRT or placebo, there was a statistically significant increase in ACP resistance with HRT.[38] However, in five women who developed recurrent VTE (all were receiving HRT), there was no significant difference in APC resistance between these women and those who were receiving HRT and did not develop recurrent VTE. In a randomized controlled trial of 196 postmenopausal women who received combined (estrogen and progestin) oral or transdermal HRT, oral but not transdermal HRT was associated with induction of resistance to APC. Other studies have provided conflicting results on the effects of HRT on APC resistance but these discrepant findings may be related to different laboratory methods used to measure APC resistance.[39–42]

Clinical significance of effects of hormone replacement therapy on biochemical indices

Although a number of studies have assessed the effects of HRT on biochemical markers and suggest that HRT may induce a prothrombotic state, what is lacking are studies that correlate these biochemical changes with clinical outcomes. Consequently, the clinical significance of the effects

Table 33.3   Effect of factor V Leiden on risk for VTE with estrogen-progestin hormone replacement therapy

Authors/study	Design	Risk of VTE according to presence or absence of factor V Leiden mutation	
		Factor V Leiden absent	Factor V Leiden present
Lowe et al.[48] Rosendaal et al.[49]	Case–control, matched, hospital based	3.9 (1.3 to 11.2)	15.5 (3.1 to 77)
Herrington et al.[50]	Nested case–control, from randomized trial	3.3 (1.1 to 9.8)	14.1 (2.7 to 72)
WHI[53]	Nested case–control, from randomized trial	2.2 (1.4 to 3.5)	6.7 (3.1 to 14.5)
Douketis[52]	Case–control, women with suspected VTE	3.2 (1.2 to 8.6)	17.1 (3.7 to 78)

VTE, venous thromboembolism.

of HRT on markers of thrombin generation, fibrinolysis, and APC remain unclear.

WHAT IS THE EFFECT OF THROMBOPHILIA ON THE RISK FOR VENOUS THROMBOEMBOLISM IN HORMONE REPLACEMENT THERAPY USERS?

Biochemical markers of thrombophilia refer to inherited or acquired prothrombotic blood abnormalities that are associated with an increased risk of developing VTE. The most common inherited prothrombotic abnormality is the factor V Leiden G1691A mutation, which occurs in 2–5 percent of Caucasian populations, and confers its prothrombotic effect by rendering factor Va resistant to degradation by activated protein C, an endogenous anticoagulant.[43] The prothrombin G20210A gene mutation, which occurs in 1–2 percent of Caucasian populations, may exert its prothrombotic effect through enhanced activation of prothrombin (or factor II).[43] Other inherited prothrombotic blood abnormalities are deficiencies in the endogenous anticoagulants protein C, protein S, and antithrombin.[43] The thermolabile variant of methylene tetrahydrofolate reductase C677T, the 4G/5G variant of PAI-1 and the factor XIII G100T variant, purported markers of thrombophilia, have not been shown to be associated with an increased risk for VTE.[44] Acquired prothrombotic abnormalities include deficiencies of hyperhomocysteinemia, usually due to vitamin B_6 or folate deficiency, and the antiphospholipid antibody syndrome, which occurs in the presence of a lupus anticoagulant or elevated anticardiolipin antibodies.[45]

In HRT users, the presence of a prothrombotic blood abnormality may further increase the risk for VTE, as has been observed in users of the oral contraceptive with the factor V Leiden or prothrombin gene mutation.[46,47] Recent studies, which have assessed this association, are summarized in Table 33.3. In the first study, a nested case–control study of the Oxford Regional Health Authority, the risk for VTE was approximately 13-fold higher in HRT users with the factor V Leiden mutation compared with nonusers of HRT without this mutation (odds ratio [OR] 13.3, 95 percent CI 4.3 to 41).[48] A further analysis that involved this

database found a similar increased risk for VTE in HRT users with the factor V Leiden mutation compared with non-users of HRT without this mutation (OR 15.5, 95 percent CI 3.1 to 77).[49] The type of HRT assessed, whether oral or transdermal, estrogen-progestin or estrogen-only, was not specified in these studies. The second study was a nested case–control study of pooled data from the HERS and ERA studies, the risk for VTE was approximately 14-fold higher in HRT users with the factor V Leiden mutation compared with nonusers of HRT without this mutation (OR 14.1, 95 percent CI 2.7 to 72).[50] In the third study, a nested case–control study of the WHI trial, the risk for VTE was approximately sevenfold higher in users of estrogen-progestin HRT with the factor V Leiden mutation compared with HRT nonusers without this mutation (OR 6.7, 95 percent CI 3.1 to 14.5).[51] This study also found a trend for an increased risk of VTE in HRT users with the prothrombin gene mutation compared to HRT non-users without this mutation (OR 2.9, 95 percent CI 0.94 to 8.7); the presence of the methylenetetrahydrofolate reductase C677T mutation, which is associated with hyperhomocysteinemia, did not confer a higher risk for VTE in HRT users compared to HRT nonusers (OR 1.8, 95 percent CI 0.77 to 4.1).

The fourth study was a prospective case–control involving postmenopausal women with suspected DVT. This study differed from the aforementioned studies in two ways. First, there was an assessment of the effects of inherited blood abnormalities (factor V Leiden and prothrombin mutations) and acquired blood abnormalities (elevated factor VIII and factor XI, hyperhomocysteinemia, antiphospholipid antibodies) modifying the association between HRT and VTE.[52] Second, there was an assessment of the effects of prothrombotic blood abnormalities in users of estrogen-progestin and estrogen-only HRT. In this study, the risk for VTE was approximately 17-fold higher in users of estrogen-progestin HRT with the factor V Leiden mutation compared with HRT nonusers without this mutation (OR 17.1, 95 percent CI 3.7 to 78). There was no statistically significant effect of the factor V Leiden mutation in users of estrogen-only HRT compared with HRT nonusers (OR 1.7, 95 percent CI 0.3 to 9.0). The other principal finding from this study was the effect of elevated factor VIII on the risk of DVT in HRT users compared with nonusers, summarized

Table 33.4 Effect of elevated factor VIII on risk for venous thromboembolism

| HRT type | Factor VIII quartiles (mmol/L) (risk ratio; 95% confidence interval) | | | |
	0.5–1.3	1.4–1.7	1.8–2.0	2.1–4.3
No HRT	1.0 (reference)	0.7 (0.2 to 2.5)	2.7 (0.9 to 8.0)	6.0 (2.1 to 17)
E-only	0.3 (0.1 to 1.3)	0.2 (0.1 to 1.5)	0.9 (0.2 to 5.4)	2.0 (0.3 to 11)
E+P	2.8 (1.0 to 7.9)	2.0 (0.4 to 11)	7.6 (1.6 to 37)	17.0 (3.6 to 80)

E, estrogen; HRT, hormone replacement therapy; P, progestin.

in Table 33.4. Thus, the risk of VTE in women with an elevated factor VIII who are using estrogen-progestin HRT is 2–17-fold higher than HRT nonusers without elevated factor VIII. The risk for VTE appears to be correlated with the level of factor VIII in users of both estrogen-progestin HRT and estrogen-only HRT.

CLINICAL MANAGEMENT SCENARIOS

Management of hormone replacement therapy users who develop venous thromboembolism

In women who develop VTE while using HRT, there are two clinical management issues that need to be addressed:

- Can HRT be discontinued?
- What is the anticoagulant management in terms of initial and long-term treatment?

With regard to the first issue, there are no prospective studies that have assessed the risk of progression of VTE or recurrent disease in women who stop HRT compared to those who continue HRT with concomitant anticoagulant therapy. However, it is generally accepted that HRT should be stopped as there are few, if any, clinical situations that would warrant ongoing treatment in the face of newly diagnosed VTE. One such situation might be patients who have debilitating climacteric symptoms in whom even temporary withdrawal of HRT may trigger recurrence of vasomotor and other climacteric symptoms. It is likely that concomitant anticoagulant therapy with warfarin, administered to achieve a target international normalized ratio (INR) of 2.0–3.0, will negate any prothrombotic effects of ongoing HRT. This assumption is based on the premise that in people in whom there is ongoing exposure to a prothrombotic stimulus, such as immobility, warfarin therapy is highly effective in preventing recurrent VTE.[53,54]

As regards the second issue, the initial anticoagulant management is the same as in women who develop VTE without associated HRT use, consisting of 4–6 days of therapeutic-dose unfractionated heparin or a low-molecular-weight heparin, overlapped with warfarin. The issue that, perhaps, is more problematic is the duration of anticoagulant therapy. In general, the duration of anticoagulant therapy for patients with VTE is determined by several factors, foremost of which

is whether the episode of VTE occurred during transient exposure to a reversible risk factor for VTE, during exposure to an ongoing risk factor for VTE, or whether the episode was unprovoked (or idiopathic). In patients who develop VTE during exposure to a transient risk factor, such as surgery, 3 months of treatment is deemed adequate, whereas in patients who develop VTE during exposure to an ongoing risk factor, such as advanced cancer or paralysis, indefinite treatment is recommended. The duration of treatment in patients with unprovoked VTE is controversial, although at least 6 months of treatment is recommended. In patients who develop VTE while using HRT (and other hormonal agents), 3 months of treatment has been recommended since such HRT is considered to be a transient (and reversible) risk factor. This approach is reasonable, particularly in women who develop VTE within months of starting HRT in whom HRT may have had a major role in the pathogenesis of VTE. On the other hand, in patients who develop VTE after they have used HRT for several years, the argument that HRT is a transient reversible risk factor is less compelling. In such patients, HRT may be an innocent bystander and there may be other factors that confer an ongoing risk for VTE even after HRT is stopped. Consequently, a 3-month course of anticoagulant therapy may be inadequate to reduce the risk for recurrent VTE. Ultimately, the duration of anticoagulant therapy in women who develop VTE in association with HRT is determined on an individual basis, and it may be reasonable to treat some patients for only 3 months and others for at least 6 months or longer.

In summary, the management of HRT-users who develop VTE involves:

- discontinuation, at least temporarily, of HRT
- 3 months of anticoagulant therapy in women who recently (within 12 months) started HRT or who had VTE occurring in the presence of a transient risk factor
- at least 6 months of anticoagulant therapy in women who were long-term users of HRT and in those with unprovoked VTE.[55]

Management of hormone replacement therapy users who require elective surgery

In users of HRT who require elective surgery, there is uncertainty as to whether HRT should be temporarily interrupted before and after surgery.[56,57] On the one hand, there is the potential that perioperative use of HRT will further increase the risk for DVT beyond that conferred by the surgical procedure and postoperative immobility. On the other hand, HRT is a relatively weak risk factor for VTE compared with the risk associated with surgery and any possible additive effect of HRT will not be important in terms of the overall risk. Thus, there is a twofold to three-fold increased in risk for VTE in users of HRT compared with nonusers, whereas there is a 40–50-fold increased risk for DVT in patients undergoing elective major orthopedic surgery compared with those not undergoing surgery.[58] Recent studies suggest that perioperative use of HRT is not associated with a significant increase in the risk for postoperative VTE. Thus, in a case–control study of 318 postmenopausal women (108 cases, 210 controls) who underwent hip or knee replacement surgery, there was no significant difference in the incidence of postoperative VTE in women who received perioperative HRT and women who did not receive perioperative HRT (17 percent vs. 23 percent; OR 0.66, 95 percent CI 0.35 to 1.18).[59] In another case–control study that assessed 1168 women with DVT (256 cases, 912 controls), a subgroup of whom had DVT occurring after exposure to a transient risk factor such as surgery or immobility, HRT use was not associated with an increased risk for DVT (OR 1.17, 95 percent CI 0.51 to 2.72).[60]

In summary, in HRT users who require elective surgery, there is no compelling evidence that HRT needs to be discontinued in the perioperative period. However, appropriate methods of thromboprophylaxis should be considered in such patients, particularly if there is anticipated postoperative immobility or in patients who are undergoing high-risk procedures such as major orthopedic surgery.

Assessment of women with prior venous thromboembolism or other venous thromboembolism risk factors who require hormone replacement therapy

GENERAL CONSIDERATIONS

The clinical management of women with previous VTE or other risk factors for VTE in whom there is a clinical indication for HRT is a relatively common clinical scenario given that VTE and risk factors for VTE are common and that 15–30 percent of postmenopausal women may require HRT for the relief of climacteric symptoms. However, few prospective studies addressing this issue are available to inform clinical practice. The overall approach to the management of such women should take into account the potential health benefits and risks of HRT and patient preference. In terms of the health benefits, the main benefit of HRT is the control of climacteric symptoms, whereas there may be several potential risks. In terms of health risks, this will depend on whether there is a personal or family history of breast cancer, coronary artery disease, stroke or other

cardiovascular disease, VTE, or other risk factors for VTE. Clinical management decisions should also take into consideration patient preferences for treatment or no treatment with HRT, and the option to reevaluate decisions about treatment over time. Finally, the issue of safety with different types of HRT warrants consideration. Although it is plausible that transdermal HRT may be associated with a lower (or no increased risk) for VTE compared to oral HRT, extrapolating this premise to women with previous VTE should be done with caution. Until there are prospective trials of different HRT preparations in women with previous VTE, all types of HRT should be used with caution in such patients.

In the context of the present review, the health risks of HRT pertain to women with previous VTE or with other VTE risk factors, and can be assessed using the following three-step approach:

1　estimating the patient's baseline risk for VTE
2　estimating the additive effect of a prothrombotic blood abnormality or exposure to HRT on the risk for VTE
3　determining the overall risk for VTE, which combines the baseline risk and the additive risk from one or more VTE risk factors.

The overall risk for VTE can be expressed as a relative risk, which compares the risk in a patient with one or more risk factors relative to the risk in a patient who does not have those risk factors. Alternatively, the overall risk for VTE can be expressed as an absolute risk, which refers to the annual or risk per year of having a VTE event.

The baseline risk for VTE will vary from patient to patient, and depends on age, sex, and the presence or absence of previous VTE or other comorbid factors, such as coronary artery disease or cancer. Thus, in healthy postmenopausal women, the annual risk for VTE, as determined from population-based epidemiologic studies, is about 0.1–0.2 percent per year. In postmenopausal women with coronary artery disease, the baseline risk for VTE, as determined from the HERS and ERA studies, is higher, at 0.5–0.6 percent per year. In postmenopausal women with previous VTE, the risk for a new or recurrent episode of VTE varies from 1–2 percent per year, in patients with secondary VTE that occurred during exposure to a transient risk factor, to 5–10 percent per year in patients who have had unprovoked (or idiopathic) VTE. These estimates pertain to the risk for recurrent VTE during the initial 1–2 years after the initial episode of VTE and may decrease over subsequent years. Suggested management options are outlined in Table 33.5.

WOMEN WITH ASYMPTOMATIC THROMBOPHILIA WHO REQUIRE HORMONE REPLACEMENT THERAPY

There is an increasing number of patients without a prior history of VTE who are undergoing testing for thrombophilia. This is usually prompted because a family

Table 33.5 Management of women with prior VTE or asymptomatic thrombophilia who require HRT

Clinical scenario	Suggested clinical management	Alternative clinical management
VTE occurring in association with HRT	Discontinue HRT permanently VTE occurring after exposure to transient risk factor (e.g., surgery, trauma) – short-term (3–6 mos) anticoagulation VTE occurring after short-term (≤12 mos) exposure to HRT and no other VTE risks – short-term (3–6 mos) anticoagulation VTE occurring after long-term (>12 mos) exposure to HRT and no other VTE risks – long-term (>6 mos) anticoagulation	Discontinue HRT temporarily and resume after ~3 months of anticoagulant therapy Long-term (>6 mos) anticoagulant therapy during coadministered HRT
Need for HRT in woman with asymptomatic thrombophilia	Coadministered HRT and oral anticoagulant therapy (target INR 2.0–3.0)	Coadministered HRT and once-daily low-molecular-weight heparin therapy Use of topical (estrogen cream) or progestin-only hormonal therapy No coadministered antithrombotic therapy and close clinical surveillance
Need for HRT in woman with previous VTE	Coadministered HRT and oral anticoagulant therapy (target INR 2.0–3.0)	Coadministered HRT and once-daily low-molecular-weight heparin therapy Use of topical (estrogen cream) or progestin-only hormonal therapy No coadministered antithrombotic therapy and close clinical surveillance

HRT, hormone replacement therapy; INR, international normalized ratio; VTE, venous thromboembolism.

member has developed VTE and testing is done to determine if a first degree relative is an asymptomatic carrier of an inherited blood abnormality such as the factor V Leiden or prothrombin mutation. There are no prospective studies that have assessed the risk for VTE with HRT use in asymptomatic women with a prothrombotic blood abnormality.

In otherwise healthy patients who are asymptomatic carriers of the factor V Leiden mutation, the risk for a first episode of VTE is fourfold to fivefold higher than the risk in patients without this mutation. In women who are asymptomatic carriers of the factor V Leiden mutation and are receiving HRT, the risk for a first episode of VTE is 7–15-fold higher than in patients without the factor V Leiden mutation who are not receiving HRT. Based on these relative risk estimates, the absolute risk for VTE can be determined based on individual patient characteristics. For example, in a patient who is a heterozygous carrier of the factor V Leiden mutation who is commencing treatment with HRT, the annual risk for VTE is estimated at 0.7–1.5 percent per year. Thus, for every 65 and 130 women treated with HRT, 1 will develop VTE per year.

Estimating the risk for VTE with HRT use in women with other prothrombotic blood abnormalities is problematic because of a lack of relevant data. Compared to heterozygous carriers of the factor V Leiden mutation, the risk for VTE appears less in carriers of the prothrombin mutation, and one can estimate the annual risk for VTE at <0.7 percent per year. In patients with deficiencies of endogenous anticoagulants (protein C, protein S, antithrombin), there are no data to provide estimates of risk for VTE. However, such patients have a high lifetime risk of developing VTE, which is up to 50 percent by the fourth or fifth decade of life. Consequently, it is likely that exposure to HRT in such women will be associated with a high absolute risk for VTE, irrespective of the additive effect of HRT on this risk. In women with elevated factor VIII, factor IX, or factor XI, or hyperhomocysteinemia, there are insufficient data to make inferences about risk for VTE, either in nonusers or users or HRT. Finally, in patients with antiphospholipid antibodies (APLA), there is also a lack of data to make inferences about VTE risk. However, such patients may be also at high risk for a first episode of VTE, particularly those with systemic lupus erythematosus, and can be considered similar to patients with deficiencies in endogenous anticoagulants.

In summary, the risk of a first VTE when starting HRT is likely to be high in women with a deficiency of endogenous anticoagulants, moderate-to-high in women with factor V Leiden or prothrombin mutations, and uncertain in women with elevated factor VIII, factor IX, or factor XI, or hyperhomocysteinemia.

WOMEN WITH PRIOR VENOUS THROMBOEMBOLISM WHO REQUIRE HORMONE REPLACEMENT THERAPY

This clinical scenario arises, typically, in women who have had prior VTE during exposure to the oral contraceptive, after surgery, or trauma, or in association with a prothrombotic blood abnormality. The risk of recurrent VTE with (re)exposure to HRT can be best estimated based on a randomized controlled trial of HRT in which 140 postmenopausal women with prior VTE received estrogen-progestin HRT (2 mg estradiol + 1 mg norethisterone).[61] In this study, there was about a fivefold higher risk of recurrent VTE in HRT users compared with nonusers (10.7 percent vs. 2.3 percent), leading to the premature termination of this study.

Overall, an estimate of the risk of recurrent VTE can be determined based on a patient baseline risk and the risk increase associated with HRT (re)exposure. In general, HRT should be avoided in women with previous VTE. If HRT is used, consideration should be given for the woman to receive coadministered antithrombotic therapy. One option is to use warfarin, administered to achieve a target INR of 2.0–3.0, in combination with HRT because the antithrombotic effects of warfarin are likely to neutralize any prothrombotic effects of HRT given that, in relative terms, HRT is a weak risk factor for VTE. However, this approach, although reasonable, has not been assessed in prospective randomized trials. An alternative management approach may be use of low-dose low-molecular-weight heparin therapy in combination with HRT, which has advantages over warfarin therapy of not requiring laboratory monitoring, but has disadvantages relating to greater costs and the potential for heparin-induced osteopenia with long-term use.[62] As with combined HRT-warfarin therapy, the efficacy and safety of this management strategy has not been elucidated.

FUTURE RESEARCH

There are several clinically important questions relating to HRT and VTE risk that warrant further investigation. First, and perhaps most importantly, is the issue of VTE risk in users of transdermal HRT. Specifically, additional studies are required to ascertain whether transdermal HRT may be a safer option in women with previous VTE or asymptomatic thrombophilia in whom HRT is needed for relief of menopausal symptoms. Second, the effect of adding progestin to estrogen on the risk for VTE warrants further investigation since progestin has, traditionally, not been associated with any prothrombotic effects. In particular, there is a need to assess whether progestin-only therapy is associated with an increased risk for VTE and may be safe to use in women at increased risk for VTE as is currently recommended. Finally, there is a need to establish consensus and uniform strategies in the assessment of women prior to the start of HRT so as to determine whether

screening for prothrombotic blood abnormalities is warranted and, if so, in which patients.

KEY LEARNING POINTS

- Clinical studies in different populations and using different designs (case–control, cohort, randomized trial) have established that users of HRT have an approximately twofold to threefold increased risk of developing VTE compared to nonusers of HRT.
- The risk of VTE may be higher in users of combined estrogen-progestin HRT than unopposed estrogen-only HRT; the former is used in women with an intact uterus and the latter is used in women who have had a hysterectomy.
- Use of transdermal (patch) HRT preparations may not be associated with an increased risk for DVT, although additional studies are warranted to further explore this observation.
- Users of HRT are at increased risk for developing VTE irrespective of the duration of HRT use although the risk appears higher during the first year of use.
- The mechanism by which HRT confers an increased risk for VTE has not been elucidated.
- In women who are carriers of the factor V Leiden mutation, the risk for VTE is markedly increased compared with the risk for VTE in women without the factor V Leiden mutation.

REFERENCES

1 Daly E, Vessey MP, Hawkins MM, *et al.* Risk of venous thromboembolism in users of hormone replacement therapy. *Lancet* 1996; **348**: 977–80.

2 Jick H, Derby LE, Myers MW, *et al.* Risk of hospital admission for idiopathic venous thromboembolism among users of post-menopausal estrogens. *Lancet* 1996; **348**: 981–3.

3 Pérez Gutthann S, Garcia-Rodriguez, Castellsague J, Duque Oliart A. Hormone replacement therapy and risk of venous thromboembolism: population based case–control study. *BMJ* 1997; **314**: 796–800.

4 Varas-Lorenzo C, García-Rodríguez LA, Cattaruzzi C, *et al.* Hormone replacement therapy and the risk of hospitalization for venous thromboembolism: a population-based study in southern Europe. *Am J Epidemiol* 1998; **149**: 387–90.

5 Grodstein F, Stampfer MJ, Goldhaber SZ, *et al.* Prospective study of exogenous hormones and risk of pulmonary embolism in women. *Lancet* 1996; **348**: 983–7.

6 Høibraaten E, Abdelnoor M, Sandset PM. Hormone replacement therapy with estradiol and risk of venous thromboembolism – a population-based case-control study. *Thromb Haemost* 1999; **82**: 1218–21.

7 Douketis JD, Julian JA, Crowther MA, *et al.* Does the type of hormone replacement therapy influence the risk of deep vein thrombosis? A prospective case-control study. *J Thromb Haemost* 2005; **3**: 943–8.

8 Grady D, Wenger NK, Herrington D, *et al.* Postmenopausal hormone replacement therapy increases risk for venous thromboembolic disease. The Heart and Estrogen/Progestin Replacement Study. *Ann Intern Med* 2000; **132**: 689–96.

9 Rossouw JE, Anderson GL, Prentice RL *et al.*; Writing Group for the Women's Health Initiative Investigators. Risks and benefits of estrogen plus progestin in healthy postmenopausal women. Principal results from the Women's Health Initiative Randomized Controlled Trial. *JAMA* 2002; **288**: 321–33.

10 Burger H. Hormone replacement therapy in the post-Women's Health Initiative era. Report of a meeting held in Funchal, Madeira, February 24, 2003. *Climacteric* 2003; **6**(Suppl 1): 11–36.

11 Solomon CG, Gluhy RG. Rethinking postmenopausal hormone therapy. *N Engl J Med* 2003; **348**: 579–80.

12 Hulley SB, Grady D. The WHI Estrogen-Alone Trial – do things look any better? *JAMA* 2004; **291**: 1769–71.

13 Humphries KH, Gill S. Risks and benefits of hormone replacement therapy: The evidence speaks. *CMAJ* 2003; **168**: 1001–10.

14 Col NF, Weber G, Stiggelbout A, *et al.* Short-term menopausal hormone therapy for symptom relief. *Arch Intern Med* 2004; **164**: 1634–40.

15 Kronenberg F. Hot flashes: epidemiology and physiology. *Ann N Y Acad Sci* 1990; **592**: 52–86.

16 Johnson SR. Menopause and hormone replacement therapy. *Med Clin North Am* 1998; **82**: 297–320.

17 Scarabin P-Y, Oger E, Plu-Bureau G, on behalf of the Estrogen and ThromboEmbolism Risk (ESTHER) Study Group. Differential association of oral and transdermal oestrogen-replacement therapy with venous thromboembolism risk. *Lancet* 2003; **362**: 428–32.

18 Herrington DM, Reboussin DM, Brosnihan KB, *et al.* Effects of estrogen replacement on the progression of coronary-artery atherosclerosis. *N Engl J Med* 2000; **343**: 5225–29.

19 Heit JA, Mohr DN, Petterson TM, *et al.* Predictors of recurrence after deep vein thrombosis and pulmonary embolism. A population-based cohort study. *Arch Intern Med* 2000; **160**: 761–8.

20 Prandoni P, Bilora F, Marchiori A, *et al.* An association between atherosclerosis and venous thrombosis. *N Engl J Med* 2003; **348**: 1435–41.

21 The Women's Health Initiative Steering Committee. Effects of conjugated equine estrogen in postmenopausal women with hysterectomy. *JAMA* 2004; **291**: 1701–12.

22 De Lignieres B, Basdevant A, Thomas G, *et al.* Biological effects of estradiol-17 beta in postmenopausal women: oral versus percutaneous administration. *J Clin Endocrinol Metab* 1986; **62**: 536–41.

23 Powers MS, Schenkel L, Darley PE, *et al.* Pharmacokinetics and pharmacodynamics of transdermal dosage forms of 17β-estradiol: comparison with conventional oral estrogens used for hormone replacement. *Am J Obstet Gynecol* 1985; **152**: 1099–106.

24 Rosendaal FR, Helmerhorst FM, Vandenbroucke JP. Female hormones and thrombosis. *Arterioscler Thromb Vasc Biol* 2002; **22**: 201–10.

25 Cano A, Van Baal WM. The mechanisms of thrombotic risk induced by hormone replacement therapy. *Maturitas* 2001; **40**: 17–38.

26 Cushman M. Effects of hormone replacement therapy and estrogen receptor modulators on markers of inflammation and coagulation. *Am J Cardiol* 2002; **90**(Suppl): 7F–10F.

27 Teede HJ, McGrath BP, Smolich JJ, *et al.* Postmenopausal hormone replacement therapy increases coagulation activity and fibrinolysis. *Arterioscler Thromb Vasc Biol* 2000; **20**: 1404–9.

28 Perry W, Wiseman RA. Combined oral estradiol valerate-norethisterone treatment over 3 years in postmenopausal women. Effect on lipids, coagulation factors, haematology and biochemistry. *Maturitas* 2002; **42**: 157–64.

29 Luyer MDP, Khosla S, Owen WG, *et al.* Prospective randomized study of effects of unopposed estrogen replacement therapy on markers of coagulation and inflammation in postmenopausal women. *J Clin Endocrinol Metab* 2001; **86**: 3629–34.

30 Van Baal WM, Emeis JJ, van der Mooren MJ, *et al.* Impaired procoagulant–anticoagulant balance during hormone replacement therapy? A randomized, placebo-controlled 12-week study. *Thromb Haemost* 2000; **83**: 29–34.

31 Høibraaten E, Os I, Seljeflot I, *et al.* The effects of hormone replacement therapy on hemostatic variables in women with angiographically verified coronary artery disease: results from the estrogen in women with atherosclerosis study. *Thromb Res* 2000; **98**: 19–27.

32 Vehkavaara S, Silveira A, Hakala-Ala-Pietila, *et al.* Effects of oral and transdermal estrogen replacement therapy on markers of coagulation, fibrinolysis, inflammation and serum lipids and lipoproteins in postmenopausal women. *Thromb Haemost* 2001; **85**: 619–25.

33 Cushman M, Psaty BM, Meilahn EN, *et al.* Post-menopausal hormone therapy and concentrations of protein C and antithrombin in elderly women. *Br J Haematol* 2001; **114**: 162–8.

34 Whiteman MK, Cui Y, Flaws JA, *et al.* Low fibrinogen level: a predisposing factor for venous thromboembolic events with hormone replacement therapy. *Am J Hematol* 1999; **61**: 271–3.

35 Nozaki M, Ogata R, Koera K, *et al.* Changes in coagulation factors and fibrinolytic components of postmenopausal women receiving continuous hormone replacement therapy. *Climacteric* 1999; **2**: 124–30.

36 Perera M, Sattar N, Petrie JR, *et al.* The effects of transdermal estradiol in combination with oral

norethisterone on lipoproteins, coagulation, and endothelial markers in postmenopausal women with type 2 diabetes: a randomized, placebo-controlled study. *J Clin Endocrinol Metab* 2001; **86**: 1140–3.

37   Braunstein JB, Kershner DW, Bray P, *et al*. Interaction of hemostatic genetics with hormone therapy: new insights to explain arterial thrombosis in postmenopausal women. *Chest* 2002; **121**: 906–20.

38   Høibraaten E, Mowinckel M-C, de Ronde H, *et al*. Hormone replacement therapy and acquired resistance to activated protein C: results of a randomized, double-blind, placebo-controlled trial. *Br J Haematol* 2001; **115**: 415–20.

39   Oger E, Alhene-Gelas M, Lacut K, *et al*. Differential effects of oral and transdermal estrogen/progesterone regimens on sensitivity to activated protein C among postmenopausal women. A randomized trial. *Arterioscler Thromb Vasc Biol* 2003; **23**: 1671–6.

40   Post MS, Rosing J, van der Mooren MJ, *et al*. Increased resistance to activated protein C after short-term oral hormone replacement therapy in healthy post-menopausal women. *Br J Haematol* 2002; **119**: 1017–23.

41   De Mitrio V, Marino R, Cicinelli E, *et al*. Beneficial effects of postmenopausal hormone replacement therapy with transdermal estradiol on sensitivity to activated protein C. *Blood Coag and Fibrinolysis* 2000; **11**: 175–82.

42   Douketis JD, Gordon M, Johnston M, *et al*. The effects of hormone replacement therapy on thrombin generation, fibrinolysis inhibition, and resistance to activated protein C: prospective cohort study and review of the literature. *Thromb Res* 2000; **99**: 25–34.

43   Crowther MA, Kelton JG. Congenital thrombophilic states associated with venous thrombosis: a qualitative overview and proposed classification system. *Ann Intern Med* 2003; **138**: 128–34.

44   den Heijer M. Hyperhomocysteinaemia as a risk factor for venous thrombosis: an update of the current evidence. *Clin Chem Lab Med* 2003; **11**: 1404–7.

45   Kearon C, Crowther M, Hirsh J. Management of patients with hereditary hypercoagulable disorders. *Annu Rev Med* 2000; **51**: 169–85.

46   Rosing J, Middeldorp S, Curvers J, *et al*. Low-dose oral contraceptives and acquired resistance to activated protein C: a randomized cross-over study. *Lancet* 1999; **354**: 2036–40.

47   Kemmeren JM, Algra A, Grobbee DE. Third generation oral contraceptives and risk of venous thrombosis: meta-analysis. *BMJ* 2001; **323**: 1–9.

48   Lowe G, Woodward M, Vessey M, *et al*. Thrombotic variables and risk of idiopathic venous thromboembolism in women aged 45–64 years. *Thromb Haemost* 2000; **83**: 530–5.

49   Rosendaal FR, Vessey M, Rumley A, *et al*. Hormonal replacement therapy, prothrombotic mutations and the risk of venous thrombosis. *Br J Haematol* 2002; **116**: 851–4.

50   Herrington DM, Vittinghoff E, Howard TD, *et al*. Factor V Leiden, hormone replacement therapy, and risk of venous thromboembolic events in women with coronary disease. *Arterioscler Thromb Vasc Biol* 2002; **22**: 1012–17.

51   Cushman M, Kuller LH, Prentice R, *et al*. Estrogen plus progestin and risk of venous thrombosis. *JAMA* 2004; **292**: 1573–80.

52   Douketis J. The effect of prothrombotic blood abnormalities on the association between hormone replacement therapy and venous thromboembolism [abstract]. *J Thromb Haemost* 2003.

53   Kearon C. Duration of therapy for acute venous thromboembolism. *Clin Chest Med* 2003; **24**: 63–72.

54   Rosendaal FR. Venous thrombosis: a multicausal disease. *Lancet* 1999; **353**: 1167–51.

55   Büller HR, Agnelli G, Hull RD, *et al*. Antithrombotic therapy for venous thromboembolic disease: The Seventh ACCP Conference on Antithrombotic and Thrombolytic Therapy. *Chest* 2004; **126**: 401S–28S.

56   Wallace WA. HRT and the surgeon. Guidelines from the Royal College of Surgeons of Edinburgh. *J R Coll Surg Edin* 1993; **38**: 58–61.

57   Ardern DW, Atkinson DR, Fenton AJ. Peri-operative use of oestrogen containing medications and deep vein thrombosis: a national survey. *N Z Med J* 2002; **115**: 1157–63.

58   Geerts WH, Pineo GF, Heit HA, *et al*. Prevention of venous thromboembolism. The Seventh ACCP Conference on Antithrombotic and Thrombolytic Therapy. *Chest* 2004; **126**: 188S–203S.

59   Hurbaneck JG, Jaffer AK, Morra N, *et al*. Postmenopausal hormone replacement and venous thromboembolism following hip and knee arthroplasty. *Thromb Haemost* 2004; **92**: 337–43.

60   Douketis JD, Julian JA, Costantini L, for the HRT-DVT Study Group. HRT and the risk of DVT: the role of progesterone and other factors in the pathogenesis of HRT-associated DVT [abstract]. *Thromb Haemost* 2001.

61   Høibraaten E, Qvigstad E, Arnesen H, *et al*. Increased risk of recurrent venous thromboembolism during hormone replacement therapy. Results of the randomized, double-blind, placebo-controlled estrogen in venous thromboembolism trial (EVTET). *Thromb Haemost* 2000; **84**: 961–7.

62   Hirsh J, Raschke R. Heparin and low-molecular-weight heparin: The Seventh ACCP Conference on Antithrombotic and Thrombolytic Therapy. *Chest* 2004; **126**: 188S–203S.

34

Practical strategies for prescribing hormone replacement therapy

MARY ANN LUMSDEN

INTRODUCTION

There are few prescribed drugs that give rise to such controversy as hormone replacement therapy (HRT). Many individuals, both professional and lay, have strong feelings either for or against it. The publication of the large studies that are discussed in this chapter and elsewhere in this book has altered the prescribing practices of virtually all doctors involved in the care of menopausal women.

Hormone replacement therapy, now often known as hormone therapy (HT), is taken by millions of women, usually for a relatively short time, the aim being to improve their quality of life. Its use in disease prevention has been advocated, but this role is currently being questioned. This chapter will consider the symptoms that lead women to request HRT, and the risks and benefits of HRT in both the short and the long term. Alternatives to HRT will also be briefly discussed. It is then possible to suggest some practical strategies for its prescription.

MENOPAUSAL SYMPTOMS

Approximately 80 percent of women in the United Kingdom will experience symptoms during the menopausal transition.

For some women these symptoms may be relatively mild and short lasting, but for others, the menopause can cause significant physical and psychological morbidity.[1] Those most frequently mentioned by women and thought to be associated with loss of ovarian function are listed in Box 34.1. Most of the physiologic changes associated with the menopause start prior to the last menstrual period, this transition often being termed the perimenopause.[2]

Box 34.1 Common menopausal symptoms

- Menstrual problems
- Hot flushes and palpitations
- Night sweats
- Sleep disturbance
- Vaginal dryness
- Urinary urgency
- Depressed mood
- Irritability
- Lethargy
- Forgetfulness and loss of concentration
- Loss of libido

VASOMOTOR SYMPTOMS

The hot flash is considered the classic menopausal symptom. It is characterized by an intermittent sensation of heat, flashes, and perspiration usually affecting the face, neck, and chest. The lack of predictability of flashes can be distressing for women who sense a lack of control and often report feelings of embarrassment. Hot flashes are experienced by up to 85 percent of women in relation to the menopause and are a significant problem for up to 45 percent. Women who undergo a surgical menopause have a precipitous fall in hormone levels and tend to experience more severe hot flashes than those who undergo a natural menopause.[3] Hot flashes are also a particular problem in those with breast cancer who are receiving hormonal therapy such as tamoxifen or an aromatase inhibitor, since severe flashes occurs in 30–50 percent of these women, and treatment is difficult as will be discussed later.[4]

When hot flashes occur at night they are known as night sweats. Insomnia is a common feature of vasomotor problems at night and in the long term, the sleep disturbance can contribute to fatigue and psychologic effects, particularly loss of concentration and mood swings.[2] Estrogen has been demonstrated by many randomized controlled trials (RCTs) to treat hot flashes effectively and remains the gold standard therapy.[5,6] Other options include progestogens, which have been shown to reduce flashes in women where estrogen is contraindicated.[7] Also clonidine[8] and venlafaxine[9] can be considered but are generally less effective than estrogen.

VAGINAL ATROPHY AND URINARY EFFECTS

Estrogen deprivation causes effects not only because of the thin vaginal mucosa and lack of lubrication, but also because of the increased susceptibility to infection. Together, these factors result in a range of symptoms including localized discomfort, a burning or itching sensation, dyspareunia, and discharge. Atrophy of the periurethral tissues can contribute to symptoms of frequency, urgency, and predispose to urinary tract infection. The timing of urogenital symptoms in relation to the menopause varies. Some women will experience atrophic changes perimenopausally. However, for the majority of women, urogenital symptoms occur several years after the menopause.

Vaginal dryness can be easily treated with topical estrogen therapy or systemic HRT.[10] For women with recurrent urinary tract infection, vaginal estrogens have been shown to significantly reduce the rate of infection when compared to placebo but it has little effect on stress incontinence.[11–14] The role of estrogen in the management of stress incontinence remains controversial.[10] The amount of topical estrogen absorbed into the systemic circulation is extremely small and there are no data to suggest that it cannot be given to women with breast cancer for the relief of urogenital symptoms.[15]

MENSTRUAL PROBLEMS

Many perimenopausal women find that their periods become irregular and may be heavy. An embarrassing problem is that of unpredictable flooding and also many complain of tiredness, which impairs their ability to function properly. Hormone replacement therapy can help regulate the periods and prevent heavy, anovulatory cycles. However, other treatments, for example, tranexamic acid, the Mirena intrauterine incision or surgical treatment may be required in addition.[16]

ANXIETY AND DEPRESSION

There is little evidence of higher rates of major depression among postmenopausal women than in premenopausal women and the levels of hormones are no different in depressed women when compared with nondepressed women.[17,18] Relatively high doses of estrogen have been shown to treat women with severe depression effectively.[19,20] Although it should not automatically be assumed that a woman is depressed because she is menopausal, there is a case for using HRT in woman in the perimenopausal or menopausal phase as a first-line option if other menopausal symptoms are present, assuming there is no contraindication. Counseling should be considered together with use of antidepressants when required.

LOSS OF CONCENTRATION/POOR MEMORY

A frequent complaint among menopausal women is an inability to concentrate and an impaired short-term memory. These are both highly subjective problems that may have a relation with other menopausal symptoms such as flashes or sleep disturbance. An improvement in cognitive functioning for women who were experiencing menopausal symptoms has been shown in RCTs, but these trials have been unable to demonstrate a clear benefit for women without menopausal symptoms.[21,22] The Women's Health Initiative (WHI) memory study failed to demonstrate an improvement in cognitive function in women over 65 years of age.[23]

SEXUAL FUNCTION

Both estrogens and androgens have a role in the control of libido and sexual function and some women with problems will benefit considerably from administration of these hormones.[24–26]

OSTEOPOROSIS

With increased life expectancy, developed societies have an ever increasing elderly population. This is associated with

Box 34.2 Most common sites at risk of osteoporotic fractures

- Vertebral bodies
- Ends of long bones in particular, hip and wrist
  - Proximal femur
  - Distal radius (Colles fracture)

degenerative diseases, one of which is osteoporosis. In the past, one of the principal reasons why HRT was advocated was the positive effect on bone metabolism and it was felt that when started at the right time, HRT could play a role in disease prevention.[27] Osteoporotic fractures typically occur in sites where there is a high proportion of trabecular bone (Box 34.2).

Epidemiology

The implications of osteoporosis, both to society and to the individual, are considerable – 1 in 3 women and 1 in 12 men will develop osteoporosis. It is estimated that 3 million patients in the United Kingdom have osteoporosis. This translates to over 200 000 fractures annually. About half of all patients who experience a fractured hip will lose the ability to live independently and a third will die within a year.[28] In the United Kingdom, the costs to National Health Service (NHS) and government currently are £1.7 billion per year.[29,30] The incidence of osteoporosis-related fracture within developed populations has been climbing and this trend is likely to continue. As bone density declines with age, it is likely that increased life expectancy is responsible for most of this increase but it may be that lifestyle changes are also contributing.

Risk factors

Osteoporosis is a multifactorial disorder and whether an individual patient develops the disease will depend on peak bone mass and the rate of its subsequent loss. In women, the peak bone mass is less than in men and a more rapid loss occurs in the 10 years after the menopause. Women have a longer life expectancy than men and together, these factors account for the female preponderance of the disease.

Prevention and treatment

Specific therapy for prevention of osteoporosis is mainly directed at preventing the accelerated loss of bone mass that occurs in the postmenopausal period. Ideally, the treatment will be tailored to the individual patient and will depend, to a degree, on the likely cause. Any reversible factors such as smoking, excessive alcohol, or lack of weight-bearing exercise should be addressed if possible. Any factors that may

increase the risk of falls, for example, sedative medication or unsafe environment, should be considered. In patients prone to falls, simple measures such as hip protectors may be helpful.

Estrogen

The relation between osteoporosis and sex steroids is well established and can result in a loss of up to 15 percent of the skeletal bone mass in the years following the menopause. Epidemiologic evidence suggests that women who experience less exposure to endogenous estrogen have a higher risk of osteoporosis, for example, women who undergo a premature menopause. Some of the earliest evidence of a protective effect of estrogen on bone was in the form of case–control studies and these with other RCTs have now been confirmed following the publication of results from the WHI.[31–38]

Recent studies have shown that lower doses of HRT are effective in improving bone density in older women (>65 years) who are also more likely to experience side effects with standard doses of HRT and opting for a lower dose may be more appropriate.[39] Current recommendations for the use of HRT in prevention and treatment of osteoporosis are considered later.

Alternative therapy for osteoporosis

There are other effective options available for the management of osteoporosis, but the options for management of menopausal symptoms are limited. Some of the progestogens can be useful for these symptoms.[40] Osteoporosis is effectively treated by the bisphosphonates but these have their own side effects and are not well tolerated by all women.[41–44] They also need to be taken on the long term and side effects with long term use are still unknown. The selective estrogen receptor modulators[45] are valuable in the older woman although hot flashes can be an unacceptable side effect. Although all elderly women are at risk of osteoporosis, those with risk factors should be particularly encouraged to take appropriate preventative measures. Parathyroid hormone, calcitonin,[46,47] strontium,[48] vitamin D,[49] and calcium[50,51] are also currently being evaluated.

HORMONE REPLACEMENT THERAPY, DEMENTIA, AND ALZHEIMER DISEASE

Dementia is a heterogeneous disorder that is present in 10 percent of the population beyond the age of 65 and 50 percent of the population beyond the age of 85. Alzheimer's disease (AD) is the most common cause of dementia and there are few therapeutic options for this disorder. Women appear to be more at risk of developing AD and prospective cohort studies have shown that estrogen use is associated with a 50 percent reduction in developing AD.[52–54] Unfortunately,

RCTs of the effect of estrogen on the cognitive abilities of women with dementia have failed to show an improvement. It may be that estrogen has a role in the prevention of Alzheimer's and this could account for the lower rates of the disease in HRT users.[55] If proven an effective therapy then this would alter the whole risk/benefit equation for postmenopausal women. The WHI failed to provide evidence for a role in prevention or treatment of women over 65 years of age.[56]

HORMONE REPLACEMENT THERAPY AND CARDIOVASCULAR DISEASE

Observational trials

Ten years ago it was believed that HRT would have a place in the prevention of chronic disease: not only osteoporosis but also both Alzheimer's and cardiovascular disease. The idea was based on observational studies such as the Nurses' Health Study, which suggested a 50 percent decrease in the incidence of cardiovascular disease in those taking HRT.[57–59] Many of the known biologic effects of estrogen on the vascular system and bone support these findings[60,61] although its effect on coagulation and fibrinolysis is less easy to interpret.[62–64] However, observational studies may demonstrate a degree of selection bias, in that women who choose to take HRT may already have a healthier lifestyle with less environmental risk behaviors than women who do not. In addition, the consistency in the gradient of the coronary heart disease (CHD) incidence curve at the time of the menopause confounds the proposed importance of estrogen deficiency. Consequently large RCTs were set up with prevention of cardiovascular disease as the primary endpoint.

Randomized controlled trials of hormone replacement therapy in heart disease prevention

The first to report was the Heart and Estrogen Replacement Study (HERS), a study of the secondary prevention of heart disease where women were randomized to receive either placebo or a combination of conjugated equine estrogen (CEE) and medroxyprogesterone acetate (MPA).[65] The results defied expectations. Overall, there was no difference in event rates in the hormone group and the placebo group over a mean follow-up of 4.1 years of the study. Moreover, there appeared to be a time trend with a greater number of coronary heart disease (CHD) events in the first year of use in women randomized to take HRT and fewer events in years 4 and 5. As a result of their findings, the authors correctly cautioned against commencing HRT in women with CHD, for the purpose of secondary prevention of acute events. However, given the favorable trend of CHD events after several years of therapy, they suggested that women with CHD, who are established on HRT could be advised to

continue. This advice had less impact in the United Kingdom than the United States as HRT was rarely used for this purpose alone in the United Kingdom. A common criticism of this paper was the advanced age and poor health of the women taking part. Consequently, the results of the primary prevention studies were eagerly awaited.

In July 2002, the WHI, a randomized, controlled trial of CEE and MPA versus placebo in healthy women was stopped because it was determined that the risks outweighed the benefits (the Writing Group of WHI).[38] Although this was the first study to demonstrate definitively that HRT prevented osteoporotic fractures and also decreased the incidence of colon cancer, these benefits were outweighed by the increased likelihood of a cardiovascular event, stroke and breast cancer, the latter reaching significance after 5 years of HRT use. Breast cancer is the most common cause of death in women of 50–56 years of age who are the most likely to take HRT for menopausal symptoms. The estrogen-only arm of WHI failed to show any significant increase in the incidence of both heart disease and breast cancer in those on HRT.[66]

Hormone replacement therapy and venous thromboembolism

Case–control studies have shown an increase in the relative risk of venous thromboembolism (VTE) in women using estrogen-containing HRT.[67–70] These studies consistently show an increased relative risk of VTE, although the absolute risk, in the absence of other risk factors, is low. The recent report from the EStrogen and THromboEmbolism Risk (ESTHER) case–control study in France,[71] showed that transdermal estrogen replacement therapy was not associated with the increased risk of VTE associated with oral preparations.[72] This may be due to the fact that transdermal HRT is not subject to first pass metabolism and has little effect on the synthesis of both coagulation factors and inflammatory mediators.[64]

The frequency of VTE in postmenopausal women is around double that of premenopausal women. In women using oral HRT there is an increased risk amounting to 4 (3–5) extra cases/1000 women aged 50–59 and 9(4–14) extra cases/1000 users in women aged 60–69.[72] It is not only the interaction of age and HRT that is responsible for the increased risk of VTE, which is now thought to be an independent risk factor to be included with obesity, varicose veins, past history of VTE, family history, and thrombophilias. Oral HRT leads to an increase in the recurrence rate of VTE[73] and should be avoided particularly when other additional risk factors are present such as a thrombophilia. This is probably because it increases activated protein C resistance, as well as having other adverse effects on both coagulation and fibrinolysis factors.[74] It is probable that oral HRT leads to an imbalance between increased coagulation factors and decreased coagulation inhibition. This may vary with the different constituents of HRT although little information is available. Oral estrogen is also known to increase inflammatory mediators such as C-reactive protein (CRP) levels. However, the significance of this in the pathogenesis of venous thromboembolism is unclear.

A recent publication from WHI indicated that the risk of VTE was doubled and increased the risk associated with age, obesity, and factor V Leiden.[75] Overall, HRT should be avoided in all women with a history of VTE unless the patient is receiving an anticoagulant

Coronary heart disease and stroke

The data relating to cardiovascular disease and the lack of any protection with HRT has already been discussed above. Both the combined arm and estrogen-only arm of WHI reported an increase in incidence in HT arm as opposed to the placebo, this being the principal reason why the estrogen-only arm was stopped prematurely.[38,66] The findings suggest that oral CEE is thrombogenic in both the arterial and venous circulation. Hormone replacement therapy is associated with an increase in stroke risk (odds ratio [OR] 1.30, confidence interval [CI] 1.09 to 1.54) and for fatal or disabling stroke 1.56 (1.11 to 2.30). This risk is confined to ischemic stroke.[76] However, all patients should be aware that the actual increase in risk is numerically extremely small, particularly in women of perimenopausal age.

The randomized trials have established that HRT does not reduce the risk of cardiovascular disease and should not be prescribed for this purpose. Whether there is an early increase in the incidence is still a matter of debate. This appeared to be the case in the combined arm but not the estrogen only. In addition, in the combined arm, HRT did not confer protection against peripheral vascular disease[77] and there was a trend towards an early increase in risk.

There are many explanations for the divergence between the observational data and those of the randomized studies. These center around the likelihood that women who choose to take HRT are generally healthier than those who choose not to. The women in the randomized studies are older since a randomized trial of heart disease prevention in peri-menopausal women would need to be very large as the event rate at this age is very low. Only one preparation was tested and this type of HRT is not commonly used in Europe. There has also been widespread discussion of the study design and interpretation of the data since the estrogen-only arm suggests that there is the possibility that some benefit may be obtained if HRT is started at the time of the menopause.

Mechanism for the increased risk of coronary heart disease and stroke in hormone replacement therapy users

The prothrombotic effects of HRT are summarized elsewhere. As mentioned above, oral HRT causes an increase

in inflammatory factors although this occurs to a much lesser extent with transdermal estradiol and the effect may also be modified by the progestogen component. It is now thought that the association of CRP with CHD risk may have been overestimated.[78]

Implications for the prescription of hormone replacement therapy

Women must be advised of the increased risk in absolute terms and should be made aware of the signs and symptoms of VTE and the implications. Those at increased risk should be prescribed a transdermal preparation and a thrombophilia screen should be considered, as additional risk factors for thrombosis appear to have a synergistic effect.[74] For those at high risk who are determined to take HRT the possibility of anticoagulation should be discussed with a hematologist. There is debate whether HRT should be stopped prior to surgery but usually this is not an issue as the women are over 40 and will usually receive antithrombotic prophylaxis as a routine. On current evidence, HRT should be avoided in women with clinical arterial disease although hypertension is not a contraindication as HRT des not have an adverse effect.

Prescribing for the women at high risk of coronary heart disease

There are, clearly, many women who would benefit from HRT for menopausal symptoms but who are at an elevated risk of CHD. From available data, it may be possible to predict HRT preparations, which may provide a more favorable physiologic response and, therefore, be more suitable for such women. Preparations that contain low-dose estradiol, rather than CEE and transdermal as opposed to oral administration, may be more suitable with potentially less effect on pathways implicated in increasing plaque instability. The North American Menopause Society reached broadly similar conclusions in a consensus statement for women with type 2 diabetes.[79] Consequently, these preparations may avoid the potential early increase in CHD risk seen with oral CEE-based preparations. The ideal choice of progestogen remains unclear.

ADVERSE EFFECTS OF HORMONE REPLACEMENT THERAPY

Long-term adverse effects: hormone replacement therapy and cancer risk

HRT AND RISK OF ENDOMETRIAL CANCER

The exposure to unopposed estrogens is a well-proved risk factor for development of endometrial hyperplasia and potentially endometrial cancer. The addition of progesterone to HRT preparations significantly reduces the risks of endometrial cancer. With regard to long-term use of sequential regimens, it appears that the risk of developing endometrial cancer increases, although to a lesser degree than if using unopposed estrogen. It may be that greater protection from endometrial cancer is provided by continuous combined preparations where the endometrium receives a daily dose of progesterone.[80,81] Long-term use of sequential preparations will require additional monitoring. The findings of the Million Women Study suggest that estrogen alone should be considered even in those with a uterus as the risk of endometrial cancer is significantly less than that of breast cancer. However, this idea has not yet become accepted clinical practice.

HRT AND RISK OF BREAST CANCER

Breast cancer is now the most commonly diagnosed malignancies in the United Kingdom and by age 74, 1 in 9 women will have developed breast cancer. Unsurprisingly, breast cancer is a major concern for women in the developed world. Observational data have shown that HRT confers a small, but significantly increased, risk of developing breast cancer with long term use (Table 34.1).[82] Women who may be considering taking HRT often overestimate this increase in risk. It is helpful to compare the background level of breast cancer when considering the additional risk that HRT confers.[83] Years of HRT use appear to equate to years of natural female hormones, that is, a woman who has an early menopause without HRT will have a lower risk of breast cancer when compared with a women who has a later menopause. These risks are generally thought to apply to years beyond the average age of menopause of 51. A woman with an early menopause may require many years of HRT before she even reaches the age of 51 but should consider this as replacement of 'normal' hormones that would have been present otherwise.

The Million Women Study[84] that included precisely the women to whom HRT is most often prescribed in terms of age demonstrated that all types of HRT increased the incidence of breast cancer, although to a variable degree, estrogen combined with progestogen having a greater effect than estrogen alone. The estrogen-only arm (CEEs versus placebo) of WHI then reported subsequently that there was a trend toward less breast cancer in those using estrogen alone.

Table 34.1 Breast cancer risk (incidence per 1000 women)[72]

No HRT	32/1000
HRT for 5 years	Additional 1.5 (±1.5) women (E alone)
	Additional 6 (±1) women (E + P)
HRT for 10 years	Additional 6 (±1) women (E alone)
	Additional 19 (±1) women (E + P)

E, estrogen alone; E + P, estrogen + progestogen; HRT, hormone replacement therapy

Short-term adverse effects

VAGINAL BLEEDING

The most common symptom to cause compliance problems is continued vaginal bleeding. The development of continuous combined no-period preparations has allowed women who find a withdrawal bleed unacceptable to continue using HRT. The drawback of these preparations is that a significant minority will have ongoing irregular vaginal bleeding. The bleeding improves within the first 6 months for the vast majority.[85,86] Bleeding can also be lessened by the use of levonorgestrel-secreting intrauterine system, the insertion of which avoids the need for systemic progestogen administration. It is associated with a significantly lower incidence of progestogen-associated side effects.

FEAR OF WEIGHT GAIN

Weight gain, or the concern over potential weight gain, is a frequently cited reason for stopping HRT. Several studies have shown that weight gain tends to occur in the middle years for both women who are on HRT, and, for women who are not on HRT. There are changes that occur in distribution of adipose tissue following menopause with an increase in the proportion of central abdominal fat. This 'android' deposition of fat is associated with a higher risk of cardiovascular disease and it may be that the use of HRT causes redistribution of fat to 'female' areas such as hips.[87, 88]

CONTRAINDICATIONS TO HORMONE REPLACEMENT THERAPY USE

The contraindications to the combined pill were, initially, used as contraindications to hormone replacement therapy, however, it has become apparent over the years that this practice is unnecessary. The doses of hormone used in HRT are much closer to physiologic levels and fewer contraindications remain. If women in the category in Box 34.3 have menopausal symptoms they should be referred to a specialist menopausal clinic where an assessment of the risks can be made with advice from appropriate sources (breast surgeons, physicians, hematologists).

Box 34.3 Absolute contraindications to use of HRT

- Breast cancer, endometrial cancer or other estrogen-dependent tumors
- Undiagnosed vaginal bleeding
- Pregnancy or breast-feeding
- Thromboembolic disease or symptomatic thrombophilia
- Severe renal or liver disease
- Acute intermittent porphyria

Box 34.4 Relative contraindications/ situations where careful monitoring of hormone replacement therapy is required

Relative contraindications
- Family history of thromboembolic disease
- Osteosclerosis
- Body mass index $> 30\,kg/m^2$
- Systemic lupus erythematosus
- Malignant melanoma

Situations where careful monitoring is required
- Severe endometriosis
- Cholelithiasis
- Hypertension
- Diabetes
- Migraine
- Epilepsy
- Multiple sclerosis

For women in the categories shown in Box 34.4, an individual assessment of the risks and benefits is required. In some cases, this will require specialist referral. Referral to a specialist menopause clinic may also be of benefit where there have been problems with several different preparations of HRT.

ALTERNATIVE REMEDIES

The alternative health options that are available often provide a more holistic approach than is offered by standard medical practice. However, there is a lack of evidence of efficacy of many of these therapies and it is unfortunate if women with significant menopausal symptoms are disillusioned by an expensive alternative option that may have few side effects but is of minimal benefit. The evidence of their effectiveness is frequently anecdotal and there are no standards of quality control as is expected of the pharmaceutical industry. Herbal remedies include black cohosh, which is a herb from the buttercup family, ginseng, and dong quai, a Chinese herbal remedy. Dietary supplements, such as vitamin E and evening primrose oil, are also recommended as treatments for menopausal symptoms. As yet, there is little trial evidence of benefit with regard to menopausal symptoms.

There is a great deal of interest in phytoestrogens,[89] which are naturally occurring substances derived from plants and have a chemical structure that is similar to estrogen. They are able to bind to estrogen receptors but are biologically much less active than estrogen and also seem to have an anti-estrogen effect. Recent RCTs have failed to demonstrate a reduction in the frequency of vasomotor symptoms when compared with placebo but as yet no comparison has been made with estrogen.[90,91] In addition, the incidence of cardiovascular disease is much lower in communities where the consumption of phytoestrogens is very high. Whether this is causally related, or whether the decreased incidence in comparison with a Western population is due to some other lifestyle factor, is unclear.

UPTAKE OF HORMONE REPLACEMENT THERAPY

Today's society expects to be well informed about health issues. Breast cancer is now the most commonly diagnosed malignancy among women in the United Kingdom and is, justifiably, a major concern to women of all ages. The potential malignant effects of steroid hormones have been of concern to the general public since high dose oral contraceptives were used in the 1960s and 1070s. The fear of breast cancer has always been one of the commonest reasons why women decide not to take HRT, however, the small increase in risk is often overestimated by the general public. As much as the medical and pharmaceutical professions have a responsibility to give accurate information regarding adverse effects of HRT, the media and other non-medical groups have a responsibility to use this information appropriately.

The level of uptake of HRT is related to the amount of information that women have access to and disparity continues to exist. Studies have shown that women with greater years of education and affluence are more likely to obtain information on menopause. The effectiveness of any health promotion regarding menopause will be affected by these factors. HRT use and long-term compliance is high among female physicians and wives of physicians. The implication being that this well-informed group could reflect greater use among the general population if understanding of the benefits and risks were higher.[92,93]

DURATION OF USE OF HORMONE REPLACEMENT THERAPY

If bone density is the only consideration and there are no increased risks with long term use of HRT, then the maximal benefit would be obtained if HRT is used lifelong. Cohort studies have shown that current and recent users have the lowest risk of osteoporotic fractures. There is also evidence that bone loss increases after HRT is stopped. Since the termination of the WHI study, the recommendation is that the lowest dose of estrogen should be used for the shortest possible time and that it should not be used as a first-line treatment in the prevention of osteoporosis (Box 34.5). The risk of an osteoporotic fracture at the age of 50 years is extremely small, whereas breast cancer causes considerable morbidity and mortality. Numerically the risks outweigh the benefits since it would be necessary to take the estrogen for 20 or 30 years to gain real benefit. Thus alternative treatments for osteoporosis should be

Box 34.5 Current recommendations regarding the prescription of HRT

- HRT is useful to treat symptoms
- The lowest dose should be used for the shortest possible time
- Alternatives should be considered in the treatment of osteoporosis
- Its use in diseases such as dementia is uncertain

carefully considered particularly in the asymptomatic women.

No one is in a position to ignore the results of the studies discussed in this chapter. There is unlikely to be another major RCT in this group of women in the near future and in addition, it would be difficult to carry out the appropriate study since it is impossible to blind a group of women starting to take hormone preparations in the perimenopausal years and also, the event rate for the primary endpoints are relatively low and would require a larger study than with the older age group. Many physicians forget the quality-of-life issues, preferring to deal with illness only. Many of the women who stopped taking HRT at the time the results of the WHI were published have started again since their symptoms were intolerable.

KEY LEARNING POINTS

- A majority of women who take HRT do so to treat menopausal symptoms, the most common being hot flashes, for which estrogen-based HRT is the most effective treatment.
- Placebo-controlled trials have shown that HRT decreases the risk of hip fracture and has a role in the prevention and treatment of osteoporosis. However, because of the risks associated with long-term use of HRT, it is not recommended as first line in the prevention and treatment of osteoporosis in women without menopausal symptoms.
- HRT does not have a role in heart disease prevention strategies. It increases the risk of venous thromboembolic disease and stroke.
- Estrogen combined with progestogen increases the risk of breast cancer whereas estrogen alone does not. The increase with combined therapy is duration dependent.
- The increase in risk of endometrial cancer with estrogen alone is minimized by the addition of a progestogen.
- Combined HRT has a protective effect against colon cancer although the reasons for this, as well as the clinical implication of the finding, are unclear.
- It is recommended that women should receive the lowest possible dose of hormones for the shortest possible duration to treat their menopausal symptoms.

REFERENCES

1 Rymer J, Morris P. Menopausal symptoms. *BMJ* 2000; **321**: 1516–19.
2 McKinlay S. The normal menopause transition: an overview. *Maturitas* 1996; **23**: 137–45.
3 Bachmann GA. Vasomotor flushes in menopausal women. *Am J Obstet Gynecol* 1999; **180**: S312–16.
4 Baum M, Buzdar A, Cuzick J, *et al.*; the Tamoxifen Alone or in Combination Trialists' Group. Anastrozole alone or in combination with tamoxifen versus tamoxifen alone for adjuvant treatment of postmenopausal women with early-stage breast cancer: results of the ATAC (Arimidex, Tamoxifen Alone or in Combination) trial efficacy and safety update analyses. *Cancer* 2003; **98**: 1802–10.
5 MacLennan A, Broadbent JL, Lester S, Moore V. Oral oestrogen replacement therapy versus placebo for hot flushes. Cochrane Review. *Cochrane Database*, 2, 2006.
6 Greendale GA, Reboussin BA, Hogan P, *et al.* Symptom relief and side effects of postmenopausal hormones: results from the postmenopausal estrogen/progestin interventions trial. *Obstet Gynecol* 1998; **92**: 982–8.
7 Loprinzi CL, Michalak JC, Quella SK, *et al.* Megestrol acetate for the prevention of hot flushes. *N Engl J Med* 1994; **331**: 347–52.
8 Nagamani M, Kelver ME, Smith ER. Treatment of menopausal hot flushes with transdermal administration of clonidine. *Am J Obstet Gynecol* 1987; **156**: 561–5.
9 Wymenga AN, Sleijfer DT. Management of hot flushes in breast cancer patients. *Acta Oncologica* 2002; **41**: 269–75.
10 Robinson D, Cardozo L. The menopause and HRT. Urogenital effects of hormone therapy. *Best Pract Res Clin Endocrinol Metab* 2003; **17**: 91–104.
11 Fantl JA, Cardozo LD, McClish DK, the Hormones and Urogenital Therapy Committee. Oestrogen therapy in the management of incontinence in postmenopausal women: a meta-analysis. First report of the Hormones and Urogenital Therapy Committee. *Obstet Gynecol* 1994; **83**: 12–18.
12 Jackson S, Shepard A, Brookes S, *et al.* The effects of oestrogen supplementation on post-menopausal urinary stress incontinence: a double blind, placebo controlled trial. *Br J Obstet Gynaecol* 1996; **106**: 711–18.
13 Samsioe G, Jansson I, Mellstrom D, *et al.* Urinary incontinence in 75-year-old women. Effects of oestradiol. *Acta Obstet Gynecol Scand* 1985; **93**: 57.
14 Sultana CJ, Walters MD. Oestrogen and urinary incontinence in women. *Maturitas* 1995; **20**: 129–38.
15 Dew JE, Wren BG, Eden JA. A cohort study of topical vaginal estrogen therapy in women previously treated for breast cancer. *Climacteric* 2003; **6**: 45–52.
16 Hurskainen RJ, Paavonen J, Teperi J. The effectiveness of the levonorgestrel-releasing intrauterine system for menorrhagia: a systematic review. *Br J Obstet Gynaecol* 2003; **110**: 87–8.

17 Ballinger CB. Psychiatric aspects of the menopause. *Br J Psychiatry* 1990; **156**: 773–87.

18 Ditkoff EC, Crary WG, Cristo M, *et al.* Estrogen improves psychological function in asymptomatic postmenopausal women. *Obstet Gynecol* 1991; **78**: 991–5.

19 Soares CN, Almeida OP, Joffe H, *et al.* Efficacy of oestradiol for treatment of depressive disorders in perimenopausal women: a double-blind, randomised, placebo-controlled trial. *Arch Gen Psychiatry* 2001; **58**; 6: 537–53.

20 Pannay N, Studd J. The psychotherapeutic effects of estrogen. *Gynecol Endocrinol* 1998; **12**: 353–65.

21 Yaffe K, Sawaya G, Leiberburg I. Estrogen therapy in postmenopausal women: effects on cognitive function and dementia. *JAMA* 1998; **279**: 688–95.

22 HRT and cognitive function: what are we to believe? [editorial]. *Menopause* 2002; **9**: 221–3.

23 Rapp SR, Espeland MA, Shumaker SA, *et al.*, and Investigators WHIMS. Effect of estrogen plus progestin on global cognitive function in postmenopausal women: the Women's Health Initiative Memory Study: a randomized controlled trial [see comment]. *JAMA* 2003; **289**: 2663–72.

24 Dennerstein L, Dudley E, Burger H. Are changes in sexual functioning during midlife due to aging or menopause? *Fertil Steril* 2001; **76**: 456–60.

25 Graziottin A. Libido: the biological scenario. *Maturitas* 2000, **34**: S9–16.

26 Hoeger K, Guzick D. The use of androgens in the menopause. *Clin Obstet Gynecol* 1999; **42**: 883.

27 Ettinger B, Pressman A, Silver P. Effect of age on reasons for initiation and discontinuation of hormone replacement therapy. *J North Am Menop Soc* 1999; **6**: 282–9.

28 Keene GS, Parker MJ, Pryor GA. Mortality and morbidity after hip fractures. *BMJ* 1993; **307**: 1248–50.

29 Donaldson IJ, Cook A. Incidence of fractures in a geographically defined population. *J Epidemiol Comm Health* 1991; **44**: 241–5.

30 Cummings SR, Melton LJ. Epidemiology and outcomes of osteoporotic fractures. *Lancet* 2002; **359**: 1761–7.

31 Adami S, Suppi R, Bertoldo F, *et al.* Transdermal estradiol in the treatment of postmenopausal bone loss. *Bone Min* 1989; **7**: 79–86.

32 Hutchinson TA, Polansky SM, Feinstein AR. Postmenopausal oestrogens protect against fractures of hip and distal radius. A case–control study. *Lancet* 1979; **2**: 705–9.

33 Kiel DP, Felson DT, Anderson JJ, *et al.* Hip fracture and the use of estrogens in postmenopausal women, The Framingham Study. *N Engl J Med* 1987; **317**: 1 169–74.

34 Lindsay R, Hart DM, Forrest C, *et al.* Prevention of spinal osteoporosis in oophoorectomised women. *Lancet* 1980; **2**: 1151–4.

35 Stevenson JC, Cust MP, Gangar KF, *et al.* Effects of transdermal versus oral hormone replacement therapy on bone density in spine and proximal femur in postmenopausal women. *Lancet* 1990; **336**: 265–9.

36 Lufkin EG, Wahner HW, O'Fallon WM, *et al.* Treatment of postmenopausal osteoporosis with transdermal oestrogen. *Ann Int Med* 1992; **117**: 1–9.

37 Paganini-Hill A, Ross RK, Gerkins VR, *et al.* Menopausal estrogen therapy and hip fractures. *Ann Intern Med* 1981; **95**: 28–31.

38 Writing Group for the Women's Health Initiative (WHI) Investigators. Risks and benefits of estrogen plus progestin in healthy post menopausal women. *JAMA* **288**: 321–33.

39 Delmas PD, Confavreux E, Garneo P, *et al.* A combination of low doses of 17 beta-oestradiol and norethisterone acetate prevents bone loss and normalises bone turnover in postmenopausal women. *Osteoporos Int* 2002; **11**: 177–87.

40 Horowitz M, Wishart JM, Need AG, *et al.* Effects of norethisterone on bone related biochemical variables and forearm bone density in postmenopausal osteoporosis. *Clin Endocrinol* 1993; **39**: 649–55.

41 Cummings SR, Black DM, Thompson DE, *et al.* Effect of alendronate on risk of fracture in women with low bone density but without vertebral fracture – results from the Fracture Intervention Trial. *JAMA* 1988 **280**: 2077–82.

42 Black DM, Cummings SR, Karpf DB, *et al.* Randomised trial of effect of alendronate on risk of fracture in women with existing vertebral fractures. *Lancet* 1996; **348**: 1531–41.

43 Harris ST, Watts NB, Genant HK, *et al.* Effects of risedronate treatment on vertebral and non-vertebral fractures in women with postmenopausal osteoporosis: a randomised controlled trial. Vertebral Efficacy With Risedronate Therapy (VERT) Study Group. *JAMA* 1999; **282**: 1344–52.

44 Pols HAP, Felsenberg D, Hanley DA, *et al.* Multinational, placebo-controlled, randomised trial of the effects of alendronate on bone density and fracture risk in postmenopausal women with low bone mass, results of the FOSIT study. *Osteoporos Int* 1999; **9**: 461–8.

45 Ettinger B, Black DM, Mitlak BH, *et al.* Reduction of vertebral fracture risk in postmenopausal women with osteoporosis treated with raloxifene: results from a 3 year randomised clinical trial. *JAMA* 1999; **282**: 637–45.

46 Overgaard K. Effect of intranasal salmon calcitonin therapy on bone mass and bone turnover in early postmenopausal women: a dose response study. *Calc Tiss Int* 1994; **55**: 82–6.

47 Reginster JY, Dennis D, Deroisy R, *et al.* Long term (3 years) prevention of trabecular postmenopausal bone loss with low-dose intermittent nasal calcitonin. *J Bone Min Res* 1994; **9**: 69–73.

48 Meunier PJ, Roux C, Seeman E, *et al.* The effects of strontium ranelate on the risk of vertebral fracture in women with postmenopausal osteoporosis [see comment]. *N Engl J Med* 2004; **350**: 459–68.

● 49   Komulainen MH, Kroger H, Tuppurainen MT, *et al.* HRT and Vit D in the prevention of non-vertebral fractures in postmenopausal women; a 5-year randomised trial. *Maturitas* 1998; **31**: 45–54.

● 50   Chevalley T, Rizzoli R, Nydegger V, *et al.* Effects of calcium supplements on femoral bone density and vertebral fracture rate in vitamin D replete elderly patients. *Osteoporos Int* 1994; **4**: 245–52.

● 51   Reid IR, Ames RW, Evans MC, *et al.* Long-term effects of calcium supplementation on bone loss and fractures in postmenopausal women: a randomised controlled trial. *Am J Med* 1995; **98**: 332–5.

◆ 52   Le Blanc ES, Janowsky J, Chan BK, *et al.* Hormone replacement therapy and cognition: systematic review and meta-analysis. *JAMA* 2001; **285**: 1489–99.

● 53   Paganini-Hill A, Henderson VW. Estrogen deficiency and risk of Alzheimer's disease in women. *Am J Epidemiol* 1994; **140**: 256–61.

● 54   Henderson W, Paganini-Hill A, Miller BL, *et al.* Estrogen for Alzheimer's disease in women. *Neurology* 2000; **54**: 195–201.

● 55   Kawas C, Resnick S, Morrison A, *et al.* A prospective study of estrogen replacement therapy and the risk of developing Alzheimer's: the Baltimore Longitudinal Study of Ageing. *Neurology* 1997; **48**: 1517–21.

● 56   Shumaker SA, Legault C, Rapp SR, *et al.*, and Investigators WHIMS. Estrogen plus progestin and the incidence of dementia and mild cognitive impairment in postmenopausal women: the Women's Health Initiative Memory Study: a randomized controlled trial [see comment]. *JAMA* 2003; **289**: 2651–62.

● 57   Grodstein F, Stampfer MJ, Manson JE, *et al.* Postmenopausal estrogen and progestin use and the risk of cardiovascular disease [see comments]. *N Engl J Med* 1996; **335**: 453–61.

● 58   Grodstein F, Stampfer M. The epidemiology of coronary heart disease and oestrogen replacement in post menopausal women. *Prog Cardiovasc Dis* 1995; **38**: 199–210.

● 59   Barrett-Connor E, Grady D. Hormone replacement therapy, heart disease, and other considerations. *Annu Rev Pub Health* 1998; **19**: 55–72.

◆ 60   Stevenson JC. Mechanisms whereby oestrogens influence arterial health. *Eur J Obstet Gynecol Reprod Biol* 1996; **65**: 39–42.

◆ 61   Stevenson JC. Cardiovascular effects of oestrogens. *J Steroid Biochem Mol Biol* 2002; **74**: 387–93.

◆ 62   Lowe GD. Hormone replacement therapy: prothrombotic vs. protective effects. *Pathophysiol Haemost Thromb* 2002; **32**: 329–32.

● 63   Lowe GD. Hormone replacement therapy and cardiovascular disease: increased risk of venous thromboembolism and stroke and no protection for coronary heart disease. *J Intern Med* 2004; **256**: 361–74.

● 64   Kroon UB, Tengborn L, Rita H, Backstrom AC. The effects of transdermal oestradiol and oral progestogens on haemostasis variables. *Br J Obstet Gynaecol* 1997; **104**: 32–7.

● 65   Hulley S, Grady D, Bush T, *et al.* Randomized trial of estrogen plus progestin for secondary prevention of coronary heart disease in postmenopausal women. Heart and Estrogen/progestin Replacement Study (HERS) Research Group. *JAMA* 1998; **280**: 605–13.

● 66   The Women's Health Initiative Steering Committee. Effects of Conjugated Equine Estrogen in Postmenopausal Women With Hysterectomy: The Women's Health Initiative Randomized Controlled Trial. *JAMA* 2004; **291**: 1701–12.

◆ 67   Castellsague J, Pereez Guttann S, Garcia Rodriguez LA. Recent epidemiological studies of the association between hormone replacement therapy and venous thromboembolism. A review. *Drug Saf* 1998; **18**: 117–23.

● 68   World Health Organisation. Venous thromboembolic disease and combined oral contraceptives: results of international multicentre case-control study. *Lancet* 1995; **346**: 1575–82.

● 69   Jick H, Jick S, Gurewich V, *et al.* Risk of idiopathic cardiovascular death and nonfatal venous thromboembolism in women using oral contraceptives with differing progestagen components. *Lancet* 1995; **346**: 1589–93.

● 70   Oger E, Scarabin PY. Assessment of the risk for venous thromboembolism among users of hormone replacement therapy. *Drugs Aging* 1999; **14**: 55–61.

● 71   Scarabin P-Y, Oger E, Plu-Bureau G, on behalf of the Estrogen and Thromboembolism Risk (ESTHER) Study Group. Differential association of oral and transdermal oestrogen-replacement therapy with venous thromboembolism risk. *Lancet* 2003; **362**: 428–32.

★ 72   UK Committee for Safety of Medicines. HRT: update on the risk of breast cancer and long-term safety. Anonymous. *Curr Prob Pharmacovigil* 2003; **29**: 1–3.

● 73   Hoibraaten E, Qvigstad E, Arnesen H, *et al.* Increased risk of recurrent venous thromboembolism during hormone replacement therapy – results of the randomized, double-blind, placebo-controlled estrogen in venous thromboembolism trial (EVTET). *Thromb Haemost* 2000; **84**: 961–7.

● 74   Lowe G, Woodward M, Vessey M, *et al.* Thrombotic variables and risk of idiopathic venous thromboembolism in women aged 45–64 years. Relationships to hormone replacement therapy. *Thromb Haemost* 2000; **83**: 530–5.

● 75   Cushman M, Kuller LHM, Prentice R, *et al.*, and for the Women's Health Initiative Investigators. Estrogen plus progestin and risk of venous thrombosis. *JAMA* 2004; **292**: 1573–80.

◆ 76   Gray LJ, Bath PMW. The effect of hormone replacement therapy on stroke risk, type and outcome: a systematic review of data from randomized controlled trials. *Cerebrovasc Dis* 2004; **17**(Suppl 5): 18.

77 Hsai J, Criqui MH, Rodabough RL, *et al.* Estrogen plus progestin and the risk of peripheral arterial disease. The Women's Health Initiative. *Circulation* 2004; **109**: 620–6.

78 Danesh J, Wheeler JG, Hirschfield GM, *et al.* C-reactive protein and other circulating markers of inflammation in the prediction of coronary heart disease. *N Engl J Med* 2004; **350**: 1387–97.

79 The North American Menopause Society. Effects of menopause and oestrogen replacement therapy or hormone replacement therapy in women with diabetes mellitus: consensus opinion of The North American Menopause Society. *Menopause* 2000; **7**: 87–95.

80 Weiderpass E, Adami HO, Baron JA, *et al.* Risk of endometrial cancer following estrogen replacement with and without progestins. *J Natl Cancer Inst* 1999; **91**: 1131–7.

81 Wells M, Sturdee DW, Barlow DH, *et al.* Effect on endometrium of long term treatment with continuous combined oestrogen-progestogen replacement therapy: follow-up study [see comment]. *BMJ* 2002; **325**: 239.

82 Colditz GA, Hankinson SE, Hunter DJ, *et al.* The use of estrogens and progestins and the risk of breast cancer in postmenopausal women. *N Engl J Med* 1995; **332**: 1589–93.

83 Beral V, *et al.* The Collaborative Group on Hormonal Factors in Breast Cancer. Breast cancer and hormone replacement therapy: collaborative reanalysis of data from 51 epidemiological studies of 527 505 women with breast cancer and 108 411 women without breast cancer. *Lancet* 1997; **350**: 1047–59.

84 Beral V, Study Collaborators Million Women. Breast cancer and hormone-replacement therapy in the Million Women Study. *Lancet* 2003; **362** : 419–27.

85 Archer DF, Pickar JH, Bottiglioni F. Bleeding patterns in postmenopausal women taking continuous combined or sequential regimens of conjugated equine estrogens and medroxyprogesteroneacetate. *Obstet Gynecol* 1994; **83**: 686–92.

86 Udoff L, Langenberg P, Adashi EY. Combined continuous hormone replacement therapy: a critical review. *Obstet Gynecol* 1995; **86**: 306–16.

87 Crawford SL, Casey VA, Avis NE, *et al.* A longitudinal study of weight and the menopause transition: results from the Massachusetts Women's Health Study. *Menopause* 2000; **7**: 96–104.

88 Norman RR, Flight I.HK, Rees MCP. Oestrogen and progestogen hormone replacement therapy for peri-menopausal and postmenopausal women: weight and body fat distribution. *Cochrane Database Syst Rev 2*, 2006.

89 Davis SR. Phytoestrogen therapy for menopausal symptoms?: there's no good evidence that it's any better than placebo. *BMJ* 2001; **323**: 354–5.

90 Penotti M, Fabio E, Modena AB, *et al.* Effect of soy-derivative isoflavones on hot flushes, endometrial thickness and the pulsatility index of the uterine artery and cerebral arteries. *Fertil Steril* 2003; **79**: 1112–17.

91 Tice JA, Ettinger B, Enstrud K, *et al.* Phytoestrogen supplements for the treatment of hot flushes: The isoflavone Clover Extract (ICE) Study. *JAMA* 2003; **290**: 207–14.

92 McNagny SE, Wenger NK, Frank E. Personal use of postmenopausal hormone replacement therapy by women physicians in the United States. *Ann Intern Med* 1997; **127**: 1093–109.

93 Isaacs AJ, Britton AR, Mcpherson K. Why do doctors in the UK take hormone replacement therapy? *J Epidemiol Comm Health* 1997; **51**: 373–7.

Index

Note – bold page numbers refer to figures, tables and boxes.